A Comprehensive Textbook of Midwifery and Gynecological Nursing

2011 - A (Nursing batch)

NTS -

A Comprehensive Textbook of Midwifery and Gynecological Nursing

THIRD EDITION

Annamma Jacob MSc (N)

Formerly
Professor, St Philomina's College of Nursing, Mother Theresa Road
Bengaluru, Karnataka, India
Principal, Graduate School for Nurses BNE, SIB, CMAI
Nurse Supervisor, Suburban Medical Center, Paramount, Southern California, USA
Assistant Director of Nursing, Al-Sabah Hospital, Ministry of Public Health, Kuwait
Sister Tutor, LT College of Nursing, SNDT Womens' University, Mumbai, Maharashtra, India
Junior Tutor, College of Nursing, CMC Hospital, Vellore, Tamil Nadu, India

Principal
Bhagwan Mahaveer Jain College of Nursing
Millers Road, Vasanthanagar
Bengaluru, Karnataka, India

JAYPEE BROTHERS MEDICAL PUBLISHERS (P) LTD
New Delhi • Panama City • London

Jaypee Brothers Medical Publishers (P) Ltd.

Headquarter
Jaypee Brothers Medical Publishers (P) Ltd
4838/24, Ansari Road, Daryaganj
New Delhi 110 002, India
Phone: +91-11-43574357
Fax: +91-11-43574314
Email: jaypee@jaypeebrothers.com

Overseas Offices

J.P. Medical Ltd.,
83 Victoria Street London
SW1H 0HW (UK)
Phone: +44-2031708910
Fax: +02-03-0086180
Email: info@jpmedpub.com

Jaypee-Highlights Medical Publishers Inc.
City of Knowledge, Bld. 237, Clayton
Panama City, Panama
Phone: 507-317-0160
Fax: +50-73-010499
Email: cservice@jphmedical.com

Website: www.jaypeebrothers.com
Website: www.jaypeedigital.com

© 2012, Jaypee Brothers Medical Publishers

Inquiries for bulk sales may be solicited at: jaypee@jaypeebrothers.com

A Comprehensive Textbook of Midwifery and Gynecological Nursing

First Edition: 2005
Second Edition: 2008
Third Edition: **2012**

ISBN 978-93-5025-557-5

Printed at: Ajanta Offset & Packagings Ltd., New Delhi

Editor's Remarks

A Comprehensive Textbook of Midwifery and Gynecological Nursing offers a unique opportunity to midwifery students as well as teachers, to assimilate an evergrowing body of scientific knowledge and to develop the technical and analytical skills necessary to apply the same into practice.

The book strives to provide the students with various aspects of midwifery to become competent and caring midwives. It includes the most accurate and clinically relevant information available, in a clearly written, visually appealing and logical format.

The book includes 12 sections and 71 chapters with an Appendix and exhaustive Glossary at the end. Each chapter is ending with a list of bibliography which are useful to find out detailed information. In addition, a number of diagrams, tables, illustrations and nursing processes have been presented, wherever necessary. The book is in simple language.

The current concept on Community Midwifery has been included, which stresses on Preventive Obstetrics and Domiciliary Care in Maternity Nursing. A detailed discussion on Primary Health Care, the Organization of Maternal and Child Health Programs and the Current Evolution of Reproductive and Child Health Programs is included which is of much use to the students to deliver Community, Maternal and Child Health Services.

I hope and trust that this midwifery textbook will be of a great help not only to midwifery students, but also to midwifery teachers, for study as well as for ready-reference.

With best wishes,

TM Krishnaveni PHN
Former Assistant Director
Directorate of Health and Family Welfare Services
Government of Karnataka
Bengaluru, Karnataka, India

Preface to the Third Edition

The goal of nursing education in general and midwifery education in particular is to prepare nurses/midwives who combine the highest level of scientific knowledge and technological skills with responsible caring practice. To that end we need to challenge students to identify and master the cognitive and technical skills as well as the interpersonal and ethical skills they will need to effectively nurse the mothers and newborns in their care.

The author has identified that addition of more information in certain topics and more chapters on Obstetric and Gynecological Nursing would further assist nursing students to expand their knowledge of maternal-newborn nursing and make the textbook more student and teacher friendly. Three more chapters are added in the midwifery section and eleven chapters in gynecological nursing section.

I am grateful to all the midwifery teachers who have given feedback on earlier editions of the book, which helped me to incorporate their suggestions in this third edition of the *A Comprehensive Textbook of Midwifery and Gynecological Nursing.*

I sincerely thank Mrs N Christina Jonathan, Lecturer of Nursing for her suggestions and assistance in preparing the matter and getting the photographs done.

I express my appreciation of the patient forbearance of Mr A J Jacob my husband who helped me to complete the work.

I am grateful to the team of M/s Jaypee Brothers Medical Publishers (P) Ltd. at Bengaluru branch and New Delhi for their prompt and high-level performance in getting this and other titles printed and published.

Annamma Jacob

Preface to the First Edition

The book is the culmination of ideas of a nurse educator who has practiced and taught maternal-neonatal nursing in India and in the United States of America. It is the fulfillment of the often stated need among nurse educators and nursing students in India. Since long, teachers of midwifery have been relying on books written with an orientation for practice in the developed countries or those written by physician authors. As a midwifery educator, I became aware of the frustrations of students in trying to piece together the information from English and American midwifery texts or from physician-authored book. The former were too much indepth and generally oriented to conditions in the developed countries while the latter lacked nursing care aspects in order to plan and provide comprehensive care to maternity clients and newborns.

As the concept of nursing process has been incorporated into midwifery education, a chapter on nursing process is included to familiarize midwifery students to the appropriateness of using the problem-oriented approach with their maternity and newborn clients. With a few selected topics, the nursing processes that can be carried out are included which are hoped to serve as guidelines. In the chapter on drugs, nursing considerations are included with a view to foster the use of nursing process in drug administration. Pertinent information from other health sciences is included throughout the book, particularly as it relates to the childbearing and child-rearing periods in the life of the family and from preconception through the first six weeks' postpartum.

This book is organized into 11 sections in logical sequence including all the units outlined in the syllabus prescribed by the Indian Nursing Council for Midwifery Course (INC syllabus, 1986). Additional information includes the chapters on Nursing Process, Childbirth Education and Preparation and the current trends in National Reproductive and Child Health (RCH) Program. This book is written completely in the Indian context and in a simple style and easy to understand language for the benefit of Indian nursing students. Practicing nurses will also find the content understandable and useful. Advances in the field of obstetrics and practice of midwifery in the developed countries are included wherever relevant.

Each chapter begins with a list of learning objectives. These tells the reader specifically what she or he should know after reading the chapter. The students can use this as a study aid. A large number of informative diagrams, tables and illustrations have been included. They have been designed to convey information in readily comprehensible form.

I sincerely hope that this book will greatly benefit the midwifery teachers, students and nurses practicing maternal-child nursing.

Annamma Jacob

Acknowledgments

One of the most pleasant parts of writing a book is the opportunity to thank those who have contributed to it.

I am deeply appreciative of Dr TM Krishnaveni, Consultant to the Government of Karnataka Institute of Health and Family Welfare Services, for the patient and wholehearted efforts in editing the book.

Special acknowledgment and thanks to Mr Joji George RN and Miss Aswathy Alexander BSc(N) who drew a many figures in this book.

There have been many people who have touched and shaped my life and beliefs in maternal-child nursing. I am indebted to Mrs Nesamoni Lazarus, my teacher at College of Nursing, CMC Hospital, Vellore, from whom I learned a lot and Mrs Phyllis Berg and Miss Chris Hamilton, Nursing Managers at Suburban Medical Center, Paramount, California, USA who have influenced me profoundly.

I am thankful to my personal friends and professional colleagues in the institutions I had worked and with whom I shared my knowledge and aspirations. The inspiration for writing this book came as a result of my association and involvement with my former students at LT College of Nursing, SNDT Women's University, St Philomina's College of Nursing and Graduate School for Nurses, BNE, SIB, CMAI.

My special thanks go to my niece Pinky Ann Thomas, nephew Pinku Cherian Thomas and brother-in-law Mr George K Cherian for their suggestions, support and assistance in ways big and small.

Finally, not least but most, I acknowledge my husband A J Jacob who encouraged me and worked with me tirelessly to complete this book and in whose honor I have decided to publish this book.

Contents

Section 4: Normal Pregnancy

Section 5: Normal Labor

PLATE 1

Figs 9.4A and B: The placenta at term: (A) Maternal surface of the placenta; (B) Fetal surface of the placenta

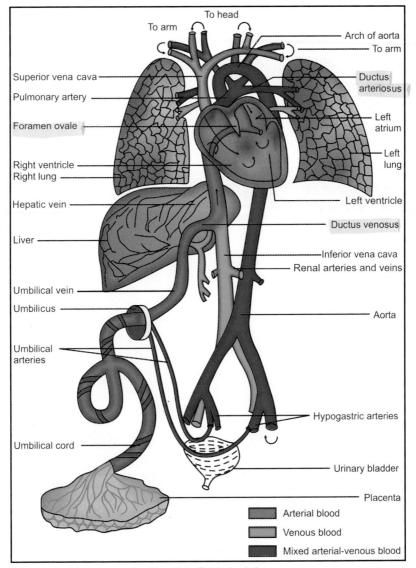

Fig. 10.1: Fetal circulation

PLATE 2

Fig. 15.3: Measuring fundal height with tape measure

Fig. 15.7: Ultrasonic Doppler device

Fig. 18.2: Electronic fetal monitor

Fig. 24.8: A post vasectomy scrotum showing the incision site

Fig. 39.1: A healthy newborn

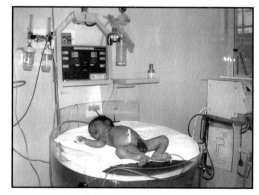

Fig. 39.4: Newborn in radiant warmer

PLATE 3

Fig. 40.1: The Moro reflex

Fig. 40.4: Stepping reflex

Fig. 40.3A: Palmar reflex

Fig. 41.2A: Feeding in side lying position

Fig. 40.3B: Plantar reflex

Fig. 41.2B: Feeding in sitting position

PLATE 4

Fig. 41.2C: Sitting position with the baby in football hold

Figs 41.3A to D: Swaddle wrapping

PLATE 5

Fig. 41.4: Initiating sucking with a drop of milk on nipple

Fig. 41.8: Burping the baby

Fig. 41.6: Baby's lips in contact with areola

Fig. 41.9: Applying warm towel to engorged breast

Fig. 41.7: Breaking suction before removing the baby from breast

Fig. 42.2A: Appearance of a SGA newborn

PLATE 6

Fig. 42.2B: Appearance of a preterm newborn

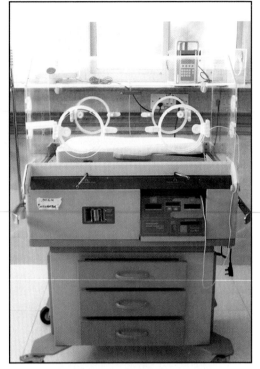

Fig. 42.3: An isolette/Incubator for care of preterm baby

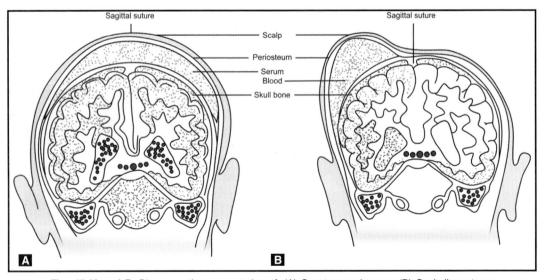

Figs 45.4A and B: Diagrammatic representation of: (A) Caput succedaneum; (B) Cephalhematoma

PLATE 7

Fig. 47.2: Baby undergoing photography

Figs 62.3A and B: (A) Cystocele and uterovaginal prolapse; (B) Cystocele and enterocele

Fig. 62.4: Rectocele

PLATE 8

Figs 62.5A and B: Complete uterine prolapse

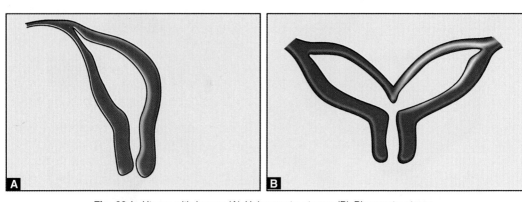

Fig. 66.1: Uterus with horns: (A) Unicornuate uterus; (B) Bicornuate uterus

Figs 66.2A and B: Septate uterus: (A) Partial septum; (B) Complete septum

SECTION

1

Midwifery

1

Historical Review

Learning Objectives

Upon completing this chapter, the learner will be able to:
- ❖ Identify the early recordings of midwifery practice
- ❖ Appreciate the early foundations of modern midwifery
- ❖ Appreciate the contributions to midwifery by various physicians through the centuries.

Midwifery is as old as the history of human species. Archeological evidence of a woman squatting in childbirth supported by another woman from behind demonstrates the existence of midwifery in 5000 BC. There are references to the midwives in the *Old Testament*. Genesis 35:17 "And it came to pass, when she was in hard labor, that the midwife said unto her, fear not Rachel, it is another boy". In Exodus 1:15, it is recorded that the King of Egypt spoke to Shiprah and Puah, the two midwives, who helped Hebrew women when they gave birth. These two Hebrew midwives are the first midwives found in the literature. Through the centuries, midwifery, the art of assisting women in childbirth has grown fulfilling its meaning "with woman" at birth.

Hippocrates (460 BC), the father of scientific medicine, organized trained and supervised midwives. Hippocrates believed that the fetus had to fight its way out of the womb and the membranes. The efforts of Hippocrates were not appreciated by the midwives.

Aristotle (384-322 BC), the father of embryology, described the uterus and the female pelvic organs. He also discussed the essential qualities of the midwife. Soranus, in the second century, was the first to specialize in Obstetrics and Gynecology. His book was used for 1,500 years.

He used a vaginal speculum, advised on cord care, and wet nursing. From the fifth to the fifteenth centuries, which was the period of decline of the Roman Empire, untrained midwives controlled the practice of midwifery.

Leonardo da Vinci (1452–1519) made anatomical drawings of pregnant uterus. In 1513, the first book on midwifery was printed in Germany, based on the teachings of Soranus. In 1540, the book was translated into English. For a century and half it was the only book on midwifery in English. During this period, doctors were rigidly excluded from labor rooms and midwives assisted women in labor. Vesalius in 1543, opened the full term pregnant uterus in a lower animal, extracted the fetus, and demonstrated uterus as a single chamber organ.

Ambroise Pare (1510–1590) laid the foundations of modern obstetrics. He performed internal podalic versions and skillfully delivered women. He was the first to deliver a woman in bed instead of the birthing-stool. He also sutured perineal lacerations. Ambroise Pare founded a school for midwives in Paris, France. Louise Bourgeois, a midwife trained by Pare, attended the ladies of the French court. She warned midwives against getting infected with syphilis and transmitting it to other women. She recommended induction of labor for pelvic contraction.

Julius Caesar Aranzi wrote the first book for Italian midwives, which ran seventeen editions. He advised cesarean section for contracted pelvis. William Harvey (1578–1657), the father of British midwifery, wrote the first English textbook on midwifery. He described the fetal circulation and the placenta and was the first to deliver the placenta by massaging the uterus. He described the raw placental surface and initiated the study of uterine sepsis. Women remained largely reluctant to be delivered by men during this period. Midwives did not usually seek medical aid until the labor was hopelessly obstructed, as in the case of gross pelvic deformity. The resultant death of the mother or the baby gave the physicians unwarranted reputation.

The French King Louis XIV in 1663, employed a Paris surgeon to attend one of his mistresses in labor and pleased with the result the King honored the surgeon with the title "accoucheur" (a person who assists women in childbirth). The French accoucheurs built a school of midwifery, which attracted doctors from all over Europe. Mauricieau in 1668, published a treatise on midwifery. Hugh Chamberlen translated it into English, which greatly assisted the advance of midwifery in Britain. Mauricieau was the greatest physician of the 17th century. He described the attitude of the fetus in uterus as that of one of squatting down to pass stools and lowering his head to see what he has done.

Chamberlen in 1675, designed obstetric forceps. William Smellie (1697–1763) is called the father of British midwifery. He explained labor to be a mechanical process and described pelvimetry, cephalometry and forceps delivery of the after coming head of a breech. He devised a lock for the obstetric forceps, which permitted each blade to be introduced separately. The chair of midwifery was founded in 1726 in the University of Edinburgh. In 1772, John Leake replaced the obstetric stool by special delivery beds.

Charles White in 1773, stated that puerperal fever was infectious. He used lime as disinfectant, and clean linen, isolation, adequate ventilation and sitting posture to facilitate drainage. Fielding Ould (1710–1789) described the mechanism of normal labor and performed the first episiotomy. Gordon in 1795, described puerperal sepsis as a wound contamination of the placental site.

Laennec in 1816, invented a stethoscope and Francois in 1818, first recognized fetal heart sounds in the pregnant uterus. James Young Simpson in 1847, used chloroform first in obstetrics for anesthesia. Florence Nightingale in 1862, organized a small training school in connection with King's College Hospital where she conducted training for midwives.

Semmelweiss in 1861, demonstrated the cause of puerperal sepsis and suggested preventive measures. His students practiced scrubbing their hands in chloride of lime, which reduced maternal mortality rate in the words. Louis Pasteur in 1879, wrote a thesis on puerperal sepsis demonstrating the presence of streptococci in the lochia, blood and in fatal cases in the peritoneal cavity. Spencer and Ballantyne promoted the concept of antenatal care for pregnant women. The first antenatal clinics was started about the time of the First World War.

The history of cesarean section dates back to 715 BC and the operation derives its name from the notification *lex cesarea*—a Roman law, which was followed even during Caesar's reign. The law provided for an abdominal delivery either in a dying woman with a hope to get a live baby or to perform postmortem abdominal delivery for a separate burial. The operation does not derive its name from the birth of Caesar, as his mother lived long time after his birth. The origin of the word cesarean is also related to a Latin verb *caedere,* which means 'to cut'.

A French obstetrician, Francois Mauricieau first reported cesarean section in 1668. In 1876, Porro performed subtotal hysterectomy. Max Sanger in 1882, first sutured the uterine walls. In 1912, Kronig introduced lower segment vertical incision and it was popularized by De Lee (1922). Munro Kerr in 1926 introduced the present technique of lower segment cesarean operation and popularized it.

BIBLIOGRAPHY

1. Bullog Vern, Bannie Bullough. The emergency of modern nursing, New York: Macmillan; 1969.
2. Davis Fred. The Nursing Profession, Five Sociological Essays, New York: Wiley; 1966.
3. Fox CG. Toward a sound historical basis for nurse-midwifery, Bull, American College of Nurse-Midwives; 1969;14:76.
4. Parulekar V, Shashank. Textbook for Midwives, 2nd edn. Mumbai: Vora Medical Publishers; 1995.

2

Development of Maternity Services and Current Trends

Learning Objectives

Upon completing this chapter, the learner will be able to:

❖ Identify the development of maternity services through different periods
❖ Appreciate the phases of the development process of midwifery practice and midwifery education in India
❖ Discuss the philosophy of family-centered maternity care
❖ Discuss the technological advances in health care that have affected maternal-newborn nursing
❖ Discuss the concept of mother-baby couplet care and single room maternity care.

Following reformation in the 16th century, the Church of England accepted the responsibility for issuing, by the Bishops, of licenses for midwives to practice. Midwifery at that time was practiced entirely by midwives who lacked knowledge of anatomy and obstetrics. The same situation existed in India where midwifery was practiced by traditional "dais". The chair of midwifery was created in Edinburgh in 1726 for giving instructions to midwives. Courses of instruction were given to midwives in various centers throughout Britain during the 18th century and a few hospitals issued certificates.

In 1756, Dr John Douglas recommended that proper courses of instructions be given to midwives and an examination should be held before certificate to practice was given. Better midwifery practice began at this time. The Ladies' Obstetrical College, London was founded in 1864, and daughters of professional men attended lectures and became midwives. In 1902, the first English Midwives' Act was passed, and state registration of midwives became mandatory by law.

The 1700s and 1800s mark a time of rapid development in medical and nursing science, discoveries and teaching pertinent to obstetric practice. These developments include the invention and refinement of obstetrical forceps, technical advances which decreased the risks involved in cesarean section, pioneering efforts in obstetric anesthesia, conquest of puerperal fever, emergence of modern nursing and inclusion of obstetrics in medical practice. The observations and teachings of William Smellie (1697-1763), who developed teaching manikins and identified the mechanisms of labor, refuted the myths and misconceptions.

William Shippen, Jr (1736-1808), the first lecturer in obstetrics and Samuel Bard (1742-1821), author of the first American textbook on obstetrics, are attributed with promoting obstetrical teaching in the United States. However, due to lack of educational programs for midwives, these developments, new knowledge and teachings remained inaccessible to them. The first two decades of the twentieth century are notable for the recognition of inadequate maternity care and subsequent actions to improve this care in the United States. The Children's Bureau in Washington, DC, and Maternity Center Association in New York City were established which contributed greatly to the development of maternal-infant health care and midwifery.

A study conducted in 1906 in New York City on maternal and infant mortality, stated that approximately 3000 incompetent and ignorant midwives attended over forty percent of deliveries. While these midwives were not solely responsible for the high maternal and infant mortality rates at that time, they received the brunt of the blame.

Progress in improving the situation was slow. It was by 1935 that the registration of births was made mandatory in all the states. In 1915, the New York City commissioner made another study of maternal and infant mortality. The findings of this study demonstrated the connection between mortality and lack of prenatal care. Several maternity centers were established in New York City and other states followed. By 1930, obstetric care began to move out of the home into the hospital, and laws were passed to regulate the practice of the indigenous midwives. Several schools were established because of the laws to regulate midwifery practice. Two of such schools, to instruct the indigenous midwives in meeting the requirements for practice, were the Bellevue School of Midwifery in New York City and the Preston Retreat Hospital in Philadelphia. These efforts improved the practice of midwifery and resulted in better obstetric care for mothers and babies.

During this period, nurse-midwives in European countries had proved their effectiveness and they were part of the health care system. The first nurse-midwives to practice in the United States were British trained nurse-midwives, taken to there in 1925 by Mary Breckinridge as part of her plan to provide health care for the remote rural people in the Kentucky Mountains. Breckinridge's professional preparation as a registered nurse in the United States and as a certified midwife in England suited the task she initiated and undertook. Great Britain had been the provider of midwifery education for United States registered nurses until 1939 when few schools were started in the United States.

In the late 1950s and during the 1960s nurse-midwives moved into hospitals because this was where majority of births, approximately 70 percent at that time, were taking place. The movement of nurse-midwives into hospitals brought concepts of family-centered maternity care and a consumer advocate to childbearing women who delivered in hospitals.

Between 1969 and 1979, several nurse-midwifery programs were established. Nurse-midwives started functioning in the full range of possible practice arenas such as clinics, federally funded programs and hospitals. Now there are both certificate programs and higher degree programs.

In India, midwifery was practiced by traditional "dais" without any formal training. Changes in the practice began in the early part of 20th century. The health organization in India at that time had two main branches. One was for administration of medical relief and maintenance of associated institutions and the other was for the development of preventive health services. The former was under the direction of the Director General of the Indian Medical Services at the center and Surgeon General of Civil Hospitals in the states. Preventive Health Services were under the direction of Public Health Commissioner at the center and Sanitation Commissioner in the states.

The British parliament in 1921, transferred from the Central Government to the Provincial Governments, certain administrative functions, which included those relating to health, education and development of natural resources. The All India Institute of Hygiene and Public Health was established in 1930, with the aid of Rockefeller Foundation. The institution provided programs of study in maternal and child health. Maternal and infant deaths were high in all parts of the country. In 1943, the government appointed a committee, called the Bhore Committee, to survey the existing health conditions and to formulate a comprehensive plan for health administration. It suggested a short-term plan and a long-term plan. The short-term plan suggested the formation of primary health centers to serve a population of about 40,000. The staff of each unit included, among other members, one institutional nurse, four midwives and four trained dais. Programs for training dais and auxiliary nurse midwives (ANMs) were started based on this report.

Training programs for nurses were mainly in the mission hospitals. One of the early institutions, that had nurses' training programs, was the Christian Medical College Hospital, Vellore in Tamil Nadu. Nursing Superintendents of Mission Hospitals felt the need for an organization of their own by 1911. In 1931, a formal association of nurses called the Nurses Auxiliary of the Christian Medical Association of India (CMAI) was formed. The CMAI, which was registered as a nonprofit charitable organization in 1926, named the Nurses' Auxiliary as Nurses League in 1964 which had two Boards of Nursing Education; the Mid India Board of Nursing Education and the Board of Nursing Education, South India Branch. Through their affiliation to the Nursing Schools attached to Mission Hospitals, the Boards regulated nursing education, conducted examinations and issued Diplomas and Certificates to those who successfully completed the general nursing and midwifery (GNM) and the auxiliary nurse midwife (ANM) programs.

With the initiative of Nursing Administration of Mission Hospitals, the Indian Nursing Council was constituted in 1949. The Indian Nursing Council formulated standards for nursing education in the country. During the last five decades, nursing education has grown and advanced. Midwifery training is incorporated into the three-year basic general nursing program leading to diploma in nursing and midwifery. Auxiliary nurse-midwives program of two years leading to ANM certificate and, the multipurpose health workers (MHWs) program of eighteen months with midwifery training are offered in different states. Graduate programs and postgraduate specialization in maternity nursing are available in several nursing colleges. Education and practice in institutions approved by the State Nursing Council and the Indian Nursing Council followed by registration with the State Nursing Council are mandatory for practicing nursing and midwifery.

CURRENT TRENDS

Since our mothers' and grandmothers' days, enormous changes have taken place in the delivery of nursing care to the mother and the newborn. In their days, most babies were delivered at home by an untrained woman, neighbor, relative or friend or for the fortunate few, by a physician or trained midwife. Surround by loved ones, with her newborn brought promptly to her bed; the new mother received the attention and support of her family.

All that started changing in the second half of 20th century when parturition moved into the hospital setting. Within the "maternity ward", priority was often given to the institution's procedures and practices, relegating the personal needs of the mother and her newborn to second place. At that point, childbearing became far from a family affair. The mother and newborn remained isolated from the family for a week to ten days when the family had only visiting privileges. The infant, separated from its mother was placed in a newborn nursery and brought to its mother only at specified times. Nursing was separated into three subspecialities, with one nurse caring for the mother during labor and delivery, another handling postpartum mothers, and a third caring for the baby in the nursery.

By 1940s, the "rooming in" concept was devised. Full-term infants were placed in a crib at their mothers' bedsides, where the mothers provided their care. Nursing care remained fragmented, with the nursery nurse responsible for infant care and postpartum nurse attending to the mother. The advantages of the system included a reduction in neonatal infection from cross contamination, increased confidence and independence for the mother and greater breastfeeding success. The infant showed better weight gain and cried less. However, the down side was that the new mother evidenced problems in accepting full responsibility for the baby's care.

It has been established that the new mothers experience three psychological phases: taking-in, taking-hold and letting-go. During taking-in, new mothers are passive and dependent, requiring rest and supportive nursing care to promote bonding and attachment. With rooming-in, the mother lacked that supportive care. The taking-hold phase, wherein the mother is ready to learn mothering skills, had been hoisted upon her too soon. Moreover, the letting-go phase, wherein she establishes maternal role patterns and incorporates those changes into her personal and family life, was almost much neglected.

In the 1960s, the focus changed from the person giving care to the recipient of that care. With that change came a change in terminology and obstetrical care became maternity care. The broadened scope includes both prenatal and postnatal care and promotes the health and well-being of the mother, the newborn and the entire family.

The World Health Organization (WHO) offers this definition of maternity care—"The object of maternity care is to ensure that every expectant and nursing mother maintains good health, learns the art of childcare, has a normal delivery and bears healthy children. Maternity care in the narrower sense consists of the care of the pregnant woman, her safe delivery, her postnatal examination, and the care of her newly born infant and the maintenance of lactation. In the wider sense, it begins much earlier in measures aimed to promote the health and well-being of the young people who are potential parents and to help them develop the right approach to family life and to the place of family in the community. It should also include guidance to parent craft and in problems associated with infertility and family planning."

Trends

Changing Patterns of Childbirth and their Effects on Maternal-infant Mortality Statistics

Increasing number of working women defers motherhood until they are in their thirties. As early marriage practices continue, teenage pregnancies, continue to occur. At both ends of the spectrum, the older and the younger mothers face increased risks of complications during pregnancy, such as preterm delivery, low birthweight babies; maternal, fetal neonatal and postnatal mortality.

In addition, women in increasing numbers are working outside the home during pregnancy and shortly after delivery compounding the risks to themselves and the fetus of exposure to toxic chemicals, excessive noise and other workplace stress.

Perinatal Risk Factors

The problems of society are reflected in the risks to today's neonates (Styles, 1990). Among them are acquired immunodeficiency syndrome (AIDS) in mothers and newborns and birth defects resulting from sexually transmitted diseases. Low birthweight babies account for about 30 to 40 percent of live births in developing countries. Preterm babies constitute two-thirds of the low birthweight babies. In addition to maternal age, risk factors of low birth-weight infants include the mother's medical history during past pregnancies, socioeconomic status, education level, and the presence or absence of prenatal care. Sexually transmitted disease (STD) can result in infant death or in a baby born with pneumonia, cerebral palsy, epilepsy, deafness, blindness or mental retardation.

Technological Advances

Advances in technology have revolutionized the diagnosis and treatment of many health conditions. Increasingly sophisticated computers have made swifter diagnosis and continuous monitoring possible (McKenzie and Vestal, 1983). Among those with the greatest effect on maternal and newborn nursing are the instruments available for fetal monitoring and care given by highly specialized professionals in the neonatal intensive care unit (NICU). Because of these advances, it became necessary for nursing personnel to become thorough in the procedures and protocols developed for the use of these advanced equipment and treatment. Although there is concern that the technological advances discourage the "hands-on-care" of the client, the nursing process must remain the foundation of quality nursing care (May and Mahlmeister, 1994).

Fetal monitoring has progressed from the use of the fetoscope to electronic fetal monitors (EFM), which allow for observation of the baby's heartbeat during pregnancy and throughout labor, even during contractions. "Indirect" methods of EFM include ultrasound, phonocardiography and abdominal fetal electrocardiography. "Direct" (internal) fetal monitoring used during labor and delivery is done with a spiral electrode attached to the baby's scalp. The strength of labor contractions can now be measured by means of an internally placed catheter attached to a monitor. Telemetry, using radio transmission, now makes it possible to monitor contractions and fetal heartbeat even when the mother is not in the same room as the monitor. This new development allows for more comfort mobility during labor. Experts predict that in the coming years births that are even more normal would utilize "high tech" innovations, with the result of lowering perinatal mortality and morbidity. Risk assessment and genetic counseling may begin well before pregnancy. Risk situations may be monitored on a 24-hour basis, for more active obstetric management (McKenzie and Vestal, 1983). Fetal assessment tools will become more sophisticated and new corrective techniques will become increasingly available, including *in utero* surgical correction and medical management of defects, direct fetal blood transfusion and drug injection, and genetic diagnosis. The challenges for nurses will be enormous, as they will have to provide humanistic, family-oriented, care in a world of high technology.

Current Problems

Decreased Length of Hospital Stay

Our grandmothers endured a "confinement" of two weeks following childbirth. By the time our mothers had their babies the average postpartum hospital stay had declined to one week. As health care becomes increasingly ambulatory-dominant, today's new mother is up and out of the hospital or health center in two or three days.

Early discharge poses a challenge to the nurse, who must provide nursing interventions during a brief time frame and disseminate information, reinforce learning and affirm the mother's role in hours rather than days. Since early discharge often preludes extensive patient teaching, the nurse will have to become adapt in individualizing teaching based on the unique needs of each patient (Styles, 1990).

Higher Patient Acuities

Multiple socioeconomic problems coupled with lack of knowledge about prenatal care have contributed to increasing number of women who have neglected their health during pregnancy. Many have anemia, hypertension, chronic diseases and STDs. Large numbers go into premature labor, delivering at risk low birthweight babies.

Lack of Facilities in the Rural Areas

About 30 percent of all births in India are conducted by trained Dais (birth attendants), who lack scientific education. Most of the villages in India still have the traditional dais (untrained birth attendants) to help with deliveries. This results in lack of detection of prenatal problems early enough for adequate management, lack of facilities to deal with childbirth complications and inadequate reporting of morbidity.

Changes in Maternal Newborn Nursing

Social, economic, political and technological factors have contributed to the many changes that have occurred in maternal-newborn nursing within recent years. The focus is now on childbirth as a familial process, with less technical interference, greater humanism and a reaffirmation of the natural birth process. In addition, recognition of the importance of mother-baby bonding in the first hours and days of the newborn's life has led to the encouragement of maximal mother-infant contact (Cohen, 1991).

Family-Centered Care

Based on the philosophy that health includes physical, social, economic and psychological dimensions, the family-centered approach assumes that family is the basic unit of society and should be viewed as a total unit with consideration given to each member. Thus, in family-centered care, the emphasis is on the delivery of professional health care that fosters family unity while maintaining the physical safety of the childbearing unit—the mother, father and the infant. The nurse attends, educates and counsels all age groups. Integration and bonding take high priority, and much anticipatory counseling is offered. In family-centered care, the nursery and postpartum staffs are combined to form one mother-baby unit.

Labor, Delivery, Recovery and Postpartum Care (LDRP)

LDRP, also called single room maternity care, was devised as a replacement for traditional maternity unit. In it, the woman labors, delivers and recovers in the same room and in the same bed; and in most cases, the baby remains with the mother during her stay. The LDRP physical setup is generally circular, with single birthing rooms surrounding a central area that contains all the equipment necessary for routine or emergency care. From the time of mother's admission until her discharge, a primary care nurse is assigned to the family. The LDRP system has the advantage of providing comprehensive medical care within a single setting, in more homelike environment, while maintaining all the advantages of hospitalization.

Mother-baby Couplet Care

Couplet care also known as Dyad care, is a system in which one-nurse cares for the post-partum mother and her newborn as single unit. It focuses and adapts to both the physical and psychosocial needs of the mother, the family and the neonate and fosters family unity while providing a secure environment in which nurses are available for consultation, reinforcement and individual education. Nurses help both parents to assume responsibility for their baby's care and assess the family's adaptation and attachment. This system facilitates parental infant attachment, neonatal transition, lactation and involution, while supporting the taking-in and taking-hold phases of the postpartum period.

BIBLIOGRAPHY

1. Bennett RV, Linda KB. Myles Textbook for Midwives, 13th edn. Edenburgh: Churchill Livingstone; 1999.
2. Cohen S. Kenner, Hollingsworth A. Maternal, Neonatal and women's health nursing. Philadelphia: Springhouse Corporation; 1991.
3. Comeron J. The history and development of midwifery in the United States—Can maternity nursing meet today's challenge? Ohio: Ross Laboratories, Columbus; 1967.
4. May K, Mahlmeister L. Maternal and Neonatal Nursing, 3rd edn. Philadelphia: JB Lippincott; 1994.
5. McKenzie CAM, Vestal KW. High-risk Perinatal Nursing, St Louis, WB Saunders, Philadelphia; 1983.
6. Parulekar V Shashank. Textbook for Midwives. 2nd edn. Mumbai: Vora Medical Publications; 1995.
7. Styles MM. Challenges for nursing in this new decade, Maternal Child Nursing 1990;15.

3

The Midwife

Learning Objectives

Upon completing this chapter, the learner will be able to:

❖ Describe the term 'midwife' and list her activities
❖ Enumerate the skills and the responsibilities of a midwife.

The role of a midwife whether she practices in hospitals, health centers or domiciliary conditions has been recognized as one of the most rewarding jobs. Her functions carry great responsibilities and demands specific knowledge and skills.

DEFINITION

The International Confederation of Midwives (ICM) developed a definition of the term 'midwife' in 1972. The International Federation of Gynecology and Obstetrics (IFGO) and World Health Organization (WHO) adopted it in 1973. It was later amended and ratified by World Health Organization in 1992. The international definition of a midwife and her sphere of practice are as follows:

A midwife is a person who, having been regularly admitted to a midwifery educational program fully recognized in the country in which it is located, has successfully completed the prescribed course of studies in midwifery and has acquired the requisite qualifications to be registered and/or legally licensed to practice midwifery.

She must be able to give necessary supervision, care and advise to women during pregnancy, labor and postpartum period, to conduct deliveries on her own responsibility, and to care for the newborn and the infant.

The care includes preventive measures, the detection of abnormal conditions in mother and child, the procurement of medical assistance, and the execution of emergency measures in the absence of medical help.

She has an important task in counseling and education, not only for patients, but also within the family and community. The work should involve antenatal education and preparation for parenthood and extends to certain areas of gynecology, family planning and childcare. She may practice in hospitals, clinics, health units, domiciliary conditions or any other service (Bennett and Brown, 1999).

Midwifery education and practice go beyond the scope of practice outlined in the definition in the European Union and the United States of America. The European directives of 1994 outlines the following:

Member states shall ensure that midwives are at least entitled to take up and pursue the following activities:

❖ To provide sound family planning information and advice
❖ To diagnose pregnancies and monitor normal pregnancies; to carryout examinations necessary for the monitoring of the development of normal pregnancies
❖ To prescribe or advice on the examinations necessary for the earliest possible diagnosis of pregnancies at risk
❖ To provide a program of parenthood preparation and a complete preparation for child birth including advice on hygiene and nutrition
❖ To care for and assist the mother during labor and to monitor the condition of the

fetus *in utero* by appropriate clinical and technical means

❖ To conduct spontaneous deliveries including where required an episiotomy and in urgent cases a breech delivery

❖ To recognize the warning signs of abnormality in the mother or infant which necessitate referral to a doctor and to assist the later where appropriate; to take the necessary emergency measures in the doctor's absence, in particular, the manual removal of placenta, possibly followed by manual examination of the uterus

❖ To examine and care for the newborn infant; to take all initiatives which are necessary in case of need and to carry out where necessary immediate resuscitation

❖ To care for and monitor the progress of the mother in the postnatal period and to give all necessary advice to the mother on infant care to enable her to ensure the optimum progress of the newborn infant

❖ To carryout the treatment prescribed by a doctor

❖ To maintain all necessary records (Bennett and Brown, 1999).

Nurse-midwives in the United States are taught a wide range of matters covering the following topics:

❖ Normal obstetrics, gynecology and neonatal pediatrics and their medical management

❖ Knowledge, skills and judgment for the facilitation of natural process and non-intervention in these normal processes unless indicated

❖ Beliefs in continuity of care

❖ Beliefs and knowledge in the promotion and implementation of family-centered maternity care

❖ Beliefs, knowledge and skills in educating patients for knowledgeable participation and decision making in their health care and for experiencing of their bodily processes (Varney H, 1996).

Midwifery also encompasses the primary focus of medicine on the diagnosis and treatment of a condition as it pertains to the essentially normal woman and neonate. Nurse

midwifery thus, is comprised of education in two disciplines that also incorporate components of a third discipline medicine. In practice, nurse midwifery, encompasses all of midwifery plus components from both nursing and medicine. It is thus, not totally nursing, not totally midwifery and not totally medicine. It is a unique profession in its own right and the nurse-midwife a unique professional.

DEVELOPMENT OF MIDWIFERY EDUCATION IN INDIA

India with its vast population distributed in urban and rural areas, has health problems and management problems, which are different from those in European countries or the United States. In order to meet the needs of the people, with varying living and economic conditions, the Government of India implemented midwifery programs of different levels. "Dais" (untrained birth attendants) were given training to perform domiciliary midwifery. Through the rural health administration plan, their services were organized and supervised.

Another level of midwifery training was the Auxiliary Nurse Midwives (ANMs) program of two years. Auxiliary Nurse Midwives require registration to practice and they function in Primary Health Centers, District Hospitals and even in certain tertiary level hospitals with supervision. General Nursing Program of three years duration includes midwifery education and practice. The graduates are registered/licensed as nurse-midwives (RN, RM) and practice in hospitals and community set-ups. The graduate program in nursing of four years duration also includes midwifery and they are registered as RN, RM by the State Registration Councils. Training programs throughout the country is regulated by the Indian Nursing council, which prescribes the syllabus for education and training.

Textbooks written by British and American authors or physician authors are used mainly for teaching in the different programs of midwifery in undergraduate, graduate, postgraduate education. For Indian midwives, there are specific written directives for practice at the State Registration Council level and the Directives of the European Union (UKCC, 1994) are used as guidelines with additional policies at the institutional level.

Skills of the Midwife

A midwife takes responsibility for her own actions but also may initiate care by others and is able to function in a multiprofessional team. She must function within the regulations governing the profession and maintain her knowledge and skills up-to-date.

She teaches parents about healthy living both before and after the birth of the baby. The midwife must be competent to diagnose pregnancy and to carry out examinations of the woman and the baby in order to assess their condition. The midwife is an expert in normal midwifery and in caring for the mother and newborn.

When faced with emergencies, she summons medical aid and also takes immediate steps to treat mother or baby and continues to give care while help is on the way. The obstetrician or the physician incharge will be called upon to give aid when deviations from normal arise. In appropriate situations, she will utilize the assistance of neonatologists, dietitians, physiotherapists and social workers.

She is duty-bound to administer intelligently, care and treatment prescribed by obstetricians or physicians. The midwife will use her listening skills and allow her clients to voice their concern and feelings. She functions cooperatively with the multiprofessional team, which exists to care for mothers, babies and their families.

Responsibilities of the Midwife

Every midwife has a responsibility to maintain professional competence. As midwifery practice develops, she will need to integrate new skills into the range of her functions. Some of these may be specific to midwives practicing in certain settings. Midwives are to keep clear, detailed records of all relevant care activities and events as required in the institution. Records must be written in an acceptable manner, as they will be preserved for years for different purposes.

Midwives today ought to be able to carryout a problem solving process in rendering care to mothers and babies. The nursing process methodology followed for the care of medical, surgical or pediatric clients needs to be implemented in maternal and newborn care as well. These management processes are elaborated in the following chapter.

BIBLIOGRAPHY

1. Bennett R, Linda KB. Myles textbook for midwives, 13th edn. Churchill Livingstone; 1999.
2. International Confederation of Nurse Midwives, Definition of the Midwife, ICM, London; 1992.
3. Megelen MC, Burst HV. Nurse-Midwives make a difference, Nursing Outlook; 1974;22:382.
4. United Kingdom Central Council for Nursing, Midwifery and Health Visiting, The Midwife's Code of Practice, UKCC, London; 1994.
5. Warwick C. Leadership in midwifery care, British Journal of Midwives; 1996;4(5):229.

4

The Nursing Process in Maternal Newborn Care

The foundation for the practice of nursing depends upon the utilization of the nursing process in all aspects of patient care. The nursing process provides an organized and comprehensive framework for directing nursing activities. It is based on the scientific method for problem solving and follows a logical sequence, which makes it most useful to students in learning the management of care of clients. As it provides a mean of putting together isolated pieces of information, findings, judgments and skills into a meaningful whole as they perform their role of patient management, it becomes a patient centered approach.

The term 'nursing process' was originated in 1955 by Hall and later used by Johnson (1959), Orlando (1961), and Weidenbach (1963). The purpose of the nursing process is to identify a client's health status, his/her actual or potential health care problems or needs, to establish plans to meet the identified needs and to deliver specific nursing interventions to meet these needs. The client may be an individual, a family or a group. The use of nursing process in clinical practice gained additional legitimacy in 1973 when it was included in the American Nurses Association's (ANA), *Standards of Clinical Nursing Practice*. The standards of care include the five phases of nursing process: *Assessment, diagnosis, planning, implementation,* and *evaluation*. The different phases of nursing process are closely interrelated and each phase affects the others. For example, if inadequate data are obtained during assessing, the nursing diagnosis will be incomplete or incorrect; and the inaccuracy will also be reflected in the planning, implementing and evaluating phases.

The nursing process is a systematic, rational method of planning and providing nursing care. The nursing process is cyclical; that is, its components follow a logical sequence, and more than one component may be involved at one time. At the end of the cycle, care may be terminated if goals are achieved, or the cycle may continue with reassessment, or the plan of care may be modified.

THE FIVE PHASES OF NURSING PROCESS

Assessing

Assessing is the systematic and continuous collection, organization, validation, and documentation of data/information for the purpose of establishing a *database* about the client's responses to health concerns or illness and the ability to manage health care needs. In effect assessing is a continuous process carried out during all phases of the nursing process. For example, in the evaluation phase assessment is done to determine the outcomes of the nursing strategies and to evaluate goal achievement.

There are four types of assessments; initial assessment, problem-focused assessment, emergency assessment and time-lapsed assessment. Assessments vary according to their purpose, time available and client status.

* *Initial assessment* is performed within specified time after admission to a health care agency, such as the admission assessment. The purpose is to establish a complete database for problem identification, reference and future comparison.
* *Problem-focused assessment* is an ongoing process integrated with nursing care. It is done to determine the status of a specific problem identified in an earlier assessment and to identify new or overlooked problems. An example for this would be the assessment of a client's ability to perform self-care while assisting him to bathe.
* *Emergency assessment is* done during any physiologic or psychologic crisis of the client. The purpose is to identify life-threatening problems. For example, rapid assessment of a person's airway, breathing status and circulation during a cardiac arrest or assessment of suicidal tendencies or potential for violence in a psychiatric patient.
* *Time-lapsed assessment* is done several months after initial assessment. The purpose is to compare the client's current status to baseline data previously obtained. Reassessment of a client's functional health patterns in a home care or outpatient setting or in hospital at shift change are examples of time-lapsed assessment.

Collecting Data

Data collection is the process of gathering information about a client's health status. It must be both systematic and continuous to prevent the omission of significant data and reflect a client's changing status.

A Database

It is all the information about a client; it includes the nursing health history, physical assessment, the physician's health history and physical examination, results of laboratory and diagnostic tests and material contributed by other health personnel.

Client data should include past history as well as current problems. For example, a history of an allergic reaction to penicillin and chronic diseases are important historical data. Current data relate to present circumstances, such as pain, nausea and sleep patterns.

Type of Data

Data can be subjective or objective.

Subjective data are also referred to as symptoms or *covert data*. These are apparent only to the person affected and can be reported or described only by that person or client. Pain, anxiety and fear are examples of subjective data. Client's sensation, feelings, values, beliefs, attitudes and perceptions of health status are all subjective data.

Objective data are referred to as signs or overt data, which are detectable by an observer or can be measured or tested against an acceptable standard. This can be seen, heard, felt or smelled and they are obtained by observation or physical examination. For example, a discoloration of the skin or a blood pressure reading is objective data. During physical examination, the nurse obtains objective data to validate subjective data and to complete the assessment phase of the nursing process.

A complete database of both objective and objective data provides a baseline for comparing the client's responses to nursing and medical interventions.

Sources of Data

Sources of data are primary and secondary. The client is the primary source of data. Family members, other support persons, other health professionals, records and reports, laboratory and diagnostic analyses, and relevant literature are secondary sources.

The best source of data is usually the client, unless *the client* is a too ill, young, or confused to communicate clearly. The client can provide subjective data that no one else can offer. Family members, friends and care givers who know the client well often can supplement or verify information provided by the client. Support people are especially important source of data for a client who is very young, unconscious, or confused.

Client records serve as good source of data. They contain data regarding the client's occupation, religion, and marital status. Type of client records includes medical records, records of therapies and laboratory records. Medical records are often a source of a client's present and past health and illness patterns. These records can provide nurses with information about the client's coping behaviors, health practices, previous illnesses and allergies.

Records of therapies provided by other health professionals such as social workers, nutritionists, dietitians or physical therapists help the nurse obtain relevant data not expressed by the client.

Laboratory records also provide pertinent health information. For example, the determination of blood glucose level allows health professionals to monitor the administration of hypoglycemic agents.

Reports from *other health care professionals* serve as other potential sources of information about a client's health. Nurses, social workers, physicians and physiotherapists may have information from either previous or current contact with the client. Both verbal and written reports of health care professionals add to data regarding client.

Review of nursing and *related literature*, such as professional journals, and reference texts can provide additional information for the database.

Data Collection Methods

The methods used to collect data are observing, interviewing and examining. Observation occurs whenever the nurse is in contact with the client or support persons. Interviewing is used mainly while taking the nursing health history. Examining is the major method used in the physical health assessment. In reality, the nurse uses all three methods simultaneously when assessing clients. For example, during the client interview the nurse observes, listens, asks questions, and mentally retains information to explore in the physical examination.

Observing

To observe is togather data by using the senses. Observation is a conscious, deliberate skill that is developed through effort and through an organized approach.

Although nurses observe mainly through sight, most of the senses are engaged during careful observations.

Observation has two aspects (a) noticing data and (b) selecting, organizing and interpreting the data. A nurse who observes that a client's face is flushed must relate that observation to, for example, body temperature, activity, environmental temperature and blood pressure. Nursing observations must be organized so that nothing significant is missed.

Interviewing

An interview is a planned communication or a conversation with a purpose. There are two approaches to interviewing: *directive* and *nondirective*. The directive interview is highly structured and elicits specific information. The nurse establishes the purpose of the interview and controls the interview, at least at the outset. The client responds to questions, but may have limited opportunity to ask questions or discuss concerns. Nurses frequently use directive interview in emergency situations.

During a *nondirective interview*, or rapport-building interview, by contrast, the nurse allows the client to control the purpose, subject matter and pacing. Rapport is an understanding between two or more people. A combination of directive and nondirective approach is usually appropriate during the information gathering interview.

Examining

The physical examination or physical assessment is a systematic data-collection method that uses observation (i.e. the sense of sight, hearing, smell and touch) to detect health problems. To conduct the examination, the nurse uses techniques of inspection, auscultation, palpation and percussion. Alternatively, the nurse may perform a screening examination. *A screening examination*, also called *a review of systems*, is a brief review of essential functioning of various body parts or systems. An example of a screening examination is the nursing admission assessment.

Validating Data

The information gathered during the assessment phase must be complete, factual and accurate because the nursing diagnoses and interventions are based on this information. *Validation* is the act of "double-checking" or verifying data to confirm that it is accurate and factual.

To build an accurate database, nurses must validate assumptions regarding the client's physical or emotional behavior. For example, a nurse seeing a man holding his arm to his chest might assume that he is experiencing chest pain, when in fact he has a painful hand.

Documenting Data

The complete the assessment phase, the nurse records client data. Accurate documentation is essential and should include all data collected about the client's health status. Data are recorded in a factual manner and not interpreted by the nurse. In order to increase accuracy, the nurse records subjective data in the client's own words.

DIAGNOSIS

Diagnosing is the second phase of the nursing process. In this phase, nurses use critical-thinking skills to interpret assessment data and identify client strengths and problems. Diagnosis is a pivotal step in the nursing process. All activities preceding this phase are directed toward formulating the *nursing diagnosis*; all the care-planning activities following this phase are based on the nursing diagnoses.

The identification and development of nursing diagnoses began formally in 1973, when two faculty members of Saint Louis University, Kristine Gebbie and Mary Ann Lavin, perceived a need to identify nurses' roles in an ambulatory care setting. The first National Conference to identify nursing diagnoses was sponsored by the Saint Louis University School of Nursing in 1973. Subsequent national conferences occurred in 1975, 1980 and every 2 years thereafter.

International recognition came with the first Canadian Conference in Toronto in 1977 and the international nursing conference in May 1987 in Calgary, Alberta, Canada. In 1982, the conference group accepted the name "North American Nursing Diagnosis Association (NANDA)", recognizing the participation and contributions of nurses in the United States and Canada.

The purpose of NANDA is to define, refine, and promote taxonomy of nursing diagnostic terminology for general use by professional nurses. *Taxonomy* is a classification system or set of categories arranged on the basis of a single principle or set of principles. The group has currently approved more than 150 *nursing diagnosis labels* for clinical use.

Definition

The term *diagnosing* refers to the reasoning process whereas the term *diagnosis* is a statement or conclusion regarding the nature of a phenomenon. The standardized NANDA names for the diagnoses are called *diagnostic labels*; and the client's problem statement, consisting the diagnostic label plus etiology (casual relationship between a problem and its related or risk factors) is called *nursing diagnosis*.

In 1990, Nanda adopted an official working definition of nursing diagnosis; "a clinical judgment about individual, family, or community responses to actual and potential health problems or life processes. Nursing diagnosis provides the basis for selection of nursing interventions to achieve outcomes for which the nurse is accountable". This definition implies the following:

❖ Professional nurses (registered nurses) are responsible for making nursing diagnoses, even though other nursing personnel may contribute data to the process of diagnosing and may implement specified nursing care. Nurses are accountable for this phase of the nursing process

❖ The domain of nursing diagnosis includes only those health states that nurses are educated and licensed to treat

❖ A nursing diagnosis is a judgment made only after thorough, systematic data collection

❖ Nursing diagnoses describe a continuum of health states: deviations from health, presence of risk factors, and areas of enhanced personal growth (Table 4.1).

Type of Nursing Diagnoses

The five types of nursing diagnoses are *actual, risk, wellness, possible* and *syndrome.*

1. *An actual diagnosis* is a client problem that is present at the time of the nursing assessment. Examples are *Ineffective Breathing Pattern* and *pain.* An actual nursing diagnosis is based on the presence of associated signs and symptoms.

2. *A risk nursing diagnosis* is a clinical judgment that a problem does not exist, but the presence of *risk factors* indicates that a problem is likely to develop unless nurses intervene. For example, a client with diabetes or a compromised immune system is at *high-risk* for infection than others. Therefore, the nurse would appropriately use the label *Risk for* infection to describe the client's health status.

3. *A wellness diagnosis* describes human responses to levels of wellness in an individual, family or community that have a readiness for enhancement. Examples of wellness diagnosis would be "Readiness for Eenhanced Family Coping" or "Readiness for Enhanced Spiritual Well-being".

4. *A possible nursing diagnosis* is one in which evidence about a health problem is incomplete or unclear. A possible diagnosis requires more data either to support or to refute it. For example, an elderly widow who lives alone is admitted to the hospital. The nurse notices that she has no visitors and is pleased with the attention from nursing staff. A nursing diagnosis for the client may be "possible social isolation related to unknown etiology".

5. *A syndrome diagnosis* is a diagnosis that is associated with a cluster of other diagnoses. Currently six syndrome diagnoses are on the NANDA international list. For example, long-term bedridden clients may experience disuse syndrome. Clusters of diagnosis associated with this syndrome include. *Impaired physical mobility, Risk for impaired Tissue Integrity, Risk for activity Intolerance, Risk for Constipation, Impaired Gas Exchange* and so on.

Components of a NANDA Nursing Diagnosis

A nursing diagnosis has three components: (1) The problem and its definition, (2) the etiology, and (3) the defining characteristics, each component serves a specific purpose.

Problem and Definition (Diagnostic Label)

The problem statement, or diagnostic label, describes the client's health problem or response for which nursing therapy is given. It describes the client's health status clearly and concisely in a few words. The purpose of the diagnostic label is to direct the information of client goals and desired outcomes. It may also suggest some nursing interventions.

To be clinically useful, diagnostic labels need to be specific when the word *specify* follows a NANDA label. The nurse states the area in which the problem occurs, for example, *Deficient Knowledge (Medications)* or *Deficient Knowledge (Dietary Modifications).*

Qualifiers

These are words that have been added to some NANDA labels to give additional meaning to the diagnostic statement. For example:

❖ *Deficient* (inadequate in amount, quality or degree) not sufficient; incomplete

❖ *Impaired* (made worse, weakened, damaged, reduced, deteriorated)

❖ *Decreased* (lesser in size, amount or degree)

- ❖ *Ineffective* (not producing the desired effect)
- ❖ *Compromised* (to make vulnerable or threat).

Etiology (Related Factors and Risk Factors)

The etiology component of a nursing diagnosis identifies one or more probable causes of the health problem, gives direction to the required nursing interventions and enables the nurse to individualize the client's care. For example, the probable causes of *activity intolerance* include sedentary life style, generalized weakness, bed rest or immobility. Differentiating among possible causes in the nursing diagnosis is essential because each may require different nursing interventions.

Defining Characteristics

Defining characteristics are the cluster of signs and symptoms that indicate the presence of a particular diagnostic label. For *actual nursing diagnoses*, the defining characteristics are the client's *signs and symptoms*. For *risk nursing diagnoses*, *no subjective* and *objective* signs are present. Thus, the factors that cause the client to be more than "normally" vulnerable to the problem form the etiology of a risk nursing diagnosis.

Differentiating Nursing Diagnoses from Medical Diagnoses

A nursing diagnosis is a statement of nursing judgment and refers to a condition that nurses are licensed to treat.

A medical diagnosis is made by physician and refers to a condition that only a physician can treat. Medical diagnoses refer to disease processes—specific pathophysiologic responses that are fairly uniform from one client to another. In contrast, nursing diagnoses describe a client's physical, sociocultural, psychological and spiritual responses to an illness or a health problem.

A client's medical diagnosis remains the same for as long as the disease process is present, but nursing diagnosis changes as the client's responses change. Nurses have responsibilities related to both medical and nursing

diagnoses. Nursing diagnoses relate to the nurse's *independent functions*, that is, the areas of health care that are unique to nursing and separate and distinct from medical management.

The Diagnostic Process

The diagnostic process uses the critical thinking skills of analysis, and synthesis. Critical thinking is a cognitive process during which a person reviews data and considers explanation before forming an opinion. The diagnostic process has three steps:
1. Analyzing data
2. Identifying health problems, risks and strengths and
3. Formulating diagnostic statement.

Formulating Diagnostic Statements

Most nursing diagnosis are written as *two-part* or *three-part statements*.
1. Basic two-part statements include the following:
   i. *Problem (P)*: Statement of the client's response (Nanda label).
   ii. Etiology (E): Factors contributing to or probable causes of the responses.
   The two parts are joined by the words *related to* rather than *due to*. The phrase *due to* implies that one part causes or is responsible for the other part. By contrast, the phrase *related to*, merely implies a relationship. Examples of two-part nursing diagnosis are:
   – Constipation related to irregular defecation habits.
   – Ineffective breastfeeding related to breast engorgement.
   Some NANDA labels contain the word *specify*. For these, the nurse must add words to indicate the problem more specifically. For example, Noncompliance (specify). Noncompliance (Diabetic diet) related to denial of having disease.
2. *Basic three-part statements*: The basic three-part nursing diagnosis statement is the *PES format* and includes the following:
   i. *Problem (P):* Statement of the client's response (NANDA label).

ii. *Etiology (E):* Factors contributing to or probable causes of the response.

iii. *Signs and symptoms (S):* Defining characteristics manifested by the client.

Example:

❖ Ineffective coping related to labor and delivery as evidenced by fatigue and expressed inability to cope.

❖ Deficient fluid volume related to postpartum hemorrhage as evidenced by decreased pulse volume and pressure.

Actual nursing diagnoses can be documented by using the three-part statement because the signs and symptoms have been identified. The format cannot be used for risk diagnoses because the client does not have signs and symptoms of the diagnosis.

In addition to using the correct format, nurses must consider the content of their diagnostic statements. The statements should, for example, be accurate, concise, descriptive, and specific. The nurse must always validate the diagnostic statements with the client and compare the clients' signs and symptoms to the NANDA defining characteristics. For risk factors, the nurse compares the client's risk factors to NANDA risk factors.

One-part statements: Some diagnostic statements, such as wellness diagnosis and syndrome nursing diagnosis, consist of a NANDA label only. As the diagnostic labels are refined, they tend to become more specific, so that nursing interventions can be derived from the label itself. Therefore, an etiology may not be needed. For example, adding an etiology to the label Rape-Trauma Syndrome does not make the label any more descriptive or useful.

NANDA has specified that any new *wellness diagnoses* will be developed as one-part statements beginning with the words *Readiness for enhanced* followed by the desired higher level wellness. For example, *Readiness for enhanced parenting.*

Currently the NANDA list includes several wellness diagnoses. Some of these are: *Spiritual well-being, effective breastfeeding, health seeking behaviors,* and *anticipatory grieving.* These are usually accepted as one-part statements, but

may be made more explicit by adding a descriptor, for example, *Health seeking behaviors (low fat diet)* (Table 4.1).

Variations of Basic Formats

Variations of the basic, one, two and three-part statements include the following:

1. Writing the terms *unknown etiology*, when the defining characteristics are present but the nurse does not know the cause or contributing factors. For example, *Non-compliance (medication regimen) related to unknown etiology.*

2. Using the phrase *complex factors*, when there are too many etiologic factors or when they are too complex to state in a brief phrase. The actual causes of chronic low self-esteem, for instance, may be long-term and complex, as in the following nursing diagnosis *chronic low self-esteem related to complex factors.*

3. Using the word *possible* to describe either the problem or the etiology. When the nurse believes more data are needed about the client's problem or the etiology, the word *possible* is used. Examples are: *Possible low self-esteem related to loss of job and rejection by family. Altered thought process possibly related to unfamiliar surroundings.*

4. Using the word *secondary* to divide the etiology into two parts; thereby making the statement more descriptive and useful. The part following secondary to is often pathophysiologic or disease process as in *risk for impaired skin integrity related to decreased peripheral circulation secondary to diabetes.*

5. Adding a secondary part to the general response or NANDA label, to make it more precise. For example, the diagnosis *impaired skin integrity (left lateral ankle)* related to decreased peripheral circulation.

Avoiding Errors in Diagnostic Reasoning

It is important that nurses make nursing diagnoses with a high level of accuracy. Nurses can avoid some common errors of reasoning

Table 4.1 NANDA—Approved nursing diagnoses for use and research through 2007-2008

1. Activity intolerance
2. Activity intolerance, risk for
3. Airway clearance, ineffective
4. Anxiety (specify level)
5. Anxiety death
6. Aspiration, risk for
7. Attachment, parent/infant/child, risk for impaired
8. Autonomic dysreflexia, risk for
9. Blood glucose, risk for unstable
10. Body image, disturbed
11. Body temperature, imbalanced, risk for
12. Bowel incontinence
13. Breastfeeding, effective
14. Breastfeeding, ineffective
15. Breastfeeding, interrupted
16. Breathing, pattern, ineffective
17. Cardiac output, decreased
18. Caregiver role strain
19. Caregiver role strain, risk for
20. Comfort, readiness for enhanced
21. Communication: Impaired, verbal
22. Communication, readiness for enhanced
23. Confusion acute
24. Confusion, acute, risk for
25. Confusion, chronic
26. Constipation
27. Constipation, perceived
28. Constipation, risk for
29. Contamination
30. Contamination, risk for
31. Coping: Community, ineffective
32. Coping: Community, readiness for enhanced
33. Coping, defensive
34. Coping: Family, compromised
35. Coping: Family, disabled
36. Coping: Family, readiness for enhanced
37. Coping (individual), readiness for enhanced
38. Coping, ineffective
39. Decisional conflict
40. Decision-making, readiness for enhanced
41. Denial, ineffective
42. Dentition impaired
43. Development, delayed, risk for
44. Diarrhea
45. Disuse syndrome, risk for
46. Divisional activity, deficient energy field, disturbed
47. Environmental interpretation syndrome, impaired
48. Failure of thrive, adult
49. Fails, risk for
50. Family processed, dysfunctional: Alcoholism
51. Family processes, interrupted
52. Family processes, readiness for enhanced
53. Fatigue
54. Fear
55. Fluid balance, readiness for enhanced
56. Fluid volume, deficient
57. Fluid volume, deficient, risk for
58. Fluid volume, excess
59. Fluid volume, imbalanced risk for
60. Gas exchange, impaired
61. Grieving
62. Grieving complicated
63. Grieving, risk for complicated
64. Growth, disproportionate, risk for
65. Growth and development delayed
66. Health behavior, risk-prone
67. Health maintenance, ineffective
68. Health-seeking behaviors (specify)
69. Home maintenance, impaired
70. Hope, readiness for enhanced
71. Hopelessness
72. Human dignity, risk for compromised
73. Hyperthermia
74. Hypothermia
75. Immunization status, readiness for enhanced
76. Infant behavior: Disorganized
77. Infant behavior: Organized, readiness for enhanced
78. Infant feeding patent, ineffective
79. Infection, risk for
80. Injury, risk for
81. Insomnia
82. Intracranial adaptive capacity, deceased
83. Knowledge, deficient (specify)
84. Knowledge (specify), readiness for enhanced
85. Latex allergy response
86. Latex allergy, response, risk for
87. Liver function, impaired, risk for
88. Loneliness, risk for
89. Memory, impaired
90. Mobility, bed, impaired
91. Mobility: Physical, impaired
92. Mobility: Wheelchair, impaired
93. Moral distress
94. Nausea

Contd...

Contd...

95. Neurovascular dysfunction: Peripheral, risk for
96. Noncompliance (specify)
97. Nutrition, imbalanced: Less than body requirements
98. Nutrition, imbalanced: More than body requirements
99. Nutrition, readiness for enhanced
100. Oral mucous membrane, impaired
101. Pain, acute
102. Pain, chronic
103. Parenting, impaired
104. Parenting, readiness for enhanced
105. Parenting, risk for impaired
106. Perioperative positioning injury, risk for
107. Personal identify, disturbed
108. Poisoning, risk for
109. Post-trauma
110. Post-trauma syndrome risk for
111. Power, readiness for enhanced
112. Powerlessness
113. Powerlessness, risk for
114. Protection, ineffective
115. Rape-trauma syndrome
116. Rape-trauma syndrome: Compound reaction
117. Rape-trauma syndrome: Silent reaction
118. Religiosity, impaired
119. Religiosity, readiness for enhanced
120. Religiosity, risk for impaired
121. Relocation stress syndrome
122. Relocation stress syndrome, risk for
123. Role conflict, parental
124. Role performance, ineffective
125. Secondary lifestyle
126. Self-care readiness for enhanced
127. Self-care deficit: Bathing / hygiene
128. Self-care deficit: Dressing/grooming
129. Self-care deficit: Feeding
130. Self-care deficit: Toileting
131. Self-concept, readiness for enhanced
132. Self-esteem, chronic low
133. Self-esteem, situational low
134. Self-esteem, risk for situational law
135. Self-mutilation
136. Self-mutilation, risk for
137. Sensory perception, disturbed (specify: Auditory, gustatory, kinesthetic, olfactory.
138. Sexual dysfunction
139. Sexuality pattern, ineffective
140. Skin integrity, impaired
141. Skin integrity, risk for impaired
142. Sleep deprivation
143. Sleep, readiness for enhanced
144. Social interaction, impaired
145. Social isolation
146. Sorrow, chronic
147. Spiritual distress
148. Spiritual distress, risk for
149. Spiritual well-being, readiness for enhanced
150. Spontaneous ventilation, impaired
151. Stress, overload
152. Sudden infant death syndrome, risk for
153. Suffocation, risk for
154. Suicide, risk for
155. Surgical recovery, delayed
156. Swallowing, impaired
157. Therapeutic regimen management: Community, ineffective
158. Therapeutic regimen management, effective
159. Therapeutic regimen management, family, ineffective
160. Therapeutic regimen management, ineffective
161. Therapeutic regimen management, readiness for enhanced
162. Thermoregulation, ineffective
163. Thought processes, disturbed
164. Tissue integrity, impaired
165. Tissue perfusion, ineffective (specify: Cerebral, cardiopulmonary, gastrointestinal renal)
166. Tissue perfusion, ineffective, peripheral
167. Transfer ability, impaired
168. Trauma, risk for unilateral neglect
169. Urinary elimination, impaired
170. Urinary elimination, readiness for enhanced
171. Urinary incontinence, functional
172. Urinary retention
173. Urinary incontinence, overflow
174. Urinary incontinence, reflex
175. Urinary incontinence, stress
176. Urinary incontinence, total
177. Urinary incontinence, urge
178. Urinary incontinence, risk for urge
179. Ventilation, impaired, spontaneous
180. Ventilatory wearing response, dysfunctional
181. Walking impaired
182. Wandering (specify sporadic or continual)

Source: NANDA Nursing diagnoses: Definition and classification, 2007–2008. Philadelphia; North America Nursing Diagnosis Association.

by recognizing them and applying appropriate critical-thinking skills. Errors can occur at any point in the diagnostic process: data collection, data interpretation and data clustering. The following steps help to minimize diagnostic errors.

❖ *Verify:* Hypothesize possible explanations of the data, but realize that all diagnoses are tentative until they are verified. Begin and end the process by talking with the client and family. Ask them what their health problems are and what they believe the causes to be. At the end of the process have them verify your diagnoses.

❖ *Build a good knowledge base and acquire clinical experience*: Nurse must apply knowledge from many different areas (applied sciences) to recognize significant cues and patterns and generate a hypothesis about the data. For example, principles from chemistry, anatomy, and pharmacology each help the nurse understand client data.

❖ *Have a working knowledge of what is normal*: Nurses need to know the normal physiological parameters for vital signs, laboratory tests, breath sounds and so on. In addition, she must determine what is normal for a particular person taking into accounts of his or her age, physical make up, life style, and physiological changes such as pregnancy.

❖ *Consult resources*: Both freshers and experienced nurses should consult appropriate resources, whenever in doubt about a diagnosis. Professional literature, nursing colleagues and nurse educators are all appropriate resources. Use of a nursing diagnosis handbook for quick reference will be useful too.

❖ *Improve critical thinking skills*: These skills help the nurse to be aware of and avoid errors in thinking, such as over generalizing, stereotyping and making unwarranted assumptions.

Guidelines for writing nursing diagnostic statements

1. State in terms of a problem not a need.
   Correct: Deficient fluid volume (problem) related to fever.
   Incorrect: Fluid replacement (need) related to fever.

2. Word the statement so that it is legally acceptable.
   Correct: Impaired skin integrity related to immobility (legally acceptable).
   Incorrect: Impaired skin integrity related to improper positioning (implies legal liability).

3. Use nonjudgmental statements.
   Correct: Spiritual distress related to inability to attend church services secondary to immobility (nonjudgmental).
   Incorrect: Spiritual distress related to strict rules requiring regular church attendance (judgmental).

4. Make sure that both elements of the statement do not say the same thing.
   Correct: Risk for impaired skin integrity related to immobility.
   Incorrect: Impaired skin integrity related to ulceration of sacral area.
   (Problem and probable cause are the same)

5. Be sure that problem and etiology are correctly stated.
   Correct: Pain: Severe headache related to fear of addiction to narcotics.
   Incorrect: Pain related to severe headache.

6. Word the diagnosis specifically and precisely to provide direction for planning nursing interventions.
   Correct: Impaired oral mucous membrane related to decreased salivation secondary to radiation of neck (specific).
   Incorrect: Impaired oral mucous membrane related to noxious agent (vague).

7. Use nursing terminology rather than medical terminology to describe the client's response.
   Correct: Risk for ineffective airway clearance related to accumulation of secretions in lungs (nursing terminology).
   Incorrect: Risk for pneumonia (medical terminology).

8. Use nursing terminology rather than medical terminology to describe the probable cause of the client's response.

Correct: Risk for ineffective airway clearance related to accumulation of secretions in lungs (nursing terminology).

Incorrect: Risk for ineffective airway clearance related to emphysema (medical terminology).

PLANNING

Planning is the third phase of the nursing process, in which the nurse and client develop client goals/desired outcomes and nursing interventions to prevent, reduce or alleviate the client's health problems.

Planning is a deliberate, systematic process that involves decision-making and problem solving. In planning, the nurse refers to the client's assessment data and diagnostic statements for direction in formulating client goals and designing the nursing interventions required to manage the client's health problems.

A *nursing intervention* is any treatment, based on clinical judgment and knowledge that a nurse performs to enhance patient/client outcomes.

Although planning is basically a nurse's responsibility, input from the client and support person (family members) is essential if a plan is to be effective. Nurses do not plan for the client, but encourage the client to participate actively to the extent possible. In a home setting, the client's family members and caregivers are the ones who implement the plan of care, thus its effectiveness depends largely on them.

Types of Planning

Planning begins with the first client contact and continues until the nurse-client relationship ends, usually when the client is discharged from the hospital.

Initial Planning

The nurse who performs the admission assessment usually develops the initial, plan of care. This nurse uses the client's body language, as well as some intuitive kinds of information that are not solely available from written database. Planning should be initiated as soon as possible after the initial assessment.

Ongoing Planning

All nurses who work with the client do ongoing planning. As nurses obtain new information and evaluate the client's responses to care, they can individualize the initial care plan further. Ongoing planning also occurs at the beginning of a shift as the nurse plans the care to be given that day/that shift. The nurse carries out the daily planning in order to:

❖ Determine whether the client's health status has changed
❖ Set priorities for the client's care during the shift
❖ Decide which problems to focus on during the shift
❖ Coordinate nurse's activities so that more than one problem can be addressed at each client contact.

Discharge Planning

Discharge planning is the process of anticipating and planning for needs after discharge. This is a crucial part of comprehensive health care and should be addressed in each client's care plan. For patients who are discharged early – before complete recovery, such care is delivered in the home. Effective discharge planning begins at first contact with client and involves comprehensive and ongoing assessment to obtain information about client's ongoing needs.

Developing Nursing Care Plans

The end product of the planning phase of the nursing process is a *formal* or *informal plan* of care.

An *informal nursing care plan* is a strategy for action that exists in the nurse's mind. For example, the nurse may think "Mrs Ramu is very tired, I will reinforce her teaching after she is rested".

A *formal nursing care plan* is a written or computerized guide that organizes information about the client's care. The benefit of a formal written care plan is that it provides for continuity of care.

A *standardized care plan* is a formal plan that specifies the nursing cares for groups of clients with common needs (example, all clients with eclamptic fits).

An individualized care plan is tailored to meet the unique needs of a specific client–those are needs that are not addressed by the standardized plan.

Nurses use the formal care plan for direction about what needs to be documented in client progress notes and as a guide for delegating and assigning staff to care for clients. *When nursing diagnoses are used to develop goals and nursing interventions, the result is a holistic, individualized plan of care that will meet the client's unique needs.*

Care plans include the actions nurses must take to address the client's nursing diagnoses and produce the desired outcome. The nurse begins the plan when the client is admitted to the hospital and constantly updates it throughout the client's stay in response to changes in the client's condition and evaluations of goal achievement.

The complete plan of care for a client is made up of several different documents that:

a. Describe the routine care needed to meet basic needs such as bathing and nutrition.
b. Address the client's nursing diagnoses and collaborative problems and
c. Specify nursing responsibilities in carrying out the medical plan of care (e.g. scheduling laboratory tests, keeping client from eating or drinking before surgery). A complete plan of care integrates dependent and independent nursing functions.

Standardized Approaches to Care Planning

Standards of care, standardized care plans, protocols, policies and procedures are developed and accepted by nursing staff in order to ensure that minimum acceptable standards for patient care are met and to promote efficient use of nurses' time.

Standardized care plans are preprinted guides for the nursing care of a client who has a need that arises frequently in the agency (e.g. specific nursing diagnosis or all nursing diagnoses associated with a particular medical condition). They are written from the perspective of what care the client can expect.

Standardized Care Plans

❖ Are kept with the client's individualized care plan on the nursing unit, probably in the 'kardex'. When the client is discharged, they become part of the permanent medical record.
❖ Provide detailed interventions and contain additions or deletion from the standards of care of the agency.
❖ Are written in the nursing process format? Problem → Desired outcomes/goals → Nursing interventions → Evaluations.

Like standardized care plans, *protocols* are preprinted to indicate the actions commonly required for a particular group of clients. For example, a hospital may have a protocol for admitting a client to the intensive care unit, for administering magnesium sulphate to client with pre-eclampsia/eclampsia or for caring for a client receiving continuous epidural analgesia. Protocols may include both physician's orders and nursing interventions.

Policies and Procedures are developed to govern the handling of frequently occurring situations. For example, a hospital may have a policy specifying the number of visitors a patient may have. Some policies and procedures specify what is to be done, for example, in the case of cardiac arrest. If a policy covers a situation pertinent to client care, it is usually entered the care plan (e.g. make social service referral according policy manual). Policies are institutional records and do not become a part of the permanent record.

A standing order is a written document about policies, rules, regulations or orders regarding client care. Standing orders give nurses the authority to carryout specific actions under certain circumstances, often when a physician is not immediately available. In a hospital critical care unit, a common example is the administration of emergency antiarrythmic medications when a client's cardiac monitoring pattern changes.

Regardless of whether care plans are handwritten, computerized or standardized, nursing care must be individualized to fit the unique needs of each client. In hospitals/health care settings when nursing process is followed for providing holistic care to clients, care plans usually consist of both preprinted and handwritten sections. The nurse uses standardized care plans for predictable, commonly occurring problems and handwrites an individual plan for unusual problems or problems needing special attention. For example, a standardized care plan for all "clients with a medical diagnosis of pneumonia" would probably include a nursing diagnosis of *deficient fluid—volume* and direct the nurse to assess the client's hydration status. On a respiratory or medical unit, this would be a common nursing diagnosis and the nurse may incorporate it in her care plan for the client. However, a nursing diagnosis, *risk for interrupted family process* would not be common to all patients with pneumonia, it is true only to certain clients. Therefore the goals and nursing interventions for that diagnosis would need to be handwritten by the nurse.

Formats for Nursing Care Plan

Formats of care plan written by working nurses or practicing nurses in hospital units are often organized into four columns or categories. (a) *Nursing diagnoses,* (b) *Goals/desired outcomes,* (c) *Nursing orders interventions* and (d) *Evaluations.*

Student care plans are more lengthy and detailed as it is a learning activity as well as plan of care. They usually have an additional column for *"rationale"* after nursing orders column. To help students learn to write care plans, these are often handwritten as required by the educators. A rationale is a scientific principle given as the reason for selecting a particular nursing intervention. Students may also be required to cite supporting literature for their stated rationale.

Guidelines for Writing Nursing Care Plans

The nurse should use the following guidelines for writing care plans:

1. *Date and sign the plan*: The date, the plan is written is essential for evaluation. The nurse's signature demonstrates accountability to the client and to the nursing profession.

2. *Use category headings*: Different columns of the record form should have headings such as "Nursing diagnoses", "Desired outcomes/goals", "Nursing interventions" and "Evaluation". Include a date for evaluation of each goal.

3. *Use standardized words and symbols rather than complete sentences to communicate your ideas.* For example, write "Turn and reposition q2h" rather than "Turn and reposition the client every two hours".

4. *Be specific*: Write specific time or instruction for nursing interventions. For example, "change incisional dressing q shift" may mean 2 dressing changes for 12-hour duty shifts and 3 dressing changes for 8-hour duty shifts.

5. *Tailor the plan to the unique characteristics of the client by ensuring that the client's preferences and choices are considered*: This reinforces the client's individuality and sense of control. For example, the written nursing intervention "Provide coffee at breakfast rather than tea" indicates that the client was given a choice for his breakfast drink.

6. *Ensure that the nursing care plan incorporates preventive and health maintenance aspects as well as restorative ones*: For example, the nursing directive "provide active assistance for range of motion (ROM) exercises to affected limbs q2h" prevents joint contractures and maintains muscle strength and joint mobility.

7. *Ensure that the plan contains interventions for ongoing assessment of the client,* e.g. inspect incision q8h.

8. *Include collaborative and coordination activities in the plan:* For example, "administer pain medication as indicated", arrange referral service with social worker.

9. *Include plans for client's discharge and home care needs:* For example, arrangements with community health nurse, social worker or specific agencies for needed equipment. Add teaching and discharge plans.

10. *Refer to procedure books or other sources of information for writing* selected and appropriate nursing directives.

The Planning Process

The processes of developing care plans include four different activities.

Setting Priorities

This is the process of establishing a preferential sequence for addressing nursing diagnoses and interventions. The nurse and client begin planning by deciding which nursing diagnosis requires attention first, which second and so on. *Life-threatening* problems, such as loss of respiratory or cardiac function are designated as high priority. Health threatening problems such as acute illness and decreased coping ability are assigned medium priority. A low-priority problem is one that arises from normal developmental needs or that requires only minimal nursing support. Nurses use Maslow's hierarchy of needs when setting priorities. In Maslow's hierarchy, physiologic needs such as air, food and water are basic to life and receive higher priority than the need for security or activity. Thus nursing diagnoses such as *Ineffective Airway Clearance* and *Impaired Gas Exchange* would take priority over nursing diagnoses such as anxiety or ineffective coping.

It is not necessary to resolve all high-priority diagnoses before addressing others. The nurse may partially address a high-priority diagnosis and then deal with a diagnosis of lesser priority. Further, because the clients usually have several problems, the nurse often deals with more than one diagnosis at a time.

Establishing Desired Outcomes/Client Goals

After establishing priorities, the nurse and client set goals for each nursing diagnosis. The *desired outcome sentences* describe, in terms of observable client responses, what the nurse hopes to achieve by implementing the nursing interventions. The terms *desired outcomes* and *goals* are used interchangeably in this book. These are stated as specific, observable criteria and used to evaluate whether the goals have

been met. For example — "Improved nutritional status as evidenced by weight gain of 5 lb by April 25". Writing the broad general goal first, may help students to think of specific outcomes that are needed as a starting point for planning. What needs to be written on the care plan is the specific, observable, outcomes than can be used to evaluate client progress?

Purposes of Desired Outcomes/Goals

Desired outcome serve the following purposes:
1. Provide direction for planning nursing interventions. Ideas for interventions come more easily, if the desired outcomes state clearly and specifically what the nurse hopes to achieve.
2. Serve as criteria for judging the effectiveness of nursing interventions and client progress in the evaluation step.
3. Enable the client and nurse to determine when the problem has been resolved.
4. Help motivate the client and nurse by providing a sense of achievement. As goals are met, both client and nurse can see that their efforts have been worthwhile.

Guidelines for Writing Desired Outcomes/Goals

The following guidelines can help nurses write useful goals and desired outcomes:
1. Write goals and outcomes in terms of client responses, not nurse activities. Beginning each statement with the *client will* may help to focus the goal on client behaviors and responses. Avoid statements that start with *enable, facilitate, allow, let, permit* or similar verbs followed by the word client. These indicate what the nurse hopes to accomplish and what the client will do.
   Correct: Client will drink 100 ml of water per hour (client behavior).
   Incorrect: Maintain client hydration (nursing action).
2. Be sure that desired outcomes are realistic for the client's capabilities, limitations and designated time span, if it is indicated. Limitations refer to finances, equipment, family support, physical and mental condition and time. For example, the outcome

Measures insulin accurately may be unrealistic for a client who has poor vision due to cataract.

3. Ensure that the desired outcomes are compatible with the therapies of other professionals. For example, the outcome will increase the time spent out of bed by 15 minutes each day is not compatible with a physician's prescribed therapy of bed rest.

4. Use observable, measurable terms for outcomes. Avoid words that are vague and require interpretation or judgment by observer. For example, phrases such as *increases daily exercise*, and *improve knowledge of nutrition* can mean differently to different people. These are not sufficiently clear and specific to guide the nurse when evaluating client responses.

5. Make sure that the client considers the desired outcomes important and values them. Some outcomes, such as those problems related to self-esteem, parenting, and communication involve choices that are best made by the client or in collaboration with the client.

6. The nurse must actively listen to the client to determine personal values, goals, and desired outcomes in relation to current health concerns. Clients are usually motivated and expend the necessary energy to reach goals they consider important.

Computerized Care Plans

Computers are being used in recent years to create and store nursing care plans. The computer can generate both standardized and individualized care plans. Nurses access the client's stored care plan from a centrally located terminal at the nurses' station. For an individualized plan, the nurse chooses the appropriate diagnoses from a menu suggested by the computer. The computer then lists possible goals and nursing interventions for those diagnoses; the nurse chooses those appropriate for the client and types in any additional goals and interventions or nursing actions not listed on the menu. The nurse can read the plan on the computer screen or get a print out of the updated working copy.

NURSING INTERVENTIONS

Nursing interventions are the actions to achieve client goals. The specific interventions chosen should focus on eliminating or reducing the etiology of the nursing diagnosis, which is the second clause of the diagnostic, which is the second clause of the diagnostic statement.

When it is not possible to change the etiologic factors, the nurse chooses interventions to treat the signs and symptoms or the defining characteristics in NANDA terminology. Examples of this situation would be *pain* related to surgical incision and anxiety related to unknown etiology.

Interventions for risk nursing diagnosis should focus on measures to reduce the client's risk factors, which are also found in the second clause. Correct identification of the etiology during the diagnosing phase provides the framework for choosing successful nursing interventions. For example, the diagnostic label *Activity Intolerance* may have several etiologies: pain, weakness, sedentary lifestyle, anxiety, or cardiac arrhythmias. Interventions will vary according to the cause of the problem.

Types of Nursing Interventions

Nursing interventions are identified and written during the planning step of the nursing process; however, they are actually performed during the implementing step. Nursing interventions include both *direct and indirect care*, as well as *nurse-initiated, physician-initiated and other provider-initiated* treatments. Direct care is an intervention performed through interaction with the client. Indirect care is an intervention performed away from but on behalf of the client such as interdisciplinary collaboration or management of the care environment.

Independent Interventions

Independent interventions are those activities that nurses are licensed to initiate on the basis of their knowledge and skills. They include physical care, ongoing assessment, emotional support and comfort, teaching, counseling, environmental management, and making referrals to other health care professionals. In performing an autonomous activity, the nurse determines that the client requires certain nursing interventions; either carries these out or delegates them to other nursing personnel, and is accountable or answerable for the decisions and the actions. An example of an independent action is planning and providing special mouth care for a client after diagnosing *impaired oral mucous membranes*.

Dependent Interventions

Dependent interventions are activities carried out under the physician's orders or supervision, or according to specified routines. Physician's orders commonly include orders for medications, intravenous therapy, diagnostic tests, diet, and activity. The nurse is responsible for explaining, assessing the need for, and administering the medical orders. Nursing interventions may be written to individualize the medical order based on the client's status. For example, for a medical order to "progressive ambulation, as tolerated" a nurse might write the following:

❖ Dangle for 5 min, 12 hrs postoperative
❖ Stand at bedside 24 hrs postoperative: observe for pallor and dizziness
❖ Check pulse before and after ambulating
❖ Do not progress if pulse rate is > 110/min.

Collaborative Interventions

These are actions the nurse carries out in collaboration with other health team members, such as physical therapists, social workers, dieticians and physicians. Collaborative nursing activities reflect the overlapping responsibilities of and collegial relationships between, health personnel. For example, the physician might order physical therapy to teach the client crutch walking. The nurse would be responsible for informing the physical therapy department and for coordinating the client's care to include the physical therapy sessions. When the client returns to nursing unit, the nurse would assist with crutch watching and collaborate with the physical therapist to evaluate the client's progress.

Writing Nursing Orders

After choosing the appropriate nursing interventions, the nurse writes them on the nursing care plan as nursing orders. *Nursing orders* are instructions for the specific, individualized activities the nurse performs to help the client meet established health care goals. The term *order* connotes a sense of accountability for the nurse who gives the order and for the nurse who carries it out. Components of nursing orders are *Date, Action verb, Content area, Time element* and *Signature*.

Example, 15/08/2007—Palpate uterine fundus for firmness, for 2 hours, then q4h for 24 hours, A Jones, RN.

Date

Nursing orders are dated when they are written and reviewed regularly at intervals depending on the individual's needs. In an intensive care unit, for example, the plan of care will be continually monitored and revised. In a community health clinic, weekly or biweekly reviews may be indicated.

Action Verb

The action verb starts the order and must be precise. For example, Explain (to the client) the actions of insulin is a more precise statement than teach (the client) about insulin. Sometimes a modifier for the verb can make the nursing order more precise. For example, apply spiral bandage firmly to left lower leg is more precise than apply spiral bandage to left leg.

Content Area

The content is, the what and where of the order. In the preceding order, spiral bandage and left leg state, the what and where of the order. The content area in this example may also clarify whether the foot or toes are to be left exposed.

Time Element

The time element answers when, how long or how often the nursing action is to occur. Examples are Assist client with sitz bath at 10 am and 5 pm daily and administer analgesic 30 minutes prior to physical therapy.

Signature

The signature of the nurse prescribing the order shows the nurse's accountability and has legal significance.

IMPLEMENTING

The nursing process is client oriented, action oriented, and outcome directed. After developing a plan of care based the assessment and diagnosing phases, the nurse implements the interventions and evaluates the desired outcomes. On the basis of this evaluation, the plan of care is continued, modified or terminated.

In the nursing process, implementing is the phase in which the nurse implements the nursing interventions. Implementing consists of *doing* and *documenting* activities that are specific nursing actions needed to carry-out nursing orders. The nurse performs or delegates the nursing activities for the interventions that were developed in planning step and then conclude the implementing step by recording nursing activities and the resulting client responses. The degree of participation depends on the client's health status. For example, an unconscious person is unable participate in his care and therefore needs to have care given to him. By contrast, an ambulatory client may require very little care from the nurse and carry-out health care activities independently.

Relationship of Implementing to Other Phases of Nursing Process

The first three phases of nursing process assessing, diagnosing and planning provide the basis for nursing actions performed during implementing step. In turn, the implementing phase provides the actual nursing activities and client responses that are examined in the final phase, the evaluating phase.

While implementing nursing orders, the nurse continues to assess the client at every contact, gathering data about the client's responses to the nursing activities and about any new problems that may develop. A nursing activity on the client's care plan may read "Auscultate lungs q4h". When performing this activity, the nurse is both carrying-out the intervention (implementing) and performing as assessment.

Some routine nursing activities are, themselves, assessments. For example, while bathing an elderly client, the nurse observes a reddened area on the client's sacrum or, when emptying a urinary catheter bag, the nurse measures 200 ml of strong-smelling, brown urine.

Implementing Skills

To implement the care plan successfully, nurses need cognitive, interpersonal and technical skills. These skills are distinct from one another and nurses use them in various combinations and with different emphasis, depending on the activity. For instance, when inserting a urinary catheter the nurse needs cognitive knowledge of the principles and steps of the procedure, interpersonal skills to inform and reassure client and technical skills in draping the client and manipulating the articles.

The *cognitive skills* (intellectual skills) include problem solving, decision-making, critical thinking and creativity. They are crucial to safe, intelligent nursing care.

Interpersonal skills are verbal and nonverbal activities people use when interacting directly with one another. The effectiveness of a nursing action often depends largely on the nurse's ability to communicate with others. The nurse uses therapeutic communication to understand the client and in turn be understood. Interpersonal skills are necessary for all nursing activities; caring, comforting, advocating, referring, counseling and supporting. Before nurses can be highly skilled in interpersonal relations, they must have self-awareness and sensitivity to others.

Technical skills are "hands on" skills such as manipulating equipment, giving injections and bandaging, moving, lifting and repositioning clients. The skills are also called as tasks, procedures, or psychomotor skills.

Technical skills require knowledge and manual dexterity. The number of technical skills expected of a nurse has increased in the recent years because of the increased use of technology, especially in acute care hospitals.

The Process of Implementing

Implementing is the process in which the nurse implements the nursing interventions and documents the care provided. The process includes:

- ❖ Reassessing the client
- ❖ Determining the nurse's need for assistance
- ❖ Implementing the nursing interventions
- ❖ Supervising the delegated care and
- ❖ Documenting nursing activities.

Reassessing the Client

Before implementing an intervention, the nurse must reassess the client to make sure the intervention is still needed. Even though a nursing order is written on the care plan, the client's condition may have changed. For example, a directive-back message may be written for a nursing diagnosis of *Disturbed Sleep Pattern*, related to anxiety and unfamiliar surroundings. During her rounds, the nurse discovers that the client is sleeping and therefore defers the back massage that had been planned as a relaxation strategy.

At times new data may indicate a need to change the priorities of care or nursing activities.

Determining the Nurse's Need for Assistance

For implementing some nursing interventions, the nurse may require assistance for the following reasons:

- ❖ The nurse is unable to implement the nursing activity safely alone (e.g. ambulating an unsteady, obese client).
- ❖ The stress on client would be reduced if nurse arranges for assistance for the activity (e.g. turning a client who experiences acute pain when moved).
- ❖ The nurse lacks the skills or knowledge to implement a particular nursing activity (e.g. a nurse who is not familiar with the use of

an isolette needs assistance the first time it is used).

Implementing the Nursing Interventions

When implementing nursing interventions, nurses should follow certain guidelines.

- ❖ Base nursing interventions on scientific knowledge, professional standards and nursing research (evidence-based practice). The nurse must be aware of scientific rationale, as well as possible side effects or complications of all interventions.
- ❖ Understand clearly the order to be implemented and question any that are not understood. The nurse is responsible for intelligent implementation of medical and nursing plans of care.
- ❖ Adapt activities to the individual client. A client's beliefs, values, age, health status and environment are factors that can affect the success of a nursing action.
- ❖ Implement safe care by following correct steps and scientific principles.
- ❖ Provide teaching, support and comfort as required.
- ❖ View the client as whole and make the plan and implementation holistic.
- ❖ Respect the dignity of the client and enhance the client's self-esteem by providing privacy and encouraging client to make their own decisions.
- ❖ Encourage clients to participate actively in implementing the nursing interventions. Active participation enhances the client's sense of independence and control. The amount of desired involvement may be related to the severity of the illness and understanding of the intervention.

Supervising Delegated Care

If the care has been delegated to other health care personnel, the nurse responsible for the client's overall care must ensure that the activities have been implemented according to the care plan. Other caregivers are required to communicate their activities to the nurse by documenting them on the client's record, reporting verbally, or filling out a written form.

The nurse validates and responds to any adverse findings or client responses. This may involve modifying the nursing care plan.

Documenting Nursing Activities

After carrying out the nursing activities, the nurse completes the implementing phase by recording the interventions and client responses in the nursing progress notes. The nurse must record the nursing intervention immediately or as early as possible after it is implemented. The recorded data must be up to date, accurate, and available to other nurses and health care professionals.

Nursing activities are communicated verbally as well as in writing. When client's health is changing rapidly, the head nurse and/or the physician may want to be kept up to date with verbal reports. Nurses also report client status at change if shifts or on a client's discharge to another unit or institution, in person, in writing, or via a voice recording.

EVALUATING

Evaluating is the final/fifth phase of the nursing process, in which the nurse determines the client's progress toward goal achievement and the effectiveness of the nursing care plan. The plan may be continued modified or terminated after the evaluation.

To evaluate means to judge or appraise. It is a planned, ongoing, purposeful activity in which clients and health care professionals determine (a) the client's progress toward achievement of outcomes/goals (b) the effectiveness of the nursing care plans. Evaluation is an important aspect of the nursing process because conclusions drawn from the evaluation determine whether the nursing interventions should be terminated, continued or changed.

Evaluation is continuous and when carried-out during or immediately after implementing a nursing order/directive, enables the nurse to make on-the-spot modifications in an intervention. Evaluation performed at specific intervals (e.g. once a week for a home care client), shows the extent of progress toward achievement of outcome and enables the nurse to correct any deficiencies and modify the care plan as needed. Evaluation continues until the client achieves the health goals or is discharged from nursing care. Evaluation at discharge includes the status of goal achievement and the client's self-care abilities with regard to follow-up care.

Through evaluating, nurses demonstrate responsibility and accountability for their actions, and indicate interest in the results of the nursing activities carried-out.

Relationship of Evaluating to Other Nursing Process Phases

Successful evaluation depends on the effectiveness of the steps that precede it. Assessment data must be accurate and complete so that the nurse can formulate appropriate nursing diagnoses and desired outcomes. The desired outcomes must be stated in behavioral terms if they are to be useful for evaluating client responses. And without the implementing phase, in which the plan is put into action, there would be nothing to evaluate.

The evaluating and assessing phases overlap as assessment (data collection), is ongoing and continuous at every client contact. However, data are collected for different purposes at different points in the nursing process. During the assessment phase the nurse collects data for the purpose of making diagnoses. During the evaluation step, the nurse collects data for the purpose of comparing it to preselected goals and for judging the effectiveness of the nursing care.

Process of Evaluating

Before evaluating, the nurse identifies the desired outcomes (indicators), which will be used to measure client's goal achievement. Desired outcomes serve two purposes:

a. They establish the kind of evaluative data that need to be collected and

b. Provide a standard against which the data are judged. For example, given the following expected outcomes, any nurse caring for the client would know what data to be collected:

- Daily fluid intake will not be less than 2500 ml.
- Residual urine will be less than 100 ml.

The process of evaluation has five components:

- Collecting data related to desired outcomes
- Comparing data with outcomes
- Relating nursing activities to outcomes
- Drawing conclusions about problem status
- Continuing, modifying or terminating the nursing care plan.

Collection of Data

Using the clearly stated, precise and measurable desired outcomes as a guide, the nurse collects data so that conclusions can be drawn about whether goals have been met. It is necessary to collect both objective and subjective data.

Comparing Data with Outcomes

Both the nurse and client play an active role in comparing the client's actual responses with the expected outcomes. For example, did the client drink 3000 ml of fluid in 24 hours? The nurse can draw one of three of the following conclusions.

- The goal was met; that is the client response is the same as the desired outcome
- The goal was partially met; that is only the short-term goal was achieved and the long-term goal was not attained
- The goal was not met.

After determining whether a goal has been met, the nurse writes an evaluative statement in the nurse's notes. *An evaluative statement* consists of two parts; a conclusion and a supporting data.

The conclusion is a statement that the desired outcome was met or not. The supporting data are the list of client responses that support the conclusion.

For example, goal met: oral intake at 300 ml more than output; skin turgor good, mucous membrane moist. In practice (in hospital units), care plans usually do not have a column for evaluation statements; rather, these are recorded in the nurse's notes.

Relating Nursing Activities to Outcomes

The aspect of the evaluating process relates to determining whether the nursing activities had any relation to the outcomes. It should not be assumed that a nursing activity was the cause of or the only factor in meeting, partially meeting or not meeting a goal. For example, if the weight gain of a prenatal client meets the expected level as stated in the care plan she must ensure that it relates to the instructions given to the mother only, or due to fluid retention related to pre-eclamptic toxemia. It is important to establish the relationship or lack of relationship of nursing actions to the client responses.

Drawing Conclusions about Problem Status

In order to determine whether the care plan was effective in resolving, reducing or preventing client problems, the nurse uses the judgments about goal achievement. When goals have been met, the nurse can draw one of the following conclusions about the client's problem:

- The actual problem stated in the nursing diagnosis has been resolved; or the potential problem is being prevented and the risk factors no longer exist. In these circumstances, the nurse documents that the goals have been met and discontinues the care for the problem
- The potential problem stated in the nursing diagnosis is being prevented, but the risk factors are still present. In this case, the nurse keeps the problem on the nursing care plan
- The actual problem still exists even though some goals are being met. For example, a desired outcome on a client's care plan is will drink 2500 ml fluid daily. Even though the data from intake-output record shows this outcome had been achieved, other data (dry oral mucous membrane) may indicate that there is *deficient fluid volume*. Therefore, the nursing interventions must be continued even though this goal was met.

When goals have been partially met or when goals have not been met the nurse may conclude on one of the following.

- The care plan needs to be revised. The revisions may need to occur during assessing, diagnosing or planning phases as well as implementing.

❖ The care plan does not need revision, because the client merely needs more time to achieve the goals.

Continuing, Modifying and Terminating the Nursing Care Plan

After drawing conclusions about the status of the clients' problems, the nurse modifies the care plan as indicated. Depending on policies of the hospital/agency, modifications may be made by marking portions using a highlighting pen or by drawing a line through portions of the care plan or writing "discontinued" and the data. This requires a review of the entire care plan and a critique of the nursing process steps involved in its development.

In addition to evaluating goal achievement for individual clients, nurses are also involved in evaluating and modifying the overall quality of care given to groups of clients. This is an essential activity of professional accountability.

Utilizing the nursing process helps define and explain the unique practice of nursing. Its use encourages creative, comprehensive, and systematic and client oriented care that is more easily communicated to all health care team members. Its five phases assessment, diagnosis, planning, implementation and evaluation are founded in the scientific problem solving method that can be utilized in all settings where nurses practice. Standardized nursing care plans; nursing diagnoses, procedures and protocols may be used to promote quality patient health care. Knowledge of and adherence to these standards and guidelines are the responsibilities of each practicing nurse.

The material in this chapter is intended to provide theoretical knowledge as background information in the pursuit of clinical management of the client. Because nursing management is a process that takes place in the clinical setting and the last two steps of the nursing process are dependent on the client and clinical situation, it is not possible to include them realistically in a textbook. However, conceptual models of nursing process for clients with different obstetrical conditions and processes are included at the end of certain chapters.

For detailed nursing care plans that could serve as guidelines for care of mothers (in prenatal, intranatal and postnatal periods) and newborns the reader may refer to the Appendix.

BIBLIOGRAPHY

1. Carpenito L. Nursing diagnosis: Application to Clinical Practice. Philadelphia: Lippincot JB; 1993.
2. Christensen P, Kenny J. Nursing Process: Application of Conceptual Models, 3rd edn. St. Louis: Mushy CV; 1990.
3. Doenges E Marilyn, Moorhouse F Mary. Application of Nursing Process and Nursing Diagnosis, 4th edn. Philadelphia: FA Davis Company; 2003.
4. Doenges E Marilyn, Moorhouse F Mary, Murr C Alice. Nursing Care Plans: Guidelines for Individualizing Client Care Across Life Span, 7th edn. Philadelphia: FA Davis Company; 2006.
5. Karpen M, et al. Essentials of Maternal Child Nursing, 2nd edn. South Easton, MA: Western Schools Press; 1995.
6. Kozier Barbara, Erb Glenora, Borman Audrey, Burke Karen. Fundamentals of Nursing: Concepts, Process and Practice, 7th edn. New Delhi, India: Dorling Kinderly Pvt Ltd; 2004.
7. Varney Helen. Nurse Midwifery, 3rd 3dn. Boston: Jones and Barlett Publishers; 1999.

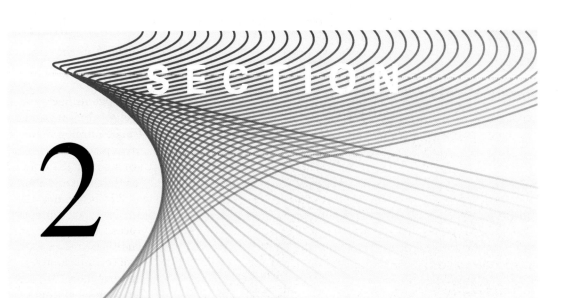

SECTION

2

Reproductive System

5

The Female Pelvis and Generative Organs

PELVIS

The female pelvis because of its characteristics, aids in childbirth. It is a skeletal ring formed by two innominate or hipbones, the sacrum and the coccyx (Fig. 5.1).

Innominate Bone

Each innominate bone is made up of three parts, the ilium, the ischium and the pubis (Fig. 5.2).

The *ilium* is the large flared out portion of the innominate bone. The upper border of it is termed iliac crest. When the hand is placed on the hip it rests on this part. The prominence at the front of the iliac crest is known as the

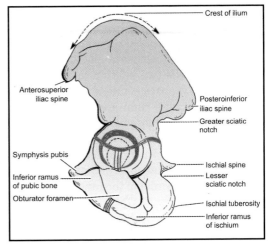

Fig. 5.2: Innominate bone showing important landmarks

Fig. 5.1: Normal female pelvis

anterosuperior iliac spine. A short distance below is the anteroinferior iliac spine. At opposite end of the iliac crest similar prominences are present which are named postero-superior and posteroinferior iliac spines. The anterior surface of the ilium is concave in shape and termed as the iliac fossa.

The *ischium* is the thick lower part of the innominate bone. It has a large prominence known as the ischial tuberosity. In sitting position, the body rests on the ischial tube-rosity. A little above and behind the tuberosity is a projection known as the ischial spine. In labor the station (level) of the fetal head is estimated in relation to the ischial spines.

The *pubic* bones form the anterior part of the innominate bone. It has a body and two oar-like projections called superior and inferior ramus. The two pubic bones meet at the sym-physis pubis. The two inferior rami form the pubic arch. The space enclosed by the body of the pubic bone, the rami and the ischium is called the obturator foramen. The innominate one has a deep cup to receive the head of the femur, which is termed as acetabulum. All three bones contribute to form the acetabulum.

On the lower border of the innominate bone are found two curves. One extends from the posteroinferior iliac spine up to the ischial spine and is called the greater *sciatic notch*. It is wide and rounded. The other lies between ischial spine and the ischial tuberosity and is the *lesser sciatic notch*.

The Sacrum

The sacrum lies between the ilia. It is a wedge-shaped bone consisting of five vertebrae fused together. The prominent upper margin of the first sacral vertebrae is called the sacral promontory. The anterior surface of the sacrum is concave and is referred to as the hollow of the sacrum. Four pairs of holes or formina pierce the sacrum and, through these, the sacral nerves pass.

The Coccyx

The coccyx is a small triangular bone with its base uppermost articulating with the lower end of the sacrum. During labor it moves backward, allowing more space for the delivery of the fetus.

Pelvic Joints

There are four pelvic joints:
1. *Two sacroiliac joints*: These are slightly movable joints, formed where the ilium joins the first-two sacral vertebrae on either side. They connect the spine to the pelvis and are the strongest joints in the body.
2. *One symphysis pubis*: It is a cartilaginous joint between the two pubic bones.
3. *One sacrococcygeal joint:* It is a hinge joint between the sacrum and the coccyx.

In the nonpregnant state, there is little arti-culation (movement) in these joints, but during pregnancy endocrine activity causes the ligaments to soften which allows the ligaments to give. During delivery this allows more room for the fetal head as it passes through the pelvis.

Pelvic Ligaments

The pelvic girdle has great strength and stability in order to fulfil its functions of support. Powerful ligaments hold the pelvic joints together.
1. *Sacroiliac ligaments*: These ligaments pass in front of and behind each sacroiliac joint.
2. *Pubic ligaments*: The superior pubic liga-ment connects the top of the pubic bones. The arcuate (arched) pubic ligament runs under the symphysis pubis.
3. *Sacrotuberous ligaments*: One ligament on each side, runs from the sacrum to the ischial tuberosity.
4. *Sacrospinous ligament*: One ligament on each side of the sacrum and the ischial spine.
5. *Sacrococcygeal ligaments*: One ligament on each side from the sacrum to the coccyx.

The True Pelvis

The true pelvis constitutes the bony passage through which the fetus must maneuver to be born vaginally. Therefore, its construction planes and diameters are of utmost interest in obstetrics.

The true pelvis has the following as its boundaries (Fig. 5.3):
* *Superiorly*: The sacral promontory, linea terminalis and the upper margin of pubic bones.
* *Inferiorly*: The inferior margins of the ischial tuberosities and the tip of coccyx.

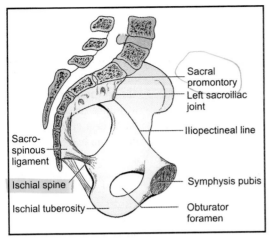

Fig. 5.3: Sagittal view of bony pelvis

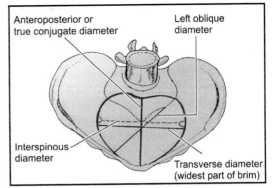

Fig. 5.4: Brim of pelvis showing diameters

❖ *Laterally*: The sacroiliac notches and ligaments, and the inner surface of ischial bones.

❖ *Anteriorly*: The obturator foramina and the posterior surface of the symphysis pubis, pubic bones and the ascending rami of ischial bones.

The true pelvis has a brim, a cavity and an outlet.

The Pelvic Brim

The brim is also termed as the inlet. Its boundaries are the sacral promontory and wings of the sacrum behind the iliac bones on the sides and the pubic bones in front.

❖ *Landmarks of the brim*: These are the fixed anatomical points on the brim.
1. Sacral promontory.
2. Sacral ala or sacral wing.
3. Sacroiliac joint.
4. Iliopectineal line: The edge formed at the inward aspect of the ilium.
5. Iliopectineal eminence: A roughened area where the superior ramus of the pubic bone meets the ilium.
6. Superior ramus of the pubic bone.
7. Upper inner border of the body of pubic bone.
8. Upper inner border of the symphysis pubis.

❖ *Diameters of the brim (Fig. 5.4)*
1. *The anteroposterior diameter of the brim*: It is a line from the sacral promontory to the upper border of the symphy-

sis pubis. When the anteroposterior diameter is measured from the sacral promontory to the uppermost point of the symphysis pubis it is called the anatomical conjugate and measures 12 cm. When it is taken to the posterior border of the upper surface, it is called the obstetrical conjugate and measures 11 cm. It is the anteroposterior diameter available for childbirth. The term *true conjugate* may be used to refer to either of these measurements.

2. *The transverse diameter of the brim of the inlet*: It is the maximum transverse diameter that can be found between similar points on opposite sides of the pelvic brim. In other words it is a line between the furthest points on the iliopectineal lines. It measures 13.5 cm.

3. *The oblique diameter*: It is a line from one sacroiliac joint to the iliopectineal eminence on the opposite side of the pelvis and measures 12.75 cm. There are two oblique diameters—right and left. Each takes its name from the sacroiliac joint from which it arises.

4. *The diagonal conjugate*: It is also measured anteroposteriorly from the lower border of the symphysis pubis to the sacral promontory. It may be estimated per vagina and should measure 12–13 cm.

The Pelvic Cavity

The cavity extends from the brim above to the outlet below. The anterior wall is formed by the pubic bones and symphysis pubis and it measures 4 cm. The posterior wall is formed by the curve of the sacrum and coccyx, which measures 12 cm. Lateral walls of the cavity are formed by the fused ilium and ischium. The pelvic cavity is short and curved with the posterior wall being considerably longer than the anterior wall resulting in a J-shaped axis with the curve directed forward called the curve of Carus.

The Pelvic Outlet

The outlets are described as the anatomical and the obstetrical outlets. The anatomical outlet is indented behind by the coccyx and the sacrum and on the sides by the ischial tuberosities.

The obstetrical outlet is of greater practical significance, because it includes the narrow pelvic strait through which the fetus must pass. The narrow pelvis strait (passage) lies between the sacrococcygeal joint, two ischial spines and the lower border of the symphysis pubis. The obstetrical outlet is the space between the narrow pelvic strait and the anatomical outlet. It is diamond shaped. Rotation of the presenting part takes place in this space.

❖ *Measurements of the pelvic outlet*
1. The anteroposterior diameter is a line from the lower border of the symphysis pubis to the sacrococcygeal joint. It measures 13 cm. As the coccyx may deflect backwards during labor, this diameter indicates the space available during delivery (Fig. 5.5).
2. The oblique diameter is the measurement between the obturator foramen and the sacrospinous ligament. The measurement is considered as 12 cm although there are no fixed points of measurement (Fig. 5.6).
3. Transverse diameter is a line between the two ischial spines and measures 10–11 cm. It is the narrowest diameter of the pelvis (Fig. 5.7).

The False Pelvis

The pelvis is divided by the linea terminalis into the false pelvis above this demarcation and

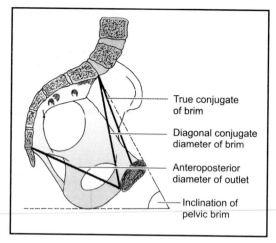

Fig. 5.5: Lateral view of pelvis showing anteroposterior diameters in different plane

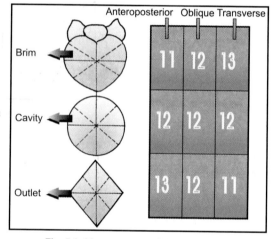

Fig. 5.6: Measurements of the pelvic canal in centimeters

the true pelvis below it. The false pelvis is the portion above the pelvic brim. It has no obstetric significance relevant to the passage of the fetus through the pelvis.

Pelvic Inclination

The longitudinal axis of the symphysis pubis is normally parallel to the longitudinal axis of the sacrum. If the symphysis pubis is not parallel to the sacrum, the anteroposterior diameter of the inlet can be changed significantly. Tilting of the superior margin of the symphysis pubis towards the sacral promontory and of the inferior margin away from the sacrum is called anterior inclination.

Fig. 5.7: Diameters of the pelvic outlet

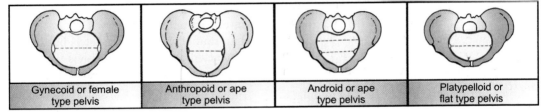

| Gynecoid or female type pelvis | Anthropoid or ape type pelvis | Android or ape type pelvis | Platypelloid or flat type pelvis |

Fig. 5.8: The four types of pelvis

Tilting of the inferior margin of the symphysis pubis towards the sacrum and the superior margin away from the sacral promontory is called posterior inclination.

TYPES OF PELVIS

There are four basic types of pelves according to the Caldwell-Moloy classification: They are (i) gynecoid, (ii) android, (iii) anthropoid and (iv) platypelloid (Fig. 5.8). These are determined by certain characteristics of the pelvis and classified according to the shape of the brim.

Many pelvis are not pure types but, rather a mixture of types. For example, a gynecoid pelvis may be said to have an android tendency. The importance of being familiar with the pelvic types lies in the fact that many of the characteristics used in determining the pelvic types affect the obstetric capacity of the pelvis, that is the adequacy of the pelvis for accommodating passage of the baby. If one of the important measurements is reduced by 1 cm

or more from the normal, the pelvis is said to be contracted and may give rise to difficulty in labor.

Gynecoid Pelvis Fifty Percent

The gynecoid pelvis is commonly known as the female pelvis because it is the type that occurs most frequently in women. This shape is ideal for childbearing. Its identifying characteristics are as follows seen in 50 percent of women:

❖ *Brim or inlet:* Well rounded with the transverse diameter about the same or slightly greater than the anteroposterior diameter
❖ *Sacrum:* Well-curved sacrum, parallel with the symphysis pubis
❖ *Sacrosciatic notch:* Well rounded and wide with an approximate distance of 2.5–3 fingerbreadths
❖ *Sidewalls:* The pelvic sidewalls are parallel or divergent
❖ *Ischial spines:* Blunt which are neither prominent nor encroaching
❖ *Pelvic arch:* Wide pubic arch of 90 degrees or more.

It is found in women of average build and height.

The Justo Minor Pelvis

This is a miniature gynecoid pelvis. All diameters are reduced but are in proportion. It is normally found in women of small stature with small hands and feet. Occasionally this type of pelvis is seen in women of normal stature. If these women have smaller babies normal labor and delivery will take place. However, if the fetus is large, a degree of cephalopelvic disproportion will result.

Android Pelvis Twenty Percent

The android pelvis is commonly known as the male pelvis because it occurs more frequently in men. However, it does occur in a small percent of women. The android pelvis is a heavy pelvis that poses difficulty for vaginal delivery and increases the incidence of posterior position and transverse arrest. The midplane and outlet contracture of the android pelvis increases the incidences of fetopelvic disproportion and cesarean sections.

Characteristics of the android pelvis are:

* *Inlet*: Heart-shaped with a narrow fore pelvis. Has a transverse diameter that is towards the back. The sidewalls converge making it a funnel shape
* *Sacrum:* Anteriorly inclined and flat thereby contributing to the shortness of the posterior sagittal diameters throughout the pelvis
* *Sacrosciatic notch:* It has a high arch and is narrow
* *Sidewalls:* The pelvic sidewalls usually are convergent
* *Ischial spines:* Usually prominent and frequently encroaching thereby decrease the transverse (interspinous) diameter
* *Pubic arch:* The angle of the pubic arch is less than 90 degrees.

It is found in short and heavy built women who have a tendency to hirsute. This type of pelvis predisposes to an occipitoposterior position of the fetal head and is the least suited to childbearing.

Anthropoid Pelvis Twenty Percent

The anthropoid pelvis, because of its characteristics, favors a posterior position of the fetus.

* *Brim*: Characteristically oval with an anteroposterior diameter much longer than the transverse diameter
* *Sacrum:* The sacrum is posteriorly inclined and deeply concave. Therefore, the space in the posterior portion of the pelvis is increased for accommodating the fetal head. The anthropoid pelvis has the longest sacrum of the four types of pelvis
* *Sacrosciatic notch:* Wide with an approximate length of four-fingerbreadth
* *Sidewalls:* Frequently somewhat divergent
* *Ischial spines:* Usually prominent but not encroaching, so the transverse diameter (interspinous) of the cavity is generally less than that of the gynecoid pelvis but not as contracted as the android pelvis
* *Pubic arch:* Somewhat narrow.

Tall women with narrow shoulders tend to have this type of pelvis. Labor does not usually present any difficulties, but a direct occipito-anterior or occipitoposterior position is often a feature.

Platypelloid Pelvis Five Percent

This type of pelvis is rare. It has a kidney shaped brim and not particularly conducive to vaginal delivery. The characteristic features are:

* *Inlet:* Short anteroposterior diameter and a wide transverse diameter
* *Sacrum:* Inclined posteriorly and quite hollow thereby presenting a short sacrum and a shallow pelvis
* *Sacrosciatic notch:* Wide and flat with an acute angle between the ischial spines and the sacrum
* *Sidewalls:* Slightly divergent
* *Ischial spines:* Somewhat blunt but, because of the flattened character of the pelvis and wide transverse diameter, this prominence has no effect. The transverse diameter of the cavity of platypelloid pelvis is the widest of all the pelves
* *Pubic arch:* Quite wide.

This pelvis is the widest of all the pelvic types. The fetal head must engage with the sagittal suture in the transverse diameter, but usually descends through the cavity without difficulty. Engagement may necessitate lateral tilting of the head known as *asynclitism*, in order to allow the biparietal diameter to pass the narrowest anteroposterior diameter of brim.

OTHER PELVIC VARIATIONS

High Assimilation Pelvis

This type of pelvis is seen when the fifth lumbar vertebra is fused to the sacrum and the angle of inclination of the pelvic brim is increased. Engagement of the fetal head is difficult, but once achieved, labor progresses normally.

Deformed Pelvis

Deformation of the pelvis may result from a developmental anomaly, dietary deficiency, injury or disease. Developmental anomalies are seen as Naegele's pelvis or Robert's pelvis. In the Naegele's pelvis one sacral ala is missing and the sacrum is fused to the ilium, causing a grossly asymmetric brim. The Robert's pelvis is similar but bilateral. In both types the abnormal brim prevents engagement of the fetal head.

Deformities due to dietary deficiencies result from deficiency of vitamins and minerals necessary for the formation of healthy bones. Rickets in early childhood can result in gross deformity of the pelvic brim. In *Rachitic pelvis* (caused by rickets), the sacral promontory is pushed downwards and forwards and the ilium and ischium are drawn outwards. This results in a flat pelvic brim similar to that of the platypelloid pelvis. The fetal head will attempt to enter the pelvis by asynclitism. Cesarean section is required to deliver the baby. Another pelvic deformity due to dietary deficiency is the *osteomalacia* pelvis. It is due to deficiency of calcium and occurs in adults. All bones of the skeleton soften and as a result of gross calcium deficiency. The pelvic canal is squashed together until the brim becomes a Y-shaped slot. Delivery impossible and a cesarean section will be performed.

Injury or disease may also cause pelvic deformities. A pelvis, which has been fractured will develop callus formation or may fail to unite correctly. This may lead to reduced measurements resulting in contraction. Fractures of pelvis or lower limbs in childhood, congenital dislocation of the hip and poliomyelitis may lead to pelvic deformity. Pelvic deformity is seen in women with spinal deformity such as kyphosis (forward angulation) and scoliosis (lateral curvature) and in women who limp. Outcome of delivery is dependent on the degree of deformity.

Muscles and Fascia

Pelvic Floor

It is a muscular partition, which separates the pelvic cavity from the perineum (Fig. 5.9). The

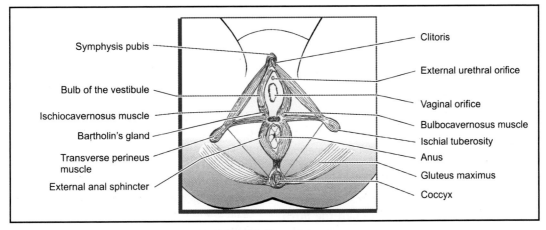

Fig. 5.9: The perineum

most important muscle supporting the pelvic organs is the levator ani, which forms the pelvic floor. The levator ani (deep layer) consists of three sets of muscles on either side.

1. The pubococcygeus muscle that passes from the pubis to the coccyx.
2. The iliococcygeus muscle that passes from the fascia covering the obturator internus muscle to the coccyx.
3. The ischiococcygeus muscle that passes from the ischial spine to the coccyx.

The superficial muscle layer of the pelvic floor is composed of five muscles:

1. The *external anal sphincter* that encircles the anus.
2. The *transverse perineal muscles* that pass from the ischial tuberosities to the center of the perineum.
3. The *bulbocavernosus muscles* that pass from the perineum forwards around the vagina and clitoris just under the pubic arch.
4. The *ischiocavernosus muscles* that pass from the ischial tuberosities along the pubic arch to the corpora cavernosa.
5. *The membranous sphincter of the urethra,* composed of muscle fibers passing about and below the urethra and attached to the pubic bones. It acts to close the urethra.

Between the muscle layers, as well as above and below them, there are layers of pelvic fascia. The muscles with the covering fascia are called the pelvic diaphragm.

Functions

❖ The pelvic floor supports the weight of the abdominal and pelvic floor organs. The pubovaginalis, which forms a 'U' shaped sling, supports the vagina, bladder and uterus. Weakness or tear of this sling during delivery is responsible for prolapse of the organs concerned

❖ The muscles are responsible for the voluntary control of micturition and defecation, and play an important role in sexual intercourse

❖ During childbirth it influences the passive movements of the fetus through the birth canal and relaxes to allow its exit from the birth canal (when the presenting part of the fetus presses on the pelvic floor, it facilitates anterior internal rotation)

❖ Maintains intra-abdominal pressure by reflexly responding to its changes

❖ Steadies the perineal body.

Nerve Supply

The 4th sacral nerve, inferior rectal nerve and a perineal branch of pudendal nerve supply it.

During pregnancy the levator ani muscle hypertrophies and becomes less rigid and more distensible. Due to water retention, it swells up and sags down.

In the second stage, the pubovaginalis and puborectalis relax and the levator ani is drawn up over the advancing presenting part. The effect of such a displacement is to elongate the birth canal.

The Perineal Body

This is a pyramid of muscles and fibrous tissue situated between the vagina and the rectum. It is the central point of the perineum and is called the obstetrical perineum. It measures 4 cm × 4 cm with the base covered by the perineal skin and the apex is pointed and is continuous with the rectovaginal septum. The apex is formed from the fibers of the pubococcygeus muscle; the base is formed from the transverse perineal muscles together with the bulbocavernosus in front and the external anal sphincter behind.

The perineal body helps to support the levator ani, which is placed above it. It is vulnerable to injury during childbirth. Deliberate cutting of these structures during delivery is called episiotomy.

Evaluation of Pelvis

Clinical evaluation of pelvis and pelvimetry are usually included as part of the initial antepartal examination and depending on the circumstances, repeated again either late in the third trimester or at the time of the initial intrapartal pelvic examination.

The woman needs to be prepared for this procedure as for the pelvic examination: Empty bladder, lithotomy position, proper draping and instruction about the procedure and relaxation techniques to help her cope with the examination.

Evaluation of the bony pelvis is often done as a part of the total pelvic examination. The pelvic measurements are then weighed against the estimated size of the fetus at term, the type of presenting part and its position. A determination of pelvic adequacy is made from these findings. When evaluation of the bony pelvis is done early in pregnancy it is often evaluated as adequate for a certain size baby. For example, charting may show a summary statement such as adequate for a 2.5 kg baby. At term if the estimated fetal weight is 3 kg, one is alerted to a potential problem requiring re-evaluation of labor status with this concern in mind.

GENERATIVE ORGANS

The generative (reproductive) organs in the female are those concerned with copulation, fertilization, growth and development of the fetus, its subsequent exit into the outer world and nurture following birth. The generative organs constitute the external genitalia, the internal genital organs and the accessory reproductive organs.

The External Genitalia (Vulva) (Fig. 5.10)

The external female genital organs (vulva) consists of the following structures:

The Mons Pubis or Mons Veneris

It is a pad of subcutaneous adipose connective tissue lying over the symphysis pubis. It is

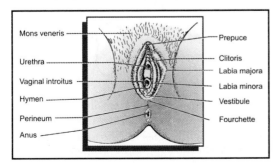

Fig. 5.10: Female external genitalia

covered with pubic hair from the time of puberty.

The Labia Majora (Greater Lips)

These are two folds of fat and areolar tissue, covered with skin and pubic hair on the outer surface. The inner surfaces of the labia majora are hairless. The labia majora are covered with squamous epithelium and contain sebaceous glands, sweat glands and hair follicles. The adipose tissue is richly supplied with venous plexus, which may produce hematoma, if injured during childbirth. The labia majora arise from the mons veneris and merge into the perineum behind. The round ligaments terminate at its upper borders.

The Labia Minora (Lesser Lips)

These are two thin folds of skin lying between the labia majora. Anteriorly they divide to enclose the clitoris; posteriorly they fuse, forming the *fourchette*. It is usually lacerated during childbirth. Between the fourchette and the vaginal orifice is the *fossa navicularis*. The labia minora do not contain hair follicles. The folds contain connective tissue, numerous sebaceous glands, erectile muscle fibers and numerous vessels and nerve endings.

The Clitoris

It is a small cylindrical, erectile body, measuring about 2.5 cm situated in the most anterior part of the vulva. It is a rudimentary organ corresponding to the male penis, but differs basically in being entirely separate from the urethra. It is attached to the under surface of the symphysis pubis by the suspensory ligament. It is extremely sensitive and highly vascular and plays a role in the orgasm of sexual intercourse.

The Vestibule

It is a triangular space bounded anteriorly by the clitoris, posteriorly by the fourchette and on either side by the labia minora. There are four openings into the vestibule.

1. *The urethral opening:* The opening is situated in the midline just in front of the vaginal orifice about 2.5 cm posterior to the

clitoris. The *Skene's glands* open on either side of the urethral orifice.

2. *The vaginal orifice or introitus:* It occupies the posterior two-thirds of the vestibule and is of varying size and shape. In virgins and nulliparae, the opening is closed by the labia minora, but in parous women, it may be exposed. It is completely closed by a septum of mucous membrane, called hymen. The membrane varies in shape, but is usually circular or crescentic in virgins. The hymen is usually ruptured at the consummation of marriage. During childbirth, the hymen is extremely lacerated and is known as the *carunculae myrtiformes.* On both sides it is lined by stratified squamous epithelium.

3. *Openings of Bartholin's glands:* There are two Bartholin's glands (greater vestibular glands), one on each side. They open on either side of the vaginal orifice and lie in the posterior part of the labia majora. They are pea-shaped and yellowish white in color. During sexual excitement, it secretes abundant alkaline mucus, which helps in lubrication. Each gland has a duct, which measures about two centimeters and opens into the vestibule outside the hymen. The duct is lined by columnar epithelium.

Blood Supply

This comes from the internal and external pudendal arteries. The blood drains through the corresponding veins.

Lymphatic Drainage

Lymphatics drain into the inguinal lymph nodes and internal iliac lymph nodes.

Nerve Supply

This is from the branches of pudendal nerve. Anterior part is supplied by the genito-femoral nerve (L-1 and L-2) and postero–inferior part by the pudendal branches from the posterior cutaneous nerve of thigh (S 1, 2 and 3). The vulva is supplied by the labial and perineal branches of the pudendal nerve (S 2, 3 and 4).

The Internal Genital Organs

The Vagina

Vagina is a fibromusculo-membranous sheath connecting the uterine cavity with the exterior at the vulva. It is a passage, which allows the escape of menstrual flow and uterine secretions. It receives the penis and the ejected sperm during sexual intercourse and provides an exit for the fetus during delivery. The canal is directed upward and backward forming an angle of 45 degrees with the horizontal in erect posture. The long axis of the vagina almost lies parallel to the plane of the pelvic inlet and at right angles to that of the uterus. The diameter of the canal is about 2.5 cm, being wider in the upper part and narrowest at the introitus. It has enough power of distensibility as evident during childbirth.

Vaginal Walls

Vagina has an anterior, a posterior and two lateral walls. The anterior and posterior walls are apposed together but the lateral walls are comparatively stiffer specifically at its middle, as such it looks "H"shaped on transverse section. The length of the anterior wall is about 7 cm and that of the posterior wall is about 9 cm.

Relations

❖ *Anterior:* In front lie the bladder and urethra, which are closely connected to the anterior vaginal wall.
❖ *Behind*: The pouch of Douglas, the rectum and the perineal body each occupy approximately one-third of the posterior vaginal wall.
❖ *Lateral:* Beside the upper two-thirds are the pelvic fascia and ureters, while beside the lower third are the muscles of the pelvic floor.
❖ *Superior:* Above the vagina lies the uterus.
❖ *Inferior:* Below the vagina lies the external genitalia.

Structures

The posterior wall is 10 cm long while the anterior wall is only 7 cm because the cervix projects at right angles into its upper part. The upper part of the vagina is known as the *vault.*

Where the cervix projects into it, the vault forms a circular recess, which is described as its four *fornices*. The posterior fornix is the largest of these because the vagina is attached to the uterus at a higher-level behind than in front. The anterior fornix lies in front of the cervix and the lateral fornices lie on either side. The vaginal walls are pink in appearance and thrown into small folds known as *rugae*. These allow the vaginal walls to stretch during intercourse and childbirth.

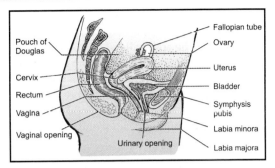

Fig. 5.11: Sagittal section of the pelvis showing generative organs

Layers

The lining of the vagina is made of squamous epithelium. Beneath the epithelium lies a layer of vascular connective tissue. The muscle layer has a weak inner coat of circular fibers and a stronger outer coat of longitudinal fibers. Pelvic fascia surrounds the vagina, forming a layer of connective tissue.

Contents

There are no glands in the vagina. It is moistened by mucus from the cervix and a transudate, which seeps out from the blood vessels of the vaginal wall. The vaginal fluid is strongly acid (pH 4.5) due to the presence of lactic acid formed by the action of Doderlein's bacilli on glycogen found in the squamous epithelium of the lining. These bacilli are the normal inhabitants of the vagina. The acid deters the growth of pathogenic bacteria.

Blood Supply

This comes from the branches of the internal iliac artery and includes the vaginal artery and a descending branch of the uterine artery. The blood drains through the corresponding veins.

Lymphatic Drainage

This is via the inguinal, the internal iliac and the sacral glands.

Nerve Supply

Sympathetic and parasympathetic nerves from the pelvic plexus (Lee Frankenhauser plexus) supply the vagina. The pudendal nerve supplies the lower part.

The Uterus (Fig. 5.11)

Position

It is situated in the cavity of the true pelvis, behind the bladder and in front of the rectum. It leans forward which is termed as *anteversion* and it bends forwards on itself, which is termed as *anteflexion*. In standing position, a woman's uterus is in horizontal position with the fundus resting on the bladder.

Relations

The structures surrounding the uterus are as follows:
- *Anterior:* The uterovesical pouch and the bladder
- *Posterior:* The rectouterine pouch of Douglas and the rectum
- *Lateral*: The broad ligaments, the uterine tubes and the ovaries
- *Superior:* The intestines
- *Inferior:* The vagina.

Supports

The uterus is supported by the pelvic floor and maintained in position by several ligaments.
- The transverse cervical ligaments extend from the sides of the cervix to the sidewalls of the pelvis. They are known as the cardinal ligaments or the Mackenrodt's ligaments
- The uterosacral ligaments pass backward from the cervix to the sacrum
- The pubocervical ligaments pass forward from cervix under the bladder to the pubic bones
- The broad ligaments formed from the folds of peritoneum, which are draped over the

uterine tubes. They hang down like a curtain and spread from the sides of the uterus to the sidewalls of the pelvis
* The round ligaments arise from the cornua of the uterus in front and from below the insertion of each fallopian tube, and pass between the folds of the broad ligament through the inguinal canal and are inserted into each labium majus
* The ovarian ligaments also begin at the cornua of the uterus but behind the tubes and pass down between the folds of the broad ligament to the ovaries.

Structure

The nonpregnant uterus is a hollow, muscular, pear-shaped organ situated in the true pelvis. It is 7.5 cm long, 5 cm wide and 2.5 cm deep. Each wall measures 1.25 cm. The uterus has the following parts:
* *The body* or *corpus:* Makes up the upper two-thirds of the uterus
* *The fundus:* The domed upper wall between the insertions of the uterine tubes
* *The cornua:* The upper outer angles of the uterus where the fallopian tubes join
* *The corpus or the body*: Lies between the openings of the two tubes and the isthmus
* *The cavity:* A potential space between the anterior and posterior walls. It is triangular in shape, the base of the triangle being uppermost
* *The isthmus:* It is a narrow area between the cavity and the cervix, which is 7 mm long. It enlarges during pregnancy to form the lower uterine segment
* *The cervix:* Protrudes into the vagina. The upper half, which is above the vagina, is termed as the supravaginal portion while the lower half is the infravaginal portion
* *The internal os:* It is the narrow opening between the isthmus and the cervix
* *The external os:* A small round opening at the lower end of the cervix. After childbirth this is seen as a transverse slit
* *The cervical canal:* Lies between the internal os and external os. This canal is a continuation of the uterine cavity and is shaped like a spindle (slender pin), narrow at each end and wider in the middle.

Layers

The uterus has three layers, of which the middle muscle layer is the thickest. The layers from inside outwards are endometrium, myometrium and perimetrium.
* *Endometrium:* This forms a lining of ciliated epithelium (mucous membrane) on a base of connective tissue or stroma. As there is no submucous layer, the endometrium is directly apposed to the muscle coat. In the uterine cavity, the endometrium is constantly changing in thickness through the menstrual cycle. The basal layer does not alter, but provides the foundation from which the upper layers regenerate. The surface epithelium is a single layer of ciliated columnar epithelium. The basal layer contains stromal cells, endometrial glands, vessels and nerves. The glands are simple tubular structures, which penetrate the stroma and sometimes even enter the muscle coat and secrete an alkaline muscles. The endometrium changes to decidua during pregnancy.
* *Myometrium:* It consists of thick bundles of smooth muscle fibers held by connective tissues and are arranged in various directions. It is thick in the upper part of the uterus and is more sparse in the isthmus and cervix. Its fibers run in all directions and interface to surround the blood vessels and lymphatic, which pass to and from the endometrium. During pregnancy, however, three distinct layers can be identified— Outer longitudinal middle interlacing and the inner circular.
  In the cervix, the muscle fibers are embedded in collagen fibers, which enable it to stretch in labor.
* *Perimetrium:* It is a double serous membrane, an extension to the peritoneum, which is draped over the uterus, covering all but a narrow strip on either side and the anterior wall of the supravaginal cervix from where it is deflected up over the bladder.

Blood Supply

Blood supply to the organs is through the uterine artery and ovarian artery. The uterine artery is a branch of the internal iliac artery and enters at the level of the cervix. The ovarian artery is a branch of the abdominal aorta. It supplies the ovaries and uterine tubes. The blood drains through corresponding veins.

Lymphatic Drainage

Lymph from the uterine body drains to the internal iliac glands, and from the cervix to several other pelvic lymph glands. This provides an effective defense against uterine infection.

Nerve Supply

This is mainly from the autonomic nervous system, the sympathetic and parasympathetic system via pelvic plexus.

Functions

The uterus serves to shelter the fetus during pregnancy. It prepares for this possibility each month. At the termination of pregnancy it expels the uterine contents.

The Uterine Tubes

Position

The uterine tubes or fallopian tubes extend laterally from the cornua of the uterus towards the sidewalls of the pelvis. They arch over the ovaries the fringed ends hovering near the ovaries in order to receive the ovum. They are attached to the broad ligament by two layers of peritoneum, called the mesosalpinx. Each tube is about 10–11.5 cm long.

Relations

* *Anterior, posterior and superior:* The peritoneal cavity and the intestines
* *Lateral:* The sidewalls of the pelvis
* *Inferior:* The broad ligaments and the ovaries
* *Medial:* The uterus lies between the two uterine tubes.

Supports

The uterine tubes are held in place by their attachment to the uterus. The broad ligaments and the infundibulopelvic ligaments support them.

Structure

Length of each tube is 10 cm. The lumen of the tube provides a pathway to the peritoneal cavity. The uterine tube has four portions (Fig. 5.12).

* *The interstitial portion*: It is 1.25 cm long and lies within the wall of the uterus. The lumen is 1 cm wide.
* *The isthmus*: The narrow part that extends from the uterus and measures 2.5 cm.
* *The ampulla*: The wider portion that is 5 cm long. Fertilization usually occurs in ampulla.
* *The infundibulum*: The funnel-shaped, fringed end of the tube, which is composed of many processes known as *fimbriae*. One fimbria is attached to the ovary.
* *The intramural part*: 1 cm long and runs through the uterine wall.

Blood Supply

This is via the uterine and ovarian arteries, returning by the corresponding veins.

Lymphatic Drainage

This is to the lumbar glands.

Functions

The uterine tube propels the ovum towards the uterus, receives the spermatozoa as they travel upward and provide a site for fertilization.

The Ovaries

Position

The ovaries or the female gonads are situated one on each side of the uterus and are attached to the back of the broad ligament within the peritoneal cavity (Fig. 5.12).

Relations

* *Anterior*: The broad ligaments
* *Posterior*: The intestines
* *Lateral*: The infundibulopelvic ligaments and the sidewalls of the pelvis
* *Superior*: The uterine tubes
* *Medial*: The uterus and the ovarian ligament.

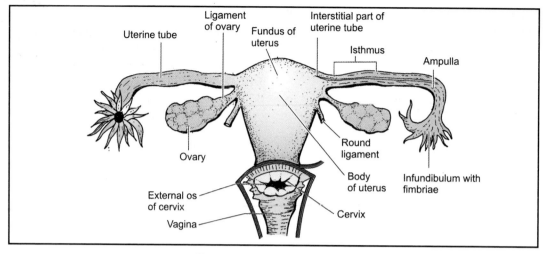

Fig. 5.12: Uterus tubes and ovaries

Supports

The ovarian ligaments from above and the infundibulopelvic ligaments laterally support the ovaries. They are attached to the broad ligament.

Structure

The ovary is almond shaped and is about 3 cm long, 1.5 cm wide and 1 cm thick. It is composed of a medulla and a cortex and is covered with germinal epithelium. The ovarian blood vessels, lymphatics and nerves pass through medulla. The hilum (opening), where the vessels enter the ovary, is called the mesovarium. The cortex is the functioning part of the ovary. It contains the ovarian follicles in different stages of development surrounded by stroma (supporting framework of connective tissue). The outer layer is formed of fibrous tissue and is known as the tunica albuginea. Over this lies the germinal epithelium.

Blood Supply

The blood supply is from the ovarian arteries and venous drainage through the ovarian veins. The right ovarian vein joins the inferior vena cava and the left returns its blood to the left renal vein.

Lymphatic Drainage

This is to the lumbar glands.

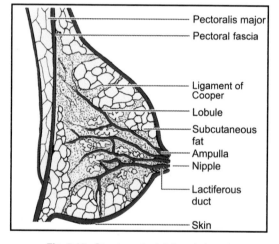

Fig. 5.13: Structure of adult female breast

Nerve Supply

This comes from the ovarian plexus.

Functions

The ovaries produce ova and the hormones estrogen and progesterone.

Accessory Reproductive Organs

Breasts

The breasts are bilateral glandular structures, which are concerned with lactation following childbirth. The shape of breasts varies in women and in different periods of life. They usually extend from the second to the sixth rib in the midclavicular line. They lie in the subcutaneous tissue over the fascia covering the pectoralis major and in some women beyond that over the serratus anterior and external oblique.

Structures (Nonlactating Breasts) (Fig. 5.13)

The areola is situated about the center of the breast and is pigmented. It is about 2.5 cm in diameter and has numerous sebaceous glands over it. The nipple is a muscular projection covered by pigmented skin. It is vascular and surrounded by unstriped muscles that make it erectile. The nipple contains about 15 to 20 lactiferous ducts and their openings. The whole breast is embedded in the subcutaneous fat. The fat is absent beneath the nipple and areola.

Each breast has 15 to 20 lobes, which are divided by fibrous tissue septa, which radiate from the center. The glandular tissue—Consists mainly of duct system and each lobe has a lactiferous duct. Each duct divides, subdivides and ultimately ends in alveoli which number from 10-100. Each alveolus is lined by columnar epithelium where milk secretion occurs. A network of longitudinal striated cells called myoepithelial cells surround the alveoli and smaller ducts. There is a dense network of capillaries surrounding the alveoli. Behind the nipple, the main duct (lactiferous duct) dilates to form ampulla where the milk is stored in lactating mothers. The interlobular ducts eventually end in the openings in the nipples, and muscle cells surround these ducts.

Blood Supply

Blood supply to the breasts is from the branches of the internal mammary artery, the axillary artery and the intercostal arteries. Superficial veins of the breasts drain into the internal mammary veins. Veins emptying into internal mammary, axillary and intercostal veins serve deep breast tissue.

Nerve Supply

The third and fourth branches of the cervical plexus provide the cutaneous nerve supply to the upper breast and thoracic intercostals nerves to the lower breast.

BIBLIOGRAPHY

1. Bennett R, Linda KB. Myles Textbook for Midwives, 13th edn. Edinburgh: Churchill Livingstone; 1999.
2. Fogel CI, Woods NF. Healthcare of Women A Nursing Perspective, St. Louis: The CV Mosby Company; 1981.
3. Rutishauser S. Physiology and Anatomy; A Basis for Nursing and Health Care, Edinburgh: Churchill Livingstone, 1994.
4. Smith A. The Body, Harmondsworth: Penguin Books; 1985.
5. Thibodeaux GA. Anatomy and Physiology, St. Louis: Mosby; 1987.

6

Hormonal Cycles

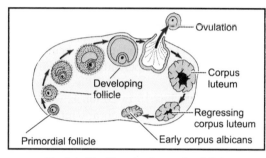

Fig. 6.1: The lifecycle of a graafian follicle

The biological cycles in a woman are controlled by the hypothalamus. It governs the anterior pituitary gland by hormonal pathways. The anterior pituitary gland in turn governs the ovaries by hormones. The hormones, produced in the ovaries, control changes in the uterus. All the changes occur simultaneously and in harmony. A woman's mood may change along with the cycle and emotional influences can alter the cycle.

THE OVARIAN CYCLE

The ovarian cortex at birth contains about 200,000 primordial (rudimentary) follicles. From puberty onwards certain follicles enlarge and one matures each month to liberate an ovum. A mature ovarian follicle is called a Graafian follicle.

Graafian Follicle (Fig. 6.1)

The ovum is situated at one end of the graafian follicle and is encircled by the narrow perivitelline space. Surrounding this lies, a clump of cells called the discus proligerus which radiate outward to form the corona radiata. The innermost cells of the corona are referred to as the zona pellucida. The whole follicle is lined with granulosa cells and contains follicular fluid. The outer coat of the follicle is the *external limiting membrane* and around this lies, an area of compressed ovarian stroma known as the theca.

Ovulation

The graafian follicle grows and matures to a size of 10 to 12 mm under the influence of follicle stimulating hormone (FSH) and later luteinizing hormone (LH). It moves to the surface of the ovary and finally protrudes above it. At the same time it swells and becomes tense, finally ruptures to release the ovum into the fimbriated end of the fallopian tube, which is cupped beneath the ovary. This is ovulation and it occurs on day 14 of 28 days cycle, or 14 days before menstruation in any cycle. A small loss of blood into the peritoneal cavity occurs at this time, which is termed as *mittelschmerz*. Some women feel pain at this time. The empty follicle is known as the corpus luteum (yellow body).

Corpus Luteum

After ovulation, the follicle collapses. Over the next 14 days it goes through the stages of proliferation, vascularization, maturity and regression and becomes an irregular yellow, structure. If fertilization does not take place, the corpus luteum will atrophy and become the corpus albicans (white body), which is the corpus luteum of menstruation. If fertilization takes place, it develops into a corpus luteum of pregnancy due to a surge of hyperplasia. In the absence of pregnancy, the corpus albicans gets broken down into small hyaline masses, which ultimately get completely reabsorbed.

Hormonal Control (Fig. 6.2)

The hypothalamus synthesizes and releases Gonadotrophin-Releasing Hormone (GnRH). It reaches the pituitary through portal circulation and causes the release of follicle stimulating hormone (FSH) and luteinizing hormone (LH). In other words under the influence of GnRH, the pituitary releases FSH and LH which are termed as gonadotrophins. The gonadotrophic activity of the hypothalamus and pituitary is influenced by positive and negative feedback mechanisms from the ovarian hormones.

FSH causes graafian follicles to develop and enlarge one of them more than all others each cycle. It stimulates the granulosa cells and theca to secrete estrogen. The level of FSH rises during the first half of the cycle and when the estrogen level reaches a certain point, its production ceases.

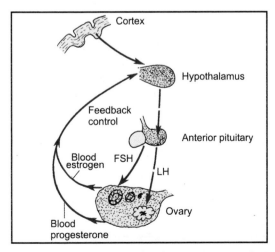

Fig. 6.2: Hormonal control of ovulation and menstruation

LH production starts a few days after the anterior pituitary starts producing FSH. Rising estrogen causes a surge (an up rush) in both FSH and LH levels resulting in the rupture of a ripened follicle-ovulation. Levels of both gonadotrophins then fall rapidly. If no pregnancy occurs the corpus luteum degenerates after 14 days. The negative feedback effect of progesterone ceases and FSH and LH levels rise again to begin a new cycle.

Prolactin

The hormone is produced in the anterior pituitary gland. It does not play a role in the control of ovarian hormones. If produced in excessive amounts, it will inhibit ovulation that is the natural phenomenon during lactation.

Ovarian Hormones

Estrogen

The granulosa cells and theca of the ovaries, under the influence of FSH produce this hormone. It comprises several compounds including estriol, estradiol and estrone.

Estrogen is responsible for the secondary sex characteristics such as the female shape, the growth of the breasts and the uterus and the female distribution of hair. It influences the production of cervical mucus. This in turn encourages the growth of Doderlein's bacilli, which are responsible for the acidity of the vaginal fluid. During the uterine cycle, estrogen causes the proliferation of the uterine endometrium. It inhibits FSH and encourages fluid retention.

Progesterone

Progesterone is produced by the corpus luteum under the influence of LH. It acts only on the tissues, which have previously been affected by estrogen. During the second half of the cycle, it causes secretory changes in the lining of the uterus as the endometrium develops tortuous glands and an enriched blood supply in readiness for the possible arrival of a fertilized ovum. It causes the body temperature of the woman to rise by 0.5 degrees C (0.5°C) after ovulation and causes tingling and a sense of fullness in the breasts prior to menstruation.

Relaxin

This hormone is secreted in the corpus luteum and is at its maximum level, after 38 weeks of pregnancy. It relaxes the pelvic girdle, softens the cervix and suppresses uterine contractions.

MENSTRUAL CYCLE

Menstruation refers to the monthly discharge through the vagina of blood and other substances from the uterus in nonpregnant adult females. Although every woman has an individual cycle of menstruation, which varies in length, the average cycle is taken to be 28 days long and recurs from puberty to menopause except when pregnancy intervenes.

During the life of a woman, the endometrium is shed and degenerated no fewer than 400 times. The menstrual cycle occurs in four phases and they affect the tissue structure of the endometrium, in response to the ovarian hormones (Fig. 6.3). The first day of the cycle is the day on which menstruation begins.

Early Proliferative Phase

This phase follows menstruation and lasts up to 9 days (5–9 days). The endometrium is less than 2 cm thick. The glands are narrow and straight. The blood vessels are numerous and prominent. Under the control of estrogen regrowth and thickening of endometrium begins.

Late Proliferative Phase

Proliferative phase continues up to 14 days until ovulation. The endometrium in this period is thicker, due to glandular hyperplasia and an increase in the stromal ground substance. At the completion of this phase the endometrium consists of three layers.

1. The *basal layer*—This lies immediately above the myometrium, about 1 mm in thickness. This layer does not undergo any change during the menstrual cycle and it contains the rudimentary structures for building up new endometrium.
2. The *functional layer*—This contains tubular glands of about 2.5 mm in thickness. This layer changes constantly according to the influences of ovarian hormone.
3. The *spongy layer*—This has cuboidal ciliated epithelium and covers the functional layer.

The Secretory Phase

This follows ovulation and is under the influence of progesterone and estrogen from the corpus luteum. This phase lasts up 26 days. The functional layer thickens to 3.5 mm and becomes spongy in appearance. The endometrium is extremely vascular and rich in glycogen in this phase. Spiral or coiled arteries develop which become tortuous.

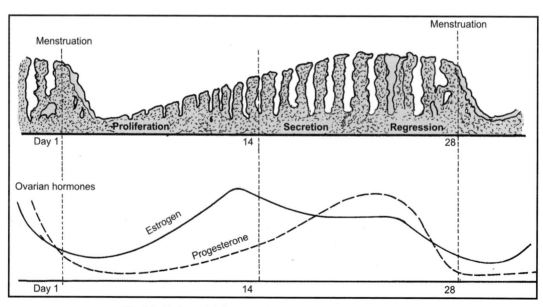

Fig. 6.3: Endometrial changes related to ovulation and menstruation

The Premenstrual Phase

It corresponds to the regression of the corpus luteum and declines in the levels of ovarian hormones and lasts from day 27 to 28.

The Menstrual Phase

This phase is characterized by vaginal bleeding and lasts for 3 to 5 days. Physiologically this is the last phase of the menstrual cycle. The endometrium is shed up to the basal layer along with blood from capillaries and the unfertilized ovum. Bleeding stops when the coiled arteries return to a state of constriction.

Clinical Aspects of Menstruation

Menarche and Puberty

Menarche is the first menstruation of a girl. It occurs at the age of 12 or 13 years, although it may occur as early as 10 years or as late as 16 years. Puberty refers to the period in life during which the reproductive organs develop and reach maturity, which is from childhood to sexual maturity. In females, the first signs are breast development and the appearance of pubic hair. The body grows considerably and takes on the female shape. Puberty culminates in the onset of menstruation. The first few cycles are not usually accompanied by ovulation.

Menopause and Climacteric

Menopause is the cessation of menses. Cessation of menstruation occurs gradually with the periods first becoming irregular and then stopping altogether marking the end of a woman's reproductive life. This is often accompanied by physical symptoms such as hot flushes and emotional changes such as mood swings. With menopause there is a fall in the production of estrogen that may lead to an increased tendency to obesity and changes such as signs of aging. The sexual drive may not diminish though some women may find it difficult to accept that they are no longer fertile. Menopause occurs between 45 and 50 years in most women. Climacteric refers to the entire transitional phase between sexual maturity and menopause.

Normal Menstrual Cycle

Menstrual cycles occur at an interval of 28 years, though this period is not same for all women. The length of cycle, vary from 22 to 35 days. The duration of menstrual flow also varies from 2 to 8 days with the usual duration ranging from 4 to 6 days. The blood flow is of liquid consistency and the amount about 25 to 60 ml for each menstruation.

BIBLIOGRAPHY

1. Bennett RV, Linda KB. Myles Textbook for Midwives, 13th edn. Edinburgh: Churchill Livingstone; 1999.
2. Rutishauser S. Physiology and Anatomy; A Basis for Nursing and Health Care, Edinburgh: Churchill Livingstone; 1994.
3. Smith A. The Body, Harmonds-worth: Penguin Books; 1985.
4. Thibodiacix GA. Anatomy and Physiology, St. Louis; Mosby; 1987.

7

The Male Reproductive System

Learning Objectives

Upon completing this chapter, the learner will be able to:
* Name the different parts of the male reproductive system
* Describe the process of spermatogenesis and sperm maturation
* List and describe the male hormones.

The parts of male reproductive system (Fig. 7.1) are described below:

The Scrotum

The scrotum is a pouch of pigmented skin in which the testes are suspended outside the body. It lies below the symphysis pubis between the upper parts of the thighs behind the penis. It has two compartments, one for each testis.

The Testes

These are the male gonads (male reproductive gland) and produce spermatozoa and testosterone. Testosterone is the hormone responsible for the secondary sex characteristics. Along with the follicle stimulating hormone, it promotes the production of sperm.

In order to achieve their function, the testes must remain below body temperature and hence they are situated outside the body. Each testis is a rounded body measuring 4.5 cm long, 2.5 cm wide and 3 cm thick.

It is composed of several layers of tissue.
* *Tunica vasculosa*: An inner layer of connective tissue containing a network of capillaries
* *Tunica vaginalis*: The outer layer which is made of peritoneum

Fig. 7.1: Male reproductive system

❖ *The seminiferous ('seed carrying') tubules*: The portion where spermatogenesis or production of sperms takes place. There are about three of them in each lobule. Between the tubules there are interstitial cells that secrete testosterone. The tubules join together to form a system of channels that lead to the epididymis.

❖ *Epididymis*: A comma-shaped, coiled tube that lies on the superior surface and extends down the posterior aspect to the lower pole of testis, where it leads into the vas deferens or deferent duct.

The Spermatic Cord

The spermatic cord consists of the vas deferens, the testicular blood vessels and nerves. It transmits the vas deferens with its blood vessels and nerves up into the body. The vas deferens carries the sperm to the ejaculatory duct. The cord passes upward through the inguinal canal from where the vas deferens continues upward over the symphysis pubis and arches backward beside the bladder. Behind the bladder it merges with the duct from the seminal vesicle and passes through the prostate gland as the ejaculatory duct to join the urethra.

The Ejaculatory Ducts

These are small muscular ducts that carry the spermatozoa and the seminal fluid to the urethra.

The Prostate Gland

This gland lies between the rectum and the symphysis pubis and surrounds the urethra at the base of the bladder. It is 4 cm long, 3 cm wide and 2 cm deep. It is composed of columnar epithelium, a muscle layer and an outer fibrous layer. It produces a thin lubricating fluid, which enters the urethra through ducts.

The Penis

The root of the penis lies in the perineum from where it passes below the symphysis pubis. The lower two-thirds is outside the body in front of the scrotum.

It carries the urethra, which is a passage for both urine and semen. During sexual excitement it stiffens (an erection) in order to be able to penetrate the vagina and deposit the semen near the woman's cervix. There are three columns of erectile tissue. Two are lateral columns called the *corpora cavernosa,* one on either side and in front of the urethra. The posterior column is termed *corpus spongiosum* contains the urethra. The posterior column is termed corpus spongiosum contains the urethra. The tip is expanded to form the glans penis.

The lower two-thirds of the penis is covered in skin. At the lower end the skin is folded back on itself above the glans penis to form the prepuce, which is a movable double fold. The penis is extremely vascular and during an erection the blood spaces fill and become distended.

The Male Hormones

The hypothalamus produces gonadotropin releasing factors. These stimulate the anterior pituitary gland to produce follicle stimulating hormone (FSH) and luteinizing hormone (LH). FSH acts on the seminiferous tubules to bring about the production of sperm, while LH acts on the interstitial cells that produce testosterone.

Testosterone is responsible for the secondary sex characteristics, namely deepening of the voice, growth of hair on the chest, pubis, axilla and face. The control of male hormones is similar to that of female except that it is not cyclical.

Formation of the Spermatozoa

Production of sperm begins at puberty and continues throughout the adult life. Spermatogenesis takes place in the seminiferous tubule under the influence of FSH and testosterone. The process of maturation requires few weeks. The mature sperm are stored in the epididymis and vas deferens until ejaculation. If ejaculation does not happen, they degenerate and get absorbed. At each ejaculation, 2 to 4 ml of semen is deposited in the vagina. The seminal fluid contains about 100 million sperm per ml, of which 20 to 35 percent are likely to be abnormal. The normal sperm move at a speed of 2 to 3 mm per minute.

The individual spermatozoon (Fig. 7.2) has a head, a body, and a long, mobile tail that lashes

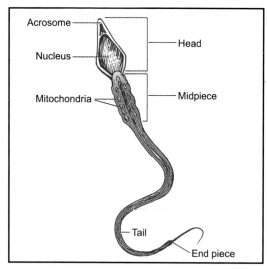

Acrosome

Nucleus

Head

Mitochondria

Midpiece

Tail

End piece

Fig. 7.2: Parts of a sperm cell

(makes flicking movement) to propel the sperm along.

The tip of the head is covered by an acrosome, which contains enzymes to dissolve the covering of the ovum in order to penetrate it.

BIBLIOGRAPHY

1. Bennett R, Linda KB. Myles Textbook for Midwives, 13th edn. Edinburgh; Churchill Livingstone: 1999.
2. Fogel CI, Woods NF. Healthcare of Women A Nursing Perspective, St. Louis; The CV Mosby Company: 1981.
3. Rutishauser S. Physiology and Anatomy, A Basis for Nursing and Health Care. Edinburgh; Churchill Livingstone; 1994.
4. Smith A. The Body, Harmondsworth; Penguin Books; 1985.
5. Thibodeaux GA. Anatomy and Physiology, St. Louis; Mosby; 1987.

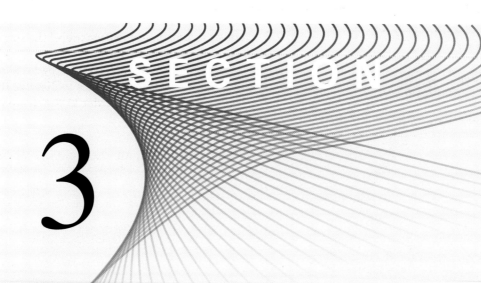

SECTION

3

Embryology
and Fetology

8

Fertilization, Implantation and Development of the Fertilized Ovum

Learning Objectives

Upon completing this chapter, the learner will be able to:
❖ Describe the process of fertilization and the development of the fertilized ovum
❖ Describe the process of implantation and the postimplantation changes in the uterus.

FERTILIZATION

The ovum, which is about 0.15 mm in diameter, passes into the uterine tube and moves towards the uterus after ovulation. Transport of the ovum through the tube is brought about by the cilia and the peristaltic muscular contraction of the tube. At this time the cervix, under the influence of estrogen, secrets a flow of alkaline mucus that attracts the spermatozoa. At an intercourse about 60 to 120 million sperm are deposited in the posterior fornix of the vagina. Those that reach the loose cervical mucus, survive to propel (drive forward) themselves towards the uterine tubes while the remainder are destroyed by the acid medium of the vagina. During the journey through the uterus, more sperm die, only thousands reach the tube, where they meet the ovum usually in the ampulla. The sperm mature and become capable of releasing an enzyme called hyaluronidase, which allows penetration of the zona pellucida and the cell membrane surrounding the ovum. Many sperm are needed for this to take place but only one will enter the ovum. After this, the membrane is sealed to prevent entry of any further sperm. The tail of the sperm is left behind. Nuclei of the two cells fuse resulting in the formation of a zygote. The sperm and ovum are known as the male and female gametes.

Neither the sperm nor the ovum can survive for longer than 2 to 3 days and hence fertilization is most likely to occur when intercourse takes place around the time of ovulation, within 48 hours prior to or 24 hours following ovulation.

Development of Fertilized Ovum (Fig. 8.1)

The fertilized ovum (zygote) continues its passage through the fallopian tube and reaches the uterus in 3 to 4 days. During this time it undergoes segmentation or cell division to form *blastomeres*. The ovum divides into two cells, then four, eight and sixteen and so on until a mulberry-like ball of cells is formed, known as the *morula*. The divisions occur quite slowly, about once in every 12 hours. Gradual accumulation of fluid in the morula results in the formation of the blastocyst. At one pole of

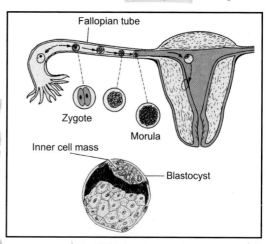

Fig. 8.1: Development of the fertilized ovum

Inner cell mass → fetus, Amnion.   Troophoblast
                                    → Placenta, Chorion.

62   SECTION 3: EMBRYOLOGY AND FETOLOGY

the blastocyst there is a compact mass of cells, called the inner cell mass. Around the outside of it there is a single layer of cells, known as the trophoblast. The trophoblast will form the placenta and chorion while the inner mass will become the fetus and the amnion. On its journey, the zygote is nourished by glycogen from the goblet cells of the uterine tubes and later the secretory glands of the uterus.

IMPLANTATION

When the blastocyst falls into the uterus, it lies free for 2 to 3 days. The part of the tropho-blast, that lies over the inner cell mass, then becomes quite sticky and adheres to the endo-metrium. It then begins to secrete enzymes

that cause erosion of the epithelium (endo-metrial cells) allowing the blastocyst to sink into the endometrium. This is called embedding or nidation (nesting) and it normally is complete by the 11th day after ovulation. The endometrium closes over it completely and the only evidence of the presence of the blastocyst will be a small bulge on the surface (Fig. 8.2). Implantation usually occurs on the posterior uterine wall, though it may sometimes occur on the anterior wall of the fundus.

Postimplantation Changes in the Uterus

Decidua is the name given to the uterine endometrium during pregnancy. It differs from the nonpregnant endometrium because of the changes it undergoes in pregnancy. Increased

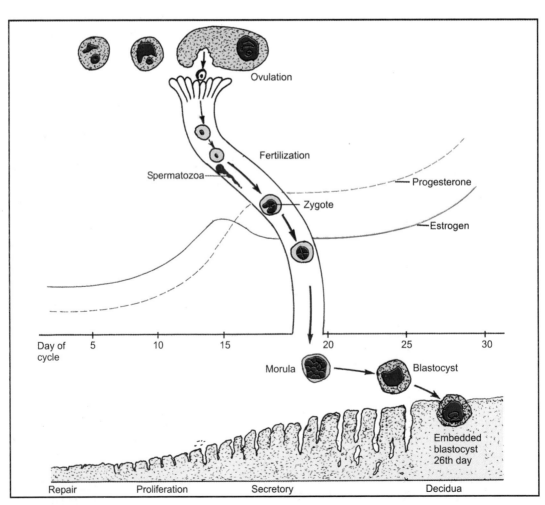

Fig. 8.2: Fertilization and nidation

secretion of estrogens causes the endometrium to grow to four times its original thickness. Progesterone from the corpus luteum stimulates the endometrial glands and increases the size of the blood vessels. It becomes a soft, vascular and spongy bed in which the fertilized ovum implants. With the exception of the zona basalis, the decidua is shed after birth giving meaning to the Latin origin of the word *deciduous* meaning 'a falling off. There are three areas of decidua.

1. *Decidua basalis*: This is the decidua beneath the site of implantation of the embryo. It lies immediately above the myometrium and remains unchanged. This part of the decidua is the maternal contribution to the placenta. It regenerates to form the new endometrium during the puerperium.

2. *Decidua capsularis*: The decidua surrounding the remainder of the embryo that serves as a covering between the embryo and the uterine cavity. With fetal growth, the decidua capsularis bulges into the uterine cavity and fuses with the decidua parietalis. The uterine cavity is thus obliterated by the end of the fourth month.

3. *Decidua parietalis* or *decidua vera*: This is the decidua lining the rest of the uterine cavity.

DEVELOPMENT OF THE FERTILIZED OVUM

The Trophoblast

Small projections begin to appear all over the surface of the trophoblast becoming most abundant at the area of contact. These trophoblastic cells differentiate into three layers— The outer syncytiotrophoblast (syncytium), the inner cytotrophoblast and below that the primitive mesenchyme or mesoderm.

The *syncytiotrophoblast* erodes the walls of the blood vessels of the decidua, to make the nutrients in the maternal blood accessible to the developing embryo.

The *cytotrophoblast*, which is a well-defined single layer of cells, produces a hormone known as human chorionic gonadotropin (hCG). This hormone is responsible for informing the corpus

luteum that pregnancy has begun. As a result corpus luteum continues to produce estrogen and progesterone. Progesterone maintains the integrity of the decidua so that menstruation does not occur. The high level of estrogen suppresses the production of FSH stopping further follicle development in the ovary.

The *mesenchyme* develops to chorionic vesicle with its membrane called chorion. It condenses about the embryo to form the body stalk that connects the embryo to the nutrient chorion and forms the umbilical cord later on.

The Inner Cell Mass

While the trophoblast develops to form the placenta, which will nourish the fetus, the inner cell mass develops to form the fetus itself. The cells differentiate into three layers— ectoderm, endoderm and mesoderm—Each of which will form particular parts of the fetus (Fig. 8.3).

The *ectoderm* develops into the central and peripheral nervous systems and the epidermis with its appendages.

The *endoderm* forms the dermis, the skeleton, the connective tissue, vascular and the urogenital systems and most skeletal, and smooth muscles.

The *mesoderm* forms certain internal organs such as the heart and blood vessels, liver, pancreas and also the bones and the muscles. The three layers together are termed as the embryonic plate. As the development continues, two cavities appear in the inner cell mass, one on either side of the embryonic plate. These are termed the *amniotic* cavity and the yolk sac.

The amniotic cavity is lies on the side of the ectoderm. It is filled with fluid and gradually enlarges to envelop the embryo. The amnion forms from its lining.

The yolk sac is lies on the side of the ectoderm and provides nourishment for the embryo until the trophoblast is sufficiently

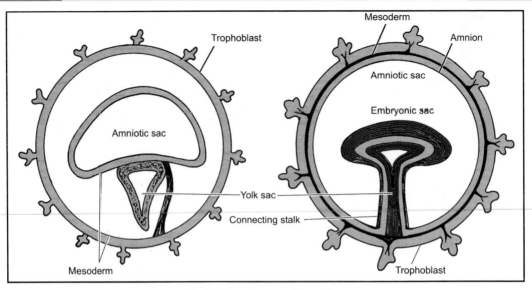

Fig. 8.3: Development of the embryo

developed to take over. Part of it forms the primitive gut and remainder atrophies under the amnion on the surface of the placenta.

The Embryo

The developing offspring is termed as embryo until eight weeks after implantation. During this period all the organs and systems of the body are laid down in rudimentary form, which in further months grow and mature. After eight weeks until term, the conceptus is known as fetus.

BIBLIOGRAPHY

1. Bennett RV, Linda KB. Myles textbook for midwives, 13th edn. Edinburgh: Churchill Livingstone; 1999.
2. Fox HA. A contemporary view of the human placenta, Midwifery; 1991:7(1).
3. Llewellyn Jones D. Fundamental of obstetrics and gynecology, faber, 5th edn. London; 1990.
4. Stein MA, Judith CM. NCLEX-RN Review, 4th edn. New York: Delmar Thomson Learning; 2000.
5. Varney Helen. Nurse midwifery, 2nd edn. Boston: Jones and Barlett Publishers; 1999.

9

Development of the Placenta and Fetus

Learning Objectives

Upon completing this chapter, the learner will be able to:
- ❖ Enumerate the developmental stages of the fertilized ovum
- ❖ Describe the development of the placenta and circulation through the placenta
- ❖ List the functions, variations, anomalies and abnormalities of placenta.

The placenta is partly fetal and partly maternal in origin. It connects closely with the mother's circulation to carry-out functions, which the fetus is unable to perform for itself during intrauterine life. The survival of the fetus depends on the integrity and efficiency of the placenta.

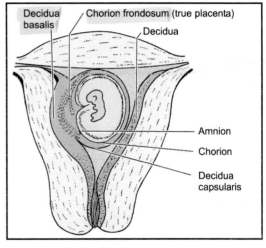

Fig. 9.1: Development of placenta

DEVELOPMENT OF THE PLACENTA (FIG. 9.1)

The small projections that appear on the trophoblastic layer of the blastocyst proliferate (grow by multiplication) and branch from about three weeks after fertilization, forming the chorionic villi. The villi become most profuse in the area where the blood supply is richest, that is, in the basal decidua. This part of the trophoblast is known as the chorion frondosum. It will eventually develop into the placenta. The villi under the capsular decidua gets less nourishment and gradually atrophy and form the chorionic laeve or bald chorion, which is the origin of the chorionic membrane.

The villi erode the walls of maternal blood vessels as they penetrate the decidua, opening them up to form a lake of maternal blood in which they float. The opened blood vessels are known as sinuses and the area surrounding the villi as blood spaces. Maternal blood circulates slowly in these vessels, enabling the villi to absorb food and oxygen and to excrete waste. A few villi are attached more deeply to the decidua and are called the anchoring villi. Placental circulation is established by the 17th day.

Each chorionic villus is a branching structure. Its center consists of mesoderm and branches of umbilical vein and artery. Four layers of tissue separate the maternal blood from the fetal blood making it impossible for the two circulations (maternal and fetal) to mix unless the villi are damaged (Fig. 9.2).

The placenta is completely developed and functioning from the 10th week after gestation. In its early stages, it is a relatively loose structure, but becomes more compact as it matures. Between 12 and 20 weeks of gestation, the placenta weighs more than the fetus. At this stage the fetal organs are insufficiently

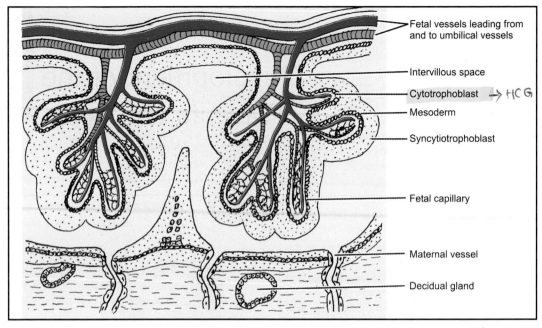

Fetal vessels leading from and to umbilical vessels

Intervillous space

Cytotrophoblast → HCG

Mesoderm

Syncytiotrophoblast

Fetal capillary

Maternal vessel

Decidual gland

Fig. 9.2: The diagrammatic representation of the chorionic villi

developed to cope with the metabolic processes of nutrition. Later in pregnancy as the fetus matures some of the fetal organs, such as the liver, begin to function resulting in easier exchange of oxygen and carbon dioxide.

Each mainstem villus and its branches form a cotyledon. The total number of cotyledons remains constant, but the individual cotyledons continue to grow until term.

Circulation through the Placenta (Fig. 9.3)

Fetal blood, that is low in oxygen, is pumped by the fetal heart towards the placenta along their branches to the capillaries of the villi. The blood returns to the fetus via umbilical vein after giving up carbon dioxide and absorbing oxygen.

Maternal blood is delivered to the placental bed in the decidua by the spiral arteries that flow into the blood spaces surrounding the villi. The blood enters the sinuses in a funnel-shaped stream similar to a fountain and as it passes upwards, bathes the villus and drains back into a branch of uterine vein.

The Mature Placenta

The normal term placenta is a flattened disc-like mass with a circular or oval outline. Its average volume is 500 ml and ranges from 200 to 900 ml. Average weight of the placenta is 500 gm and the range is 200 to 800 gm. It often weighs approximately one-sixth of the baby's weight at term. Average diameter is 20 cm and thickness 2.5 cm.

The fetal surface of the placenta is smooth, shiny and transparent. The underlying chorion can be seen through it. The umbilical cord is attached to the fetal surface near the center and branches of the umbilical vessels radiate out under the amnion at this point, the veins being larger and deeper than the arteries. The amnion can be peeled off the surface, leaving the chorionic plate (Fig. 9.4).

The maternal surface is finely granular and divided into 15 to 30 lobes (average 20) that are called cotyledons by a series of fissures or furrows termed as sulci. The lobes are made up of lobules, each of which contains a single villus with its branches (Fig. 9.4).

Functions of the Placenta

The placenta truly is an organ of life with a number of functions designed to provide for and protect the fetus. Its functions include respiration, nutrition, storage, protection and endocrine.

Fig. 9.3: Placental circulation

Figs 9.4A and B: The placenta at term: (A) Maternal surface of the placenta; (B) Fetal surface of the placenta (*For color version see Plate 1*)

Respiration

The fetus obtains oxygen and excretes carbon dioxide through the placenta. Oxygen from the mother's hemoglobin passes into the fetal blood by simple diffusion and similarly the fetus gives off carbon dioxide into the maternal blood.

Nutrition

The fetus requires all the nutrients like anyone. Amino acids, glucose, vitamins, minerals, lipids, water and electrolytes are transferred across the placental membrane. Food from the maternal diet gets broken down into simpler forms by the time it reaches the placental site. The placenta selects those substances required by the fetus. It can breakdown complex nutrients into compounds that can be used by the fetus. Protein gets transferred as amino acids, carbohydrates as glucose, and fats as fatty acids.

Storage

The placenta stores glucose, iron and vitamins. Glucose stored in the form of glycogen gets reconverted to glucose when required.

Excretion

Carbon dioxide is the major substance excreted from the fetus. Other substances include bilirubin from the breakdown of red blood cells and small amounts of urea and uric acid.

Protection

The placental membrane has a limited barrier function. Certain antibodies, which the mother possesses gets passed on to the fetus to provide immunity for the baby for three months after birth. Certain viruses such as the rubella virus, and bacteria such as *Treponema pallidum* of syphilis and *Mycobacterium* of tuberculosis also cross the barrier. Most drugs given to mother also cross the barrier and reach the baby. However, most bacteria and certain drugs do not cross the barrier. It is important for the midwife to know which substances cross or does not cross the placental membrane.

Endocrine

The cytotrophoblastic layer of the chorionic villi produces human chorionic gonadotropin (hCG). It is present in large quantities between the seventh and tenth week when the production is at its peak and then gradually decreases as the pregnancy advances. hCG forms the basis of many pregnancy tests as it is excreted in the mother's urine. Estrogens are produced by placenta in large amount throughout pregnancy. The amount of estrogen produced is an index of fetoplacental wellbeing.

Progesterone is produced in the syncytial layer of the placenta in increasing quantities until immediately before the onset of labor, when its level falls.

Human placental lactogen (HPL) is another hormone produced by the placenta. It is involved in lactogenic and metabolic processes in pregnancy. The production of HPL increases as the level of hCG falls and continues throughout pregnancy.

Mechanisms of Transfer of Materials

As an organ of transfer, the placenta has several mechanisms by which to transfer materials between the maternal and fetal circulations in the intervillous space across the placental membrane. These include the following:

1. *Diffusion*: The transfer of substances across a membrane from an area of higher concentration to an area of lower concentration. Low molecular weight substances diffuse readily across the placental membrane. Substances concerned with biochemical homeostasis are transferred by diffusion, e.g. water, oxygen, carbon dioxide, urea and certain simple amines.
2. *Active transport*: This transfer is against usual physiological principles. It includes the transfer of substances, which are in low

concentration in the maternal blood and in high concentration in the fetal blood. It is a metabolic process requiring energy and enzymatic transfer systems. The transport of iron and ascorbic acid from the mother to the fetus are examples.

3. *Pinocytosis* or *phagocytosis*: A substance is taken and moved across the cells of the fetal membrane to the fetal bloodstream by invaginations (infoldings) of the chorionic villi simply engulfing the material. Large protein molecules with a higher molecular weight, such as immune gamma globulin G, are thought to be taking place by this mechanism. The direction of cellular transfer may depend on such factors as whether the mother is erect or supine.
4. *Breaks between cells*: A break in the chorionic villi allows for the direct transfer of cells. An example of this, is the sensitization of an Rh-negative woman from the receipt of erythrocytes from her Rh-positive fetus.
5. *Placental infection*: Conditions in which the placenta is infected and the lesions in the placenta caused by the infectious organisms serve as a means of access into the fetal bloodstream. Protozoal and bacterial infections are transferred this way. Viral infections may pass through the placental membrane and infect the fetus without infecting the placenta.

Amniotic Fluid

Amniotic fluid, also termed as liquor amnii, is the fluid which distends the amniotic sac and allows for the growth and free movement of the fetus. It equalizes pressure and protects the fetus from jarring (sudden vibrations) and injury. The fluid maintains a constant temperature for the fetus and provides small amounts of nutrients. In labor, it aids effacement of cervix and dilatation of the os. As long as the membranes remain intact the amniotic fluid protects the placenta and umbilical cord from pressure of uterine contractions.

Constituents

Amniotic fluid is a clear, pale straw colored fluid, consisting of 99 percent water. The remaining 1 percent is dissolved in solid matter including food substances and waste products. It contains fetal urine, respiratory tract secretions, and skin cells shed by the fetus, vernix caseosa and lanugo.

Source

Amniotic fluid comes from both maternal and fetal sources. Some fluid is exuded from
i) maternal vessels in the decidua and some from
ii) fetal vessels in the placenta. It is also secreted by the amnion and umbilical cord. Fetal urine also contributes to the volume from the tenth week of gestation.

1000 ml → Normal
1500 ml → Polyhydramnios
↓ 300 ml → Oligohydramnios.

Volume

The volume of amniotic fluid increases throughout pregnancy. At 38 weeks, it is about one liter (1000 ml). Then it diminishes slightly and at term the amount is about 800 ml. If the total amount exceeds 1500 ml, the condition is termed as polyhydramnios (often referred to as hydramnios) and if less than 300 ml, the term oligohydramnios is used. Such abnormalities are often associated with congenital malformation of the fetus. As the normal fetus swallows amniotic fluid, conditions which interfere with swallowing increases the amount of fluid. Similarly, the normal fetus passes urine and when urine production is affected due to congenital problems, amount of liquor tends to be less.

The Umbilical Cord (Fig. 9.5)

The umbilical cord or funis extends from the fetus to the placenta. It transmits the umbilical blood vessels, which are two arteries and one vein.

These are enclosed and protected by a gelantinous substance known as Wharton's jelly. The whole cord is covered in a layer of amnion continuous with that covering the placenta.

The length of the average cord is 50 cm. A cord is considered to be short when its length is less than 40 cm. Certain cords are longer and with longer cords, problems can arise. It may become wrapped round the neck or body of the fetus or become knotted. A true knot occurs when the fetus has passed through a

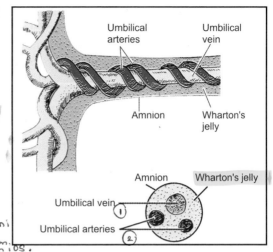

Fig. 9.5: The umbilical cord

loop in the cord and a real knot has been created. False knotting of the cord occurs when the cord appears to be knotted but instead has kinking of the blood vessels within the cord or accumulation of lumps of Wharton's jelly on the side of the cord. True knotting is most likely to occur in one of two situations.

a. *Small fetus, long cord and large amount of amniotic fluid*: The higher ratio of amniotic fluid to fetal size in early pregnancy makes this the time of greatest incidence. These knots are usually benign because they are kept from tightening by pulsations in the blood vessels. However, with true knots there is possibility of occlusion of blood vessels during labor.

b. *Multiple gestation within a single amnion*: All sorts of cord entanglements and knots are possible because the fetuses have greater freedom of movement within the fetal sac thereby increasing the chance of knot forming and its tightening.

Variations, Anomalies and Abnormalities of Placenta

1. Larger and heavier than normal placentas are seen with excessively large fetuses, fetal syphilis and erythroblastosis.

2. Smaller and lighter than normal placentas may occur with general systemic diseases or local uterine conditions which cause

undernourishment of the placenta and resultant intrauterine growth retardation.

3. Color of placental tissue markedly lighter. This condition may be caused by fetal anemia, such as those found in erythroblastosis.

4. *Excessive infarct formation*: Infarction of cotyledons happen due to disease processes, such as severe maternal hypertension, severe pre-eclampsia or eclampsia. Extensive infarcting reduces effective placental functioning, which may result in intrauterine growth retardation or if a substantial portion of the placenta is infarcted, may result in fetal death.

5. *Edema of the placenta*: Edematous placenta is mushy, thick and pale, and fluid can be squeezed from it. This may be caused by severe maternal heart disease, diabetes or nephritis and by severe erythroblastosis. The fetus usually dies *in utero* either as a stillbirth or earlier as an abortion.

6. Tumors are found in association with prematurity and polyhydramnios. Perinatal mortality and maternal hemorrhage are both increased.

7. *Syphilitic placenta*: It is abnormally large, pale, yellow gray placenta.

8. *Succenturiate placenta* or *placenta succenturiata (Fig. 9.6)*: One or more separate accessory lobes in the membranes a variable distance away from the main placental mass. These accessory lobes are usually connected to the main placental mass.

The primary significance of this anomaly lies in the possibility that the succenturiate lobe(s) will be retained in the uterus after expulsion of the main placental mass. Retained succenturiate lobes may cause severe postpartal hemorrhage. The retention of succenturiate lobes can be detected during inspection of the placenta and membranes by noting:

a. Torn blood vessels at the margin of the placenta or extension of blood vessels into the membranes.

b. Rough or torn roundish defects or holes in the membranes at a short distance from the placenta. The midwife must

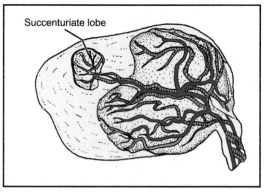

Fig. 9.6: Succenturiate lobe of placenta

examine every placenta for evidence of a retained lobe. Manual exploration of the uterus and removal of the succenturiate lobe(s) is indicated if retention has occurred.

9. *Extrachorial placentas*: A placental anomaly observed on the fetal surface as a thick white ring which gives the impression that the central portion is somewhat depressed. There are two varieties of extrachorial placentas, which are determined by the location of the ring. Both may be complete or incomplete as dictated by whether or not the ring circumscribes a full circle.

a. *Placenta circumvallata or circumvallate placenta*: The ring situated at a variable distance between the margin and center of the placenta. A double fold of both chorion and amnion, with fibrin and degenerated decidua forms the ring giving it a raised appearance (Fig. 9.7).

b. *Placenta marginata or circummarginate placenta*: The ring is located at the edge or margin of the placenta and is raised by the presence of degenerated decidua and fibrin.

10. *Lobulated placenta*: There appears to be multiple placentas for a single baby. In fact, it is one placenta divided into two or more parts either completely separated or joined in part. Either way, the lobes are held together by the one set of membranes and blood vessels. The number of lobes determines the name as bipartite placenta (placenta Duplex) (Fig. 9.8) or tripartite

Fig. 9.7: Circumvallate placenta

Fig. 9.9: Battledore insertion of the cord

Fig. 9.8: Bipartite placenta

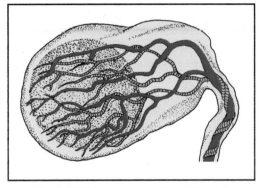

Fig. 9.10: Velamentous insertion of the cord

placenta (placenta triplex). This anomaly is thought to be due to abnormalities in the blood supply to the decidua. Its main significance is that the midwife must be alert to make sure that all lobes have been expelled from the uterus.

Variations, Anomalies and Abnormalities of the Umbilical Cord and Its Insertion

1. *Battledore placenta*: A variation in which the umbilical cord is inserted at the edge or margin of the placenta (Fig. 9.9). Marginal insertion of the cord occurs in less than 10 percent of placentas and it is considered a normal insertion (Varney, 1997).
2. *Velamentous insertion*: The cord is inserted into the membranes at some distance from the edge of the placenta (Fig. 9.10). The umbilical vessels from the cord run through the membranes for a variable distance before each enters the placenta. Velamentous

insertion occurs approximately one percent of the time, with an increased incidence in the event of multiple gestation (Varney, 1997).

A velamentous insertion can be dangerous for the fetus. Rupture of the membranes may also rupture a fetal blood vessel because their portion is flimsy since they are covered only with amnion. A ruptured vessel may cause hemorrhage and exsanguination (without blood) of the fetus.

A velamentous insertion when noticed upon inspection of the placenta after its delivery, a disaster that might have happened will have already happened. In such cases, noting the anomaly would be of diagnostic value.

3. *Vasa previa*: It is a dangerous anomaly with a high perinatal mortality if rupture occurs. Vasa previa refers to blood vessels, covered only with amnion and running between the

chorion and amnion, which present first at the cervical os by crossing it ahead of the fetal presenting part. With fetal descent and rupture of the membranes, the vessels are subject to compression and rupture with resulting exsanguinations and anoxia of fetus.

Vasa previa occurs in conjunction with a velamentous insertion of the cord. Vasa previa may also occur when there is a succenturiate placenta since the vascular connections to the succenturiate lobe are also unprotected vessels coursing between the chorion and amnion.

Vasa previa is extremely rare. However, it should be thought of as a possibility when the midwife is not sure of what is felt at the cervical os on vaginal examination. Examination should include feeling for pulsations synchronous (coinciding) with the fetal heart, in questionable presenting part.

4. Abnormal number of blood vessels in the umbilical cord has high correlation with fetal anomalies. About one-third of babies born with only one umbilical artery will have multiple and severe malformations.

5. *Short cord* (relative or absolute): An absolute short cord is one that is short in length. A relative short cord is one of average length (or, more likely, excessively long), which has become short because of looping around the body or neck of the fetus. It is short in terms of reaching from its placental insertion to the umbilicus of the newborn outside the maternal vulva as is necessary for normal delivery. A short cord may be a causative factor in failure of the fetus to descend. In such an event it might additionally cause abruptio placentae, umbilical hernia, fetal distress, rupture of the cord, shoulder dystocia, or a combination of these. Recognition of a short cord usually does not take place until there is evidence of a problem. Therefore, it should be considered as a possibility whenever descent does not take place in the presence of an adequate pelvis and good contractions. Fetal distress in such situations compounds the urgency for action.

6. *Excessively long cord*: Long cords are more common than short cords. Generally it has no significance. However, a long cord becomes looped around the fetal body or neck causing a relative short cord. It can also become knotted or prolapsed in front of the presenting part.

7. *Cord looping*: The average length of a cord is 50 to 55 cm. Cords longer than 100 centimeters will become looped. Single or multiple looping may cause a short cord with all its complications. Looping of the cord around the neck may cause fetal distress due to tightening of the cord around the neck during descend, especially if the distance is short between the loop and the placental insertion. Therefore, it is important to check for a cord around the neck as soon as the baby's head is born.

8. *Cord knotting*: False knotting occurs when the cord appears to be knotted, but instead has kinking of the blood vessel within the cord or accumulation of Wharton's jelly on the cord.

A true knot occurs when the fetus has passed through a loop in the cord and a real knot has been created. True knots are liable to occur with small fetus, long cord, large amount of amniotic fluid and multiple gestation within a single amnion.

9. Markedly decreased amount of Wharton's jelly may be seen in malnourished and post-mature newborns.

10. *Rarities*: Other conditions that may occur in the umbilical cord are hematomas, tumors, cysts and edema. Hematomas usually are the result of rupturing of the umbilical vein. Edema is common with an edematous or macerated fetus.

DEVELOPMENT OF THE FETUS (FIG. 9.11)

First Trimester

Growth and development begins with the moment of fertilization and the fusing of the female and male pronuclei from the ovum and sperm. This fusion produces what is called a zygote. At this moment a new individual is fertilization

10th to 11th day.

↓

Implantation.

7th week

Embryonic period.

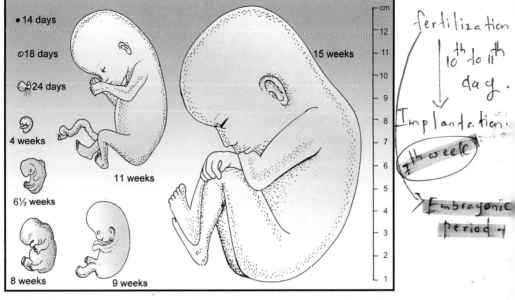

• 14 days
○18 days
○24 days
4 weeks
6½ weeks
8 weeks
9 weeks
11 weeks
15 weeks

cm: 12, 11, 10, 9, 8, 7, 6, 5, 4, 3, 2, 1

Fig. 9.11: Changes in the body size of the embryo and fetus during development in the uterus

created with his or her own unique make up, as determined by the totally new combination of chromosomes and genes. This unique combination results because the pronucleus (fully matured nucleus of a germ cell) of each gamete (sex cell, i.e. ovum and sperm) contains only half (23) of the total number (46) of chromosomes in human beings. The halving of the chromosome number is a result of gameto-genesis, the process by which mature ova and spermatozoa are developed. At the moment of fertilization, the fusion of the pronucleus of the two gametes restores the diploid (doubled) number of chromosomes. As a result of this fusion and restoration of the diploid number, the sex of the new individual is determined at the moment of fertilization. The males determine the sex as they carry two dissimilar sex chromosomes XY. Females carry two similar sex chromosomes XX. Each spermatozoa will carry either an X or a Y chromosome, whereas the ovum always carries an X chromosome. Upon fusion an XX combination normally develops into a female, while and XY combi-nation normally develops into a male. Imme-diately following fertilization, the resulting zygote begins to undergo mitotic cellular divi-sion called cleavage. Going through sequential stages, the dividing cellular mass is called a morula. With cellular reorganization and the entry of fluid, the morula becomes a blastocyst. It is the blastocyst which implants in the uterine lining. The process of implantation is completed on the tenth or eleventh day after fertilization after which the embryonic period begins.

Embryonic period is roughly the period of life from the second through seventh week after fertilization. At the time of implantation (6th week), the embryo known as a bilaminar embryo because the embryonic disk arising from the inner cell mass has two layers of cells: (1) the embryonic ectoderm and (2) the embryonic endoderm. The embryonic endoderm is the first of the three germ layers from which all tissues (e.g. bone, muscle, connective, skin), organs, and structures derive. Structures such as the fetal membranes, the umbilical cord, and part of the placenta also develop from these layers.

From the beginning of the third week, the primitive stalk, arising from the embryonic disk, is the growth center for the embryo for about two weeks after which it disintegrates. During the third week, the neural tube (rudiment of the brain and spinal cord), notocord (rudiment of the vertebrae), coelomic spaces (rudiment of body cavities), and primitive blood cells develop.

The heart starts to beat at the beginning of the fourth week. During the fourth week, a longitudinal and transverse folding of the embryonic disk takes place. The longitudinal folding, involving a head fold and a tail fold, converts the embryo from a straight form to a curved form. The transverse folding involving right and left transverse folds, folding towards the midline converts the embryo from a flat form to a cylindrical form. By the end of the fourth week, the embryo has assumed it's often called salamander look and has the rudiments of ears (otic pit), arms (arm buds), legs (leg buds) and facial and neck structures.

During the fifth week rapid development of the brain results in extensive growth of the head and makes it much larger in relation to the rest of the body. Development takes place from cephalic to caudal, with development of the legs almost a week behind development of the arms. The eyes begin development with lens, vesicles, optic cups and retinal pigment.

During the sixth week nose, mouth and palate begin to take form and the eyelids become visible. Arms and legs undergo extensive development and by the end of seventh week. Arms and legs are formed with clearly defined fingers and toes.

During the seventh week, the neck region is established, the abdomen is less protuberant and urogenital development begins. The external ears are evident although they are not fully developed. The embryo by the end of seventh week has distinctive human characteristics. The end of the seventh week also marks the end of the embryonic period. All essential internal and external structures are formed. They undergo further elaboration and growth, including the replacement of cartilage with bone cells. The embryonic period is a critical period during which any teratogen (e.g. drugs, X-rays, viruses) may either be lethal (deadly) or cause major congenital malformations.

By the end of the first trimester or the 12th gestational week calculated from the LMP, the intestines are fully into the abdomen, the external genitalia have male or female characteristics but neither are fully formed, the anus has formed and the facial characteristics of the fetus now look undeniably human. The fetus at this stage weighs about 0.5 to 1 ounce, can swallow and make respiratory movements, urinate, move specific parts of limbs and open and shut his or her mouth.

Second and Third Trimester

The second trimester which is fifteen weeks long includes weeks 13 through 27 by gestational age. The third trimester of 13 weeks includes weeks 28 through 40 by gestational age.

Fourth Month (13 to 16 Weeks)

Head growth slows while the ears move to a higher elevation on the sides of the head and the chin becomes evident. Eyes remain closed and body growth accelerates. Reflex responses and muscular activity begin. Sex is clearly distinguishable by fourteenth week. Bone development takes place by 16th week and they could be seen with roentgenography. The average crown-rump (top of head to buttocks) length is 11.5 cm (4.5 inches), and the fetus weights between 99 to 113 gm (3.5 to 4 ounces) by the end of 16th week.

Fifth Month (17 to 20 Weeks)

Rapid body growth continues; legs reach their full length and toe nails develop. The eyelids remain fused. The fetus moves freely inside the uterus. Stronger fetal movements and thinner uterine wall result in the mother's experiencing quickening around the 18th week. The fetus hiccups and the mother may feel it as a series of slight rhythmic jerks or jolts. By the end of the 5th month the vernix caseosa covers the entire body. Vernix caseosa, a mixture of sebum (secretion from the sebacious glands) and surface epithelial cells, is a thick cheesy substance that is protective to the delicate skin of the fetus. The fetal heart may be heard with a fetoscope by the end of the month. By the end of the twentieth week the average crown-rump length of the fetus is about 16.5 cm (6.5 inches) and the average weight is almost 341 gm (0.75 lbs).

Sixth Month (21 to 24 Weeks)

Hair growth is prominent. The fetus is completely covered with lanugo, a fine downy (soft) hair. Eyebrows, eyelashes, and head hair are present. The head remains large compared to the rest of the body. The skin is wrinkled, translucent (imperfectly transparent) and red, giving an aged appearance to the fetus. Buds for the permanent teeth are present. The fetus being small has room in the uterus to somersault (turn heels over head) and can make motions of crying and sucking. The hands make fists. Brown fat, which is a source of energy, heat production and heat regulation in the newborn forms. The average crown-rump length of the fetus reaches just over 20 cm (8 inches) and the weight is approximately 568 gm (1.25 lbs).

Seventh Month (25 to 28 Weeks)

The fetus continues to look old and wrinkled though a little fat storage begins. By the end of the month, the body becomes better proportioned because of weight gain. The hair on the baby's head is longer, the sucking reflex is stronger, the eyes begin to open and shut, and the fingernails are present. The average crown-rump length is approximately 22.5 cm (9 inches) and the weight is about 1023 gm (2.25 lbs) by the end of the 28th week. Survival may be expected if born.

Eighth Month (29 to 32 Weeks)

Subcutaneous fat begins to smooth out some of the wrinkles and the body begins to store fat and iron. Thick vernix caseosa covers the entire fetus. The hair on the head continues to grow and the lanugo is plentiful except on the face from where it has now disappeared. Fingernails reach the ends of the fingers; toenails are present but do not reach the ends of the toes. The fetus has control of rhythmic breathing and body temperature. The eyes are open. The average crown-rump length is about 27.5 cm (11 inches) and weight is approximately 1.7 kg (3.75 lbs).

Ninth Month (33 to 36 Weeks)

By the end of ninth month the skin is smooth and without wrinkles as the subcutaneous fat becomes thicker from additional deposits. The baby is rounder, the hair is larger, the toenails have reached the ends of the toes, and the left testicle has usually descended into the scrotum and plantar creases are visible. The average crown-rump length is a little over 31 cm (12.5 inches) and the weight is approximately 2.5 kg (5.5 lbs) in the thirty-six weeks.

37 to 40 Weeks

The fetus receives the finishing touches during this period. Full growth and development are attained. The fetus is now well rounded with a prominent chest and protuberant mammary glands in both sexes. Both testes are in the scrotum. The lanugo has disappeared from most of the body. The nails project beyond the tips of both fingers and toes. The skull is firm. The skin varies in color from white to pink to bluish-pink regardless of race because the melanin that colors the skin is produced only after exposure to light. The crown-rump length now averages 31 cm (14 inches). The weight depends on a number of variables but has a general average of 3.2 kg (7 lbs). Term is reached and birth is due.

An understanding of fetal development is essential for the midwife in order to estimate the approximate age of a baby born before term. It is also helpful to know the outline of organogenesis in order to appreciate the ways in which developmental abnormalities arise. When making reference to the age at which various events happen, it is important for the midwife to distinguish between the gestational age (the time since the first day of last menstrual period) and the conceptional age (the interval since fertilization). In obstetric practice, gestional age is commonly used.

BIBLIOGRAPHY

1. Bennett RV, Linda KB. Myles Textbook for Midwives, 13th edn. Edinburgh: Churchill Livingstone; 1999.
2. Dutta DC. Textbook of obstetrics, 5th edn. Calcutta: New Central Book Agency; 2001.
3. Johnson M, Evereitt B. Essential Reproduction, 4th edn. Oxford: Blackwell Science; 1995.
4. Moore KL. Before we are Born, 5th edn. London: Sounders; 1998.
5. Varney Helen. Nurse-Midwifery, 2nd edn. Boston: Jones and Barlett Publishers; 1999.

10

Fetal Organs and Fetal Circulation

[handwritten: 3rd 6th month RBC Production. After 6th month → (red bone marrow/spleen)]

Learning Objectives

Upon completing this chapter, the learner will be able to:

❖ Describe the fetal development and fetal circulation
❖ Describe the features of fetal skull, its regions, diameters and the mechanism of moulding.

FETAL ORGANS

Blood

The origin of fetal blood is from the inner cell mass. The fetus will inherit the genes, which determine its blood group from both its parents. The ABO group and Rhesus factor may therefore be the same or different from those of its mother.

The fetal hemoglobin termed as HbF is of a different type from adult hemoglobin. It has a much greater affinity for oxygen and is found in greater concentration (18-20 g/dl) at term. Towards the end of pregnancy the fetus begins to make adult-type hemoglobin (HbA). *In utero* the red blood cells have a shorter lifespan. This is about 90 days by the time the baby is born.

The Urinary Tract

The kidneys begin to function and fetus begins to pass urine from tenth week. The superior vesical arteries arise from the hypogastric arteries, which lead to the umbilical arteries. If a single umbilical artery is found instead of the normal two, abnormalities of the renal tract are suspected.

[handwritten: Urine production start at 10th week.]

The Liver

The fetal liver is comparatively large in size, occupying much of the abdominal cavity, especially in the early months. From the third to the sixth month, the liver is responsible for the formation of red blood cells, after which they are produced in the red bone marrow and the spleen.

The Alimentary Tract

[handwritten: non functional, 2. Amniotic fluid, Swallowing begins after 12 week]

The digestive tract is nonfunctional before birth. It forms from the yolk sac as a straight tube first, later growing out into the base of the umbilical cord and finally rotating back into the abdomen. Sucking and swallowing of amniotic fluid begins about 12 weeks after conception. Most digestive juices are present before birth and they act on the swallowed substances (shed skin cells and other debris) and discarded intestinal cells to form meconium. This is normally retained in the gut until after birth when it is passed as the first stool of the newborn.

The Lungs

The lungs originate from a bud growing out of the pharynx, which divides and subdivides repeatedly to form the bronchial tree. The process continues until about eight years of age when the full number of bronchioles and alveoli will have developed. The chances of survival are reduced for babies born before 24th week of gestation because of the immaturity of lungs. At this stage the alveolar surface is limited, the capillary system is immature and surfactant is insufficient. Surfactant is a lipoprotein, which reduces the surface tension in the alveoli and assists gaseous exchange. At term the lungs contain about 100 ml of lung fluid. About one-third of this is expelled during delivery and the rest is absorbed and carried away by the lymphatics and blood vessels as air takes its place.

There is some movement of the thorax from the third month of fetal life and more definite diaphragmatic movements from the sixth month.

The Central Nervous System

This is derived from the ectoderm. It folds inwards to form the neural tube, which is then covered over by skin. This process is occasionally incomplete, leading to open neural tube defects.

The fetus is able to perceive strong light and to hear external sounds. Periods of wakefulness and sleep occur.

The Skin

The fetus is covered with a white, creamy substance called *vernix caseosa* from 18th week onwards. At 20th week the fetus will be covered with a fine downy hair called *lanugo* and at the same time the head hair and eyebrows begin to form.

Fingernails develop from about 10th week and toenails from about 18th week.

FETAL CIRCULATION (FIG. 10.1)

Fetal circulation differs from adult circulation in several ways and is designed to ensure a high oxygen blood supply to the brain and myocardium.

Characteristics

a. Placenta is the source of oxygen for the fetus.
b. Fetal lungs receive less than 1 percent of the blood volume; lungs do not exchange gas.
c. Right atrium of fetal heart is the chamber with the highest oxygen concentration.

Structures

Fetal circulation contains five unique structures:

a. *Umbilical vein*: Carries oxygen and nutrients to the fetus.

b. *Two umbilical arteries*: Carry deoxygenated blood and waste products from the fetus.
c. *Ductus venosus (from a vein to a vein)*: Shunts blood from the umbilical vein to the interior vena cava, bypassing the liver and organs of digestion.
d. *Foramen ovale (oval opening)*: Shunts blood from the right atrium to the left atrium, bypassing the lungs.
e. *Ductus arteriosus (from an artery to an artery)*: Shunts blood from the pulmonary artery to the aorta, bypassing the lungs.

Pattern of Altered Blood Flow

Blood is carried from the placenta through the umbilical vein and enters the inferior vena cava through the ductus venosus. This permits most of the highly oxygenated blood to go directly into the right atrium, bypassing the liver. This right atrial blood flows directly into the left atrium through the foramen ovale, an opening between the right and left atria. From the left atrium, blood flows into the left ventricle and aorta and through the subclavian arteries, to the cerebral and coronary arteries resulting in the brain and heart receiving the most highly oxygenated blood. Deoxygenated blood returns from the head and arms through the superior vena cava, enters the right atrium and passes into the right ventricle.

Blood from the right ventricle flows into the pulmonary artery, but because fetal lungs are collapsed, the pressure in the pulmonary artery is very high. Because pulmonary resistance is high, most of the blood passes into the distal aorta through the ductus arteriosus, which connects the pulmonary artery and the aorta distal to the origin of the subclavian arteries. From the aorta, blood flows to the rest of the body.

Normal Circulatory Changes at Birth

When the umbilical cord is clamped or severed, the blood supply from the placenta is cut off and oxygenation must then take place in the newborn's lungs. As the lungs expand with air, the pulmonary artery pressure decreases and circulation to lungs increases. This leads to the following structural changes to occur in the vascular system.

Fig. 10.1: Fetal circulation (*For color version see Plate 1*)

Closure of the Umbilical Arteries

Functional closure is almost instantaneous. Actual obliteration takes place in about 2 to 3 months. The distal parts form the *lateral umbilical ligaments*.

Closure of the Ductus Arteriosus

The increased pulmonary blood flow increases arterial oxygen, causing vasoconstriction of ductus arteriosus within hours of birth. Functional closure occurs soon after the establishment of pulmonary respiration and anatomical closure occurs when there is growth of fibrous tissue in the lumen by 1 to 3 months. The ductus arteriosus then becomes *ligamentum arteriosum*.

Closure of the Umbilical Vein

Obliteration of the umbilical vein occurs a little later than the arteries, allowing a little extra volume of blood (80–100 ml) to be received by the baby from the placenta. After obliteration, the umbilical vein forms the *ligamentum teres*.

Closure of the Ductus Venosus

When the umbilical cord is severed, blood flow through the ductus venosus decreases and eventually ceases. It constricts in 3 to 7 days and eventually becomes *ligamentum venosum*.

Closure of Foramen Ovale

Expansion of pulmonary artery and increased pulmonary blood flow increases the left ventricular and left atrial pressure. Functional close of this valve-like opening occurs when the pressure in the left atrium exceeds pressure in the right. The anatomical obliteration occurs in about 12 months with deposits of fibrin and becomes *fossa ovalis*.

BIBLIOGRAPHY

1. Bennett RV, Linda KB. Myles Textbook for Midwives, 13th edn. Edinburgh: Churchill Livingstone; 1999.
2. Dutta DC. Textbook of Obstetrics (5th Edn). Calcutta: New Central Book Company; 2001.
3. Fox HA. A contemporary view of the human placenta, Midwifery; 1991:7(1).
4. Llewellyn Jones D. Fundamental of Obstetrics and Gynecology, 5th edn. London: Faber;1990:1.
5. Stein MA, Judith CM. NCLEX-RN Review, 4th edn. New York: Delmar Thomson Learning; 2000.
6. Varney Helen. Nurse Midwifery, 2nd edn. Boston: Jones and Barlett Publishers; 1999.

11

The Fetal Skull

Learning Objectives

Upon completing this chapter, the learner will be able to:

❖ Identify the bones of the vault of the fetal skull
❖ List and explain the sutures of the fetal skull
❖ Identify and describe the regions and diameters of the fetal skull in the mechanism of moulding
❖ Explain the mechanism of moulding.

The fetal skull is oval shaped. At term, it is larger in proportion to the fetal body and in comparison with the true pelvis. The baby's head is wider than its shoulders and one quarter of its length.

The bones of the fetal head originate in two different ways. The face is laid down in cartilage and is almost completely ossified at birth, the bones being fused together and firm. The bones of the vault are laid down in membrane and are much flatter and pliable. They ossify from the center onwards and this process is incomplete at birth leaving small gaps, which form the sutures and fontanelles. The ossification center on each bone appears as a protuberance.

Bones of the Vault

There are five main bones in the vault of the skull.

Two Frontal Bones

The two frontal bones form the forehead or sinciput. At the center of each is a frontal eminence. The frontal bones fuse into a single bone by 8 years of age.

Two Parietal Bones

The two parietal bones lie on either side of the skull. The ossification center of each is called the parietal eminence.

Occipital Bone

The occipital bone lies at the back of the head and forms the region of the occiput. Part of it contributes to the base of the skull as it contains foramen magnum, which protects the spinal cord as it leaves the skull. At the center is the occipital protuberance.

Sutures

Sutures are cranial joints and are formed where two bones adjoin. They are composed of fibrous tissue and allow mobility between the cranial bones. There are four sutures in the vault, which are of obstetrical significance (Fig. 11.1).
1. *Frontal suture:* It is between the two frontal bones.
2. *Sagittal suture:* It is between the two parietal bones.
3. *Coronal suture:* There are two coronal sutures, each between the frontal and parietal bones on either side of the head.
4. *Lambdoidal suture:* There are two lambdoidal sutures, each between the parietal bones and the upper margin of the occipital bone on either side of the head. It is shaped like the Greek letter lambda (λ).

Fontanelles

These are areas of fibrous tissue membrane found at the angles of the parietal bones where ossification is incomplete at birth (Fig. 11.1).

Frontal eminence, Parietal eminence, Occipital protuberance, Mentum, Bregma, Sinciput, Glabella → Landmarks of the

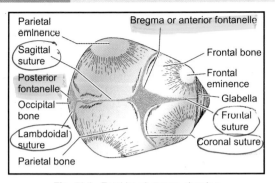

Fig. 11.1: Fetal head at term showing fontanelles and sutures

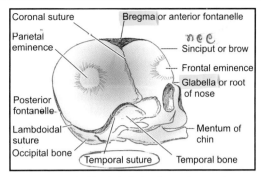

Fig. 11.2: Fetal skull showing regions and landmarks of obstetrical importance

Anterior Fontanelle or Bregma

The anterior fontanelle or bregma is formed by the meeting of the frontal, sagittal and two coronal sutures. This is roughly in the shape of a diamond (◊) and four sutures can be felt leading from the anterior fontanelle in four different directions, as indicated by the points on the diamond. It measures 3 to 4 cm long and 1.5 to 2 cm wide and normally closes by the time the child is 18-month-old. Pulsations of cerebral vessels can be felt through it.

Posterior Fontanelle

The posterior fontanelle is formed by the meeting of the sagittal and the two lambdoidal sutures. This is roughly in the shape of a triangle (Δ) and three sutures can be felt leading from the posterior fontanelle in three different directions as indicated by the points of the triangle. It is small and normally closes by 6 weeks of age.

Regions of the Fetal Skull (Fig. 11.2)

1. *Vertex* is bounded by the anterior fontanelle, the two parietal eminences and the posterior fontanelle. Of the 96 percent of babies born head first, 95 percent present by the vertex.
2. *Sinciput* or brow extends from the anterior fontanelle and the coronal suture to the orbital ridges.
3. *Face* extends from the orbital ridges and the roof of the nose to the junction of the chin and the neck. The point between the eyebrows is known as the *glabella*. The chin is termed mentum and is an important landmark.

4. *Occiput* lies between the foramen magnum and the posterior fontanelle. The part below the occipital protuberance is known as the suboccipital region.

Landmarks of the Skull

The skull is considered as divided into three parts—vault, face and base. The vault is the large, dome-shaped part above the imaginary line, drawn between the orbital ridges and the nape of the neck. In the vault, the bones are relatively thin and pliable, which allows the skull to alter slightly in shape during birth. The face is composed of 14 small bones, which are also firmly united and noncompressible. The facial part forms 1/3rd of the cranium compared to 1/2 in an adult. The base is comprised of bones, which are firmly united to protect the vital centers in the medulla (Fig. 11.3).

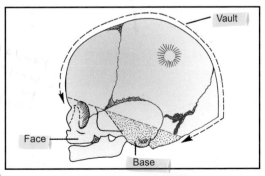

Fig. 11.3: Regions of the skull showing the vault, face and base

The fetal head is large in comparison with the true pelvis; therefore some adaptation between skull and pelvis must take place during labor. The head is the most difficult part to deliver, whether it comes first or last. The knowledge of the landmarks and measurements of the skull enables the midwife to recognize normal presentations and positions, and to facilitate delivery with the least possible trauma to mother and baby. Where malpresentation or disproportion exists, she will be able to identify it and alert the physician.

Diameters of the Fetal Skull (Fig. 11.4)

1. *Biparietal diameter (9.5 cm)*: It lies between the two parietal eminences.
2. *Bitemporal diameter (8.5 cm)*: It lies between the furthest points of the coronal suture.
3. *Suboccipitobregmatic (9.5 cm)*: From below the occipital protuberance to the center of the anterior fontanelle or bregma.

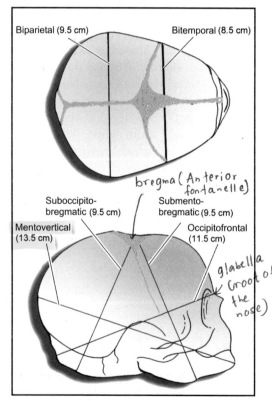

Fig. 11.4: Diameters of the fetal skull

4. *Suboccipitofrontal (10 cm)*: From below the occipital protuberance to the center of the frontal suture.
5. *Occipitofrontal (11.5 cm)*: From the occipital protuberance to the glabella.
6. *Mentovertical (13.5 cm)*: From the point of the chin to the highest point on the vertex.
7. *Submentovertical (11.5 cm)*: From the point where the chin joins the neck to the highest point on the vertex.
8. *Submentobregmatic (9.5 cm)*: From the point where the chin joins the neck to the center of the bregma.

Knowledge of the measurements of the skull is important for the midwife, because some diameters are more favorable for easy passage through the pelvic canal.

Attitude of the Fetal Head

A term used to describe the degree of flexion or extension of the head on the neck. The attitude of the head determines which diameters will present in labor.

Presenting Diameters

The presenting diameters are those, which are at right angles to the curve of Carus. Presenting diameters are always two—a longitudinal diameter and transverse diameter. The diameters presenting in cephalic or head presentations are the following (Figs 11.5A to E).

Vertex Presentation

When the head is well flexed, the suboccipitobregmatic diameter and the biparietal diameter present. As those two diameters are more or less the same length (9.5 cm), the presenting area is round and most favorable for dilating the cervix. The diameter distending the vaginal orifice will be suboccipitofrontal 10 cm. When the head is erect and not flexed, the presenting diameters are the occipitofrontal (11.5 cm) and the biparietal (9.5 cm). This situation often arises when the occiput is in a posterior position. The diameter distending the vaginal orifice will be occipitofrontal (11.5 cm).

Brow Presentation

When the head is partially extended, the mentovertical diameter (13.5 cm) and the bitemporal diameter (8.5 cm) present. With these diameters vaginal delivery is unlikely.

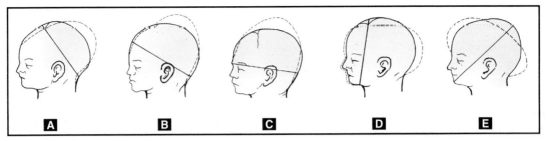

Figs 11.5A to E: Diagrams illustrating moulding when the head presents in varying degrees of flexion; (A) Vertex presentation, head well flexed; (B) Vertex presentation, head partially flexed; (C) Vertex presentation, head deflexed; (D) Face presentation; (E) Brow presentation

Face Presentation

When the head is completely extended, the presenting diameters are the submento-bregmatic (9.5 cm) and the bitemporal (8.5 cm). The submentovertical diameter (11.5 cm) will distend the vaginal orifice.

Presenting diameters of the fetal trunk are the following:

1. *Bisacromial diameter (12 cm)*: This is the distance between the acromion processes on the two shoulder blades and is the dimension that needs to pass through the pelvis for the shoulders to be born.
2. *Bitrochanteric diameter (10 cm)*: This is the distance between the greater trochanters of the femurs and is the presenting diameter in breech presentation.

Moulding

This is the term applied to the change in shape of the fetal head that takes place during its passage through the birth canal. Alteration in shape is possible because the bones of the vault allow a slight degree of bending and the skull bones are able to override at the sutures (Fig. 11.6).

In a normal vertex presentation with the fetal head in a fully flexed attitude the suboccipitobregmatic and the biparietal diameters will be reduced as much as 1.25 cm and the mentovertical will be lengthened (Fig. 11.7). The skull of the preterm infant, being softer and having wider sutures, may mould excessively. The skull of the postmature infant does not mould well and its greater hardness tends to make labor more difficult. Moulding is a protective mechanism and prevents the fetal

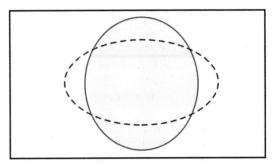

Fig. 11.6: Illustration of the principle of moulding of fetal skull

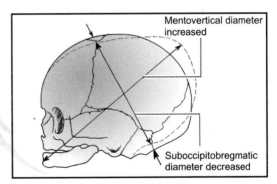

Fig. 11.7: Moulding in a normal vertex presentation

brain from being compressed as long as it is not too excessive or too rapid.

BIBLIOGRAPHY

1. Barnet CWF. Anatomy and Physiology of Obstetrics, 6th edn. London: Faber and Faber; 1979.
2. Bennett RV, Linda KB. Myles Textbook for Midwives, 13th edn. Edinburgh: Churchill Livingstone; 1999.
3. Dutta DC. Textbook of Obstetrics, 5th edn. Calcutta: New Central Book Company; 2001.
4. Wolpert L. The Triumph of the Embryo, Oxford: Oxford Universuty Press; 1991.

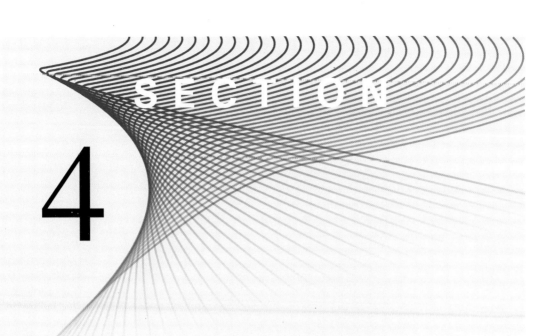

4

Normal Pregnancy

12

Physiological Changes due to Pregnancy

Physiological changes that take place in a mother's body during pregnancy are associated with and caused by the effects of specific hormones (Case and Waterhouse, 1994). These changes enable her to nurture the fetus, prepare her body for labor and develop her breasts for production of milk during the puerperium.

CHANGES IN THE REPRODUCTIVE SYSTEM

The changes in pregnancy that take place in the reproductive system are a temporary adaptation to meet the needs and demands of the fetus.

The Body of Uterus

After conception the uterus develops to provide a nutritive and protective environment in which the fetus will develop and grow (Nilsson, 1990).

Changes in Uterine Shape

The uterus changes to a globular shape to accommodate the growing fetus, increasing amounts of liquor and the placental tissue.

The lower part of the uterus, consisting of the isthmus, softens and elongates to three times its original length during the first trimester, giving the appearance of a stalk below the globular upper segment. This is the beginning of the upper and lower segments of the uterus.

By 12th week of pregnancy, the uterus rises out of pelvis and becomes upright. It is no longer anteverted and outflexed. It is about the size of a grape fruit and may be palpated abdominally above the symphysis pubis (Bennett and Brown, 1999).

By 16th week, the conceptus has grown enough to put pressure on the isthmus, causing it to open out so that the uterus become more globular in shape.

By 20th week of pregnancy, the uterus becomes spherical in shape and has a thicker, more rounded fundus. As the uterus continues to rise in the abdomen, the uterine tubes, being restricted by attachments to the broad ligaments, become progressively more vertical. At 20th week, the fundus of the uterus may be palpated at or just below the umbilicus.

By 30th week, the lower uterine segment can be identified. It is the portion of the uterus above the internal os of the cervix. The fundus can be palpated midway between the umbilicus and the xiphisternum (Miller and Hanretty, 1997).

The uterus reaches the level of the xiphisternum by 38th week. A reduction in fundal height, known as *lightening*, may occur at the end of pregnancy when the fetus sinks into the lower pole of the uterus. This is due to softening of the tissues of the pelvic floor and further formation of the lower uterine segment. In the primigravida, this also encourages the beginning of a gradual descend of the fetus into the pelvis and the head becomes engaged. In the multiparous women, descend often does not occur until labor begins (Murray, 1999).

When the formation of the lower uterine segment is complete in labor it measures approximately one-third of the body of the uterus.

Decidua

The decidua is the name given to the endometrium during pregnancy. Estrogen and progesterone, produced by the corpus luteum, causes the decidua to become thicker, richer and more vascular at the fundus and in the upper body of the uterus, which are the usual sites of implantation. The decidua provides a glycogen rich environment for the blastocyst until the placenta is formed. Once the placenta is formed, it is able to produce its own hormones. After 13th to 17th week of pregnancy the corpus luteum atrophies and becomes the corpus albicans (Findlay, 1984).

Myometrium

The myometrium is made up of smooth muscle fibers, held together by connective tissue. The muscle fibers grow up to 15 to 20 times their non-pregnant length.

The hypertrophy (increase in size) and hyperplasia (increase in number) of the uterine muscle is due to the effects of estrogen and progesterone. The uterus continues to grow in this way for the first three months, after which the growth is related to distention by the growing fetus (Llewellyn Jones, 1994). At term the uterus measures 30 × 23 × 20 cm and weights 750 to 1000 gm. Individual muscle cell grows 17 to 40 times (Verrals, 1993). The walls of the myometrium becomes thicker in the first few months of pregnancy, and as gestation advances, the walls become thinner owing to the gross enlargement of the uterus, being only 1.5 cm thick or less at term (Cunningham et al, 1989).

Throughout most of the pregnancy, the uterus generates small waves of irregular and usually painless contractility known as Braxton Hicks contractions. These are infrequent and nonrhythmic and facilitate the formation of the lower uterine segment (McFadyen, 1995). They usually increase in frequency and intensity from about 36th week of pregnancy, causing some discomfort. These prelabor contractions are associated with 'ripening' of the cervix and eventually become the contractions of labor as the effects of estrogen supersede those of progesterone (progesterone normally suppresses myometrial activity). During pregnancy, the muscle layers become more differentiated and organized for their part in expelling the fetus.

Muscle Layers (Fig. 12.1)

The outer longitudiual layer of muscle fibers is thin. The middle layer of spiral myometrial fibers is thick. During labor the synchronous contraction and retraction of these fibers cause them to become heaped up in the upper uterine segment making it thicker and shorter in length while the lower uterine segment becomes thinner and more stretched (Chamberlain et al, 1991).

The thickness of the upper uterine segment acts as a piston to force the fetus into the receptive, passive lower uterine segment. Contraction of these muscle fibers is necessary to entrap and enmesh bleeding vessels and ligate them after the placenta is delivered.

The inner circular layer is thin and forms sphinters around the openings of the uterine tubes at the cornua, and around the lower uterine segment and cervix (McFadyen, 1995). During labor, the stretching and pulling up of the circular layer of muscles around the cervix into the lower uterine segment causes the cervix to become effaced and dilated (Chamberlain et al, 1991).

Blood Supply

The uterine blood vessels increase in diameter and new vessels develop under the influence of estrogen. The blood supply to the uterus through the uterine and ovarian arteries increases to about 750 ml per minute at term to keep pace with its growth and also to meet the needs of the functioning placenta (Bissonette, 1991).

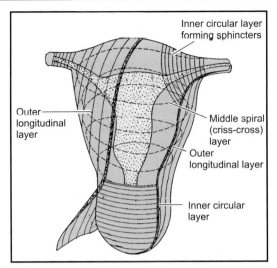

Fig. 12.1: Muscle layers of the uterus in pregnancy

The Fallopian Tubes

The fallopian tubes on either side are more stretched out in pregnancy and is much more vascular. The uterine end of the tube is usually closed and the fimbriated end remains open.

The Cervix

The cervix remains tightly closed during pregnancy, providing protection to the fetus and resistance to pressure from above when the woman is in standing position. It acts as an effective barrier against infection during pregnancy. The mucus secreted by the endo-cervical cells become thicker and more viscous during pregnancy. The thickened mucus forms a cervical plug called the *operculum*, which provides protection from ascending infection (McFadyen, 1995).

Cervical vascularity increases during pregnancy and if viewed through a speculum, it looks bluish in color. The cervix remains 2.5 cm long throughout pregnancy. In late pregnancy softening, or ripening of the cervix occurs making it more distensible. The muscles of the fundus enhance tension in the outer longitudinal layer of muscles of the cervix contributing to the process of effacement. Effacement or taking up of the cervix normally occurs in the primigravida during the last two weeks of pregnancy but does not usually take place in the multigravida until labor begins (Verralls, 1993).

The Vagina

Estrogen causes changes in the muscle layer and epithelium of the vagina. The muscle layer hypertrophies and the capacity of the vagina increases (McFadyen, 1995). Changes in the surrounding connective tissue make it more elastic. These changes enable the vagina to dilate during the second stage of labor. The epithelium becomes thicker with marked desquamation (peeling off) of the superficial cells, which increases the amount of normal vaginal white discharge, known as *leukorrhea* (Beischer et al, 1997).

The epithelial cells have high glycogen content. These cells interact with Doderlein's bacillus, which is normally found in vagina and produce a more acid environment (McFadyen, 1995). The acid environment provides an extra degree of protection against some organisms and an increasing susceptibility to others, such as *Candida albicans* (Symmonds, 1992).

The vagina becomes more vascular and appears violet in color, probably due to increased blood supply (Cunningham et al, 1989).

CHANGES IN THE CARDIOVASCULAR SYSTEM

In the cardiovascular system, profound changes take place during pregnancy. For the care of women with normal pregnancies as well as for the management of women with pre-existing cardiovascular diseases, an understanding of these changes is important.

The Heart

The heart muscle, particularly the left ventricle, hypertrophies leading to enlargement of the heart. The growing uterus pushes the heart upwards and to the left. During pregnancy the heart rate and stroke volume (the amount of blood pumped by the heart with each beat) increases. This is due to the increased blood volume and increased oxygen requirements of the maternal tissues and the growing fetus (Symmonds, 1992).

The cardiac output (the rate at which blood is pumped by the heart expressed as liters per minute) increases markedly by the end of the first trimester. In the third trimester, a rise, fall or no change at all has been shown to occur, depending on individual variations (Van Oppen et al, 1996).

Although the cardiac output is increased in pregnancy, the blood pressure does not rise because of the reduction in peripheral resistance. The capacity of veins and venules increases. Arterial walls relax and dilate due to the effect of progesterone. The increased production of vasodilator prostaglandin also contributes to this (Cunningham et al, 1989).

During the midtrimester, changes in blood pressure may occur causing fainting. In later pregnancy, hypotension may occur in 10 percent of women in unsupported supine position. This is termed as the supine hypotensive syndrome. The pressure of the gravid uterus compresses the vena cava, reducing the venous return. Cardiac output is reduced by 25 to 30 percent and the blood pressure may fall by 10 to 15 percent, which produces the feelings of dizziness, nausea and even fainting (Cruikshank and Hays, 1991).

Poor venous return in late pregnancy along with increased distensibility and pressure in the veins of the legs, vulva, rectum and pelvis can lead to edema in the lower leg, varicose veins and hemorrhoids (Case and Waterhouse, 1994).

Blood flow increases to the uterus, kidneys, breasts and skin during pregnancy. Much of the increased cardiac output goes to the utero-placental circulation, which is about 750 ml per minute at term (Bissonette, 1991).

Regulation of uterine blood flow is of critical importance to the welfare of the fetus. Hemorrhage, uterine contractions and lying in the supine position in late pregnancy can all reduce uterine blood flow. Chronic impairment can lead to intrauterine growth retardation and ultimately fetal death. Renal blood flow increases during pregnancy. Blood flow to the capilla-

ries of the skin and mucous membranes, and in particular to hands and feet increases. The associated peripheral vasodilatation causes the women to sweat profusely at times. Some may suffer nasal congestion.

There is increased blood flow to the breasts throughout pregnancy and dilated veins may be seen on the surface of the breasts along with enlargement and tingling from early pregnancy (Llewellyn-Jones, 1994).

The Blood Volume

The increase in blood volume in pregnancy varies according to the size of the woman, the number of pregnancies she has had, her parity and whether the pregnancy is singleton or multiple. The increase begins at about 10th week gestation and progresses up to 30th to 34th week of gestation. The increase may be as much as 100 percent in some women. A higher circulating volume is required for the following functions:

❖ To provide extra blood flow for placental circulation
❖ To supply the extra metabolic needs of the fetus
❖ To provide extra perfusion of kidneys and other organs
❖ To counterbalance the effects of increased arterial and venous capacity
❖ To compensate for blood loss at delivery (Cruikshank and Hays, 1991).

There is increase in plasma volume, which reduces the viscosity of the blood and improves capillary blood flow.

The total volume of red cells in the circulation (red cell mass) increases as a result of increased production in response to the extra oxygen requirements of maternal and placental tissue. There is constant increase throughout the pregnancy from about tenth week resulting in a total increase of 18 to 25 percent (Cruikshank and Hays, 1991).

As the increase in plasma volume is much greater than that of the red cell mass, hemodilution occurs. It is characterized by a lowered red cell count and hemoglobin level (in spite of the rise in total circulating hemoglobin).

The hematocrit concentration or packed cell volume falls from an average non-pregnant figure of 35 percent to 29 percent at around 30th week. The effect is referred to as *physiological anemia*.

Plasma Protein

During the first 20 weeks of pregnancy, the plasma protein concentration reduces as a result of the increased plasma volume. This leads to lowered osmotic pressure, contributing to edema of the lower limbs seen in late pregnancy (Case and Waterhouse, 1994). In the absence of disease, moderate edema is seen as physiological.

Iron Metabolism

Iron requirement increases significantly in the last trimester, during which time iron absorption from the gut is enhanced. The purpose of iron supplementation in pregnancy is to prevent iron deficiency in the mother, not to raise the hemoglobin.

Clotting Factors

The clotting and fibrinolytic systems undergo major changes during pregnancy. Plasma fibrinogen (factor 1) increases from the third month of pregnancy progressively until term. Prothrombin (factor 2) increases only slightly. Factors 7, 8, 9 and 10 increase leading to change in coagulation time from 12 to 8 minutes (Cunningham et al, 1989).

The capacity for clotting is thus increased, in preparation for the prevention of hemorrhage at placental separation. However, there is a higher risk of thrombosis, embolism.

White Blood Cells

The neutrophils increase in pregnancy, which enhances the blood's phagocytic and bactericidal properties. In the second and third trimester the action of the polymorphonuclear leukocytes may be depressed, perhaps accounting for the increased susceptibility of pregnant women to infection (Moore, 1994). The lymphocyte and monocyte numbers remain the same throughout pregnancy.

Immunity

Immune response is reduced in pregnancy. Levels of immunoglobulins IgA, IgG and IgM decrease steadily from the 10th week to the 30th week and then remain at these levels until term resulting in reduced immune response (Llewellyn-Jones,1994). Antibody titers against viruses, such as measles, influenza virus A and herpes simplex, are reduced in proportion to the hemodilution effect, therefore viral resistance is unchanged (Cunningham et al, 1989).

CHANGES IN THE RESPIRATORY SYSTEM

The shape of the chest changes and the circumference increases in pregnancy by 6 cm. As the uterus enlarges the diaphragm is elevated as much as 4 cm, and the rib cage is displaced upwards. The lower ribs flare out and may not always fully recover their original position after pregnancy (de Swiet, 1991).

There is a progressive increase in oxygen consumption, which is caused by the increased metabolic needs of the mother and fetus.

The mucosa of the respiratory tract becomes hyperemic and edematous, with hypersecretion of mucus, which can lead to stuffiness and epistaxis. As a result women may suffer chronic cold during pregnancy. Long-term use of nasal decongestant sprays should be avoided because of their effect on the mucosa (Cruikshank and Hays, 1991).

Progesterone causes an increase in the sensitivity of the respiratory center to stimulation by carbon dioxide. This causes a little hyperventilation and lowering of blood PCO_2. The alveolar CO_2 concentrations are lower than that in the non-pregnant woman, that causes the maternal CO_2 tension to be lower, leading to a respiratory alkalosis. The mild alkalemia (arterial pH 7.44) facilitates oxygen release to the fetus (Cunningham et al, 1989). The maternal PCO_2 is lower (5 kPa-4 kPa) than that in the fetus (6 kPa). This facilitates transfer of CO_2 from the fetus to the mother (Case and Waterhouse, 1994).

Hyperventilation (over breathing) can lead to discomfort, dyspnea and dizziness. Women may complain of shortness of breath, when their need to breathe become a conscious one.

The stress on respiratory system, imposed by pregnancy, is very little in comparison with the cardiovascular system. The changes however, can cause some discomfort or inconvenience to the pregnant woman and diseases of the respiratory tract may be more serious during pregnancy.

CHANGES IN THE URINARY SYSTEM

Renal blood flow increases by as much as 70 to 80 percent by the second trimester (Davison and Dunlop, 1995). After 30 weeks it decreases slowly although it is still above nonpregnant levels at term. The kidneys enlarge and glomerular filtration increases. The increase is maintained throughout the second trimester but decreases significantly during the last weeks of pregnancy.

Plasma levels of urea, uric acid and creatinine fall in pregnancy although uric acid level return to nonpregnant level in late pregnancy (Cunningham et al, 1989).

Protein and amino acids are less efficiently reabsorbed and as a result found in much greater amounts in the urine of pregnant women. Proteinuria does not usually occur in normal pregnancy.

Glucose excretion increases as a result of increased glomerular filtration rate of glucose. Glycosuria is therefore, quite common in pregnancy and is not usually related to a high blood glucose level. Glycosuria can be a cause of urinary tract infection. It should, however, be monitored to exclude diabetes mellitus.

Urinary output is diminished because of an enhanced tubular reabsorption of water. An accompanying increase in the reabsorption of sodium is seen, which is possibly due to hormonal effect.

The urine of pregnant women is more alkaline due to the alkalemia of pregnancy. In early pregnancy, increased production of urine causes frequency of micturition. In later pregnancy, frequency is caused by pressure of the growing uterus on the bladder.

The ureters become relaxed, and are dilated, elongated and curved above the brim of the pelvis due to the influence of progesterone. This, along with compression of the ureters against the pelvic brim, can result in stasis of urine in the ureters leading to bacteriuria and infection of the urinary tract. Hydroureter and hydronephrosis may be associated with stasis of urine.

The muscle of the bladder is relaxed owing to raised levels of progesterone. Bladder vascularity increases and bladder capacity is reduced. Towards the end of pregnancy, as the head engages, the entire bladder may be displaced upwards.

CHANGES IN THE GASTROINTESTINAL SYSTEM

In the mouth, the gums become edematous, soft and spongy which can bleed when mildly traumatized as with a toothbrush. Increased salivation (ptyalism) is a common complaint in pregnancy. This problem seems to be associated with nausea, which prevents women from swallowing their saliva.

Around 4 to 8 weeks, most women (about 70%) start complaining of nausea and vomiting, which may continue until about 14 to16 weeks. Relaxation of the smooth muscles of the stomach, and hypomotility may also contribute to this problem. It can be quite distressing and sometimes causing weight loss in early pregnancy. It occasionally causes nutritional or electrolyte imbalance.

Occasionally vomiting may become excessive. Excessive vomiting is common in multiple pregnancy or hydatidiform mole, and hence excessive hormone levels are thought to be the cause for it.

In earlier period of pregnancy, a change in the sense of taste can occur. It can be metallic taste in the mouth, distaste for something usually enjoyed or craving for a food usually not eaten. Craving for bizarre substances such as coal, wall plaster, mothball, mud, etc. may be seen occasionally. This is termed as pica.

Many women notice an increase in thirst during pregnancy. This may be due to the fall in plasma osmolarity and rising levels of prolactin. An increase in appetite is also experienced by most of women, which may be due to the fall in plasma glucose and amino acids in early pregnancy (Hytten, 1990).

The enlarging uterus misplaces the stomach and intestines. Raised intragastric pressure without accompanying increase in tone of the cardiac sphincter, causes reflux of acid mouthfuls with epigastric pain. The resulting symptom of heartburn is quite common in pregnancy.

The tendency to constipation is more in pregnancy, as the passage of food through the intestines is so much slower that there is increased absorption of water from the colon. This probably is due to raised levels of aldosterone and angiotensin. A high residue diet, which helps to hold water in its passage through the colon, will help to relieve this problem (Hytten, 1990). Constipation may also be caused by mechanical obstruction by the uterus and by the relaxing effect of progesterone on smooth muscle. Oral iron may also contribute to the problem (McFadyen, 1995). Constipation may worsen hemorrhoids, which are caused by the increased pressure in the veins below the level of the enlarged uterus.

The gallbladder increases in size and empties more slowly during pregnancy. Stagnation of bile, which is almost physiological in pregnancy, is probably a hormonal effect and can lead to pruritis or gallstone formation (McFadyen, 1995). There are many changes in liver function that mimic liver disease; therefore liver function tests in pregnancy should be interpreted with caution. Following are the common alterations:

* Serum albumin levels fall progressively throughout pregnancy and at term are 30 percent lower than the non-pregnant level
* Serum alkaline phosphatase levels rise progressively and at term are at two to four times the nonpregnant values
* Serum cholesterol levels are raised two-fold by the end of pregnancy
* Many liver proteins are raised
* Fibrinogen levels are increased 50 percent by the end of the second trimester (Cruikshank and Hays, 1991).

CHANGES IN METABOLISM

There is increased food intake during pregnancy. This, along with the gastrointestinal changes, lead to characteristic alteration in the metabolism of carbohydrate, protein and fat. These changes, which are brought about by human placental lactogen, ensure that glucose is readily available for body and brain growth in the developing fetus, and protects against nutritional deficiencies (Case, 1985).

Fasting plasma glucose concentration falls during the first trimester, rises between 16 and 32 weeks, then falls again towards term (Cruikshank and Hays, 1991).

Insulin secretion correspondingly rises in the second trimester and then falls to non-pregnant levels towards term. As human placental lactogen levels rise with advancing pregnancy, insulin resistance increases leading the diabetogenic effect of pregnancy. As a result a glucose load takes longer time to reach a maximal plasma concentration. When the maximum concentration is reached, it is higher than normal and remains elevated for longer allowing more time for placental exchange (Case and Waterhouse, 1994).

A continuous supply of glucose must be available to transfer to the fetus. Pregnant women should not fast or skip meals for the following reasons:
* Maternal blood glucose levels are critically important for the fetal well-being
* Fasting in pregnancy produces a more intense ketosis, known as accelerated starvation, that may be dangerous to fetal health (Cruikshank and Hays, 1991).

As the nutritional demands of the fetus increases in the second half of pregnancy and insulin resistance increases, mobilization of fat stores laid down in the first half of pregnancy occurs providing the mother with extra energy. However, because of the increased concentration of fatty acids resulting from this process, the mother is more prone to ketosis. Even an overnight fast of 12 hours will result in hypoglycemia and increased production of ketone bodies (Miller and Hanretty, 1997).

Restriction of carbohydrate in any diet may be avoided and the mother may be encouraged to take bed time snacks.

Plasma albumin concentration is reduced due to increased plasma volume. This causes reduction of colloid osmotic pressure resulting in limb edema in late pregnancy. Plasma amino acid concentrations also fall because amino acids are used to make glucose (Case and Waterhouse, 1994).

Plasma calcium concentrations fall as a result of both fetal needs and the normal hemo-dilation of pregnancy. If the intake of vitamin D is sufficient, calcium absorption from the intestines increases by the end of second tri-mester, which provides for fetal needs as well as protecting the mother's skeleton. Pregnant clients should therefore be advised to increase their calcium intake by about 70 percent (Case, 1985).

Maternal Weight Changes

A continuing weight increase in pregnancy is considered to be a favorable indicator for maternal adaptation and fetal growth. Ana-lysis of studies on weight gain in pregnancy suggests the following as the expected increase in primigravida.

- ❖ 4.0 kg in first 20 weeks
- ❖ 8.5 kg in second 20 weeks (0.4 kg per week in the last trimester)
- ❖ 12.5 kg approximate total (Murray, 1999).

The average weight gain in multigravida is approximately 1 kg less than in the primi-gravida.

There is a wide range of normality in weight gain and many factors influence it which include maternal edema, maternal metabolic rate, dietary intake, vomiting or diarrhea, amount of amniotic fluid and size of the fetus.

Maternal age, prepregnancy body size, parity and diseases like diabetes and hyperten-sion also seem to influence the pattern of weight gain (Hytten, 1990). Distribution of average weight gain in pregnancy is illustrated in Figure 12.2.

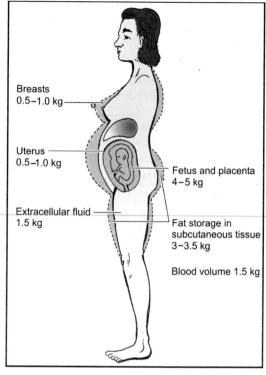

Fig. 12.2: Distribution of average weight gain in pregnancy

Breasts 0.5–1.0 kg

Uterus 0.5–1.0 kg

Fetus and placenta 4–5 kg

Extracellular fluid 1.5 kg

Fat storage in subcutaneous tissue 3–3.5 kg

Blood volume 1.5 kg

Skeletal Changes

Relaxation of pelvic ligaments and muscles occurs because of the influence of estrogen and relaxin. This reaches the maximum during the last weeks of pregnancy allowing the pelvis to increase its capacity in readiness to accommo-date the fetal presenting part at the end of pregnancy and in labor.

The ligaments of the symphysis pubis and the sacroiliac joints loosen. The symphysis pubis widens by about 4 mm by 32 weeks gestation and the sacrococcygeal joint loosens, allowing the coccyx to be displaced backwards. Increased mobility of the pelvic joints facilitates vaginal delivery. It also results in a rolling gait in late pregnancy, which is the likely cause of backache and ligamental pain (Cruikshank and Hays, 1991).

Posture of the pregnant woman alters to compensate for the enlarging uterus anteriorly. The woman leans backwards exaggerating the

normal lumbar curve and causing a progressive lordosis (an abnormal curvature of the spinal column with convexity towards the front), which shifts her center of gravity back over her legs. The side effect of this; is low back pain and sometimes shoulder pain, which most women suffer during pregnancy. Relaxation of the joints and lordosis can also lead to unsteadiness of gait and the tendency to fall.
The teeth are prone to decay during pregnancy, perhaps due to calcium deficiency resulting from increased demand for it by the growing fetus.

Skin Changes

Increased activity of the melanin-stimulating hormone from the pituitary causes varying degrees of pigmentation in pregnant women from the end of second month until term. The depth of pigmentation varies according to skin color and race.

The areas most commonly affected are the areolae of breasts, the abdominal midline, the perineum and the axillae. On the breasts, darkening of the nipple, primary areola (areola around the nipple), and secondary areola (mottling of the skin around and beyond the primary areola) are seen. The face is less frequently involved. It is speculated that these areas become more pigmented than others, either because of increased sensitivity of the melanocytes to the hormone or because of a greater number of melanocytes in these areas (Wade, 1984).

The irregular brownish discolorations of the forehead, nose, cheeks and neck known as the 'mask of pregnancy' or *chloasma* usually develops in the second half of pregnancy in about 50 to 70 percent of women. Chloasma is most noticeable in dark-haired, brown-eyed women. It regresses completely after delivery. In the most pregnant women, a narrow line of dark skin pigmentation appears in the midline of the abdomen from the symphysis to the umbilicus called as *linea nigra*.

As maternal size increase, stretching occurs in the collagen layer of the skin, particularly over the breasts, abdomen, thighs and occasionally buttocks. The areas of maximum stretch become thin and stretch marks known as *striae gravidarum* appear as red stripes during the pregnancy. Hair growth increases during pregnancy over face, scalp and body. The excess hair is shed after delivery.

A rise in body temperature of 0.5°C with an increased blood supply causing vasodilatation makes women feel hotter and sweaty. Many women develop angiomas during pregnancy, which are red elevations on the skin of the face, neck, arms and chest. Palmar erythema, which is reddening of the palms, is another frequent occurrence. Both are likely to be due to high levels of estrogen and disappear after delivery.

Breast Changes

Marked changes take place in the breasts. The changes are more obvious in primigravidae than in multiparae. The breasts increase in size and sensitiveness, and bluish discoloration appears in the form of streaks. The nipple becomes more erectile with the areola more deeply pigmented. Prominent tubercles, Montgomery's follicles appear in the primary areola. About the fifth month a less pigmented area forms around the primary areola, which is known as the secondary areola and on this also some Montgomery's tubercles may be seen. After the first trimester, a little clear, sticky fluid may be expressed from the nipples, which later becomes yellowish in color. This is known as colostrums.

CHANGES IN THE ENDOCRINE SYSTEM

Placental Hormones

Placenta produces several hormones. These hormones cause a number of physiological changes that aid in the diagnosis of pregnancy. The high levels of estrogen and progesterone produced by the placenta are responsible for breast changes, skin pigmentations, and uterine enlargement in the first trimester. Chorionic gonadotropin is the basis for the immunologic pregnancy tests. Human placental lactogen stimulates the growth of the breasts, has lactogenic properties and effects a number of metabolic changes. The secretion of HPL and hCG by the fetoplacental unit alters the function of the mother's endocrine organs either directly or indirectly. Raised estrogen levels increase production of globulins that bind thyroxine and corticosteroids and the sex steroids. As a result, the total plasma content of these hormones is increased but the levels of free (physiologically active) hormones are not necessarily raised (McFadyen, 1995).

Pituitary Hormones

The secretion of prolactin, adrenocorticotropic hormone, thyrotropic hormone and melano–cyte-stimulating hormone increases. Follicle stimulating hormone and luteinizing hormone secretion is greatly inhibited by placental pro-gesterone and estrogen (Case and Waterhouse, 1994).

The effects of prolactin secretion are suppressed during pregnancy. Following delivery of placenta, plasma concentrations of prolactin decrease, but is subsequently secreted in pulsatile bursts with sucking to stimulate milk production (Cunningham et al, 1989).

The posterior pituitary gland releases oxytocin in low frequency pulses throughout pregnancy. At term the frequency of pulses in-creases which stimulates uterine contractions.

Thyroid Function

In normal pregnancy the thyroid gland increases in size by about 13 percent due to hyperplasia of glandular tissue and increased vascularity (Cunningham et al, 1989). There is normally an increased uptake of iodine during pregnancy, which may be to compensate for renal clearance of iodine leading to a reduced level of plasma iodine.

Although pregnancy can give the impre-ssion of hyperthyroidism, thyroid function is basically normal. The basal metabolic rate is increased mainly because of increased oxygen consumption by the fetus and the work of the maternal heart and lungs. Rising levels of T4 (Thyroxin) and T3 (triiodothyronine may also

contribute to the increased metabolic rate (Guyton, 1991).

Adrenal Glands

The adrenal gland is stimulated by estrogen to produce increasing levels of total and free plasma cortisol and other corticosteroids including ACTH from 12th week to term.

It is thought that the raised levels of free cortisol have an antagonistic action to insulin. More glucose is made available to the fetus by raising the levels of glucose in the blood, mobilizing maternal fatty acids and amino acids for production of glycogen and decreasing the uptake of glucose by muscle (De Sweit and Chamberlain, 1992).

The increase in free plasma cortisol may also be responsible for some of the cushingoid features of normal pregnancy such as fat deposition and striae gravidarum (Davey, 1995).

Because of the stimulus of progesterone and estrogen there is large increase in the con-centration of renin by the adrenal cortex in the first 12 weeks of pregnancy. This activates the renin angiotensin system, which is associated with maintaining blood pressure. It also balances the salt-losing effect of progesterone by enhancing aldosterone secretion from the adrenal cortex (Cunningham et al, 1989). Aldosterone's effects of promoting sodium absorption is most likely to be the key factor in maintaining the delicate balance of salt and water excretion (Cruikshank and Hays, 1991).

Imbalance of these substances can cause pregnant women to reabsorb excess sodium from renal tubules and therefore to retain fluid, which can cause hypertension. High levels of angiotensin II would also cause the blood pressure to rise.

Nervous System

The nervous system is in a more excitable condition in pregnant women. Temperamental changes are frequently noticed. Mood changes and symptoms of psychosis may develop in those with a family history.

BIBLIOGRAPHY

1. Beischer N, Mackay E, Colditz P. Obstetrics and the Newborn, 3rd edn. London: WB Saunders; 1997.
2. Bissonette J. Placental and fetal physiology. In: Gabbe S, Niebyl J, Simpson J (Eds) Obstetrics-normal and Problem Pregnancies, 2nd edn. Edinburgh: Churchill Livingstone; 1991.
3. Case R. Variations in Human Physiology, Manchester: Manchester University Press; 1985.
4. Case R, Waterhouse J. Human Physiology, 2nd edn. Oxford: Oxford University Press; 1994.
5. Chamberlain G. The changing body in pregnancy. British Medical Journal, 1991;302(23):719-2.
6. Cruikshank D, Hays P. Maternal Physiology in Pregnancy. In: Gabbe S, et al (eds). Obstetrics-Normal and Problem Pregnancies, Edinburgh: 2nd edn. Churchill Livingstone; 1991.
7. Cunningham F, McDonald P, Gant N. William's Obstetrics, 18th edn. London: Prentice Hall; 1989.
8. Davison J, Dunlop W. Urinary Tract in Pregnancy, In: Chamberlain G (Eds). Turnbulls Obstetrics, 2nd edn. Edinburgh: Churchill Livingstone; 1995.
9. De Swiet M. The Cardiovascular System. In: Hytten F, Chamberlain G (Eds). Clinical Physiology in Obstetrics, 2nd edn. Oxford: Blackwell Scientific Publications; 1991.
10. Findlay A. Reproduction and the Fetus. London: Edward Arnold; 1984.
11. Guyton A. Textbook of Medical Physiology, 8th edn. London: Saunders; 1991.
12. Hytten F. The Alimentary System in Pregnancies. Midwifery 1990;6:201-4.
13. Llewellyn-Jones D. Fundamentals in Obstetrics and Gynecology, 6th edn. St. Louis: Mosby; 1994.
14. McFadyen. Maternal Physiology in Pregnancy, In: Chamberlain G (Ed). Turnbulls Obstetrics, 2nd edn. Edinburgh: Churchill Livingstone; 1995.
15. Miller A, Hanretti K. Obstetrics Illustrated, 4th edn. Edinburgh: Churchill Livingstone; 1989.
16. Moore P. Maternal Physiology During Pregnancy, In: De Cherney A. Pernoll M (Eds). Current Obstetric and Gynecologic Diagnosis and Treatment, 8th ed. London:Prentice Hall; 1994.
17. Murray Irene. Change and Adaptation in Pregnancy, In: Bennett RV, Linda KB (Eds). Myles Textbook for Midwifes, 13th edn. Edinburgh:Churchill Livingstone; 1999.
18. Nilsson L. A child is born. London: Doubleday;1990.
19. Symmonds E. Essential Obstetrics and Gynecology. Edinburgh: Churchill Livingstone; 1992.
20. Van Oppen A, Stigler R, Bruins H. Obstetrics and Gynecology; 1996;87:(2)310-7.
21. Verralls S. Anatomy and Physiology Applied to Obstetrics, 3rd edn. Edinburgh:Churchill Livingstone; 1993.
22. Wade T. Skin disorders. In: Brudenell M, Wilds P. Medical and Surgical Problems in Obstetrics. Bristol: John Wright; 1984.

$T_1 \rightarrow 1^{st} - 12^{th}$ weeks
$T_2 \rightarrow 13^{th} - 27^{th}$ weeks
$T_3 \rightarrow 28^{th} - 40^{th}$ weeks.

13

Diagnosis of Pregnancy

Learning Objectives

Upon completing this chapter, the learner will be able to:
- List the signs of pregnancy and explain the changes evident in the mother's body
- Diagnose pregnancies at different stages of gestation based on the findings of examination
- Explain the different pregnancy tests.

The antepartum period covers the time of pregnancy from the first day of the last menstrual period (LMP) to the start of true labor, which marks the beginning of the intrapartum period.

The antepartal period is divided into three trimesters, each consisting of approximately 13 weeks or 3 calendar months. This derives from the calculation of pregnancy as being approximately 280 days, or 40 weeks from the first day of last menstrual period. In reality gestation is not that long. Fertilization takes place at the time of ovulation, that is approximately 14 days after the last menstrual period. This makes actual gestation approximately of 266 days or 38 weeks. Adding 14 days gives a total of 280 days from the last menstrual period. In practice, the first trimester is generally considered to be of 1st to 12th (12 weeks), the second trimester to be of 13th to 27th week (15 weeks) and third trimester to be of 28th to 40th week (13 weeks) (Varney, 1987).

DIAGNOSIS OF PREGNANCY

Pregnancy may be diagnosed by the woman herself even before she has missed a period because she feels different. Changes in the breasts can occur as early as 5 to 6 weeks after conception.

Diagnosis of pregnancy, in the first trimester and early second trimester, is based on a combination of presumptive and probable signs of pregnancy. Pregnancy is self-evident later in gestation, when the positive signs of pregnancy are readily observed.

Presumptive signs of pregnancy are maternal physiological changes, which the woman experiences and which, in most cases, indicate to her that she is pregnant.

Probable signs of pregnancy are maternal physiological changes other than presumptive signs, which are detected upon examination and documented by the examiner.

Positive signs are those directly attributable to the fetus as detected and documented by the examiner.

Following is an outline of all the presumptive, probable and positive signs of pregnancy.

Presumptive Signs

- Abrupt cessation of menstruation (amenorrhea) at 4th week
- Nausea and vomiting (morning sickness) from 4th to 14th week
- Tingling, tenseness, nodularity and enlargement of the breasts and enlargement of the nipples around 3rd to 4th week
- Increased frequency of micturition (bladder irritability) around 6th to 12th week
- Fatigue
- Color changes of breasts, i.e. darkening of the nipples and primary and secondary areolar change

- Appearance of Montgomery's tubercles
- Continued elevation of basal body temperature in the absence of an infection
- Expression of colostrum from nipples
- Excessive salivation
- Quickening (the first movement felt by the mother around 18th to 20th week)
- Skin pigmentation and conditions such as chloasma, breast and abdominal striae, linea nigra and palmar erythema.

Probable Signs

- Enlargement of the uterus
- Change in shape of the uterus
- Presence of human chorionic gondotropin in blood 4th to 12th week) and in urine 6th to 12th week)—positive pregnancy tests
- *Hegar's sign:* Softening and compressibility of the isthmus (6th to 12th week)
- *Jacquemier's sign / Chadwick's sign:* The violet-blue discoloration of the vulva and vaginal mucosa including the vaginal portion of the cervix due to increased vascularity evident by about 6 weeks gestation
- *Osiander's sign:* Pulsation in the lateral fornices (8th week)
- *Goodell's sign:* Softening of the cervix from a nonpregnant state of firmness similar to the tip of a nose to the softness of lips in the pregnant state
- Presence of Braxton Hicks contractions (16th week)
- Ballottement of fetus (16th–28 week).

Positive Signs

- Visualization of fetus by ultrasound (6th week +)
- Visualization of fetal skeleton by X-ray (16th week)
- Fetal heart sounds by ultrasound (6th week)
- Fetal heart sounds with fetoscope (20th week)
- Palpable fetal movements (22th week)
- Visible fetal movements (late pregnancy) ·
- Palpation of fetal parts (24th week +).

It is not always appropriate to seek findings regarding all of the signs of pregnancy outlined here when examining a woman who thinks she is pregnant. This is because of not all the signs are manifested at the same time. It is also important to know that the majority of these signs can be due to other conditions, and a diagnosis of pregnancy can be made only in the presence of several of these changes.

Uterine Enlargement

Estrogen and progesterone are primarily responsible for the hypertrophy of the uterine wall during the early months of pregnancy. Uterine enlargement is the result of a considerable increase in the size and stretching of the muscle cells. The hypertrophy of the muscle cells is accompanied by a marked increase in the elastic and fibrous tissue, which strengthens the uterine wall.

After the third month of pregnancy the uterine enlargement is also due to the mechanical effect of inside pressure on the uterine wall by the growing products of conception. In the early months of pregnancy there is a marked increase in the size of the uterine blood vessels and lymphatics. The resulting vascularity, congestion and edema most likely account for the overall softening of the uterus. This along with hypertrophy of the cervical glands, give rise to Chadwick's/Jacquemier's sign and Hegar's sign.

The softness and compressibility of the uterine isthmus (Hegar's sign) has the effects of nonsupport to the enlarging body of the uterus with its increasing heaviness in the fundus. The result is an exaggerated uterine anteflexion during the first-three months of pregnancy while the uterus is still a pelvic organ. This causes the fundus to press on the bladder resulting in urinary frequency. Urinary frequency is relieved early in the fourth month of pregnancy as the uterus rises out of the pelvis.

As the uterus enlarges it changes from its nonpregnant pear-shape to globular and then to ovoid. Early uterine enlargement may not be symmetrical. The ovum implants in the upper uterine wall, more frequently on the posterior side.

Uterine enlargement contributes to two other maternal signs of pregnancy—The Braxton Hicks contractions and abdominal enlargement. Braxton Hicks contractions are nonrhythmic, sporadic, painless uterine contractions that start about the 6th week of pregnancy. These are detectable on bimanual examination in the second trimester and during abdominal examination in the third trimester. They increase in frequency, duration and intensity as well as attain some degree of rhythm and regularity close to term at which time they are frequently misinterpreted as labor contractions.

Abdominal enlargement begins at the fourth month of pregnancy, as the uterus becomes an abdominal organ. The abdomen is more prominent when the woman is standing than when she is supine. Abdominal enlargement is also more noticeable in multiparas than in primigravidas, because of the loss of muscle tone of the abdominal wall, which was not exercised back into shape after each previous pregnancy. A pendulous abdomen results as the uterus sags forward and downward.

Other Signs of Pregnancy

It is thought that the basal metabolic rate (BMR) initially falls during pregnancy and then progressively rises throughout the pregnancy as a direct result of the metabolic activity of the products of conception (Varney, 1996).

The initial fall in the BMR might account for the fatigue often encountered during the first trimester. Nausea and vomiting have been attributed to a number of possible causes, but their actual etiology is not yet known. Normal nausea and vomiting in pregnancy rarely extend beyond the first trimester. Excessive salivation (ptyalism) is an unusual occurrence, which may be caused either by increased acidity in the mouth or by the intake of starch stimulating the salivary glands in women who are susceptible to excessive secretion. Women who have ptyalism frequently, are nauseated also.

Fetal Contributions to the Diagnosis of Pregnancy

Anatomic

The combination of uterine enlargement, thinning of the uterine wall and the uterus becoming an abdominal organ enable the detection of a number of signs of pregnancy in the second trimester which were previously inaccessible. The precise time, when the fetal heart tones are heard and the quickening is felt, vary with the thinness or obesity of the individual woman as well as with parity. In multiparous women, as the abdominal musculature have hypertrophied and stretched earlier, it may be thin enough to facilitate eliciting of the following signs of pregnancy a week or two earlier than in a primigravida.

The fetal heart starts beating at the sixth week (4th week postfertilization) and can be heard by 20th week with a fetoscope during abdominal examination of the mother. However, it can be heard between 12th and 20th week with ultrasonic instruments. Fetal heart tones must be differentiated from two other sound—(1) *The uterine souffle*—A soft blowing and systolic murmur heard low down at the sides of the uterus, best on the left side. The sound is due to increase in blood flow through the dilated uterine vessels and is synchronous with the maternal pulse. (2) *The funic souffle*—The sound of blood rushing through the umbilical arteries. It is a soft blowing murmur synchronous with the fetal heart sounds.

Weak fetal movements start in the 3rd month of pregnancy, and by 20th week they are strong enough and the uterine wall is thin enough for them to be felt and properly diagnosed during abdominal examination. The mother may be aware of fetal movements around 18th week. These movements, increase in intensity over the weeks from gentle flutterings to unmistakable fetal kicks. The time when she feels the first fetal movement is called *quickening*, meaning the perception of life.

After the 20th week, fetal outline can be palpated during abdominal examination. This is not a definitive diagnostic sign, because subserous myomas may feel like fetal parts. Ballottment can be elicited abdominally around the same time. In this sign, a sudden tap on the uterus causes the fetus to sink in the amniotic fluid and rebound to strike gently against the fingers of the examiner. Ballottment is possible at this time because there is a large volume of amniotic fluid in relation to the size of the still small fetus. This proportion grossly changes later in pregnancy.

Hormonal Pregnancy Tests

Pregnancy tests are based on the production of chorionic gonadotropin by the syncytiotrophoblastic cells during early pregnancy. Human chorionic gonadotropin (hCG) is secreted into the maternal bloodstream where it is present in the plasma. It is then excreted in the mother's urine.

Human chorionic gonadotropin is first detected in the urine about 26 days after conception and is excreted at rates, which increases rapidly between 30 to 60 days. Peak levels occur between 60 and 70 days of gestation. The level then gradually decreases to a low between 100 and 130 days and is maintained at this level throughout the remaining weeks of gestation.

Quantitative assays of hCG are of diagnostic significance in pregnancy. They are abnormally low in ectopic pregnancies and threatened abortions, and abnormally high in women with multiple pregnancy, hydatidiform mole, or choriocarcinoma. Human chorionic gonadotropin in the urine has been used for pregnancy tests since the late 1920s when Aschheim and Zondek originated *biologic assay* of its presence (Varney, 1989). These tests utilized small immature animals such as mice, rabbits, frogs and toads and were based on the response of the animals' ovaries or testes after being injected with either serum or urine of the woman suspected of being pregnant.

These tests have been largely superseded by the immunologic assays of hCG. The immunologic assays of hCG test utilizes specific antisera, obtained from animals (rabbits) in which antibody response to hCG has been stimulated. It is based on the fact that hCG is a protein and therefore antigenic. The antisera are mixed with urine of the woman suspected of being pregnant. This mediates the response of the antisera when mixed with either latex particles coated with hCG or with erythrocytes, which have been sensitized to hCG. This will neutralize the antibodies in the antiserum and inhibit agglutination, which is a positive pregnancy test. If the woman is not pregnant her urine does not contain hCG and agglutination will occur which is a negative pregnancy test.

More recently, radioreceptoassay and radioimmunoassay tests have become available. Both require expensive equipment and trained technicians. These are extremely sensitive tests, able to detect hCG at far lower levels than previous tests. The radioimmunoassay blood test commonly known as beta-preg; can be used as early as one week after conception if laboratory facilities are available. Because the radioreceptoassay test cross-reacts with luteinizing hormone, it is more limited in its sensitivity than the radioimmunoassay.

BIBLIOGRAPHY

1. Dutta DC. Textbook of Obstetrics, 5th edn. Calcutta: New Central Book Company; 2001.
2. Ladewig PW, London ML, Old SB. Essentials of Maternal-Newborn Nursing, New York: Addison-Wesley; 1990.
3. Murray Irene. Change and Adaptation in Pregnancy, In: Bennett RV, Linda KB (Eds). Myles Textbook for Midwives, 13th edn. Edinburgh: Churchill Livingstone; 1999.
4. Neeson JD. Clinical Manual of Maternity Nursing, Philadelphia:JB Lippincot; 1989.
5. Varney Helen. Nurse-midwifery, 2nd edn. Boston: Jones and Barlett Publishers; 1996.

14

Minor Disorders in Pregnancy

Learning Objectives

Upon completing this chapter, the learner will be able to:

❖ List the disorders of pregnancy
❖ Explain the causes and measures for the relief of discomforts
❖ Outline the disorders that can possibly escalate requiring immediate intervention.

Many women experience some minor disorders during pregnancy. These disorders should be treated adequately as they may escalate and become life-threatening.

Minor disorders may occur due to hormonal changes, accommodation changes, metabolic changes and postural changes. Every system of the body is affected by pregnancy. The mother needs knowledge to cope with the experience of pregnancy. She also needs knowledge when she presents with discomforting or worrying symptoms.

DIGESTIVE SYSTEM

Nausea and Vomiting

It is a common disorder seen in about 50 percent women between 4th and 16th week of gestation. Hormonal influences are thought to be the most likely cause. Human chorionic gonadotropin, that is present in large amounts in the first trimester, estrogen and progesterone are all contributors to this. The sickness is confined to "early morning" but can occur at any time in the day. The smell of food cooking will often cause the mother to retch.

The midwife can explain the probable reasons and encourage the mother to look positively towards the resolution of the problem, which may happen between 12th and 16th week. Women have found the following as helpful practices:

❖ Salads and light snacks are more tolerable than full meals
❖ Carbohydrate snacks at bedtime can prevent hypoglycemia, which is often shown as a cause of nausea and vomiting
❖ Dry toast or biscuit on waking up and breakfast after half an hour.

If vomiting becomes severe, the mother may lose weight and become dehydrated and ketotic. This condition is called hyperemesis gravidarum and warrants specialized care and appropriate referral.

Heartburn

This is a burning pain in the mediastinal region caused by reflux of stomach contents into the esophagus. It occurs because the cardiac sphincter relaxes during pregnancy due to the effect of progesterone. The condition tends to worsen as pregnancy advances, because the stomach is displaced upward by the enlarging uterus. Heartburn is most troublesome at about 30th to 40th week of gestation, because at this stage the stomach is under pressure from the growing uterus.

The advice varies according to the severity of the condition.

❖ If the heartburn is occasional, the reflux can be prevented by avoiding bending and kneeling while doing household chores
❖ Small meals take less room in the reduced stomach space and are digested more easily
❖ Fried and fatty foods should be avoided

❖ Sleeping with more pillows than usual and lying on the right side semi reclining can sometimes help

❖ For persistent heartburn antacids may be prescribed by the physician.

Excessive Salivation (Ptyalism)

This occurs from 8th week of gestation and it is thought that the hormones of pregnancy are the cause for it. It may accompany heartburn.

Pica

This is the term used when the mother craves certain foods or unnatural substances such as coal. The cause is unknown but hormones and changes in metabolism are thought to contribute to this. If the substances craved are harmful to the unborn baby, the mother must be helped to seek medical advice.

Constipation

This is due to smooth muscle relaxant effect of progesterone causing decreased peristalsis of the gut. Pressure of the gravid uterus on the colon near term makes it worse as the colon gets displaced. It is usually overcome by adjusting the diet. The women may be advised to:

❖ Increase the intake of water

❖ Add green leafy vegetables, fruits and bran cereals to her diet

❖ Take a glass of warm water in the morning before tea or breakfast which would activate the gut and help regular bowel movements

❖ Exercise by regular walking.

Constipation is sometimes associated with taking oral iron and it can aggravate hemorrhoids.

MUSCULOSKELETAL SYSTEM

Backache

The gradual weight gain and the change in the body's center of gravity combined with the stretching of weak abdominal muscles often lead to a hollowing of the lumbar spine. There is a tendency for back muscles to shorten as the abdominal muscles stretch and extra strain is put on the ligaments. This results in backache, usually of sacroiliac or lumbar origin.

Women with this problem must be helped with:

❖ Postural re-education, including correction of the "pelvic tilt"

❖ Advice relating to comfortable positions in sitting, standing, lying, general mobility and how to lift correctly.

Lying on the side away from the discomfort, with the affected leg uppermost may relieve the problem. Pillows should be placed to support the whole limb.

Backache must never be dismissed lightly as it is associated with urinary tract infection and with the onset of labor, especially when the fetal occiput is posterior.

Cramps

These are quite common, usually in the leg. They are worse at night. The cause of leg cramps in pregnancy is not known, but has been attributed to deficiency of vitamin B₁ and decreased levels of calcium. It may be due to ischemia or changes in pH or electrolyte status. It may be helpful to:

❖ Make gentle leg movements whilst in a warm bath prior to settling for the night

❖ Sleep with the foot end of the bed elevated by 20 to 25 cm

❖ Take vitamin B complex and calcium supplements.

An attack can be aborted by sharply stretching the involved muscle. Once a cramp has occurred, gentle kneading is effective.

GENITOURINARY SYSTEM

Frequency of Micturition

This occurs in the first trimester when there is pressure of the gravid uterus on the urinary bladder. It is spontaneously relieved when the uterus rises up in the abdomen. It may recur late in pregnancy when the fetal head descends into the pelvis. Urinary tract infection should always be ruled out before attributing the frequency to pregnancy. Reassurance is sufficient.

Leukorrhea

This is the term used for the increased white, nonirritant vaginal discharge in pregnancy. If the mother finds the discharge disturbing, it is helpful to offer simple advice of personal hygiene.

Frequent washing of the vulva (3-4 times a day) with plain water would be sufficient. She should wear cotton underwear and avoid tights. The midwife should exclude the possibility of infection such as thrush and *Trichomonas*.

CIRCULATORY SYSTEM

Fainting

In early pregnancy fainting may occur due to vasodilation under the influence of progesterone. It may subside following the compensatory increase in blood volume. Measures for relief include avoiding long periods of standing as well as sitting or lying down when she feels slightly faint.

Later in pregnancy, a mother may feel faint while lying flat on her back. This is because the weight of the uterine contents presses on the inferior vena cava and slows the return of blood to the heart. Turning the mother quickly on to her side will bring rapid recovery. She should be advised not to lie on her back except during abdominal examination.

Varicosities

Progesterone relaxes the smooth muscles of the veins and results in sluggish circulation (slow moving). The valves of the dilated veins become inefficient and varicosities result. Varicose veins occur in legs, anus (hemorrhoids) and vulva. The situation is often compounded by pelvic congestion.

Mothers with a family history of varicose veins and those doing work, which demands long periods of standing and sitting usually, develop varicose veins. Measures to reduce the discomfort of leg varicosities include:

- Exercising the calf muscles by rising onto the toes or making circling movements with the ankles
- Resting with the legs vertical against the wall for a short time
- Wearing support tights before rising or after resting with legs elevated.

Those with hemorrhoids or tendency to develop them should be advised about:

- Avoidance of constipation by including fiber in the diet and adequate fluids
- Seeking medical advice for topical applications.

Vulvar varicosities are rare and very painful. A Panty Girdle or sanitary pad may give support. Vulval varicosities may rupture and bleed during delivery. Occasionally numerous spider varices develop on the skin. Most of those enlarged veins disappear after delivery.

Edema

It is the result of venous and lymphatic stasis. Additional factors responsible are—Changes in osmotic pressure of blood and tissue fluids, and altered capillary permeability. The blood pressure should be checked to see if the patient has pregnancy induced hypertension. The treatment of gestational edema of feet is elevation of legs, sleeping in left lateral position and avoiding sitting with the feet hanging down.

INTEGUMENTARY SYSTEM

Skin

Some mothers complain of generalized itching, which often starts over the abdomen. This is thought to have some connection with the liver's response to the hormones in pregnancy and with raised bilirubin levels. It clears soon after the baby is born and comfort can be gained from local applications. An antihistamine is often prescribed. If a mother complains of vulvar irritation, infection such as thrush, and glycosuria as a result of diabetes must be excluded. Washing with mild soap and cotton underwear might help to ease the irritation.

NERVOUS SYSTEM

Carpal Tunnel Syndrome

Mothers complain of numbness and pins and needles in their fingers and hands. This usually happens in the morning, but it can occur at any time of the day. It is caused by fluid retention, which creates edema and pressure on the median nerve. Wearing a splint at night, with the hands resting on two or three pillows sometimes help. Restriction of salt intake and flexing the fingers while the arm is held above the head can be recommended. Carpal tunnel syndrome usually resolves spontaneously following delivery.

Intercostal neuralgia may develop in late pregnancy due to muscle spasm. It may be unilateral or girdle type. Sitting in a straight-backed chair, using a cushion for lumbar support and lateral flexion exercises relieves it.

Bell's palsy may rarely develop in the last trimester due to edema compressing the facial nerve. It is relieved spontaneously in 3 to 4 weeks following delivery.

Insomnia

This is relatively common in late pregnancy owing to the discomfort caused by the fetal movements, frequency of micturition and difficulty in finding a comfortable position. It may also be due to some deep-seated anxiety or fear. Women with such problems can be advised to:

❖ Take rest in the afternoon
❖ Drink a glass of warm milk at bed time
❖ Tuck a pillow under the abdomen when lying in a lateral position
❖ Talk about her fears and anxieties so that she can have a sense of normality and lightness.

DISORDERS THAT REQUIRE IMMEDIATE ACTION

Most minor disorders can escalate into a more serious complication of pregnancy. Mothers should be encouraged to seek advice if at any time they feel unwell or the signs exceed what they have been led to expect. In addition there are incidents, which should always be reported to the physician. These are:

❖ Vaginal bleeding
❖ Reduced fetal movements
❖ Frontal or recurring headaches
❖ Sudden swelling/edema
❖ Rupture of the membranes
❖ Premature onset of contractions
❖ Sudden nausea or sickness
❖ Epigastric pain.

Mothers must be reassured about their pregnancy status. Knowledge that the pregnancy proceeds without complications, would add to their security and confidence. They should also know when to seek the help of a professional.

BIBLIOGRAPHY

1. Jamieson L. Preparing for Parenthood: Daily Life in Pregnancy, In: Bennett RV, Linda KB (Eds). Myles Textbook for Midwives, 13th edn. Edinburgh: Churchill Livingstone; 1999.
2. Karpen M, Conrad L, Chitwood L. Essentials of Maternal Child Nursing; 1995.
3. Light HK, Fenster C. Maternal Concerns during Pregnancy, American Journal of Obstetrics and Gynecology 1974;118: 46.
4. Moore P. Maternal Physiology during Pregnancy, In: De Cherney A, Pernol M, (Eds). Current Obstetric and Gynecologic Diagnosis and Treatment, 8th edn. London: Prentice Hall; 1994.
5. Parulekar SV. Textbook for Midwives, 2nd edn. Mumbai: Vora Medical Publications; 1998.
6. Varney Helen. Nurse-Midwifery, 2nd edn. Boston: Jones and Barlett Publishers; 1996.

15

Antenatal Care

Learning Objectives

Upon completing this chapter, the learner will be able to:

- Explain the meaning and objectives of antenatal care
- List the objectives and procedure of initial assessment and review of body systems
- Describe the physical examination of the mother during the initial and subsequent visits
- Describe the steps of abdominal examination
- Enumerate the steps of nursing process for an antenatal mother.

MEANING

Antenatal care refers to the care given to an expectant mother from the time the conception is confirmed until the beginning of labor. It includes monitoring the progress of pregnancy, providing appropriate support to the woman and her family and providing information, which will assist them to make sensible choices.

OBJECTIVES

The objectives of prenatal care are to:

- Promote, protect and maintain the health of the mother during pregnancy
- Detect "high-risk" pregnancies and give the mothers special attention
- Foresee complications and take preventive measures
- Remove anxiety and fear associated with pregnancy
- Reduce maternal and infant morbidity and mortality
- Teach the mother elements of nutrition, personal hygiene and newborn care

- Sensitize the mother to the need of family planning.

ANTENATAL VISITS

Ideally the antenatal mother should visit the antenatal clinic once a month during the first seven months; twice a month during the eighth month, and there after once a week if everything is normal. A large proportion of mothers in India are from lower socioeconomic group and many are working women. For women who find regular attendance at the clinic difficult due to economic reasons, if the pregnancy is uncomplicated, a minimum of three visits covering the entire period of pregnancy should be the target as outlined below (Park, 2000). First visit at 20th week or as soon as the pregnancy is known. Second visit at 32nd week and third visit at 36th week.

THE INITIAL EXAMINATION

The first visit, irrespective of when it occurs, should include the client's health history, obstetric history, physical and pelvic examinations and laboratory examinations.

Health History

- Identifying information
- Chief complaints in her own words. Medical conditions that affect pregnancy may vary from common urinary tract infections to severe cardiac conditions. Some of the medical conditions that require special care are:
  - Urinary tract infection
  - Essential hypertension that may lead to pregnancy induced hypertension

– Asthma, epilepsy, psychiatric disorders
– Medical conditions such as diabetes and cardiac conditions.

Family History

❖ History of conditions that are genetic in origin, familial or have racial characteristics such as:
  – Diabetes in a first degree relative
  – Hypertension
  – Multiple pregnancies
  – Conditions like spina bifida, sickle cell anemia and thalassemia.

Menstrual History

❖ Age at menarche
❖ Frequency, duration and amount of menstrual flow
❖ Dysfunctional uterine bleeding, i.e. menorrhagia, metrorrhagia or intermenstrual spotting
❖ Premenstrual spotting.

Obstetric History

This includes obtaining the date of her last menstrual period (LMP), calculation of her expected date of delivery (EDD), determination of the present number of weeks' of gestation and calculation of her gravida and para status.

Gravida

Gravida refers to the number of times a woman has been pregnant. It does not take into account at what time during pregnancy it (the pregnancy) was terminated. Nor does it matter how many babies were born from the pregnancy. It is the pregnancy that counts and not the number of babies. A woman who had one pregnancy from which she issued triplets would still be a gravida 1 until she becomes pregnant again, at which time she would be gravida 2. A woman who is pregnant for the first time is called a *primigravida* and a woman who is pregnant for the second time is called a *secondigravida*. There after, if she becomes pregnant again, she is called a *multigravida*. A woman who has never been pregnant is called a *nulligravida*.

Para

Para refers to the number of pregnancies that terminated in the birth of a fetus or fetuses that reached the point of viability (the ability of the fetus to survive if born). This point is considered to be 28 weeks of gestation or 1,000 gm (in India). It is the number of pregnancies carried to the point of the fetus or fetuses reaching the point of viability that determines parity and not the number of fetuses reaching the point of viability. Para is not affected whether the fetus or fetuses are born alive or are stillbirths.

A *primipara* is a woman who has given birth to a fetus or fetuses that has reached the point of viability. A *multipara* is a woman who had given birth to two or more babies live or still excluding abortions.

A *grandmultipara* is a woman who has given birth five times or more. A woman who has not carried a pregnancy to the point of viability is called *nullipara*. The items to be included in obstetric history are:

❖ Gravida, para
❖ Rh and ABO blood type
❖ Previous pregnancy and delivery
  – Weeks of gestation and dates of termination
  – Delivery in the hospital or at home
  – Length of labor
  – Type of delivery, i.e. spontaneous, instrumental or cesarean section
  – RhoGAM received
  – Any obstetric, medical problems during pregnancy, labor or delivery.
❖ Status of newborn at birth
  – Cried immediately, problems, death
  – Sex and weight of the baby
  – Any congenital anomalies or neonatal problems.

PRESENT PREGNANCY

History of the present pregnancy is designed to detect complications, discomforts and any complaints about pregnancy the woman may have experienced since her last menstrual period (LMP).

The date of the first day of the last normal menstrual period is used as the baseline for determining gestational age and estimated date of delivery (EDD). Hence, it is important to obtain the accurate date of this event. When the accuracy of pinpointing the LMP is impossible, other parameters may be used to arrive at the expected date of delivery. Ascertaining the approximate date, on which the baby was conceived, is important to predict the date of giving birth and to calculate the gestational age at any point of pregnancy.

The EDD is calculated by *Naegele's* rule, in which seven days are added to the date of the first day of LMP and three months are subtracted from that date. It is also calculated by adding nine calendar months and seven days to the date of the first day of the woman's last menstrual period.

The actual period of gestation is from the time of fertilization. Since ovulation is generally considered to occur approximately 14 days before the next menstrual period, the length of a woman's menstrual cycle will affect the accuracy of the EDD. A woman with a longer menstrual cycle (more than 28 days) will actually begin her pregnancy later in relation to her LMP and subsequently will deliver at a correspondingly later date. The reverse is true for women with shorter menstrual cycle. The majority of women will deliver within 10 to 14 days either earlier or later of their EDD, and this is considered physiologically normal.

It is useless to calculate the EDD by Naegele's rule in the presence of the following situations:

❖ Irregular menstrual periods in which one or more months are amenorrheic
❖ Conception occurring while the mother is breastfeeding and ovulating but amenorrheic
❖ Conception occurring before regular menstruation is established after termination of pregnancy or discontinuation of oral contraceptive pills.

In such instances an estimated date of delivery is arrived at, based on clinical findings and if indicated an ultrasound scan is taken between 18th to 26th week of gestation. The woman may be seen for her initial antenatal examination at any time during the present pregnancy, and therefore the present pregnancy history here covers the symptoms of possible problems in all three trimesters of pregnancy.

– Headache, dizziness, visual disturbances
– Syncope, fatigue
– Nausea, vomiting, heartburn
– Breast changes
– Shortness of breath
– Abdominal pain, back pain, dyspareunia
– Vaginal discharge, vaginal bleeding
– Dysuria, urinary frequency
– Constipation, hemorrhoids
– Leg cramps, varicosities
– Edema—ankles, pretibial, face, hands
– Feelings about pregnancy—body image, feeling about the baby.

PHYSICAL EXAMINATION

A complete screening physical examination is done during the initial antepartal examination in order to ascertain whether the woman has any medical disease or abnormalities. It includes a structured review of body systems through observation, inspection, examination and measurements. The physical examination should be carried-out in an organized manner. As the midwife begins the procedure she should be respectful to the client and gentle. The components of physical examination are:

❖ *Physical measurements,* i.e. temperature, pulse, respirations and blood pressure
❖ *General observations and client's own evaluation*
– Appropriateness of appearance
– Apparent state of health
– Mental and emotional state
– Posture, gait and body movements
– Striking obvious findings such as pallor, cyanosis or respiratory distress
– Client's own evaluation of health, dietary patterns and ability to carry-out daily living activities.

Review of Systems

❖ *Integumentary system*
Rashes, moles, lesions, pruritis, bruises, hirsutism, pigmentation, moisture, scars, tumors, and turger.

❖ *Hair and scalp*
General character, scalp infections, lice, dandruff, alopecia, and lumps.

❖ *Head*
Headache, dizziness, fainting, sinusitis, involuntary movements.

❖ *Eyes*
Blurring of vision, blind spots in vision, diplopia, photophobia, lacrimation discharge, redness, burning, glasses or contact lenses, injuries, infection, color of conjunctiva, pupillary size and reaction to light.

❖ *Ears*
Hearing acuity, ear aches or discharges, tinnitus, vertigo, infection, mastoid, tenderness, lesions, and placement on head.

❖ *Nose*
Size, placement, patency of nostrils, epistaxis, discharge, sense of smell, and septal deformity.

❖ *Mouth and throat*
Condition of lips, gum, teeth, tongue and mucosa; sense of taste, voice, speech, odor of breath, any inflammation or surgery.

❖ *Neck*
Movement, lymph node enlargement, vein distention, position of trachea.

❖ *Breasts*
Nipples—Normal flat or inverted, discharge, skin and glandular changes.

❖ *Gastrointestinal system*
Appetite, nausea, vomiting, heartburn, belching, flatulence, bowel pattern, hemorrhoids, food allergies, hernias.

❖ *Cardiorespiratory system*
Breathing pattern, cough, wheezing, infection, respiration rate and rhythm, auscultation findings.

❖ *Genitourinary system*
Urination difficulties and deviations, genital lesions and infections, history of hormone therapy.

❖ *Muscular, skeletal and vascular systems*
Status of joints, muscles and extremities, appearance of nails and fingers.

❖ *Central nervous system*
 – Speech and memory, complaints of vertigo, convulsions or loss of consciousness
 – Mental status
 – Motor symptoms
 – Sensory symptoms.

❖ *Lymphatic and hematopoietic system*
Lymph nodes, bruising tendencies, blood dyscrasias.

Assessments and Laboratory Tests

❖ *Height*
Height of the woman is checked at the time of first visit. Height over 160 cm is an indication of normal pelvis. A woman who is short in stature may belong to a small-sized race or family or may be stunted because of poor nutrition *in utero* or childhood. In individual situations, the size of the fetus will determine the adequacy of the pelvis. At about 36th week when the fetus is almost fully-grown the pelvic size is reassessed. If the fetal head will engage in the pelvic brim, there is little cause for concern about cephalopelvic disproportion.

❖ *Weight*
Weight must be checked at every visit and the rate of gain to be assessed. Obesity is associated with an increased risk of gestational diabetes and pregnancy induced hypertension.

❖ *Blood pressure*
Blood pressure is checked to provide a baseline reading for comparison throughout pregnancy. An adequate blood pressure is required to maintain placental perfusion. A blood pressure of 140/90 mm Hg at the first visit is indicative of hypertension.

Urinalysis

This is done to exclude certain abnormalities. Pyelonephritis can readily develop because of changes in the renal tract during pregnancy. Possible findings in urinalysis include:

❖ Ketones due to increased maternal metabolism or vomiting
❖ Glucose caused by higher circulating blood levels, reduced renal threshold or disease
❖ Protein due to contamination by vaginal leukorrhea, diseases such as UTI or PIH.

Blood Tests

❖ *ABO blood group and Rh factor*
Blood tests are done as part of the initial assessment to determine ABO blood group

and Rhesus (Rh) factor. Antibody screening is done followed by titration, if present. Follow-up of a woman, whose blood group is Rh-negative, will include further blood tests at 28th, 32nd, 36th and 40th week for Rh antibody titer to ensure that the pregnancy is not stimulating antibody activity. If the titration demonstrates a rising antibody response, more frequent assessment will be done in order to plan the management.

❖ *Hemoglobin and hematocrit*

These are performed in order to assess the adequacy of iron stores. Hemoglobin estimation is repeated at 28th week, when the physiological effects of hemodilution become more apparent, and at 36th week to ensure that any anemia is treated prior to delivery. The decision to use supplements is made on an individual basis. However, most women in the rural population are given iron and folic acid supplements. Health education about including iron-rich foods in diet should also be given.

❖ *Venereal disease research laboratory (VDRL) test*

This test is done for all pregnant women. Early testing will allow the women to be treated adequately in order to prevent infection of the fetus. It is to be remember that all positive results do not indicate active syphilis.

❖ *Human immunodeficiency virus (HIV) test*

Routine screening to detect HIV infection is done in many centers. It is important to gain informed consent prior to the blood test and to offer appropriate counseling.

❖ *Rubella immune status*

This is done by measuring the rubella antibody titer. Women who are not immune must be advised to avoid contact with anyone suffering from the disease. Other blood tests, such as screening for blood disorders or hepatitis, are done on individual cases based on the history.

Abdominal Examination

An abdominal examination of the pregnant woman should be done in addition to the physical examination and assessment. The examination includes:

❖ Observation of the size of the uterus, the shape of the uterus, the contour of the abdominal wall, any scar or injury marks, linea nigra and striae gravidarum

❖ Determination of the lie, presentation, position and variety of the fetus

❖ Measurement of fundal height, abdominal girth, palpation of fetal position and auscultation of fetal heart tones.

Each of these items provides informative data useful in diagnosis of pregnancy, evaluation of fetal well-being and growth, and serve as indicators of possible problems.

INSPECTION

The examiner's eyes assess the size of the uterus roughly. A distended colon or obesity may give a false impression. Multiple pregnancy or polyhydramnios will enlarge both the length and breadth of the uterus, whereas a large baby increases only the length.

The shape of the uterus is longer than it is broad when the lie of the fetus is longitudinal. If the lie of the fetus is transverse, the uterus is low and broad which occurs only in small percentage (0.5%). The multiparous uterus lacks the sung avoid shape of the primigravid uterus. Occasionally it is possible to see the shape of the fetal back or limbs. In posterior positions of the occiput a saucer-like depression is seen at or below the umbilicus.

A full bladder may be visible and may be more obvious in the later weeks of pregnancy. The umbilicus becomes less dimpled as pregnancy advances and may protrude lightly in later weeks. Lightening may be evident when the woman is erect. The uterus may sag forwards in multiparous women with lax abdominal wall. This is known as pendulous abdomen or anterior obliquity. In the primigravida, it is a sign of pelvic contraction.

Observation of *linea nigra* and *abdominal striae* are presumptive signs of pregnancy. Observation or palpation of fetal movement and hearing fetal heart sounds (FHS) are positive signs of pregnancy. The normal range of fetal heart tones is 120 to 160 per minute.

Determination of the lie, presentation, position and variety of the fetus varies in importance with the length of pregnancy. Prior to the 20th week of gestation, it is not possible to ascertain these informations because of the smallness of the fetus, the thickness of the uterus, and the high ratio of amniotic fluid to baby in the amniotic sac. The baby will continue to turn and somersault in the amniotic sac until the bulk of the baby's body is far greater than the amount of fluid and there is no longer room for the fetus to turn easily. By the 36th week, most babies have settled into what will be their lie and presentation for the intrapartal period. This is not absolute, however, as some babies will turn again. Malpresentation prior to 36 weeks is not a cause for concern because the baby is still turning. Malpresentation after this time, however, may be cause for possible concern and intervention. Lie, presentation, position and variety (anterior or posterior) are informations obtained by doing Leopold's maneuvers of abdominal examination by palpation.

Measurements of the Fundal Height (Table 15.1 and Fig. 15.1)

It provides information regarding the progressive growth of the fetus as a gross screening tool for detection of problems related to fundal height, which is too large or too small for the presumed gestational age by dates.

This method of assessment does not always produce an accurate result because the size and number of fetuses and the amount of amniotic fluid vary. A fundal height that is not increasing but remains the same over a period of time is ominous. Signs and symptoms of possible intrauterine fetal growth retardation or fetal death must be looked for and these possibilities ruled out.

The fundal height can be measured in one of three methods. All have an inherent degree of inaccuracy because each depends on the examiner's identifying the top of the fundus correctly.

First Method

The first method combines knowledge of where to expect the fundal height to be at various weeks of gestation in relation to the woman's symphysis pubis, umbilicus, and the tip of the xiphoid process and the use of the examiner's fingerbreadths as the measuring tool.

Table 15.1	Approximate expected locations of the fundal height at various weeks of gestation
Weeks of gestation	*Approximate expected location of fundal height*
12	Level of the symphysis pubis
16	Half way between symphysis pubis and umbilicus
20	1–2 fingerbreadths below the umbilicus
22–24	1–2 fingerbreadths above the umbilicus
28–30	1/3 of the way between umbilicus and xiphoid process (3 fingerbreadths above the umbilicus)
32	2/3 of the way between umbilicus and xiphoid process (3–4 fingerbreadths below the xiphoid process)
38	Level of the xiphoid process
40	2-3 fingerbreadths below the xiphoid process if lightening occurs

Fig. 15.1: Approximate height of the fundus as the uterus enlarges

In order to determine the height of the fundus, the midwife places her hand just below the xiphisternum pressing gently she moves her hand gently down the abdomen until she feels the curved upper border of the fundus. She notes the number of fingerbreadths, which can be comfortably accommodated between the two.

This method of measuring the fundal height combines a knowledge of where to expect the fundal height to be at various weeks of gestation in relation to the woman's symphysis pubis, umbilicus and tip of the xiphoid process and the use of the examiner's fingerbreadths as the measuring tool. Though it is a time-honored method, it has inherent inaccuracies. First, there is considerable variation between women in the distance from their symphysis pubis to their xiphoid process and in the location of the umbilicus between these two points. Second, there is a considerable variation between examiners in the width of their fingers. For example, two fingerbreadth of a thick-fingered person can be the same as three fingerbreadths of a thin-fingered person.

Second Method

The caliper method of measuring fundal weight is probably the most accurate method of measuring the fundal height after the 22nd to 24th week of gestation. In order to use a caliper or external pelvimeter (Fig. 15.2), place one tip on the superior boarder of the symphysis pubis and the other tip at the top of the fundus. Both placements are in the abdominal midline. The measurement is then read on a centimeter scale located on an arc close to where the two ends of the calipers come together. The number of centimeters should be equal approximately to the week of gestation after about 22nd to 24th week of gestation.

Fig. 15.2: External pelvimeter

Third Method (Fig. 15.3)

Measuring fundal height with a tape measure is the most frequently used method for obtaining an exact measurement. It is probably the second most accurate method of measuring fundal height after 22nd to 24th week of gestation. The zero line of the tape measure is placed on the superior border of the symphysis pubis and the tape measure stretched across the contour of the abdomen to the top of the fundus. The abdominal midline is used as the line of measurement. In order to avoid error in locating the

Fig. 15.3: Measuring fundal height with tape measure
(*For color version see Plate 2*)

superior border, you must palpate for the symphysis pubis. The number of centimeters measured should be approximately equal to the weeks of gestation after about 22nd to 24th week of gestation.

All of the three methods described above have an inherent degree of inaccuracy because each depends on the examiner's identifying the top of the fundus correctly. Some unidentifiable point on the anterior slope of the fundus is often mistaken for the top of the fundus. This error can be avoided by doing the following:

Facing the woman's head, as she lies supine, place your hands on each lateral side of the uterus approximately midway between the symphysis pubis and the fundus. Ballotte the uterus between your hands with gentle pressure and, being sure to stay on the lateral portion of the uterus, palpate up to the fundus. As you near the top your hands will begin to come together and they will meet at the top of the fundus. Staying on the lateral portion of the uterus assures reaching the actual top of the fundus and keeping off its anterior slope.

ABDOMINAL PALPATION AND LEOPOLD'S MANEUVERS

The term abdominal palpation is often used to mean doing Leopold's maneuvers for determining fetal lie, presentation, position and engagement. While doing Leopold's maneuvers, other information is also obtained and further palpation may be involved than that strictly needed for doing Leopold's maneuvers. The following information is obtained from abdominal palpation.

- ❖ Evaluation of uterine irritability, tone, tenderness, consistency, and any contractility present
- ❖ Evaluation of abdominal muscle tone
- ❖ Detection of fundal movement
- ❖ Estimation of fetal weight
- ❖ Determination of fetal lie, presentation, position and variety
- ❖ Determination of whether the head is engaged.

Before performing abdominal palpation and Leopold's maneuvers, several preparatory steps are done (Table 15.2).

Inspection of the Abdomen

Before actual palpation, the abdomen should be inspected for what its contours can tell you about the fetal lie, presentation and position. Palpation then gives you further information with which to confirm or rule out this initial impression (Table 15.3).

Leopold's Maneuvers
(Figs 15.4A to D and Table 15.4)

There are four maneuvers starting at the fundus and ending at the pelvic brim. It is suggested that learners go through the steps sequentially due to the fact that, in this pattern, they form a thought process and create a mental image for determining fetal position that will most quickly aid in developing skill and accuracy. Consistently following an orderly

Table 15.2	Preparation for abdominal palpation

Preparatory steps of the procedure	Rationale
1. The woman's bladder should be empty.	1. A full bladder makes abdominal palpation very uncomfortable for the woman as pressure is applied to it. It is difficult to feel fetal structures beneath the bladder, thereby obscuring findings pertaining to the presenting part.
2. The woman's abdomen is completely exposed from just below the breasts to the symphysis pubis.	2. Complete exposure of the abdomen at one time is essential for visual observation of the contours of the abdomen. Expose no more than that necessary for examination.
3. The women's abdominal muscles should be relaxed. This is achieved by the following: a. Placing a pillow under her head and upper shoulders. b. Having her arms by her sides. c. Explaining what you will be doing. d. Helping her with relaxation breathing. e. Having her bend her knees slightly.	3. Palpation is difficult for both the woman and the examiner if the abdominal muscles are contracted. It is difficult for the examiner to feel the fetus and therefore leads to longer and more forcible palpation. This causes the woman discomfort and she tenses her muscles more. This is avoided by starting with relaxed abdominal muscles, with warm hands and with smooth and gentle, but firm palpation.
4. Be sure your hands are warm. If not, rub them together or dip in warm water.	4. Cold hands are uncomfortable to the woman. They may cause muscle contraction.
5. Before palpating, lightly rest your hands on the woman's abdomen. A good time for this is while you are explaining what you are going to do.	5. This action gives the woman an opportunity to adjust to and become acquainted to your touching her. Since this is not uncomfortable to her, the initial muscle-tightening reaction gets dissipated.
6. The technique of palpation is as follows: a. Use the flat palmar surface of your fingers for palpating, not your fingertips. b. Keep the fingers of your hands together. c. Apply smooth, deep pressure as firm as necessary to obtain accurate findings. d. Avoid any sudden movement, jabbing, poking, or prodding.	6. This technique is designed for the least possible discomfort for the woman and the gathering of the greatest amount of information for the examiner.

Table 15.3   Inspection of abdomen

Observations	Significance
1. A longitudinal ovoid, fundal height as expected for gestational age.	1. Indicative of a longitudinal lie.
2. A transverse ovoid, fundal height lower than expected for gestational age.	2. Indicative of a transverse lie.
3. Long smooth curve prominent on one side of the abdomen.	3. Indicative that the fetal back is on that side of the abdomen.
4. A saucer like depression just below the umbilicus and a bulge like a full bladder above the symphysis pubes.	4. Indicative of a posterior position.
5. Movement of fetal small parts all over the abdomen.	5. Indicative of a posterior position.

Figs 15.4A to D: Abdominal palpation: Leopold's maneuver: (A) First maneuver (Fundal palpation); (B) Second maneuver (Lateral palpation); (C) Third maneuver (Pawlik's grip/second pelvic grip); (D) Fourth maneuver (Pelvic palpation/first pelvic grip)

sequence will also aid in remembering to include all the maneuvers and gathering all necessary information. In doing the Leopold maneuvers, stand on the side of the bed, most convenient and comfortable for you. Right-handed people usually stand on the right side of the women.

The findings from the first and third maneuvers must be compared and final determination made of the lie and presentation before proceeding to the fourth maneuver. For a final determination of the fetal lie and presentation a combined Pawlik grip may be performed. In this, Pawlik's grip is done with

Table 15.4	Abdominal palpation: Leopold's maneuvers

Procedure steps	Findings and significance
1. *First maneuver/Fundal palpation* (Fig. 15.4A) • Face the woman's head. Place both hands on the woman's fundus and curve the fingers around the top of the fundus. • Palpate for shape, size, consistency and mobility of the fetal part in the fundus.	• Fetal parts, that feel round and hard which are readily movable and ballotable between fingers of two hands is indicative of fetal head. The mobility is due to the head being able to move independently of the trunk. The lie is longitudinal. • Fetal part that feels irregular, large or bulkier, and less firm than a head, which cannot be readily moved or balloted, is indicative of fetal breech. The breech cannot move independently of the trunk. The lie is longitudinal. • If neither of the above is felt in the fundus, it is indicative of transverse lie.
2. *Second maneuver/lateral palpation* (Fig. 15.4B) • Continue to face the woman's head. Place your hands on both sides of the uterus about midway between the symphysis pubis and the fundus. • Apply firm gentle pressure with one hand against the side of the uterus, thereby pushing the fetus to the other side of the abdomen and with your examining hand, stabilizing it there. Maintaining pressure on one side, palpate the other side of the uterus. • With the examining hand, palpate the entire area from the abdominal midline to the lateral side and from the symphysis to the fundus. Use firm, smooth pressure and rotary movement. • Reverse the procedure for examination of the other side of the uterus.	• A firm convex, continuously smooth and resistant mass extending from the breech to the neck is indicative of the fetal back. The location of the back in the left or right side of the woman's abdomen determines the position in a longitudinal lie. • Small knobby, irregular masses, which move when pressed or may kick or hit your examining hand is indicative of the small parts—hands, feet, knees and elbow. • These should be felt in the opposite side of the abdomen than the side where the fetal back is in. • Small parts all over the abdomen and the fetal back difficult to feel as it may seem just out of reach in the posterior portion of the abdomen is indicative of a posterior position.
*3. *Third maneuver/Pawlik's maneuver/second pelvic grip* (Fig. 15.4C) • Continue to face the woman's head. Have her to bend her knees in order to avoid discomfort during this maneuver. • Grasp the portion of the lower abdomen immediately above the symphysis pubis between the thumb and middle finger of one of your outstretched hands. Press gently into the abdomen in order to feel the presenting part below and between your thumb and finger. • As in the first maneuver, palpate for size, shape, consistency and mobility in order to differentiate if it is the head or breech in the lower pole of the abdomen.	• A movable mass will be felt if the presenting part is not engaged. • If the presenting part is the head that is engaged, it may not be readily movable.
*4. *Fourth maneuver/Pelvic palpation/first pelvic grip* (Fig. 15.4D) • Turn and face the woman's feet. • Make sure that the woman's knees are bent to avoid pain during the maneuver. • Place your hands on the sides of the uterus with the palms of your hands just below the level of the umbilicus and your fingers directed towards the symphysis pubis. • Press deeply with your fingertips into the lower abdomen and move them towards the pelvic inlet. • Continue to move your hands towards the pelvic inlet.	• If the head is the presenting part, one of your hands will make contact with a hard round mass while your other hand continues in the direction of the pelvis. This is the cephalic prominence and if it is on the same side of the woman as the fetal back, the prominence is occiput and indicates a face presentation with the head extended. • If the cephalic prominence is on the same side of the woman as are the fetal small parts, it is the sinciput and indicates a vertex presentation with the head well flexed. If both hands will encounter simultaneously a hard mass, which is equally prominent on both sides, it is indicative of brow presentation due to partial flexion of the head. The occiput and sinciput are felt at the same time.

Contd...

Contd...

	• At the brim of the pelvis your hands will *converge* around the presenting part with the fingertips of your two hands touching in the midline indicating the presenting part is not engaged. It is above the pelvic brim or floating.
	If the presenting part is the breech, it will be readily movable.
	• The hands will *diverge* away from the presenting part and the midline indicating the presenting part is either engaged or dipping.
• Share your findings with the woman.	If the presenting part is the breech it will have a feeling of give along with the trunk of the fetus.
• Offer to help her feel and identify various fetal parts if she would like to.	• If you are unable to feel the cephalic prominance because it is out of reach in the pelvis, the head is engaged.

Note: *Leopold's maneuvers 3 and 4
• Performing the 3rd maneuver/Pawlik's grip/second pelvic grip, following lateral palpation (2nd maneuver), enables the midwife to complete this stage without taking her hands off the woman's abdomen and still facing her head.
• Performing the 4th maneuver/pelvic palpation/first pelvic grip, following the 3rd maneuver enables the midwife to change her position to face the woman's feet and place her hands with fingers directed towards the woman's symphysis pubis in order to palpate and feel the degree of flexion and descend of fetal presenting part.
  The maneuver that might give more discomfort to the client is then performed last

one hand and the fundus is grasped in the same way with the other hand at the same time. This combination enables you to compare simultaneously what are in the two poles for final determination of the fetal lie and presentation.

Auscultation (Fig. 15.5)

Auscultation usually forms part of each abdominal examination and follows any procedure in order to assess fetal well-being. Abdominal palpation determining the lie, presentation and position of the fetus enable you to locate the fetal heart tones. This is because the sound of the fetal heart is transmitted through the convex portion of the fetus closest to the anterior uterine wall. Therefore, the fetal heart tones are best heard through the fetal back in vertex and breech presentations and through the chest in face presentations. Thus, if you know the position you can readily locate the fetal heart tones, allowing for some variation depending on the amount of descend of the fetus into the pelvis.

Conversely, location of the fetal heart tones is an additional piece of data that serves to confirm or question your diagnosis of the fetal position. If you find the fetal heart tones loudest in a location different from where you expect

Fig. 15.5: Auscultation of the fetal heart sounds

to find them, then the question is raised, if you were in error in findings or in your interpretation of your findings from abdominal palpation.

Like all heartbeats, it is a double sound but more rapid than the adult heart. Pinard's fetal stethoscope (Fig. 15.6) is commonly used to hear the fetal heart. It is placed on the mother's abdomen and at right angles. The

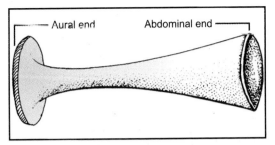

Fig. 15.6: Pinard's fetal stethoscope

Table 15.5	Location of fetal heart tones in various fetal presentations and positional varieties
Presentations and positional varieties	*Location*
• Cephalic	• Midway between umbilicus and level of anterosuperior iliac spine.
• Breech	• At the level or above umbilicus.
• Anterior	• Close to abdominal midline.
• Transverse	• In lateral abdominal area.
• Posterior	• In flank area or close to abdominal midline on other side of abdomen.

Fig. 15.7: Ultrasonic Doppler device
(*For color version see Plate 2*)

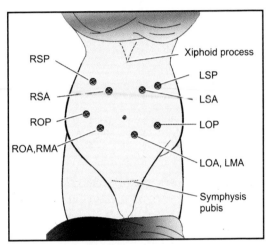

Fig. 15.8: Location of the point of maximum intensity of the fetal heart tones for specific fetal positions

ear must be in close, firm contact with the stethoscope, but the hand should not touch it while listening because extraneous sounds are produced. The fetal stethoscope (fetoscope) should be moved about until the point of maximum intensity is located where the fetal heart is heard more clearly. In recent times, increasingly, ultrasound equipment such as ultrasonic Doppler device (Fig. 15.7) and fetal monitor are used for this purpose. When the monitor is used the woman may also hear the fetal heartbeat.

In a full-term infant with an unengaged presenting part, the fetal heart tones are best heard in the following locations in relation to presentations and positions (Table 15.5) (Fig. 15.8).

The nurse-midwife in making her diagnosis must assess all the information she had gathered from inspection, palpation and auscultation, and draw the conclusion, which accounts for all the factors. If one factor does not fit in with the rest she must think again.

Other Findings

Gestational Age

During pregnancy uterine size will usually equate with the gestation estimated by dates (*see* Table 15.1). Later in pregnancy, increasing uterine size gives evidence of continuing fetal growth but is less reliable as an indicator of gestational age.

Multiple pregnancy increases the overall uterine size and should be diagnosed by 24th week of gestation. In a singleton pregnancy the fundus reaches the umbilicus at 22nd to 24th week and the xiphisternum at 36th week. In the last month of pregnancy lightening occurs and the fetus sinks down into the lower pole of the uterus. The uterus becomes broader and the fundus lower.

Lie

Lie is the relationship of the long axis of the fetus to the long axis of the uterus. There are three possible lies—longitudinal, transverse and oblique (Fig. 15.9).

In 95 percent of cases the lie is longitudinal owing to the ovoid shape of the uterus; the remainder are oblique or transverse. Oblique lie that results when the fetus is diagonally across the uterus must be distinguished from obliquity of the uterus, when the whole uterus is tilted to one side (usually right) and the fetus lies longitudinally within it. When the lie is transverse the fetus lies at right angles across.

Presentation

Presentation refers to the part of the fetus, which lies at the pelvic brim or in the lower pole of the uterus. This is the first portion of the fetus to enter the pelvic brim or inlet. There are three possible presentations—cephalic, breech and shoulder. The first two are further subdivided—Cephalic into vertex, sinciput, brow and face, and Breech into frank, full (or complete) and footling, which can be single or double (Figs 15.10A to F).

When the head is well flexed the vertex presents; when it is fully extended the face presents and when partially extended the brow presents. It is common for the head to present because the bulky breech finds more space in the fundus, which is the widest diameter of the uterus and the head lies in the narrower lower pole.

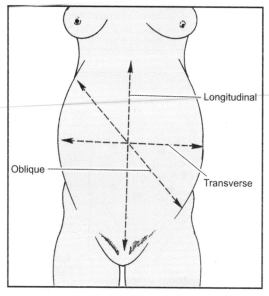

Fig. 15.9: The fetal lie

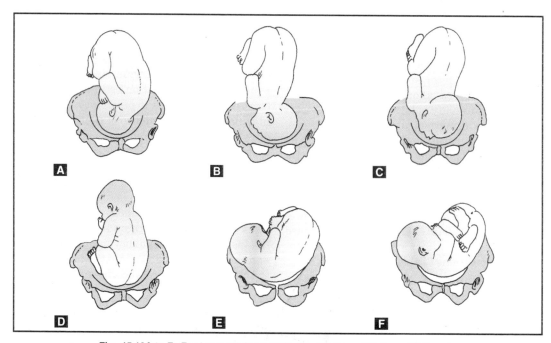

Figs 15.10A to F: Fetal presentations: (A) Vertex; (B) Brow; (C) Face; (D) Breech; (E) Shoulder—dorsoanterior; (F) Shoulder—dorsoposterior

Figs 15.11A to D: Attitude of the fetus in vertex, brow and face presentations:(A) Vertex well–flexed head; (B) Vertex deflexed head; (C) Brow military attitude; (D) Face extended head

Attitude

Attitude is the relationship of the fetal head and limbs to its trunk. The attitude of the fetus varies according to its presentation. For example, a fetus in a vertex presentation has a well-flexed head, flexion of the extremities over the thorax and abdomen, and a convex curved back; while a fetus with a face presentation has a head, which is acutely extended, flexion of the extremities on the thorax and abdomen, and a vertebral column which not only is straightened but also has some degree of arching. Flexion of the fetal head enables the smallest diameters to present to the pelvis and results in an easier delivery (Figs 15.11A to D).

Denominator

The denominator is the name of the part of the presentation that is used when referring to fetal position. Each presentation has a different denominator, which are as follows:

❖ *Occiput* in vertex presentation
❖ *Sacrum* in breech presentation
❖ *Mentum* in face presentation
❖ *Acromion process* in shoulder presentation.

In brow presentation no denominator is used.

Position

Position is the arbitrarily chosen point on the fetus for each presentation in relation to the left or right side of the mother's pelvis. It is also expressed as the relationship between the denominator and six points on the pelvic brim (Figs 15.12A to F).

Figs 15.12A to F: Diagrammatic presentation of six positions of the vertex: (A) ROT; (B) LOT; (C) ROA; (D) LOA; (E) ROP; (F) LOP

Anterior positions are more favorable than posterior positions because when the fetal back is in front, it conforms to the concavity of the mother's abdominal wall and can therefore flex

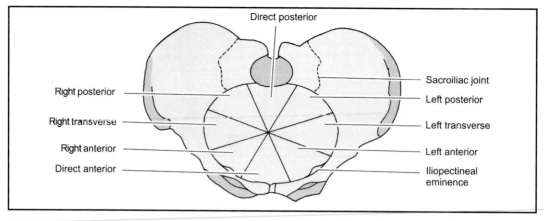

Fig. 15.13: Segments of pelvis showing positions of fetus

Table 15.6	Possibilities of fetal relationship to the maternal pelvis (positions)	
Lie	*Presentation*	*Position and variety*
Longitudinal	Cephalic Vertex	Left occipitoanterior (LOA), Right occipitoanterior (ROA) Left occipitotransverse (LOT), Right occipitotransverse (ROT) Left occipitoposterior (LOP), Right occipitoposterior (ROP)
	Sinciput, brow	These two usually convert to either vertex or face presentation
	Face	Left mentoanterior (LMA), Right mentoanterior (RMA) Left mentotransverse (LMT), Right mentotransverse (RMT) Left mentoposterior (LMP), Right mentoposterior (RMP)
	Breech; frank, full and footling	Left sacroanterior (LSA), Right sacroanterior (RSA) Left sacrotransverse (LST), Right sacrotransverse (RST) Left sacroposterior (LSP), Right sacroposterior (RSP)
Transverse	Shoulder	Left acromion anterior (LAA), Right acromion anterior (RAA) Left acromion posterior (LAP), Right acromion posterior (RAP)
Oblique		Nothing is felt at the inlet. There is no presentation, position or variety associated with this lie. An oblique usually is a transitory condition.

better. When the back is flexed, the head also tends to flex and a smaller diameter presents to the pelvic brim. There is more room in the anterior part of the brim for the broad biparietal diameter of the head.

Engagement

Engagement is said to have occurred when the widest presenting transverse diameter of the fetal part has passed through the brim of the pelvis (Fig. 15.13). In head presentations this is biparietal diameter. Engagement is an important sign that the maternal pelvis is adequate for the particular fetus and that a vaginal delivery may be expected (Table 15.6).

In a primigravid woman, the head normally engages between about the 36th and 38th week of pregnancy but in a multipara, this may not occur until after the onset of labor.

When the vertex presents and the head is engaged the following will be evident on clinical examination.
- ❖ The head is not mobile
- ❖ Less than half the head is palpable above the brim
- ❖ The anterior shoulder is little more than 5 cm above the brim

If the head is not engaged, the findings are as follows:
- ❖ More than half the head is palpable above the brim
- ❖ The head may be high and freely movable
- ❖ The sinciput may be 7.5 cm above the brim.

If the head remains unengaged in a primigravid woman at 38th week, the possibility of cephalopelvic disproportion should be ruled out.

Transverse and oblique lies in labor are abnormal conditions and they require cesarean

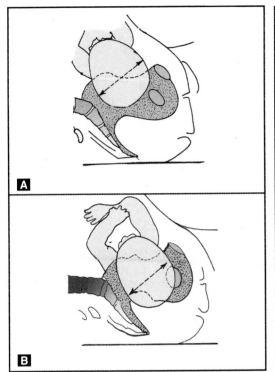

Figs 15.14A and B: Engagement of fetal head, diagrammatic presentation: (A) Head fixed, not engaged; (B) Head engaged

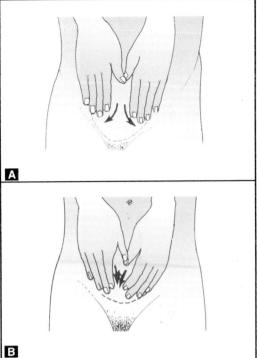

Figs 15.15A and B: Pelvic palpation: (A) Fingers diverge when head is engaged; (B) Fingers converge when head is not engaged

section. Approximately 0.5 to 3.5 percent of women will enter labor with a breech presentation and 0.5 percent with a face presentaion (Varney, 1996).

Although the breech of the fetus (podalic pole) is smaller than the fetal head (cephalic pole), the combination of the breech and the flexed lower extremities is bulkier because the flexed lower extremities are kept close to the breech (Figs 15.14A and B).

Pelvic Examination

A complete pelvic examination is done during the initial antepartal examination. This includes speculum examination, bimanual, and retrovaginal examination as well as evaluation of the bony pelvis for assessment of pelvic capacity (Figs 15.15A and B).

Ongoing Antenatal Care

All the information gathered during the first visit will enable a decision to be made for subsequent visits. The timing and number of visits may vary for different mothers depending on the risk factors identified during the initial

visit. Someone who develops complications during pregnancy will have more frequent visits.

Each revisit consists of:
❖ A chart review
❖ A history and physical examination geared toward evaluation of the well-being of mother and fetus
❖ A speculum and/or pelvic examination when indicated
❖ Laboratory and adjunctive studies when indicated
❖ Explanations and teaching appropriate to the patient's needs and her baby's gestational age.

NURSING PROCESS FOR THE ANTENATAL MOTHER

Step 1: Collection of the Database

Data may be collected from the following:
❖ Chart review for evaluation of preceding concerns and their management

❖ History of any symptoms of complications or discomforts, use of medicines, and any medical care

❖ Physical examination

❖ Pelvic examination

❖ Laboratory studies.

Step 2: Interpretation of Database

Interpretation of database to identify the client's problems and needs to:

❖ Determine normality

❖ Identify discomforts and possible complications

❖ Identify signs and symptoms of complications.

Step 3: Development of a Comprehensive Plan of Care

Development of a comprehensive plan of care, includes the following components:

❖ Measures for dietary re-evaluation and intervention

❖ Instructional measures for meeting learning needs

❖ Measures for relief of any discomfort

❖ Measures for treatment of minor complications (e.g. vaginitis, urinary tract infection, anemia)

❖ Measures for referrals to other health professionals (e.g. nutritionist, social worker)

❖ Measures for special counseling or anticipatory guidance by the physician

❖ Schedule for the next revisit.

Revisits for a woman who is progressing normally through her pregnancy are usually scheduled as follows:

❖ Up to 28th week of gestation: Every 4 weeks

❖ Between 28th and 36th week: Every 2 weeks

❖ Between 36th week and delivery: Every week.

Though there is a general pattern recommended for prenatal visits to the clinic, if the mother develops any risk factors during pregnancy, she must be advised to visit more frequently.

Risk Factors

Following risk factors can arise during the course of pregnancy:

❖ Change in fetal movement pattern

❖ Weight loss or poor weight gain

❖ Proteinuria, glycosuria

❖ Hypertension

❖ Uterus large or small for dates

❖ Excess or decreased liquor

❖ Malpresentation

❖ Head not engaged by 38 weeks in primigravid women

❖ Vaginal bleeding

❖ Vaginal or urinary infection

❖ Premature labor.

Record Keeping

In order to evaluate the effectiveness of advice and treatment during prenatal period, good record keeping is essential. Legibly written and signed entries are important for different health workers to know the well-being of mother and baby.

Indicators of Fetal Well-being

❖ Increasing maternal weight in association with increasing uterine size compatible with the gestational age of the fetus

❖ Fetal movements which follow a regular pattern throughout pregnancy

❖ Fetal heart rate between 110 and 150 beats per minute.

Evidence of at least ten movements a day is considered normal. The movements are usually observed for 12 hours starting at 9 am. The same time period should be used each day to allow for comparison. If the fetus takes longer time to achieve these ten movements, this indicates that the fetus is becoming compromised *in utero*. It is important that the woman is asked to seek help if the fetus has not moved ten times in the twelve hours labor period or if its pattern of activity changes greatly (fetal activity is often greatest during late afternoons). She should not wait for the next clinic appointment.

Preparation for Labor

During the last weeks of pregnancy, labor should be discussed with the mother. A woman who has decided to give birth at home must be visited by the public health nurse or the female health worker to help her make the final arrangements. Most women choose hospital delivery and they should be explained how to recognize the onset of labor, emphasizing the normal pattern of events, with clear instructions as to when they should reach the hospital.

BIBLIOGRAPHY

1. Das S. Antenatal Care. In: Bennett RV, Linda KB (Eds). Myles Textbook for Midwives, 13th edn. Edinburgh: Churchill Livingstone; 1999.
2. Dutta DC. Textbook of Obstetrics, 5th edn. Calcutta: New Central Book Company; 2001.
3. Park K. Park's Textbook of Preventive and Social Medicine, 16th edn. Jabalpur: M/s Banarasidas Bhanot Publishers; 2000.
4. Varney Helen. Nurse-Midwifery, 2nd edn. Boston: Jones and Barlett Publishers; 1996.

16 Specialized Investigations and Fetal Evaluation in the Antenatal Period

Learning Objectives

Upon completing this chapter, the learner will be able to:

❖ Describe the screening methods for congenital abnormalities
❖ Discuss the technologies used to screen and diagnose anomalies of the fetus
❖ Describe the procedures for fetal evaluation in the antenatal period.

The fetal evaluation measures are used when the fetus is suspected of being at risk. Because many of them are expensive or carry with them an element of risk in the procedure involved, or both, the value of their use must be weighed against any possible risk and the expense in each given situation.

ULTRASONOGRAPHY

Ultrasound is the production of high frequency sound waves which are reflected or echoed when beamed into the body and an interface is encountered between different types of tissues or structures with different densities. These echoes can be translated into visible images of the tissues or structures encountered. When the transducer, which transforms electrical energy to sound is placed on the body, a sound wave passes into the body and encounters a structure; a fraction of that sound is reflected back. The amount of sound from each organ varies according to the type of tissue encountered.

❖ Strong echoes give bright white dots, for example bone

❖ Weaker echoes give various shades of gray according to their strength
❖ Fluid-filled areas cause no reflexion and give rise to a black image.

The procedure is simple and painless. Prior to 20th week of gestation, it is necessary to have a full bladder for the procedure.

Diagnostic Uses in Obstetrics

1. *Early pregnancy*: Pregnancy can be diagnosed by ultrasound by 5th week of gestation.
2. Ectopic pregnancy.
3. *Hydatidiform mole*: Produces a characteristic image of scattered echoes. Diagnosis is reliable to the exclusion of other tests.
4. *Gestational age and fetal maturity*: An approximated fetal age is determined by using specific measurements at different stages:
   ❖ At 5 to 10 weeks, by measuring the gestational sac
   ❖ At 8 to 14 weeks, by measuring the crown-rump length—This is the length of the embryo from the top of the head to the rump or base of the sacrum
   ❖ At 14 to 20 weeks, by measuring the length of the femur
   ❖ At 18–26 weeks, by measuring the biparietal diameter
   ❖ The fetal head is demonstrable by ultrasound by the 12th week of gestation.
5. *Multiple gestation:* Multiple gestation may be diagnosed as early as first trimester.
6. Localization of placenta:
   ❖ Aids in diagnosis of third trimester bleeding

❖ Useful to locate placenta prior to amniocentesis.

7. *Fetal anomalies*: A number of fetal anomalies can be identified including, abnormalities of the head and spine, the genitourinary tract, gastrointestinal defects, cardiac, thoracopulmonary and musculoskeletal anomalies.

8. *Fetal death*: Separation and overlapping of skull bones will be evident (Spalding's sign).

9. Estimated fetal weight.

10. Fetal lie and presentation.

11. Intrauterine growth retardation.

12. *Polyhydramnios*: Indicated by a large intrauterine space that projects no echos.

13. Oligohydramnios.

14. *Placental grading*: Used for estimating fetal maturity and fetal pulmonary maturity.

15. *Biophysical profile*: This is used to evaluate the fetal well-being, e.g. in postdated pregnancy:
    ❖ Biparietal diameter
    ❖ Fetal movement
    ❖ Respiratory movements
    ❖ Amniotic fluid volume
    ❖ Height-weight ratio (Ponder's index)
    ❖ Heart rate pattern.

16. Localization of intrauterine contraceptive devices.

Ultrasonography is reliably replacing former diagnostic methods, especially roentgenography as a far safer methodology. Ultrasound does not carry the known risks that accompany irradiation. Ultrasonography is still in its developmental period and data are inconclusive about any adverse or long-term effects, which would develop or evidence themselves years later.

AMNIOCENTESIS AND AMNIOTIC FLUID STUDIES

Amniocentesis is the aspiration of amniotic fluid by way of a needle passed transabdominally into the gestational (amniotic) sac. The technique of amniocentesis can also be used for the injection of solutions into the amniotic sac. It is generally not possible to perform an amniocentesis until the second trimester, when the uterus has enlarged to become readily accessible to abdominal organ and the entire uterine cavity is filled with the amniotic sac. This change occurs when the chorionic laeve fuses with the decidua parietalis around the uterine cavity other than the site of implantation, at approximately the third or fourth month of gestation.

The ratio of amniotic fluid to fetus is high in the first trimester, about 3:2 by 20th week of gestation, and decreases thereafter as the fetus grows. The average fluid volume during the third trimester is 800 ml; this quantity decreases to around 450 ml by term and further decreases post-term.

Amniocentesis is performed by physicians and usually is indicated when the fetus is in jeopardy or suspected of being at high risk. The physician weighs the reason for performing amniocentesis against the risks involved in the technique. These include the following:

1. Perforation of the placenta or fetal placental vessels which may result in:
   a. Hemorrhage.
   b. Transfer of fetal cells, which could cause or aggravate isoimmunization and hemolytic disease in the newborn.
   c. Fetal death.

2. Infection which may result in:
   a. Maternal morbidity or mortality.
   b. Fetal or neonatal morbidity or mortality.

3. Abortion.

4. Premature labor or premature rupture of membranes.

5. Fetal trauma resulting from needle puncture.

6. Trauma to the umbilical cord or umbilical vessels.

7. Amniotic fluid leakage.

8. Hematoma.

The risk of amniocentesis is reduced when performed after the 20th week of gestation. RhoGAM is given to Rh-negative women when the amniotic fluid is bloody and there is the possibility of an Rh-positive fetus.

Early in pregnancy, amniotic fluid is light yellow or straw-colored with slight turbidity. It then becomes essentially colorless and clear, reflecting light and containing white particulate matter (*vernix caseosa*). The color of the amniotic fluid thus may indicate conditions or diseases even before definite testing is done. The following are examples:

1. *Opaque with green-brown discoloration:* May be thick depending on the amount of meconium in the amniotic fluid. May indicate fetal distress.
2. *Yellow with slight turbidity:* Colored by products of hemolysis especially bilirubin. May indicate hemolytic disease of the newborn.
3. *Opaque with some degree of dark red:* Indicates the presence of blood in the amniotic fluid. May indicate perforation of a placental vessel.
4. *Opaque, yellow-brown fluid:* Referred to as tobacco juice characteristic of fetal intrauterine death.

Reasons for Amniocentesis

1. Diagnosis of genetic disorders or abnormalities. Early amniocentesis is done when ultrasound scan suggests a fetus having Down syndrome. Fetal cells can be extracted from very small amounts of fluid and used to determine the karyotype. If a fetal abnormality is detected and the mother wishes to terminate the pregnancy, it can be undertaken at an early stage.
2. Maternal illness, which may affect the fetus, for example, rubella infection.
3. Parents being carriers of genetic disease, for example, cystic fibrosis.
4. Suspected infection of the fetus, for example, toxoplasmosis.
5. Assessment of lecithin-sphingomyelin ratio to determine fetal maturity.
6. Determination of the severity of fetal hemolytic disease (erythroblastosis fetalis).
7. Determination of fetal maturity by measurement of the creatinine level in the amniotic fluid.

Technique of Amniocentesis

An ultrasound examination is performed, the placenta localized, and a pool of liquor is found. The woman's bladder should be empty and strict asepsis to be observed throughout the procedure. The skin is cleaned and dried and the physician inserts a needle and a stilette through the abdominal wall into the uterus under direct ultrasound guidance. The needle is inserted under direct ultrasound visualization into the pool of liquor identified, so that the tip is seen to be in the center of the pool. The needles most commonly used are 20- or 22- gauge spinal needles. A local anesthetic may be used, but is not always considered necessary. 10 to 20 ml of amniotic fluid is withdrawn for analysis or a smaller amount if the amniocentesis is performed in the first trimester.

Following the procedure, the fetal heart must be auscultated, if necessary with a sonicaid, or demonstrated on scan.

Diagnostic Studies Possible with Amniotic Fluid

1. *Diagnosis of genetic disorders and abnormalities:* Amniocentesis for this purpose is done sometime between 14th and 18th week of gestation, when there is sufficient number of shed fetal cells in the fluid. For diagnosis of chromosomal abnormality, the amniotic fluid is centrifuged, the cells cultured and karyotyping done. For abnormalities caused by biochemical disorders, amniocentesis is done around the 20th week of gestation.

2. *Measurement of the lecithin-sphingomyelin (L/S) ratio:* The L/S ratio is used to determine fetal maturity. It is used to predict the potential development of respiratory distress syndrome (RDS), since lecithin is essential to preventing collapse of the alveoli during respiratory expiration after birth. Prior to the 34th week of gestation, lecithin and sphingomyelin are present in the amniotic fluid in approximately equal amounts. Thereafter, lecithin increases in relation to sphingomyelin when the proportion becomes 2:1 or 2:0, the chance of RDS is slight unless the mother is diabetic. An L/S ratio of 2, or above is considered indicative of a mature fetus.

3. *Determination of fetal maturity by the "rapid surfactant test":* It is also called the "shake test", or the "foam test". This test is used to determine

the amount of surfactant properties of lecithin present as an indicator of fetal maturity. This is determined by, whether or not there is a complete circle of foam or bubbles around the circumference of a test tube in which amniotic fluid has been shaken with ethanol and isotonic saline for 15 seconds and then allowed to sit for 15 minutes. A complete ring of bubbles is interpreted as fetal maturity.

4. *Determination of the severity of fetal hemolytic disease (erythroblastosis fetalis)*: It is done when the result of maternal indirect Coombs test is positive and an antibody titer indicates the possibility of severe hemolytic disease in the fetus.

ALPHA-FETOPROTEIN (AFP) TESTING

Alpha-fetoprotein testing is done to identify women at risk for having a baby with a neural tube defect (e.g. spina bifida, anencephaly) or a number of other congenital defects.

AFP is a normally occurring fetal protein. It is found in abnormally concentrated amounts in the amniotic fluid of a fetus with a neural tube defect and in the mother's blood. AFP testing is most accurate between 15th and 18th week of gestation. AFP testing is a sequence of tests. The first-two are of maternal serum and the final test is of amniotic fluid. An elevated AFP level is indicative of significant fetal pathology. A low level of AFP may be associated with Down syndrome. The normal AFP concentration in liquor amnii at the 16th week is about 20 mg/L.

AMNIOSCOPY AND FETOSCOPY

Amnioscopy and fetoscopy both involve direct visualization through the fetal membranes. In amnioscopy, the amniotic fluid is viewed through the fetal membranes at the cervical os. In fetoscopy, the fetus and placenta are visualized through the fetal membranes with an endoscope inserted through a small abdominal incision.

Amnioscopy can be done only when the cervix is fully dilated. It is possible that the membranes will be ruptured inadvertently during the procedure. It may also be uncomfortable for the woman. Amnioscopy may be done during late pregnancy in multiparas with patulous cervices, or during labor. Detection of meconium stained amniotic fluid indicates a probable episode of fetal hypoxia and need for a closely monitored delivery.

ESTRIOL LEVEL DETERMINATION

Normal estriol production is dependent on a physiologically normal fetus and placenta since the fetal adrenal gland provides the precursor for the production of estrogens by the placenta. Measurement of estriol in either blood or urine and comparison of the findings with the established normal values for the time in gestation, therefore, gives an indication of the functioning of the fetoplacental unit. The level of estriol increases throughout pregnancy, especially in the last trimester, to a peak at term. There is a wide range of normal values between women and further variation in the daily values of the same woman. Therefore, a series of values is needed in order to assess the well-being of the fetus and to determine whether there is any compromise in feto-placental functioning. Compromise is determined by a decrease in estriol as reflected in a curve of descending values from a series of measurements.

A value above 12 mg indicates fetal well-being. Values between 4 and 12 mg may indicate fetal jeopardy if late in pregnancy, with the probability of jeopardy being higher the closer the value is to 4 mg. Values below 4 mg indicate severe fetal jeopardy or even impending death of fetus.

Estriol series may be ordered when there is a potential concern such as in the following conditions.

- ❖ Postmaturity by dates
- ❖ Unsure dates and possibility of post-maturity
- ❖ Elderly primigravida
- ❖ Toxemia/hypertensive disorders of pregnancy
- ❖ Diabetes
- ❖ Intrauterine growth retardation
- ❖ Suspected fetal death

❖ Suspected fetal abnormality such as anencephaly.

FETAL BLOOD SAMPLING (CORDOCENTESIS)

This technique is used to take a sample of fetal blood during pregnancy in order to screen for chromosomal abnormalities, hemoglobinopathies and other disorders affecting blood or cells. Under ultrasound guidance, a needle is passed into the base of the umbilical cord and samples are drawn. These samples are then sent for fetal karyotyping.

FETAL EVALUATION PROCEDURES

Fetal Movement

Fetal movement is generally thought to be an indication of fetal well-being. The obvious and ideal person to count fetal movement is the mother; but two difficulties have been encountered. One is the variation in maternal sensitivity to fetal movements and the other is the wide range of factors, which affect fetal movement, sound, touch and external stimulation.

Therefore, parameters have been set for the lower limits of normal, within established time-periods during which the mother counts and records daily fetal movements. The lower limit of normal is generally agreed to be 10 movements in 12 hours. Fewer than this constitutes a movement alarm signal (MAS). If the mother's count results in MAS, she immediately reports this and a nonstress test (NST) and/or a contraction stress test (CST) is arranged. The absence of MAS correlates well with good outcomes in over 90 percent of mothers. When there is an MAS, special note must be made of any progressive decrease in fetal movement: Progressive decrease is ominous. A sudden or progressive fall in the movement count, even if it stays within normal range, may not be normal for a particular fetus and may be an indicator of fetal distress and impending death.

Nonstress Test (NST)

The nonstress test monitors the fetal heart rate in response to fetal movement in order to assess fetal well-being. It has the advantage of involving no external stimulation (e.g. oxytocin stimulation) in the conduct of the test. Because of this, it can be done for women for whom the CST might be contraindicated. Such women include those with previous cesarean section, placenta previa, or threatened premature labor. Otherwise, the indications for an NST are the same as those for CST. The other advantage is that its simplicity and absence of risk factors allow it to be done in an outpatient setting.

The preparation and positioning of the woman are the same as for the CST. The fetal heart rate is then monitored for approximately 20 to 30 minutes. It is important that the fetus not be in a fetal sleep state for the entirety of the test as sleep may cause decreased fetal heart rate variability. If necessary, an abdominal palpation can be used to rouse the fetus. During the test, the woman presses a button whenever she feels fetal movements which produce marks on the monitor strip so that fetal movements and fetal heart rate can be correlated.

Interpretation of the nonstress test is based on patterns of fetal heart rate reactivity to fetal movement. Normally the fetal heart rate decreases (within the normal range of 120 to 160 beats per minute) and variability increases with gestational age, probably in relation to the development of the central nervous system. The fetus normally has a transient accelerated heart rate with average baseline variability when moving or to external stimuli such as abdominal palpation. An abnormal fetal heart rate reactivity response to fetal movement is evidenced by a persistent reduction in baseline variability with an absence of fetal heart rate acceleration. This pattern may indicate a distressed fetus and occurs when the fetal central nervous system is depressed by drugs, hypoxia or acidosis.

A *reactive test* is one in which a normal fetal reactivity pattern is demonstrated. This is evidenced by fetal heart rate acceleration of 15 beats per minute above the baseline lasting for 15 to 30 seconds in association with fetal movement. Two or more occurrences of this acceleration pattern within a 10-minute period or five or more accelerations within a 20-minute period are considered normal. A normal fetus near term will also evidence a baseline fetal heart rate between 120 and 160 beats per minute, variability between 10 and 25 beats per minute and no deceleration of any type.

A *nonreactive test* is one in which there is a persistent decreased variability with an absence of accelerations in fetal heart rate in response to fetal movement. This is evidenced by fetal heart rate accelerations of less than 15 beats per minute above the baseline or lasting less than 15 seconds in association with fetal movement.

A *suspicious (equivocal) nonstress test* is one in which there are definite fetal heart rate accelerations associated with fetal movements but the number of accelerations, the increase in beats per minute above the baseline, or the length of their duration does not meet the criteria for being either reactive or non-reactive.

A reactive test indicates fetal well-being and predicts a good outcome if birth were to occur within one week. If the test is non-reactive, further assessment of fetal status should be initiated to aid in determining fetal well-being. If the test is suspicious, it should be repeated in 24 to 48 hours. The nonstress test can be repeated or continued at any desired frequency without concern for adverse effects to the fetus.

Contraction Stress Test (CST)

Contraction stress test assesses fetal placental functioning and the fetus's projected ability to cope with the continuation of a high-risk pregnancy and the stress of labor. It aids the physician in selecting the optimal time for delivery of a high-risk fetus. The underlying physiological and technological bases for the CST are as follows:

1. Contractions decrease the blood flow through the intervillous space.
2. If the uteroplacental reserve is normal, this intermittent decrease in blood flow by contractions will not negatively affect the fetus.
3. If the uteroplacental reserve is diminished or suboptimal, the intermittent decrease in blood flow by contractions will affect the fetus.

4. This negative effect on the fetus is reflected as a fetal heart pattern of late deceleration.
5. A fetal heart pattern of late deceleration is thought to be due to uteroplacental insufficiency.

CST is a test that ascertains the fetus's response to contractions—Naturally occurring, or induced by nipple stimulation or oxytocin—By using external fetal monitoring to record simultaneously the fetal heart rate and the uterine contractions.

Some of the conditions in which a CST might be helpful in selection of an optimal time for delivery include the following:

- Postmaturity—Suspected or actual
- Intrauterine growth retardation as suspected by a small for gestational age (SGA) fetus
- History of previous stillbirth
- Meconium stained amniotic fluid obtained at amniocentesis
- Falling or abnormal estriol values
- Diabetes
- Toxemia/hypertensive disorders of pregnancy
- Chronic hypertension
- Chronic lung disease
- Cyanotic heart disease
- Chronic renal disease
- Hyperthyroidism
- Collagen disease
- Severe isoimmunization
- Sickle cell disease or other hemoglobinopathies.

Procedure

The woman's bladder should be empty (to promote comfort and avoid disruption) and she should be in either a semi-Fowler's or left lateral position (to avoid supine hypotensive syndrome). Her blood pressure should be checked to obtain a baseline recording. There are two methods of inducing the contractions needed for a contraction stress test—Nipple stimulation and intravenous oxytocin administration.

Nipple Stimulation Test

Nipple stimulation causes the neurohypophysis to release endogenous oxytocin. This method of producing naturally occurring oxytocin avoids the risks, discomfort and expenses associated with the intravenous infusion of oxytocin. At the beginning of the test, warm washcloths are applied to the breasts. A & D ointment or K-Y lubricating jelly is applied to the nipples to prevent soreness. The woman then stimulates her nipples by either rolling them or gently pulling them. Stimulation is initially unilateral. If contractions are inadequate (fewer than three contractions in the first 10 minutes), the woman then simultaneously stimulates both nipples for another 10 minutes. If contractions are still inadequate, intravenous oxytocin is used. Nipple stimulation provides adequate contractions approximately in 75 percent of women using this method.

Oxytocin Challenge Test

The administration of oxytocin to induce contractions is called an oxytocin challenge test or oxytocin contraction test (OCT). A venipuncture is done, an intravenous line is established, and a very dilute solution of oxytocin, controlled by an infusion pump, is administered via a piggyback set up to another bag of intravenous solution. The rate of infusion is increased at intervals until the contractions are occurring at a frequency of at least three in a 10-minute period and lasting at least 30 seconds (preferably 40 to 60 seconds). The recording is then interpreted and the infusion stopped. Both the monitoring and the intravenous solution, without oxytocin in it, are continued until the contractions have diminished to their baseline activity. This is to assure that the OCT has not put the woman into labor without your knowing about it.

A negative CST is one in which no late decelerations occur with contractions as frequent as three in a 10-minute period. A negative CST indicates fetal well-being and predicts that the fetus will continue to be alright for another week without needing the intervention of delivery, if the woman's clinical status does not change. Negative CSTs are repeated weekly or sooner depending on the continuing clinical status.

A positive CST is one in which there have been repeated late decelerations of fetal heart rate patterns during the test. A positive CST indicates that the fetus may not withstand continuation of the pregnancy. Serious consideration needs to be given to immediate termination of the pregnancy by delivery. A positive CST is a valuable piece of information in decision-making but urge caution and encourage use of a total picture of assessment methods and clinical judgment, as there can be a 25 percent rate false-positive results.

Other Categories of Interpretation of CST

1. *Hyperstimulation,* in which the contractions are more frequent than 2 minutes or have a duration of more than 90 seconds. This is more apt to occur with the use of oxytocin than with nipple stimulation. Hyperstimulation renders the test invalid. The late decelerations in the presence of hyperstimulation may not be due to uteroplacental insufficiency. The test should be repeated within 24 to 48 hours with an even more dilute solution of oxytocin.
2. *Suspicious (equivocal),* in which there has been an occasional late deceleration but this is not repetitive and does not occur with continued contractions. The CST should be repeated within 24 to 48 hours.
3. *Unsatisfactory,* in which the recording (tracing) is not of good enough quality to be interpreted. This may be due to the problems inherent with external fetal monitoring.

BIBLIOGRAPHY

1. Das S. Antenatal Care. In: Bennett RV, Linda KB (Eds). Myles Textbook for Midwives, 13th edn. Edinburgh: Churchill Livingstone; 1999.
2. Dutta DC. Textbook of Obstetrics, 5th edn. Calcutta: New Central Book Company; 2001.
3. Park K. Park's Textbook of Preventive and Social Medicine, 16th edn. Jabalpur: M/s Banarasidas Bhanot Publishers; 2000.
4. Varney Helen. Nurse-Midwifery, 2nd edn. Boston: Jones and Barlett Publishers; 1996.

SECTION

5

Normal Labor

17

Physiology of the First Stage of Labor

Learning Objectives

Upon completion of this chapter, the learner will be able to:

❖ Define the term labor and describe the onset and stages of labor
❖ Describe the signs and symptoms of impending labor
❖ Enumerate the physiological changes in the uterus as labor progresses
❖ Explain the mechanical factors that contribute to the progress of labor
❖ Describe the assessment of a pregnant client for evaluation of maternal and fetal conditions
❖ Explain the procedure of vaginal examination and enumerate the probable findings.

The first stage of labor usually starts with the onset of regular uterine contractions and culminates in the complete dilatation of the cervix. There are number of premonitory signs and symptoms that may alert a midwife to a woman's approaching labor. A woman may exhibit any, all or none of these but it is useful to keep them in mind when seeing a woman late in pregnancy so that appropriate counseling, guidance and care can be given.

Definition of Labor

Labor may be defined as rhythmic contraction and relaxation of the uterine muscles with progressive effacement (thinning) and dilatation (opening) of the cervix, leading to expulsion of the products of conception (Clausen et al, 1973).

Labor is described as the process by which the fetus, placenta and membranes are expelled through the birth canal (Cassidy, 1999).

Labor can and does occur at any time during pregnancy but takes place most frequently at term, or about 40 weeks after the normal menstrual period.

Normal Labor

Normal labor occurs at term and is spontaneous in onset with the fetus presenting by the vertex. The process is completed within 18 hours and no complications arise (Cassidy, 1999).

The Three P's of Normal Labor

The labor process involves a relationship between the three P's: The *powers* or uterine contractions; the *pelvis* including the size and shape; and the *passenger*, which includes the size, position and presentation of the fetus as well as the bag of waters or amniotic sac. Normal labor assumes that the powers are sufficient, the pelvis is adequate and passenger is of average size and is in a normal position. Complications of labor occur when there are problems with one or more of the P's.

STAGES OF LABOR

Labor is divided into four stages:

The *first stage* is that of dilatation of cervix. It begins with regular rhythmic contractions (true labor) and is complete when the cervix is fully dilated and effaced.

The *second stage* is the stage of expulsion of the fetus. It begins with complete dilation of the cervix through complete birth of the baby.

The *third stage* of labor is that of separation and expulsion of the placenta and membranes. It lasts from the birth of the baby through the delivery of the placenta and membranes with contraction and retraction of uterus.

The fourth stage is the first four hours after delivery of the placenta. This is an arbitrary time during which, the vital signs must stabilize and any tendency for immediate hemorrhage must be controlled. This is a critical period for every mother.

The First Stage

The first stage of labor begins with the onset of regular contractions and ends when the cervix is fully dilated. The stage is divided into three phases: Latent, active and transition phases.

Latent Phase

The latent phase of labor begins with the onset of true labor contractions, which are usually mild. During this phase, contractions may be 15 to 20 minutes apart, lasting 20 to 30 seconds. As this phase progresses, however, the contractions will occur every 5 to 7 minutes and the duration will lengthen to 30 to 40 seconds. This phase usually begins with little or no cervical dilation and ends when the cervix is 3 to 4 cm dilated. For the primigravida, the latent phase lasts an average of 9 hours; whereas in the multigravida, the latent phase generally lasts an average of 5 hours. Although the woman may exhibit some anxiety during this phase, she often is comfortable enough to verbalize her concerns.

Active Phase

The active phase of labor begins when the woman is 3 to 4 cm dilated and ends when she is 8 cm dilated. During this phase, contractions occur every 3 to 5 minutes and last up to 60 seconds. The intensity of each contraction begins as moderate and continues to increase as the woman gets closer to transition phase. The average length of the active phase in the primigravida is 6 hours and in the multigravida 4 hours. Dilation rate should be at least 1.2 to 1.5 cm/hr.

Transition Phase

The last and shortest part of the first phase of labor is transition, which typically is the most intense phase for the laboring woman. In transition, contractions occur every 2 to 3 minutes lasting 60 to 90 seconds. The intensity of contractions is very strong in the transition phase. The woman often becomes restless and agitated, may have difficulty focusing during contractions. They hyperventilate, complain of nausea and vomiting, tremble and experience rectal pressure. During this time the nurse will need to prepare the women for the second stage of labor. The average length of transition phase is 2 hours in primigravidae and 1 hour in multigravidae.

Second Stage

The second stage of labor with the cervix completely dilated and effaced and ends when the fetus is expelled; it is also known as the expulsion stage. The average length of the second stage of labor in primigravida is 1 hour and in the multigravida 25 minutes. Many factors influence the length of the second stage of labor, including maternal parity, fetal size, uterine contractile force, presentation, position, pelvic size, method of anesthesia (if used), and magnitude of maternal expulsive effort. During contractions, the woman will bear down, causing the abdominal muscles to contract and helping the fetal head to descend though the birth canal. As the fetal head continues into the birth canal, the perineum begins to bulge. Crowning is defined as the point at which the fetal head is visible at the vulval opening. When crowning occurs, birth is imminent. At this time, women develop an urge to push. Some women describe intense pain and burning of the perineum as the pressure increases on the vulva. Nurses need to be aware of prolonged second stage of labor, because intervention may be required.

Third Stage

The third stage of labor or placental stage begins as soon as the fetus is delivered and lasts until the placenta is delivered. The mechanism of placental separation is a combination of uterine

Table 17.1 Average length of labor stages

Characteristic	First stage Latent phase	First stage Active phase	Transition phase	Second stage	Third stage	Fourth stage	Total duration
Primigravida	6–10 hrs	5–6 hrs	2 hrs	1–1½ hrs	10–15 min	1 hr	16–24 hrs
Multigravida	5 hrs	3–4 hrs 10–12 hrs	1–1½ hrs	25–30 min	10–15	1 hr	8–10 hrs
Cervical dilation	0–4 cm	4–8 cm	8–10 cm	---	---	---	---
Contractions frequency	15–20 min progressing to 5–7 min	3–5 min	2–3 min	1.5–2.0 min	---	---	---
Duration of contractions	10–20 sec progressing to 30–40 sec	40–60 sec	60–90 sec	60–90 sec	---	---	---
Intensity	Mild progressing to moderate	Moderate progressing to strong	Strong	Strong	---	---	---

contractions and involution. After expulsion of the fetus, the uterus continues to contract every 3 to 4 minutes. As the uterus contracts and begins the process of involution (reduction in size) shrinkage of the site of implantation of the placenta occurs. Within 10 to 15 minutes after delivery of the infant, most of the placenta gets detached from the uterine wall. At this point, vaginal bleeding from the uncovered implantation site increases, and delivery of the placenta generally follows.

The classic signs of placental separation are founding up of the uterus, upward movement of the fundus, lengthening of the umbilical cord, and a rush of blood from the vagina. Once the placenta is delivered, the uterus continues to contract, closing the spiral arterioles. As the uterus continues to shrink, the bleeding decreases.

Fourth Stage

The *fourth stage of labor* or recovery stage is defined as the first one hour after delivery of the placenta. During this time, many internal physiologic readjustments occur. The average blood loss from a vaginal delivery is 250 to 300 ml. Because of the blood loss and the return of a more normal abdominal anatomy as the uterus returns to a more normal size (involution), there is a decreased in blood pressure and pulse rate. The fundus is in midline and at the level of the umbilicus. The fundus should remain firm, contracted, and midline. Most of the discomforts of labor, such a nausea and vomiting should be subsiding.

Signs and Symptoms of Impending Labor

The signs and symptoms of impending labor are lightening, cervical changes, false labor, premature rupture of membranes, bloody show, energy-spurt, and gastrointestinal upsets. The last weeks of pregnancy during which these changes occur is termed as *prelabor*.

Lightening

Two to three weeks before the onset of labor, the lower uterine segment expands and allows the fetal head to sink lower. The baby's head,

if there is a cephalic presentation, usually is fixed or engaged afterwards. The symphysis pubis widens and the pelvic floor becomes more relaxed and softened, allowing the uterus to descend further into the pelvis.

In a primigravid woman when the abdominal muscles are in good tone, the uterus will be braced into an upright position, which helps the fetal head to engage. The increasing intensity of the Braxton Hick's contractions in late pregnancy may also contribute to lightening. In the multigravida the abdominal muscles tend to be more lax and as a result, the abdomen becomes somewhat pendulous so that the fetal head may not engage.

The woman will experience a decrease in the minor discomfort of shortness of breath she has had during the third trimester, because lightening will give her more room in the upper abdomen for lung expansion. However, lightening will cause other discomforts due to the pressure of the presenting part on structures in the area of the true pelvis. Specifically, she will have:

- ❖ Frequency of urination, because the bladder feels pressure and has less room for expansion
- ❖ An uncomfortable feeling of generalized pelvic pressure, which may make her feel awkward and produces the constant sensation that something needs to come out or that a bowel movement is needed
- ❖ Leg cramps, which may be caused by the pressure of the presenting part on the nerves that course through the foramen obturator and lead to the legs
- ❖ Increased venous stasis producing dependent edema because the pressure of the presenting part inhibits blood return from the lower extremities
- ❖ Vaginal secretion becomes more profuse at this time.

Lightening lowers the height of the fundus to a position similar to that of the eighth month of pregnancy, and the ballottement of fetal head is no longer possible.

The nurse's knowledge of lightening is of value in being able to reassure the woman of the normality of the bodily changes she is experiencing and explain why they are occurring. This also provides a good opportunity to review with the woman her plans for labor. It provides an indication of the adequacy of the pelvic inlet. Lightening tends to encourage the woman that the long-awaited end of pregnancy is within sight.

Cervical Changes

As labor approaches the cervix becomes "ripe". The cervix becomes softer, like the consistency of pudding, and evidences some degree of effacement and perhaps slight dilatation. Evaluation of ripeness is relative to the individual woman for example, a grand multipara's cervix may normally be 2 cm dilated as opposed to a Primigravida's normally closed cervix.

Ripeness indicates a readiness of the cervix for labor. It is of value in assuring the patient that she will go into labor with the onset of labor contractions and that the time of labor is relatively close.

False Labor

False labor consists of painful uterine contractions that have no measurable progressive effect on the cervix and are in actuality an exaggeration of the usually painless Braxton Hick's contractions, which have been occurring since about six weeks of gestation.

False labor may occur for days or intermittently even 3 to 4 weeks before the onset of true labor. False labor is genuinely painful and a woman may loose sleep and energy coping with it. She has no way of knowing for sure whether she is in true labor since this can be determined only by vaginal examination. Such women need a great degree of understanding, patience, support, reassurance and explanation from the midwife, as they may get frustrated of making trips to the hospital. False labor, however, does indicate the approach of labor.

Premature Rupture of Membranes

Normally the membranes rupture at the end of the first stage of labor. When rupture occurs before the onset of labor, it is termed as premature rupture of membranes and occurs in about 12 percent of women. Approximately 80 percent of women with premature rapture of membranes begin labor spontaneously within 24 hours.

Bloody Show

A mucus plug, created by cervical secretions from proliferation of the glands of the cervical mucosa early in pregnancy, serves the function of a protective barrier and closes the cervical canal throughout pregnancy. Bloody show is the expulsion of this mucus plug. Bloody show is most often seen as a tenacious, blood tinged mucus discharge, which must be carefully differentiated from frank bleeding. Bloody show is a sign of imminent labor, which usually takes place within 24 to 48 hours.

Energy Spurt

Many women experience an energy spurt approximately 24 to 48 hours before the onset of labor. After days or weeks of feeling tired (physically tied and tired of being pregnant) they get up one day to find themselves full of energy and vigor. Typically these women do lot of household tasks which they either have not had the energy to do or now feel need doing before the baby's arrival.

There is no known explanation for this energy spurt other than it is a nature's way of giving the woman the energy she needs for the work of labor. Women should be informed of the possibility of their having this energy spurt and advised to deliberately refrain from expending it and instead to conserve it for use during labor.

Gastrointestinal Upsets

In the absence of any causative factors for the occurrence of diarrhea, indigestion, nausea and vomiting, it is thought that they might be indicative of impending labor. No explanation for this is known, but some women do experience one to all of these signs.

Causes for the Onset of Labor

Theories regarding initiation of labor include the following:

❖ *Oxytocin stimulation theory*: Although the mechanism is unknown, the uterus becomes increasingly sensitive to oxytocin as the pregnancy progresses

❖ *Progesterone withdrawal theory*: A decrease in progesterone production may stimulate prostaglandin (PG) synthesis and enhance the effect of estrogen, which has a stimulating effect on uterine muscles

❖ *Estrogen stimulation theory*: Estrogen stimulates irritability of uterine muscles and enhances uterine contractions.

❖ *Fetal cortisol theory*: Cortisol may affect maternal estrogen levels.

❖ *Prostaglandin stimulation theory*: Prostaglandin stimulates smooth muscle to contract.

Labor is likely initiated by a combination of all the above mechanisms.

Fig. 17.1: Contraction and restraction of uterine muscle fibers during labor

PHYSIOLOGICAL PROCESSES IN THE FIRST STAGE OF LABOR

Uterine Action

Fundal Dominance

Each uterine contraction starts in the fundus near one of the cornua and spreads across and downwards. Each contraction is longest and intense in the fundus, but the peak is reached simultaneously over the whole uterus and fades from all parts together. This pattern permits the cervix to dilate and the fundus to expel the fetus.

Polarity

A neuromuscular harmony prevails between the two poles or segments of uterus throughout labor, which is termed as polarity. During each contraction, these two poles act harmoniously. The upper pole contracts stronger and retracts to expel the fetus; the lower pole contracts slightly and dilates to allow expulsion to occur. If polarity is disorganized, the progress of labor is inhibited.

Contraction and Retraction (Fig.17.1)

During labor the contraction does not pass off entirely, the muscle fibers retain some of the shortening of contraction instead of becoming completely relaxed. This is termed retraction, which is a unique property of the uterine muscle. Because of this, the upper segment of the uterus becomes gradually shorter and thicker and its cavity diminishes assisting in the progressive expulsion of the fetus.

When labor begins, uterine contractions occur every 15 to 20 minutes and may last for 30 seconds. They are weak to begin with and occur with rhythmic regularly and intervals between them gradually lessen while the length

and strength of the contractions gradually increase. By the end of first stage, they occur at 2 to 4 minute interval, last for 50 to 60 seconds and are very powerful.

Formation of Upper and Lower Uterine Segments

By the end of pregnancy, the body of the uterus has divided into two anatomically distinct segments—Upper and lower uterine segments. The upper uterine segment is mainly concerned with contraction, and is thick and muscular. The lower segment is prepared for distension and dilatation, and is thinner. The lower segment develops from the isthmus and is about 8 to 10 cm in length.

The Retraction Ring

A ridge forms between the upper and lower uterine segments, which is known as the retraction ring (Fig. 17.2). The physiological retraction ring gradually rises as the upper uterine segment contracts and retracts and the lower uterine segment thins out to accommodate the descending fetus. Once the cervix is fully dilated and the fetus can leave the uterus, the retraction ring rises no further.

The retraction ring is normally not visible over the abdomen. When the phenomenon is exaggerated in an obstructed labor, the retrac-

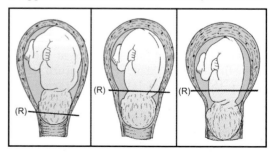

Fig. 17.2: Formation of retraction ring

tion ring becomes visible above the symphysis pubis; it is termed as *Bandl's ring*.

Cervical Effacement

Cervical effacement is defined as the thinning of the cervix and shortening of the cervical canal from its usual length of 2 to 3 cm to one in which the cervical canal is obliterated leaving only the external os as a circular orifice with thin edges.

This shortening results from the lengthening of the muscular fibers around the internal os as they are taken up into the lower uterine segment. Effacement is facilitated by the cleft like arrangement of the endocervix, which in effect unfolds like an accordion as it is stretched and taken up to become part of the lower uterine segment. The process of effacement is also facilitated by the expulsion of the mucus plug. Effacement is clinically evaluated in terms of percentages, e.g. 50 percent effaced, 80 percent effaced or completely effaced, which is often paper thin. The degree of effacement depends upon the examiner's evaluation and judgment, and the estimation varies among examiners. In the primigravida, this usually

Fig. 17.3: Dilatation and effacement of the cervix

occurs prior to the onset of labor, while in the multigravida, this occurs simultaneously with cervical dilatation (Fig. 17.3).

Cervical Dilatation

Dilatation of the cervix is the process of enlargement of the external cervical os from an orifice of a few millimeters to an opening large enough for the baby to pass through. Dilatation is effected primarily by the action of contractions and facilitated by the hydrostatic action of the amniotic fluid under the influence of contractions, causing the membranes to serve as a dilating wedge in the area of least resistance in the uterus. If the membranes have ruptured, the pressure of the presenting

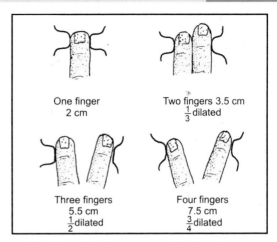

One finger 2 cm

Two fingers 3.5 cm $\frac{1}{3}$ dilated

Three fingers 5.5 cm $\frac{1}{2}$ dilated

Four fingers 7.5 cm $\frac{3}{4}$ dilated

Fig. 17.4: Clinical estimation of dilatation of cervix

part on the cervix and the lower uterine segment has a dilating effect.

Dilatation is clinically evaluated by measuring the diameter of the cervical opening in centimeters, with 0 centimeter being a closed external cervical os and 10 centimeters being complete dilatation (Fig. 17.4).

Because of the dilatation of the cervix, the operculum, which formed the cervical plug during pregnancy, is lost. This blood stained mucoid discharge is termed as the *show*. The blood comes from the ruptured capillaries in the parietal decidua where the chorion has become detached from the dilating cervix.

Ripening of the Cervix

The term "ripe" cervix is often used. It is believed that the Braxton Hick's contractions help prepare the cervix, or ripen it for the job ahead. The cervix moves from its posterior position during pregnancy to an anterior position, and the normally firm tissue softens considerably. The cervix may be described as "pudding soft", "butter soft", or "very pliable".

A certain number of contractions and time are required to first ripen the cervix and then to efface and dilate it.

Mechanical Factors that Contribute to the Progress of Labor in the First Stage

Formation of the Forewaters (Fig.17.5)

As the lower uterine segment stretches, the chorion becomes detached from it and the

Fig. 17.5: Formation of bag of membranes and forewaters

increased intrauterine pressure causes this loosened part of the sac of fluid, to bulge downwards into the dilating internal os, to the depth of 6 to 12 mm. The well-flexed head fits snugly into the cervix and cuts off the fluid in front of the head from that, which surrounds the body. The fluid in front of the head is termed *forewaters* and that which surrounds the body as *hindwaters*.

The effect of separation of forewaters is to keep the membranes intact during the first stage by preventing the pressure applied to the hindwaters during uterine contractions from being applied to the forewaters.

General Fluid Pressure

While the membranes remain intact, the pressure of the uterine contractions is exerted on the fluid and, as fluid is not compressible, the pressure is equalized throughout the uterus and over the fetal body, which is known as general fluid pressure. This equalization of pressure is lost when the membranes rupture and a quantity of fluid escapes causing compression of the placenta between the uterine wall and fetus during contractions lending to diminution of oxygen supply to the fetus. Preserving the integrity of the membranes, therefore, optimizes the supply of oxygen to the fetus and helps to prevent intrauterine infection.

Rupture of the Membranes

The physiological moment for the membranes to rupture is at the end of the first stage of labor when the cervix becomes fully dilated and no longer supports the bag of waters.

Spontaneous rupture of membranes may sometimes occur days or hours before labor begins or during the first stage. With a badly fitting presenting part, the forewaters are not cut off effectively and the membranes rupture early. In some cases, it happens without any apparent reason. It may sometimes rupture during the second stage just before the delivery of the head. Occasionally the membranes do not rupture even in the second stage and appear at the vulva as a bulging sac covering the fetal head as it is born; this is known as the *caul*.

Fetal Axis Pressure

During each contraction the uterus rears forward (becomes upright) and the force of the fundal contraction is transmitted to the upper pole of the uterus, down the long axis of the fetus and is applied by the presenting part to the cervix. This is known as fetal axis pressure. It becomes more significant after rupture of the membranes and during the second stage of labor.

Descent of the Presenting Part

Descent of the presenting part refers to the downward and outward movement of this part through the pelvis. The normal well-flexed head (vertex) twists and turns, flexes and extends to maneuvre through the pelvis just as one might twist and turn a hand and flex and extend the fingers to get the hand into a jar. There are three planes or obstacles involved in the process of descend—The pelvic inlet, the pelvic brim and the pelvic outlet. When the examiner can feel the presenting part at the level if the ischial spines, a midplane (pelvic brim) mark, it indicates the largest part of the head has come through the inlet. The head is thus

Fig. 17.6: Diagrammatic representation of the stations of presenting part stations of presenting part

engaged. The presenting part is now at zero (0) station. When the vertex has descended to the perineum, the largest part has passed the ischial spines, another obstacle. The head is now at + 2 station. Delivery of the head brings it past the third obstacle—The outlet, which is under the pubic arch, between the ischial tuberosities and over the coccyx. Station is the relationship of the lowermost part of the presenting part to an imaginary line drawn between the ischial spines of the woman's pelvis. The lowermost part at the level of the ischial spines is called a '0' station. Station is measured in terms of centimeters above or below the level of ischial spines with above being designated as –1, –2, –3, – 4, and –5 station, and below being designated as + 1, +2, +3, +4 and +5 station. A, –5 station, is equivalent to a floating head and a, +5 is equivalent to a head at the perineum (Fig. 17.6).

Station is at times difficult to ascertain if there has been considerable molding of the fetal skull and development of caput succidaneum. In cephalic presentation, the skull bones may be a centimeter or so higher than the caput, which is what an examiner's fingers may feel.

INITIAL ASSESSMENT AND DIAGNOSIS

When a woman presents herself for examination, thinking that she is in labor, the midwife needs to evaluate her possible labor status, assess the well-being of both mother and baby and screen for immediate complications. On the basis of these findings and other related factors, a decision of whether or not the woman is in labor or needs any medical help or intervention is made.

Evaluation of labor status refers to that information needed to determine whether a woman is in the progress of her labor and to anticipate her continued progress. Requirements for this are history, physical examination (general and abdominal) and pelvic (vaginal) examination. Steps of the evaluation process with the significance of each are explained below.

History

Age

An age under 16 or over 35 predisposes the woman to a number of complications.

Gravida and Para

Parity has an effect on both duration of labor and on the incidence of complications. A cervix which has been completely dilated in a previous labor offers less resistance to being dilated again, thereby shortening the length of labor. In addition multiparas have more relaxed pelvic floors, which offer less resistance to the passage of the baby and decreases the length of labor. However, in grand multiparas the duration of labor may be longer—Exhaustion of uterine muscle due to changes in the uterine musculature. Increased parity increases the incidence of complications.

Time of onset of contractions and the frequency and duration of the contractions: This information is necessary in order to establish the start of labor, usually timed from when the contractions became regular, and to differentiate between false and true labor. False labor contractions do not increase in frequency, duration and intensity; are irregular and are of short duration. True labor contractions may start as irregular and of short duration, but then become regular with increased frequency, duration and intensity.

Intensity of contractions when lying down contrasted to when walking around: This information helps to differentiate between true and false labor contractions. Walking intensifies true labor contractions, whereas false labor contractions are rarely intensified by walking and may actually be relieved.

Description of the location of discomfort or pain felt with contractions: This information also helps to differentiate between false and true labor contractions. False labor contractions are usually felt in the lower abdomen and groin. True labor contractions are usually felt as radiating across the uterus from the fundus to the back.

Length of previous labor: If a previous labor has been within the past few years, the length of that labor is a good indication of the potential length of this labor.

Number of years since the last baby: If there are a number of years between babies, a woman may have a length of labor more similar to her first one. If ten or more years have passed since her last baby, she is predisposed to prolonged labor and to the complications of antepartum hemorrhage and perinatal mortality.

Delivery method of previous deliveries: This is to rule out previous cesarean section and instrumental deliveries.

Size of the largest and smallest previous babies: The size of the largest baby delivered vaginally assures the adequacy of the woman's pelvis for up to that size baby. It also provides baseline information for anticipating possible complications when compared with the estimated fetal weight of this baby. History of a baby over 4 kg and/or abortions and preterm babies are an indication to screen the woman for diabetes.

Expected date of delivery and present weeks of gestation: This is baseline data for evaluating gestational size and if labor is at term or premature.

Absence, presence or increase in bloody show: Bloody show is a premonitory sign of labor. An increase in bloody show is indicative of impending second stage of labor.

Absence or presence of vaginal bleeding: Bleeding is abnormal. Any frank bleeding requires immediate consultation and attention.

Membranes ruptured or not: Rupture of membranes is a premonitory sign of labor. Because ruptured membranes predispose both mother and baby to high risk factors due to the increased risk of intrauterine infection. A history of ruptured membranes demands determining by examination whether or not they have indeed ruptured. Women are not always clear as to whether their membranes have ruptured or not because a slow leak can always be confused with incontinence of urine. A history of sudden gush of water, which ran down her legs wetting her clothes, is a good history that the membranes have ruptured. A definitive test may be done to confirm the history. A strongly alkaline reaction or deep blue color on nitrazine test paper indicates a positive result. A fern test may also be done, which is a microscopic examination of a fern-like crystallization of the sodium chloride in amniotic fluid on a slide on which it is allowed to dry.

Any prenatal problems: It is essential to screen the woman quickly for antepartal complications, which may affect the intrapartal period, e.g. pre-eclampsia and anemia.

Physical Examination

Vital Signs

Temperature, pulse, respiration and blood pressure: An elevated temperature is indicative of an infectious process. An elevated pulse may indicate infection, shock or anxiety. An elevated respiratory rate may indicate shock and anxiety. An elevated or lowered blood pressure is indicative of hypertensive disorders of pregnancy or shock respectively. An elevated systolic but normal diastolic blood pressure may indicate anxiety.

Physical Measurements

Height and weight.

Fetal Heart Tones

To assess the status of the baby—Normal fetal heart rate is 120 to 160 beats per minute. A fetal heart rate below 120 or above 160 may be indicative of fetal distress and warrants immediate evaluation.

Contraction Pattern

The frequency, duration and intensity of the contractions must be accurately assessed to determine labor status.

Engagement

This is determined by abdominal palpation. An unengaged or unfixed head in a primigravida in labor is indicative of possible cephalopelvic disproportion. Such finding requires repeating clinical pelvimetry during vaginal examination.

Estimated Fetal Weight (EFW) and Fundal Height

A smaller than expected estimated fetal weight and fundal height indicates either that the woman's dates are incorrect or that she has a small for date baby.

A larger than expected EFW and fundal height indicates that the woman's dates are in error, or a large baby indicative of diabetes, or multiple gestation or polyhydramnios. A large baby also forewarns of the possibility of postpartum uterine atony producing hemorrhage or possible shoulder dystocia.

Lie, Presentation, Position and Variety

To ascertain an abnormal lie (i.e. transverse), presentation (i.e. breech) or position (i.e. mentum or brow): Also to determine variety, as a posterior variety may lengthen or increase the discomfort of the first stage of labor. A woman in even early labor must be admitted, if she has a transverse lie. A primigravida with a breech presentation is also at risk and should be admitted.

Edema of Extremities

This is one of the classic signs of pre-eclampsia. Ankle, pretibial, finger and facial edema is checked for and evaluated. Ankle edema alone may simply be dependent edema resulting from the decrease in venous blood flow caused by pressure from the enlarged uterus.

Pelvic Examination/Vaginal Examination

Effacement and dilatation: To determine if progressive cervical changes have occurred and to diagnose labor. Also to determine what stage and phase of labor the woman is in, if in labor.

To confirm abdominal findings: Sometimes it is easier to obtain these findings upon vaginal examination, e.g. suture lines, fontanels and skull bones in cephalic presentation, a hand or foot in podalic presentation.

Position of the Cervix

The cervix is usually directed posteriorly prior to labor. Movement of the cervix anteriorly so that it is in the midline indicates readiness for or entry into labor.

Station

To determine descent of the fetal head—Descend of the fetal head is one of the mechanisms of labor and is indicative of progress and pelvic adequacy.

Whether or not the Membranes have Ruptured

To confirm or rule out a history of ruptured membranes or to detect a rupture of membranes not reported.

If the membranes are not easily felt over the presenting part or as bulging, it is helpful to have the woman bear down or to apply fundal pressure, which may cause the membranes to bulge if they are there. Membranes in close contact with a head feel smooth and slick to the touch.

Diagnosis is definitive for ruptured membranes when the amniotic fluid is seen escaping from the cervical os and pooled in the vaginal vault or when the membranes are not felt over the presenting part at the cervical os.

When you feel the membranes bulging against your examining fingers during vaginal examination of the cervix, other possibilities must also be considered. They are: (1) unruptured membranes, (2) a high leak that is occluded by pressure from the presenting part, or escape of fluid trapped between the membranes with rupture of the chorion only and not amnion.

Vaginal Examination for the Woman in Labor

A vaginal examination must follow an abdominal examination so that the midwife can combine the external and internal findings to arrive at a clearer picture of the progress of labor.

Purposes

A vaginal examination for the client in labor will help to:

- Make a positive diagnosis of labor
- Make a positive identification of the presentation
- Determine if the presenting part is engaged
- Ascertain if the forewaters have ruptured or rupture them artificially
- Exclude cord prolapsed after rupture of the forewaters
- Assess progress or delay in labor
- Apply fetal scalp electrode.

Under no circumstances should a midwife make a vaginal examination if there is any frank bleeding.

Procedure

Prepare the client for the procedure by giving adequate explanation. This would enable her to relax and cooperate during the examination.

- The bladder must be empty so that discomfort during the procedure will be minimized
- Assemble sterile articles such as a vaginal examination pack containing sterile swabs and bowls along with sterile disposable gloves. This is important to avoid introducing microorganisms into the vagina
- Position the woman on her back with thighs separated and knees bent, taking care to avoid unnecessary exposure
- Be sure that the woman's arms are down by her sides or across her abdomen to aid relaxation of her abdominal muscles
- Wash hands thoroughly and put on sterile gloves
- Swab the client's vagina
- Dip the first two fingers of the dominant hand in the antiseptic cream to get them lubricated
- Holding the labia apart with the thumb and index fingers of the other hand, insert the lubricated fingers into the vagina palm side down, pressing downwards. Direct the fingers along the anterior vaginal wall and should not be withdrawn until the required information has been obtained. With the fingers inside, explore the vagina for required data, taking care not to touch the clitoris where it may cause great discomfort or the anus where it may be contaminated.

Findings

External genitalia: Before cleansing the vulva, observe and note the following:

- Any sign varicosities, edema, vulval warts or sores
- Scar from previous episiotomy or tear
- Any discharge or bleeding from the vaginal orifice
- Color and odor of amniotic fluid if the membranes have ruptured. Offensive liquor suggests infection and green fluid indicates the presence of meconium, which may be a sign of fetal distress.

Condition of the Vagina

- The vagina should feel warm and moist and the walls soft and distensible. A hot dry vagina is a sign of obstructed labor. If the woman has raised temperature, the vagina will feel hot but not dry
- Firm and rigid wall may suggest a longer labor
- Presence of scars from previous perineal wound may cause delay in the second stage
- In a multiparous woman, a cystocele may be found through the anterior wall
- A loaded rectum may be felt through the posterior wall.

The Cervix

As the examining fingers reach the end of the vagina, they are turned so that the sensitive pads face upwards and come in contact with cervix.

- Palpate around the fornices and sense the proximity of the presenting part of the fetus to the examining finger. A spongy feeling between the fingers and presenting part may indicate the possibility of a placenta previa
- The cervical os is located by sweeping the fingers from side to side. It will normally be situated centrally, but sometimes in early labor, it will be posterior
- Length of the cervical canal must be assessed
- A long tightly closed cervix indicates that labor has not yet started. The cervical canal may be obliterated (without margins), partially or completely depending on the degree of effacement. In a primigravida, the cervix may be completely effaced but still

closed. As it will be closely applied to the presenting part, the os may be felt as a small depression in the center

❖ The consistency of the cervix is then noted. It should be soft, elastic and applied closely to the presenting part. If it is tight, rigid or unyielding, labor may be prolonged or it may be poor application associated with an ill-fitting presenting part.

The uterine os: Dilatation of the cervix, that is the distance across the opening is estimated in centimeters. Ten centimeters dilatation equates to full dilatation. At the point where the maximum diameters of the fetal head have passed through the os, the cervix can no longer be felt. It is important that the midwife feel for the cervix in every direction as a lip of cervix frequently remains in one quarter only, usually anteriorly.

The forewaters: Intact membranes can be felt through the dilating os. Between contractions, they feel slack but will become tense when the uterus contracts. The consistency of the membranes will be similar to thin plastic film. When forewaters are very shallow, it may be difficult to feel the membranes.

If the presenting part does not fit well, some of the fluid from the hindwaters escape into the forewaters, causing the membranes to protrude through the cervix. This will be more exaggerated in obstructed labor. Bulging membranes are more likely to rupture early and in such case they will not be felt at all. Following rupture of membranes, there is possibility that the cord may prolapse and the midwife must feel for any cord. Following leakage of amniotic fluid, if forewaters are felt, it may be supposed that the hindwaters have ruptured.

Level or Station of the Presenting Part

In order to assess descend of the fetus in labor, the level of the presenting part is estimated in relation to the maternal ischial spines. The distance of the presenting part above or below the ischial spines is expressed in centimeters.

As a caput succedaneum may form over the presenting part, care must be taken to relate the bony part of the spines and not the edematous swelling. Moulding of the fetal skull can also result in the presenting part becoming lower without any appreciable advance of the head as a whole. It is not possible to make an accurate judgment of the station vaginally. The purpose of making this estimate is to assess progress and it is therefore valuable for the same person to make all the vaginal examinations on any particular mother.

Identity of the Presentation

In 96 percent of cases, the vertex presents and is recognized by feeling the hard bones of the vault of the skull and the fontanelles and sutures. For details of finding in other presentations, *see* Chapter 15.

Position

By feeling the features of the presenting part, the position of the presentation can be derived. In vertex presentations the first feature to be felt even in early labor, is the sagittal suture. It may be felt in the right or left oblique diameter of the pelvis, or it may be transverse. Later, as further descent occurs, it rotates to the anteroposterior diameter of the pelvis.

The sagittal suture is to be followed with the finger until a fontanelle is reached. If the head is well flexed, the posterior fontanelle will be felt. The location of the fontanelle(s) in relation to the pelvis, give information as to the whereabouts of the occiput.

Moulding

This can be judged by feeling the amount of overlapping of the skull bones and can give additional information as to position. The parietal bones override the occipital bone.

Completion of the Examination

As the midwife withdraws her fingers from the vagina, she should note any blood or amniotic fluid and compare this with the observations made earlier. Finally, she should remove her gloves and auscultate the fetal heart prior to assisting the mother to find a comfortable position.

The woman must be kept informed of her progress in labor. Findings of examination must be recorded accurately after each examination.

BIBLIOGRAPHY

1. AJN/Mosby, Nursing Board's Review for NCLEX-RN Examination, 10th edn. St. Louis, Baltimore: Mosby; 1997.
2. Cassidy P. Management of the First Stage of Labor, In: Bennet RV, Linda KB (Eds). Myles Textbook for Midwives, 13th edn. Edinburgh: Churchill Livingstone; 1999.
3. Dick-Read G. Childbirth without Fear, 2nd edn. Harper and Row; 1957.
4. Freidman EA. Labor: Clinical Evaluation and Management, 2nd edn. New York: Meredith; 1978.
5. Pritchard JA, McDonald PC, Gant N. Williams Obstetrics, 17th edn. Connecticut: Appleton Century Crafts; 1885.
6. Varney Helen, Nurse-Midwifery, 2nd edn. Boston: Jones and Barlett Publishers; 1996.

18

Management of the First Stage of Labor

Management of the first stage of labor includes the diagnosis of labor, management of false labor, management of early labor and initial evaluation and care of mother and fetus.

ADMISSION TO LABOR AND DELIVERY UNIT

When the woman is admitted, she undergoes an admission procedure. This procedure may not be same in all the hospitals or health care centers, but generally includes the following:
❖ Changing from street clothing to a hospital gown
❖ Safeguarding the woman's personal belongings or returning them to family
❖ Applying identification band for the woman
❖ Filling out the chart forms
❖ Carrying-out the admission orders
❖ Carrying-out an evaluation of the woman and fetus including history, physical and pelvic examinations and laboratory tests.

Admission orders and procedures for a woman in labor include enema, perineal shave, oral or intravenous fluids, ambulation, medication and monitoring of maternal and fetal well-being.

Enema

The purposes of an enema are:
❖ To stimulate uterine contractions
❖ To assure a clean field without fecal contamination at the time of delivery
❖ To eliminate a possible deterent to accurate and comfortable examination.

Though most women require an enema for the above reasons, it is to be avoided in the following situations:
1. A woman in the late first stage of labor or in rapidly progressive labor, especially a multipara. Expulsion of the enema may be accompanied by expulsion of the baby.
2. The membranes are ruptured; if the membranes are ruptured, there is an increased risk of possible intrauterine infection.
3. Unengaged presenting part.
4. The presence of complications, such as vaginal bleeding with suspected placenta previa or abruptio placentae (danger of severe bleeding), premature labor (to avoid stimulating labor) and severe pre-eclampsia (need for the woman to be as quiet and undisturbed as possible).

Perineal Shave

The purpose of a perineal shave is to prevent infection. Preparation of the perineum involving the shaving of the mons pubis, vulva, and anal region, provides for cleanliness and easy viewing of the perineum. The decision about shaving may be made according to the practice established in the particular institution or setting. There are practitioners today who believe in no preparation at all, especially if delivery over an intact perineum is expected. There are others, who believe that long hairs, which extend to the vulval area, can be clipped.

Food and Fluids by Mouth

A woman in labor, even in early labor, should not eat solid food. If she does, it will most likely remain in her stomach throughout labor or be vomited during transition. This is because of the severe decrease in secretion of gastric juice, gastric motility and absorption during labor. These decreases do not affect liquids, which leave the stomach in the usual amount of time. Liquids therefore may be ingested during labor.

The best liquids for women to have are clear liquids to which sugar (for energy) has been added, such as tea or coffee and water to provide fluid. Excessive fluids are not desirable as they may produce nausea. Most women want to only moisten their dry mouths and parched throats and should be given the means for continuing relief.

If general inhalation anesthesia is anticipated, restrict even fluids.

Intravenous Infusion

Intravenous infusion serves as a means to maintain maternal nutrition and as a lifeline for medications, fluid or blood in the event of an obstetric disaster. An intravenous infusion is mandatory if one of the following conditions is present:

❖ Gravida 5 or greater
❖ An over distended uterus for any reason including multiple gestation, polyhydramnios and excessively large baby
❖ A pitocin induction or augmentation
❖ Maternal dehydration or exhaustion
❖ Any obstetric or medical condition which is life-threatening, such as abruptio placentae, placenta previa pre-eclampsia, or eclampsia
❖ History or presence of any other condition that predisposes an immediate postpartum hemorrhage.

Some obstetricians want all their clients to have an IV and some want none of their clients to have an IV unless there is an indication for it.

The usual intravenous solution for a woman in labor consists of D5W or D5RL. An intravenous intracatheter is used to permit the woman more free movement of her arm without trauma to the involved blood vessel and has the best chance of staying in the vein if she becomes physically active during labor.

Position and Ambulation

A woman in labor should assume a position, that is comfortable for her, provided there are no contraindications to it. Positions may include supine or flat, lateral recumbent, sitting, standing or walking. If the membranes have ruptured and the fetus presents problems such as transverse lie, breech presentation or small size (less than 2000 gm), it poses a risk of prolapsed cord. Then the positions are to be supine or lateral recumbent.

The lateral recumbent position has several beneficial effects, which are as follows:
❖ Better coordination and greater efficiency of uterine contractions
❖ Facilitation of kidney function (urine flow is increased in lateral position)
❖ Facilitation of fetal rotation in posterior positions
❖ Relief of uterine pressure on, and compression of, the major maternal blood vessels (the inferior vena cava and the aorta).

In order to avail these benefits, women with the following conditions should be instructed to assume lateral recumbent position during first stage of labor.
❖ Maternal supine hypotensive syndrome
❖ Fetal distress (to reduce uterine activity and pressure on the umbilical cord)
❖ Severe pre-eclampsia (for best urine flow)
❖ Mild hypertonicity or ineffectual uterine contractions.

A woman in labor should be allowed to ambulate for as long as she desires, provided there are no complications. Walking in early labor may stimulate labor. Many women cope with their labor better when they can walk. The woman's freedom to walk, sit in a chair, and use the toilet is certainly more conducive to normal process than the sickness orientation of being confined to bed.

There are however, times when the woman should not be out of bed or ambulating. These are:

1. When the membranes are ruptured and the fetus is either small or in a footling or ill-fitting breech presentation or transverse lie. In such events, there is a risk of cord prolapse, which is increased when the woman is upright.
2. When the woman has been medicated with any drug which might make her light headed, dizzy, or unsteady on her feet.
3. During rapidly progressive labor, or late first stage labor in multiparas.
4. Any obstetric or medical complication requiring that the woman remain in bed (e.g. abruptio placentae, placenta previa, severe pre-eclampsia).

Medication

Medications used during labor are for the following purposes.

- ❖ Pain relief
- ❖ Decrease of anxiety and apprehension
- ❖ Sedation
- ❖ Control of vomiting.

The commonly used drugs are demerol (maperidine), phenargan (promathazine), vistaril (hydroxyzine) and seconal (secobarbital). The midwife may have to administer these drugs combined (adding them together) in divided doses and repeat doses. It is to be remembered that tranquilizers (ataractics) potentiate the action of analgesics.

In making decisions regarding medication administration, the midwife must consider the following factors:

Woman's Desire for Medication

Some women want as much medication as they can get. Usually such women do not understand why you can't give them enough to take the pain away even after explanation. On the other hand there are women who want to experience or tolerate as much as they can without medication. There may be women, who have had some preparation for labor. The art of administering medication during labor compri-

ses achieving a balance on the woman's desire, need and facilitation of her coping abilities within the parameters of safety.

Timing of Medication

This is important in the care of women in labor. The following principles should be observed.

1. The progress of labor evaluated carefully and the giving of medication timed so that it will not be at its peak action at the time of baby's birth. Otherwise, the baby might be sleepy and have some respiratory depression. This principle does not apply if a single small dose (e.g. 25 mg of Demerol) given early in labor.
2. A narcotic analgesic should not be given until the woman is in active labor. If given before the contractions are well established, as in the latent phase of labor, the drug will most likely render the contractions ineffectual by diminishing their frequency, duration and intensity. The total labor may be lengthened. After the woman is in well-established active labor, a narcotic analgesic will not affect the contraction pattern.
3. Tranquilizers do not affect uterine contractions and will not slow down or delay the progress of labor. Because of their calming effect on the woman, progress of labor is often facilitated.
4. The sedatives are for use:
   - ❖ When the woman is in false labor
   - ❖ When the woman is in early labor, and exhausted and needs a rest
   - ❖ As part of the treatment for hypertonic uterine dysfunction and to stop the present labor with its abnormal contraction pattern.

Fetal Size

Because of developmental immaturity and a high risk of respiratory distress in a preterm (premature) or small-for-gestational age fetus, all medications are withheld from the woman during labor in order not to distress the baby. Unlike full-term babies, small or premature babies cannot handle any amount of drugs crossing the placental barrier.

Fetal Condition

If there is any fetal distress, regardless of fetal age and size, all medications are withheld from the woman in order not to further stress the fetus, which no longer is able to handle drugs crossing the placental barrier.

For any fetus at risk, such as those of diabetic mothers, pre-eclamptic mothers or those who are post-term, judicious very small dosages must be tried and fetus carefully monitored for the drugs' effect. In such cases, internal fetal monitoring will be used for comprehensive monitoring of the fetal response.

Maternal Size

The amount of medication is limited by the fact that the fetus cannot tolerate the levels it would take to totally alleviate the woman's pain. Thus, if a woman is large, additional medication cannot be given in accordance with her increased body size. On the other hand, you need to consider the body size of the small, petite woman in determining the amount of medication within the limits imposed by the fetus.

Woman's Response to Support in Labor

Women who have undergone preparation for childbirth and have practiced relaxation and breathing exercises often require less medication. The presence and help of a significant other (spouse or coach) during labor where it is permitted or possible, makes coping easier and such women require less medication generally.

Need for Medication

In addition to and underlying all the factors discussed is the amount of real pain or discomfort the woman is feeling. This varies in each woman depending on her pain threshold and on the amount of anxiety and tension she has and their effect on intensifying the amount of pain. For some women, supportive care alone or in conjunction with a small dose of tranquilizer would be sufficient to cope with labor. In medicating a woman in labor, the midwife should always be anticipating when she is going to really need it most, which is during transition and plan to give it accordingly. A woman's pain in labor, as she is experiencing it, should never be scoffed at regardless of your findings, she is feeling it and needs to have it respected.

Monitoring Maternal Physiological Changes

In order to plan the care during the first stage, the midwife needs to know the normal physiologic changes that take place during labor and their significance. This knowledge is important to accurately interpret certain signs, symptoms and laboratory findings as normal or abnormal during the first stage of labor. They may also be significant factors to consider in the management of care of the woman.

Vital Signs

Blood pressure rises during contractions with the systolic rising an average of 15 to 20 mm Hg and the diastolic rising an average of 5 to 10 mm Hg. Between contractions the BP returns to its pre-labor level. A shift of the woman's position from supine to lateral eliminates the change in BP during contractions. Pain, fear and apprehension may also raise the blood pressure. In order to ascertain the true BP, it is to be checked between contractions.

An increase in pulse rate during the increment of contractions, a decrease during the acme and an increase during the decrement are usual. A slightly elevated pulse may be normal.

A slight increase in respirations may be due to the increased metabolism. Prolonged hyperventilation may result in alkalosis.

Renal System

Bladder distention commonly occurs due to increased glomerular filtration. The bladder must be evaluated and emptied every two hours to prevent obstruction of labor and trauma to the bladder. Slight proteinuria (trace to +1) is common in a third to half of women in labor. This is seen more frequently in women who have anemia or are in prolonged labor.

Gastrointestinal Changes

Gastric motility and absorption of solid foods taken are severely reduced. Secretion of gastric juice is reduced. Digestion is stopped and gastric emptying is prolonged. Oral intake should be limited to liquids. Nausea and vomiting are not uncommon during the transition stage. Pain medications, fear and apprehension may be the contributing factors.

Hematological Changes

Blood coagulation time decreases and plasma fibrinogen level increases. These changes decrease the risk of postpartum hemorrhage. The white cell count increases during the first stage.

Blood glucose decreases during labor dropping markedly in prolonged and difficult labors probably as a result of the increased uterine and skeletal muscle activity.

Monitoring of Fetal Well-being

Assessment of fetal well-being includes continuing evaluation of the following:
* Normality of the fetal lie, presentation, attitude, position and variety
* Fetal adaptation to pelvis
* The fetal heart rate and pattern.

Evaluation of the fetal lie, presentation, attitude, position and variety is done first by abdominal palpation and confirmed by vaginal examination. Information needed to evaluate fetal adaptation to the pelvis includes synclitism/asynclitism, moulding of the fetal skull, the formation of caput succedaneum and the parameters of normal for each.

All the information in these two categories of evaluating fetal well-being is obtained when the client is evaluated upon admission to the labor and delivery suite and at any other time a vaginal examination is done during labor.

The fetal heart rate and pattern are checked by any one of the following methods:
* Intermittent auscultation of the fetal heart
* Intermittent external fetal monitoring
* Continuous external fetal monitoring
* Continuous internal fetal monitoring.

The decision should be based on the indicated need and the established policy of the institution (Table 18.1).

The frequency of evaluation of the fetal heart rate and the pattern, using auscultation with a fetoscope or ultrasonic method (e.g. Doptone/Dopler) is every 30 minutes during active labor. In addition, the fetal heart rate is checked at other times during the course of a normal labor, including the following:
* When the membranes rupture
* After expulsion of an enema
* Whenever there is sudden change in the contraction or labor pattern
* After giving medication, at its peak action time
* Whenever there is any indication that an obstetric or medical complication is developing.

In using a fetoscope, it helps to be able to hear the fetal heart if you remember that the fetoscope is constructed to take advantage of bone conduction of sound. For this reason, keep your fingers off the fetoscope while listening. Fingers on the fetoscope disrupt the conduction of sound.

External and internal fetal monitoring is discussed on pages 152 and 153 in this chapter.

CONTINUING CARE AND EVALUATION

As the mother continues in labor, the midwife is responsible for carrying out all of the following, which may be going on simultaneously.
* Evaluation of the maternal well-being
* Evaluation of the fetal well-being
* Evaluation of the progress of labor
* Screening for maternal or fetal complications
* Bodily care of the woman
* Supportive care of the woman and her significant other/family.

Evaluation of Maternal Well-being

This includes continuing evaluation of the following:
* Vital signs
  a. Blood pressure
  b. Temperature
  c. Pulse
  d. Respiration.
* Bladder care
* Urine testing
  a. Protein
  b. Ketones.
* Hydration
  a. Fluids
  b. Nausea/vomiting.

Table 18.1　FHR pattern, significance and nursing interventions

Pattern	Features and causes	Significance	Nursing intervention
1. Normal pattern	– Baseline rate 120–160 bpm – Average variability – Absence of late or variable decelerations	– Fetus can respond to environment – A reassuring pattern	None needed
2. Acceleration	– Increased FHR during contractions – Fetal movement can also cause acceleration	– Response to stress – Lowered oxygen, or fetal movement	None needed
3. Variability of FHR	– Beat to beat variation (short term) – 3–5 fluctuations per minute (long–term)	– Indicates fetus can respond to environment	None needed
4. Early deceleration	– Uniform – Inversely mirrors uterine contractions – Starts and ends with uterine contractions – Caused due to compression of fetal head associated with contractions	– Caused by head compression	None needed
5. Late deceleration	– Inversely mirrors contractions – Occurs after the peak of contraction – Does not end until after contraction ends – Cause may be uteroplacental insufficiency	– May indicate fetal distress	– Turn mother to left side (to maximize uteroplacental perfusion) – Administer oxygen at 7–10 L/min by face mask – Increase IV fluids (to treat hypotension and to decrease intensity of contractions) – Discontinue IV oxytocin (if it is being used) – Maintain continuous monitoring
6. Variable deceleration	– Varies in onset, occurrence and waveform – Cause may be umbilical cord compression	– Indicates compression of umbilical cord – May be associated with fetal distress	– Change maternal position – Administer oxygen at 7–10 L/min via face mask – Look for prolapsed cord
7. Decreased variability	– Minimal variations – Causes may be anoxia, fetal sleep and CNS depression due to medications taken by mother	– Short term if associated with fetal sleep or medications – If pattern persists more than 30 minutes or variability continues to decrease, it is ominous	– Carefully evaluate pattern – Maintain continuous FHR monitoring – Notify physician

❖ General condition
   a. Fatigue
   b. Behavior and response to labor
   c. Pain and coping ability.

Vital Signs

All of the vital signs are checked upon admission to the labor and delivery suite. Thereafter, the frequency of checking vital signs may vary with the hospital since each may have a policy regarding this to assure a minimum standard. A generally accepted norm of frequency for a normal laboring woman during the active phase of first stage is as follows:

❖ Blood pressure—Every hour
❖ Temperature, pulse and respirations:
   a. Every two hours (or every four hours) when the temperature is normal and the membranes are intact.
   b. Every hour (or every two hours) after, the membranes have ruptured.

Bladder Care

During the active phase of first stage of labor, the woman's bladder should be evaluated for distention, at least every two hours. With the descent of the fetal presenting part into the true pelvis, the bladder is compressed so that distention occurs even with 100 ml of urine in the bladder. This distention is visible above the symphysis pubis. If the bladder is not carefully attended to and emptied, the following may result:

❖ *Obstructed labor*—An overdistended bladder can impede the progress of labor by preventing fetal descend.
❖ *Difficulty in management of an immediate postpartal hemorrhage resulting from uterine atony*—An overdistended bladder displaces the postpartal uterus, thereby inhibiting its ability to contract and effect uterine haemostasis.
❖ *Difficulty in delivering the shoulders*—An overdistended bladder interferes with descend of the shoulders and decreases the amount of room in the true pelvis (shoulder dystocia).
❖ *Discomfort to the woman*—A distended bladder increases the discomfort or pain in the lower abdomen that women frequently experience during labor.

❖ Bladder hypotonicity, urine stasis, and infection during postpartal period resulting from trauma due to pressure exerted on the distended bladder during labor.

Every time the woman's abdomen is uncovered for abdominal examination or taking fetal heart tones, the contour of her abdomen should be noted for bladder distention. A distended bladder appears as a bulge above the symphysis pubis and, in severe cases, may extend as high as the umbilicus. When the fetus is in a posterior position, the contour of the woman's abdomen may look as though she has a full bladder; distention must then be excluded.

If bladder distention occurs, all measures must be taken to facilitate the woman's efforts to void. The best method is to make her walk to the toilet if there are no contraindications to her ambulating. If she is unable to be out of bed, following measures can be tried:

❖ Having her listen to the sound of running water
❖ Dabbling her fingers in water
❖ Running warm water over her perineum.
❖ Applying light suprapubic pressure.

If these measures do not result in her voiding, then the midwife must decide for catheterization. The decision for catheterization is to be taken on the basis of the severity of the distention, her labor status, and her progress in labor.

Urine Testing

Subsequent to the initial specimen collected at the time of admission for a routine microscopic examination, when a woman voids during labor, the urine should be examined for protein and ketones. Dipstick may be used if available for this test. If there is protein in the specimen it is vital to know whether or not this is proteinuria. Urine, contaminated with bloody show, may have positive result due to the contamination of blood protein. The results from carefully collected clean-catch specimens may be considered valid.

Examination of the urine for ketones is for the purpose of screening the patient for maternal exhaustion and distress due to dehydration, electrolyte imbalance, and nutritional deficiency during labor. It is most important to use dipstick testing of the urine for ketones to evaluate the well-being of a laboring woman who does not have an intravenous infusion in order to evaluate the adequacy of her oral intake of liquids for maintenance of hydration. Ketonuria would indicate the need for an IV infusion.

Hydration

The maintenance of hydration throughout labor is essential for the well-being of the woman. Signs of dehydration, such as dry or cracked lips, a dry mouth or a parched throat may not always be due to dehydration at all in a woman in labor but may instead be due to the type of breathing she is doing with her contractions. Evaluation thus, is based on the screening for ketonuia and knowledge of the woman's intake (by whatever route) and loss (output). Concentration of the urine should also be noted.

Excessive nausea or vomiting in a woman with or without IV fluids must be counterbalanced with IV fluids. While strict intake and output record need fluid intake, urinary output and the amount of any emesis.

Evaluation of Fetal Well-being

Assessment of fetal wellbeing includes continuing evaluation of the following:

❖ Normality of the fetal lie, presentation, attitude, position and variety
❖ Fetal adaptation to pelvis
❖ The fetal heart rate and pattern.

Evaluation of the fetal lie, presentation, attitude, position and variety is done first by abdominal palpation and confirmed by vaginal examination. Information needed to evaluate fetal adaptation to the pelvis includes synclitism/asynclitism, moulding of the fetal skull, the formation of caput succedaneum and the parameters of normal for each.

All the information in these two categories of evaluating fetal well-being is obtained when the client is evaluated upon admission to the labor and delivery suite and at any other time a vaginal examination is done during labor.

The fetal heart rate and pattern are checked by any one of the following methods:

❖ Intermittent auscultation of the fetal heart
❖ Intermittent external fetal monitoring
❖ Continuous external fetal monitoring
❖ Continuous internal fetal monitoring.

The decision should be based on the indicated need and the established policy of the institution.

The frequency of evaluation of the fetal heart rate and the pattern, using auscultation with a fetoscope or ultrasonic method (e.g. Doptone/Doppler) in every 30 minutes during active labor. In addition, the fetal heart rate is checked at other times during the course of a normal labor, including the following:

❖ When the membranes rupture
❖ After expulsion of an enema
❖ Whenever there is sudden change in the contraction or labor pattern
❖ After giving medication, at its peak action time
❖ Whenever there is any indication that an obstetric or medical complication is developing.

In using a fetoscope, it helps to be able to hear the fetal heart if you remember that the fetoscope is constructed to take advantage of bone conduction of sound. For this reason, keep your fingers off the fetoscope while listening. Fingers on the fetoscope disrupt the conduction of sound.

Electronic Fetal Monitoring

External Method (Fig. 18.1)

Electronic monitoring is the use of electronic devices for monitoring frequency, intensity and duration of contractions and, for continuous recording of fetal heart rate patterns. It should be obvious that continuous monitoring of the fetus is more accurate, in terms of detecting fetal distress, than is periodic evaluation with fetoscope. Intermittent stethoscopic monitoring during labor and delivery, when the fetus is at the highest risk of the entire pregnancy, allows detection of only gross changes in the fetal heart rate and therefore provides little useful information. Only ominous changes are likely to be detected by fetoscopic or stethoscopic monitoring as usually practiced. It has been established that

Fig. 18.1: External monitoring

Fig. 18.3: Internal monitoring

Fig. 18.2: Electronic fetal monitor
(*For color version see Plate 2*)

simultaneous graphic recording of the fetal heart rate and uterine activity can give an accurate picture of the status of the fetus (Fig. 18.2).

Continuous recording of the uterine activity and response of the fetal heart are done using an electronic apparatus in the form of a fetal heart monitor. The recording combines a fetal cardiograph and a maternal tocograph.

The ultrasound transducers are strapped on the abdomen, one over the uterine fundus and the other at the point where the fetal heart is heard at a maximum intensity. This method is noninvasive and does not require rupture of membranes. One drawback to external monitoring is that women doing abdominal breathing to help them cope with their contractions find it difficult to breath deeply. If the straps are too loose, however, the transducer will not pick up the contraction or monitor the fetus. Correct placement of the transducers for comfort and accuracy is a legitimate nursing function. The quality of the recording on the graph paper may be affected by the thickness of the abdominal wall, fetal position and maternal or fetal movement.

Internal Monitoring (Fig. 18.3)

Internal monitoring means the sensing devices are introduced directly into the uterus. The contraction transducer is a special fluid-filled catheter, which transmits exact pressure in terms of centimeters of water to the monitor. The fetal monitoring device is a pronged scalp electrode, which is applied to the fetal scalp over a bone by the physician and transmits the electrocardiogram of the fetus to the graphic display.

In order to achieve this the membranes must be ruptured and the cervix be at least 2 to 3 cm dilated. A small scalp wound is inevitable, but this rarely causes problems.

Internal monitoring is more comfortable for the patient insofar as breathing and position are concerned. However, she must use a bedpan to empty her bladder when the intrauterine catheter is used (Figs 18.4 and 18.5).

Nursing Care of the Monitored Patient

Before caring for expectant mothers who are to have fetal monitoring during labor, it is of utmost importance for the nurse to be acquainted with the proper application and operation of the particular monitor in use and how to read the monitor strips.

Continuous electronic monitoring of the labor contractions and the fetus should free the nurse to give more and better direct assistance to the expectant mother. Explanation of the monitor, emphasizing the benefits to be gained

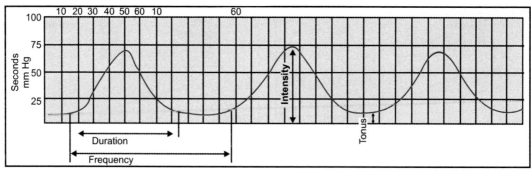

Fig. 18.4: Terms used in describing uterine contractions

Fig. 18.5: Tracing of normal fetal heart rate and uterine contractions

by its use, is essential to the psychological well-being of the client. Although readjustments of the transducers, is a common necessity with external monitoring, when the woman moves, the monitoring should not be affected. Nurses should readjust the abdominal transducers and note on the graph paper any changes in position.

Evaluation of the Progress of Labor

In the continuing evaluation of the progress of labor, the following items of information are used:

❖ Contraction pattern, frequency, duration, intensity
❖ Maternal behavior changes
❖ Signs and symptoms of transition and impending second stage
❖ Position of low back pain
❖ Position of location of maximum intensity of fetal heart tones.

Vaginal Examination

Vaginal examinations are done to determine the dilatation and effacement of cervix and the level of presenting part (fetal station).

For the normal intrapartal woman, vaginal examinations are indicated.

❖ Upon admission, to establish an informational baseline
❖ Before administering medication
❖ As labor progresses, to verify complete dilatation in order to either encourage or discourage maternal pushing effort
❖ After spontaneous rupture of membranes if a prolapsed cord is suspected or is a possibility.

If the membranes have ruptured prematurely, vaginal examinations are restricted to none except by the obstetrician. This is because of the increased risk of introducing contaminants and the development of intrauterine infection.

PARTOGRAPH (FIG. 18.6)

Definition

Partograph is a record of all the observations made on a woman in labor; the central feature of which is the graphic recording of the dilatation of the cervix as assessed by vaginal examination.

Principal Features

1. The active phase of labor commences at 3 cm cervical dilation
2. The latent phase of labor should last no longer than 8 hours.
3. During active labor, the rate of cervical dilatation should not be lesser than 1 cm/ hour
4. A lag time of 4 hours between slowing of labor and interventions is unlikely to compromise the fetus or mother
5. 4-hourly vaginal examination is recommended.

Purposes

1. To record the clinical observations accurately.
2. To identify the difference between latent phase and active phase of labor.
3. To interpret the recorded partograph and to identify any deviation from normal.
4. To monitor the progress of labor and to recognize the need for action at the appropriate time for timely referral.
5. To monitor the well-being of mother as she goes through labor.

Use of Partograph

The Partograph should have all data related to the client in labor and the physiological changes during the process. It is recommended to be used in the following manner.

Patient Information

Name, obstetric score, Hospital Number, Date and time of admission, status of membranes on admission to labor room.

Fetal Condition

1. **Fetal heart rate (FHR)**
   FHR is recorded hourly during 1st stage and half hourly in 2nd stage of labor.

2. **Liquor amnii**
   Amniotic fluid is observed and recorded as:
   "I" If the membranes are intact,
   "C" If liquor is clear
   "B" For blood stained liquor
   "R" If membranes are ruptured
   "M" For meconium stained liquor.

3. **Moulding**
   (O) Sutures felt easily
   (-) Absence of moulding
   (+) Bones are touching each other
   (++) Bones are overlapping.

Progress of Labor

1. **Cervical dilatation:** The dilatation is plotted with the zero time on the graph and further examinations are made at least every four hours. A line joins the points of each dilatation. The cervical dilatation is divided into two phases.

   Latent Phase
   Dilatation 4 cm to 10 cm, at the rate of 1 cm per hour in primigravida and 1.5 cm per hour in multipara.

   Alert Line
   The alert line drawn from 4 cm to 10 cm represents the rate of dilatation. If the line marked for the patient moves to the right of the alert line, dilatation is slow and an indication of delay in progress of labor.

   Action Line
   Action line is drawn 4 hours to the right of the alert line. It is suggested that if the cervical dilation reaches this line, there should be a critical assessment of the cause of delay and a decision about appropriate management should be taken.

2. **Station of the head:** Station of the head identified and noted on vaginal examination are to be marked on the right end of the partograph and points to be joined.

3. **Time:** This is recorded with time of admission as zero time. The actual time of day is recorded below the hours. For induced labour, the time of starting the induction is recorded as zero time and further recordings are at hourly intervals.

Patient Name: ....
Age: ....
Ward: ....
Gravida: ....Para: ....
EDD: ....
Onset of labor: Date: ....
                             Time: ....
Obstetrician: ....

Date & Time of Admission: ....

Fig. 18.6: Partograph

4. **Uterine contractions:** The contractions are recorded at 10 minutes interval in the appropriate square box.
5. **Oxytocin, drugs and IV fluids:** These are recorded in the space provided.

Maternal Condition

1. **Blood pressure, pulse and temperature**: These are recorded in the space provided, BP every 4 hours, pulse every 30 minutes and temperature 2 hourly. Systolic and diastolic markings are joined with a vertical line. Pulse is marked by placing dots.
2. **Urine:** The amount is recorded every time urine is passed. Acetone (Ketone) and protein are tested and recorded.

Screening for Maternal and Fetal Complications

Interpretation of Cardiotocograph Recordings

The cardiotocograph provides information on:
* Baseline fetal heart rate
* Baseline variability
* Response of fetal heart to uterine contra-dictions.

Baseline fetal heart rate: It is the fetal heart rate between uterine contractions. A rate more than 160 bpm is termed *baseline tachycardia*. A rate slower than 120 bpm is called *baseline bradycardia*. Either may be indicative of fetal hypoxia. Fetal tachycardia may be associated with maternal ketosis also. A constant baseline rate between 110–120 bpm may indicate cord compression as in cord prolapse.

Baseline variability: The tracing on the graph paper appears uneven due to the minute variations in the length of each beat. The baseline rate should normally vary by at least five beats over a period of one minute. Loss of this variability may indicate fetal hypoxia. It may also be seen for a short period after the administration of pethidine to mothers, which depresses the cardiac reflex center in the fetal brain. Periods of 'fetal sleep' also cause reduction in variability, which usually last for 20 to 30 minutes during labor.

Response of the fetal heart to uterine contractions: The fetal heart rate will normally remain steady or accelerate during contractions (Fig. 18.7). Decelerations (slow down) of fetal heart rate, if recorded must be assessed for their relationship to uterine contractions.

Early deceleration begins at or after the onset of a contraction and returns to the baseline rate by the time the contraction has finished. An early deceleration is commonly associated with compression of the fetal head, for example as it engages, but may also indicate early fetal hypoxia (Fig. 18.8A).

Late deceleration begins during or after a contraction, reaches its lowest point after the peak of the contraction and has not recovered by the time that contraction has ended. Sometimes the deceleration has barely recovered by the onset of the next contraction. The time lag between the peak of the contraction and the lowest point of the deceleration is more significant of severity than the drop in the fetal heart rate. This always indicates fetal hypoxia and the physician must be informed. A vaginal examination should be performed to exclude prolapse of the cord, as late decelerations are suggestive of cord compression (Fig. 18.8B).

Variable deceleration varies in onset, occurrence and waveform. The cause may be fetal distress (Fig. 18.8C).

While reading the cardiotocograph the midwife must be careful not to be confused with the artifacts, which may appear on the tracing if the contact is lost. An attempt should be made to improve the quality of recording by repositioning the electrodes and maternal position and the fetal heart rate should be checked using a Doppler apparatus (*see* Table 18.1).

Fetal Blood Sampling

The fetus that has become hypoxic will also become acidotic as the pH of the blood is lowered. The normal pH of fetal blood is 7.35 or above. If it falls below 7.25 in the first stage of labor, careful surveillance is required. Cardiotocograph recording of the fetal heart may suggest hypoxia but acidosis can only be confirmed by fetal blood sampling.

Fig. 18.7: Acceleration of the fetal heart rate in response to uterine activity

In order to collect fetal blood, an amnioscope is passed through the cervix to obtain access to the fetal scalp. A small puncture is made on the fetal scalp and 0.5 ml of blood is collected in a heparinized capillary tube. The specimen must be analyzed immediately for accurate result. Care must be taken to prevent clotting of blood while transporting the sample to the laboratory.

Observation of Amniotic Fluid

Following rupture of membranes amniotic fluid escapes from the uterus continuously and may provide information about the condition of the fetus. The fluid should normally remain clear. If the fetus becomes hypoxic, meconium may be passed as hypoxia causes relaxation of the anal sphincter. As a result of meconium staining, the amniotic fluid becomes green. Amniotic fluid, which is a muddy yellow color or which is only slightly green, may signify previous distress from which the fetus has recovered.

If the fetus presents by breech and is compacted in the pelvis, the fetus may pass meconium because of the compression of abdomen. Thus, green amniotic fluid with the fetus in the breech presentation is considered normal. However, a fetus presenting by the breech is also prone to fetal distress and may pass meconium as a result of hypoxia.

If a fetus is severely affected by Rhesus iso-immunization the amniotic fluid may be golden-yellow due to an excess bilirubin.

In case of a vasa previa, at the time of rupture of membranes the blood vessel may also become torn causing bleeding. Blood in the amniotic fluid is an acute emergency.

Fetal Distress

Fetal distress occurs when the fetus suffers oxygen deprivation and becomes hypoxic. In

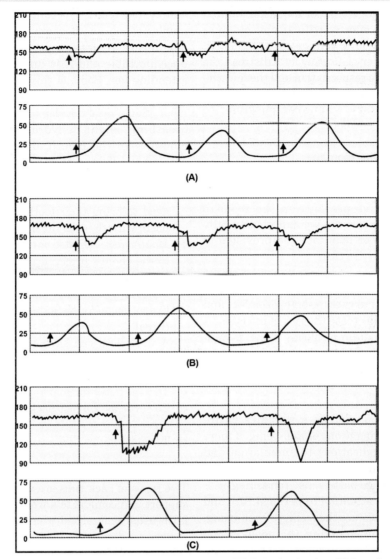

Figs 18.8A to C: Types of decelerations in fetal heart rate: (A) Early deceleration; (B) Late deceleration; (C) Variable deceleration

severe hypoxia the baby may be asphyxiated at birth and suffer brain damage or result in stillbirth.

Signs of Fetal Distress

❖ Fetal tachycardia, which is an early sign of oxygen deprivation
❖ Fetal bradycardia, which may be shown as fetal heart rate deceleration in the monitor tracing
❖ Passage of meconium stained amniotic fluid.

Management of Fetal Distress

When signs of fetal distress are noticed, the midwife must call the physician. If pitocin is being administered, it must be stopped and the woman placed on her left side. The mother may be given oxygen via a facemask especially in cases of maternal oxygen lack such as eclampsia or antepartum hemorrhage. Fetal blood sample may need to be taken.

If the fetal distress does not get corrected, delivery will be expedited. In the first stage of labor, this will necessitate cesarean section.

In the second stage of labor a quicker vaginal delivery may be effected with an episiotomy, a forceps delivery or a ventouse extraction. In all cases of delivery following fetal distress, the baby will require resuscitation and the midwife must be prepared for it. Presence of a pediatrician is necessary whenever possible, to resuscitate the newborn.

Bodily Care of the Woman

A woman in labor needs constant care throughout labor. This care refers to an active and participative presence in the room to manage the care of the woman obstetrically and to provide or facilitate the provision of indicated supportive care.

Keeping Clean and Dry

Cleanliness and dryness promote comfort and relaxation and decrease the risk of infection. A possible combination of bloody show, perspiration, amniotic fluid, solutions for vaginal examinations, and feces creates a feeling of messiness, discomfort and general misery for the woman.

A shower can change a woman's entire outlook and feeling to one of well-being, if there are no contraindications to ambulation and there are available facilities. If a shower is not possible, a sponge bath is also refreshing.

Subsequent attention to perineal care and keeping dry continues the feeling of well-being. This is done by changing the gown if one becomes damp with perspiration, changing sheets if they become wet from solutions, discharges, or perspiration; giving perineal care to remove any solutions or discharges and frequently changing the absorbent pad beneath her buttocks. Emphasis on cleanliness of the perineum and anything that comes close to the perineum, as well as scrupulous attention to handwashing by both the woman and all in contact with her decreases the chance for intrauterine infection developing from contamination at the vaginal introitus.

Mouth Care

A woman in labor will develop bad breath, a dry mouth, dry or cracked lips, a parched throat, and coated teeth, especially if in labor for a number of hours without oral fluids and without mouth care. If all these develop the woman is uncomfortable and it is unpleasant to those attending her. Some of this can be avoided if the woman is able to ingest liquids during her labor. Some of it develops because of mouth breathing, slight dehydration, and lack of moisture in the mouth or passage of time without mouth care. Mouth care consists of the following:

❖ *Brushing teeth*—Women should be encouraged to bring their toothbrush and toothpaste with them to the hospital
❖ *Mouthwash*—Diluted or undiluted according to the client's preference
❖ Glycerin swabs or Vaseline for lips
❖ Sips of water or clear liquids with sugar for hydration and moistening of the mouth and throat.

A washcloth can save several useful purposes for a woman in labor:

❖ To refresh by cleaning/washing
❖ To wipe away facial perspiration
❖ To serve as a moist pack or as a cold compress
❖ To moisten dry lips.

Back Rub

Two types of back rubs are useful in providing support and comfort to a woman in labor. One is the usual generalized, overall back rub, which is used to promote relaxation. The second is called the OB back rub. This is done just during contractions, when the woman experiences the greatest discomfort or pain in her lower back. Some women experience localized pain caused by the pressure of the fetal head against her spine. This pain is exaggerated if the fetus is in an occipital posterior position. The OB back rub is application of external pressure on the spine to counteract the internal pressure on the spine by the fetal head and thus reduces the pain. You will need to recheck with the woman frequently about the proper location of the pressure you are applying as the pain will move downwards as descent of fetal head occurs.

The OB back rub is offered by placing the palm of your hand against the spot identified by the woman and applying pressure. You can massage the spot and adjacent area at the same time by circularly moving your palm on that spot without lifting your palm or moving it off the identified spot. The woman can also guide you as to the proper amount of pressure. Too much pressure is painful and too little pressure is ineffective. In order to give the rub effectively and without strain for the midwife, the client needs to be in lateral position. Lotion or powder should be used to reduce friction and prevent skin irritation.

Both types of back rubs have the effect of expressing care for the woman and assuring a sustaining human presence for as long as the back rub is given. At times, some degree of relief can be obtained by folding a small towel and placing it at the specific spot where the woman feels pain, so she lies on it. It will provide counter pressure.

Abdominal Rub

The abdominal rub is a light rubbing (massage) of the entire abdomen usually done in a circular fashion. The midwife or attendant/significant other can do it while using one hand for feeling a contraction or holding the woman's hand. This is very comforting to the woman and it expresses caring in a strange environment. It also increases circulation to the area, thereby dilating blood vessels, which have become constricted from contractions and caused tissue anoxia. The increased blood flow combats the tissue hypoxia and provides a physiological basis for a decrease in pain.

Effleurage

Effleurage is a technique used in the Lamaze and other psychoprophylactic methods of childbirth preparation. By definition effleurage means "feather-touch" which describes the amount of pressure to be used in doing it. It is usually done by the laboring woman, using both hands and following definite pattern over primarily her lower abdomen (symphysis pubis to just above her umbilicus) as illustrated in Figure 18.9. Using all her fingers of both hands, with the fingers loosely separated, the woman covers the entire lower abdominal area with the two circular patterns—up and outwards

Fig. 18.9: Effleurage pattern

from her umbilicus, down and around or in a reverse pattern. Its effectiveness is both psychological and physiological.

Psychological in that it is one more thing to concentrate on along with her breathing, other than discomfort, and physiologic in that the action also increases circulation to the area, combating tissue hypoxia and thus decreasing pain.

Alleviation of Leg Cramps

Leg cramps during labor are usually so acute they capture the woman's total attention and demand immediate relief. Cramps probably are caused by pressure of the presenting part on the nerves of the extremities as they cross through the obturator foramen in the pelvis.

The woman's legs must never be massaged because of the risk of unwittingly dislodging unknown thrombi developed during months of trouble with venous return and possible varicosities. In order to obtain immediate relief straighten the woman's leg and dorsiflex her foot. Alternating relaxation with dorsiflexion of her foot increases the rapidity of the effectiveness. The dorsiflexion should be forcibly exaggerated to effect relief.

Supportive Care of the Woman and her Significant Other

Use of Physical Touch

This means the touching of the woman by the midwife (e.g. on her leg, head or arm) for no other reason than to touch her. Most people who touch mean to convey caring, comfort and understanding in an effort to soothe, calm, dispel loneliness, and so forth. However, touching is effective only if the one touching is comfortable with touching others and if the woman is comfortable with being touched. Touching can be extremely effective when both the toucher and the touched are comfortable with it. Some clients who are extremely frightened, especially young women may throw their arms around your neck and forcibly hang onto you during a contraction. It is important that you do not reject such a client because her touch is more like a cry for help. Between contractions, ascertain the problems and location of pain and either find a significant other for her to hang on to (if it is possible) or tell her you have to be free bodily to do other things to help her, but she can hang on to one of your hands.

Significant Others

In places where a significant other is allowed to stay with the laboring woman, it is found as the most important of all support and comfort measures. The first step is to identify the woman's significant other who she wants with her during the childbirth process—spouse, parent, sibling, friend, or relative. In hospitals where it is practiced, the woman has to identify one person who is so designated and accepted as the person who will be with her in the labor room.

The family member should be made to feel welcome and wanted in the labor room by the staff and viewed as important participants in the ongoing events. They should be given territorial space at the side of the woman. Unprepared significant others usually are glad to do anything you suggest and show them how to do. Prepared significant others have probably planned beforehand with the woman what they will do. Find out their plans so that you will facilitate rather than frustrate them.

They will do anything within their capacity that is agreeable to the laboring women, themselves and the midwife. The woman will respond to the prepared significant other with whom she has practiced and on whom she relies for coaching. Unprepared

attendants usually learn quickly and do well in coaching breathing. The significant other can be involved in such activities as the use of a wet washcloth, hand holding, fanning and abdominal rubbing. Men usually make the best back rubbers.

The most important thing in working with women and their significant others is to facilitate their relationship as it involves a continuing commitment in their daily life.

Records

Throughout the first stage of labor, the midwife must keep meticulous records of all the events of the woman's physical and psychological condition and the condition of the fetus. While observing the progress of labor, she should be alert for signs of second stage of labor. A comprehensive record of the progress of the labor must be evident. Vital parameters, treatments and nursing care must be clearly documented.

NURSING PROCESS DURING THE FIRST STAGE OF LABOR

Assessment

Nursing History (On Admission)

1. Name and age
2. Personal data—Blood type, Rh, current weight and amount of weight gain, allergies to medications and other substances.
3. Data regarding this pregnancy—Gravida, para.
4. Status of labor— Characteristics of contractions and whether membranes have ruptured.

Physical Assessment

1. Assess maternal vital signs.
2. Assess uterine contractions, determine frequency, duration and intensity.
3. Assess contractions either by palpation or by an electronic monitor.
4. Assess fetal station, presentation and position by Leopold's maneuvers and/or vaginal examination.
5. Assess cervical dilatation and effacement.
6. Assess fetal heart rate.

7. Evaluate FHR pattern—Variability, acceleration, deceleration.
8. Assess coping skills, level of anxiety and response to labor.

Analysis/Nursing Diagnosis

1. Anxiety related to knowledge deficit
2. Risk for infection
3. Pain
4. Fatigue
5. Impaired skin integrity
6. Anxiety
7. Ineffective individual coping
8. Powerlessness
9. Impaired adjustment
10. Self-care deficit: Bathing/hygiene.

Planning

1. Orient the client and significant other to surroundings.
2. Promote physical comfort and safety.
3. Promote maternal-fetal well-being during the birth process.
4. Provide support and counseling to client and spouse/significant other during labor.
5. Encourage self-care activities and support measures during labor and delivery.
6. Monitor woman and fetus.

Implementation

1. Complete maternal-fetal physical assessment:
   a. Maternal vital signs
   b. Determine if membranes are ruptured
   c. Assess FHR.
2. Evaluate uterine contractions.
3. Evaluate progression of cervical dilatation, effacement and fetal descend.
4. Provide support measures for mother:
   a. Quiet environment
   b. Reassurance and encouragement
   c. Rest between contractions.
5. Maintain comfort measures.
6. Support breathing methods.
7. Provide teaching and associated nursing care.

8. Identify signs of any developing complications:
   a. Decreased fetal movement
   b. Abnormalities in FHR
   c. Meconium—stained liquor
   d. Abnormal presentation and position
   e. Maternal fever, PIH, diabetes
   f. Bleeding.
9. Encourage woman to empty bladder every two hours.
10. Provide clear fluids and/or IV fluids.
11. Monitor labor for signs of fetal distress:
    a. Meconium stained amniotic fluid
    b. Fetal hyperactivity or lack of activity
    c. Fetal tachycardia or bradycardia
    d. Loss of baseline variability
    e. Presence of late or variable decelerations.

Note: Items d and e for clients on continuous fetal monitoring.

Evaluation

Ensure that:

1. The woman and significant other has knowledge regarding the surroundings and labor process.
2. The woman understands and practices safety measures.
3. The woman and her fetus experiences a safe labor and birth.
4. The woman acknowledges that support was received during labor and birth.

BIBLIOGRAPHY

1. AJN/Mosby. Nursing Board's Review for NCLEX-RN Examination, 10th edn. St. Louis, Baltimore: Mosby; 1997.
2. Cassidy P. Management of the First Stage of Labor. In: Bennet RV, Linda KB (Eds). Myles Textbook for Midwives, 13th edn. Edinburgh: Churchill Livingstone; 1999.
3. Dick-Read G. Childbirth without Fear, 2nd edn. Harper and Row; 1957.
4. Freidman EA. Labor: Clinical Evaluation and Management, 2nd edn. New York: Meredith; 1978.
5. Pritchard JA, McDonald PC, Gant N. Williams Obstetrics, 17th edn. Connecticut: Appleton Century Crafts; 1885.
6. Varney Helen. Nurse-Midwifery, 2nd edn. Boston: Jones and Barlett Publishers; 1996.

19

Physiology of the Second Stage of Labor

Learning Objectives

Upon completion of this chapter, the learner will be able to:

❖ Explain the second stage of labor
❖ Describe the physiological processes during the second stage of labor
❖ Enumerate the presumptive signs and differential diagnosis of second stage
❖ Describe the mechanisms of labor
❖ Describe the maternal physiological changes and the limits of normality for each.

The second stage of labor begins with complete dilatation of the cervix and ends with the birth of the baby. It is known as the stage of expulsion. It is the period when the baby descends from the uterus through the birth canal and is expelled.

PHYSIOLOGICAL PROCESSES

The physiological changes result from a continuation of the same forces, which have been at work during the first stage of labor.

Descend

Descend of the fetal presenting part, which began during the first stage of labor and reached its maximum speed toward the end of the first stage of labor, continues its rapid pace through the second stage of labor until reaching the pelvic floor. The average maximum rate of descend is 1.6 cm per hour in nulliparas and 5.4 cm per hour in multiparas.

Uterine Action

Contractions during the second stage are frequent, strong and slightly longer that is

approximately every two minutes, lasting 60–90 seconds. They are of strong intensity and become expulsive in nature. After the painful contractions she experienced during the transition, the woman usually feels relief to be in second stage and be able to push if she so desires.

In the natural course of labor, there is often a lull, or quiet period, between first and second stage. The hard contractions of transition are now past and the cervix is fully dilated. The woman's body seems to "take a breath" before starting expulsive efforts. The contractions space out and are not so intense. The woman rests and may even nap. This quiet period may last as long as an hour and is longer in primigravidae than in multigravidae. Gradually momentum builds as the fetal head descends through the pelvis, the contractions become more forceful and the woman begins to voluntarily bear down with expiratory, grunty, short pushes.

Rupture of Membranes

The membranes often rupture spontaneously at the onset of the second stage. The consequent drainage of liquor allows the hard, round fetal head to be directly applied to the vaginal tissues and aid distention. Fetal axis pressure increases flexion of the head, which results in smaller presenting diameters, more rapid progress and less trauma to both mother and fetus. As the fetus further descends into the vagina, pressure from the presenting part stimulates nerve receptors in the pelvic floor and the woman experiences the need to push.

Soft Tissue Displacement

As the hard fetal head descends, the soft tissues of the pelvis become displaced. Anteriorly, the bladder is pushed upwards into the abdomen where it is at less risk of injury during fetal descent. Posteriorly, the rectum becomes flattened into the sacral curve and the pressure of the advancing head expels any residual fecal matter. The levator ani muscles dilate, thin out and become displaced laterally, and the perineal body is flattened, stretched and thinned. The fetal head becomes visible at the vulva, advancing with each contraction, and receding during the resting phase until crowning takes place and the head is born.

PRESUMPTIVE SIGNS OF SECOND STAGE AND DIFFERENTIAL DIAGNOSIS

Expulsive Contractions

The woman's verbal expression: "My baby is coming" often signals an imminent delivery. It is possible for a woman to feel strong desire to push before the cervix is fully dilated if the fetus is in an occipitoposterior position, the rectum is full or the woman is highly parous.

Rupture of Membranes

Membranes normally rupture at the onset of second stage. However, this may occur at any time during labor.

Dilatation and Gaping of Anus and Perineal Bulging

Deep engagement of the presenting part and premature maternal effort may produce this sign during the latter part of the first stage.

Progressive Visibility of the Fetal Head at the Introitus

Excessive moulding may result in the formation of a large caput succedaneum, which can protrude through the cervix prior to full dilatation. Similarly, a breech presentation may be visible when the cervix is only 7 to 8 cm dilated.

Congestion of the Vulva

Enthusiastic premature pushing may also cause this.

❖ The average length of the second stage is one hour for primigravidas and 15 minutes for multiparas (Friedman, 1978). Generally, a second stage that lasts longer than two hours for a primigravida or one hour for a multipara is considered abnormal.

MATERNAL PHYSIOLOGICAL CHANGES IN THE SECOND STAGE

The normal physiological changes that occur in the first stage of labor continue through the second stage of labor.

Blood Pressure

Blood pressure may rise another 15 to 20 mm of mercury with contractions during the second stage. Maternal pushing effort affects the blood pressure, causing variation from an increase to a decrease and ending at a level slightly above normal. It is important therefore, to evaluate the blood pressure well between contractions. A rise of 10 mm of mercury between contractions, when a woman has been pushing, is normal.

Metabolism

The steady rise in metabolism continues through the second stage. The maternal pushing effort adds further skeletal muscle activity that contributes to the increase in metabolism.

Pulse Rate

Pulse rate increases during each pushing effort. It is elevated throughout the second stage with a definite tachycardia reaching a peak at the time of delivery.

Temperature

The highest elevation of temperature is at the time of delivery and immediately thereafter. An increase of 0.5 to 1°C is considered normal.

Gastrointestinal Changes

The reduction in gastric motility and absorption continues through the second stage. Usually, the nausea and vomiting of transition subside during the second stage but they may persist for some women.

Renal and Hematological Changes

These are same as discussed for the first stage of labor.

THE MECHANISM OF NORMAL LABOR

The mechanisms of labor are the positional movements that the fetus undergoes to accommodate itself to the maternal pelvis. This is necessary in as much as the larger diameters of the fetus must be in alignment with the larger diameters of the maternal pelvis in order for the full term fetus to negotiate its way through the pelvis to be born.

At the onset of labor, the most common presentation is the vertex and the most common position is either, left or right occipitoanterior; therefore it is this mechanism that will be described below. When the fetus presents in left or right occipitoanterior position, the way the fetus is normally situated can be described as follows:

❖ The lie is longitudinal
❖ The presentation is cephalic
❖ The position is right or left occipitoanterior
❖ The attitude is one of flexion
❖ The denominator is the occiput
❖ The presenting part is the posterior part of the anterior parietal bone.

Positional Movements (Figs 19.1A to G)

There are several basic positional movements, which take place when the fetus is in a cephalic vertex presentation. These are as follows:

❖ Engagement
❖ Descend throughout
❖ Flexion
❖ Internal rotation of the head
❖ Crowning
❖ Birth of the head by extension
❖ Restitution
❖ Internal rotation of the shoulders
❖ External rotation of the head
❖ Birth of the shoulders and body by lateral flexion.

Although the mechanisms of labor are listed separately, some of these overlap or occur simultaneously (internal rotation of shoulders and external rotation of the head).

Engagement

Engagement takes place when the biparietal diameter of the fetal head has passed through the pelvic inlet. In primigravidae it usually occurs during the latter weeks of pregnancy. In multigravidae, as the muscle tone is lax engagement may not occur until labor actually begins.

Descend

Descend occurs throughout the mechanisms of labor and is therefore both requisite to and simultaneous with the other mechanisms. Descend is the result of a number of forces including contractions (which straighten the fetal spine, bring the fundus into direct contact with the breech, and exert pressure of the fundus on the breech) and maternal pushing effort with contraction of her abdominal muscles.

Flexion

Flexion is essential to further descend. The pressure exerted down the fetal axis will be transmitted to the occiput. The effect is to increase flexion, which results in the substitution of the smaller suboccipitobregmatic diameter of 9.5 cm for the larger suboccipitofrontal diameter of 10 cm. The occiput becomes the leading part. Flexion occurs when the fetal head meets resistance; this resistance increases with descend. It is first met from the cervix, then the sidewalls and finally the pelvic floor.

Internal Rotation of the Head

Internal rotation brings the anteroposterior diameter of the fetal head into alignment with the anteroposterior diameter of the maternal pelvis. This is accomplished by rotation of the occiput to the anterior portion of the maternal pelvis. During a contraction the leading part (occiput) is driven downwards on to the pelvic floor. The slope of the pelvic floor determines the direction of rotation. In a well-flexed vertex presentation, the occiput leads and meets the pelvic floor first and rotates anteriorly through one-eighth of a circle (45 degrees). This causes a slight twist in the neck of the fetus (45 degrees), as the head is no longer in direct alignment with the shoulders. As the fetal head

Figs 19.1A to G: Mechanisms of labor: (A) Engagement descent, flexion; (B) Internal rotation; (C) Extension beginning; (D) Extension complete; (E) Restitution; (F) External rotation; (G) Lateral flexion (expulsion)

now lies in the widest (anteroposterior) diameter of the pelvic outlet, an easy escape is facilitated. The occiput slips under the pubic arch and *crowning* occurs when the head no longer recedes between contractions and the widest transverse diameter (biparietal) is born.

Internal rotation is essential for vaginal birth to occur except for abnormally small babies. Internal rotation is effected by the 'V' shape of the pelvic floor musculature and the decreased dimensions of the pelvic cavity due to the ischial spines. The distance the occiput has to travel from its original position upon entering the pelvis to the occiput anterior or occiput posterior position determines the amount of internal rotation. The distance is described as the degrees in a circle, which is being traversed.

Crowning

After internal rotation of the head, further descent occurs until the subocciput lies underneath the pubic arch. At this stage, the maximum diameter of the head (biparietal diameter) stretches the vulval outlet without any recession of the head even after the contraction is over. This is called "crowning of the head".

Birth of the Head

Once crowning has occurred, the fetal head can extend. The suboccipital region, or nucha impinges under the symphysis pubis and acts as a pivotal point. The fetal head is now positioned so that further pressure from the contracting uterus and maternal pushing serves to further extend the head as the vaginal orifice opens. Thus, the head is born by extension as the sinciput face and chin sequentially sweep over the perineum.

Restitution

Restitution is the rotation of the head either, to the left or right depending on the direction from which it rotated into the occiput anterior position. In effect, restitution untwists the neck so that the head is again at right angle with the shoulders. With restitution, the occiput moves 45 degrees or one-eighth of a circle towards the side from which it started.

Internal Rotation of Shoulders

The anterior shoulder reaches the pelvic floor and rotates anteriorly one-eighth of a circle (45 degrees). The shoulders come to lie in the anteroposterior diameter of the pelvic outlet (under the symphysis pubis).

External Rotation of the Head

External rotation of the head occurs as the shoulders rotate 45 degrees internally causing the head to rotate another 45 degrees (as the shoulders rotate towards the symphysis pubis from the oblique diameter it carries the head in a movement of external rotation). The movement can be seen clearly as the head turns at the same time. External rotation occurs in the same direction as restitution and the occiput of the fetal head now lies laterally (LOT or ROT).

Birth of the Shoulders and Body by Lateral Flexion

The anterior shoulder comes into view at the vaginal orifice, where it impinges under the symphysis pubis, while the posterior shoulder distends the perineum. This enables a smaller diameter to distend the vaginal orifice than if both shoulders were born simultaneously. After the shoulders are delivered, the remainder of the body is born by lateral flexion following the curve of Carus.

Degrees of Internal Rotation in Transverse and Posterior Positions

When the occiput rotates from an LOT, ROT, LOP or ROP position, the shoulders also rotate with the head until the LOA or ROA position has been reached. As the occiput rotates the final 1/8th of a circle (45 degrees) into the occiput anterior position, the shoulders do not continue their rotation with the head, but instead enter the pelvic inlet in one of the oblique diameters (the left oblique diameter for an LOA and the right oblique diameter for an ROA). The entire mechanism therefore, has the effect of twisting the neck 1/8th of a circle (45 degrees).

Internal rotation in transverse positions (LOT and ROT) is 90 degrees and in posterior positions (LOP and ROP) 135 degrees. When the rotation is 135 degrees, it is termed as *long arc rotation*.

The Curve of Carus

The curve of Carus is the pelvic curve at its lower end as determined by the pelvic structure. The products of conception must follow this curve for birth. The pelvic cavity actually resembles a curved cylinder, so that the direction of either the baby or the placenta coming through it is first downward from the axis of the inlet to just above the tip of the sacrum and then forward, upward and outward to the vaginal orifice.

SUMMARY OF MECHANISMS IN LEFT OCCIPUT ANTERIOR (LOA) POSITION (FIGS 19.2A to H)

❖ Lie is longitudinal
❖ Presentation is cephalic
❖ Position is left occipitoanterior
❖ Attitude is one of flexion
❖ Denominator is the occiput
   Presenting part is the posterior part of the anterior parietal bone.
❖ Engagement takes place with sagittal suture of the fetal head in the right oblique diameter of the pelvic inlet and the biparietal diameter of the fetal head in the left oblique (opposite) diameter of the pelvis. The occiput points to the left iliopectineal eminence and the sinciput to the right sacroiliac joint
❖ Descend occurs throughout
❖ Flexion substitutes the suboccipitobregmatic diameter for the diameter, which entered the pelvic inlet (suboccipitofrontal)
❖ Internal rotation takes place and the occiput turns 1/8th of a circle (45 degrees) to the

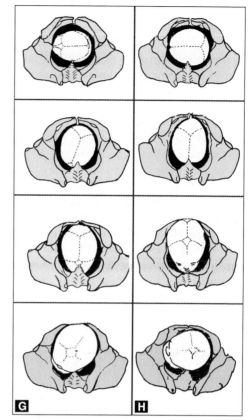

Figs 19.2A to H: Diagrammatic representation of the positions of fetal skull in LOT to LOA mechanism: (A) At onset of labor; (B) Descend and flexion; (C) Internal rotation: LOT to LOA; (D) Internal rotation: LOT to OA; (E) Extension beginning; (F) Extension complete; (G) Restitution: OA to LOA; (H) External rotation: LOA to LOT

right. The sagittal suture comes to the anteroposterior diameter of the mother's pelvis
❖ The occiput escapes under the symphysis pubis and crowning occurs when the head no longer recedes between contractions
❖ The head is born by extension, pivoting on the suboccipital region around the pubic arch
❖ Restitution—The occiput turns 1/8th of a circle (45 degrees) to the left to undo the twist on the neck
❖ Internal rotation of the shoulders. The anterior shoulder reaches the pelvic floor and rotates anteriorly to lie under the symphysis pubis. This movement can be seen as the head turns at the same time (external rotation of the head)

❖ External rotation of the head. The head turns another 1/8th of a circle (45 degrees) to the mother's left. The bisacromial diameter of the shoulders comes into the anteroposterior diameter of the maternal pelvis. This occurs in the same direction as restitution and at the same time as internal rotation of the shoulders

❖ The anterior shoulder escapes under the symphysis pubis and the body is born by lateral flexion.

For every presentation and position that is delivered vaginally, there is a mechanism. These are the series of passive movements taken by the fetus to negotiate the birth canal. Knowledge of these movements enables the midwife to recognize the level of descend and anticipate the next step in the process. Monitoring of the movements, aids in assessment of the progress, safe completion of delivery and intervention for any delay.

Principles

Principles are common to all mechanisms:

❖ Descend occurs throughout

❖ The part that leads and first meets the resistance of the pelvic floor will rotate forwards until it comes under the symphysis pubis

❖ The part that escapes under the symphysis pubis will pivot around the pubic bone

❖ During the mechanism, the fetus turns slightly to take advantage of the widest available space in each plane of the pelvis, i.e. transverse at the brim and antero-posterior at the outlet.

FETAL NORMALITY DURING THE SECOND STAGE

Evaluation of the fetus during the second stage of labor includes evaluation of the amount of caput succedaneum and moulding as well as the normalcy of progress being made in the mechanisms of labor and the fetal heart tones.

Periodic fetal heart rate—changes of the early deceleration type may occur as delivery nears. Early deceleration caused by compression of the head, is a uniform shaped pattern reflecting the uniform shape of the contractions. Head compression occurs at this time, because of the pressure exerted on the fetal head by the pelvic floor and perineum during contractions and further exaggerated by the woman's pushing effort. Usually the fetal heart rate does not fall below 100 beats per minute during the deceleration period, and the baseline fetal heart rate is usually within normal range in an early deceleration pattern. Early deceleration is not considered an indication of acute fetal distress but needs to be differentiated carefully from a late deceleration pattern, which is due to uteroplacental insufficiency. A baseline bradycardia may occur when the fetal head descends rapidly into the pelvis and needs to be carefully evaluated.

DURATION OF THE SECOND STAGE

The duration of the second stage is difficult to predict with any degree of certainty. In multigravidae, it may last as little as 5 minutes; in primigravidae, the process may take 2 hours (average length for multigravidae is 15 minutes and for primigravidae 1 hour). More important than the time factor is the evidence of progressive descend and the condition of mother and fetus. Once the onset of second stage has been confirmed, a woman should not be left without a midwife in attendance.

BIBLIOGRAPHY

1. Caldero Barcia P, et al. Effects of position changes on the intensity and frequency of uterine contractions during labor. American Journal of Obstetrics and Gynecology 1971;109:274.
2. Dutta DC. Textbook of Obstetrics, 5th edn. Calcutta: New Central Book Company 2001.
3. Friedman EA. The functional divisions of labor, American Journal of Obstetrics and Gynecology, 1971;109:274.
4. Hillan EM. Physiology and management of the second stage of labor. In: Bennett RV, Brown KB (Eds) Myles Textbook for Nurses, 13th edn. Edinburgh: Churchill Livingstone; 1999.
5. Hon EH. An Introduction to Fetal Monitoring, 2nd edn. North Haven Corometrics. Connecticut: Medical Systems; 1971.
6. Peterson G. Birthing Normally, A Personal Growth Approach to Childbirth, 2nd edn. Berkeley, California: Mind-Body Press; 1984.
7. Schrag K. Maintenance of Pelvic Floor Integrity during Childbirth. Journal of Nurse-Midwifery 1979;24(6).
8. Varney Helen. Nurse-Midwifery, 2nd edn. Boston: Jones and Barlett Publishers; 1996.

20

Management of the
Second Stage of Labor

Learning Objectives

Upon completing this chapter, the learner will be able to:
- Enumerate the nursing care activities for a woman in the second stage of labor
- Describe the sequence of events during the second stage in a normal labor
- Describe the process and conduct of delivery
- Discuss the rationale for an episiotomy and explain its risks and benefits
- Describe the midwife's role in the immediate care of the newborn.

Management of the second stage of labor is a continuation of the responsibilities included in the management of the first stage of labor and additional responsibilities for preparation for delivery and management of delivery.

EVALUATION OF MATERNAL WELL-BEING

Continuing evaluation of maternal well-being during the second stage of labor includes the following items:
- Vital signs
- Bladder care
- Hydration and general condition
- Maternal pushing effort
- Analgesia and anesthesia
- Perineal integrity.

Vital Signs

The frequency, with which vital signs are checked, is increased during the second stage of labor. This frequency may vary somewhat from hospital-to-hospital or from obstetrician-to-obstetrician but the following schedule reflects generally accepted standards for a normal woman during the second stage of labor. Temperature, pulse and respirations are to be evaluated every hour and blood pressure every 15 minutes. It is important to remember that the blood pressure should be taken between contractions and it is normally increased by an average of 10 mm of mercury if the woman has been pushing.

Bladder Care

Management of the woman's bladder during the second stage of labor and the rationale for this management is same as discussed for the first stage of labor.

In addition, a decision may have to be made about catheterizing the woman immediately prior to delivery, which is towards the end of the second stage of labor. If catheterization is to be done it is usually done after the woman is scrubbed and draped and before any other procedure such as pudendal block or cutting of an episiotomy. This timing is important so that the catheter can be inserted before the fetal head gets any lower in the pelvis, since further descend makes the catheterization more difficult.

In making a decision whether or not to catheterize a woman at this time, the following factors are considered:
1. Whether or not the bladder needs emptying
   a. Is it distended?
   b. Has the woman voided within the last two hours?
   c. What has been her fluid intake since her last voiding?

2. There is increased risk of bladder infection with catheterization.
3. Whether or not a possible potential complication is being anticipated:
   a. Immediate postpartum hemorrhage.
   b. Shoulder dystocia.
   (Management of both of these complications includes having an empty bladder. Precious time can be gained if an empty bladder is already assured).

Careful monitoring of the bladder during the first and second stage of labor and use of all measures to get the woman void naturally, often avoids the need for catheterization. However, if the bladder is obviously distended, a decision must be made to catheterize the woman in order to avoid further trauma to the bladder, decrease the discomfort in her lower abdomen and circumvent a problem with the bladder in the event of aforementioned complications. A high probability for complications warrants catheterization, even if a distended bladder is not obvious, as the woman should end this phase of labor with an empty bladder.

Catheterization for a client in the second stage of labor with the fetal head in the true pelvis is different from usual as regards the direction of the catheter is concerned. The urethra is displaced to conform to the contour of the fetal head, which is displacing it.

Therefore, immediately upon entry of the catheter into the urethra, it is necessary to direct the catheter upward and over the fetal head while going inward. Otherwise, by going straight in as usual, the catheter simply will not go in and the urethra will be traumatized. Going up and over the fetal head also means that more than usual length of the catheter will be inserted before reaching the bladder.

Hydration and General Condition

Management of these three areas during the second stage of labor and the rationale for their management is the same as for the first stage of labor.

Hydration, however, is further affected during the second stage of labor by fluid loss through the skin in the form of perspiration. The woman may perspire profusely from the effort of pushing.

The general condition of the woman in the second stage of labor depends on the manner in which it was maintained in the first stage of labor. If she enters the second stage of labor exhausted, she is going to have difficulty in mustering the energy required for pushing, especially if she is a primigravida. This is because the average length of a primigravid second stage is longer than that of a multipara.

Maternal Pushing Effort

The maternal pushing effort occurs in response to a reflex mechanism, which is initiated when the head is pressing against and distending the pelvic floor. The reflex mechanism is thereafter triggered with each contraction; the maternal response of pushing is activated shortly after the onset of the contractions, after it has started to build toward its acme.

The maternal pushing effort must be evaluated for effectiveness. Proof of effectiveness is the progressive descend and sequence of mechanisms of labor by the fetus. The sequential bulging of the rectum, then the perineum, and finally visualization of an ever-increasing amount of the fetal presenting part at the enlarging vulval orifice generally evidence this. In the absence of progress, it is essential to re-evaluate pelvic adequacy and rule out arrest in the mechanisms of labor by careful vaginal examination. If neither of these difficulties exists, the problem is probably either ineffectual pushing or a psychological obstacle (e.g. a frightened woman).

There are those who believe that the word pushing should never be used and the woman should bear down only as she feels like it. There are others, who believe in vigorously encouraging the maternal pushing effort as soon as the cervix is completely dilated. Management by most obstetricians and midwives lies some where between these two extremes.

The breathing used in the natural pushing effort is that of a series of short pushes often during the expiratory phase of respiration. This reduces the possibility of fetal hypoxia and acidosis, which may result from repeated breath holding after inspiration and prolonged bearing down. Natural bearing down and slow distension of the perineal musculature serves the following advantages:

1. Reduced possibility of lacerations or the need for an episiotomy.
2. Lessened incidence of uterine prolapse and cystocele because of less strain on the cardinal ligaments.
3. Lessened trauma to the fetal head because of gradual even pressure against the head.

Taking all these into consideration, it seems reasonable to use an approach that combines the best of the two methods. In this approach, the "natural" method is used unless or until there is evidence of a need for the woman to push deliberately, as in the case of spinal anesthesia.

Women, who have not had preparation for childbirth in the prenatal period, must be taught the techniques of breathing and bearing down before she reaches the second stage of labor. If the natural efforts of pushing are ineffectual, such women should be taught how to push effectively.

Analgesia and Anesthesia

Analgesia, during the second stage of labor, usually is the continuation of analgesia given during the first stage of labor.

Anesthesia is achieved by one of the following methods.

Local Infiltration

Local infiltration of the perineal body is carried out to provide anesthesia when an episiotomy is planned.

Pudendal Block

Pudendal block is used when a larger area of the perineum is to be anesthetized. It anesthetizes the perineum and vulva including the clitoris, labia majora, perineal body and rectal area without tissue distortion.

Lumbar Epidural Block

For lumbar epidural block, the anesthetic is introduced between lumbar vertebrae two and three or three and four as a single shot, intermittent technique or continuous technique.

Perineal Integrity

Evaluation of perineal integrity is for determining if delivery can possibly occur over an intact perineum or if episiotomies are needed.

This decision is continually re-evaluated until the baby is born. There are several techniques, which facilitate delivery over an intact perineum. The commonly used techniques include:
1. "Ironing out" the perineum by sweeping the midwife's fingers back and forth from side-to-side in the vagina just ahead of the fetal head. The pressure applied to iron out, or stretch the muscles also stimulate the pushing reflex.
2. Perineal support at the time of birth: Some midwives do this by directly bracing the perineal body with their hand. Other midwives place their thumb and middle finger across from each other in the left and right groin and press inward to provide a little extra support across the perineal body.
3. Fetal head control by asserting pressure against the fetal head to keep it well-flexed and then allowing gradual extension as the perineum stretches. This is essential in lithotomy and dorsal positions in order to prevent tears.

Some midwives believe that if fetal head control is done properly, there is no need to touch the perineum. Others combine fetal head control and perineal support.

Maternal self-control is the key to whatever method of delivering over an intact perineum is used. A woman, who is out of control, is more likely to tear or need an episiotomy.

EPISIOTOMY

An episiotomy is a surgical incision of the perineal body. The perineum is evaluated prior to the time of delivery to determine whether or not an episiotomy is indicated and, if so, what kind of episiotomy. The perineum is evaluated for its length, thickness and distensibility. A short perineum may indicate performing a mediolateral episiotomy rather than a median episiotomy, in order to avoid injury to the rectal sphincter and wall.

Indications

Any condition that places the woman at risk for perineal tearing:
1. Large size baby: A baby estimated to be 4,000 gm or more may cause need for an episiotomy either to prevent laceration or in anticipation of a possible shoulder dystocia.

2. Preterm or small for gestational age (SGA) baby in order to minimize the risk of intracranial hemorrhage.
3. An uncontrolled woman who is unable to respond to instructions as to when to push and when to breathe, in order to slowly ease the head out.
4. Anticipation of shoulder dystocia.
5. Fetal malpresentations and malpositions. In these situations, the widest diameter of the fetal head coming through the pelvic outlet and vaginal orifice is larger than usual.
6. A thick perineum, which is rigid and resistant to distention.
7. An inevitable laceration evidenced by narrow white lines resembling stretch marks and visible just beneath the skin. These appear just prior to laceration and probably represent beginning of tearing of the underlying tissues. A quick episiotomy prior to the moment of crowning is indicated to avoid an inevitable tear.
8. Prior to an assisted delivery such as forceps or vacuum extraction.
9. To speed up delivery if there is fetal distress.

Types of Episiotomies (Fig. 20.1)

There are two main types of episiotomies:
1. Midline or median
2. Mediolateral, which may be to the right or left.
3. Lateral and 'J' shaped episiotomies are mentioned in the literature. Both are not done currently due to several drawbacks.

Midline or Median

Midline episiotomy is cut into the central tendinous point of the perineum. It follows the natural line of insertion of the pectineal muscles.

Advantages
❖ Easily repaired
❖ Generally less painful
❖ Minimal blood loss.

Disadvantage
❖ Higher incidence of damage to the anal sphincter.

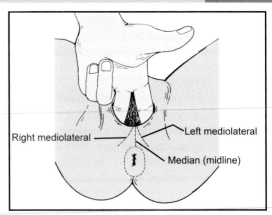

Right mediolateral — Left mediolateral

Median (midline)

Fig. 20.1: Types of episiotomies

Mediolateral Episiotomy

Mediolateral episiotomy is cut at a slant, starting at the midpoint of the posterior forchette and is directed at 45 degrees angle towards a point midway between the ischial tuberosity and the anus. The cut may be to either the left or right and about 2.5 cm.

Advantages
❖ Extension into the rectum is less likely
❖ Avoids danger of damage to anal sphincter and Bartholin glands

Disadvantages
❖ Blood loss is greater
❖ Repair is more difficult
❖ During healing the area is more painful
❖ Possible damage to pubococcygeal muscle.

Principles

The following principles should be observed regardless of which type of episiotomy is cut.
1. The presenting part of the fetus is protected from injury.
2. A single cut in any direction is far preferable to repeated snipping because the latter will leave jagged ends.
3. The episiotomy should be large enough to meet the purpose for deciding to cut it.
4. The timing of the cut should be such that lacerations are prevented (too late) and unnecessary blood loss avoided (too early). The perineum should be bulging, the vaginal orifice distended by approximately a 3 cm diameter of presenting part between

contractions, and delivery of the presenting part should be expected to occur within the next two to four contractions.

Perineal Tears

Spontaneous trauma may be of the labia anteriorly, the perineum posteriorly or both. A gentle and thorough examination must be carried out to assess accurately the trauma and to determine whether a physician should carry-out the repair.

Anterior Labial Tears

The labia are vascular and hence control of bleeding is important. A suture may be necessary to secure hemostasis.

Posterior Perineal Trauma

Spontaneous tears of the perineum are usually classified in degrees, which are related to the anatomical structure, which have been traumatized. This classification only serves as a guideline because it is difficult to identify the structures precisely.

1. First degree tear involves the forchette only.
2. Second degree tear involves the forchette and the superficial perineal muscles. Namely, the bulbocavernous and the transverse perineal muscles and in some cases the pubococcygeus.
3. Third degree tear involves damage to the anal sphincter in addition to the above structures.
4. Fourth degree tear is one, which extends into the rectal mucosa.

Note: Third and fourth degree tears should be repaired by an experienced obstetrician under a general anesthetic or effective epidural or spinal anesthetic.

EVALUATION OF THE FETAL WELL-BEING

Continuing evaluation of the fetal well-being during the second stage of labor is a continuation of the evaluation of the well-being of the fetus during the first stage of labor. It consists of evaluating the following:

1. Normalcy of the fetal lie, presentation, attitude and position.
2. Fetal adaptation to the pelvis (synclitism or asynclitism, moulding, formation of caput succedaneum).
3. Fetal heart rate pattern.
4. The normalcy of progress being made in the mechanisms of labor.

Progress in the mechanisms of labor is determined during vaginal examinations done prior to delivery. The frequency for checking fetal heart rate is increased to every 15 minutes during the second stage. Some obstetricians believe that it should be checked at the end of, and after each contraction during which the woman pushes.

In interpreting the fetal heart rate and pattern, it must be remembered that towards the end of second stage when the resistance on the fetal head from pelvic floor and perineum increases there may be a resultant early deceleration pattern. This is not considered an indication of acute fetal distress. Increased pressure on the head occurs as the delivery nears.

EVALUATION OF THE PROGRESS OF LABOR

Continuing evaluation of the progress of the second stage of labor is based on the following:

1. Contraction pain
2. Length of second stage
3. Descend and station
4. Progress through the mechanisms of labor.

The decisions regarding moving the woman to the delivery room (timing) and consulting with the physician be made, based on evaluation of progress.

Evaluation of the progress through the mechanisms of labor is essential to detecting deep transverse arrest and concomitant second stage hypotonic uterine dysfunction. The fetus is in danger in the situation in which there are strong expulsive contractions and maternal pushing effort but failure to progress because of some fetopelvic disproportion including deep transverse arrest.

Detection of progressive descend includes the following:

1. Progressively lower location (on the woman's spine) of back pain due to pressure from the fetal head.
2. Progressively lower location in the woman's abdomen of the maximum point of intensity of the fetal heart tones.
3. Increasing desire of the woman to push, which indicates descend of the fetal head to the pelvic floor and subsequent initiation of the reflex mechanism for pushing.
4. Change in station of the presenting part noted during vaginal examination.
5. Rectal and perineal bulging.
6. Appearance of the presenting part at the vaginal orifice.
7. The woman's assertion that the "baby is coming", confirmed by either observation or examination.

Engagement should have occurred during the active phase of the first stage of labor in the primigravida and by the onset of the second stage of labor in the multipara. Failure of engagement if noted in the second stage, is a signal of a potential problem.

BODILY AND SUPPORTIVE CARE OF THE WOMAN

Bodily and supportive care during the second stage of labor are continuations of the care begun during the first stage of labor, modified to meet the woman's changing needs as she progresses through labor. Additional measures specific to the second stage of labor are breathing and pushing. The woman's significant other may be permitted if the policy of the institution permits it.

Breathing

The usual instruction for the woman is to take one or two cleansing breaths (a deep breath in and out) when she feels the start of the contraction and while the contraction is building. A controlled form of breathing should be used through the contractions if the woman does not yet feel like pushing. A woman needs help with her breathing and in making effective use of either her natural pushing desire or a deliberate pushing effort.

The woman needs to be instructed to pant if she feels like pushing and you do not want her to push. Panting may be a quick inhalation followed by a forcible exhalation and repeated immediately. It may also be rapid, shallow throat breathing. The woman's ability to pant and not push can be critical in the second stage and should be taught when she enters this stage of labor as a form of anticipatory instruction if it has not been taught before.

Pushing

A woman who feels like or needs to push can be helped in a number of ways in order to make her effort as effective as possible. Her significant other (if present) can also be involved in helping her push in a way that will make the person feel important, contributing and participating in the experience.

The urge to push may come before the vertex is visible. In order to conserve maternal energy and to allow vaginal tissues to stretch passively, the mother should be helped to avoid pushing at this stage. She should be instructed to lie in left lateral position and take breathing exercise at this time.

When the head becomes visible, the woman should be encouraged to follow her own inclinations in relation to expulsive effort. The usual instruction for the woman is to take one or two deep breaths when she feels the start of the contraction and while the contraction is building, to hold the breath and push as long as she could. However, it is possible that this kind of breath holding, combined with prolonged bearing down, may produce fetal hypoxia and acidosis because the breath holding closes the glottis while bearing down and increases the intrathoracic pressure. This combination results in a drop in arterial pressure caused by decreased cardiac output leading to decreased blood flow to the placenta and decreased oxygen content in the placental circulation causing fetal hypoxia (Nikodem, 1995).

In cases where there is delay in the delivery of the fetus the woman may be given a different instruction, which is to push after expiration, as forced exhalations, for short periods of time (5 to 6 seconds). This often will be accompanied by a grunt. In such an effort, the glottis is at least partially open and the intrathoracic pressure does not increase to interfere with venous return to the heart that produce its resulting effect on cardiac output and arterial pressure.

PREPARATION FOR DELIVERY

Location of the Delivery

Once the onset of second stage has been confirmed, it is the midwife's responsibility to assure that all is in readiness for the delivery, when managing the labor and delivery of the woman. The alternatives for delivery within a hospital are the delivery room, the labor room or a birthing room. Newer hospitals often are designed for combination of labor and delivery rooms or birthing rooms for normal women. The planned location of the delivery may change due to unforeseen circumstances such as development of fetal distress and need for forceps delivery and availability of immediate newborn resuscitation equipment.

Positions for the Delivery

The usual positions, in a hospital delivery room, are lithotomy or dorsal. Other positions used for delivery are left lateral, supported sitting, squatting, kneeling, standing and knee-chest. When the dorsal position is the choice, the woman can be encouraged to be in a semisitting or back up and legs down modification.

In deciding which of the two positions to utilize for the delivery of a woman in the hospital, the following should be considered.

- A woman with varicosities should be delivered in dorsal rather than lithotomy position. This position avoids pressure on the legs in the popliteal space, which is exerted by stirrups and cause circulatory interference. The risk of thrombophlebitis would be quite high with the woman in stirrups.
- A dorsal delivery is more effective when the woman is cooperative and in control.

- The lithotomy position gives the midwife better control in the event the woman is out of control.
- In the event of any existing complications (e.g., malpresentations, multiple gestation) or anticipated complications (e.g. shoulder dystocia), the woman should be in lithotomy position, because the obstetrician needs all possible visualization and room in which to function with ready, direct access to the woman.

General Preparation

- The room in which the delivery is to take place should be warm with a spotlight available so that the perineum can be easily observed
- A clean area should be prepared to receive the baby and waterproof covers provided to protect the bed and floor
- A sterile delivery pack, which includes articles for cutting and suturing an episiotomy, two cord clamps, a pairs of scissors for cutting the cord and a bulb syringe for oropharyngeal and nasal suctioning of the baby are placed at hand
- An oxytocic agent (methergine, ergometrine or syntometrine) is prepared in readiness for the active management of third stage or for use during an emergency. It must be kept separate from any neonatal drugs to avoid risk of error
- A warm cot and blankets should be prepared for the baby. In hospital a warmed mattress, a radiant warmer or an incubator may be used. At home, a warm (not hot) water bottle can be placed in the cot
- Neonatal resuscitation equipment must be thoroughly checked and readily available
- A cap and a mask must be worn in the delivery room (if available) prior to opening the sterile packs
- A surgical hand scrub is done as soon as the head becomes visible for a multigravid woman. In primigravida, the head usually takes a little longer to advance over the perineum

❖ Once, she has put on her sterile gown and gloves (after hand scrub), the midwife must prepare her sterile articles on the instrument table. This includes antiseptic solution, cotton wool and pads.

During delivery, both mother and baby are particularly vulnerable to infection. Care must be taken to observe meticulous aseptic technique when preparing sterile equipment. Sterile surgical gloves must be worn during the delivery for the protection of both mother and the midwife.

Figs 20.2A to J: Hand maneuvers for delivery of the baby in occiput anterior position: (A and B) Controlling the head; (C) Feeling for nuchal cord; (D) Wiping the baby's face and head; (E) Delivery of the anterior shoulder; (F and G) Delivering of the posterior shoulder; (H and I) Delivery of the trunk; (J) Safety hold

CONDUCTING THE DELIVERY

Management of the delivery includes the hand maneuvers used to assist the baby's birth, the immediate care of the newborn, and the following management decisions (Figs 20.2A to J).

Delivery of the Baby's Head (Figs 20.2A to J)

In preparation for the delivery of the baby, the mother's perineum needs to be swabbed, the delivery area draped with sterile linen and a pad used to cover the anus.

Delivery of the Head between Contractions

The idea behind delivering the baby's head between contractions is that the combination of the contractions and the maternal pushing effort actually constitutes exertion of a double force at the moment of birth. This makes the birth of the head more rapid and the release of restraining pressure more abrupt both of which increase the risk of intracranial damage to the baby and laceration to the woman. If the woman is in control of herself, it is possible for her to follow the midwife's instructions and then gently push in between contractions, an action that will ease the baby's head out with the least amount of trauma to the baby and woman.

Ritgen's Maneuver

The midwife or obstetrician controls the delivery of the head by this technique. It is performed as follows:

1. Place the pads of your fingertips on the portion of the vertex showing at the vaginal introitus. As more of the head is accessible at the vaginal introitus, spread your fingers over the vertex of the baby's head with the fingertips pointing towards the as yet unseen face and your elbow pointing upward towards the mother.
2. Allow the head to gradually extend beneath your hand by exerting control, but not prohibitive, pressure with your hand. Use the length of your fingers in doing this and not just the fingertips. Proper control of the head in this manner

will prevent explosive crowning and preserve the perineum.

3. An additional maneuver of supporting the perineum may also be used. For this, cover the hand not being used on the baby's head with a towel. Place the thumb in the crease of the groin midway on one side of the perineum. Place the middle finger in the crease of the groin midway on the other side of the perineum. Apply pressure with the thumb and finger downward and then inward toward each other across the perineal body.

4. While doing this combination of head control and perineal support, observe the perineum in the space between the thumb and middle finger. As the perineum distends, the decision is made as to whether an episiotomy is required.

5. Infiltrate the perineum, cut a mediolateral episiotomy and secure hemostasis if required.

6. Watch the perineum, while the head born by extension.

7. As soon as the head is born, (during the resting phase before the next contraction) place the fingertips of one hand on the occiput and then slide them down the curve of the baby's head at the level of the top of the shoulders and sweep them in both directions, feeling for the umbilical cord (nuchal cord). Most midwives use their dominant hand for this maneuver, as it is the hand most accustomed to and sensitive for touching.
   Management of a nuchal cord is as follows:
   a. If the cord is loose, slip it over the baby's head.
   b. If the cord is too tight to slip over the baby's head but not tight around the neck, slip it back over the shoulders as the baby's body is born.
   c. If the cord is tight, immediately clamp (about 3 cm apart) and cut the cord at the neck before the baby's body is born. Tell the mother to pant while you are clamping, cutting, and unwinding the cord.

8. Wipe the baby's face and head and wipe off fluid from the nose and mouth with a soft absorbent cloth.

9. Suction the nasal and oral passages of the baby with a soft, rubber bulb syringe or mucus sucker.

10. *Delivery of the shoulders*: Wait for a contraction and watch the head return to anatomical alignment with the body (restitution) and external rotation. External rotation shows that the shoulders are rotating into the anteroposterior diameter of the pelvic outlet, which is the largest space. The midwife proceeds to deliver one shoulder at a time to avoid overstretching of the perineum.

11. A hand is placed on each side of the baby's head, over the ears and downward traction is applied. This allows the anterior shoulder to slip beneath the symphysis pubis while the posterior shoulder remains in the vagina.

12. When the axillary crease is seen the head and trunk are guided in an upward curve to allow the posterior shoulder to escape over the perineum. The baby is then grasped around the chest to aid the birth of the trunk and lift the baby towards the mother's abdomen. This allows the mother immediate sighting of the baby and provides close skin contact. The time of birth is noted.

Clamping and Cutting the Umbilical Cord

Clamping the umbilical cord is done by placing two instrument clamps on the cord about 8 to 10 cm from the umbilicus with enough room between them to allow for easy cutting of the cord. Application of a gauze swab over the cord while cutting it will prevent blood spraying the delivery field. The timing of clamping the cord is not crucial unless asphyxia, prematurity or Rhesus incompatibility is present. Some centers advocate delay until respirations are established and cord pulsation has ceased, thus ensuring that the infant receives a placental transfusion of some 70 ml of blood. This view is countered by those who maintain that the placental transfusion so acquired may predispose to neonatal jaundice.

Immediate Care of the Newborn

After the cord is severed at whatever time is considered appropriate, the baby is dried and warmly wrapped to prevent cooling. Subsequent actions vary but may include the use of:

- Bodily contact with the mother
- Radiant warmer
- Warmed blankets.

The baby is then shown to the mother and her significant other. A one minute Apgar score must also be done by the midwife. If the baby is taken to a warmed crib or radiant warmer, the bulb syringe is also taken as well as the cord clamp and scissors for the final clamping and cutting of the cord. During this minute of life while doing the above, the baby must be grossly examined for any visible deformities or congenital defects. When the cord will be shortened, care must be taken to apply the clamp nearer the baby, 3 to 4 cm clear of the abdominal wall to avoid pinching the skin. A greater length of the cord is left when the umbilical vessels are expected for needed transfusion as in cases of preterm and Rhesus hemolytic disease.

Records

It is the responsibility of the midwife conducting the delivery to complete the labor record. This should include details of any drugs administered, the duration and progress of labor and if an episiotomy was performed and repaired. The information is entered in the mother's records as well as in the birth register. Details of the baby's condition including Apgar score are also recorded.

NURSING PROCESS DURING THE SECOND STAGE OF LABOR

Assessment

1. Maternal blood pressure, pulse and respiration every 5 to 15 minutes.
2. FHR every 10 to 15 minutes.
3. Labor progress
   a. Cervical dilatation.
   b. Fetal descent.
   c. Uterine contractions.
   d. The amount of bloody show.
   e. The woman's urge to bear down.
4. The woman's response to labor.
5. The woman's coping pattern.

Analysis/Nursing Diagnosis

1. Anxiety related to knowledge deficit.
2. Risk for infection
3. Pain
4. Fatigue
5. Impaired skin integrity
6. Anxiety related to outcome
7. Ineffective individual coping
8. Powerlessness
9. Impaired adjustment
10. Self-care deficit: bathing/hygiene.

Planning

1. Promote a quiet, focused environment to enhance pushing efforts.
2. Monitor maternal and fetal status.
3. Provide encouragement for pushing efforts.
4. Support ongoing comfort measures and pushing efforts.

Implementation

1. Continue assessment of maternal blood pressure, FHR and uterine contractions.
2. Assist laboring woman into position of comfort and pushing efforts.
3. Observe for approaching birth such as:
   a. Perineal bulging.
   b. Appearance of the fetal head.
4. Provide comfort measures such as:
   a. Wiping face with wet washcloth
   b. Moistening the lips
   c. Supporting the woman's body and/or extremities during pushing efforts.
5. Prepare for the delivery.
6. Complete perineal cleansing.

Evaluation

Ensure that:
1. The laboring woman is able to remain focused on pushing.
2. The woman and the fetus maintain physical parameters within normal limits.
3. The woman feels encouragement.
4. The woman feels comfortable.

BIBLIOGRAPHY

1. Caldero Barcia P, et al. Effects of position changes on the intensity and frequency of uterine contractions during labor. American Journal of Obstetrics and Gynecology. 1971;109:274.
2. Dutta DC. Textbook of Obstetrics, 5th edn. Calcutta: New Central Book Company; 2001.
3. Friedman EA. The Functional Divisions of Labor, American Journal of Obstetrics and Gynecology. 1971;109:274.
4. Hillan EM. Physiology and Management of the Second Stage of Labor. In: Bennett RV, Brown KB (Eds). Myles Textbook for Nurses, 13th edn. Edinburgh: Churchill Livingstone; 1999.
5. Hon EH. An Introduction to Fetal Monitoring (2nd Edn). North Haven Corometrics, Connecticut: Medical Systems; 1971.
6. Peterson G. Birthing Normally, A Personal Growth approach to Childbirth, 2nd edn. Berkeley, California: Mind-Body Press; 1984.
7. Schrag K. Maintenance of Pelvic Floor Integrity during Childbirth, Journal of Nurse-Midwifery, 1979;24(6).
8. Varney Helen. Nurse-Midwifery, 2nd edn. Boston: Jones and Barlett Publishers; 1996.

21

Physiology and Management of the Third Stage of Labor

Learning Objectives

Upon completing this chapter, the learner will be able to:

❖ Describe the mechanism of placental separation, descend and the physiological factors that ensure hemostasis
❖ Enumerate the use of oxytocic drugs in third stage management
❖ Outline the nursing management of the mother immediately after delivery of the placenta and membranes
❖ Describe the causes and management of postpartum hemorrhage.

The third stage of labor begins upon completion of the birth of the baby and ends with the birth of the placenta. It is known as the placental stage of labor. The third stage of labor averages between five and fifteen minutes but any period up to one hour may be considered within normal limits.

PHYSIOLOGICAL PROCESSES OF PLACENTAL SEPARATION AND EXPULSION

These are a continuation of the processes and forces at work during the earlier stages of labor. The processes of the third stage of labor and parameters of normal for this period must be known by the midwife for effective practice.

The third stage of labor consists of two phases. The first phase is the placental separation and the second phase is that of placental expulsion. Both separation and expulsion are brought about by contractions, which begin again after a brief pause at birth. The contractions must have been approximately every 2 to 2½ minutes apart during the second

stage of labor. After the birth of the baby, the next contraction may not occur for 3 to 5 minutes. Contractions then follow every 4 to 5 minutes until there has been separation and expulsion of the placenta and membranes. After that, the emptied uterus contracts down on it and remain contracted if the muscle tone is good. Otherwise, recurrent contraction and relaxation constitute after birth pains if the muscle tone is not as good.

Placental Separation (Figs 21.1A and B)

Placental separation is the result of the abrupt decrease in size of the uterine cavity during and following delivery of the baby. As the uterine cavity empties progressively, the retraction process accelerates (the unique characteristic of the uterine muscle). This decrease in uterine size necessarily means a concomitant decrease in the area of placental attachment. The placenta, however, remains the same size and at the site of attachment, it is unable to withstand the stress and buckles. The result is a separation of the placenta from the uterine wall, which takes place in the spongiosa layer of the decidua.

Separation usually begins at the center so that a retroplacental clot is formed. This may further aid separation by exerting pressure at the midpoint of placental attachment so that the increased weight helps to strip the adherent lateral borders. This increased weight also helps to peel the membranes off the uterine wall.

While the formation of the retroplacental clot is the result rather than the cause of placental separation, it does facilitate the completion of placental separation.

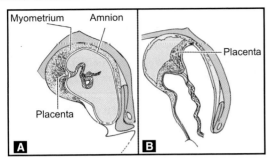

Figs 21.1A and B: The mechanism of placental separation: (A) Placenta attached to the uterine wall; (B) Placenta separated from the uterine wall

Descend of the Placenta

After the placenta has separated, it descends into the lower uterine segment or into the upper vaginal vault, causing the clinical signs of placental separation to become evident. These are as follows:

1. Sudden trickle or gush of blood.
2. Lengthening of the amount of umbilical cord visible at the vaginal introitus.
3. Change in the shape of the uterus from a discoid (circular) to globular, as the uterus now contracts upon itself.
4. Change in the position of the uterus as it rises in the abdomen, because the bulk of the placenta is in the lower uterine segment or upper vaginal vault.

Expulsion of the Placenta

Placental expulsion begins with descend of the placenta into the lower uterine segment (Fig. 21.2). It then passes through the cervix into the upper vaginal vault from where it is expelled. Expulsion of the placenta is by one of two mechanisms.

1. The Schultz mechanism of placental expulsion is delivery of the placenta with the fetal side presenting (Fig. 21.3A). This is thought to occur when separation begins centrally with corresponding formation of a central retroplacental clot, which weights the placenta so the central portion descends first. This in effect inverts the placenta and amniotic sac, and causes the membranes to peel off the decidua and trail behind the placenta. The majority of bleeding occurring with this mechanism of placental separation is not visualized until the placenta and membranes are delivered, since the inverted membranes catch and hold the blood. This method is more common of the two.

2. The Duncan mechanism of placental expulsion is delivery of the placenta with the maternal side presenting (Fig. 21.3B). This is thought to occur when separation first takes place at the margin or periphery of the placenta. Blood escapes between the membranes and uterine wall and is visualized externally. The placenta descends sideways and the amniotic sac, therefore, is not inverted but trails behind the placenta for delivery.

The memory aid for correctly identifying the mechanisms of placental expulsion is based on the appearance of two different sides of the

Fig. 21.2: Placenta in the lower uterine segment

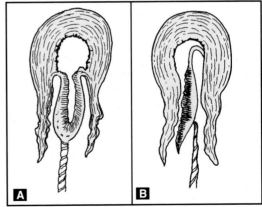

Figs 21.3A and B: Methods of placental expulsion: (A) Schultz method; (B) Matthew's Duncan method

placenta. The fetal side is shiny and glistening, because it is covering the fetal membranes, while the maternal side is rough and red-looking. Hence, the sayings "shiny Schultz" and "dirty Duncan".

Hemostasis

The normal volume of blood flow through the placental site is 500 to 800 ml per minute. At placental separation, this has to be arrested within seconds to prevent serious hemorrhage. The interplay of three factors within the normal physiological processes, which control bleeding occurs to control bleeding. They are:

1. Retraction of the oblique uterine muscle fibers in the upper uterine segment through which tortuous blood vessels intertwine. The resultant thickening of the muscles exerts pressure on the torn vessels, acting as clamps, thus securing a ligature action. Oblique fibers are absent in the lower uterine segment that explains the greatly increased blood loss in placenta previa when placental separation occurs.
2. The presence of vigorous uterine contraction following placental separation brings the walls into apposition so that further pressure is exerted on the placental site.
3. The achievement of hemostasis: There is a transitory activation of the coagulation and fibrinolytic systems during and immediately following, placental separation (Bonner et al, 1970). This protective response is especially active at the placental site so that clot formation in the torn vessels is intensified. Following separation, the placental site is rapidly covered by a fibrin mesh utilizing circulating fibrinogen.

MANAGEMENT OF THE THIRD STAGE OF LABOR

Care of the mother in the third stage of labor should be based on an understanding of the normal physiological processes at work. Prompt nursing actions can reduce the risk of hemorrhage, infection, retained placenta and shock. Management of the third stage can make considerable difference for blood loss by the mother. Mismanagement of third stage is the largest single cause of third stage hemorrhage. Mismanagement can also be the cause of uterine inversion and life-threatening shock. Such complications can be readily avoided by strict adherence to the following rules:

1. Guard the uterus to keep yourself and anyone else from massaging it prior to placental separation.
2. Do not massage the uterus before placental separation, except when partial separation has occurred by natural processes and excessive bleeding is evident.
3. Do not pull on the umbilical cord before the placenta separates or ever with an uncontracted uterus.
4. Do not try to deliver the placenta prior to its complete separation unless in the emergency of third stage hemorrhage.
5. Wait for the natural process to occur and do not interfere.

During the third stage of labor, the nurse is also responsible for initial management of the baby (i.e. drying the baby, providing for warmth, assuring a clear airway) and for the initial mother-baby bonding unless there is another nurse to receive and attend the baby soon after its birth. During the initial care of the baby, the nurse-midwife must keep one eye on the mother's perineum in order to watch for signs of placental separation and for excessive bleeding (By the same token, when she returns to the mother's perineum to manage third stage, she must keep one eye on the baby to continually evaluate the baby's well-being). Upon return to the mother to evaluate the progress of labor and the mother's condition, she places one hand on the mother's abdomen to feel, without massaging, the shape and position of the uterus and whether or not it is contracted.

If cord blood is to be collected, she can guide the cut end of the umbilical cord into the open end of the blood tube and hold it in position with the fingers of the same hand, that is holding the blood tube. The other hand may release the clamp on the cord. The cord can be reclamped as soon as the tube is filled. This procedure is repeated for more blood tubes, if required. Care must be taken to hold the umbilical cord in position in the upper end of the blood tube to avoid sudden spray of blood when the clamp is released due to the sudden pressure of blood flowing through the depleted cord. The sample may also be collected using a syringe and needle from the fetal surface of the placenta where the blood vessels are congested and easily visible. This must be done before the blood clots.

The cord is wound around the clamp until the clamp is at the vaginal introitus, so that traction can be effectively exerted on the cord when needed. This clamp is held with one hand while the other hand continues to guard the uterus. Guarding the uterus from massaging is essential to avoid partial separation of the placenta and resulting hemorrhage. Normal placental separation from the uterine wall is accomplished by the effect of uterine contractions.

If you are unsure whether the placenta has separated, it can be checked by using a modification of the Brandt-Andrews maneuver. For this, hold the cord taut at the vaginal introitus with one hand, using the clamp for leverage. With the fingers of the abdominal hand held together press down into the lower abdomen above the symphysis pubis. If the cord recedes into the vagina, the placenta is not separated (Fig. 21.4).

If the cord has a feeling of give and remains the same or lengthens beyond its position at the vaginal introitus, then the placenta has separated and you may proceed with facilitating placental expulsion.

Fig. 21.4: Checking for placental separation

Delivery of the Placenta and Membranes

At the beginning of the third stage, the fundus is palpable below the umbilicus. It feels broad as the placenta is still in the upper segment. As the placenta separates and falls into the lower segment the following signs are evident:

a. A small fresh blood loss.
b. Lengthening of the cord.
c. Fundus becoming rounder, smaller and more mobile in the abdomen.

It is important not to manipulate the uterus until a strong contraction is palpable. In the management of third stage, strict vigilance and correct practice are important to prevent disastrous consequences. The following methods are generally followed:

1. Expectant management
2. Assisted expulsion
   a. Controlled cord traction (modified Brandt-Andrews method).
   b. Expression by fundal pressure.

Expectant Management

In this method of management, the placental separation and its descend into the vagina are allowed to occur spontaneously. Mother's efforts are used to aid the expulsion. Minimal assistance is given if the mother's efforts fail to expedite the expulsion. This method can be practiced when the mother has not received any anesthesia, or an oxytocic drug has not been administered at the delivery of the anterior shoulder.

Steps of the Method

1. A hand is placed over the fundus to feel the signs of placental separation, the state of uterine activity—Contraction and relaxation, and any collection of blood in the uterine cavity. The placenta generally separates within minutes and 15 to 20 minutes may be allowed for the separation to occur.

2. When the features of placental separation and its descend into the lower segment are confirmed, the client is asked to bear down simultaneously with the hardening of the uterus. With a good uterine contraction, mother's bearing down effort will usually bring about expulsion of the placenta. The tendency to massage the uterus must be avoided. If the placenta fails to expel, one

can wait for up to ten minutes if there is no bleeding. With another contraction and bearing down by the mother, it is likely to be expelled.

3. As soon as the placenta passes through the introitus, it is grasped by both hands and twisted round and round or slightly up and down with gentle traction applied as the membranes are stripped off intact. If the membranes threaten to tear, they are to be held by an artery forceps and gentle traction applied to deliver the rest of the membranes. Gentleness and patience are important in delivering the membranes completely.

Controlled Cord Traction (Modified Brandt-Andrews Method) (Fig. 21.5)

This method is used after an oxytocic drug has been administered and given time to act. The uterus must be well contracted and signs of placental separation must be evident.

The left hand is placed above the level of the symphysis pubis with the palmar surface facing towards the umbilicus to exert pressure in an upward direction. The body of the uterus is displaced upwards and towards the umbilicus while, with the right hand, steady tension is given in a downward and backward direction following the line of birth canal (curve of Carus), by holding on the clamp placed on the cord at the vulva. It is important to apply steady traction by pulling the cord firmly and maintaining the pressure. Force and jerky movements must be avoided.

Fig. 21.5: Controlled cord traction (Brandt-Andrews method)

If the maneuver is not immediately successful, there should be a pause before another contraction is palpated and further attempt is made. Great care should be taken to avoid tearing the membranes. Tension on the umbilical cord without uterine contraction can cause inversion of the uterus, partial separation of placenta and hemorrage or detachment of cord from the placenta, thereby requiring manual removal.

This method when used properly achieves reduced blood loss, shorter third stage of labor and as a result less risk of postpartum hemorrhage.

Expression by Fundal Pressure

This is done by placing four fingers of the hand behind the fundus and the thumb in front of the uterus to use as a piston. The uterus is made to contract by gentle rubbing. When the uterus becomes hard, it is pushed downwards and backwards. The pressure is to be withdrawn as soon as the placenta passes through the introitus. This method is preferred in cases where the baby is premature or macerated, as the cord in such cases tends to have reduced tensile strength.

A sterile receiver should be placed against the woman's buttocks to catch blood and to hold the placenta when it is born. If the woman is in a lithotomy position, the basin is braced between the woman's buttocks and the midwife's body because the midwife needs both her hands free to manage the third stage of labor. Use of placenta basin to catch the blood makes it possible to measure the majority of the blood loss and minimize mess.

As the placenta is born it is allowed to slide gently down the side of the placenta basin, which is positioned more on its side at the vaginal introitus for this purpose or is delivered into the midwife's hands at the vaginal introitus. Either way, the purpose is not to let the placenta drop any distance from the level of the introitus, since this might cause the after coming membranes, which may still be peeling off the uterine wall as the placenta is delivered, to tear and break off and retained.

Third stage has ended if the membranes follow the placenta immediately, and are delivered with the placenta. However, sometimes the membranes trail behind and threaten to break off, if tension is applied to them. In such an instance, they may be teased out in one of the following two ways.

1. One way is to take a clamp (large Kelly clamp or large ring forceps) and place it on the membranes at the vaginal introitus. One hand continues to support the placenta or the basin with the placenta in it, in order to prevent tension on the membranes. The other hand manipulates the clamped membranes by gently rocking them up and down and side-to-side while exerting the slightest bit of traction on them. The appropriate amount of traction can be judged by the feeling of steady "give" of the membranes being teased out. As the membranes are gradually teased out, the clamp moves away from the vaginal introitus. Therefore, it needs to be periodically reclamped on the membranes at the introitus whenever it gets an inch or two away, because you have better control of manipulating the membranes the closer the clamp is to the vaginal introitus. The process is continued until the membranes are delivered.

2. The other way to tease out the membranes is to hold the placenta in your hands and turn it repeatedly. This causes the membranes to twist, thereby having the effect of gradually teasing them out until they are delivered. This method may be more difficult for inexperienced hands because the placenta is slippery and it is not as easy to control the amount of tension on the membranes as it is in the first method.

If the membranes do break off while you are trying to tease them out, third stage is considered ended. Sometimes the torn end of the membranes may be visualized during the cervical inspection and more teased out. The generally accepted management, if a portion of the membranes is retained, is that it does not warrant uterine exploration to remove them. Retention of a portion of the membranes is not a cause of hemorrhage as is true for retained placental fragments. The retained portion of the membranes will eventually be expelled with lochia. They need to be expelled as soon as possible as their retention increases the risk of endometritis. To achieve this more rapid expulsion, a full series of Methergin or Ergometrine is usually ordered (Methergin or Ergometrine 0.2 milligrams every 4 hours for 6 doses or t.i.d for 3 days). If the estimated amount of membranes retained was a large amount, some obstetricians also give an immediate dose of Methergin 0.2 mg or Ergometrine 0.5 mg intramuscularly unless the mother is hypertensive in which case it would be contraindicated. A uterine exploration is not done to remove the fragments of membranes as it is traumatic to the woman and increases the risk of intrauterine infection.

USE OF OXYTOCIC AGENTS

These drugs stimulate the uterus to contract. They may be administered at crowning of the baby's head, at delivery of the anterior shoulder of the baby, at the end of second stage of labor or following the delivery of the placenta.

Prophylactic Use

This is the routine administration of an oxytocic at the time of birth of the baby, given as a precautionary measure for the prevention of postpartum hemorrhage regardless of the assessed risk status of the woman. This is a part of active management, a policy of labor management practiced in developed countries. It usually comprises the administration of an oxytocic drug at the time of delivery of the anterior shoulder, clamping to the umbilical cord immediately following birth of the baby and delivery of the placenta by controlled traction.

Therapeutic Administration

This method implies the use of an oxytocic either to stop the bleeding once it has occurred or to maintain the uterus in a contracted state when there are indications that excessive bleeding is likely to occur. This oxytocic administration practice is more consistent with a physiological or expectant philosophy of care. In this event, routine administration of an oxytocic drug is withheld, the umbilical cord is left unclamped until cord pulsation has ceased and the placenta is expelled by use of gravity and maternal effort. A procedure generally practiced in midwife managed deliveries is the administration of ergometrine 0.5 mg or methergin 0.2 mg intramuscularly soon after the expulsion of the placenta.

FUNDAL HEIGHT DURING THIRD STAGE

At the beginning of the third stage, the fundus is palpable below the umbilicus. It feels broad as the placenta is still in the upper segment. As the placenta separates and falls into the lower uterine segment, there is a small fresh blood loss, the cord lengthens, and the fundus becomes rounder, smaller and more mobile as it rises in the abdomen to the level of the umbilicus or just above the umbilicus. At the end of third stage following the expulsion of the placenta, the fundus is about 4 cm below the umbilicus (Fig. 21.6).

COMPLETION OF THE THIRD STAGE

Continuing evaluation is essential at the completion of third stage. The midwife must ensure that the uterus is well contracted and fresh blood loss is minimal. Careful inspection of the perineum and lower vagina under good light is important. Slight lacerations are usually repaired immediately. If repair of a more extensive wound, such as an episiotomy or a second degree tear, is necessary, the mother should be made comfortable by changing soiled bed linen while preparations are made for suturing.

The vulva and perineum are gently cleansed using antiseptic solution, softly dried and a clean pad placed in position. The mother's blood pressure, pulse and temperature should be taken and recorded at least once. Once the mother is comfortable, examination of the placenta and membranes is the next priority.

Examination of Placenta and Membranes

This should be performed as soon as after delivery as possible, so that if there is doubt about their completeness, further action could be taken before the mother leaves the labor room or the midwife leaves the home in case of home delivery. A thorough inspection must be carried-out in order to make sure that no part of the placenta or membranes has been retained. The membranes often become torn during delivery and may be ragged and hence, care must be taken to piece them together to have an overall picture of their completeness. This is easier to see if the placenta is held by the cord, allowing the membranes to hang. The hole through which the baby was delivered can usually be identified and a hand spread out inside the membranes to aid inspection. The placenta should then be laid out on a flat surface and both placental surfaces examined carefully (Fig. 21.7). The amnion should be peeled from the chorion right up to the umbilical cord, which allows the chorion to be fully viewed.

Assessment of the Placenta

Any clots from the maternal surface must be removed and kept for measuring. Broken fragments of cotyledons must be carefully replaced before an accurate assessment is made.
- ❖ *Infarctions that are recent or old*—These areas on the placental surface indicate deprivation of blood supply. Recent infarctions

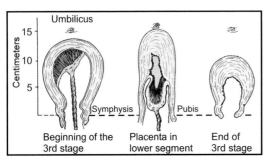

Fig. 21.6: Fundal height relative to the umbilicus and symphysis pubis

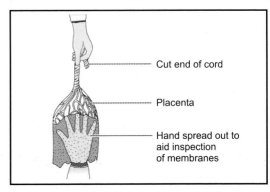

Fig. 21.7: Examination of membranes

appear bright red and old infarctions as gray patches.

- ❖ *Localized calcifications*—These are seen as flattened white plaques that feel gritty (as small hard particles of sand) to the touch.
- ❖ *Lobes*—The lobes of a complete placenta fit neatly together without any gaps, the edges forming a uniform circle.
- ❖ *Blood vessels*—They should not radiate beyond the placental edge. If they do, this denotes a succenturiate lobe. If the lobe has been retained, the vessels will end abruptly at a hole in the membrane.
- ❖ *Insertion of the cord (on the fetal surface)*— Normal insertion is central. Lateral insertion is abnormal.
- ❖ *Umbilical vessels*—Two umbilical arteries and one vein should be present. The absence of one artery may be associated with congenital abnormality, particularly renal agenesis.
- ❖ *Cord length*—Average length is 50 cm.
- ❖ *Weight of placenta*—Approximately one-sixth of the baby's weight.

Immediate Care to Mother and Baby

The mother and baby should remain in the midwife's care for at least an hour after delivery. In some hospitals, the baby may be in a nursery unit and cared for by another nurse. Both need careful observation and specific care during this period.

The mother should receive cleansing body wash, mouthwash and perineal care. She should be encouraged to empty her bladder and a bedpan offered. Blood pressure, pulse, uterine contraction and bleeding should be checked every 15 minutes.

The baby's general well-being and security of the cord clamp needs to be checked. As the baby will quickly chill after birth, it is important to thoroughly dry and wrap the baby in a clean, dry towel or blanket. A full neonatal examination is done at an early stage and the baby is kept in a warm crib, or cuddled close to the mother.

Mothers intending to breastfeed may be encouraged to put their babies to the breast during early contact. Babies are usually alert and their sucking reflex strong at this time. For the mother, early breastfeeding causes a reflex release of oxytocin from the posterior lobe of the pituitary gland that stimulates the uterus to contract. The mother may experience a sudden fresh blood loss as the uterus empties and she should be reassured.

Records

The midwife is responsible for documentation of all the events of labor and observations. Her recording should include the following details— all the drugs administered, examination of the placenta, membranes and cord with attention drawn to any abnormalities and the amount of blood loss.

After the specified period of observation, the mother and baby are transferred to the postnatal ward.

COMPLICATIONS OF THE THIRD STAGE

Postpartum Hemorrhage

Postpartum hemorrhage is defined as excessive bleeding from the genital tract at any time following the baby's birth to six weeks after delivery. If it occurs during the third stage of labor or within 24 hours of delivery, it is termed *primary postpartum hemorrhage.*

If bleeding occurs subsequent to the first 24 hours following birth until the sixth week postpartum, it is termed *secondary postpartum hemorrhage.*

Primary Postpartum Hemorrhage

During the first hour or two after birth when blood loss is excessive, it is difficult to measure it accurately, especially when the fluid has soaked into dressings and linen. The measurable solidified clots only represent about half the fluid loss. If measured blood loss reaches 500 ml, it is treated as postpartum hemorrhage. Another yardstick is maternal condition and states that any blood loss, however, small which adversely affects the mother's condition, constitutes a postpartum hemorrhage. Causes of primary postpartum hemorrhage are atonic uterus, retained placenta, trauma and coagulation disorders.

Atonic uterus: This is a failure of the myometrium at the placental site to contract and retract and to compress torn blood vessels and control blood loss by a living ligature action. The volume of blood flow at the placental site, when the placenta is attached, is approximately 500 to 800 ml per minute. Upon separation, the efficient contraction and retraction of the uterine muscle stops the flow of blood and prevents hemorrhage. Factors that interfere with this phenomenon and cause bleeding are listed below.

1. *Incomplete placental separation*: If placental tissue remains partially embedded in the spongy decidua, efficient contraction and retraction are interrupted. If the placenta remains fully adherent to the uterine wall, it is unlikely to cause bleeding. However, once separation has begun, maternal vessels are torn open.

2. *Retained cotyledon, placental fragment or membranes*: These will similarly impede efficient uterine action.

3. *Precipitate labor*: When the uterus has contracted vigorously resulting in a short duration of labor, that is less than one hour, the muscle may have insufficient opportunity to retract.

4. *Uterine inertia due to prolonged labor*: In a labor where the active phase lasts more than 12 hours, uterine inertia may result owing to muscle exhaustion.

5. *Uterine over distension due to polyhydramnios, multiple pregnancy or large baby*: The myometrium becomes excessively stretched and therefore less efficient.

6. *Placenta previa*: The placental site is partially or wholly in the lower uterine segment where the muscle layer contains few oblique fibers. This results in poor control of bleeding.

7. *Uterine relaxant anesthetic agents*: Volatile inhalational agents, such as halothane, cause uterine relaxation.

8. *Mismanagement of the third stage of labor*: Manipulation of the uterus or "fundus fiddling" may precipitate arrhythmic contractions so that the placenta separates only partially and retraction is lost.

9. *A full bladder may interfere with uterine action*: This is also considered as mismanagement.

10. *Grand multiparity*: With each successive pregnancy fibrous tissue replaces muscle fibers in the uterus, reducing its contractility and the blood vessels become more difficult to compress. Women who have had five or more deliveries are at increased risk.

11. *Uterine fibroids*: These may impede efficient uterine action.

12. *Anemia*: Women who enter labor with reduced hemoglobin concentration (below 10 gm/dl) are more prone to bleed more.

13. Retention of the placenta or a part of the placenta due to:
    ❖ Cornual implantation
    ❖ Constriction ring below the placenta
    ❖ Placenta membranacea
    ❖ Placenta accreta, increta or percreta
    ❖ Placenta in one horn of the uterus, with the fetus in the other horn
    ❖ Firm adhesion of extraplacental chorion to the decidua.

14. Abruptio placentae.

15. *Traumatic conditions*: These include perineal tears, vaginal tears, cervical tears, lower segment tears and uterine rupture.

16. *Previous history of postpartum hemorrhage or retained placenta*: In such clients, there is a risk for recurrence in subsequent pregnancies.

17. *Coagulopathy*: Conditions such as disseminated intravascular coagulation, excessive fibrinolysis, inherited coagulation disorders and idiopathic thrombocytopenic purpura.

Clinical Features

1. Visible bleeding per vaginum, which may be in the form of copious, continuous ooze, or intermittent gushes.

2. *Enlarged uterus*: Sometimes there may be little or no visible loss of blood. Blood accumulates within the uterus and the fundal height increases. Uterus feels "boggy" on palpation, i.e. soft and distended lacking tone.

3. Pallor

4. Rising pulse rate

5. Falling blood pressure (severe hypotension)

6. Altered level of consciousness: May become restless or drowsy.
7. Metabolic acidosis and shock.

Prophylaxis

1. Women, who are identified as having risk factors, should be instructed to have delivery in a unit where facilities for dealing with emergencies are available.
2. Anemia should be detected and corrected so that women enter labor with a hemoglobin level in excess of 10 gm/dl.
3. During labor, good management practices should be followed to prevent prolonged labor and ketoacidosis.
4. A woman should not enter the second or third stage of labor with a full bladder.
5. Prophylactic administration of oxytocic agent is recommended for the third stage either by intramuscular or intravenous infusion.
6. Two units of cross-matched blood should be kept available for any woman known to have a placenta previa.

Management of Postpartum Hemorrhage

Primary postpartum hemorrhage is an emergency, which requires prompt and efficient management. As soon as the midwife recognizes the occurrence, she must call the physician, if one is not already present in the delivery room. This initial step is important because the mother's condition can deteriorate very rapidly.

1. *Stop the bleeding*: Feel the fundus with the fingertips. If it is soft and relaxed (atonic), massage the fundus with a smooth, circular motion to make it contract. When a contraction occurs, the hand is to be held still.
2. *Give an oxytocic to sustain the contraction*: In many cases, syntocinon 10 units must have already been administered and this may be repeated. Alternatively, ergometrine 0.25 to 0.5 mg may be given intravenously, which will be effective in 45 seconds.
3. *Resuscitate the mother*: An intravenous line should be commenced while peripheral veins are easily negotiated. Fluid replacement and administration of oxytocics are

done. Ringers lactate and blood may be administered. As an emergency measure, the mother's legs may be lifted up in order to allow blood to drain from them into the central circulation. The foot of the bed should not be raised as this encourages pooling of blood in the uterus, which prevents uterus from contracting
4. *Empty the uterus*: Once the midwife is satisfied that the uterus is well contracted, she should ensure that it is emptied. With firm gentle pressure on the fundus expel residual clots. If the placenta is still in the uterus, it should be delivered by applying suprappubic pressure and controlled cord traction. If this fails, the placenta is removed manually.
5. *Bimanual compression*: If bleeding continues, bimanual compression of the uterus may be necessary in order to apply pressure to the placental site. In order to do this, the fingers of the right hand are inserted into the vagina like a cone, the hand is formed into a fist and placed in to the anterior vaginal fornix, the elbow resting on the bed. The left hand is placed behind the uterus abdominally, the fingers pointing towards the cervix. The uterus is brought forward and compressed between the palm of the left hand and the fist in the vagina.
6. *Removal of the retained placenta*: If the placenta is retained by a constriction ring, it is removed manually after relaxing the ring with general anesthesia. Placenta accreta, increta and percreta require total abdominal hysterectomy. Very rarely, a totally adherent placenta that does not cause bleeding is left *in situ* to be absorbed during puerperium.
7. *Genital tract injuries or trauma*: If bleeding continues despite a well-contracted uterus, it may be due to trauma. In order to identify the source of bleeding, the mother must be placed in lithotomy position under good directional light. Any torn vessels identified must be clamped and ligated. Internal trauma to vagina, cervix or uterus, which may have occurred following instrumental

or manipulative delivery, must be visualized through a speculum and suturing done under general anesthesia. If bleeding persists when the uterus is well contracted and no evidence of trauma can be found, uterine rupture must be suspected. This needs repair following laparotomy or hysterectomy.

8. *Blood coagulation disorders*: Postpartum hemorrhage may be the result of coagulation failure. It can occur following severe pre-eclampsia, antepartum hemorrhage, amniotic fluid embolism, intrauterine death or sepsis. Transfusion of fresh blood is usually the best treatment, as this will contain platelets and coagulation factors. Fresh frozen plasma and fibrinogen are also transfused.

Observations of the Mother Following Postpartum Hemorrhage

The woman will usually remain in the labor ward until her condition is stable. This allows her progress to be monitored closely.

Once bleeding is controlled, the total volume lost must be estimated as accurately as possible. Pulse and blood pressure are recorded every 15 to 30 minutes and temperature every 4 hours. The uterus must be palpated frequently to ensure that it remains well contracted. Intravenous fluid replacement must be carefully monitored. Monitoring of central venous pressure, fluid intake and output are done hourly and recorded. All records should be meticulously completed. Continued vigilance will be required for 24 to 48 hours.

Secondary Postpartum Hemorrhage

Secondary postpartum hemorrhage is bleeding from the genital tract more than 24 hours after delivery of the placenta and may occur up to 6 week later. It is most likely to occur between 10 and 14 days after delivery. Bleeding is usually due to retention of a fragment of the placenta or membranes, or the presence of blood clots. Subinvolution, infection and estrogen withdrawal following its use for suppression of lactation have also been identified as causes.

Clinical Manifestations

1. The lochia are heavier than normal and recurrence of bright red flow.
2. Offensive lochia if infection is a contributory factor.
3. Subinvolution of uterus.
4. Pyrexia and tachycardia.

Management

1. Massage the uterus if it is still palpable to bring about a contraction.
2. Express any clots.
3. Encourage the mother to empty her bladder
4. Give an oxytocic drug such as ergometrine by intravenous or intramuscular route.
5. Save all pads and linen to assess the volume of blood loss.
6. If retained products of conception are not seen on an ultrasound scan, the mother may be treated conservatively with antibiotic therapy and oral ergometrine.
7. If bleeding persists an exploration of the uterine cavity under general anesthesia and a blunt curettage is done. The material obtained by curettage is to be subjected to histopathological examination if a choriocarcinoma is suspected.
8. Anemia is treated with iron supplement and in severe cases, blood is transfused

Hematoma Formation

Postpartum hemorrhage may also be concealed because of hematoma formation. These form at sites such as the perineum, lower vagina, the broad ligament or vault of the vagina. A large volume of blood (up to 1 liter) may collect insidiously. Involution of the uterus and lochia are usually normal. The main symptom is increasingly severe pain. The hematoma has to be drained in the operating room under general anesthetic. Secondary infection is a high possibility and broad spectrum antibiotics are generally administered.

NURSING PROCESS DURING THE THIRD STAGE

Assessment

1. Determine that normal third stage progress is occurring.
   a. Rhythmic contractions until the placenta is born.
   b. Birth of placenta occurs 5 to 30 minutes after birth of the baby.
   c. Signs of placental separation is seen:
      ❖ Fundus rises slightly in abdomen
      ❖ Uterus changes shape
      ❖ Umbilical cord lengthens
      ❖ Slight gush of blood noted.
   d. Placental expulsion occurs:
      ❖ Schultz mechanism
      ❖ Duncan's mechanism.
   e. Following birth of placenta, the uterine fundus remains firm and is located two fingerbreadths below the umbilicus.
   f. The mother may experience chills or shivering.
2. Assess maternal blood pressure following birth of the baby.
3. Assess status of the uterus: Contractions will continue until birth of the placenta.
4. Assess the newborn's Apgar score and complete newborn assessment.
5. Examine placenta to document that all cotyledons and membranes are present.

Analysis/Nursing Diagnosis

1. Anxiety related to knowledge deficit
2. Risk for infection
3. Pain
4. Fatigue
5. Impaired skin integrity
6. Anxiety
7. Ineffective individual coping
8. Powerlessness
9. Impaired adjustment
10. Self-care deficit: Bathing/hygiene.

Planning

1. Complete initial assessment of the newborn.
2. Monitor maternal and newborn status.

3. Provide support in parental newborn interactions.
4. Provide support and comfort measures during the third stage.

Implementation

1. Observe and record birth of placenta
2. Monitor maternal blood pressure
3. Dry the baby completely
4. Complete initial newborn assessments
5. Provide initial newborn care
   a. Provide warmth
   b. Prevent infection
   c. Promote mother-baby attachment
6. Administer oxytocic drugs as per physician's order.

Evaluation

1. See that the newborn establishes and maintains adequate respiratory pattern.
2. Be sure that mother and newborn maintain normal physical parameters.
3. Monitor mother-baby attachment/bonding.
4. Make sure that mother feels comfortable and supported during the third stage.

BIBLIOGRAPHY

1. Klaus M, Kennel JH. Maternal Infant Bonding, St. Louis: Mosby; 1976.
2. Ladipo OA. Management of Third Stage of Labor with particular reference to fetomaternal transfusion, British Medical Journal 1972;1:721-3.
3. Levy V, Moore J. The Midwife's Management of the Third Stage of Labor. Nursing Times 1985; 81 (5):47-50.
4. McDonald S. Physiology and Management of the Third Stage of Labor, In: Bennett BV, Linda KB (Eds). Myles Textbook for Midwives, 13th edn. Edinburgh: Churchill Livingston; 1999.
5. Oliver CM, Oliver GM. Gentle birth, its safety and its effect on neonatal behavior. Journal of Obstetrics. Gynecology and Neonatal Nursing. 1978;7:35.
6. Phillips CR. The essence of birth without violence, American Journal of Maternal-Child Nursing 1976;1:162.
7. Varney Helen. Nurse-Midwifery, 2nd edn. Boston: Jones and Barlett Publishers; 1996.

22

Management of the Fourth Stage of Labor

Learning Objectives

Upon completing this chapter, the learner will be able to:

❖ Explain the physiological changes during the fourth stage of labor
❖ Describe the nursing actions required in the fourth stage of labor
❖ Describe the observations and checks to be done on the mother.

The fourth stage of labor begins with the birth of the placenta and ends one hour later. This stage marks the completion of the tasks associated with the first-three stages of labor. The mother may have expressions of relief and accomplishment, intermingled with excitement.

EVALUATION AND INSPECTION

The first postpartal hour is a critical time of initial recovery from the stress of labor and delivery and requires close observations of the mother. A portion of this hour will be spent in activities directly related to the intrapartal period. These activities may include the following:

1. Evaluation of the uterus.
2. Inspection and evaluation of the perineum, vagina and cervix.
3. Inspection and evaluation of the placenta, membranes and umbilical cord.
4. Repair of episiotomy and laceration, if any.

In addition to these, vital signs and other physiologic manifestations are checked and evaluated as indicators of recovery from the stress of labor. This period is the beginning of family relationships and mother-baby bonding.

The mother, and perhaps father, may want to see, hold and fondle the baby. Facilitation of this phase and encouraging the mother's participation in it are vital to the bonding process. Continuing evaluation of the baby's vital signs and physiologic manifestations are important and should be ongoing during the fourth stage of labor. Evaluation of the baby is discussed in Chapter 39.

Evaluation of the Uterus

After delivery of the placenta, the uterus is normally found in the midline of the abdomen approximately two-thirds to three-fourths of the way up between the symphysis pubis and umbilicus. A uterus found above the umbilicus is indicative of blood clots inside, which need to be expressed and expelled. A uterus found above the umbilicus and to one side, usually the right side, indicates a full bladder. In such an instance, the bladder must be emptied. A full bladder displaces the uterus from its position and prevents its contracting as it should, thereby allowing a greater amount of bleeding.

The uterus should be firm to touch. A soft, boggy uterus is a hypotonic uterus that is not contracting as it should and therefore, more bleeding is occurring than should be. Uterine atony is the major cause of immediate postpartum hemorrhage. A firm uterus is indicative of effective uterine hemostasis.

Hemostasis

Uterine hemostasis occurs as a result of the interplay of certain physiological processes.

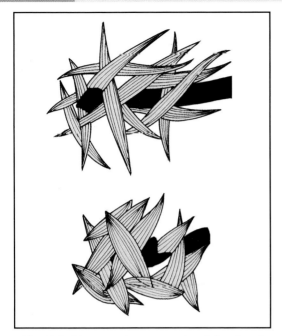

Fig. 22.1: Diagrammatic representation of clamping of blood vessels by the contracting muscle fibers

1. Retraction of the oblique uterine muscle fibers in the upper uterine segment through which the tortuous blood vessels intertwine. When contracted the entwining muscle fibers in the myometrium serve as ligatures to the open blood vessels at the placental site and bleeding is controlled (Fig. 22.1). It is the absence of oblique fibers in the lower uterine segment that contributes to increased blood loss following placental separation in placenta previa.
2. The vigorous uterine contraction that occurs following separation of placenta brings the walls into apposition exerting further pressure on the placental site.
3. The third mechanism that contributes to the achievement of hemostasis is the transitory activation of the coagulation and fibrinolytic system during and immediately following placental separation. This protective response is especially active at the placental site so that clot formation in torn vessels is intensified.

Inspection of the Cervix and Upper Vaginal Vault

The cervix and upper vaginal vault must be inspected in the presence of any (or a combination) of the following indications.

❖ The uterus is well contracted but there continues to be a steady trickle or flow of blood from the vagina
❖ The mother was pushing prior to complete dilatation of the cervix
❖ The labor and delivery were rapid and precipitous
❖ There was manipulation of the cervix during labor, such as manually pushing back an edematous anterior lip of cervix
❖ Traumatic procedures were necessary such as forceps application
❖ Traumatic second stage of delivery such as prolonged shoulder dystocia or large baby.

Following normal, spontaneous, vaginal deliveries, if none of these indications is present, it is not necessary to do a cervical and upper vaginal vault inspection. However, some obstetricians advocate routine inspection of these structures in order to rule out the possibility of a cervical laceration as the cause, if the woman bleeds excessively after an hour or two after the delivery.

Repairs

The repair of any laceration or an episiotomy is done after the examination of the placenta and membranes. If a uterine exploration for retained placental fragments is necessary, it is done prior to the repair. The uterus is checked again for consistency and repair is begun.

Inspection and evaluation of the placenta, membranes and umbilical cord are done before repairing any laceration or an episiotomy. This is because, if during the examination of the placenta, the midwife determines that the uterus needs to be explored manually because of a retained placental fragment, it needs to be done as soon as possible since it has the potential for causing hemorrhage.

Perineal Cleansing and Positioning of Legs

When all the inspections and repairs if necessary, are completed the midwife must recheck the uterus for consistency, watch the effect of uterine massage on the amount of vaginal blood flow, and express any blood clots.

The next nursing action is to wash off the mother's entire perineal area including the perineum, vulva, inner thighs, buttocks and the rectal area.

A perineal pad is then placed against the perineum and the mother assisted to put her legs together. If the woman was in lithotomy position it is important to remove both legs from the stirrups at the same time in order to avoid undue back strain and discomfort which may occur if one leg is down and the other is still up in a stirrup. It is also helpful to have put her legs together while they still are in the air with the midwife supporting them and bicycle them down with help to a resting position. This stimulates circulation to the legs and makes the transition of position less abrupt and more comfortable.

CONTINUING CARE AND MONITORING

Throughout the remainder of the fourth stage of labor the mother's vital signs, uterus, bladder, lochia and perineum are monitored and evaluated. This monitoring is maintained until all are stabilized within normal range. The technique of monitoring should be organized and include the following:

❖ Vital signs check
❖ Palpation of the fundus of the uterus for contractility
❖ Massage of the fundus and expression of clots and free blood from the uterus
❖ Measurement of the fundus in relation to the umbilicus
❖ Inspection of the perineum for discoloration and swelling
❖ Inspection of the bladder
❖ Inspection of the perineal pad and change if necessary
❖ Offering food and fluids if allowed and comfort, and safety measures.

Vital Signs

The mother's blood pressure, pulse and respirations are evaluated every 15 minutes until stable at prelabor levels. The temperature is taken at least once during the fourth stage of labor. The temperature continues to be elevated with normal being less than 2°F increase, or below 100.4°F (38°C).

In assessing the blood pressure and pulse rate, it must be remembered that, the excitement after delivery may cause an elevation in some mothers. Injection of oxytocic drugs may also cause some women to experience elevated blood pressure and pulse rate. The optimum postpartum blood pressure and pulse rate is that which most closely approximates the mother's blood pressure and pulse rate prenatally, provided these were within normal limits at that time.

A common complaint of mothers after delivery of the baby and placenta is a feeling of chill (the postpartum chill). It often occurs while the mother is being prepared for transfer from the recovery room, while she is being transferred or immediately after transfer. The mother actually shakes as a manifestation of chill. The chill and the overt shaking usually do not last over 15 minutes. Some of the hypotheses regarding the cause of the chill are the following:

1. The mother's nervous reaction and exhaustion related to childbearing.
2. An aftermath of and due to release of nervous tension and energy put out during labor and delivery.
3. The muscular exertion during labor and delivery cause disequilibrium between the external and internal body temperature.
4. The sudden release of intra-abdominal pressure after the uterus is emptied.
5. Previous maternal sensitization to elements of fetal blood, as well as maternal fetal transfusions at the time of delivery causing a reaction in the mother manifested as chills (Hellmann and Jack, 1971).

Whether this reaction is emotional, physiological or an interaction of the two, the midwife can be helpful by reassuring the mother that chills are not uncommon after delivery and that it will quickly pass. Comfort measures should be provided and include warm blankets, gown and warm fluids by mouth if not contraindicated.

Palpation of the Fundus of Uterus for Contractility

During the fourth stage of labor, the uterus continues to contract and relax. The uterus controls postpartum hemorrhage by contracting and compressing the patent blood vessels at the site where the placenta was implanted. Therefore, the immediate precaution to postpartum hemorrhage is sustained contraction of the uterus.

Medications such as ergometrine, methergine, pitocin or syntocinon may have been given to the mother intramuscularly or intravenously during the delivery of the anterior shoulder or immediately after the placenta is delivered. These medications stimulate uterine contractions, the effect of which may last several hours. Oxytocics work well in the prevention of uterine atony—The most common cause of postpartum hemorrhage. However, the tone of the uterus is dependent on many factors other than whether the mother has had oxytocics. Contractions of the uterus occur when the mother hears her newborn baby's cry or when she can see or hold the baby. These contractions are brought about by the sympathetic nervous system, which is activated by the mothers' emotions. In some hospitals, the baby is put to breast on the delivery table. This action tends to cause the uterus to contract and is prophylactic to postpartum hemorrhage.

The fundus of the uterus is palpated by placing the side of one hand on top of, and slightly cupped above the fundus, while the other hand is placed suprapubically with the exertion of slight pressure. Ideally, the fundus should lie on the mid-plane of the pelvis at or below the umbilicus (Fig. 22.2).

Fig. 22.2: Hand maneuver involved in palpation of the fundus of uterus

Massage of the Uterus and Expression of Clots

If the fundus is found boggy on palpation, it is massaged until it contracts and becomes firm. Care must be taken not to over massage or over stimulate the fundus. Over stimulation can result in undue muscle fatigue with subsequent relaxation of the organ and possible hemorrhage.

Expression of the fundus is done by utilizing the same maneuvers as shown in Figure 22.2. In addition, during expression, pressure is applied to the fundus with one hand while equal pressure is applied suprapubically with the other hand. Expression is done in sequential 3 to 5 seconds, with several seconds rest between, until the nurse is sure that clots and free blood held in the uterus is expressed sufficiently. After palpation, massage and expression have been completed, the uterus usually stays firm for a period. However, there is always possibility that it may not remain contracted. If there is any doubt in the midwife's mind regarding the tone of the uterus or if during the check it is believed that bleeding and clotting is heavier than what it should be, the nurse should repeat the maneuvers more frequently than the suggested every 15 minutes and notify the physician.

Measurement of the Fundus

A measurement of the height of the fundus is taken after the fundus is expressed, measuring from the top of the fundus to the umbilicus using fingerbreadths. The fundus of the uterus tends to lie closer to the umbilicus in mother's who are multiparous than in those who are primiparous. Some factors which affect the size, placement and muscular tone of the uterus include presence of antepartum hydramnios, multiple births, uterine inertia during labor, effects of oxytocic and the amount of urine in the bladder.

Inspection of the Perineum

Perineal discomfort is a common complaint of mothers during the first hour postpartum, particularly after the period of time during which the anesthetic used for perineal repair looses its effect. Some physicians order an ice bag placed to the perineum for several hours postpartum. The cold lessens the edema in the episiotomy area and tends to numb the area so that the mother's discomfort is not as pronounced. This is especially useful if there has been extensive repair, such as third or fourth degree perineal repair or repair of an exceptionally sensitive area, such as the clitoris. If chemical perineal "ice" packs are not available, adequate ice packs can be created by putting crushed ice in a rubber glove or a sandwich bag. All ice packs should be covered with some form of clean cloth before being placed on the perineum.

Fig. 22.3: Palpation of a full bladder on a postpartum client

While inspecting the perineal area, during the postpartum check, the nurse may observe swelling or echymosis. This is indicative of the formation of a perineal or perineal-vaginal hematoma. The midwife can make a positive nursing diagnosis of a hematoma by touching the area *very lightly* with sterile gauze or with the patient's perineal pad. If the swelling is more than edema and is in fact the beginning of a hematoma, the mother will complain of extraordinary tenderness when touched. The physician should be notified immediately. A hematoma should not be left unattended for it may continue to enlarge, causing the mother increasing pain. Continued extravasations can lead to circulatory shock.

Inspection of the Bladder (Fig. 22.3)

The bladder must be evaluated and emptied if it is full and displacing the uterus. In the event that the bladder is filling or full, a bladder bulge will be evident. It feels, and appears as a spongy, fluid filled mass below the uterus and above the symphysis pubis. A hypotonic bladder with urinary retention and bladder enlargement is common. This is due to trauma caused by pressure and compression placed on the bladder and urethra during labor and delivery. It is important for the bladder to be emptied, because a full bladder displaces the uterus and decreases its ability to contract properly. A poorly contracted uterus increases the amount of bleeding and the severity of after pains. On examination, the uterus can be seen elevated in the pelvis and displaced from the midline.

Bladder hypotonicity may cause the woman not to feel a desire to void. Catheterization which carries with it significant risk of infection, is to avoided except when all inducements to void fail and it is essential to empty the bladder in order for the uterus to better contract and reduce bleeding. Putting the woman on a bedpan, running water over the perineum, having her fingers dabble in water, having her listen to the sound of running water, applying light suprapubic pressure, or having her practice perineal relaxation may work in getting her to void, but the most effective and comfortable method is simply to assist her to the bathroom. There is no contraindication to walking with assistance at this time, if she is not heavily medicated, did not have spinal anesthesia, or has not had an excessive blood loss.

Inspection and Change of Perineal Pad

It is not necessary to perform any particular type of perineal care during the first hour postpartum except to keep the area as clean and dry as possible. Regular change of perineal pad and linens under her buttocks is required in order to keep the lochia from becoming dry and adhering to mother's body. It is necessary to wash the perineal area and buttocks with mild soap and water to remove lochia not absorbed by the perineal pad.

When checking the perineal pads for lochia, the mother is rolled on her side so that the midwife can better determine the amount of bleeding. The lochia is prone to collect under the buttocks and is obscured from sight if the patient is not turned on her side during the check.

The lochia during the fourth stage of labor is rubra, neither dark red nor bright red. Normally it has a fleshy odor, similar to that of fresh blood. The lochia consist of blood from the placental site, shreds of membranes, vernix, lanugo, decidua and meconium. Size and consistency of lochial clots are to be observed and noted in the chart. If the midwife has any doubt as to whether the clots contain placental tissue, they should be saved for inspection by the physician.

A constant bright red trickle of lochia from the vagina in the presence of a contracted uterus is an indication of fresh bleeding. This is the result of cervical or vaginal laceration or both. The physician is to be notified immediately so that the laceration can be repaired as soon as possible.

If the bleeding is more than normal, the midwife must keep a perineal pad count, so that the estimation of blood loss is more accurate. Notations must be made in the mother's chart of how many pads were used, the degree of saturation of each pad, the size and character of clots and the color of lochia.

Fluids and Food

Any previous nausea and vomiting should have subsided and the mother most likely will be thirsty and if all is progressing normally, she should be encouraged to take water, juices and tea or coffee with sugar. After her condition has stabilized within the limits of normal, which will usually be by the end of the first hour postpartum, she may also eat solid foods. Mothers must be encouraged to eat a small amount first and to eat slowly. Comfort measures should be supplied and include warm blankets, gown and warm fluids by mouth if not contraindicated.

USE OF OXYTOCIC DRUGS

Oxytocic drugs stimulate uterine contractions. A number of factors should be considered in

using oxytocics during the immediate postpartum period. They include—Determination of the need, action and effect, and dosage and route.

Determination of the Need

Determination of whether or not there is a need for an oxytocic drug is based on the following:
1. Uterine consistency: The uterus should be well contracted, feeling firm and hard to touch in the immediate postpartum period.
2. Potential for the uterus to relax even if it is presently firm. A uterus is more likely to relax if:
   a. It has been over distended due to multiple gestation, polyhydramnios or large baby.
   b. The patient had a pitocin induction or augmentation.
   c. Labor and delivery have been rapid and precipitous.
   d. The patient is a grand multipara.
   e. There is a history of uterine atony during previous childbearing experience.
   f. The first and second stages of labor were prolonged.
3. Whether or not the membranes were delivered completely.
4. Whether or not the mother initiates breastfeeding immediately.

Action and Effect

The action and effect of different oxytocic drugs must be considered. The synthetic forms of oxytocin, such as *pitocin* and *syntocinon* stimulate intermittent contractions. They have little or no effect on the blood pressure if given intramuscularly or added to IV fluids. These are the drugs of choice in most situations.

The natural and synthetic ergot preparations—*ergotrate* and *methergine* respectively—stimulate a sustained, tetanic contraction. Both of these drugs potentiate a hypertensive condition and may cause blood pressure increase in normotensive women because of their vasoconstrictive effect. However, of the two drugs, methergine causes lesser elevation. Therefore, if the woman is bleeding excessively due to atony of uterus (which indicates a need for a drug that will stimulate a sustained contraction) but there is concern for a possible hypertensive effect, methergine would be the drug of choice.

Drugs with the action of stimulating intermittent contractions may be used to supplement those effecting a sustained contraction by adding them to an IV infusion which will last over time or may be used by themselves when the bleeding is not excessive, but the uterus has a tendency to relax.

Dosage and Route

The standard single dose for each oxytocic drug is as follows:

Ergotrate (ergometrine)
Injection: 0.2 mg (1 cc),
Tablets: 0.2 mg per tablet

Methergine (methylergonovine)
Injection: 0.2 mg (1 cc),
Tablets: 0.2 mg per tablet

Pitocin—Injection: 10 USP units (1 cc)

Syntocinon—Injection: 10 USP units (1 cc)

The use of oxytocic drugs is invaluable in controlling postpartal uterine bleeding. The desired action, however, can be obtained rapidly by way of intramuscular route for the ergot preparations or by way of intramuscular or diluted intravenous infusion routes for the synthetic oxytocic drugs. *At no time should any of these drugs be given IV push (direct intravenous administration) because of the danger of cardiovascular complications.*

SUMMARY

The first hour postpartum is of critical importance to the well–being of the newly delivered mother. The uterus continues to relax and contract just as it did during the first three stages of labor. The newly delivered mother is a biopsychosocial being. Consequently, nursing care appropriate to the integration of these components must be rendered.

NURSING PROCESS DURING THE FOURTH STAGE OF LABOR

Assessment

1. *Physical Assessment*
   Determine that fourth stage is progressing within normal limits.

   a. Blood pressure returns to prelabor state.
   b. Pulse is slightly lower than in labor.
   c. Fundus remains contracted in the midline and is located 1 to 2 fingerbreadths below the umbilicus.
   d. Lochia is scant to moderate.
   e. Bladder is nonpalpable
   f. Perineum is intact.
2. *Psychosocial Assessment*
   a. Assess the mother's emotional state. May vary from exhaustion to euphoria.
   b. Some mothers may want to interact with their baby, and others may wish to rest at this time.

Nursing Diagnosis

1. Rest and sleep deprivation.
2. Altered parenting.
3. Altered nutrition.
4. Pain.
5. Anxiety.
6. Risk for altered homeostasis.

Planning

1. Frequent assessments to monitor maternal recovery from delivery.
2. Enhance maternal-newborn attachment.
3. Teach self-care measures to prevent bleeding and enhance comfort.

Implementation

1. Complete maternal assessment every 15 minutes for the first hour, every 30 minutes for the second hour and then hourly for the next 2 hours.
2. Provide comfort measures:
   a. Provide warm blankets and/or hot drinks for shivering or chilling.
   b. Place ice packs on perineum to decrease swelling and increase comfort.
   c. Carry out perineal cleansing.
   d. Offer sponge bath.
   e. Provide clean linen.
3. Massage and express fundus.

Evaluation

Ensure that the mother:
1. Has physical parameters monitored at frequent intervals.

2. Had uneventful recovery period and does not develop complications.
3. Has opportunity to interact with newborn as desired.
4. Can demonstrate fundal massage and practice comfort measures.

BIBLIOGRAPHY

1. Klaus M, Kennel JH. Maternal Infant Bonding, St. Louis: Mosby; 1976.
2. Ladipo OA. Management of Third Stage of Labor with particular reference to fetomaternal transfusion. British Medical Journal 1972;1:721-3.
3. Levy V, Moore J. The Midwife's Management of the Third Stage of Labor, Nursing Times 1985; 81(5):47-50.
4. McDonald S. Physiology and Management of the Third Stage of Labor, In: Bennett BV, Linda KB (Eds). Myles Textbook for Midwives, 13th edn. Edinburgh: Churchill Livingstone 1999.
5. Oliver CM, Oliver GM. Gentle birth, its safety and its effect on neonatal behavior. Journal of Obstetrics, Gynecology and Neonatal Nursing 1978;7:35.
6. Phillips CR. The essence of birth without violence American Journal of Maternal-Child Nursing 1976;1:162.
7. Varney Helen. Nurse-Midwifery, 2nd edn. Boston: Jones and Barlett Publishers; 1996.

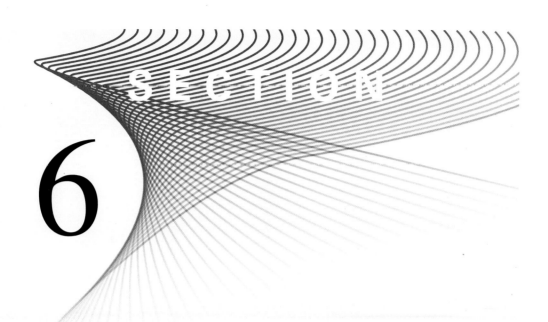

6

The Normal Puerperium

23
Physiology and Management of the Normal Puerperium

Learning Objectives

Upon completing this chapter, the learner will be able to:
* Discuss the anatomical and physiological changes of the puerperium
* Describe the physical signs, symptoms and discomforts in the puerperal period
* Describe the postnatal assessment as a basis for exploring normal physiology and potential complications
* Enumerate the responsibilities of the midwife in managing the care of postnatal clients.

DEFINITION

Puerperium is the period following childbirth during which the body tissues, especially the pelvic organs, revert approximately to the pre-pregnant state both anatomically and physiologically. The retrogressive changes are mostly confined to the reproductive organs with the exception of the mammary glands, which show features of activity.

DURATION

The puerperium (postpartal period) is the time from the delivery of the placenta and membranes to the return of the woman's reproductive *tract to its nonpregnant condition and lasts for approximately six weeks.* The woman progressing through the puerperium is called a puerpera. The postpartum period is arbitrarily divided into: (a) *immediate—the first 24 hours,* (b) *early—up to 7 days* and (c) *remote—up to 6 weeks.*

ANATOMICAL AND PHYSIOLOGICAL CHANGES OF THE PUERPERIUM

The term *involution* is used to refer to the *retrogressive changes taking place* in all of the organs and structures of the reproductive tract.

Uterus

Immediately following delivery, the uterus becomes firm and retracted with alternate hardening and softening. It weighs approximately *1,000 gm and measures 15 × 12 × 8 to 10 cm* in length, width and thickness, respectively. This is roughly about two to three times the size of the nonpregnant, multiparous uterus. Subsequently, the uterus weights approximately 500 gm by the end of the first postpartal week, *early* 300 to 350 gm by the end of the second week, *100 gm by the sixth postpartal week* and its usual nonpregnant weight of 60 gm by the eighth week postpartum. This rapid decrease in size is reflected in the changing location of the uterus as it descends out of the abdomen and *returns to being a pelvic organ. Immediately after delivery, the top of the fundus is approximately two-thirds to three-fourths of the way up between the symphysis pubis and the umbilicus.* It then rises to the level of the umbilicus *within a few hours.* It remains at approximately the level of or *one fingerbreadth below the umbilicus for a day then involutes at the rate of 1-2 cm / day (one fingerbreadth per day) and then* gradually descends into the pelvis, being abdominally nonpalpable above the symphysis pubis after *the tenth day.* The uterine descend is illustrated in Figure 23.1.

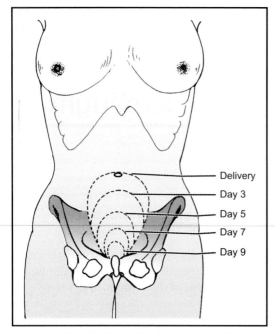

Fig. 23.1: Fundal height and uterine involution

If at any postpartal time, the top of the fundus is above the umbilicus, the following should be considered—Filling of the uterus with blood or blood clots in the early postpartal hours or displacement of the uterus by a distended bladder especially if also displaced to the right upper quadrant.

Involution of the uterus involves the re-organization and shedding of the decidua/endometrium and the exfoliation of the placental site as evidenced by the decrease in size and weight and change in location of the uterus and by the color and amount of the lochia. Involution is hastened if the mother is breastfeeding.

The placental site contracts rapidly presen-ting a raised surface, which measures about 7.5 cm. It remains elevated even at six weeks when it measures about 1.5 cm. By this time, complete regeneration of the endometrium at the placental site takes place.

The blood vessels degenerate and become obliterated followed by thrombosis. New blood vessels grow inside the thrombi.

Cervix

Immediately after delivery, the cervix is ex-tremely soft, flabby and floppy. It may be bruised and edematous, especially anteriorly if there was an anterior lip during labor. It looks congested and readily admits two to three fingers. The cervix contracts slowly, the ex-ternal os admits two fingers for a few days and by the end of first week, narrows down to admit the tip of a finger only. The contour of the cervix takes longer time to regain (six weeks) and the external os never reverts to the nulliparous state.

The broad and round ligaments, which accompanied the uterus during its increase in size, are now lax because of the extreme stret-ching. This accounts for the easy displacement of the uterus by the bladder. By the end of the puerperium the ligaments regain their non-pregnant length and tension.

Lochia

Lochia is the name given to the uterine discharge that escapes vaginally during the puerperium. As it changes color, it changes its descriptive name, i.e. rubra, serosa and alba.

Lochia rubra is red as it contains blood. It is the first lochia that starts immediately after delivery and continues for the first 3 to 4 days postpartum. Lochia rubra contains primarily blood and decidual tissue.

Lochia serosa is the next lochia. It is paler than lochia rubra and is serous and pink as it contains less RBCs but more leukocytes, wound exudates, decidual tissue and mucus from the cervix. Lochia serosa lasts for 5 to 9 days.

Lochia alba is the last lochia. It starts about the 10th postpartum day and dwindles to nothing in about a week or so (10 to 15 days). It is pale, creamy-white and consists primarily of leukocytes, decidual cells and mucus.

Lochia has a characteristic odor, which is heavy but not offensive. The odor is strongest in the lochia serosa. It is still stronger if mixed with perspiration, and must be carefully differentiated from a foul odor indicative of infection.

Lochia begins as a heavy discharge in the early postpartum hours. Subsequently it decreases to a moderate amount as lochia rubra, a small amount as lochia serosa and a scant amount as lochia alba. It is common for a woman to have small amount of lochia while lying down and to flood when she gets out of bed. This occurs because the discharge pools in the upper vaginal vault in the recumbent position and then drains out of the vagina with the positional change of standing up. Pooling may cause some clotting, particularly on the day of delivery. A slight increase in the amount or in the blood content may be seen when the mother becomes more active and during breast-feeding. The average lochial discharge for the first 5 to 6 days is estimated to be approximately 250 ml.

The normal duration of lochial discharge may extend up to three weeks. The discharge may be scanty following premature labor or may be excessive in twin delivery or hydramnios.

Vagina and Perineum

The immediate postdelivery vagina remains quite stretched, may have some degree of edema and bruising, and gapes open at the introitus. In a day or so it regains enough tone that the gaping reduces and the edema subsides. It is now smooth-walled, larger than usual and lax. Its size decreases with the return of the vaginal rugae by about the third post-partal week. It will always be a little larger than it was prior to the first childbirth. Perineal muscle tightening exercises will restore its tone. This can be accomplished by the end of the puerperium with daily practice. The torn hymen heals by scar formation, leaving several tissue tags called myrtiform caruncles (carunculae myrtiformes). Abrasions and lacerations of the vulva and perineum heal readily including those requiring repair.

Breasts

For the first two days following delivery, no further anatomic changes occur in the breasts. The secretion from the breasts called colostrum, which starts during pregnancy, becomes more abundant during this period.

Colostrum is a deep yellow, serous fluid that is alkaline in reaction. It has higher specific gravity, protein, sodium, chloride and vitamin-A content than breast milk. Carbohydrates, fat and potassium content are lower than in the breast milk. It contains antibodies (IgA, IgG and IgM) and humoral factors (lactoferrin) that provide immunological defence to the newborn. Colostrum has a laxative action on the baby because of the large fat molecules in it and facilitates passage of meconium.

Physiology of Lactation

Lactation is initiated in all puerperal women normally and naturally unless effectively prohibited by a lactation suppressant. Though some secretary activity is present (colostrum) during pregnancy, it is accelerated following delivery and milk secretion actually starts on third or fourth postpartum day. Around this time, the breasts become engorged, tense and tender and feel warm. In spite of a high prolactin level during pregnancy, milk secretion is kept in abeyance. The steroids estrogen and progesterone circulating during pregnancy are thought to make the breast tissues unresponsive to prolactin. When estrogen and progesterone are withdrawn following delivery of the placenta, prolactin begins its milk secretary activity in previously fully developed mammary glands. The secretary activity (lactogenesis) is enhanced by growth hormone, thyroxin, glucocorticoids and insulin.

Discharge of milk from the mammary glands (galactokinesis) depends on the suction exerted by the baby during suckling and the contractile mechanism, which expresses the milk from the alveoli into the ducts.

After initiation of lactation, its subsequent continuation is dependent on the suckling stimulus of the baby to the breast. During suckling, a conditioned reflex is set-up. The ascending impulses from the nipples cause the posterior pituitary to liberate oxytocin, which enters the circulating blood in the breasts and causes contraction of the myoepithelial cells surrounding the alveoli and ducts. The contraction of these cells expels the milk out of the alveoli, through the ductile to the lactiferous (storage) sinuses where it is readily accessible to the baby by compression of the sinuses as the baby sucks.

The milk ejection reflex is inhibited by factors such as pain, breast engorgement or adverse psychic condition. The ejection reflex may be deficient for several days following initiation of milk secretion in some women and results in breast engorgement.

Maintenance of lactation (galactopoiesis) is achieved by the continued release of prolactin from the anterior pituitary. For maintenance of effective and continuous lactation, sucking is essential. It is not only essential for the removal of milk from the glands, but also causes the release of prolactin. Secretion of milk is a continuous process unless suppressed by congestion, emotional disturbances or medication. Milk pressure reduces the rate of production and hence periodic breastfeeding is necessary to relieve the pressure, which in turn maintains the secretion.

The sucking propels the milk the final distance through the lactiferous ducts into the baby's mouth. The movement of milk from the lactiferous sinuses is called the "let-down" or "milk ejection", and is felt by the woman as a specific event. Eventually the let-down can be triggered without the actual sucking of the baby, by the mother's simply hearing the baby cry or thinking about the baby. This is due to the influence of emotions on this mechanism. In such an event, the milk may stream from the breasts and leak on to the mother's clothing. As the demand and supply of milk stabilizes and lactation is well established, this profuse ejection of milk from the breasts is less apt to happen.

Milk Production

In the first postpartum week, the total amount of milk yield in 24 hours is calculated to be 60 multiplied by the number of postpartum days and is expressed in terms of milliliters. Thus, the milk yield on the fourth day is about 60 × 4 = 240 ml. A milk yield of 120–180 ml per feeding is usual by the end of second week (Dutta, 2001).

Stimulation of Lactation

The methods that can be adopted during pregnancy include:
❖ Improving the maternal desire to breast-feed the baby through education regarding breastfeeding
❖ Care and preparation of the nipple.

Following delivery the mother should be encouraged to:
❖ Put the baby to breast as soon as possible after delivery
❖ Nurse the baby every 2 to 3 hours without missing any feeding
❖ Take plenty of oral fluids.

Suppression of Lactation

Suppression becomes necessary if the baby is born dead or dies in the neonatal period or when the woman does not want to breastfeed her baby or if breastfeeding is contraindicated. Either hormones or mechanical means may be used to achieve suppression.

Drugs

1. Bromocriptine (parlodel) 2.5 mg orally twice daily for two weeks. This inhibits prolactin secretion.
2. Ethynyl estradiol 0.05 mg twice daily for five days.
3. Combination of estrogen and testosterone preparation (mixogen), intramuscularly soon after delivery.

Use of parlodel may be associated with early return of ovulation and hormonal preparations carry the risk of thromboembolic complication.

Mechanical methods can be used effectively when lactation is to be suppressed after the establishment of milk secretion. For this the woman should:
❖ Stop breastfeeding
❖ Not express or pump out milk from breasts
❖ Apply a tight compression bandage or binder for 2 to 3 days.

Analgesic tablets may be given to relieve pain.

GENERAL PHYSIOLOGICAL CHANGES

Vital Signs

The blood pressure should be stabilized within the realm of normal. The pulse rate is likely to be raised for a few hours after normal delivery, which settles down to normal during the second day. In some mothers it may be slowed down for 1 to 2 days, may be due to rest, diminished fluid intake and excessive fluid excretion. The pulse rate is often unstable and often rises with after pains or excitement. Any pulse rate above 100 during the puerperium is abnormal and may be indicative of infection or delayed postpartal hemorrhage.

Respirations should be within the realm of normal. The temperature should return to normal from its slight elevation during the intrapartal period and stabilized within the first 24 hours postpartum. There may be slight reactionary rise following delivery by 0.5°F but comes down to normal within 12 hours. The temperature should not be above 37.2°C (99°F) within the first 24 hours. However, on the third day, there may be slight rise of temperature due to breast engorgement, which should not last for more than a day.

Renal System Changes

The renal pelvis and ureters, which were stretched and dilated during pregnancy, return to normal by the end of the fourth postpartum week.

Immediately postpartum, the bladder is edematous, congested and hypotonic which may result in overdistention, incomplete emptying and excessive urine residual, unless care is taken to encourage periodic voiding even when the woman does not feel like it. The urethra is insensitive because of trauma during labor. Unless urinary tract infection develops, the effects of trauma during labor on the bladder and urethra diminish within the first 24 hours.

Approximately 40 percent of postpartal women have nonpathologic proteinuria from immediately after delivery up to the second day postpartum. To avoid contamination with protein-laden lochia, only "clean catch" sample of urine should be collected for examination. A nonpathologic condition of proteinuria can be assumed only in the absence of signs and symptoms of a urinary tract infection or pre-eclampsia. Stagnation of urine along with a devitalized bladder wall contributes to the urinary tract infection in puerperium.

There is considerable diuresis starting shortly after delivery and lasting up to fifth day postpartum. The urine output may be more than 3,000 ml per day. This is thought to be one of the means the body uses in ridding itself of the increased extracellular water (interstitial fluid) that is a normal part of pregnancy. Other routes are also used for this purpose and this is the explanation for a rather profuse perspiration that may occur during the early postpartum days.

Gastrointestinal Changes

In early puerperium there is increased thirst, due to loss of fluid during labor, in the lochia, diuresis and perspiration. Women are usually hungry and ready for a regular meal an hour or two after delivery.

Constipation may be a problem in the early puerperium due to lack of solid foods during labor and self-restraint because her perineum is sore. Lack of tone of the perineal and abdominal muscles and reflex pain in the perineal region are contributing factors for constipation.

Weight Loss

In addition to the weight loss because of the expulsion of the uterine contents, a further loss of about 2 kg (5 lbs) occurs during the first postpartal week because of fluid loss through diuresis. Most women return to their pre-pregnant weight by the end of the puerperium.

Fluid Loss

There is a net fluid loss of about two liters during the first week and an additional 1.5 liters during the next five weeks. The amount of loss depends on the amount retained during pregnancy, dehydration during labor and blood loss during delivery.

Abdominal Wall

The abdominal striae are never eradicated completely but they do change to fine, silvery white lines. The abdominal walls are flabby after delivery because of their stretching during pregnancy. All puerperal women have some degree of diastasis recti, which is the separation of the rectus muscles of the abdomen. Women who take exercises regain their abdominal muscle tone and close the diastasis to some extend, however regaining complete muscle tone becomes difficult with increasing parity. If the abdominal wall muscle tone is not regained, the space between the rectus muscles fills in with peritoneum, facia and fat. Subsequent pregnancies do not have the necessary muscle support, which accounts for the pendulous abdomen often seen in multiparas. The rapidity of pregnancies, where there is no time to regain the muscle tone before being into another pregnancy and over distention in conditions such as multiple gestation, also contribute to pendulous abdomen. This condition may lead to extreme back pain for the woman and difficulties with fetal engagement at the time of labor and delivery.

Hematologic Changes

Immediately following delivery, there is slight decrease of blood volume due to dehydration and blood loss. The blood volume returns to the nonpregnant level by the second week. Cardiac output rises soon after delivery to about 60 percent above the prelabor value but gradually returns to normal within one week.

RBC volume and hematocrit values return to normal by the end of first week after the hydremia disappears. Leukocytosis to the extent of 30,000 per cubic mm occurs following delivery probably in response to the stress of labor. However, the various types of possible infections should be ruled out in the presence of such a finding. Platelet count decreases soon after separation of the placenta but secondary elevation occurs with increase in platelet adhesiveness between 4 to 10 days. Fibrinogen level remains high up to the second week puerperium, resulting in persistent high level of ESR in puerperium as during pregnancy. A hypercoagulable state persists and fibrinolytic activity is enhanced.

Normal nonpregnant levels for all the constituents of the blood are reached by the end of the puerperium.

Menstruation and Ovulation

The onset of the first menstrual period following delivery is very variable and depends more than anything on lactation. If the woman does not breastfeed her baby, the menstruation returns by sixth week following delivery in about 40 percent and by twelfth week in 60 percent of cases. If the woman breastfeeds her baby, the menstruation may be suspended in about 70 percent until the baby stops breastfeeding. However, menstruation may start even before cessation of breastfeeding in the remaining 30 percent.

In nonlactating mothers, ovulation may occur as early as four weeks and in lactating mothers about ten weeks after delivery. Thus, lactation provides a natural method of contraception and contributes to spacing of pregnancies. However, ovulation may precede the first menstrual period in about one-third and it is possible for the woman to become pregnant before she menstruates following her delivery.

MANAGEMENT OF EARLY PUERPERIUM

The principles in management of postpartal clients are:
- To restore the health of the mother
- To prevent infection
- To take care of the breasts
- To motivate the mother for contraceptive acceptance.

Immediate Attention

Immediately following delivery, the mother should be closely observed as outlined in the management of the fourth stage of labor. She may be given a drink or something to eat if she is in hungry. Measures to promote sleep must be instituted.

Rest and Ambulation

Physician's order for rest and ambulation may vary by virtue of the intrapartal course, the mother's condition, type of analgesia and anesthesia used and so on. For example, a woman who had a long, difficult labor, and is exhausted, who hemorrhaged or who is still groggy from medication may be ordered bed rest for a specified period. A woman who has had spinal or epidural anesthesia may be ordered 6 to 8 hours flat in bed to prevent spinal headache. For a woman who entered labor rested, progressed normally and is alert, the order may be ambulate pro re nata (PRN) with assistance at first.

Each woman should be assisted and accompanied the first time she gets up and thereafter as indicated until she feels no dizziness, weak knees, light headedness or any other indication that she might faint or fall. For most women 8 to 10 hours of rest is sufficient, after which they become fresh and can breastfeed the baby or move about. The practice of early ambulation decreases the incidence of postpartal thrombophlebitis, bladder complications and constipation. It facilitates uterine drainage and hastens involution of the uterus.

Diet

The woman may be given regular diet (normal diet) after delivery. For a woman who hemorrhaged, high protein diet may be given to promote tissue healing. Women who breastfeed require high calories, adequate protein, plenty of fluids, minerals and vitamins.

Perineal Care

Routine perineal care varies from setting to setting. An elaborate washing of the perineum using sterile equipment 2 to 3 times is practiced in some settings.

At its minimum, the woman should be instructed clearly about how to cleanse herself after urination, defecation, and provision of supplies and equipment made available. Basics related instructions to patients should include:

- ❖ Washing her hands before and after giving herself, perineal care
- ❖ Not touching her stitch area with her fingers—if uncomfortable or concerned, she should call for help
- ❖ Wipe with wet cotton or disposable wipe from front to back across the stitches, rinse and pat dry from front to back
- ❖ Application of perineal pads snugly enough so it would not move back and forth with movements
- ❖ Application and removal of perineal pad from front to back
- ❖ Not to touch the side of the perineal pad that will be worn next to her perineum.

Care of the Bladder

The anatomical changes described earlier necessitate extra attention to the urinary bladder, especially in the early puerperium. The woman is encouraged to pass urine 6 to 8 hours following delivery and thereafter at 4 to 6 hours interval. At times, the woman fails to pass urine due to unaccustomed position or reflex from perineal injuries. Allowing the woman to use the toilet if not contraindicated, usually serves the purpose. If measures such as running water, pouring water on her perineum and perineal relaxation fail, catheterization should be done. Catheterization is also indicated in case of incomplete emptying of the bladder evidenced by the presence of residual urine of more than 60 ml. The principle of bladder care is to ensure adequate drainage of urine so that infection may not occur.

Care of the Bowel

The problem of constipation is much less because of early ambulation and liberalization of dietary intake. A diet containing sufficient roughage and fluids is enough to move the bowel. If necessary, mild laxatives such as milk of magnesia may be given at bedtime.

Sleep

The postpartal woman is in need of rest both physical and mental. She should be protected against undue fatigue and worries as she is in a hypersensitive state of the nervous system. Sleep may be ensured by administering diazepam 5 mg or phenobarbitone 30 to 60 mg orally at bedtime. If she has discomfort due to after pains, painful piles or engorged breasts, they should be dealt with adequate analgesics such as aspirin with codeine orally (30 to 60 mg) 4 to 6 hours as necessary.

Care of the Breasts

The breasts should be examined daily, regardless of the chosen feeding method. Following enquiry as to any discomfort or concerns, the midwife should inspect the breasts for areas of redness. Then proceed to gently palpate the breasts to exclude areas of heat, redness or pain. The mother should be instructed to give scrupulous attention to hand washing and hygiene to prevent infection, which is a serious and painful complication of the puerperium. The nipples should be washed before each feeding, cleansed and dried after the feeding is over. A nursing brassiere provides comfortable support.

Uterus and Involution

The uterine fundus should be carefully palpated each postnatal day to ensure adequate involution. It is helpful if the woman has emptied her bladder prior to the palpation as a full bladder may make the uterine fundus appear high and deviated to one side. On palpation, the uterus should feel evenly contracted, smooth and firm and it should not be painful. Specific daily measurement of fundal descend, either by tape measure or manual palpation is done in some settings though it is of questionable value (Montgomery and Alexander, 1994). Subinvolution is identified if the uterus remains the same size for several days. Uterine fibroids could also lead to delayed involution. Tenderness of the uterus is suggestive of infection.

Rooming-in or Bedding-in

Following a normal delivery, the baby should be kept with the mother in a cot (basinet) beside her bed or, when the mother is awake in her bed. This not only establishes mother-child relationship but the mother is conversant with the art of baby care so that she can take full care of the baby while at home.

Immunization

Unimmunized Rh-negative mothers who delivered Rh-positive babies are given anti-D-gamma globulin. Women who are susceptible to rubella infection must be vaccinated and instructed about postponement of pregnancy for at least two months. The booster dose of tetanus toxoid should be given at the time of discharge, if it is not given during pregnancy.

Monitoring and Charting of Postpartum Events

During the postpartum period, assessment of maternal condition must be done on a regular basis and a progress record to be maintained noting the following:
1. Blood pressure, pulse, respiration and temperature recording every 4 to 6 hours.

2. Measurement of the height of the uterine fundus above the symphysis pubis once a day at a fixed time with prior evacuation of the bladder and preferably the bowel too.
3. Character, color and amount of lochia.
4. Voiding and bowel movement.
5. Perineal status such as healing, edema, inflammation, hematomas and bruising.
6. Extremities for varicosities, calf tenderness and heat, edema and reflexes.

Postpartum Exercises

The objectives of postpartum exercise are: (1) To improve the tone of abdominal and perineal muscles which were stretched during pregnancy and labor, (2) To educate the mother about correct posture in different working positions, while lifting during day-to-day activities.

Practicing the exercises would help the mother: (1) To minimize the risk of puerperal venous thrombosis by preventing venous stasis, (2) To prevent backache, (3) To prevent uterine prolapse and stress incontinence of urine.
1. Initially, the mother is taught *deep abdominal breathing* to strengthen the diaphragm. This may be begun on the first postpartum day. She is taught to take a deep breath raising her abdominal wall, and exhale slowly. To ensure exercise is being done correctly, place one hand on the chest and one on the abdomen. When inhaling, the hand on the abdomen should be raised and the hand on the chest should remain stationary. Repeat the exercise five times.
2. To tone up the abdominal muscles, she may be taught head and shoulder raising exercise, leg raising exercise, pelvic tilt exercise and sit-ups.
   ❖ *Head and shoulder raising*: On the second postpartum day, lie flat without pillow and raise head until the chin is touching the chest. On the third postpartum day raise both head and shoulders off the bed and lower them slowly. Increase gradually until able to do ten times.
   ❖ *Leg raising*: This exercise may be begun on the 7th postpartum day. Lying down on the floor with no pillow under the head, point toe and slowly raise one leg

keeping the knee straight. Lower the leg slowly. Gradually increase to ten times each leg. On the ninth postpartum day, slowly raise both legs together.

❖ *Pelvic tilt*: Lie flat on the floor with knees bent, inhale, and while exhaling, flatten the back against the floor so that there is no space between the back and the floor. While doing this, tighten abdominal muscles and the muscles of the buttocks.

❖ *Sit-ups*: In two weeks, the mother may begin sit-ups, slowly increasing the number until she is able to do at least ten times. Lie flat on the back with hands on hips. Slowly raise head, shoulder and trunk until attaining a sitting position.

3. Kegel exercise: This exercise is used to strengthen and tone the muscles of the pelvic floor. The mother should be instructed to do this daily for the rest of her life. Exercise can be done lying on the floor with ankles crossed or sitting in a chair with knees apart and feet flat on the floor. Tighten the muscles around the anus as if to control a bowel movement and then tighten the muscles around the vagina and urethra as if to stop urine in midstream. Now hold these muscles tightly to the count of six and then relax. This exercise can be done on the first postpartum day. It also increases the circulation to the perineal region, hence promoting faster healing of the episiotomies.

After two weeks, the mother may do almost any exercise she chooses. She must be reminded that if she notices that the lochia turns bright red after she has been exercising, she should stop for a few days until the bleeding is no longer bright red. If the mother does these six exercises faithfully and follows a sensible diet, she will most likely be able to regain her figure quickly (Joseph and Peck in Clausen et al, 1973).

CONTINUING PHYSICAL ASSESSMENT AND DAILY CARE

The nurse should follow an organized method when examining the postpartum client, which provides a consistent, quality approach to nursing care. The acronym, BUBBLEHE can serve a helpful reminder of the elements in a postpartum assessment.

BUBBLEHE stands for:

❖ Breasts
❖ Uterus
❖ Bladder
❖ Bowel
❖ Lochia
❖ Episiotomy
❖ Homan's sign
❖ Emotional status

The nurse should assess these elements every 8 hours along with vital signs.

Breasts

On palpation after delivery, breasts usually are enlarged, soft and warm and contain only small amount of colostrum. The nipples should be intact without redness, tenderness, cracks or blisters. Colostrum may be expressed. If the mother is not breastfeeding, the breast changes that occurred as a result of pregnancy regress in 1 to 2 weeks postpartum.

The mother may experience breast engorgement (enlargement and filling of the breasts with milk), which may begin as a tingling sensation in her breasts, 2 to 4 days after delivery. The breasts feel very full, tender and uncomfortable until the milk is released through infant sucking, manual expression, or pumping. The discomfort from engorgement normally subsides once stimulation to produce milk is decreased. The nursing mother's breasts should be inspected for the presence of inverted nipples, cracks, blisters, fissures and palpated for fullness and tenderness.

For nonbreastfeeding mothers, suppression can be achieved through a variety of methods that decrease simulation to the breasts such as securely binding the breasts with a snug support bra or a binder, avoiding warmth (e.g. hot shower water) on breasts, and applying ice packs to the breasts. The mother may be prescribed analgesics for breast discomfort and manual expression of milk and simulation of nipples to be avoided. These methods can be used until milk production stops.

Uterus

Immediately after delivery, the uterus begins the process of involution or reduction in size. It generally takes 6 weeks for complete physiologic involution and for the reproductive system to be restored to its nonpregnant state, except for the nursing mother's breasts. Subinvolution, or the failure of the uterus to return to a nonpregnant state, occurs when the process of involution is prolonged or stopped as a result of hemorrhage, infection or retained placental parts.

Uterine involution involves diminishing in size and weight, and anatomic location back into the pelvis. The endometrial decidua is shed as the lochial vaginal bleeding. By the end of 3 weeks postpartum, the endometrial lining and site of placental attachment return to a non-pregnant state. The placental site usually is completely healed without scarring by 6 weeks postpartum.

Immediately after delivery, the uterus weighs about 100 g, measuring 8 to 10 cm, which is 2 to 3 times the nonpregnant size. At the end of 6 weeks postpartum, the uterus weighs 50 to 100 g. Breastfeeding assists in hastening the speed of uterine involution. There generally is no difference between primiparas and multiparas regarding healing time. Multiparas may have less abdominal muscle tone and their cervix does not completely return to its closed, nonpregnant appearance. The parous cervix is easily distensible and appears as a slit.

Assessment of Fundus

For assessing the location and firmness of the uterine fundus (the top portion of the uterus), the nurse should place the client in a supine position with the bed flat. Immediately after delivery, the fundus usually can be located midline at the level of or one to two finger-breadths below the umbilicus. The fundus is approximately 1 cm below the umbilicus at 12 hours after delivery. After the first postpartum day, the fundus descends or involutes 1 to 2 cm (one finger breadth) each day. The fundus becomes nonpalpable on or about 9 days postpartum as it gradually descends into the true pelvis.

Immediately after delivery of the placenta, the fundus should be firm upon palpation. If the fundus is not firm or palpable, it may feel soft or boggy. A boggy uterus may be related to an over distended uterus or structural anomalies (e.g. fibroid uterus). A fundus that remains boggy is a warning sign of uterine atony and potential postpartal hemorrhage. Assessment will also include monitoring for risk factors for hemorrhage such as tocolytics, high parity and prolonged labour.

The position of the fundus should also be noted. An overfilled bladder easily displaces the uterus. It is palpated above the umbilicus and deviated to the right. This displacement interferes with the ability of the uterus to contract after delivery, resulting in uterine atony and hemorrhage.

Management of Bleeding

After delivery of the placenta 20 to 40 units of oxytocin (Pitocin) often is added to the intravenous solution if an IV line is in place, oxytocin is prescribed to hasten uterine contractility and control bleeding. When IV access is not present, other options such as administering oxytocin intramuscularly (10 units IM), initiating early breastfeeding or performing nipple stimulation is employed.

When the uterus remains boggy despite massage and oxytocin administration, other reasons for bleeding must be determined. When bleeding continues, a second pharmacological agent such as methylergonovine (Methergine) 0.12 mg IM may be given to clients who do not have a current history of high blood pressure. Another medication used for controlling bleeding is a prostaglandin called carboprost trome-thamine (Hemabate), which can be given when methergine does not stop bleeding or is contraindicated. If the fundus is firm and Lochia is heavy, the nurse should suspect cervical laceration. Common causes of postpartum hemorrhage are (1) Uterine atony, (2) Retained placenta, (3) Cervical or perineal laceration, and (4) Subinvolution and bleeding disorders.

Assessment of Uterine Pain

Abdominal cramping or afterpains are caused by uterine tonic contractions, which are the efforts of the uterus to expel blood clots and placental fragments. The contractions are enhanced with oxytocin and breastfeeding. Afterpains usually will seem more intense and occur at regular intervals in multiparous women. The cramping becomes milder after 3 days. When the pain becomes significantly more intense or the uterus tender to palpation, the nurse should assess for problems such as endometritis (an infection of the uterine lining).

Bladder

In the immediate postpartum period, the bladder is congested, edematous, and hypotonic from the effects of labor. Unless a urinary tract infection is present these effects should resolve within 24 hours of delivery. Diuresis up to 3000 ml per day occurs in the first 2 to 3 days postpartum due to decreasing production of aldosterone causing removal of excess fluid. In the immediate postpartum period, bladder distension, incomplete emptying and residual urine may occur due to edematous perineum, pain, reflex spasms and bladder desensitization.

Nursing responsibilities include teaching the newly delivered mother to empty the bladder often after birth to assist in controlling pain and bleeding. After delivery the client should be assisted to the toilet the first two to three times to protect against falls due to orthostatic hypotension and dizziness. Early ambulation and comfort facilitate urination. After delivery, the client should be able to urinate within 4 hours, at least 300 ml, with complete empting of the bladder. Complaints of urinary frequency, dysuria, retention and inability to void for 6 to 8 hours after delivery should be noted and informed to the physician.

After urination the fundus should be palpated for location and bladder for appropriate emptying. The bladder normally should be nonpalpable. Presence of residual urine (palpable bladder) can result in urinary infection. For clients who cannot urinate, a straight catheterization mat be done after considering individual circumstances such as the degree of bladder distention, location of the displaced uterus, amount of bleeding, amount of fluid or IV intake since the last voiding and the techniques used to encourage voiding.

An indwelling catheter inserted before cesarean delivery generally is kept in place for 24 hours. For the client who cannot empty her bladder completely, an indwelling catheter may be inserted and retained for the minimum required period as it carries the risk of bacteriuria.

Bowels and Gastrointestinal System

The client's appetite typically will return to normal in 1 to 2 hours after delivery. If there are no complications from anesthesia, regular food may be resumed. The client who had vomited during labor may not have an appetite. She should be encouraged to increase her fluid intake. The new mother after a long and difficult labor will need food and fluids to regain her strength. Diet rich in protein and iron is needed to promote tissue healing and to restore iron levels due to blood loss.

Following vaginal delivery, bowel movement normally occurs 2 to 3 days later. When gastric motility does not return by 2 to 3 days, constipation occurs. Causes of constipation include increase in progesterone levels in late pregnancy, decreased bowel motility and fluid intake during labor, side effects of medications, and hesitancy to defecate owing to perineal discomfort. In order to avoid this problem, the client should be encouraged to drink six to eight glasses of fluids daily and eat a high fiber diet (e.g. whole grains, legumes, vegetables and fruits). Sitz baths, topical medications and stopping medications that cause constipation are helpful.

When constipation is severe administering an analgesic and a stool softener before ambulation may facilitate bowel movement by 2 to 3 days postpartum. Mineral oil, bisacodyl (Dulcolax) suppository or Fleet enema (evacuant enema) may be given to stimulate intestinal activity.

Examination of the bowels includes assessment for the presence of hemorrhoids. Haemorrhoids present during pregnancy may enlarge during labor. If the hemorrhoids are large, they may cause pain if they become thrombosed and may subsequently cause constipation. Treatment with topical ointment or spray may relieve discomfort.

Lochia

The usual uterine discharge of blood, mucus, and tissue after childbirth is called lochia. Lochia contains the sloughing of decidual tissues, including erythrocytes, epithelial cells, and bacteria. Lochia is assessed according to its amount, color and change with activity and time.

The descriptive name of lochia changes with the change in color. Lochia rubra is the term given for the discharge in the first 3 days after delivery. Lochia rubra has bright red colour and consists mainly of decidual tissue and blood.

Lochia serosa, which occurs 4 to 10 days after delivery, is watery, pink or brown-tinged and lesser in amount than lochia rubra. Lochia serosa primarily contains serous fluid, leukocytes, erythrocytes, and decidual tissue. The lochia changes into lochia alba, a whitish-yellow creamy discharge in 10 to 15 days. Many women may have minimal discharge by day 14; however, it is not uncommon for lochia alba to last until 6 weeks postpartum. Lochia alba consists of a mixture of leukocytes, decidual tissue and decreasing fluid content.

When the client is bleeding heavily, the nurse needs to ensure that the bleeding is not coming from another source such as cervical or vaginal laceration. Lacerations are highly suspected when heavy bleeding continues despite a firm uterus. Saturation of a perineal pad within 15 to 30 minutes may indicate hemorrhage. A complete blood count (CBC) may indicate a 1.0 to 1.5 g/dl decrease in hemoglobin and a 3 to 4% decrease in hematocrit, which is consistent with a loss of 500 ml of blood.

The amount of lochia varies with position changes, but should continually decrease throughout the first 4 to 6 weeks postpartum.

Blood pools in the vaginal vault when the client is recumbent and drains when standing up. Clot formation occurs as a result of the pooling in the uterus or vagina. An increase in bright red bleeding and the passage of clots may also occur during physical activity or breastfeeding. Lochia with a reddish color that persists after 2 weeks of delivery may indicate subinvolution of the placental site or retained placental parts.

The client should be instructed to report to the physician if blood clots larger than 1 cm are passed. Nursing actions include assessing the fundus for firmness and amount of lochia. Further examination may be required to evaluate for other sources of continued bleeding.

Lochia has a characteristic menstrual—like musky or fleshy smell. A foul-smelling discharge, along with other indicators, such as fever or uterine tenderness, may suggest an infection such as endometritis. Because lochia is an excellent medium for bacterial growth, clients should be taught to change the perineal pad after each voiding.

The first menstrual period usually begins within an average of 8 weeks after delivery for most nonlactating women. The timing may be delayed from 2 to 18 months in breastfeeding mothers, and ovulation may occur without the onset of first menstrual period. Thus, it is possible for a woman to become pregnant before the return of menses. Consistent, continuous breastfeeding increases prolactin levels, thus postponing the resumption of ovulation. Once breast stimulation decreases, prolactin levels decrease and FSH and LH hormone levels increase, inducing ovulation.

Episiotomy

An episiotomy is the surgical incision made to enlarge the vaginal opening for delivery of the baby's head. The episiotomy may be incised midline down the center of the perineum, or mediolaterally, which extends in a diagonal angle to either the left or right side. With or without episiotomy, the perineum may suffer from lacerations during childbirth. Lacerations are classified as first, second, third or fourth degree. First degree involves only the skin and superficial structures above the muscle. Second degree extends to the perineal muscles. Third degree reaches into the anal sphincter muscles. Fourth degree continues into the anterior rectal wall.

To assess an episiotomy and condition of the perineum, it is best to have the client lie on her side, flexing her upper leg toward her hip. The nurse can then lift her buttocks examine the perineum. Using a good light source facilitates visualization of incision and for inspection. The REEDA (redness, edema, echymosis, discharge and approximation) scoring scale can be used when assessing the episiotomy.

Care of the vulva includes applying ice packs to the perineum, for the first 24 hours, to help decrease edema and pain. Ice packs also assist in constricting blood vessels, minimize the risk of hematoma formation and decrease muscle irritability and spasm. Ice packs should not be applied directly to the skin; they should be wrapped with an absorbent disposable type of covering.

After the first 24 hours following delivery, a sitz bath with warm water may be used to reduce the local discomfort, increase circulation and healing. Use of heat lamp or infra red lamp two to three times a day also will assist in the healing process. The client should be taught perineal hygiene, including daily washing with warm water and mild soap. The perineum should be cleansed after each voiding and bowel movement. The perineum should be wiped from front to back (anterior to posterior) to avoid contamination from the anal region. Practices such as changing the perineal pad frequently after each voiding and bowel movement or at least 4 times a day, removing pad from front to back, and hand washing will help decrease the risk of infection. Soiled pads should be placed in appropriate disposal container. Pain should be assessed and medication provided as needed.

Immediately after delivery, the vagina appears edematous, bruised, and stretchable and may gape at the introitus. By 4th week, the vaginal rugae return. The vagina returns to its prepregnant state (except for a slightly larger size than in pregnant state) by 6 to 8 weeks postpartum. The nurse should reach the client how to perform perineal exercises such as Kegel exercises to assist in restoring vaginal perineal tone and elasticity and to help reduce urinary incontinence.

Extremities

Assessment of the extremities should include examination of varicosities, deep tendon reflexes (DTRs), tenderness, and presence of edema or nodular areas on the legs. DTRs should be no greater than +1 to +2. Brisk DTRs (+3 to +4) or hyperactive reflexes are suggestive of PIH. Pretibial or pedal edema may be present, especially in the client with PIH.

Risk factors for developing deep vein thrombosis are severe anemia, traumatic delivery and obesity. Pain, erythema, or local swelling on the legs, especially the calves may signify thrombophlebitis.

The client's legs should be assessed for sensation and mobility, when epidural anesthesia has been administered. With appropriate return of mobility, the client should be able to move her toes and lift her buttocks off the bed within 2 to 4 hours after discontinuation of anesthesia.

Homan's Sign (Fig. 23.2)

Assessment of Homan's sign must be done for all postpartum clients, to check for presence of thrombophlebitis. In order to perform the test, have the client straighten her legs flat on the bed. Place one hand under the knee in the popliteal region for support. Place the other hand on the foot and dorsiflex (flexing the foot towards the body) it. Presence of calf pain during sharp dorsiflexion in either foot is a sign of deep vein thrombosis.

Prevention of Thrombophlebitis

Clients who remain in bed up to 8 hours should perform leg exercises to prevent formation of clots (thrombus) in the legs, which can develop into thrombophlebitis or thromboembolism. A clot formed in the deep leg vein may fragment from the original clotted site and lodge in the lungs as pulmonary embolus, which is a serious complication. Superficial thrombophlebitis is

Fig. 23.2: Homan's sign check to identify thrombosis in the calf

noted as hard, painful, warm and red vein. Unlike DVT, there is little potential for pulmonary embolism with superficial thrombophlebitis.

It is important to teach clients to flex and extend both feet and legs alternatively while in bed. In a rhythmic motion, press and then relax the backs of the knees into the mattress. Clients should also be taught other ways to prevent thrombus formation, such as:

❖ Keeping the legs uncrossed while seated,
❖ Not flexing the legs at the groin,
❖ Resting the legs without putting pressure on the back of the knees,
❖ Wearing support hose or antiembolism stockings when varicosities are present and
❖ Padding pressure points during lithotomy position.

Examine the calves for redness, hardness or nodules along leg veins. In addition, check the ankles and pretibial areas for edema. Assess the client for signs of pulmonary embolism such as dyspnea, cough and chest pain.

Emotional Status

The immediate postpartum period is an emotional roller coaster, and almost any emotion may be observed. The nurse should b continually assessing the mother for appropriate responses to her infant. Clients often experience a sense of elation immediately after the birth of their babies. They are excited and relieved that labor is finally over. They may want to relive the experience by talking about the process of labor and delivery. However, they may also be exhausted and need sleep and rest to restore their bodies to health.

In this "taking in phase", mothers wish to meet their own rest and nutritional needs before focusing their energy on newborns. The attainment of parental roles, infant care and family adaptations should also be assessed.

OTHER ASSESSMENTS

In addition to the basic postpartum assessments addressed in the approach using the acronym BUBBLEHE, other important body systems need to be assessed.

Hemodynamic Status

Blood values return to normal within the first six weeks after delivery. A CBC may show marked leukocytosis, predominantly neutrophils, both during and after labor. The leukocyte count may increase during labour up to 25,000/mm^3 and up to 30,000/mm^3 during a prolonged labour and remain elevated for the first 2 days postpartum. The average leukocyte count is 14,000 to 16,000/mm^3. A possible infectious process must be ruled out in the presence of such increased counts, especially during the first 6 hours after delivery.

Hemoglobin, hematocrit and erythrocyte levels may fluctuate during the first postpartum days. When considerable blood loss occurs, the levels may decrease below those measured before labor. Immediately after delivery, the hematocrit level begins to rise owing to hemodilution, increase in plasma volume and dehydration. By 4 to 5 weeks, the hematocrit returns to normal values.

Blood coagulation normalizes a few days after delivery. Depending on the amount of blood lost during delivery, it takes 3 to 4 weeks for the blood volume to return to prepregnant levels. Cardiac output remains increased for at least 48 hours after delivery.

Integumentary System

The striae on breasts, thighs and abdomen eventually fade to a pale color but may never completely disappear. Skin discolorations that appeared during pregnancy such as chloasma usually disappear toward the end of pregnancy. However, hyperpigmentation of the areolae and linea nigra may be permanent.

After giving birth, the mother may complain of profuse perspiration, especially at night, which is normal during the first week as the body rids itself of excess fluid from pregnancy. Some women may have a mild eruption of acne from hormonal changes. Other changes include hair loss for the first two months after delivery. The nurse should reassure her that this is normal owing to hormonal changes. The rapid decrease in estrogen also induces the regression of vascular abnormalities such as palmar erythema and spider angiomas.

Musculoskeletal System

Because the abdomen stretches during pregnancy the mother's abdominal wall relaxes or becomes flaccid after delivery. When visually assessing and palpating the abdomen and fundus, the nurse may notice some degree of muscle separation, called diastasis recti, along the center of the abdomen. This separation occurs due to pressure from an enlarging uterus and may increase with each subsequent pregnancy. The severity depends on the client's general physical condition, muscle tone, timing between pregnancies, parity and other circumstances that distend the uterus and abdomen. Conditions such as multiple gestation, macrosomia, and hydramnios also distend

the uterus to a larger than average size, making it difficult for the client to regain her prepregnant muscle tone.

Activity

After childbirth many mothers complain of fatigue and require time to recuperate and recover from the effects of labor and delivery. Once the mother is stable, the nurse should encourage her to ambulate often. Women who deliver vaginally often are able to ambulate to the toilet within few hours of delivery.

Before rising from the bed, the client should be assessed for dizziness and motor weakness from weak knees or legs. When assisting the client in getting up from bed for the first time, the nurse should accompany her because she may experience orthostatic hypotension and be at risk of falling. When the mother is very tired or has received an epidural or analgesic that may cause drowsiness, she may not have the ability to stand and walk independently.

The client should be encouraged to return to normal activities of daily living as soon as possible. She should be able to provide independent self-care before going home. After going home she may perform light household chores depending on physician's instructions.

The client would feel better and stronger if she ambulates early after delivery. Specific medical advantages of early ambulation are:

- ❖ Fewer bladder infections
- ❖ Less frequent constipation
- ❖ Decreased incidence of deep vein thrombosis and
- ❖ Decreased incidence of pulmonary embolism.

Exercise

A woman who has had an uncomplicated vaginal delivery can begin moderate exercise soon afterward. Vigorous exercise should be delayed until 6 to 8 weeks because joints do not stabilize earlier. She may be instructed to perform mild stretching and flexing of muscles especially abdominal muscles, which may relieve tension and muscle strain. These include deep breathing, head raising, arm raising, knee flexes and leg raising. Other safe exercises include Kegel exercises, and pelvic tilts. Exercising too much and too soon may result in bright-red vaginal flow. The client must not lift anything heavier than her baby for the first 2 weeks after childbirth. She should avoid climbing stairs for 2 to 3 weeks.

Pain Management

After delivery, the mother is at risk for various types of discomfort. She may complain of perineal discomfort, uterine cramping, sore nipples, or a headache if she received incorrectly administered spinal anesthesia. The most common discomfort is from the *afterpains* related to uterine contractions.

Analgesics may be administered orally every 4 to 6 hours as needed. Emptying the bladder every 1 to 2 hours or so is an effective measure to relieve afterpains. Another useful method is for the client to lie on her abdomen with a pillow against her lower abdomen because this creates pressure that keeps the uterus contracted.

Topical anesthetics provide temporary relief from episiotomy pain. Ice packs and sitz baths also provide relief for the mother. When medications do not relieve complaints of perineal pain, the site should be assessed more carefully. Pain not relieved by the usual means may indicate a possible hematoma. Episiotomy pain normally is relieved by 3 weeks.

Sexuality

Mothers must be instructed to avoid sexual activity until their episiotomy has healed, which may take 6 weeks or more, or until they are comfortable and desire to have sex. Because of perineal discomfort or swelling, most mothers wait to resume sexual intercourse until after the six-week check-up.

Contraception

The decision about contraception depends on many things; the client's and her spouse's motivation, the number of children desired, the state of the child's health, whether she is breastfeeding and the couple's religious beliefs.

If an intrauterine device is the method of choice, it usually is inserted after the 6-week postpartum check-up. Some physicians may decide to insert it in the immediate postpartum period; however, the risk of expulsion is higher with rates from 10 to 20%.

For clients who prefer to go on oral contraceptives it may be prescribed to start after breastfeeding has been firmly established. The mother who is not breastfeeding can begin to take oral contraceptives as early as 2 to 3 weeks after delivery.

If the couple is sure about permanent sterilization, this can often be accomplished during a cesarean delivery or 24 to 48 hours following vaginal delivery.

Immune System

Unsenstized mothers who are Rh (D) - negative and have given birth to an infant who is Rh - positive should receive 300 μg of Rh (D) immune globulin (RhoGAM) within 72 hours of delivery. RhoGAM is administered even if the mother received RhoGAM in the antepartum period. Depending on the extent of hemorrhage and exchange of maternofetal blood, a larger dose may be necessary in some instances.

Before discharge, the client's rubella status needs to be checked. If the mother is rubella nonimmune with a titer below 1:8, she should be vaccinated before leaving the hospital. It is important to counsel the woman against becoming pregnant again for next 4 weeks after receiving the vaccine. The client should also be informed that she might experience a brief period of rubella like symptoms such as a rash, lymphadenopathy, joint symptoms and low-grade fever for 5 to 21 days after vaccination. The vaccine is safe to be given to breastfeeding mothers. If the client declines to receive the vaccine in the hospital, she should be counseled about the devastating teratogenic effects on the fetus if she conceives before receiving the vaccine.

Documentation

Careful documentation is the closing step of each assessment encounter. Daily care of the woman after delivery includes the parameters such as episiotomy, lochia, and breastfeeding. If written in narrative format, the nurse may use the acronym BUBBLEHE to assist her in ensuring that all pertinent assessment are charted completely at least every shift, or more frequently depending on the client's acuity. Nursing documentation should follow the nursing process and the facility's policy on documentation.

Discharge Preparation

Client education comprises much of the nurse's responsibilities throughout the postpartum stay with shortened hospital stays. The nurse must streamline her teaching methods, assessing the new mother's and her family's personal teaching needs. Focused client interactions should be directed toward desired client outcomes, empowering the woman and her family. The nurse should assess the mother's current knowledge regarding self-care and infant care because the mother's prior experiences with pregnancy and infant care may change the direction of the nurse's teaching plans. New mothers must learn how to care for herself and her infant. Self-care topics include those activities that help her to manage, anticipate and recognize health problems and danger signs. Infant care encompasses activities such as feeding, dressing, and recognition of health problems.

General instructions in addition to self and infant care activities include the following:
* Do not lift anything heavier than the baby for the first 2 to 3 weeks
* Do not move furniture or vacuum for the first few weeks
* Get lots of rest and sleep when the baby sleeps
* Get help from family for household chores for first few weeks and enjoy the baby
* If an episiotomy is present, avoid having sexual intercourse until it heals or the bottom feels better
* Take medications as prescribed
* Keep the postpartum follow-up appointment
* Seek medical help if any warning sign of sickness occurs.

A postpartum follow-up examination usually is scheduled for 6 weeks after delivery, or earlier depending on the agency policy.

DISCOMFORTS OF THE PUERPERIUM AND RELIEF MEASURES

There are number of discomforts of the puerperium. While they are considered normal, there is no reason for a woman to have to suffer with them.

Afterbirth Pains

Afterbirth pains, sometimes called afterpains, can be quite painful. They are continuing sequential contraction and relaxation of the uterus. They are much more common with increasing parity and in women who breastfeed. With increased parity, there is decrease in uterine muscle tone, which causes the uterus to relax thereby subject it to recontraction. In the instance of breastfeeding women, the suckling of the baby stimulates the production of oxytocin by the posterior pituitary. The release of oxytocin not only triggers the let-down reflex in the breasts but also causes the uterus to contract—Even the well-contracted uterus of a primipara will contract even more.

The key to effective relief from afterbirth pains is an empty bladder. The reason for this is the fact that a full bladder displaces the uterus from its normal and proper position. When the uterus is so displaced, it is unable to contract as it should and tends to relax, thus prohibiting relief from afterpains. Sometimes afterbirth pains are totally relieved just by the act of emptying the bladder.

Once the bladder is empty, the woman may lie prone with a pillow under her lower abdomen. The prone position places constant pressure against her uterus (the pillow creates even greater pressure), which keeps it contracted and thus eliminates afterbirth pains since there is no uterine relaxation. The woman needs to be forewarned that when she first lies on stomach, she will have severe cramps or pain for about five minutes before she experiences complete and total relief.

Analgesia can be effective for afterbirth pains, but not for very long if the woman's bladder is not emptied. For nonbreastfeeders analgesia generally is not needed because the prone position usually alleviates the discomfort even in multipara. It is important to remember that the let-down essential to breastfeeding is inhibited by pain. The amount of analgesic that gets into the milk will not hurt the baby.

Excessive Perspiration

Excessive perspiration is due to the body's using this route as well as diuresis to rid itself of the excess interstitial fluid that resulted from the hormonal effect during pregnancy. Keeping the mother clean and dry will provide comfort. The woman may want to change her gown frequently. Bed sheets should be changed as necessary. Care must be taken to assure that the woman is hydrated. Drinking a glass of water or any fluid of her liking during each hour she is awake, will assure this.

Breast Engorgement

It is thought that engorgement of the breasts is due to a combination of milk accumulation and stasis and increased vascularity and congestion. It occurs on approximately the third postpartal day in both breastfeeding and non-breastfeeding mothers and lasts approximately 24 to 48 hours. Signs and symptoms of engorgement include the following, which are experienced to a greater or lesser degree by individual woman.

❖ Sense of increasing breast heaviness or filling on the day prior to engorgement
❖ Enlargement of breasts from distention
❖ Skin becomes tight, shining and reddened
❖ Breasts are warm to touch
❖ Veins become visible
❖ Breasts are tender, throbbing and painful
❖ Breasts feel firm, full and hard.

Because this is not an inflammatory process, there is no temperature elevation caused by breast engorgement.

Relief measures for a woman who is not breastfeeding are geared toward relief of discomfort and cessation of lactation. Relief for a breastfeeding woman aims for relief of discomfort and continuation of lactation. Treatment of breast engorgement is important to the breastfeeding mother as unrelieved breast engorgement suppresses the milk supply. With the current short hospital stay, many women will be home before breast engorgement occurs and need to be instructed about what to do when it happens.

Relief Measures for Nonbreastfeeding Mothers

❖ Give the breasts good support. A breast binder should be used to provide upward and inward thrust and support. If a binder is not available, one may be prepared using a pillowcase or towel, which will go around the woman and two shorter strips to be used as shoulder straps. The binder has to be secured with safety pins to fit each woman. A tuck is to be given beneath each breast to provide support and the ends are overlapped and fitted in front. Applied this way a breast binder is extremely comfortable for the woman because it imparts support and prevents painful movement.
❖ Apply ice bags or packs to the breasts. Ice relieves discomfort, has a certain numbing effect, and does not encourage milk flow.
❖ Take analgesics such as aspirin or paracetamol to relieve pain.
❖ *Avoid massaging* the breasts in an effort to get the milk out. Such actions will only extend the length of time of breast engorgement. Any emptying of the breasts by any means stimulates the breasts to further lactation.
❖ *Do not apply heat* to breasts as heat dilates the blood vessels and ductile system causing the milk to flow. This causes partial emptying and stimulates the breasts to further lactation.

Relief Measures for Breastfeeding Mothers

Relief measures for the breastfeeding woman are designed to get the milk flow and empty the breasts. This also alleviates the mother's discomforts. The following are the relief measures.

❖ Carry-out breast massage, manual expression and nipple rolling
❖ Nurse the baby every 2 to 3 hours without missing any feeding or using any supplements.
❖ Use both breasts at each feeding. Start on the breast which is used last during the previous feeding. The baby should be on each

breast for 5 to 10 minutes to start with and then build-up to complete emptying of one breast which may take about 20 minutes before switching to the other to finish the feeding. Sucking for shorter period initially helps to accustom the nipples to the baby's sucking and minimize soreness.

Many breastfeeding mothers, who had antenatal breast preparation, begin breastfeeding within an hour of delivery, feed frequently thereafter and use both breasts to avoid undue breast engorgement.

❖ Apply warmth to the breasts, prior to each breastfeeding to promote milk flow. This can be accomplished with warm washcloth on breasts or warm shower

❖ Manually express the milk if there is engorging of the areola, to soften the area prior to nursing the baby. This will help the baby latch on to the nipple properly and easily

❖ Use manual expression of milk to empty the breasts after the baby has nursed if they are still uncomfortably full and engorged

❖ Maintain good support to the breasts without any pressure points. A nursing brassier may be worn for this purpose

❖ Ice bags may be used between feedings to deduce swelling and pain

❖ Analgesics may be used if needed.

Perineal (Stitch) Pain → (due to episiotomy suture.)

Before any measures are instituted, it is essential to examine the perineum to ascertain if the woman is experiencing normal pain or if a complication, such as hematoma or infection, is developing. Perineal comfort measures are as following:

❖ Ice pack or ice bags, or rubber gloves filled with crushed ice or ice chips can be applied. Ice bags or packs should be wrapped in sterile towel or any clean disposable soft material. These are most useful in reducing the swelling and numbing the area in the immediate postpartum period especially if the woman had a third or fourth degree laceration

❖ Topical anesthetic spray or ointment may be used as ordered. If an ointment is to be used the woman should be instructed to wash her hands before applying it

❖ Sitz bath 2 to 3 times a day.

Many women consider the sitz bath most soothing of all the measures. A modification of the same idea is to pour warm water over the perineum. This can be a part of routine perineal care after voiding and defecation. The warmth of the water increases circulation and promotes healing. The warmth and motion of the water are soothing.

Constipation

Stool softeners or mild laxatives are usually ordered for women with third or fourth degree repair of perineum. Multiparas with lax abdominal wall may also require measures to avoid constipation.

Hemorrhoids

If the woman has hemorrhoids, they may be quite painful for a few days. Relief measures include the following:

❖ Ice bags or packs
❖ Medicated compresses
❖ Analgesic or anesthetic spray or ointment
❖ Heat lamp
❖ Warm water compresses
❖ Stool softeners
❖ Rectal suppositories
❖ Replacement of external hemorrhoids inside the rectum.

BREASTFEEDING DIFFICULTIES AND MANAGEMENT

A mother who is breastfeeding for the first time is in a vulnerable position and requires support, encouragement and knowledgeable assistance. She has to make the transition from being insecure, anxious and self-doubt to being self-assured and confident in herself and her abilities. The mother should be prepared for each breastfeeding and helped with the following measures:

❖ Assume a comfortable position, which also allows proper positioning of the baby. Side lying, reclining or sitting position with generous use of pillows for support and comfort

❖ Her bladder should be empty and should have received comfort measures for any afterpains or perineal discomfort prior to breastfeeding time

Personal Hygeine, Baby care, nutrition, rest & sleep, elimination, breast feeding, family planning, Immunization, Lochia, How to prevent discomfort

226   SECTION 6: THE NORMAL PUERPERIUM

* Assure of available help as necessary
* Rested and relaxed
* Hands should be washed and nipples cleansed by gently wiping them off with plain water.

The baby's immediate preparation includes having a clean diaper and if absolutely necessary to be swaddle wrapped.

Position the baby so that he or she will not be doubled up or have a twisted neck when sucking and the head and body are supported.

In bringing the baby and breast together, the following steps are helpful:

* Let the baby find the breast and grasp the nipple. Do not thrust the breast in the baby's face
* Help the mother to hold the breast beyond the areolar area so her fingers will not interfere with proper positioning of the baby's mouth and gums on the nipple
* Touch the baby's cheek with the nipple so the baby will turn towards the breast (use the rooting reflex)
* Express few drops of colostrum, so they are on the surface of the nipple. This provides the baby with instant gratification and reinforces learning
* As the baby grasps the nipple, the mother must make sure that the baby has enough of it for proper positioning in the mouth. The baby must grasp more than just the end of the mother's nipple to compress the lactiferous sinuses located beneath the areolae in order to obtain colostrum or milk
* Once the baby's mouth is properly positioned well on to the areola, the mother releases her grasp of her breast. As the baby starts sucking and swallowing, she must provide breathing space for the baby if needed, by pressing with a finger on her breast where the baby's nose is. This is needed only during the learning period, and when the breast is engorged. Babies usually suck a bit, rest a bit (maintaining their hold on the nipple while they rest), and then suck some more. The mother must be prepared for this
* Suction must be broken before trying to remove the baby from the breast by slipping a finger into the corner of the baby's mouth and between the baby's gums. Once the suction is broken, the baby is removed from the breast without injury to the nipple. The baby is then burped and put to the other breast

Lactation is established by a combination of the following:

a. Starting breastfeeding as soon as possible after delivery.
b. Frequent feedings during the first few days, using both breasts.
c. No missed feedings.
d. No supplementary feedings. Rotation of breasts as the starting and ending breasts to provide for complete emptying of both breasts.
e. Tension-free, painless, rested, relaxed mother during feeding times.
f. Baby properly positioned on the breast.
g. Supportive spouse.

After the first few days, the baby will settle into his or her own pattern of feeding frequency. A self-demand scheduling (i.e. feeding the baby when he or she is hungry) can be adopted rather than a rigid scheduling.

The final factor in successful breastfeeding is effective breast care. Breast care and preparation for breastfeeding begin in the antenatal period. Breast care while breastfeeding is as follows:

a. Wash the nipples only with water. Soap, alcohol or any other drying agent can lead to cracking of the nipples.
b. Expose the nipples to air for 15 to 30 minutes after a feeding.
c. While exposing the nipples to air, expose them also to a 25-watt light bulb or sunshine.
d. Following exposure, rub in a nipple cream, A and D ointment or other prescribed ointment.
e. Provide good support to the breasts.
f. If breasts become engorged, care for them, as discussed earlier in this chapter.
g. If the nipple becomes tender:
   * Enhance the let-down before feeding with warmth, as discussed for care of the breast during engorgement.
   * Nurse on the less sore nipple first until there is let-down, then switch the baby

to the sorest nipple to empty that breast, then switch back to the less sore nipple to finish the feeding
- ❖ Use a pacifier to meet the baby's sucking needs rather than the end of feedings on the nipple
- ❖ Breastfeed more frequently for shorter periods of time
- ❖ Be sure to use a combination of exposure to air and heat after each breastfeeding, followed by thorough application of nipple cream

h. Be sure to break the suction, before removing the baby from the breast.

Guidance and Instructions in Preparation for Home Care

Following normal delivery, mothers are discharged on the second or third postpartum day. Prior to discharge from the hospital, the midwife must appraise the mother's need for instructions and guidance for the care of self, baby and self in relation to others.

Self

a. Measures to improve her general health
b. Perineal care
c. Breast care
d. Care of breasts during breast engorgement
e. Postnatal exercises (abdominal muscle tightening and perineal muscle tightening)
f. Gradual return to day-to-day activities
g. Return for six week postpartum check-up.

Baby

a. Breastfeeding (as discussed earlier in this chapter)
b. If being bottle fed:
- ❖ Care and preparation of formula
- ❖ Care and preparation of bottles and nipples or container and spoon or feeding dish
- ❖ How to hold the baby during feeding
- ❖ How to hold the feeding bottle to prevent the baby sucking air (the nipple to be full).
c. Burping
d. Baby bathing and dressing including care of genital area.

e. Cord care.
f. Prevention and treatment of diaper rash.
g. Checking baby's temperature.
h. Recognizing baby's needs.
i. Check-up and immunization for the baby.

Self in relation to others:
- ❖ Sibling and husband rivalry
- ❖ Family planning
- ❖ Resumption of sexual intercourse after six weeks.

NURSING PROCESS DURING THE PUERPERIUM

Assessment

Assess for the following manifestations:
1. Vital signs—BP, pulse, temperature, respirations.
2. Breasts—Soft or engorged.
3. Abdomen—Soft and loose.
4. Gastrointestinal system.
   a. Appetite (increased normally)
   b. Thirst (more thirst)
   c. Bowel movements (sluggish).
5. Uterus
   a. Location on different days
   b. Consistency (firm normally)
   c. Rate of involution
   d. Afterpains especially for multiparas and breastfeeding mothers.
6. Lochia
   a. Color—Rubra to serosa to alba.
   b. Smell—Any foul smell indicates infection.
7. Small clots
8. Urinary output
   a. Large amounts normal
   b. Difficulty in emptying.

Analysis/Nursing Diagnosis
- ❖ Ineffective individual management of therapeutic regimen
- ❖ Impaired home maintenance management
- ❖ Altered nutrition
- ❖ Pain
- ❖ Altered sexuality pattern
- ❖ Anxiety
- ❖ Altered family process
- ❖ Altered parenting

Planning

❖ Create an environment to parent—newborn interaction/bonding
❖ Promote maternal-neonatal well-being
❖ Provide support and counseling to new mothers
❖ Provide teaching regarding postpartal self-care measures and newborn care.

Implementation

1. Complete postpartum assessment every 4 to 6 hours. Include the following areas:
   a. Take and record vital signs.
   b. Palpate breasts. Note firmness and complaints of breast tenderness. Assess nipples for tenderness/soreness, blisters and cracking in breastfeeding mothers.
   c. Palpate abdomen and note any tenderness.
   d. Palpate fundus. Note height, position (midline or to the side) and firmness.
   e. Inspect perineum for bruising, edema, and hematoma. Note presence of hemorrhoids.
   f. Inspect legs for reddened, tender areas, and inquire about areas of tenderness. Check Homan's sign.
   g. Inquire about urinary and bowel elimination.
   h. Assess comfort level and need for pain medication.
2. After initial recovery period, assess vital signs every eight hours according to the protocol.
3. Promote urinary and bowel function.
   a. Urine elimination.
      ❖ Encourage voiding within 6 to 8 hours. Catheterization to relieve bladder distention.
      ❖ Measure urinary output for the first three voidings.
      ❖ Note frequent voidings of small amounts (less than 100 ml), which may indicate retention with overflow.
      ❖ Teach woman regarding
         – Adequate fluid intake
         – Emptying bladder on regular basis
         – Wiping from front to back.
   b. Feces elimination.
      ❖ Encourage adequate fluid intake.
      ❖ Administer stool softeners as needed and desired.
      ❖ Teach client regarding
         – Daily exercise
         – Adequate fluids
         – Including fiber and roughage in diet.
4. Promote perineal healing and teach self-care measures.
   a. Apply ice packs for 6 to 12 hours.
   b. Cleanse perineum by applying warm water rinse.
   c. Offer sitz baths 2 to 4 times a day.
   d. Use local anesthetics.
   e. Apply perineal pads from front to back and change after each voiding.
   f. Teach client to report:
      ❖ Blood clots
      ❖ Foul smelling lochia
      ❖ Change from lochia alba to serosa back to lochia rubra.
5. Provide breast care and teach self-care measures.
   a. Breastfeeding mothers should:
      ❖ Cleanse breast with warm water (no soap)
      ❖ Wear a supportive bra
      ❖ Apply cream (as prescribed) for nipple soreness
      ❖ Be taught breast massage
      ❖ Be assisted with breastfeeding technique
   b. Nonbreastfeeding mothers should:
      ❖ Wear a supportive bra
      ❖ Use a breast binder if desired
      ❖ Avoid breast stimulation
      ❖ Be offered cold /ice packs to decrease swelling and inflammation from engorgement.
6. Teach abdominal and pelvic strengthening exercises.
   a. Modified sit-ups.
   b. Woman should be advised that increase in vaginal flow or return to lochia rubra may occur if activity becomes excessive.

7. Provide information regarding sexual activity.
   a. Sexual activity may be resumed in about six weeks postdelivery.
   b. Ovulation may occur, so contraceptive measures are needed to prevent pregnancy.
8. Provide infant-care teaching
   a. Common variations in infants
   b. Cord care
   c. Elimination
   d. Diapers
   e. Feeding
   f. Temperature
   g. Signs of illness should be reported to the physician/pediatrician
   h. Newborn bath
   i. Formula preparation and feeding
   j. Breastfeeding.

Evaluation

1. Ensure that parents have opportunities for interaction with their baby.
2. Ensure that mother and baby remain within normal physiological parameters.
3. Provide parents with support and counseling.
4. Confirm that mother is able to demonstrate self-care measures and infant care.

BIBLIOGRAPHY

1. Hynes L. Physiology, complications and management of the puerperium, In: Bennett RV, Linda KB. Myles Textbook for Midwives, 13th edn. Edinburgh: Churchill Livingstone; 1999.
2. Kitzinger S. The Complete Book of Pregnancy and Childbirth, New York: Knopf; 1980.
3. Llewellyn Jones D. Fundamentals of Obstetrics and Gynecology, 6th edn. London: Mosby; 1994.
4. Montgomery E, Alexander J. Assessing Postnatal Uterine Involution, a Review and Challenge, Midwifery 1994;10:73-6.
5. Royal College of Midwives, Successful breastfeeding, 2nd edn. Edinburgh, London: Churchill Livingstone; 1991.
6. Varney Helen. Nurse-Midwifery, 2nd edn. Boston: Jones and Barlett Publishers; 1996.

24

Family Planning

Learning Objectives

Upon completing this chapter, the learner will be able to:

❖ Describe the magnitude of population increase and the urgency for measures to reduce the rate of growth
❖ Describe the concept and objectives of family planning
❖ Describe the contraceptive methods
❖ Explain the role of the midwife regarding family planning and related issues
❖ Explain the provision of family planning services.

People throughout the world are becoming increasingly aware of and concerned about the steadily rising population and the inherent effect this will have on the quality of life and the delicate balance of nature. Man continues to seek for answers to the question of how a level of population can be maintained through reproduction that will not exploit the environment.

The disparity between the death rate and the birth rate results in the rapid rise of population. This is specially pronounced in the developing countries comprising about 70 percent of the total world population.

MAGNITUDE OF THE PROBLEM

In the beginning of the 20th century, the rate of population increase was about ten million per year. It is now increasing at a much faster rate of 100 million per year. As the population growth continues unabated, India's population has reached 1027 million in 2001 from 944.5 million in 1996.

India with 2.5 percent of the world's land surface area has to accommodate about 16 percent of the world population. India is the second most populous country in the world, next to China. The density of the population is 267 per sq. kilometer. The death rate was nine per 1,000 in 1997. Thus, there is a wide gap between births and deaths resulting in rapid rise of population.

Impact of Population Increase

The rapid increase of population has an adverse effect on the national economy. The benefits of improvement in the different sectors are being eroded by the growing population. At the level of families, the increasing number of births has a deleterious effect on the health of the mother and the child, and hinders social and economic upliftment of the family. High parity is associated with increased maternal and infant mortality and various other obstetric and gynecological complications and nutritional problems. For these reasons, population control by appropriate family welfare program is considered a branch of preventive and social medicine. Many developing countries, India in particular, have taken family planning as a national program of vital importance.

FAMILY PLANNING

Definition

An expert committee of WHO (1971) defined family planning as "a way of thinking and living that is adopted voluntarily, upon the basis of knowledge, attitudes and responsible decisions by individuals and couples, in order to promote the health and welfare of the family group and thus contribute effectively to the social development of the country".

Another expert committee defined and described family planning as follows:

Family planning refers to practices that help individuals or couples to attain certain objectives:

a. To avoid unwanted births.
b. To bring about wanted births.
c. To regulate the interval between pregnancies.
d. To control the time at which births occur in relation to the ages of the parent
e. To determine the number of children in the family (Park, 2000).

BASIC HUMAN RIGHTS

The United Nations Conference on human rights in 1968 recognized family planning as a basic human right. The 1974 conference on world population endorsed the same view and stated in its "plan of action" that all couples and individuals have the basic human right to decide freely and responsibly the number and spacing of their children and to have the information, education and means to do so. The world conference of the International Women's Year in 1975 also declared the right of women to decide freely and responsibly on the number and spacing of their children and to have access to the information and means to enable them to exercise that right. Thus, family planning has become the focus of international concern as a basic human right and a component of family health and social welfare (Park, 2000).

Modern Concept of Family Planning

Family planning is not synonymous with birth control. A WHO expert committee in 1970 has stated that family planning in its purview includes all the following:

* The proper spacing and limitation of births
* Advice on sterility
* Education for parenthood
* Sex education
* Screening for pathological conditions related to the reproductive system (e.g. cervical cancer)
* Genetic counseling
* Premarital consultation and examination

* Carrying-out pregnancy tests
* Marriage counseling
* The preparation of couples for the arrival of their first baby
* Providing services for unmarried mothers
* Teaching home economics and nutrition
* Providing adoption services.

These activities vary from country to country according to national objectives and policies with regard to family planning.

Health Aspects of Family Planning

The principal health outcomes of family planning, as listed by a WHO scientific group on health aspects of family planning, include women's health, fetal health and child health.

Women's Health

Pregnancy can mean serious problems for women. It may damage the mother's health or even endanger her life. The risk increases as the mother grows older and after she has had three or four children. Family planning by intervening in the reproductive cycle of women helps them to control the number, interval, timing of pregnancies and births, and thereby reduces maternal mortality and morbidity and improves health (Park, 2000).

The health impact of family planning occurs through the avoidance of unwanted pregnancies, limiting the number of births and proper spacing, and timing the births, particularly the first and last in relation to the age of the mother.

Fetal Health

A number of congenital anomalies are associated with advancing maternal age (e.g. Down's syndrome). Such congenital anomalies can be avoided by timing the births in relation to the mother's age. Further, the "quality" of population can be improved only by avoiding unwanted pregnancies.

Child Health

Mortality among children is high when pregnancies occur in rapid succession. A birth interval of two to three years is considered desirable to reduce child mortality. Family planning is therefore an important means for birth spacing and limiting family size thereby insuring the survival of all children in the family.

Small Family Norm

The objective of family welfare program in India is that people should adopt the "small family norm" to stabilize the country's population at the level of some 1,533 million by the year 2050 AD. In the 1970s and 1980s, the models adopted in India for family size were three children and two children respectively. The current emphasis is on three themes: "Sons or Daughters—two will do"; and "Second child after three years"; and "Universal immunization".

The national target is to achieve a Net Reproduction Rate of one, by the year 2006, which is equivalent to attaining approximately the two-child norm.

Objectives of Family Planning Program in India

Conception Control

1. To bring down the birth rate to a realistic minimum during a given period. There were about 168 million eligible couples in India in 1999. These are couples with wives in the reproductive age group of 15 to 45 years and who require the use of some sort of family planning method. According to the latest available report, about 44 percent of the eligible couples in the country are practicing effective methods of contraception.
2. To bring about certain special changes such as:
   - To educate and motivate the sexually active and fertile couples to accept the small family norm
   - To increase the literacy rate especially among women in rural areas
   - To raise the marriageable age of both boys and girls. Low age of marriage not only contribute to the increased birth rate but adversely affects the health of the

woman. In 1948, the Indian parliament approved the bill fixing the minimum age of marriage at 21 years for men and 18 years for women
- To maximize the access of good quality family planning services.

Maternity and Child Health Services

- To extend maternity services through antenatal, intranatal and postnatal care with immunization against tetanus and prevention, and correction of anemia.
- To offer protection to children through immunization schedule and vitamins supplement program.

Other Services

- To provide sex education and marriage guidance
- To promote research on normal reproduction, investigation and treatment of infertility and recurrent abortion. It also includes evaluation of pregnancy termination as a method of family limitation.

Birth Control, Contraception and Family Planning

The words birth control, contraception and family planning are often used interchangeably although they are not identical in meaning. The term birth control refers to regulation of the number of children that are conceived or born. Contraception refers to the prevention of pregnancy, which is accomplished by specific contraceptive or birth control methods. Family planning has the broadest connotation. It encompasses the additional considerations of the physical, social, psychological, economic and theological factors that govern the family's attitudes and influence decisions pertaining to the size of the family, the spacing of children and the selection and utilization of a contraceptive method.

Contraception plays an important role in the lives of many women. It should be viewed in the wider context of sexual and reproductive health. The capacity to enjoy and control sexual and reproductive behavior is a key element of sexual health (WHO, 1992).

Role of the Midwife in Family Planning

The role of the midwife in family planning has been acknowledged by the World Health Organization and the International Confederation of midwives. She must be able to facilitate client knowledge and choice by providing valid, current information in a way, which is easily understood by the woman and possibly by her partner or spouse. Her counseling skills, attributes such as being non-judgmental and positive listening skills are of supreme importance.

Discussion regarding family planning may well be appropriate at all stages of reproductive period. Preconceptionally, contraception is advocated for two months after rubella vaccination. Antenatally, the woman and her partner may wish to have information on which to base future choices and following delivery they may require further information.

A mother who has chosen not to breastfeed will need to commence contraception so that it is effective before postpartum ovulation that occurs on an average between 40 and 50 days after delivery (Wang and Fraser, 1994). The midwife needs to be aware that general factors governing individual contraceptive choices vary greatly and can include religion and culture, relationship, age, motivation to avoid pregnancy, lifestyle and socioeconomic considerations. After childbirth, these may be compounded by issues such as breastfeeding, because their chosen method of contraception must not affect lactation, health of their baby, body image and adjustment to motherhood.

The midwife will also need to be aware of the family planning services available in the area where she practices. Guilleband (1993) suggested that the ideal contraceptive would be 100 percent effective, perfectly safe, reversible, inexpensive, free of side effects, simple to obtain and use, and not related to the time of coitus. Although, some of these ideal standards have been achieved, no single method meets all the criteria.

METHODS OF CONTRACEPTION

1. Temporary methods
   a. Barrier methods
   b. Natural contraception
   c. Intrauterine contraceptive devices (IUCDs)
   d. Steroidal/hormonal contraception.
2. Permanent methods
   a. Female: Tubal occlusion/tubal ligation
   b. Male: Vasectomy

Temporary Methods of Contraception

These are commonly used to postpone or to space births. However, these are also used frequently by couples who desire to have no more children.

Barrier Methods

These methods prevent sperm deposition in the vagina or sperm penetration through cervical canal. The objective is achieved by mechanical devices or by chemical means, which produce sperm immobilization, or by combined means. The following are included:

❖ Mechanical
  – Male: Condom
  – Female: Condom, diaphragm, cervical cap
❖ Chemical (vaginal contraceptives)
  – Creams—Delfen
  – Jelly—Preceptin, volpar paste
  – Foam tablets—Aerosol foams, clorimin T or contab
  – Sponge—Today
❖ Combination—Combined use of mechanical and chemical methods.

Male Condom

Condoms are made of polyurethane or latex. Polyurethane condoms are thinner and suitable to those who are sensitive to latex rubber. It is the most widely practiced method used by the male. A widely marketed brand in India is "Nirodh". The efficacy of condoms can be augmented by adding spermicidal agents during its use. Protection against sexually transmitted disease is an additional advantage. The method is suitable for couples who want to space their pregnancies and who have contraindications for the use of oral contraceptive or IUCD. These are also suitable to those who have infrequent sexual intercourse.

Instructions for Use

The condom is unrolled over the erect penis before any genital contact. The rim of the condom should be held against the base of the penis during withdrawal making sure the condom does not become dislodged from the penis. The condoms are tested for holes electronically by the manufacturer and need not be tested before use. The condom should be grasped at its open end and held in place during withdrawal of penis. However, after use it should be checked for tears before throwing it away. If it is found torn, a spermicidal jelly should be put into the vagina immediately. The condom should be thrown away after single use.

Use of Condom

1. As an elective contraceptive method.
2. As an interim form of contraception during pill use, following vasectomy operation and if an IUCD is thought lost, until a new IUCD can be fitted.
3. During the course of treatment of the wife for *Trichomonas vaginitis*.

Advantages

1. Easily available and inexpensive.
2. No contraindications or side effects.
3. Easy to carry, simple to use and disposable.
4. Protection against sexually transmitted diseases like *Chlamydia*, gonorrhea and HIV.
5. Protection against pelvic inflammatory diseases.
6. Suitable for use during lactation, for teenagers and in cases where pills and IUCDs are contraindicated.
7. Useful where sexual intercourse is infrequent and irregular.

Disadvantages

1. It reduces sexual pleasure to a small extent due to reduced sensitivity for the male and interruption of sexual act.
2. May accidentally break or slip off during coitus.

Fig. 24.1: Female condom: "Femidom"

Female Condom (Fem Shield) (Fig. 24.1)

It is a pouch made of polyurethane, which lines the vagina and external genitalia. It is about 15 cm in length with one flexible polyurethane ring at each end. The condom is inserted into the vagina in such a manner that the closed inner end is anchored in place by the polyurethane ring, whilst the open outer edge lies flat against the vulva. The inner ring at the closed end is smaller compared to the outer ring. It gives protection against sexually transmitted disease and pelvic inflammatory disease.

Female condoms were not accepted well though they were not expensive or required no prescription from physician (Ford and Mathie, 1993).

Diaphragm (Figs 24.2A and B)

Diaphragm is an intravaginal device made of rubber with flexible metal or spring ring at the margin. Its diameter varies from 5 to 10 cm. It is not a popular method. It requires a medical person to measure the size required.

Instructions for Use

The diaphragm of the right size is selected, that is of the same length as the distance between the top of the posterior fornix and the under surface of the symphysis pubis. It is inserted dome down with some spermicidal jelly within the cup and along the rim. The diaphragm is pinched between the thumb and index finger and released only after insertion into the vagina. The device should be introduced up to three hours before intercourse and kept for at least six hours after the last coital act. Ill fitting and accidental displacement during intercourse increase the failure rate.

Figs 24.2A and B: Diaphragm—insertion and checking: (A) Insertion of a diaphragm; (B) Checking the position of diaphragm using finger

Advantages

1. Inexpensive
2. Can be used repeatedly for long-time
3. Highly effective if used properly
4. No interruption in love making as with condom.

Disadvantages

1. Requires help of a physician to measure the size required.
2. Risk of vaginal irritation and urinary tract infection.
3. More difficult to use than condom and requires high degree of motivation for the user.
4. Not suitable for women with uterine prolapse.

Vaginal Contraceptives

Chemicals: Several spermicidal agents are available in the market in the form of cream, jelly or foam tablet. These agents mostly cause sperm immobilization when they come in contact and to some extent prevent sperm penetration through the cervical canal. The cream or jelly is introduced high in the vagina with plastic applicators at least fifteen minutes

before sexual intercourse. Foam tablets are to be introduced high in the vagina at least five minutes prior to intercourse. No douching should be done within eight hours to avoid dilution of the spermicide, which would decrease its potency. In isolation, these are not very effective, but enhance the efficacy of condom or diaphragm when used along with it. There may be occasional allergic manifestations in either the vulva or vagina. Spermicides are messy to use and are not acceptable to couples that are unwilling to interrupt lovemaking or prepare in advance.

Vaginal Contraceptive Sponge (Today)

The sponge is made of polyurethane impregnated with a spermicide—nonoxynol-9, which acts as a surfactant. It is to be worn by the woman in the vagina during coitus. It is shaped like a mushroom cap, the concave surface facing the cervix. The sponge is moistened with water, squeezed gently to remove excess water and inserted high in the vagina manually or with an applicator. It is not removed for at least 6 to 8 hours after coitus. The sponge absorbs semen as it is deposited in the vagina, prevents its entry into the cervix and releases nonoxynol-9 during coital thrust, which inactivates sperm. The sponge measures about 2 cm in diameter and is made for single use. It does not require fitting by physician. It is less effective and more expensive. Allergic reactions and soreness are common.

NATURAL CONTRACEPTION

Rhythm Method

The rhythm method is the only birth control method (besides total abstinence), which is officially approved by the Roman Catholic Church. It is also referred to as "safe period" or "temporary abstinence".

This method is based on the fact that a woman is fertile only around the time of ovulation and if she abstains from intercourse during that time, she is unlikely to conceive. Usually a woman ovulates once during each menstrual cycle. The ovum has an active life of 12 to 24 hours during which it can be fertilized. Sperm cells, once within the birth canal are viable for 72 hours during which they can fertilize the ovum. Thus, there is a minimum total of 96 hours (4 days) during each cycle when conception is possible. To these 4 days, an additional margin of several days is added to allow for variation in the exact day of ovulation.

The method to determine the approximate time of ovulation and the fertile period include:

a. Recording of the previous menstrual cycles (calendar rhythm)
b. Recording the basal body temperature (temperature rhythm)
c. Taking note of the excessive mucoid vaginal discharge (mucus rhythm).

The users of the calendar method obtain the period of abstinence from calculations based on the previous twelve menstrual cycle records. From this record the number of days in each cycle is listed. From this list the longest cycle and the shortest cycle are noted. The number 20 is subtracted from the number of days in the shortest cycle to get the first day of the fertile or unsafe period and the number 10 is subtracted from the number of days in the longest cycle to get the last day of the fertile or unsafe period. Thus, if a woman had cycles ranging from 25 to 31 days, she would abstain from intercourse from the 5th day of her current menstrual cycle (25 – 20 = 5) until the 21st day of her current cycle (31 – 10 = 21).

Users of the temperature rhythm require abstinence until the third day of the rise of temperature. This is because the basal temperature (taken immediately on awakening and before any activity) of a woman is more or less constant during the first part of menstrual cycle until the day of ovulation. At that time, it drops slightly and then rises to a level somewhat higher (usually five-tenths to seven-tenths of a degree) than it has been and remains at that higher level for the rest of the cycle. If there is no cold or infection to account for this elevation, the woman can consider beyond the fertile period when the elevation has persisted for three days.

Users of mucus rhythm require abstinence on all days of noticeable mucus and for three days thereafter.

The effectiveness of rhythm method can be considered satisfactory for highly motivated, carefully selected women with fairly regular cycles, who have the intelligence and self-discipline as well as cooperative marital partner to understand and practice it correctly. However, many couples find it difficult to have sex by the calendar instead of by inclination.

Advantages

1. No cost
2. No side effects.

Disadvantages

1. Difficult to calculate the safe period.
2. Compulsory abstinence from sexual act during certain periods.
3. Not applicable during lactational amenorrhea or when periods are irregular.
4. Higher rate of ectopic or congenital abnormality of the fetus because of chances of the union of aging sperm and ovum.

Coitus Interruptus

It is the oldest and probably the most widely accepted contraceptive method used by man. It necessitates withdrawal of penis shortly before ejaculation. It requires sufficient self-control by the man so that withdrawal of penis precedes ejaculation.

Disadvantages

1. Requires sufficient self-control by the men.
2. The woman may suffer anxiety, vaginismus or pelvic congestion.
3. Chance of pregnancy is more.
   - Precoital secretion may contain sperm.
   - Accidental chance of sperm deposition in the vagina.

Breastfeeding

Prolonged and sustained breastfeeding offers a natural protection of pregnancy. This is more effective in women who are ammenorrheic than those who are menstruating. The risk of pregnancy to a woman who is fully breastfeeding and ammenorrheic is less than 2 percent in the first six months.

Contraceptive Effectiveness of Conventional Methods of Contraception

Conventional methods of contraception are: (1) Condoms, (2) Vaginal diaphragms, (3) Spermicides, and (4) Rhythm method.

The failure rate of any contraceptive is calculated in terms of pregnancy rate per hundred women years (HWY) of use. It is calculated according to the following formula (Pearl Index).

Pregnancy failure rate

$$= \frac{\text{Number of accidental pregnancies} \times 1200^*}{\text{Number of patients observed} \times \text{months of use}}$$

* 1200 = Number of months in 100 years.

Example: If 100 couples have used a method for a period of two years (24 months) and have resulted in 20 pregnancies, the pregnancy rate is calculated to be:

$$\frac{20 \times 1200}{100 \times 24} = 10$$

When the pregnancy rate is below 10, the effectiveness of the particular method is considered to be high. If it is more than 20, it is said to be low. The following are the failure rates of the commonly used contraceptive methods (Table 24.1).

Table 24.1	Failure rate of contraceptive methods

Method of contraception	*Failure rate*
• Condom	14 (HWY)
• Diaphragm	12 (HWY)
• Vaginal contraceptives (spermicides)	9–27 (HWY)
• Rhythm method	20–30 (HWY)
• Coitus interruptus	18 (HWY)

INTRAUTERINE CONTRACEPTIVE DEVICES (IUDs)

Intrauterine devices often referred to, as IUDs are small plastic or metal forms to which a 'tail' of nylon threads is usually attached. These are worn by women in their uterine cavity. During the last couple of decades, there has been a significant improvement in its design and content.

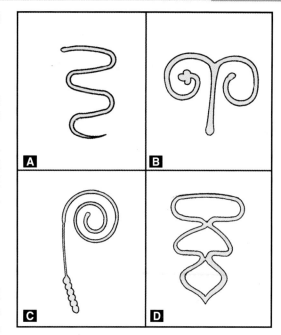

Figs 24.3A to D: First generation IUDs: (A) Lippes loop; (B) Safe T-coil; (C) Margulies spiral; (D) Dana super

Types of IUD

There are two basic types of IUD, non-medicated and medicated. Both are usually made of polyethylene or other polymers; in addition, the medicated or bioactive IUD, release either metal ions (copper) or hormones (progestogens).

The nonmedicated IUDs are often referred to as *first generation* IUDs. The copper IUDs comprise the *second* and the hormone releasing IUDs the *third generation* IUDs. The medicated IUDs were developed to reduce the incidence of side effects and to increase the contraceptive effectiveness.

First generation IUDs: Include Lippes loop, Margulies spiral, Safe-T-coil and Dana super (Figs 24.3A to D). Of these, the Lippes loop was widely used in India since 1965 when it was introduced in the national family planning program.

Second generation IUDs: Were introduced in the 1970s. It was found that metallic copper had a strong antifertility effect (Zipper, 1969). The addition of copper has made it possible to develop smaller devices, which are easier to fit, even in nulliparous women. A number of copper bearing devices are now available (Fig. 24.4).

Fig. 24.4: Second generation IUDs

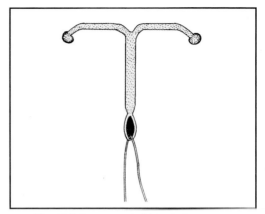

Fig. 24.5: Levonorgestrel intrauterine system

❖ Earlier devices:
    Copper-7
    Copper T-200

❖ Newer devices:
    – Variants of the T device
      (i) Cu T-220 C
      (ii) Cu T-380 A or Ag
    – Nova T
    – Multiload devices
      (i) ML-Cu-250
      (ii) ML-Cu-375

The numbers included in the names of the devices refer to the surface area (in sq mm) of the copper on the device. Nova T and Cu T-380 Ag are distinguished by a silver core over which is wrapped the copper wire.

According to recent reports, copper devices have become very popular in India, accounting for 99.7 percent of the total IUD insertions in 1990–91. Lippes loop, which was widely used in the 1970s, and 1980s is being phased out.

Advantages of copper devices
❖ Lower expulsion rate
❖ Lower incidence of side effects, e.g. pain and bleeding
❖ Easier to fit even in nulliparous women
❖ Better tolerated by nullipara
❖ Increased contraceptive effectiveness.

Third generation IUDs: These are based on still another principle, i.e. release of a hormone. The most widely used hormonal device is *progestasert*. It has a direct local effect on the uterine lining, on the cervical mucus and possibly on the sperms. Because the hormone supply is gradually depleted, regular replacement of the device is necessary.

Another hormonal device that has been tested is a T-shaped IUD, the *Levonorgestrel intrauterine system* (Levonorgestrel-IU) releasing 20 µg of the potent synthetic steroid (Fig. 24.5).

Long-term clinical experience with levonorgestrel releasing IUD has shown to be associated with lower menstrual blood loss and fewer days of bleeding than the copper devices.

Description of Devices

Copper T-200: This is the widely used medicated device. It carries 215 sq mm surface area of fine copper wire wounded round the vertical stem of the device. The stem of the T-shaped device is made of a polyethylene frame. It has a polyethylene monofilament tied at the end of the vertical stem. These two threads are used for detection and removal. The device contains 120 mg of copper. The device is to be removed after three years.

Copper 380-A: Carries 380 mm^2 surface area of copper wire wound around the stem (175 mg) and sleeves on the horizontal arms (66.5 mg). Replacement is after ten years (copper is lost at the rate of 50 µg per 24 hours during a period of one year).

Multiload Cu-250: The device is available in a sterilized, sealed packet with an applicator. The device emits 60 to 100 µg of copper per day during a period of one year. The device is to be replaced every three years.

Multiload Cu-375: It has 375 mm^2 surface area of copper wire wound around its vertical stem. Replacement is every five years.

Progestasert: Bioactive core containing microcrystals of progesterone (38 mg) enclosed within the plastic wall, which releases about 65 µg of progesterone daily into the uterine cavity. It should be replaced after one year.

Levonorgestrel Intrauterine System (LNG-IUS)

This is a T-shaped device, with a polydimethyl-siloxane membrane around the stem, which contains levonorgestrel (a potent synthetic steroid). It releases the hormone at the rate of 20 µg/day. The device is to be replaced every five years. The third generation devices are more expensive, to be used on a wider scale.

Mode of Action of IUDs

The precise mode of action of IUDs by which they prevent pregnancy, is not clear even after three decades of use and study. At present, the most widely accepted views are the following:

❖ The IUD causes a foreign body reaction in the uterus causing cellular and biochemical changes in the endometrium and uterine fluids, and it is believed that these changes impair the viability of the gamete and thus reduce its chance of fertilization rather than its implantation (Luskin, 1982).

❖ Medicated IUDs produce other local effects that may contribute to their contraceptive action. Copper seems to enhance the cellular response in the endometrium. It also affects the enzymes in the uterus. By altering the biochemical composition of cervical mucus, copper ions may affect sperm motility, capacitation and survival (Hutchins, 1985).

❖ Hormone releasing devices increase the viscosity of the cervical mucus and thereby prevent sperm from entering the cervix. They also maintain high levels of proges-terone and low levels of estrogen in the endometrium, thereby sustaining it unfavo-rable to implantation (Hutchins, 1985).

Time of Insertion

1. During menstruation or within ten days of the beginning of a menstrual period (Gray, 1980). During this period, insertion is technically easy because the diameter of the cervical canal is greater at this time than during the secretary phase. The uterus is relaxed and myometrial contractions, which might tend to cause expulsion, are at a minimum (Hawkins, 1979). In addition, the risk that a woman is pregnant is remote at this time.

2. Postpartum insertion is done six to eight weeks after delivery. Postpuerperal inser-tion has several advantages. It can be combined with the follow-up examination of the woman and her child.

3. Postabortion insertion can be taken-up immediately after a legally induced first trimester abortion.

4. Immediate postpartum insertion IUD insertion can also be done during the first week after delivery before the woman leaves the hospital. Special care is required with insertions during the first week after delivery because of the greater risk of perforation during this time. Furthermore, immediate insertion is associated with a high expulsion rate.

Follow-up and Client Instructions

The objectives of follow-up examination are:
1. To provide motivation and emotional support.
2. To confirm the presence of IUD
3. To diagnose and treat any side effects or complication.

The IUD wearer should be examined after her first menstrual period, for chances of expulsion of the device are high during this period; and again after the third menstrual period to evaluate the problems of pain and bleeding and thereafter annually. The IUD wearer should be given the following instruc-tions:

1. She should regularly check the threads or "tail" to be sure that the IUD is in the uterus. If she fails to locate the thread, she must consult the physician.

2. She should visit the clinic whenever she experiences any side effects such as fever, pelvic pain or bleeding.

3. If she misses a period, she must consult the physician.

Side Effects and Complications

Bleeding

The most common complaint of women, fitted with IUD (inert or medicated), is increased vaginal bleeding. It may be greater volume of blood loss during menstruation, longer menstrual periods or midcycle bleeding (Liskin, 1982). Copper devices and hormone-releasing devices cause less average blood loss.

If the bleeding is heavy or persistent or if the woman develops anemia despite the iron supplement, the IUD should be removed. In most women, removal of the device is rapidly followed by a return to the normal menstrual pattern.

Pain

Pain is the second major side effect leading to IUD removal. Pain may be experienced during IUD insertion and for a few days thereafter, as well as during menstruation (Hutchings, 1985). It may manifest itself as low backache, cramps in the lower abdomen and occasionally pain down the thighs. These symptoms usually disappear by the third month (Gray, 1980).

Slight pain during insertion can be controlled by analgesic or antispasmodic drugs. If pain is intolerable, the IUD should be removed.

Pelvic Infection

Pelvic inflammatory disease (PID) is a collective term that includes acute, subacute and chronic conditions of the ovaries, tubes, uterus, connective tissue and pelvic peritoneum and is usually the result of infection. IUD users are about two to eight times more likely to develop PID than noncontraceptive users.

The clinical manifestations of PID are vaginal discharge, pelvic pain and tenderness, abnormal bleeding, chills and fever. Even one or two episodes of PID can cause infertility, permanently blocking the fallopian tubes. Therefore, young women should be fully counseled on the risks of PID before choosing an IUD.

When PID is diagnosed, it should be treated promptly with broad-spectrum antibiotics. Most clinicians recommend removing IUD if infection does not respond to antibiotics within 24 to 48 hours.

Uterine Perforation

The reported incidence ranges from 1:150 to 1:9,000 insertions depending upon the time of insertions, design of IUD, technique of insertion and operator's experience. In the hands of experienced physicians, it should not be higher than 0.3 percent. Perforations occur more frequently when insertions are performed between 48 hours and 6 weeks postpartum.

The device may migrate into the peritoneal cavity causing serious complications such as intestinal obstruction. The perforation may be completely asymptomatic and discovered only when searching for a missing IUD. The conclusive diagnosis of perforation is usually made by a pelvic X-ray. Any IUD that has perforated the uterus should be removed because the risks of intra-abdominal inflammatory response, leading to adhesions or perforation of organs within the abdominal cavity outweigh the risks associated with removal.

Pregnancy

Pregnancy may occur in three to five per hundred users per year. About fifty percent of uterine pregnancies occurring with the device in situ end in a spontaneous abortion. Removal of the IUD in early pregnancy has been found to reduce this abortion rate by half. In women who continue the pregnancy with the device in situ, a four-fold increase in the occurrence of premature births has been reported (WHO Offset Publication, 1983).

Lowest pregnancy rates are observed with Cu T 380 A and LNG-IUS. Should pregnancy occur with a device in situ, there is risk of ectopic pregnancy (1–2%).

If the thread is visible through the cervix, it is best to remove the device. However, if the thread is not visible it is better to leave it alone after counseling the woman about the risks involved in continuing the pregnancy. The device may be expelled spontaneously with the delivery of the placenta.

Ectopic Pregnancy

Ectopic pregnancies among IUD users are estimated at 3 to 4 percent of all pregnancies, while among nonusers, the estimate is 0.8 percent of all pregnancies. Women using IUDs must be taught to recognize the symptoms of ectopic pregnancy— Lower abdominal pain, dark and scanty vaginal bleeding or amenorrhea. Women with previous ectopic pregnancy or PID should not use IUD if other methods are feasible. Studies indicate that the rate of ectopic pregnancies is higher among users of hormone-containing devices than among women using other IUDs (Hutchings, 1985).

Expulsion

Expulsion rate vary between 4 to 30 percent. It can be partial or complete. Partial expulsion can be diagnosed on speculum examination by observing the stem of the IUD protruding through the cervix. Spontaneous expulsion occurs during the first few weeks or during menstruation. Expulsion is more common among young women, nulliparous women and women who have postpartum insertion. Expulsion rates are somewhat lower for copper than for inert devices. In general, expulsion in itself is not a serious problem, but if expulsion is unnoticed, pregnancy may occur.

Fertility after Removal

Fertility does not seem to be impaired after removal of a device provided there has been no episode of PID, whilst the device was *in situ*. Over 70 percent of IUD users conceive within one year of removal (Hutchings, 1985). It is now established that PID is a threat to woman's fertility.

Mortality

Mortality with IUD use is extremely rare and has been estimated to be one death per 100,000 woman-years of use. The deaths usually occur following complications such as septic spontaneous abortion or ectopic pregnancy. In this regard, IUD is safer than oral contraceptive, particularly in older or high-risk women.

Cancer or Teratogenesis

There is no evidence to date that IUD use increases cancer risks. Nor there is any evidence of developmental abnormality or congenital malformations among the offspring of either former IUD users or those who conceive with an IUD *in situ* (WHO Offset Publication, 1985).

Indications for Removal of IUD

The indications for removal are:
1. Persistent excessive regular or irregular bleeding and/or severe cramp like pain in the lower abdomen.
2. Flaring up of salpingitis.
3. Perforation of the uterus with the device in the peritoneal cavity.
4. Downward displacement of the device into the cervical canal or partly protruding outside into the vagina.
5. Patient desirous of a baby.
6. Missing thread.

Missing Thread

The thread may not be visible through the cervical os due to:
1. Thread coiled inside.
2. Thread torn through.
3. Device expelled outside unnoticed by the woman.
4. Device perforated the uterine wall and lying in the peritoneal cavity.
5. Device pulled up by the growing uterus in pregnancy.

Identification of the missing IUD is done by straight X-ray or ultrasonography.

Removal may be done with a specially designed hook, an artery forceps or by uterine curette. Removal under hysteroscopic visualization is the best procedure.

Advantages of Third Generation IUDs Over the Others (Cu T-380 A, Multiload 375, Levonorgestrel IUS)

1. Higher efficiency with lower pregnancy rate (less than one percent women years).
2. Significant reduction in menorrhagia, dysmenorrhea and premenstrual tension syndrome is observed with LNG-IUS.
3. Risk of ectopic pregnancy is significantly reduced (0.02/HWY).
4. Risk of PID is reduced.
5. Longer duration of action (5–10 years).
6. Low expulsion rate and fewer indications for medical removal.

Disadvantages of Third Generation IUDs

1. Expensive.
2. Not available through government channel in India currently.
3. Deposition of calcium salts over the device on prolonged use may prevent the diffusion of copper.

Cu T is distributed free of cost through government channel in India. Because of the prolonged contraceptive protection, it is suitable for the rural population of developing countries. With Cu T, there are no systemic side effects and reversibility to fertility is prompt soon after removal. Local reactions include menstrual abnormalities, pelvic pain, heavy period and pelvic inflammatory disease. Ectopic pregnancy is a risk and failure rate is 0.1 to 2.0 HWY.

HORMONAL CONTRACEPTIVES

Hormonal contraceptives when properly used are the most effective spacing methods of contraception. Oral contraceptives of the combined type are almost 100 percent effective in preventing pregnancy. More than 65 million people in the world are estimated to be taking the "pill", of which about 10 million are estimated to be in India.

Gonadal Steroids

Estrogens and progestogens are the gonadal steroids used for contraception.
a. *Synthetic estrogens*: Two synthetic estrogens are used in oral contraceptives. These are ethinyl estradiol and mestranol. Both are effective.
b. *Synthetic progestogens*: These are classified into three groups—pregnanes, estranes and gonanes.
    Estranes, which are also known as 14-norestosterones, and gonanes, are used in oral contraceptives.

CLASSIFICATION OF HORMONAL CONTRACEPTIVES

Hormonal contraceptives currently in use and/or under study are classified as follows:
A. Oral pills
  ❖ Combined pill
  ❖ Progestogen-only pill (minipill)
  ❖ Postcoital pill
  ❖ Once a month (long acting) pill.
B. Depot (slow-releasing) formulations
  ❖ Injectables
  ❖ Subcutaneous implants
  ❖ Vaginal rings.

Combined Pill

The combination pill is one of the major spacing methods of contraception. Most formulations of the combined pill of the present time contain 30 to 35 µg of synthetic estrogen, and 0.5 to 1.0 mg of progestogen.

The pill is given orally for 21 consecutive days beginning on the 5th day of the menstrual cycle, followed by a break of 7 days of no hormonal intake (seven pills contain no hormones and are inert) during which menstruation occurs. When bleeding occurs, this is considered the first day of the next cycle. The bleeding is not like normal menstruation, but is an episode of uterine bleeding from an incompletely formed endometrium caused by the withdrawal of exogenous hormones. Therefore, it is called "withdrawal bleeding" rather than menstruation. The loss of blood, which occurs, is about half that occurring in a woman having ovulatory cycle. If bleeding does not occur, the woman is instructed to start the second cycle one week after the preceding one. Ordinarily, the woman menstruates after the second course of pill intake.

The pill should be taken every day at a fixed time, preferably before going to bed at night. The first course should be started strictly on the fifth day of the menstrual period, as any deviation in this respect may not prevent pregnancy. If the user forgets to take a pill, she should take it as soon as she remembers, and that she should take the next day's pill at the usual time. If she forgets her pill for two days in a row, she should be advised to continue the daily schedule, but to use an additional contraceptive, such as condom for the remainder of the cycle. Cessation of pill taking at any point prior to completion of the full cycle of pills will result in withdrawal bleeding.

Biphasic and triphasic preparations are two different formulations of the combined pills. In these pills, there are two and three different levels of progestogens respectively during a 21-day cycle of pills followed by 7 days of no hormonal pills. These are prepared to mimic the natural hormonal fluctuations during the menstrual cycle.

Types of Pills

The department of family welfare, in the Ministry of Health and Family Welfare, Government of India has made available two types of low dose oral pills under the brand names of Mala N and Mala D.

Mala N: Norgestrel 0.3 mg, and Ethinyl estradiol 0.03 mg.

Mala D: Norgestrel 0.3 mg, and Ethinyl estradiol 0.03 mg.

Mala D is available in a package of 28 pills (21 of oral contraceptive pills and 7 brown, ferrous fumerate coated tablets at a price of rupees two per packet. Mala N is supplied free of coast through all Primary Health Centers and Urban Family Welfare Centers.

Mode of Action

The probable mechanisms of contraception are:

a. *Inhibition of ovulation*: Both the hormones act synergistically on the hypothalamo-pituitary axis. The release of gonadotropic releasing hormones from the hypothalamus is prevented through a negative feedback mechanism. There is thus no peak release of FSH and LH from the anterior pituitary, so the follicular growth is not initiated.

b. *Production of static endometrial hypoplacia*: There is stromal edema, residual reaction and regression of glands.

c. *Alteration of the character of the cervical mucus*: Thick, viscid and scanty, to prevent sperm penetration.

Contraindications

The contraindications are either absolute or relative.

Absolute

a. Circulatory diseases (past or present).
   - ❖ Arterial or venous thrombosis
   - ❖ Severe hypertension
   - ❖ Vulvular disease, ischemic heart disease, angina
   - ❖ Hyperlipidemia
   - ❖ Focal migraine.

b. Diseases of the liver
   - ❖ Active liver disease
   - ❖ History of cholestatic jaundice in pregnancy
   - ❖ Liver adenoma, carcinoma.

c. Others
   - ❖ Pregnancy
   - ❖ Genital tract bleeding
   - ❖ Breast cancer.

Relative

- ❖ Obesity
- ❖ Varicosities
- ❖ Epilepsy
- ❖ Bronchial asthma
- ❖ Depression, mood fluctuation
- ❖ Age over 35
- ❖ Smoking
- ❖ Nursing mothers who are in the first six months.

Follow-up

The woman should be examined after three months, six months and then once a year. Women above 35 years should be checked more frequently. Any adverse symptoms are to be noted at each visit. Examinations of breasts, weight, blood pressure, pelvic examination including cytology are to be done and compared with the previous records.

Length of Pill Use

For spacing of births, use of 3 to 5 years is considered adequate and safe. However, with careful monitoring, pill use may continue until the age of 40. Beyond 40 years, pills may not be continued because of the risk of cardiovascular complications.

Beneficial Effects

The most important benefit is prevention of unwanted pregnancy (failure rate is 0.1 per 100 women years).

Noncontraceptive Benefits

Relief of:
- ❖ Menorrhagia (less by 50%)
- ❖ Dysmenorrhea (less by 40%)
- ❖ Premenstrual tension syndrome
- ❖ Mittelschmerz syndrome.

Improvement of:
* Iron deficiency anemia
* Endometriosis
* Hirsutism
* Rheumatoid arthritis.

Reduction in risk of:
* Pelvic inflammatory disease
* Benign breast disease
* Fibroid uterus
* Functional ovarian cysts
* Carcinoma of endometrium and ovary
* Osteoporosis.

Adverse Effects

a. Nausea, vomiting, and headache—These are transient and often subside following continuous use.
b. Mastalgia—Heaviness and tenderness of breasts are transient.
c. Weight gain and edema of legs.
d. Cloasma and acne.
e. Menstrual abnormalities—Breakthrough bleeding, hypomenorrhea, menorrhagia, amenorrhea.
f. Reduced libido.
g. Leukorrhea.

Major Complications

a. Depression, change of mood and sleep disturbances.
b. Hypertension (less than 1% of cases).
c. Vascular complications—Venous thrombo-embolism, arterial thrombosis.
d. Cholestatic jaundice (due to stasis of bile).

Effects on Reproduction

* Ovulation returns within three months of withdrawal of the drug in 90 percent of cases.
* Lactation may be affected by a reduction in the milk production.

Progestogen-only Pill (POP)

This pill is commonly referred to as the mini-pill or micropill. It contains only progestogen, which is given in small doses throughout the cycle. The commonly used progestogens are norethisterone (350 µg) and levonogestrel (30 µg).

Mechanism of Action

It works mainly by making cervical mucus thick and viscous, thereby prevents sperm penetration. Endometrium becomes atrophic. In about 2 percent of cases, ovulation is inhibited.

Advantages

a. No adverse effects on lactation and hence, can be suitably given to lactating women and as such is known as lactation pill.
b. It can be given to women having hyper-tension, fibroid, diabetes or epilepsy.

Drawbacks

a. There may be breakthrough bleeding or at times amenorrhea in about 20 to 30 percent of cases.
b. Simple cysts in ovary may be seen.
c. Failure rate is about 0.5 to 2 per HWY.

Postcoital Contraception

Postcoital (or "morning after") contraception is recommended within 48 hours of unprotected intercourse. Two methods are available.

a. IUD, especially a copper device.
b. Hormonal: More often, a hormonal method may be preferable.

The combined oral pill has been generally accepted as the preparation of choice for post-coital contraception, as it is less likely to cause adverse side effects. The method is to give a double dose of the standard combined pill. The recommended regimen is to take two pills immediately, followed by another two pills 12 hours later, if pills containing 50 µg, are used. If pills containing 30 to 35 µg estrogen are available, four of these must taken at one time rather than two in each dose.

Postcoital contraception is advocated as an emergency method, for example, after un-protected intercourse, rape or contraceptive failure. Although the failure rate of postcoital contraception is less than one percent, some experts think, a woman should not use this method unless she intends to have an abortion, if the method fails. Though there is no evidence of fetal abnormalities, some doubts remain regarding this.

Once a Month (Long Acting) Pill

Experiments with once a month pill in which quinestrol, a long acting estrogen is given in combination with a short acting progestrogen, have been disappointing. The pregnancy rate was too high to be acceptable.

DEPOT (SLOW-RELEASING) FORMULATIONS

The need for depot formulations, which are highly effective, reversible, long acting and estrogen free for spacing pregnancies in which a single administration suffices for several months or years led to the development of injectable contraceptives and subdermal implants.

Injectable Contraceptives

There are two types of injectable contraceptives:
a. DMPA (Depot medroxyprogesterone acetate) or Depot provera.
b. Net-En (Norethyisterone Enanthate).
   Both are administered intramuscularly. DMPA is given in a dose of 150 mg every three months or 300 mg every six months. Net-En is given in a dose of 200 mg at two-monthly intervals.

Mechanism of Action
1. Inhibition of ovulation by suppressing the midcycle LH peak.
2. Cervical mucous becomes thick and viscid thereby prevents sperm penetration.
3. Endometrium becomes atrophic preventing blastocyst implantation, if fertilization occurs, which is extremely unlikely.

Advantages
1. It eliminates regular medication as imposed by oral pill.
2. It can be used safely during lactation.
3. No estrogen related side effects.
4. Menstrual symptoms such as menorrhagia and dysmenorrhea are reduced.
5. Protective against endometrial cancer.
6. Can be used as an interim contraception before vasectomy becomes effective.

Fig. 24.6: Subdermal implant—Norplant

Drawbacks
1. Failure rate for DMPA is 0-1 (HWY).
2. There are chances of irregular bleeding and an occasional phase of amenorrhea.
3. Return of fertility after their discontinuation is usually delayed for several months (4–8 months).
4. The preparations are available only in selected centers in India. The potential long-term effects of DMPA and Net-En are not yet known.

Subdermal Implants (Fig. 24.6)

The population council, New York has developed a subdermal implant known as *Norplant* for long-term contraception. It consists of six silastic (silicone rubber) capsules containing 35 mg (each) of levonorgestrel (100). More recent devices comprise fabrication of levonorgestrel into two small rods, *Norplant (R)–2*, which are comparatively easier to insert and remove. It initially releases 80 µg and later on reduced to 30 µg levonorgestrel per day over 5 years.

Norplant capsules measure 34 mm × 24 mm and provide effective contraception for five years.

Insertion
The capsules are inserted subdermally, in the inner aspect of the nondominant arm, 6 to 8 cm above the elbow fold. It is done under local anesthetic. It is ideally inserted on day one of menstrual cycle, immediately after abortion and three weeks after delivery.

Removal
Norplant should be removed within five years of insertion. Loss of contraceptive action is immediate.

Advantages

Advantages are same as with DMPA, and additional ones are:

1. Improvement of anemia due to control of menorrhagia.
2. Suitable for women who have completed their family and do not desire permanent sterilization.

Efficacy is comparable to the combined pills. Failure rate is 0.7 per 100 women years (Newton, 1993).

Disadvantages

1. Frequent irregular, menstrual bleeding, spotting, especially in the first year.
2. Surgical procedure necessary to insert and remove implants.

Implanon

Single implant rod of 4 cm long, containing 60 mg of ketodesogestrel is used. It releases the hormone about 60 µg per day over three years. Use of single rod makes implanon easier for insertion and removal. Efficacy and side effects are the same as that of Norplant.

PERMANENT METHODS (STERILIZATION)

Voluntary sterilization is a well-established contraceptive procedure for couples desiring no more children. Currently female sterilizations account for 85 percent and male sterilizations for 10 to 15 percent of all sterilizations in India (Government of India Yearbook, 1983–1984). Voluntary sterilization is a surgical method whereby the reproductive function of an individual male or female is destroyed purposefully and permanently. The operation done on male is vasectomy and that on female is tubal ligation or tubal occlusion.

Sterilization offers many advantages over other contraceptive methods:

❖ It is a one-time method
❖ It does not require sustained motivation of the user for its effectiveness
❖ It provides the most effective protection against pregnancy
❖ The risk of complications is small if the procedure is performed according to accepted medical standards
❖ It is most cost-effective.

Guidelines for Sterilization

Sterilization services are provided free of charge in government institutions. Guidelines issued by the Government of India covers various aspects of sterilization. These are:

1. The age of husband should not ordinarily be less than 25 years or more than 45 years.
2. The age of wife should not be less than 20 years or more than 45 years.
3. The motivated couple must have two living children at the time of operation.
4. If the couple has three or more living children, the lower limit of age of the husband or wife may be relaxed at the discretion of the operating surgeon.
5. The couple knows that for all practical purposes, the operation is reversible.

Vasectomy or Male Sterilization

It is a permanent sterilization operation done in the male where a segment of vas deferens of both the sides are resected (1 cm) and the cut ends are ligated. The ligated ends are then folded back on them and sutured into position so that the cut ends face away from each other. This will reduce the risk of recanalization later.

Following vasectomy, sperm production and hormone output are not affected. The sperm produced are destroyed intraluminally by phagocytosis. This is a normal process in the male genital tract, but the rate is increased after vasectomy. The vasectomized person is not immediately sterile after operation, usually until approximately thirty ejaculations have taken place, as the semen is stored in the distal part of the vas deferens for about two to three months. During this period, another contraceptive must be used.

Advantages

1. The vasectomy operation is simple and can be performed as an outpatient or outdoor procedure.
2. Complications—Immediate or late, are few.
3. Failure rate is about 0.15 percent and there is a fair chance of success of reversal anastomosis (recanalization) operation (50%).
4. The overall expenditure is minimal in terms of equipment, hospital stay and doctor's

training. Cost wise the ratio is about five vasectomies to one tubal ligation.

Drawbacks

1. Additional contraception is needed for about two to three months following operation, i.e. until the semen becomes free of sperm.
2. Frigidity or impotency when occurs is mostly psychological.

Selection of Candidates

Sexually active and psychologically adjusted husband having the desired number of children is an ideal candidate. Any misconception about the fear of castration, loss of hormones and impotency are to be removed by sympathetic explanation. Eczema or scabes in the scrotal area is a temporary contraindication. In the presence of hydrocele or inguinal hernia, vasectomy can be done only along with the operative correction of these conditions.

Postoperative Advices

1. Antibiotic (injection penidure) is administered as a routine and an analgesic is prescribed.
2. Weight lifting, heavy work and cycling are restricted for about two weeks while usual activities can be performed forthwith.
3. To wear a scrotal support (T-bandage) for 15 days.
4. The patient should report for check-up after one week or earlier, if any complication arises.
5. To have the stitches removed on the fifth day.
6. Additional contraceptive should be used for three months.
7. Semen should be examined once a month and if two consecutive semen analyzes show an absence of spermatozoa, the man is declared sterile. Until then additional contraceptive (condom or DMPA) should be adviced.

Complications

- ❖ Immediate
  1. Wound sepsis, which may lead to scrotal cellulitis or abscess.
  2. Scrotal hematoma.
- ❖ Remote
  1. *Frigidity or impotency*: It is mostly psychological in origin. They may complain of diminution of sexual vigor, impotence, headache or fatigue.
  2. *Sperm granuloma or sperm granules* caused by accumulation of sperm. They appear in 10 to 14 days after the operation. The most frequent symptoms are pain and swelling. The mass is hard and approximate size is 7 mm. The sperm granules eventually subside. This can be prevented by cauterization or fulguration of the cut ends.
  3. *Autoimmune response*: Vasectomy is said to cause an autoimmune response to sperm. Blocking of the vas causes reabsorption of spermatozoa and subsequent development of antibodies against sperm in blood. Normally 2 percent of men have circulating antibodies against their sperm. In vasectomized men, the figure can be as high as 54 percent. Such antibodies are harmless to physical health. It is likely that they can cause a reduction in subsequent fertility despite successful reanastomosis of the vas (Belsky Reymond, 1973).
  4. *Spontaneous recanalization*: The incidence of recanalization is variously placed between 0 to 6 percent. Its occurrence is serious. Therefore, the surgeon should explain the possibility of this complication to every acceptor prior to the operation and have written consent acknowledging this fact. Regular follow-up for up to three years is recommended to avoid this possibility.

No-scalpel Vasectomy (Figs 24.7 and 24.8)

No-scalpel vasectomy is a new technique that is safe, convenient and acceptable to males. This new method is now being canvassed for men as a special project, on a voluntary basis under the family welfare program. This method, which is popular in China, is performed under local anesthetic. Stretched skin over the vas is punctured with one blade of a sharp pointed dissecting scissors, instead of using a scalpel. Then the hole is increased and the vas is dissected out by using the tip of the scissors. The testicular end is dropped back into the scrotum and the upper end is cauterized. The

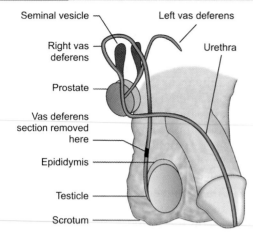

Fig. 24.7: Vasectomy operation showing the site of vasectomy

Fig. 24.8: A post vasectomy scrotum showing the incision site *(For color version see Plate 2)*

procedure is repeaked for the second vas through the same incision. The rest of the steps are same as for the regular vasectomy procedure.

Open-ended Vasectomy

The abdominal end of the resected vas is coagulated. The testicular end is left open. This will prevent congestive epididymitis.

Female Sterilization

Occlusion of the fallopian tubes in some form is the underlying principle to achieve female sterilization. It is the most popular method of terminal contraception, specially adopted in the developing countries, where high parity births prevail in a comparatively younger age group. It is also widely accepted in the affluent countries.

Female sterilization also known as *tubal ligation* or *tubectomy* is a surgical procedure in which the fallopian tubes are severed and sealed or "pinched shut" in order to prevent fertilization. It is a highly effective, safe and simple procedure that involves cutting, tying or removing a part of the fallopian tubes. Consequently the passage of eggs from the ovaries to the uterus is blocked, and sperm will not be able to reach the eggs. The eggs released from the ovaries after tubal ligation break and get absorbed harmlessly by the body. Tubal ligation is preformed in a hospital as inpatient or outpatient procedure under general or regional anesthesia, using various techniques.

Methods of Tubal Ligation

a. *Occlusion method*: Occlusion methods for tubal ligation are typically carried out on the isthmic position of the fallopian tube that is the thin portion of the tube closest to the uterus.
   ❖ *Partial salpingectomy*: The Pomeroy technique is widely use for achieving partial salpingectomy. This method involves tying a small loop of the tube by suture and cutting off the top segment of the loop. This can be done via laparoscopy or laparotomy (Fig. 24.9).
   ❖ *Clips*: Clips clamp the tube and inhibit blood flow to that portion causing a small amount of scarring or fibrosis, in turn preventing fertilization. The most commonly used clips are *Filshie clip*

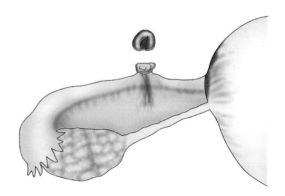

Fig. 24.9: Partial salpingectomy, Pomeroy method

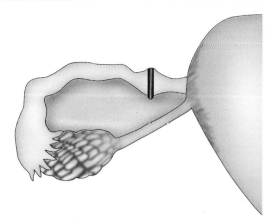

Fig. 24.10: Hulka clip on fallopian tube

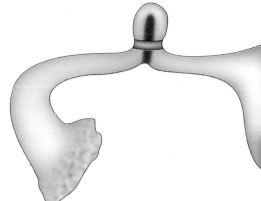

Fig. 24.11: Falope ring on fallopian tube

made of titanium and the *Hulka clip* or *Wolf clip* made of stainless steel and spring loaded. Clips are simple to insert, but require a special instrument to put it in place (Fig. 24.10).

The clip is introduced into the abdominal cavity via laparoscopic clip applicator. It is placed across the fallopian tube and when closed, a small spring holds it firmly. The Hulka clip has the advantage of damaging only a very small portion of the fallopian tube–approximately 7 mm. The squeezed portion is deprived of its blood supply and eventually undergoes a vascular necrosis.

❖ *Falope rings*: Tubal rings are similar to clips and they are used to block the tube mechanically. When placed, it encircles a small loop of the fallopian tube, blocking the blood supply to that small loop, resulting in scarring that blocks passage of sperm or egg. A commonly used type of ring is the *Yoon ring* made of silicone. The procedure is performed by inserting a laparoscope just under the umbilicus. After identifying the fallopian tube, the device with the ring is slid over 2–3 cm "knuckle" of tube that is kinked off by the ring. This is done once for each side (Fig. 24.11).

❖ *Electrocoagulation or cauterization*: Electric current is used to coagulate or burn a small portion of each fallopian tube. It mostly uses bipolar coagulation, where electric current enters and leaves through two ends of a forceps applied to the tubes. The procedure is usually done via laparoscopy.

b. Method of tubal ligation by entry sites or routes.

1. Laparotomy method:

❖ *Pomeroy method*: An occlusion type procedure in which a part of the fallopian tube on each side is elevated to create a loop or knuckle. An absorbable suture is tied around the base of the elevated segment and the segment is severed (same as shown in Figure 24.9).

In modified Pomeroy method, a silk stitch is applied medial to the tubal stump after the conventional steps. Pomeroy method is usually performed after delivery by cesarean section.

❖ *Irving tubal ligation*: In this procedure two ligatures are placed around the tube in its proximal to mid segment and a tubal segment between the two ligatures is removed. The tied end of the tube attached to the uterus is then sutured into the back side of uterus and the other end is buried in the connective tissue underlying the fallopian tube. This method keeps the two cut ends of the tubes healthy, should reversal microsurgery become a need.

❖ *Uchida method*: The fallopian tube is dissected at the midpoint and the proximal end is ligated and allowed to drop back into a sac that has been created in the serosa. The distal end is tied and left to project into the abdominal cavity. This method has been abandoned as it was associated with higher failure rates. Earlier techniques that used fimbriectomy were also abandoned.

2. *Laparoscopic tubal ligation*: The procedure is done under general or regional anesthesia. The surgeon makes an incision of about 1½ inches just inside the naval. The laparoscope (a fine tube that conducts light connected to a telescope) is inserted through the opening. The instrument for blocking the tube is then introduced through another opening on the side. Application of clips, rings or cauterization is then performed.

3. *Minilaparotomy*: This procedure is done under general anesthesia and involves making a small incision just above the pubic hairline. The surgeon lifts the fallopian tubes through the incision and blocks them using electrocoagulation, clips or rings. This method differs from laparoscopy that no visualizing instrument is inserted.

This method is recommended for women for whom laparoscopy is contraindicated such as those who had previous abdominal surgery for other reasons, recent or chronic tubal infections or serious heart or respiratory illness.

4. *Vaginal tubal ligation (Colpotomy)*: This procedure is done for women who cannot have a laparoscopy or laparotomy. This involved making a small incision in the vaginal wall through which the surgeon can draw the tubes and ligate them using suture material.

The procedure can be performed under local anesthesia and there will be no visible scar. However, the woman is more susceptible to infection because of high bacterial count in vagina. Some women find sexual intercourse painful for several months after surgery.

Timing for Tubal Ligation

1. *Postpartum or puerperal tubal ligation*: This procedure is basically a minilaparotomy done following childbirth. It is done through a small incision just below the umbilicus. Ths operation may be performed any time within the first three days of childbirth.

2. *Cesarean ligation*: The procedure is done, following cesarean childbirth for women who have completed their families.

3. *Interval tubal ligation*: The operation is done beyong three months following delivery or abortion. The ideal time of procedure is following the menstrual period in the proliferative phase.

4. *Concurrent with MTP*: Sterilization is done along with termination of pregnancy.

Advantages of Female Sterilization

❖ Very effective as a method of contraception
❖ Gives permanent or lifelong protection
❖ Nothing to remember, no supplies needed and no repeated clinic visits required
❖ No interference with sex
❖ No known long-term side effects or health risks.

Disadvantages or Possible Problems

❖ Pain for few days after surgery
❖ Infection or bleeding at the incision site
❖ Injury to internal organs
❖ Anesthetic risks:
  − Allergic reaction or overdose of local anesthesia or sedation.
  − Delayed recovery and side effects of general anesthesia.
❖ Reversal surgery is difficult and expensive.

Failure Rate

The overall failure rate for tubal ligation is about 0.7 percent, the Pomeroy technique being the lowest 0.1 to 0.3 percent.

Mortality rate following tubal ligation is estimated to be 72 per 100,000 for all methods. Laparoscopic procedures carried a mortality rate of 5 to 10 per 100,000 compared to 7 per 100,000 for puerperal ligations (ICMR, 1982).

POSTCONCEPTION METHODS OF BIRTH CONTROL (TERMINATION OF PREGNANCY)

Menstrual Regulation

Menstrual regulation is a relatively simple method of birth control. It consists of aspiration of the uterine contents 6 to 14 days of a missed period, but before most pregnancy tests can accurately determine whether a woman is pregnant (Robinson, 1975). Cervical dilatation is indicated only in nullipara or in apprehensive subjects. No after-care is necessary as a rule.

The immediate complications are uterine trauma and perforation. Late complications (after six weeks) include a tendency to abortion or premature labor (if the aspiration was not successful), infertility, menstrual disorders and an increase in ectopic pregnancies. Menstrual regulation differs from abortion in three respects:

* The lack of certainty if a pregnancy is being terminated
* The lack of legal restrictions
* Increased safety as the procedure is done early in pregnancy.

Menstrual Induction

This is based on disturbing the normal progesterone prostaglandin balance by intrauterine application of 1 to 5 mg solution (or 2.5–5 mg pellet) of prostaglandin F_2. Within a few minutes of the prostaglandin impact, performed under sedation, the uterus responds with a sustained contraction lasting about seven minutes, followed by cyclic contractions continuing for 3 to 4 hours. The bleeding starts and continues for 7 to 8 days (Robinson, 1975).

Abortion

Abortion is defined as termination of pregnancy before the fetus becomes viable (capable of living independently). This has been fixed administratively at 28 weeks, when the fetus weighs approximately 1,000 gm. Abortion is sought by women for a variety of reasons including birth control.

Abortions usually are categorized as *spontaneous and induced*.

Spontaneous abortions occur once in every 15 pregnancies (Vlugt et al, 1973). They may be considered "Nature's method of birth control" (Park, 2000).

Induced abortions are deliberately induced—They may be legal or illegal. Illegal abortions are usually the last resort of women determined to end their pregnancies at the risk of their own lives.

In India, about six million abortions take place every year of which four million are induced and two million spontaneous.

Abortion Hazards

Abortions, whether spontaneous or induced, whether in the hands of skilled or unskilled persons are usually fraught with hazards, resulting in maternal morbidity and mortality. The mortality ratio ranges from 1 to 3.5 per 100,000 in developed countries (WHO technical report, 1978). In India, mortality is reported to be 7.8 per 1,000 "random abortions" (Lahiri and Konar, 1976). This is because most of the random abortions are illegally induced.

The early complications of abortion include: hemorrhage, shock, sepsis, uterine perforation, cervical injury, thromboembolism and anesthetic and psychiatric complications.

The late complications include infertility, ectopic gestation, increased risk of spontaneous abortion and reduced birth weight of newborns. The optimum time for termination of pregnancy is the seventh and eighth weeks of gestation. Studies indicate that the risk of death is seven times higher for women who wait until the second trimester to terminate pregnancy. The Indian law (MTP Act, 1971) allows abortion only up to twenty weeks of pregnancy.

The Medical Termination of Pregnancy Act is a health care measure, which helps to reduce maternal morbidity and mortality resulting from illegal abortions. It also affords an opportunity for motivating such women to adopt some form of contraception.

Although abortion has been greatly liberalized, the annual number of legal abortions are about 0.6 million, which contribute hardly ten percent of the abortions done in the country (Park, 2000). The numerous abortion hazards, which are inherent, should serve as a warning that abortions even under the best of circumstances can never be as safe as efficient contraception.

BIBLIOGRAPHY

1. Bounds W. Contraceptive efficacy if the diaphragm and cervical caps are used in conjunction with spermicides-A fresh look at the evidence". British Journal of Family Planning 1994;20:84-7.
2. Calderone MS. Manual of Contraceptive Practice. Williams and Wilkins, Baltimore, 1964.
3. Dutta DC. Textbook of Obstetrics 5th edn. Calcutta: New Central Book Company, 2001.
4. Ford N, Mathie E. The acceptability and experience of the female condom, British Journal of Family Planning. 1993;19:187-92.
5. Franey J. Family Planning. In: Bennett RV, Linda KB (Eds). Myles Textbook for Midwives, 13th edn. Edinburgh: Churchill Livingstone, 1999.
6. Government of India, Yearbook-Family Welfare Program in India. New Delhi: Ministry of Health 1983-1984.
7. Guilleband J. Combined hormonal contraception. In: Londen N, Glasier A, Gebbie A. Handbook of Family Planning and Reproductive Health Care 3rd edn. Edinburgh: Churchill Livingstone, 1995.
8. Hawkins DF, Elder MC. Human Fertility Control: Theory and Practice London: Butterworth, 1979.
9. Huchings JE, et al. International Family Planning Perspectives 1985;11(3):77-85.
10. ICMR Bulletin 1983.
11. Lahiri D, Conar M. Journal of Indian Medical Association 1976;66:288.
12. Liskin L. Intrauterine Devices. The John Hopkins University, Population Report Series B:4, 1980.
13. Park K. Park's Textbook of Preventive and Social Medicine, 16th edn. Jabalpur; Banarasidas Banot Publishers 2000.
14. Vlugt T. et al. Pregnancy Termination. The George Washington University Population Report Series F: 1973.
15. WHO. Global Health Situations and Projections, 1992.

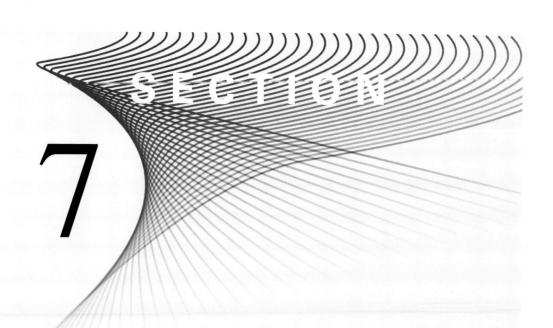

Abnormalities of Pregnancy, Labor and Puerperium

25

Abnormalities of Early Pregnancy

Learning Objectives

Upon completing this chapter, the learner will be able to:
- ❖ Discuss the types of spontaneous and induced abortions, and the medical and nursing management of patients
- ❖ Describe the varieties of ectopic gestation, their presentation, outcome and management
- ❖ Enumerate the pathology, clinical presentation and treatment of hydatidiform mole in pregnancy
- ❖ Discuss the clinical presentation and management of clients who suffer hyperemesis in pregnancy
- ❖ Describe ABO and Rh disease and retroversion.

CLASSIFICATION OF ABORTION

The classification of abortion is given in Flow chart 25.1.

ABORTION

Any bleeding in pregnancy is abnormal. Vaginal blood loss in early pregnancy should be thought of as a threatened miscarriage until shown otherwise. The term miscarriage and spontaneous abortion are synonymous.

DEFINITION

Abortion is the process of partial or complete separation of the products of conception from the uterine wall with or without partial or complete expulsion from the uterine cavity before the age of viability.

The age of viability is 28 weeks in India. Abortions are usually categorized as spontaneous and induced.

Flow chart 25.1: Classification of abortion

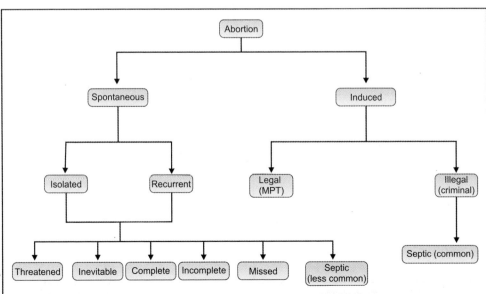

SPONTANEOUS ABORTION

Spontaneous abortion is defined as the involuntary loss of the products of conception prior to 28 weeks of gestation, when the fetus weights approximately 1,000 gm or less.

Spontaneous abortions occur once in every 15 pregnancies (Park, 2000). In India it has been computed that about 6 million abortions take place, every year of which 2 million are spontaneous and the 4 million are induced.

Causes

The causes of spontaneous abortion in most cases are not known. Where a cause is determined, 50 percent of miscarriages are due to chromosomal abnormalities of the conceptus. Genetic and structural causes are also attributed to pregnancy loss. Maternal causes are:

❖ Structural abnormalities of the genital organs such as retroversion of uterus, bicornate uterus and fibroids
❖ Infections such as rubella and chlamydia
❖ Medical conditions such as diabetes, renal disease and thyroid dysfunction, when not well-controlled.

Types of Spontaneous Abortions
Threatened Abortion (Fig. 25.1)

It is an abortion characterized by vaginal bleeding with or without recognizable uterine contractions. The blood loss may be scanty with or without accompanying backache and cramp-like pain. The pain may resemble dysmenorrhea or period pains. The cervix remains closed and the uterus soft with no tenderness when palpated.

The outcome of a threatened abortion could be either stoppage of bleeding and continuance of pregnancy to term or continuance of bleeding and uterine contractions to expel the products of conception.

Management: General and systemic examination may reveal the cause of threatened abortion. Investigations include hemoglobin, ABO grouping and Rh, VDRL, urine routine and blood glucose. Thyroid function tests are done if thyroid dysfunction is suspected. Plasma progesterone estimation is done if corpus luteum insufficiency is suspected. The patient is admitted and given complete rest in bed. If any specific cause is found, it is treated accordingly. If pregnancy continues, the possibility of intrauterine growth retardation, due to poor placental function must be considered. There is also an increased risk of preterm labor.

Inevitable Abortion (Fig. 25.2)

The woman presents with bleeding, often heavy, with clots or products of conception. Blood loss may be heavy and the mother in a shocked state. The cervix is dilated and on examination, products may be seen in the vagina or pro-

Fig. 25.1: Threatened abortion

Fig. 25.2: Inevitable abortion

truding through the os. The uterus if palpable may be smaller than expected.

Management: Blood loss may be controlled by administering injection syntocinon or ergometrine.

The pain may be intense and appropriate analgesics are prescribed.

The woman and her family must be given information and reassurance.

Incomplete Abortion (Fig. 25.3)

In this type of abortion, remnants of placenta remain within the uterine cavity, contributing to heavy and profuse bleeding. Intravenous or intramuscular ergometrine is given to control bleeding. Evacuation of the uterus to remove any retained tissue should be done under general anesthesia, when the mother is in a stable condition. Incomplete miscarriage is a cause of maternal mortality.

Complete Abortion (Fig. 25.4)

The conceptus, placenta and membranes are expelled completely from the uterus. The pain stops. Signs of pregnancy will regress. The uterus on palpation is contracted. No further medical intervention is required.

Missed Abortion

In missed abortion, the embryo dies despite the presence of a viable placenta and the sac is retained. Death of the embryo occurs before 8

Fig. 25.4: Complete abortion

weeks of gestation but the mother's body fails to recognize the demise.

A brown discharge from the degeneration of placental tissue may present and threatened miscarriage is suspected. There may be a regression of signs and symptoms of pregnancy. Often there is failure to gain weight. The uterus is smaller than expected for the period of amenorrhea, firm rather than soft in consistency.

Thromboplastin may be liberated from the placental bed into the maternal circulation causing disseminated intravascular coagulation (DIC) usually about five weeks after fetal death.

Ultrasonography will show smaller than expected uterus with distorted or broken sac and an absence of fetal heart movements.

A coagulation profile is done because of the risk of hypofibrinogenemia. Treatment of a missed abortion of first trimester is evacuation of the uterus by dilatation and curettage. In the second semester, it is achieved by administration of prostaglandins intramuscularly.

Habitual Abortion

It is an occurrence of spontaneous abortions in three or more successive pregnancies. Usually abortions occur at the same gestational age. Cervical incompetence occurs when painless dilatation of the cervix occurs as pregnancy progresses, allowing the membranes to bulge through the cervical os into the vagina. As the intrauterine pressure increases, the membranes may rupture, resulting in miscarriage.

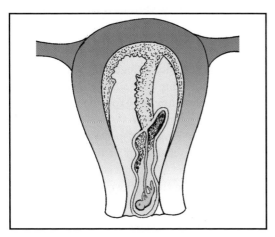

Fig. 25.3: Incomplete abortion

Abortions due to incompetent os, usually occurs after 16 weeks.

Causes of incompetence are uncertain. Genetic causes, endocrine factors and immunological factors are thought as possible causes.

Treatment
* The patient is given complete bed rest from before the time of occurrence of the earliest abortion to after the time of occurrence of the latest abortion
* Specific treatment is given for any cause identified
* Cervical circlage at 14 weeks gestation by Shirodkar's or McDonald's method; Nonabsorbable suture is inserted at the level of the cervical os. This remains *in situ* until 38 weeks or the onset of labor, when it is removed.

INDUCED ABORTION

This is deliberate interruption of an intact pregnancy. Induced abortions are performed legally in India since the Medical Termination Pregnancy (MTP) Act of 1971 (revised in 1975).

Medical Termination of Pregnancy (Legal Abortion)

It is the deliberate induction of abortion prior to 20 weeks gestation by a registered medical practitioner in the interest of mother's health and life.

Provisions for MTP Under the MTP Act
* The continuation of pregnancy would involve serious risk of life or grave injury to the physical and mental health of the pregnant woman
* There is substantial risk of the child being born with serious physical and mental abnormalities so as to be handicapped in life
* The pregnancy is the result of rape
* The pregnancy is caused as a result of failure of contraceptive
* Where there are actual or reasonably foreseeable environments (social or economic), which could lead to risk or injury to the health of the mother.

Indications for MTP
Therapeutic
* Deteriorating health due to pulmonary tuberculosis
* Cardiac diseases grade III and IV with history of decompensation
* Chronic glomerulonephritis
* Malignant hypertension
* Intractable hyperemesis gravidarum
* Cervical or breast malignancy
* Diabetes mellitus with retinopathy
* Psychiatric illness.

Social indications
* Parous women having unplanned pregnancy with low socioeconomic status
* Pregnancy caused by rape
* Pregnancy due to failure of contraceptive.

Eugenic indications
* Risk of baby being born with various physical and mental abnormalities and include:
  - Inherited chromosomal and gene disorders
  - Exposure to teratogenic drugs or radiation
  - Rubella infection in first trimester
  - One or both parents being mentally defective
  - Congenital malformations for siblings.

Consultation with geneticists will be required prior to deciding on MTP.

Conditions to be Met Prior to the Procedure

1. The act provides safeguards to the mother by authorizing only a registered medical practitioner having experience in gynecology and obstetrics to perform abortion where the length of pregnancy does not exceed 12 weeks. In order to terminate pregnancies, which exceed 12 weeks and are not more than 20 weeks the opinion of two registered medical practitioners is necessary.

2. The procedure can only be performed in hospitals established or maintained by the government or places approved by the government for this purpose.
3. A pregnancy can be terminated only with the written consent of the woman.
4. Pregnancy in a minor (below the age of 18 years) or lunatic can only be terminated with the written consent of parents or legal guardians.
5. The procedure has to be reported to the Directorate of Health Services of the state.

Methods of Termination in the First Trimester

❖ Menstrual regulation
❖ Suction evacuation and curettage
❖ Dilatation and evacuation
❖ Pharmacological methods.

Menstrual regulation: This is aspiration of uterine cavity and extraction of endometrium within 14 days of the missed period, when the presence of an early pregnancy is suspected. The procedure is performed by introducing a 4 to 5 mm flexible plastic canula into the uterine cavity and sucking out the endometrium with a 50 ml plastic syringe attached to it. Menstrual regulation is done as an outpatient procedure.

Suction evacuation and curettage: This is a procedure in which the products of conception are sucked out from the uterus with the help of a canula attached to a suction apparatus. The cervix is dilated with small metal dilators and a suction canula introduced into the uterine cavity. With the canula fitted to a suction machine, the products of conception are sucked out. With a small flushing curette, the uterine cavity is curetted and suctioned out once again for any remaining portion of the conceptus. A dose of methergine is administered intravenously to control bleeding.

Dilatation and evacuation: This is done either as a two-stage procedure (slow method) or a one-stage procedure (rapid method). For the two-stage method, slow dilatation of the cervix is achieved by introducing Laminaria tents or synthetic dilators like dilapan into the cervical canal. The woman is kept in bed for 12 hours during which time the tents swell up due to its hygroscopic property dilating the cervix. In the second stage of the procedure (after 12 hours), the tents are removed and cervix further dilated with metal dilators up to the desired extent for introduction of an ovum forceps. The products of conception are then removed and curetted with a flushing curette. Prophylactic antibiotic and methergine are administered.

For the one-stage procedure, cervical dilatation with metal dilators followed by evacuation is done at one stage. The steps of the procedure are similar to those followed in the second phase of the two-stage procedure.

Pharmacological Methods
Mifepristone (RU 486)

This is a progesterone antagonist used for termination of pregnancy up to 9 weeks. A single dose of 600 mg is given orally and abortion is likely to occur in about 36 hours. If it fails, prostaglandin E_1 methylester pessary (1 mg) is introduced vaginally to complete the abortion process. Abortion occurs within 4 hours.

Methotrexate: Termination with methotrexate has been used effectively up to 8 weeks of pregnancy. A single dose of methotrexate is given intramuscularly followed by application of prostaglandin E_1 analog (misoprostol) vaginally. The products of conception are usually expelled in 3 to 4 hours.

Second Trimester Terminations
(up to 20 weeks)

❖ Intrauterine instillation
❖ Extrauterine instillation
❖ Prostaglandins and oxytocin
❖ Hysterotomy.

Intrauterine instillation of hypertonic saline either as intra-amniotic or extra-amniotic instillation

❖ *Intra-amniotic instillation:* Hypertonic saline (20%) is instilled through a polythene tube connected to a drip set into the amniotic cavity. An amount of 10 ml multiplied by the number of weeks gestation is infused at a rate of 10 ml per minute. Uterine contraction and expulsion of the products of conception occurs in about 32 hours. Hypertonic urea (40%) with syntocinon or prostaglandin is also used for intra-amniotic instillation.

❖ *Extrauterine instillation:* This is done by instillation of ethacridine lactate 0.1 percent solution vaginally about 10 cm above the internal os. Presence of the solution between the membranes and myometrium results in stripping of the membranes and dilatation of the cervix by the catheter (No. 16 Foley's) in about 4 hours. Expulsion of the products of conception follows.

❖ *Prostaglandins:* Prostaglandins are used in women for whom hypertonic saline is contraindicated. Vaginal, intramuscular, extra-amniotic and intra-amniotic methods are used for termination of pregnancy in the second trimester.

❖ *Oxytocin:* Oxytocin is administered intravenously in conjunction with chemical agents used intra-amniotically or extra-amniotically, to augment the abortion process.

❖ *Hysterotomy:* Hysterotomy is used as a method of termination of mid trimester pregnancy where other methods of termination have failed or are contraindicated. The products of conception are extracted out of the uterus by cutting through the anterior wall of the uterus.

Septic Abortion

It is an abortion characterized by infection of the products of conception and the uterus. This condition is most commonly a complication of induced or incomplete abortion. Illegal abortions carried out in nonsterile conditions often lead to septic abortion.

Causes

❖ Criminal abortion which is inexpert attempts at termination of pregnancy by passing sticks, catheters, pastes or soap solution into the uterine cavity
❖ Inevitable abortion with infection
❖ Medical termination of pregnancy with infection.

Clinical Manifestations

The patient may present with pyrexia (fever with chills), headache, nausea and foul smelling discharge per vagina. There is tenderness in the lower abdomen.

Examination may reveal localized infection in the uterine cavity and tubes, adnexal masses and pelvic abscess or generalized septicemia with peritonitis. They may even present with signs of septic shock and gas gangrene of the uterus. Blood culture and vaginal swabs should be taken to identify the cause of infection. Ultrasonography may be done for evaluation of adnexal masses.

Treatment

Intravenous antibiotics commencing with a broad-spectrum antibiotic and one effective against anaerobic infection are given. Pelvic abscess if present will be drained. When adequate blood levels of antibiotics have been reached, uterine evacuation by gentle curettage is done. Heparinization is done to prevent intravascular coagulation and in certain cases, an exchange transfusion is given to remove damaged red blood cells.

NURSES' ROLE WITH PATIENTS UNDERGOING ABORTION

All women have an emotional response to learning or having confirmed that they are pregnant. For some it is a very happy news, perhaps a much desired and planned-for-event; for some others the news has all the events of a catastrophe; for still others the response is that of not caring one way or the other. For all women, it requires a number of adjustments. The first trimester is the period of adjustment.

For a woman in the first category who desired having a baby, symptoms of miscarriage or termination of pregnancy brings lot of anxiety and grief. She may express feelings of inadequacies and failure and even blame herself for the loss of her baby. She is incapable of bearing children. Some parents may want to see and hold the baby.

Midwives need to support the mother and her family at the time when they are grieving for their lost baby. Parents must be helped to meet their wishes. Depending on the type of abortion, they need advice regarding follow-up and future pregnancies.

The legalization of abortion means that every woman, upon being diagnosed as pregnant, now has a choice as to whether or not to carry the pregnancy to its natural conclusion. The woman's decision to have an abortion or to terminate her pregnancy is not lightly made. In many cases, she may approach the nurse for counsel, information and advice prior to the procedure. A calm and relaxed atmosphere and psychological support are import to the client during the procedure.

Women who undergo MTP as an inpatient procedure require close monitoring, support and care during therapy and as they develop uterine contractions and expel the products of conception.

It is important that all women going home after an abortion be aware of possible complications. Vaginal bleeding will continue for 1 to 3 weeks, but if it becomes heavier than a menstrual period, or if the patient passes large clots with bleeding, she should consult the physician, she should also seek medical advice if she develops fever, persistent pain or burning on micturition. The first menses usually occurs 2 to 8 weeks after the abortion. The menses may be heavier or less in quantity and may be either of a longer or shorter duration.

If lactation begins, it is usually mild and lasts less than 48 hours if the breasts are not stimulated. Using a tight brassiere or binding the breasts and using an ice bag will ease the discomfort until the engorgement decreases.

Normal physical activity can be resumed as early as desired. Increased fatigue is often noted for a few days. Tub baths or immersion baths should be avoided for at least one week.

Follow-up visits must be made in 2 to 4 weeks after abortion. It is important for the patient to have this examination to ensure that the reproductive organs have returned to the prepregnancy state.

At some time during the abortion experience, the nurse should introduce the subject of family planning if she has not already requested for information. Counseling on contraception is of importance to those women who are or have been faced with the reality of an unwanted pregnancy.

NURSING PROCESS FOR CLIENTS WITH ABORTION

Assessment

Assess for the following manifestations:
* Vaginal bleeding, spotting, clots
* Low abdominal cramping
* Passing of tissue through the vagina
* Shock-decreased blood pressure, increased pulse rate
* Woman may verbalize fear, disappointment or feelings of guilt.

Analysis/Nursing Diagnosis

* Risk for fetal injury
* Risk for infection
* Ineffective airway clearance
* Actual/risk for aspiration
* Anxiety
* Anticipatory grieving
* Altered family processes
* Actual/risk for altered parenting
* Health seeking behavior.

Planning

* Provide information regarding treatment plan
* Provide support and reassurance regarding nursing care
* Promote maternal physical well-being
* Provide opportunities for counseling and support
* Provide teaching related to self-care.

Implementation

* Observe for vaginal bleeding and cramping
* Save expelled tissue and clot for examination
* Monitor vital signs every 5 minutes to 4 hours depending on maternal status
* Maintain woman on bed rest
* Observe for signs of shock, and institute treatment measures
* Prepare for dilatation and curettage if appropriate
* Provide support, but avoid offering false assurance.

Evaluation

Ensure that the woman:
❖ Is free from anemia and/or infection
❖ Is free from vaginal bleeding
❖ Returns to normal physiological status following the abortion
❖ Verbalizes feelings regarding the event and the outcome as does her significant other/spouse
❖ Understands self-care measures.

ECTOPIC PREGNANCY/ECTOPIC GESTATION

An ectopic pregnancy is one where implantation occurs at a site other than the uterine cavity. Sites can be in the uterine tube, ovary, cervix and the abdomen (Fig. 25.5).

About 1 percent of all pregnancies are ectopic and the life-threatening outcome of this condition calls for appropriate treatment for the mother.

Tubal Pregnancy

Tubal pregnancy develops when the transport of the fertilized ovum into the uterine cavity is interfered with. Implantation can occur at any point along the tube, although the ampulla is the common site. The isthmus is next in frequency, and the interstitial portion least common.

Causes of Tubal Pregnancy

Any alteration of the normal function of the uterine tube in transporting the gametes contributes to the risk of tubal pregnancy.

❖ Congenital abnormalities of the tube such as hypoplacia, undue tortuosity and tubal diverticula
❖ Previous infection such as postabortal sepsis, puerperal sepsis, gonorrhea and tuberculosis.

This may alter the ciliated lining, or the peristaltic action of the tube. Infection can also leave adhesions both inside and surrounding the tube restricting normal function.

❖ Surgery on the uterine tube—Reconstructive surgery for infertility or reversal of tubal ligation
❖ Use of intrauterine contraceptive devices— These devices protect from intrauterine pregnancy but not from tubal pregnancy
❖ Assisted reproductive techniques like *in vitro* fertilization and embryo transfer— The transferred embryo may get injected into the tube
❖ Induction of ovulation with gonadotrophic hormones
❖ Endometriosis.

Physiology of Tubal Pregnancy

In tubal pregnancy, the blastocyst erodes the epithelium and attaches itself to the muscle layer. It grows and expands within the wall, distending the tube. Maternal vessels are exposed and the pressure caused by the resultant blood flow can destroy the embryo. The uterus enlarges in size and in the body, changes associated pregnancy occur under the influence of hormones.

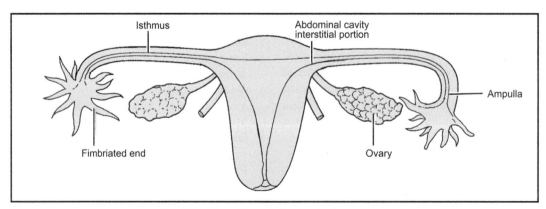

Fig. 25.5: Sites of implantation in ectopic pregnancy

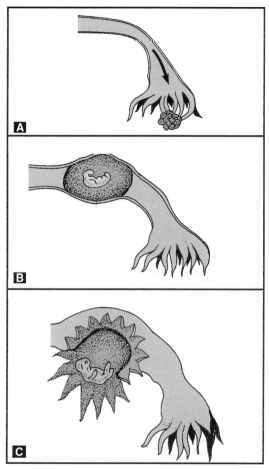

Figs 25.6A to C: Possible outcomes of tubal pregnancy: (A) Tubal abortion; (B) Tubal mole; (C) Tubal rupture

Outcomes of Tubal Pregnancy (Figs 25.6A to C)

The result of a tubal ectopic gestation may be any of the following:

❖ *Tubal abortion:* A pregnancy in the infundibulum or ampulla of the tube may be aborted into the pelvic peritoneal cavity through the fimbriated end of the tube.

❖ *Tubal mole*: Bleeding around the embryo from the site of implantation causes death of the embryo and formation of layers of organized blood clots distending the tube. The mole may need to be removed.

❖ *Tubal rupture*: The tubal wall is distended by the pregnancy and penetrated by the trophoblast to such an extent that it ruptures.

❖ *Pelvic hematocele*: A considerable collection of blood forms in the pouch of Douglas or the uterovesical pouch. Initially, it is fluid, later forms as a mass. Finally, it becomes firm as it gets absorbed

❖ *Secondary abdominal ectopic pregnancy*: If the embryo is implanted on the pelvic peritoneum after expulsion from the ruptured tube, a secondary abdominal ectopic pregnancy develops.

Clinical Presentation

Amenorrhea is present in 75 to 95 percent of pregnancies. In the remaining cases, ectopic pregnancy ruptures before the woman misses a period. The woman may give the history of some vaginal spotting.

Acute lower abdominal pain, often localized in nature is present. This may be sharp and stabbing type, the mother may have dizziness, nausea and shoulder pain indicative of bleeding into the perineal cavity.

The woman will have severe pallor, rapid and thready pulse, tachypnea and low blood pressure. Abdominal examination will show lower abdominal tenderness, rebound tenderness, guarding and shifting dullness due to hemoperitoneum. Pelvic examination will show tenderness on transverse cervical movements, lateral forniceal tenderness, adnexal mass and vascular pulsations on the side of the ectopic pregnancy. Ultrasound examination enables an accurate diagnosis.

Treatment

The patient is resuscitated if she presents with an acute rupture. An exploratory laparotomy is carried-out under controlled general anesthesia. The ruptured tube is removed by salpingotomy or salpingostomy may be done. If the tubal pregnancy is in the process of tubal abortion, the process is completed by suction of the ectopic pregnancy through the fimbriated end. The mother should be offered follow-up support and information regarding subsequent pregnancies. As with any loss during pregnancy, the client will need to grieve and the midwife must offer needed psychological support.

Abdominal Pregnancy

Abdominal pregnancy is rare. A primary abdominal ectopic pregnancy is the result of implantation of the fertilized ovum on the peritoneal surface. A secondary abdominal pregnancy forms when an embryo extruded through rupture or abortion of a tubal pregnancy. The embryo does not die because of its chorionic attachments to the uterine tube and grows by forming attachments to the pelvic peritoneum, omentum, intestines, etc. The fetus grows in the peritoneal cavity but the majority of these pregnancies do not survive. If the fetus dies early in pregnancy, it may be reabsorbed or calcification occurs.

If pregnancy continues, the woman complains of persistent lower abdominal pain, nausea, vomiting, constipation, diarrhea, distension and urinary frequency. There may be vaginal spotting or hemorrhage. Fetal movements are painful. On abdominal examination, there is tenderness and superficiality of fetal parts. Abnormal fetal lie and loud fetal heart sounds. Ultrasonography confirms the diagnosis.

Delivery is by laparotomy. Separation of placenta may be followed by major hemorrhage. If the placenta is attached to the intestines, it may be left *in situ*. When the placenta is left inside, the risk of infection is high but is considered a safer option. Fetal mortality is very high. The fetus is growth retarded and deformed in 20 to 40 percent of cases due to oligohydramnios. The fetus usually dies when the membranes rupture or in the immediate neonatal period from respiratory distress.

Cervical Pregnancy

Cervical pregnancy occurs due to implantation in the cervical canal. It may be due to rapid passage of the fertilized ovum or fertilization of the ovum after it reaches the cervical canal. It is rare and seldom lasts beyond the 20th week. Signs and symptoms include the following:

❖ Painless bleeding soon after the time of implantation
❖ Palpation of the cervical mass with distention and thinning of the cervical wall
❖ Partial dilatation of the external os and a slightly enlarged uterine fundus.

The treatment is removal of the products of conception by curettage and packing of the cervical canal or total abdominal hysterectomy.

NURSING PROCESS FOR CLIENTS WITH ECTOPIC PREGNANCY

Assessment

Assess for the following clinical manifestations:
❖ Sharp localized pain in lower abdomen
❖ Syncope and referred shoulder pain
❖ Irregular vaginal bleeding
❖ Abdominal rigidity and distention
❖ Shock-decreased blood pressure, increased heart rate
❖ Palpable mass in the cul-de-sac or adnexa
❖ Lower than normal HCG titers
❖ Disorientation and lack of cooperation due to severe pain
❖ Expression of fear if the woman was unaware of pregnancy
❖ Grief over loss of pregnancy.

Analysis/Nursing Diagnosis

❖ Risk for fetal injury
❖ Risk for infection
❖ Ineffective airway clearance
❖ Actual/risk for aspiration
❖ Anxiety
❖ Anticipatory grieving
❖ Altered family processes
❖ Actual/risk for altered parenting
❖ Health seeking behavior.

Implementation

❖ Provide pain relief
❖ Manage shock
   a. Administer oxygen, IV fluids
   b. Type and crossmatch blood.
❖ Prepare for surgery, laparotomy with removal of the ectopic pregnancy, and perhaps the affected fallopian tube.
❖ Provide postoperative care
   a. Give routine postoperative care
   b. Assess vaginal bleeding
   c. Offer emotional support.

Evaluation

Ensure that the woman

❖ Has participated in decision-making
❖ Is free from pain
❖ Is normotensive
❖ Acknowledges support through the treatment process
❖ Demonstrates knowledge of self-care measures.

HYDATIDIFORM MOLE

A hydatidiform mole, also known as vesicular mole is a gestational trophoblastic malformation in which the chorionic villi proliferate and become avascular.

The incidence of hydatidiform mole is 0.5 to 2.5 in the western world and 1:160 to 1:400 in India. The risk rises where the mother has previously had a molar pregnancy.

Incidence

❖ The incidence is high at the beginning and the end of childbearing period (under 20 and over 40 years of age)
❖ Poor nutrition: Protein deficiency
❖ Consanguinity
❖ Maternal blood group A and paternal blood group O
❖ Genetic disposition.

Pathology

The mole is usually bulky, weighing up to 2000 gm. There are bunched chains and clusters of globular and ovoid stalked vesicles looking like grapes, of size varying from pinhead to 3 cm in diameter. Blood clots usually accompany a mole and may obscure it. The vesicles appear to be loosely attached or unattached to the endometrium, and can be pulled away by gentle traction. The amniotic sac is small, flattened, displaced to one side and may not be found easily.

Ovarian changes are seen in 50 percent of cases. There are multiple cysts enlarging the ovaries. About 50 percent of molar pregnancies develop into choriocarcinoma, a malignant trophoblastic tumor. It is a dull-red, liver-like or spongy nodule in the myometrium, occasionally streaked with yellowish or greenish-white areas. It may or may not reach the endometrium. It differs from hydatidiform mole in having no villi.

Two forms of moles have been identified, one of which carries an increased risk of the mother subsequently developing choriocarcinoma, the malignant gestational trophoblastic disease.

Complete Hydatidiform Mole

This type of mole contains no evidence of embryo, cord or membranes. Death of embryo occurs prior to the development of the placental circulation (Szulman, 1988). The chorionic villi alter to form clear, hydropic, vesicles, which hang in clusters from small pedicles. The mass occupies the uterine cavity and can be large enough to mimic an advanced gestation. The developing mole penetrates the uterine wall beyond the site of implantation. Myometrium can be involved and more rarely the veins. Rupture of the uterus with massive hemorrhage is a possible outcome.

Complete moles usually have 46 chromosomes of paternal origin only. Choriocarcinoma can develop from complete mole.

Partial Mole

In this type, evidence of an embryo, fetus or amniotic sac may be found as death occurs at eighth or ninth week. Hyperplacia of the trophoblast is confined to a single syncytiotrophoblast layer and is less widespread than in complete moles. Chromosome analysis usually show this to be triploid with 69 chromosomes, i.e. three sets of chromosomes, one maternal and two paternal. The risk to the mother of developing choriocarcinoma from a partial mole is slight. Follow-up however, is still essential (Bennett and Brown, 1999).

Clinical Features

❖ Apparently normal first trimester of pregnancy
❖ Persistent nausea and vomiting
❖ Uterine bleeding evident by 20th week of pregnancy—Usually more brown than red, occurring intermittently or continuously over time
❖ Anemia: Often it is out of proportion to the amount of blood lost due to rapidly growing tumor

- A large-for-dates uterus clearly out of proportion to the presumed gestational age in about 50 percent of cases
- On palpation the uterus feels "doughy" or elastic
- Shortness of breath
- Often enlarged, tender ovaries
- No fetal heart tones
- No fetal activity
- Palpation of fetal parts impossible
- Hyperemesis gravidarum due to high levels of hCG
- Pregnancy-induced hypertension, pre-eclampsia, or eclampsia before 24 weeks of gestation
- Vaginal discharge may rarely show vesicles of the mole.

Investigations

- Urinary pregnancy test, due to the large amounts of human chorionic gonadotropin (hCG) produced by the tumor, the test is positive in a dilution 1:2000 or more after 14 weeks of gestation
- Serum levels of hCG levels is high
- Ultrasound scan shows a characteristic pattern and a snow storm appearance.

Possible Complications

- Hemorrhage and shock
- Pulmonary embolism and acute corpul-monale
- Thyrotoxicosis due to production of thyro-trophic hormone by the mole
- Rupture of an invasive mole into the peritoneal cavity
- Disseminated intravascular coagulation
- Choriocarcinoma
- Recurrence in subsequent pregnancies.

Treatment

The aim of treatment is to remove all the trophoblastic tissues. If the patient presents with bleeding and shock, she is resuscitated. Then the mole is evacuated by vacuum aspiration or dilatation and curettage. A slow dilatation of cervix may be achieved by using laminaria tends over 12 to 24 hours. Spontaneous expulsion of the mole carries less risk of malignant change.

The mole can be aborted by administration of prostaglandin intramuscularly. In about 10 percent of cases, the trophoblast tissue does not die off completely. For this reason and the possibility of developing malignancy, women confirmed as having complete mole require follow-up for over a two-year period. Follow-up examinations are done every week for 8 weeks, monthly for ten months and three monthly for two years. At each visit the patient is examined for vaginal metastasis, subinvolution of uterus and theca lutein cysts. Curettage is repeated if there is irregular vaginal bleeding, the uterus does not involute or hCG levels are still positive six weeks after evacuation. If serum hCG level is high (more than 20 IU/ml) or rising, chemotherapy is given. Usually actinomycin D or methotrexate is given for 5 days.

Pregnancy should be avoided during the follow-up period. Intrauterine contraceptive devices are contraindicated because of perforation and infection and hormonal methods of contraception are not prescribed until levels of human chorionic gonadotropin have returned to normal.

The midwife has to provide support and explanations of the importance of the prolonged period of screening. The client should be helped to plan subsequent pregnancy and care during pregnancy.

Choriocarcinoma

Choriocarcinoma is a malignant neoplasm, which can develop because of a molar pregnancy. The growth actively invades the myometrium, which can result in severe hemorrhage. The mother is also at risk for developing lung, hepatic and cerebral metastasis. Choriocarcinoma can also occur after a normal term gestation or a termination of pregnancy (Bennett and Brown, 1999).

NURSING PROCESS FOR CLIENTS WITH HYDATIDIFORM MOLE

Assessment

Assess for:
- Vaginal bleeding by the 12th week that is intermittent, bright red or dark brown, slightly or profuse in amount

- Hyperemesis
- Fundal height in relation to EDC
- hCG levels
- "Snow storm" pattern in ultrasonography
- No FHT on auscultation
- Symptoms of PIH
- Fear of pregnancy and apprehension.

Analysis/Nursing Diagnosis

- Risk for fetal injury
- Risk for infection
- Ineffective airway clearance
- Actual/risk for aspiration
- Anxiety
- Anticipatory grieving
- Altered family processes
- Actual/risk for altered parenting
- Health seeking behavior.

Planning

- Provide information regarding treatment plan
- Promote maternal physical well-being
- Provide opportunities for counseling and support
- Provide teaching related to self-care.

Implementation

- Coordinate diagnostic testing
- Prepare woman for uterine evacuation
- Observe for postprocedure hemorrhage and infection
- Instruct and facilitate follow-up care.
  a. Monitor hCG level for two years
  b. Instruct regarding birth control measures to prevent pregnancy for two years
- Provide support during family's grieving period.

Evaluation

Ensure that the woman:
- Has rapidly decreasing hCG titers
- Recovers physically after evacuation of the molar pregnancy
- Verbalizes positive self-image
- Avoids conception during the follow-up period

- Voices understanding regarding need to avoid pregnancy as per the physician's recommendations.

HYPEREMESIS GRAVIDARUM

Hyperemesis gravidarum is excessive nausea and vomiting during pregnancy. This pernicious vomiting is differentiated from the more common and more normal morning sickness by the fact that it is of greater intensity and extends beyond the first semester. Hyperemesis gravidarum may occur in any of the three trimesters. It is a condition affecting one in 1000 pregnancies.

Causes

High levels of hCG or undue sensitivity to normal levels of hCG may cause vomiting. Psychological factors are thought to play an important role. Women with a previous history of hyperemesis are likely to experience it in subsequent pregnancies (Fairweather, 1968). It is known to be associated with first pregnancies. An allergic factor may also be operative, since large amounts of histamine are found in cases of hyperemesis. The sensitizing agents possibly are the woman's own corpus luteum, syncytial cells and gonadotropic hormones.

Clinical Presentation

- Pernicious vomiting (anything taken orally is rejected)
- Poor appetite and poor nutritional intake
- Loss of more than 25 percent of body weight
- Dehydration and electrolyte imbalance
- Acidosis due to starvation
- Alkalosis resulting from loss of hydrochloric acid in the vomitus
- Occasionally jaundice develops in severe cases
- Low urine output
- Rapid pulse and low blood pressure
- Hemoconcentration with rising blood urea nitrogen and falling sodium, potassium and chloride.

The condition is said to be mild when there is loss of weight but no dehydration. Moderate cases are those characterized by dehydration and circulatory changes. Severe cases have biochemical changes with complications.

Complications

* Circulatory failure
* Jaundice due to liver involvement
* Retinal hemorrhage
* Wernicke's encephalopathy and Korsakoff's syndrome (disorientation and loss of memory)
* Renal insufficiency
* Polyneuritis
* Delirium, coma, death.

Treatment

Women with hyperemesis gravidarum are admitted to the hospital. Initially nothing is given by mouth. Hypovolemia and electrolyte imbalance are corrected by intravenous infusion. Vitamin supplements are given parenterally. Fluids and diet are gradually introduced as the woman's condition improves.

The mother should be encouraged to rest and be cared for in a single room. Some women are prescribed a mild sedative if they are agitated. Supportive psychotherapy and counseling may help.

Small palatable meals, at regular intervals may help the mother to regain her appetite. Antihistamines may be prescribed for treatment of nausea and vomiting. Patient's weight is taken twice a week to monitor the recovery.

Termination of pregnancy is recommended in severe cases with jaundice, persistent albuminuria, and polyneuritis to reverse the condition and to prevent maternal mortality.

SUMMARY OF NURSING PROCESS FOR CLIENTS WITH HYPEREMESIS

Assessment

* Intractable vomiting
* Weight loss of 25 percent or more
* Ketosis, ketonuria (alkalosis)
* Dehydration—Poor skin turger, dry tongue
* Epigastric pain
* Drowsiness and confusion
* Uncoordinated movements, jerking
* Jaundice.

Analysis/Nursing Diagnosis

* Risk for fetal injury
* Risk for infection
* Ineffective airway clearance
* Actual/risk for aspiration
* Anxiety
* Anticipatory grieving
* Altered family processes
* Actual/risk for altered parenting
* Health seeking behavior.

Planning

* Provide IV and/or oral fluids to re-establish fluid and electrolyte balance
* Create opportunities for the woman to explore feelings about pregnancy and coping abilities
* Provide teaching related to need for fluids.

Implementation

* Administer parenteral fluids, vitamins, and sedatives as prescribed
* Monitor intake, output and daily weight
* Assess state of hydration
* Begin oral feedings slowly with fluids. Progress to six small feedings a day
* Obtain psychiatric consultation if indicated.

Evaluation

Ensure that the woman:
* Is well hydrated
* Has normal electrolyte values
* Verbalizes feelings and ability to cope with the pregnancy
* Verbalizes knowledge of need for fluids.

Rh ISOIMMUNIZATION AND ABO INCOMPATIBILITY

Immunization is a process in which immune antibodies are produced in an individual in response to injection of antigens from another individual of the same species who possesses antigens that the first one lacks.

Rh antibodies develop when Rh-positive cells enter the circulation of an Rh-negative person. This may occur due to a mismatched transfusion. In obstetrics, this happens due to fetomaternal hemorrhage during abortions, childbirth, rupture of ectopic pregnancy, antepartum hemorrhage, versions, amniocentesis, etc.

To the transfer of fetal red blood cells, the mother responds by producing antibodies against the Rh factor, which on the first exposure begin to show-up in her serum a few days after the event—usually delivery. Since the production of antibodies takes time, the first Rh-incompatible fetus usually escapes disease unless the mother has been sensitized earlier by an Rh-incompatible blood transfusion.

Incompatibility of the ABO groups occurs more frequently than that caused by the Rh factor. It usually occurs when the woman is type O and the fetus is A or B. Hemolytic disease due to ABO incompatibility can occur without prior sensitization since A, B antibodies are already present in the mothers blood, and thus the first-born can be affected. However, the disease is much less severe with ABO isoimmunization.

Screening for blood incompatibility between the mother and fetus is limited to Rh-incompatibility because there is no generally accepted method for diagnosing ABO incompatibility during pregnancy. History taking which may be relevant to ABO or Rh-incompatibility includes the following:

❖ History of previous blood transfusion
❖ History of previous "yellow baby" or baby needing blood transfusion or phototherapy
❖ History of stillbirth or neonatal death from causes not known to the mother
❖ History of taking RhoGAM after previous deliveries or abortions.

If a pregnant woman is found to be Rh negative, her husband's Rh-status should be determined. If it is Rh-negative, the baby will also be Rh-negative. The baby cannot be affected and nothing further needs to be done.

Investigations

Determination of Rh type is made during the initial prenatal visit. If the woman is Rh-negative, an indirect Coomb's test is ordered. This is a screening for Rh-antibodies. If the test is positive, thereby indicating the presence of Rh-antibodies, antibody titers are then ordered.

A woman who is Rh-negative, with a negative indirect Coomb's should have the test repeated every four weeks up to 28 weeks. Increasing titer indicates that the fetus is Rh-positive.

If the Coomb's test is negative at 28 weeks, a dose of Rh immunoglobulin (Rhogam) is given to the mother to prevent the development of antibodies in the event of an antepartum hemorrhage or during intrapartum period. A dose of 300 μg offers protection against developing antibodies for approximately 12 weeks. If antibodies are found at any stage, the antibody titers are measured regularly and the fetus is monitored closely by ultrasound for any edema or hepatosplenomegaly. Rh-negative mothers are given 300 μg of RhoGam after delivery, within 72 hours, if the baby is Rh-positive. Rh-negative women who have ectopic pregnancies and evacuation of hydatidiform mole should also receive anti-D gamma globulin. The antibodies disappear from maternal blood within about 6 hours following an intramuscular administration of RhoGAM.

RETROVERSION OF THE GRAVID UTERUS

A gravid uterus is said to be retroverted when its long axis is directed backwards. In the first trimester, retroversion of the uterus occurs in 11 percent of all pregnancies (Weekes et al, 1976). It is associated with a slightly increased risk of early pregnancy—bleeding and abortion. This is due to compression of the uterine vessels, decreasing blood flow to the decidua (Gibbons and Paley, 1969). As pregnancy progresses most cases correct spontaneously, the uterus rises out of the pelvis in to the abdomen, causing no further problems.

Incarceration of the Retroverted Gravid Uterus

If the retroverted gravid uterus fails to rise out of the pelvic cavity by 14th week it is considered as incarcerated. This occurs in one to 3,000 pregnancies (Bennett and Brown, 1999). Congenital anomalies of the pelvis and uterus are identified as causes. Conditions such as pelvic adhesions, endometriosis, fibroids and ovarian tumors may contribute to incarceration.

The growing uterus is confined within the pelvis beneath sacral promontory. Pressure causes abdominal discomfort, feeling of pelvic fullness and low back pain. Frequency of micturition, dysuria and incontinence may be experienced because of the urethra being elongated. Compression of the bladder neck causes urinary retention and stasis resulting in urinary infection including pyelonephritis. The mother may complain of rectal pressure and constipation with impaction of feces.

The distended bladder will be palpable abdominally. Fetal heart sounds are difficult to auscultate. Management measures include:

❖ Catheterization to relieve the retention of urine

❖ Indwelling catheter to keep the bladder empty.

These measures may enable the uterus to rise out of the pelvis. In cases where correction does not occur, the uterus continues to expand and extend forming a pouch to accommodate the fetus. Uterine rupture can result. Rupture of the bladder can also happen due to over distension.

BIBLIOGRAPHY

1. Bracken MB. Incidence and etiology of hydatidiform mole. British Journal of Obstetrics and Gynecology 1987;94:1123-35.
2. Dutta DC. Textbook of Obstetrics (5th edn). Calcutta: New Central Book Company 2001.
3. Edmonds DK. Spontaneous and recurrent abortion. In: Shaw RW, Soutter PW (Eds). Gynecology Edinburgh: Churchill Livingstone; 1972.
4. Fairweather DI. Nausea and vomiting in pregnancy, American Journal of Obstetrics and Gynecology 1992;102:135-73.
5. Gibbons JM, Paley WB. The Incarcerated Gravid Uterus. Obstetrics and Gynecology 1969;33:842-5.
6. Shiers CV. Abnormalities early pregnancy. In: Bennett RV, Linda KB (Eds). Myles Textbook for Midwives (13th edn). Edinburgh: Churchill Livingstone 1999.
7. Szulman AE, The biology of trophoblastic disease: Complete and partial hydatidiform moles. In: Beard RW (Ed). Early Pregnancy Loss: Mechanisms and Treatment, London: Springer-Verlag, 1988.
8. Weekes ARL, et al. The Retroverted gravid uterus and its effect on the outcome of pregnancy. British Medical Journal 1976;1:622-24.

26 Sexually Transmissible and Reproductive Tract Infections

Learning Objectives

Upon completing this chapter, the learner will be able to:
* Outline the relevance of sexually transmissible infections for women of childbearing age
* Describe the local infections of the vagina and vulva and their management
* Describe the bacterial infections common in pregnancy and their impact on mother and baby
* Discuss the commonly occurring viral infections and their impact on pregnant women and their newborn babies.

Sexually transmissible diseases (STDs) are a group of communicable diseases that are transmitted predominantly by sexual contact and caused by a wide range of bacterial, viral, protozoal and fungal agents. The true incidence of STDs is not known because of inadequate reporting and the secrecy that surrounds them. Minimal estimates of yearly incidence of four major bacterial STDs worldwide are (WHO Health for all Ser. 1981):

* Gonorrhea   62 million
* Genital chlamydial infection   89 million
* Syphilis   12 million
* Chancroid   2 million

For viral STD, due to the importance of asymptomatic infection, incidence can only be very roughly estimated:

* Genital herpes   20 million
* Genital human papilloma
  virus infection   30 million

Trichomoniasis, which is of much less public health importance than the bacterial and viral STD, has an estimated annual incidence of 170 million cases (WHO, Health Situation in the South-East Asia Region, 1994).

EXTENT OF THE PROBLEM IN INDIA

Sexually transmitted diseases are becoming a major public health problem in India.

Syphilis

Serological surveys continue to be the best source of information on the prevalence of syphilis. The extent of the problem can be gauged from the reports of surveys done in Aurangabad (Maharashtra) and Kerala which showed prevalence of 2.4 and 1.4 respectively (WHO, World Health Report, 1999), which are rather high figures.

Gonorrhea

Accurate information on the morbidity of gonorrhea is lacking, as most cases are not reported. However, the general impression is that gonorrhea is more prevalent than syphilis. Eighty percent of infected women are reported to be asymptomatic carriers (Park, 2000).

Chancroid

Chancroid or soft sore is reported to be widely prevalent in India.

Chlamydia Infections

These are more prevalent in the southern states of India than in the northern states.

Donovanosis

Donovanosis or granuloma inguinale is endemic in Tamil Nadu, Andhra Pradesh, Orissa, Karnataka and Maharashtra. A greater prevalence along the coastal areas has been reported (WHO, World Health Report, 1999). Information about this disease in other states is lacking.

Other STDs

Information about other STDs in India is not readily available as there is no reporting system for these diseases.

Host Factors

Age

For most notifiable STDs, the highest rates of incidence are observed in 20 to 24 years old, followed by 25 to 29 and 15 to 19 years age groups. The most serious morbidity is observed during fetal development and in the neonate.

Sex

For most STDs, the overall morbidity rate is higher for men than for women, but the morbidity caused by infection is generally much more severe in women, for example, pelvic inflammatory disease.

Marital Status

The frequency of STD infection is higher among single, divorced and separated persons than among married couples.

Socioeconomic Status

Individuals from the lowest socioeconomic groups have the highest morbidity rate.

Social Factors

Several social and behavioral factors are involved in the spread of STDs. These include:

Prostitution

This is a major factor in the spread as prostitutes act as reservoir of infection. In Asia, most STDs are contracted from prostitutes. The male component of prostitution, the prostituant, is also equally important in the spread as prostitution supplies a demand.

Broken Homes

Social studies indicate that promiscuous women are usually drawn from broken homes,

e.g. homes, which are broken either due to death of one or both parents or their separation. Children reared in such unhappy atmosphere is likely to go astray in search of other avenues of happiness.

Sexual Disharmony

Married people with strained relation, divorced and separated persons are often victims of STDs.

Easy Money

In most of the developing world, prostitution is simply a reflexion of poverty. It provides an occupation for earning easy money. It is fostered by lack of female employment and the prospect of a financial return impossible to achieve by other means.

Emotional Immaturity

This has been often stressed as a social factor in acquiring STDs.

Urbanization and Industrialization

These are conducive to the type of lifestyle that contributes to high level of infection.

Social Disruption

Caused by disasters, wars and civil unrest have always caused an increase in the spread of STDs.

International Travel

Travelers can import as well as export infection and their role in the transmission of STD is exampled by the rapid spread throughout the world of resistant strains of *N. gonorrhoeae* and AIDS.

Changing Behavioral Patterns

In the modern society, there has been a relaxation of moral and cultural values. The tendency to break away from traditional ways of life is particularly marked among young people desiring more independence and freedom from supervision.

Social Stigma

The social stigma attached of STDs accounts for the nondetection of cases, not disclosing the sources of contact, dropping out before treatment is complete, going to quacks for treatment and self-treatment.

Relevance for Women

1. A number of sexually transmitted organisms such as *Neisseria gonorrhoeae* and *Chlamydia trachomatis* cause salpingitis, which may lead to chronic pelvic inflammation and permanent damage to the uterine tubes resulting in reduced fertility and ectopic pregnancy.
2. The presence of an organism within or around the genitalia or its presence in the blood and sexual secretions facilitate perinatal transmission of infection from the mother to her fetus or newborn baby.
3. Some perinatally acquired infections have serious and prolonged consequences for the fetus or neonate, e.g. cardiac defects, hearing problems, cataracts and developmental delay.
4. Pregnancy may have an impact on the presentation and course of infection, giving rise to difficulties in diagnosis or management. Some infections, such as human papilloma virus (HPV) become more virulent; some, such as group *B. Streptococcus* (GBS), are asymptomatic in the woman but may produce serious neonatal disease.
5. The diagnosis of a sexually transmitted infection may have stressful consequences for the relationship between the woman and her husband.
6. Women may experience high levels of anxiety and guilt about the implications for their babies of a perinatally transmissible infection.
7. Some infections, such as syphilis and cytomegalovirus infection, are important causes of stillbirths and neonatal deaths.
8. Certain carcinomas occur as sequel of STDs which include hepatocellular carcinoma caused by hepatitis B, Kaposi's sarcoma, B-cell lymphomas and primary lymphoma of the central nervous system in patients with AIDS.

Control of STDs

The aim of the control program for STDs is the prevention of ill health resulting from the above conditions through various interventions.

These interventions have a primary prevention focus (prevention of infection), a secondary prevention focus (minimizing the adverse health effects of infection) or a combination of the two.

Case Detection

Case detection is an essential part of any control program. The methods of early detection in a STD control program are:

Screening

Screening is the testing of apparently healthy volunteers from the general population for the early detection of disease. Priority is given to screening of special groups, such as pregnant women, blood donors, industrial workers, army, police, refugees, prostitutes, convicts and, restaurant and hotel staff.

Contact Tracing

Contact tracing is the technique by which the sexual partners of diagnosed patients are identified, located, investigated and treated. This is one of the best methods of controlling the spread of infection.

Cluster Testing

The patients are asked to name other persons of either sex who move in the same sociosexual environment. These persons are then screened through blood testing.

Case Holding and Treatment

Adequate treatment of patients and their contacts is the mainstay of STD control. There is a tendency on the part of patients suffering from STDs to disappear or drop out before treatment is complete. Therefore, every effort should be made to ensure complete and adequate treatment.

Epidemiological Treatment

This consists of the administration of full therapeutic dose of treatment to persons recently exposed to STD while awaiting the results of laboratory tests. It is combined with a venereological examination and the tracing of contacts revealed by that examination.

Personal Prophylaxis

Contraceptives

Mechanical barriers, such as condoms and diaphragms can be recommended for personal prophylaxis of STDs. These barrier methods, especially when used with spermicides, will minimize the risk of acquiring STD infections. The exposed parts should be washed with soap and water as soon as possible after contact. Vaccine is now available for Hepatitis B.

Health Education

Health education is an integral part of STD control programs. The principal aim of educational intervention is to help individuals alter their behavior in an effort to avoid STDs, that is, to minimize disease acquisition and transmission.

LOCAL INFECTIONS OF THE VAGINA AND VULVA

The vagina is a host to a rich variety of microorganisms. These are subject to dynamic alteration in quantity and composition, reflecting at any given time a woman's current physiological state, her immunological defense mechanisms and her past exposure. Transfer and sharing of microorganisms between partners occur during sexual intercourse, and may include the exchange of infective organisms.

Clinical disease may occur because of the introduction of organisms, which are new to the woman, or because of redistribution of existing microbiological flora due to the pathophysiological changes of pregnancy or the action of antibiotics. Changes may occur in a woman's susceptibility to, or the pathogenicity of, previously encountered organisms.

FUNGAL INFECTIONS

The most common of these is *Candida albicans (thrush)*, which accounts for the vast majority of fungal vulvovaginal infections. A minority of infections is caused by organisms such as *Torulopsis glabrata* and *Candida tropicalis* (Lossick, 1986).

Candida is a common inhabitant of the mouth, large intestine and vagina in 25 to 50 percent of healthy individuals and isolation of the organism does not correlate strongly the presence of clinical disease. Some women are more susceptible to candida infection. Predisposition to infection is associated with diabetes, pregnancy and the administration of antibiotics, particularly those, like penicillin, which are effective against vaginal lactobacilli.

Resistance to fungal infection depends on cell-mediated immunity and therefore, compromise of this by disease such as HIV infection or immunosuppressive therapy increases infection risk. Some individuals develop candida-specific reduced cell immunity. Tight clothes and mild skin abrasions may contribute to clinical presentation of infection.

Clinical Presentation and Diagnosis

The woman may complain of vulval pruritis (itchiness) and on examination, there may be evidence of vulvovaginitis and/or vulval, vaginal and cervical erythema. Dyspareunia (pain during intercourse) is a common complaint.

A vaginal discharge is common but not universal and may be scant or thick and white with a curd-like consistency.

In less than 20 percent of cases, white thrush patches may be present on the vulva or walls of the vagina.

Half of the babies born to infected women will be infected by candida, generally involving oral or gastrointestinal infection (Lossick, 1986). Treatment of the mother prior to delivery is desirable.

Treatment

Female

Vaginal infection is treated by insertion of vaginal suppositories at night with cream for application to the vulval and perineal area.
1. Clotrimazole suppositories or pessaries for 6 nights
   * Clotrimazole cream 1 percent for application to the vulva two to three times daily.

2. Miconazole pessaries 150 mg for 3 nights.
3. Nystatin pessaries × 2 of 100,000 i.u for 14 nights with Nystatin gel 100,000 i.u/g for external use.

Male

Signs of clinical infection in a man, usually small red spots or plaques on the glans penis, should be treated with cream applied to the infected area.

Instructions

❖ Avoid sexual intercourse until the treatment is complete.
❖ Avoid local irritation, which might provoke reinfection.
❖ Take daily bath to maintain cleanliness of the perineal area.
❖ Avoid the use of harsh soaps and other irritants.
❖ Wipe away from the vagina after defecation.
❖ Use cotton underwear and avoid clothing which is tight or constricting in the crotch.

PROTOZOAL INFECTIONS

The protozoan, *Trichomonas vaginalis*, is an anaerobic organism, which is highly pathogenic to the epithelium in the vagina. Its prevalence varies considerably in different populations.

The major mode of transmission is sexual intercourse. Eighty percent of women, whose partners are infected with *T. vaginalis*, become infected, although the rate of female-male transfer is lower than this (Lossick, 1986). Severe vaginitis is experienced by some women. Infection of the neonate seems to be uncommon.

Clinical Presentation and Diagnosis

About half to two-thirds of infected women will complain of symptoms. Pruritus, burning and increased vaginal discharge are commonly seen. Vaginal discharge may range from normal to copious, grayish in color and somewhat bubbly in character. The green, frothy discharge and friable erythematous cervix are the "classic" presenting features of the infection. Urethritis may also be a feature.

Asymptomatic infection may sometimes bo detected on the Papanicolaou smear. A wet swab examined immediately under a microscope will demonstrate the presence of the pear-shaped protozoan, with 3 to 5 flagellae and an undulating membrane. Swabs should be cultured to exclude the presence of gonococcal and chlamydial infection.

Treatment

A single oral dose of metronidazole 2 g or a five-day course of 400 mg twice daily is the treatment of choice. Clotrimazole may also be used as local treatment. The woman's partner should also be prescribed treatment with metronidazole.

Metronidazole potentiates the action of alcohol, anticonvulsant and warfarin. Alcohol should be avoided and use of other drugs monitored when the client is prescribed metronidazole. Because of its excretion in breast milk, it is contraindicated for breast-feeding mothers (Erikson et al, 1981).

Clients must be advised to avoid sexual intercourse until treatment is complete.

BACTERIAL INFECTIONS

Bacterial Vaginosis

Bacterial vaginosis is a term applied to vaginal discharge associated with a variety of anaerobic organisms including *Gardnerella vaginalis* and *Bacteroides* spp. It has been associated with postpartum pyrexia, amniotic fluid infection, preterm labor and pelvic inflammatory disease (Lossick, 1986).

Presentation, Diagnosis and Treatment

The infection presents with a grey or white, fishy smelling discharge which may be adherent or of normal consistency and may be more profuse than normal.

The distinctive fishy odor of the discharge and a vaginal pH of greater than or equal to 4.5 are diagnostic clues.

Treatment is with metronidazole 400 mg twice daily for five days.

Chlamydial Infection

Chlamydia trachomatis is one of a group of intracellular parasites, closely related to Gram-negative bacteria. The organism is a major cause of salpingitis and pelvic inflammatory disease (PID) with their sequelae of ectopic pregnancy and infertility, and postpartum and postabortal infection. Chlamydial infection has been associated with increased risk of low birth weight, preterm rupture of membranes and a shorter gestation (Brunham et al, 1970). It is currently the most common cause of neonatal conjunctivitis and it is estimated that from 3 to 18 percent of babies born to infected mothers will develop chlamydial pneumonia (Abel and von Unwerth, 1988).

Presentation and Diagnosis

The condition is often asymptomatic in the woman, although a mucopurulent cervicitis may be detected clinically, or the woman may present with salpingitis or the urethral syndrome (Wang and Smaill, 1989).

In the light of its association with maternal and neonatal morbidity, detection of chlamydial infection during pregnancy could offer significant benefits. The Centers for Disease Control (CDC) in the US recommended that at least one prenatal culture for C. trachomatis be undertaken for pregnant women who fall into one of the following categories:

❖ Age less than twenty years
❖ Unmarried
❖ History of other sexually transmitted disease
❖ Multiple sexual partners and a partner with multiple sexual partners (Bell and Grayson, 1986).

Treatment

Erythromycin 500 mg four times a day for 7 to 10 days is the antibiotic of choice during pregnancy. Therapy should be instituted to the husband simultaneously. As a prophylaxis to ophthalmia neonatorum, tetracycline or erythromycin ointment one percent is to be applied to the neonate's eye soon after birth. Neonatal infection is treated with erythromycin 50 mg/kg/day four times a day for 14 to 20 days.

GROUP B STREPTOCOCCUS

Group B Streptococcus (GBS, agalactiae) is part of the vaginal flora of 5 to 25 percent of women. One-third or more pregnant women may be vaginal carriers of GBS during pregnancy, with intermittent and recurring colonization.

This asymptomatic maternal infection is significant in pregnancy as the most frequent cause of overwhelming sepsis in neonates, estimated to occur from 0.6 to 3.7 cases per 1,000 live births (Wang and Smaill, 1989). The mortality rate of neonatal GBS in the US is 50 percent (Brunham et al, 1990).

GBS has been associated with early spontaneous rupture of membranes and with a three-fold increase in preterm delivery at or before 32 weeks' gestation (Brunham et al, 1990).

Of the neonates of women with GBS colonization, 65 to 75 percent will be colonized with the organism, although only 1 to 2 percent of exposed neonates will develop invasive disease (Brunham et al, 1990).

Treatment of GBS Colonization in Pregnancy

The recommended treatment is intravenous administration of ampicillin (or erythromycin if the woman is allergic to penicillin).

Gonococcal Infection

Gonorrhea is caused by Neisseria gonorrhoeae, a gram-negative Diplococcus that has an affinity for columnar epithelial tissue. In women, infection occurs in the urethra or cervix.

Incidence of maternal infection varies greatly between populations, ranging from 1 to 5 percent (Wang and Smaill, 1989). The rate of asymptomatic infection is high, and as many as 50 percent of women diagnosed are usually asymptomatic (Adler, 1995).

Effects of Gonococcal Infection in Pregnancy

Gonorrhea in pregnancy may present as local infection (arthritis) or systemic disease.

Among nonpregnant women with endocervical infection, about 1 to 20 percent show clinical evidence of pelvic inflammatory disease (PID). Acute PID is rare in pregnancy, although positive *N. gonorrhoeae* cultures are sometimes associated with fever and pain.

Manifestations of Gonococcal Infection in Pregnant Women

- ❖ Dysuria (urethral infection)
- ❖ Cervicitis (endocervical infection)
- ❖ Proctitis (rectal infection)
- ❖ Conjunctivitis (ophthalmic infection).

Less common manifestations noted include acute inflammation of the Bartholin's glands (Bartholinitis), endometritis, and salpingitis (Wang and Smaill, 1989).

Arthritis is the most common manifestation of disseminated infection. Infection usually presents with fever and rigors and there may be a characteristic purpuric petechial rash. Pregnancy complicated by gonococcal endocervicitis is associated with premature rupture of membranes, chorioamnionitis, early rupture of membranes and preterm delivery. Early infection is associated with septic abortion and chorioamnionitis.

Intrapartum infection is associated with postpartum endometritis and upper genital tract infection (Brunham et al, 1990).

Neonatal infection most commonly presents as conjunctivitis, but infection at other body sites can occur and may be associated with a higher risk of disseminated infection.

Diagnosis

Swabs should be taken from the cervix and the urethral meatus for culture. If culture is being done because of known contact with an infected partner, other sites of exposure such as the throat and anus should be swabbed.

Screening

Screening of all women for gonococcal infection in pregnancy is recommended because of its serious effects on pregnancy and the risks of neonatal and puerperal infection and the fact that a high proportion of infection in women is asymptomatic (Brunham et al, 1990; Wang and Smaill, 1989). Repeat cultures in the last trimester are suggested for women with a previous history of gonorrhea or other sexually transmitted infection.

Treatment

Single dose of procaine penicillin 4.8 million units combined with probenecid 1 g orally or Ampicillin 3 gm in a single dose orally with probenecid 1 gm orally. In cases of disseminated infection, penicillin is to be administered intravenously or intramuscularly for 10 to 14 days. If arthritis is a feature of infection, a longer therapy is indicated (Wang and Smaill, 1989).

Syphilis

Syphilis is an infection caused by *Treponema pallidum*. In pregnancy, its particular significance is the devastating effect it has on fetal wellbeing. The natural course of adult infection is divided into stages.

Early Infectious Stage

Primary stage: Nine to Sixty days after exposure.

Secondary stage: Six weeks to six months after exposure.

Early latent stage: Two years after exposure.

Late Noninfectious Stage

Late latent stage: More than 2 years after exposure.

Neurosyphilis, cardiovascular syphilis or gummatous syphilis.

Most pregnant women diagnosed are in the primary or secondary stages and untreated infection will affect almost all fetuses. Depending upon the intensity and time of occurrence of the infiltration, the fate of the fetus will be as follows:

- ❖ Abortion or intrauterine death 20 percent
- ❖ Preterm deliveries 20 percent
- ❖ Delivery of highly infected baby with neonatal death 20 percent
- ❖ Survival with congenital syphilis with resulting disability 40 percent.

Prenatal diagnosis and treatment through routine serological testing in early pregnancy is the key to prevention of congenital syphilis. This should be done as a routine in the first antenatal visit. VDRL (Venereal Disease Research Laboratory) is commonly done. A positive VDRL test has to be confirmed by fluorescent treponemal antibody (FTA) test, which is a specific test. Husband's blood should also be tested for VDRL. Detection of spirochaetes from the cutaneous lesion, if any is done by dark field examination. Fetal infection could be diagnosed by demonstration of *T. pallidum* in the amniotic fluid.

Congenital Syphilis

The syphilitic baby may appear normal at birth but shows signs of infection within one or two weeks after birth. Purulent nasal discharge—often hemorrhagic, hoarse cry, maculopapular rash and pemphigus (highly contagious vesicles) on the soles and palms are common manifestations. Ulcers can occur on the lips and mouth and, if on the larynx, the baby's cry may be thin or soundless.

Poor feeding and weight loss may be features of infection. Periostitis produces swelling of the long bones and the resulting pain may cause the baby to behave as if he or she has a fracture. The baby may also present with patchy alopecia, hepatosplenomegaly and mild jaundice.

Late signs may develop at any time from second to thirtieth year of life even if none of the early signs was exhibited. These include eighth nerve deafness, saddle nose (depression on the nasal bridge), corneal scarring causing impaired vision or blindness, and mental disability. Prognosis depends on the damage, which has occurred prior to treatment.

Treatment

Mother: Treatment should be started as soon as the diagnosis is established. The baby may have the chance of protection even if the treatment is begun late in pregnancy. For primary, secondary or latent syphilis (of less than one year duration), Benzathine penicillin 2.4 million units intramuscularly as a single dose is administered. When the duration is more than a year, Benzathine penicillin 2.4 million units weekly for 3 weeks is given. If the woman is allergic to penicillin, oral erythromycin 2 gm daily for 15 days is given. If the treatment is given in early pregnancy, the treatment should be repeated in late pregnancy. Irrespective of the serological report, treatment should be repeated in subsequent pregnancies.

Treatment for Baby

❖ Infected baby with positive serological reaction requires: (1) Isolation with the mother (2) Intramuscular administration of acqeous procaine penicillin G 50,000 units per kg body weight each day in divided doses for 10 days. In the presence of contagious lesions, the baby must be barrier nursed until antibiotics have been given for 48 hours.

❖ Babies with positive serum reaction without clinical evidences of the disease may be treated with a single intramuscular dose of penicillin G 50,000 units per kg body weight. The baby must be observed for 8 weeks and quantitative blood reactions are tested twice a week for four weeks and then at weekly intervals for another four weeks.

❖ An apparently healthy baby of a syphilitic mother should be tested for serological reaction every week for the first month and then monthly for 6 months.

VIRAL INFECTIONS

Herpes Simplex Virus (HSV)

Herpes simplex is one of a family of herpes viruses, which includes varicella-zoster, cytomegalovirus (CMV) and Epstein-Barr virus. All within this family share the ability to establish lifelong, persistent infection in their host and to undergo periodic reactivation. Reactivated infection may have characteristics different from the primary episode.

Herpes simplex virus type 1 is associated with infections of the lip and oropharynx, and type 2 associated with genital infection.

Neonatal infection is most often associated with HSV type 2. However, postnatal infection of the newborn baby with HSV type 1 from maternal or nonmaternal sources such as staff and visitors have also been documented (Bennett and Brown, 1999).

For transmission to occur the HSV virus must come into contact with mucosal surfaces or abraded skin. Viral replication occurs at the site of infection and then the virus or particles of it are transported along the neurons to the ganglia where they remain dormant until there is an alteration in the host environment that gives rise to occurrence of active infection.

Presentation of Infection with HSV

Primary infection of HSV type 1 is usually asymptomatic, though it may present with gingivostomatitis. In young adults, it is often associated with pharyngitis.

Primary infection with HSV type 2 usually presents with painful genital ulcers after an incubation period of less than 7 days. Skin lesions begin with erythema, progress to vesicles and then ulcers and finish with crusting. Local lesions with viral shedding may last about 12 days with complete healing taking another week (Adler, 1995). Both vulva and cervix are involved in most primary attacks, but single sites may be affected.

Recurrent infection involves reactivation of the same virus at the same site rather than reinfection. Clients may experience prodromal symptoms of local tingling and numbness at the site of the lesions about 24 to 48 hours prior to the onset of lesions. In recurrent attacks there may be fewer lesions, milder symptoms and a shorter duration.

Both primary and recurrent infection may be asymptomatic in pregnancy, which is the situation in which the fetus is at greater risk. Primary infection is associated with an increased risk of spontaneous abortion, prematurity and the acquisition of serious infection by the neonate. Transmission of virus to the fetus or neonate is thought to occur at delivery and only rarely trans-placentally (Brunham, 1990).

Management of HSV in Pregnancy

Because most genital herpes infection is unrecognized, it is important that a careful vulval inspection is done at the time of labor of all women, not just those with a history of genital herpes. When the infection occurs in the first or second trimester of pregnancy the women are treated with oral or intravenous acyclovir.

When the first episode occurs in the third trimester, there is an increased risk of premature labor. If labor becomes established, the recommended management is intravenous administration of acyclovir and delivery by cesarean section, on the grounds of reducing maternal viremia and reducing exposure of the fetus to virus.

In the case of women who have recovered from the first episode without going into labor, because of the high risk of continued viral shedding, an elective cesarean section at 38 weeks may be done; especially if symptoms began within six weeks of the expected date of delivery.

If following a first episode of infection in the third trimester, a vaginal delivery is unavoidable or if the membranes have been ruptured for more than four hours prior to cesarean section, the mother and baby must be treated with intravenous acyclovir to reduce the risk of neonatal infection.

Cytomegalovirus (CMV)

This is another of the herpes group of viruses, which can be found in saliva, urine, breast milk, semen and cervical secretions. Transmission between adults usually occurs by direct contact, for example by kissing and may be sexual. Primary infection may occasionally present similarly to glandular fever or influenza, with headache, sore throat and anorexia. There may be hepatitis with prolonged pyrexia. Subsequently the virus may remain dormant but be subject to reactivation and be excreted for many years.

Diagnosis is by culture of specimens of urine, blood or saliva or of a swab taken from the cervix. Serology is performed for antibody levels.

Infection in Pregnancy

At any stage of pregnancy, both primary and reactivated CMV infection can result in transplancental transmission to the fetus. The results are probably more serious in primary infection. Abortion, stillbirth, growth retardation and premature labor may result.

The incidence is estimated to be about 4 per 1000 live births. Two percent of these develop serious problems such as micro- or hydrocephaly, spastic quadriplegia, psychomotor retardation and deafness. About 8 percent develop minor problems like hepatosplenomegaly and thrombocytopenia. Ninty percent of babies are symptom-free at birth, but some will not attain their expected intellectual potential and/or will become deaf in later childhood. If transplacental infection is suspected, cord blood should be examined for specific IgM and a urine sample and nasopharyngeal swab sent for culture. Treatment is supportive only, and care should be taken to avoid infection of other babies and members of staff, particularly pregnant staff. The virus may continue to be shed by the infected infant for a prolonged period.

Whilst it is estimated that 50 percent of women of childbearing age have been infected by CMV, only about one percent of their infants will be infected.

Hepatitis B Infection

Hepatitis B virus (HBV) is the most common cause of jaundice in pregnancy. It has an incubation period of 1 to 6 months. Perinatal transmission from an infected mother to her newborn is the major mode of transmission. It can also be transmitted sexually and by means of infected blood products or parenteraly by use of unsterilized equipment contaminated by infected blood.

The risk of transmission to fetus ranges from 10 percent in the first trimester to as high as 90 percent in the third trimester and it is specially high from those mothers who are seropositive to hepatitis surface antigen (HBsAg) and 'e' antigen (HBeAg). Approximately 10 percent of the infected individuals will go to the chronic state. They are at high risk of developing chronic active hepatitis, cirrhosis and hepatocellular carcinoma. The presence of HBe antigen (HBeAg) indicates continued viral activity, although antibody to this indicates a lower level of infectivity.

Neonatal transmission mainly occurs at or around the time of birth through mixing of maternal blood and genital secretions. About 90 percent of infected babies become chronic carriers, who can infect others. About 25 percent of carrier neonates will die from cirrhosis or hepatic carcinoma between late childhood and early adulthood (Dutta, 2001). HBV is not teratogenic.

Maternal infection: The acute infection is manifested by flu-like illness as malaise, anorexia, nausea, and vomiting and mild diarrhea. There may be arthralgia, skin rashes and pain over the liver. Majority may remain asymptomatic. Jaundice is rare and fever is uncommon. Spontaneous resolution occurs in 90 percent and 1 percent may die of fulminating hepatitis (Dutta, 2001).

Diagnosis

Diagnosis is confirmed by serological detection of HBsAg, HBeAg (denote high infectivity) and antibody to hepatitis B core antigen. Chronic carriers are diagnosed by presence of HBsAg or HBeAg and anti-HBe antibodies six months after initial infection. Liver enzymes are elevated during the initial phase.

Screening

All pregnant women should be screened for HBV infection at the first antenatal visit and it should be repeated during the third trimester for "high-risk" groups (intravenous drug abusers, sexually promiscuous individuals, hemophilics or women having multiple sex partners).

Management

The babies of mothers who are chronic carriers or who have been infected with HBV during pregnancy should receive hepatitis B vaccine within 24 hours of birth which will be repeated at 1 and 6 months of age. In addition, the babies of mothers who had acute hepatitis B during pregnancy and those who do not have anti-HBe antibodies should receive 0.5 ml of hepatitis B immunoglobulin (HBIg) intramuscularly, administered in a different site from the vaccine, not later than 48 hours after birth to provide immediate passive immunity.

Infection control measures should be instituted where the mother is considered infectious. The woman should be given information about the disease and advice regarding sexual behavior. Household contacts and husband should be tested for HBsAg and offered immunization.

Rubella (German Measles)

The virus that causes rubella is particularly virulent during pregnancy. If the woman contracts rubella during the first trimester, there is approximately a 20 percent chance that her baby will be born with congenital malformations. This figure is as high as 50 percent during the first month of pregnancy.

The most common malformations are cataracts, cardiac defects and deafness. There may also be glaucoma, microcephaly and other defects involving the heart, brain and central nervous system. The most severely affected fetuses may abort spontaneously.

Diagnosis of rubella is difficult because the disease may be subclinical, thereby infecting the fetus but not exhibiting itself clinically in the mother.

Clinical signs of rubella, when they are present include the following:

❖ Low grade fever
❖ Drowsiness
❖ Sore throat
❖ Rash-pale or bright-red on the first or second day, spreading rapidly from the face over the entire body and fading rapidly
❖ Swollen neck glands
❖ Duration of 3 to 5 days.

Women who contact rubella in the first trimester are faced with the decision of whether or not to obtain a therapeutic abortion.

Genital Warts

Genital warts are caused by the human papilloma virus (HPV) and nearly always transmitted by sexual contact. Rarely, a baby may acquire laryngeal papilloma because of exposure at the time of delivery.

The significance of warts in pregnancy is that they occasionally increase very dramatically in size, which may be distressing to the woman and may occasionally jeopardize the possibility of vaginal delivery.

Women presenting with genital warts should be fully investigated to exclude other sexually transmitted infections. In addition, the cervix should be examined to exclude flat warts on the cervix, which may be associated with malignant changes. Because of the possible association between human papilloma virus (HPV) and cervical intracellular neoplasia (CIN), cytological screening is recommended for women with vulval or vaginal warts or those whose husbands have penile warts.

The treatment suggested during pregnancy includes trichloroacetic acid cryotherapy or electrocautery (Adler, 1995). Treatment with podophyllin 10 to 25 percent is recommended for nonpregnant women. In pregnancy, it is contraindicated because of its toxicity. If the warts are smaller, they may be left untreated until after delivery.

Acquired Immunodeficiency Syndrome (AIDS) in Pregnancy

Acquired immunodeficiency syndrome is caused by Human Immunodeficiency Virus (HIV), which is a group of retrovirus, HIV-1 and HIV-2. The virus specifically reduces the CD-4 receptor molecule of the T-lymphocytes, monocytes, macrophages and other antigen presenting cells leading to immunodeficiency. As a result, the individual is susceptible to infections by opportunistic microorganisms and specific tumors. The incubation period is from 2 months to 4 years. AIDS is the end stage of HIV infection.

Incidence in India

Estimate at the national level are that about 3.7 million people were suffering from HIV infection at the end of 1999. Serosurveillance findings from the states showed 98,451 persons positive for HIV by June 2000, a seropositivity rate of 26.88 per thousand (Park, 2000). The cumulative number of AIDS in the country has risen to 12,389 that include 2,632 females.

Mode of Transmission

The modes of transmission of HIV are:

* Sexual contact (homosexual or heterosexual)
* Transplacental
* Exposure to infected blood or tissue fluids
* Through breast milk.

HIV Infection in Pregnancy

The transmission from mother to fetus (vertical transmission) is about 30 percent in sero-positive mothers. The fetus may be affected through uteroplacental transfer, during delivery by contaminated secretions and blood of the birth canal and through breast milk in the neonatal period (Dutta, 2001).

Clinical Presentation

Initial presentation of an infected woman may be fever, malaise, headache, sore throat, lymphadenopathy and maculopapular rash. Primary illness may be followed by an asymptomatic period. Progression of the disease may lead to multiple opportunistic infections with candida, tuberculosis, pneumocystis and others. Patient may present with neoplasms such as cervical carcinoma, lymphomas (Hodgkin's and Non-Hodgkin's) and Kaposi's sarcoma. There may be associated constitutional symptoms like weight loss, lymphadenopathy or protracted diarrhea.

Diagnosis of HIV Infection

The diagnosis of asymptomatic adult HIV infection is made on the basis of the presence in serum of antibodies to the virus. Most individuals will produce antibodies (sero-coversion) within 3 months after the most recent exposure. During the so-called "window of infectivity" (3 months), a negative result will require a repeat test in order to account for the late sero-conversion.

Diagnostic HIV testing employs two tests. The ELISA (Enzyme-Linked Immunosorbent Assay) is highly sensitive to the presence of antibodies. Its sensitivity increases the possibility of false positive results and thus a 'Western blot' test, which has a greater specificity for HIV, is used to confirm the presence of the antibodies. A second specimen of blood may be tested to confirm the result.

Management

Prenatal care:

* All clients should be offered voluntary serologic testing for HIV infection.
* In seropositive cases, additional investigations should be done to test for other STDs. Husbands should be offered serologic testing for HIV.
* Counseling about the risk of HIV transmission to the fetus and neonates should be made and termination of pregnancy offered.
* Tuberculin test is to be done. If it is positive, a chest X-ray should be performed. Even if the chest X-ray is negative, chemoprophylaxis with isoniazid (INH) 300 mg orally daily should be administered.
* The woman should have T-lymphocyte count in each trimester. If the count falls to less than 200 cells/µL, the woman should be treated with zidovudine, the woman should receive prophylaxis against *Pneumocystis carinii* infection with trimethoprim 160 mg and sulphamethoxazole 800 mg orally thrice weekly. Nevirapine is found to reduce the viral transmission to breastfed infants (Dutta, 2001).
* The progression of the disease is assessed by CD-4 lymphocyte count (gradual fall), presence of P24 core antigen and decrease of titer of P24 antibody.

Care during Intrapartum Period

Cesarean section does not protect the baby from vertical transmission. It should only be for obstetric indications.

* Procedures that might result in break in the skin or mucous membrane of the baby such as amniotomy, attachment of scalp electrode, and fetal blood sampling (fetal scalp blood for pH) should be avoided.

❖ Health care workers should be protected from contact with potentially infected body fluids.

❖ Caps, waterproof gowns, double gloves and goggles (protective eye wear) should be worn by physicians and midwives.

❖ Disposable needles and syringes should be used and the needles should be placed in puncture proof containers.

❖ Mechanical suctioning devices should be used to remove secretions from the neonates' air passages.

❖ Any blood contamination must be washed off the skin immediately.

Postpartum Care

❖ Mothers must be counseled about the risks and benefits of breastfeeding and helped to make an informed choice.

❖ Zidovudine syrup 2 mg/kg is given to the neonate 4 times daily for first 6 weeks.

❖ Mother should be encouraged to manage the baby's care herself with the support of the midwife.

❖ Gloves must be worn for examining the perineum, lochia or cesarean wound.

❖ Disposal of sanitary napkins and disinfection and cleaning of any spilled blood must be done correctly (using recommended methods).

Contraception

Barrier methods of contraception are effective in preventing transmission of the virus. Simultaneous use of a spermicidal agent such as nonoxynol-9 is found to improve the efficacy.

Follow-up Care of the Baby

Babies born to HIV positive women will have passively acquired maternal antibodies to HIV and these may persist for as long as 18 months. Therefore, diagnosis of HIV cannot be achieved with antibody testing and confirmation of the infants infection status may not occur for an extended period. Parents must be counseled with regard to this period of uncertainty and doubt.

NURSING PROCESS FOR PREGNANT WOMEN WITH ACQUIRED IMMUNE DEFICIENCY SYNDROME

Assessment

Assess for the following clinical manifestations:

❖ History of IV drug use, prostitution or infection for spouse

❖ Malaise

❖ Progressive weight loss

❖ Lymphadenopathy

❖ Diarrhea

❖ Evidence of opportunistic infection

❖ Fever

❖ Evidence of Kaposi's sarcoma (purplish, reddish brown lesions)

❖ Anxiety about future of self and baby.

Analysis /Nursing Diagnosis

❖ Risk for fetal injury

❖ Risk for infection

❖ Ineffective airway clearance

❖ Actual/risk for aspiration

❖ Anxiety

❖ Anticipatory grieving

❖ Altered family processes

❖ Actual/risk for altered parenting

❖ Health seeking behavior.

Planning

❖ Protection from infection

❖ Isolation precautions

❖ Opportunities for counseling

❖ Education for selfcare regarding isolation precautions and prevention of infection.

Implementation

❖ Observe blood and body-secretion precautions

❖ Teach precautions to client

❖ Maintain isolation to prevent client from other organisms

❖ Follow blood and body fluid precautions during all contacts with expectant woman (antepartal, intrapartal, postpartal and for the newborn infant)

❖ Provide education regarding disease process and treatment.

Evaluation

Ensure that the expectant woman:

❖ Is protected from further infection
❖ Participates in maintaining blood and body secretion isolation
❖ Is able to verbalize feelings about her condition
❖ Verbalizes knowledge of disease condition.

BIBLIOGRAPHY

1. Abel E, von Unwerth L. Asymptomatic Chlamydia during Pregnancy. Research in Nursing and Health 1988;11(6):359-65.
2. Adler MW. The ABC of Sexually Transmitted Diseases, 5th edn. British Medical Journal, London, 1995.
3. Bell TA, Grayson JT. Centers for Disease Control; Guidelines for prevention and control of Chlamydia trachomatis infections. Annals of Internal Medicine 1986;104:524-6.
4. Brunham et al. Sexually transmitted diseases in pregnancy. In: Holmes KK, Mardh PA, et al. Sexually Transmitted Diseases, 2nd edn. New York: HcGraw Hall, 1999.
5. Erikson SH, et al. Metronidazole in breast milk", Obstetrics and Gynecology 1981;57:48-50.
6. Hankins CA, Handley MA. HIV diseases and AIDS in women. Journal of Acquired Immune Deficiency Syndrome. 1992;5(10):957-71.
7. Lossick JG. Sexually Transmitted Vaginitis". Seminars in Adolescent Medicine. 1986;2(2):131-42.
8. Park K. Park's Textbook of Preventive and Social Medicine, 16th edn. Jabalpur: M/s Banarasidas Banot Publishers, 2000.
9. Roth C. Sexually Transmissible and Reproductive Tract Infections in Pregnancy. In: Bennett RV, Linda KB. Myles Textbook for Midwives, 13th edn. Edinburgh: Churchill Livingstone, 1999.
10. Wang E, Smaill F. Infection in pregnancy. In: Chalmers J, et al, Effective Care in Pregnancy and Childbirth. Oxford: Oxford University Press, 1989.
11. WHO, Health for All Series, 1981.
12. WHO, World Health Report 1999; Report of the Director General, WHO.
13. www.unaids.org, Internet website.

27

Disorders of Pregnancy

Learning Objectives

Upon completing this chapter, the learner will be able to:

❖ Define antepartum hemorrhage and explain its causes and effects on mother and fetus
❖ Describe the role of the midwife in relation to the identification, assessement and management of clients with placenta previa and abruptio placentae
❖ Explain the disorders of amniotic fluid, their treatment and nursing care of patients admitted for management.

Medical disorders, associated with pregnancy, increase as women delay childbearing. They become more at risk with increasing age.

ANTEPARTUM HEMORRHAGE

Definition

Antepartum hemorrhage is defined as bleeding from the genital tract after 28th week of pregnancy and before the birth of the baby.

Types of Antepartum Hemorrhage

1. Placental bleeding
   a. Placenta previa
   b. Abruptio placentae
2. Extra placental bleeding
   Due to local cervicovaginal lesions

PLACENTA PREVIA

Definition

A low implantation of the placenta in the uterus causing it to lie alongside or in front of the presenting part.

Incidence

Placenta previa occurs approximately one of every 250 births. It is one in 200 in India. One-third of all antepartum hemorrhage occurs due to placenta previa.

Causes

The exact cause of implantation of the placenta in the lower segment is not known. Following are the postulated theories.

Dropping Down Theory

The fertilized ovum drops down to the lower uterine segment. Poor decidual reaction in the upper segment may be the cause.

Multiple Pregnancy

The large placental bed of the twin placenta is prone to low implantation of at least a part of the placenta.

Defective Decidua

This causes spreading of the chorionic villi over a wide area in the uterine wall encroaching on to the lower segment.

Degrees of Placenta Previa (Fig. 27.1)

Type 1: The lower margin of the placenta dips into the lower segment (lateral).

Type 2: The placenta reaches the internal os when closed, but does not cover it (Marginal).

Type 3: The placenta covers the internal os when closed, but not when fully dilated (partial or incomplete).

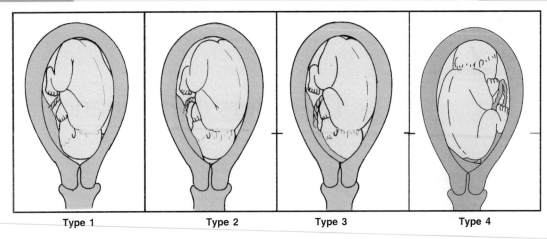

Fig. 27.1: Types of placenta previa

Type 4: The placenta completely covers the internal os even when the cervix is fully dilated (central or complete).

Predisposing Factors

❖ Increased placental size, e.g. twin placenta
❖ Previous uterine scar, e.g. previous cesarean or myomectomy scar
❖ Multiparity
❖ Advanced maternal age, over 35 years
❖ Previous reproductive surgery, e.g. dilatation and curretage *(D&C) 3x in the cervix*
❖ Placental abnormality, e.g. succenturiate lobe
❖ Leiomyomas distorting the uterine cavity
❖ Congenital malformations of the uterus.
  fibroids (Glyomyoma)

[handwritten left margin: Current — spoon like instrument; Removal of any material after miscarriage. Obtaining a endometrial biopsy]

Signs of Placenta Previa

❖ Painless vaginal bleeding in the third trimester of pregnancy
❖ The bleeding is usually bright red and the amount varies with the proportion of separation of placenta. Bleeding occurs as the lower segment of the uterus begins to pull upward with cervical effacement and dilatation in late pregnancy, causing the placental villi to tear away from the uterine wall *good and odor*
❖ The bleeding may be scant at first and then become more profuse as more and more of the placenta separates *bleeding from gum*
❖ There is no way that the bleeding from the placenta can be arrested other than delivering the fetus and complete removal of the placenta.

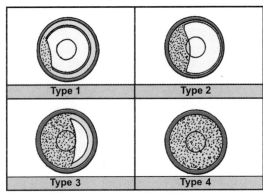

Fig. 27.2: Relationship of placenta previa to cervical os

Risk to Mother and Fetus

The mother is at risk for severe hemorrhage, embolism and endometritis. The fetus is at risk for prematurity, asphyxia or hemorrhage.

Diagnosis

❖ Clinical diagnosis is reached by an ultrasound examination in which the placenta is localized in relation to the cervix (Fig. 27.2).
❖ The placenta may be visualized by means of an examination with a sterile speculum. This should be done only with a "double set-up" with personnel and equipment available for immediate cesarean delivery, should a sudden hemorrhage occur.
❖ The midwife should not attempt to do a vaginal examination as this could precipitate severe hemorrhage.

Management

After a diagnosis of placenta previa is established by ultrasonography, the gestational age is calculated. Management depends on the gestation of pregnancy.

❖ If the gestational age is early, an attempt is made to prolong the pregnancy with the intention of optimizing the neonatal outcome. The woman is usually hospitalized to try and avoid preterm labor or hemorrhage

❖ Her mobility is usually restricted to bedrest at first

❖ Activity may be gradually increased as the pregnancy progresses to term

❖ The hemoglobin and hematocrit values are monitored

❖ Blood replacement therapy or iron therapy is instituted if anemia is present

❖ The pulmonary maturity of the fetus is monitored at appropriate intervals

❖ Unless an emergency situation arises, delivery is planned for some point after the fetus has reached 37 weeks gestation and lung maturity is assured.

A vaginal delivery would be considered only if the placenta previa were 1st degree or very marginal, the fetal head has descended low enough to act as a tampon placing pressure against the placenta, active labor has begun and no other complications were evident. Vaginal delivery would also be considered if the fetus were dead. In most situations however, surgical intervention is the delivery method of choice.

The women are at increased risk of postpartum hemorrhage because the lower uterine segment, where the placenta was attached, does not have the number of interlacing muscle fibers found in the upper portion of the uterus and thus is not as efficient in contraction to control bleeding in the early postpartum period.

Possible Complications

❖ Maternal shock resulting from blood loss and hypovolemia.

❖ Anesthetic and surgical complications in women with major placenta previa. Preparation for surgery may be suboptimal due to the urgency of the situation

❖ Placenta accreta in small percentage of women with placenta previa

❖ Air embolism when the sinuses in the placental bed have been broken

❖ Postpartum hemorrhage

❖ Puerperal sepsis

❖ Fetal hypoxia due to placental separation

❖ Fetomaternal hemorrhage and Rh-iso-immunization if the mother is Rh-negative and the fetus is Rh-positive

❖ Fetal death depends on gestation and amount of blood loss

❖ Maternal death—A very rare outcome.

SUMMARY OF NURSING PROCESS

Assessment

Assess for:

1. Painless unexplained vaginal bleeding after the 20th week (usually around week 27).
2. Intermittent gushes of blood.
3. Placental placement revealed by ultrasound.
4. Maternal apprehension caused by the bleeding episode.

Analysis/Nursing Diagnosis

1. Risk for fetal injury.
2. Risk for infection.
3. Ineffective airway clearance.
4. Actual/risk for aspiration.
5. Anxiety.
6. Anticipatory grieving.
7. Health promotion/maintenance.
8. Altered family process.
9. Actual/risk for altered parenting.
10. Health seeking behavior.

Planning

1. Monitor for bleeding episodes.
2. Monitor maternal and fetal status.
3. Provide opportunities for support and counseling.
4. Provide education for self-care.

Implementation

1. Do not perform vaginal or rectal examinations or give enemas.

2. Monitor FHR and prepare client for ultrasound test.
3. Facilitate 'double set-up', vaginal examination by the obstetrician
   a. Prepare for cesarean section before vaginal examination.
   b. Vaginal examination is done in operating room.
   c. Type and crossmatch for possible blood transfusion.
4. Manage bleeding episodes
   a. Keep woman NPO.
   b. Monitor vital signs and FHR (by continuous Electronic Fetal Monitor).
   c. Maintain woman on absolute bed rest.
   d. Start and/or maintain IV
   e. Maintain perineal pad count to estimate amount of bleeding (1 gm of weight is approximately 1 ml).
   f. Prepare for cesarean delivery.
   g. Maintain meticulous sterile techniques.
5. Support mother, spouse and family, and encourage them to verbalize feelings.
6. Provide parents information about the nature of problem.
7. Prepare women for vaginal birth, if pregnancy is near term, the cervix is favorable, and marginal placental placement is identified.

Evaluation

Ensure that the woman:
1. Maintains normal vital signs, Hct and hemoglobin.
2. Verbalizes her apprehension and feelings.
3. Demonstrates FHR between 120 to 160 bpm with average variability and no late or variable decelerations.

ABRUPTIO PLACENTAE

Definition

Abruptio placentae is defined as premature separation of a normally situated placenta after 28 weeks gestation and before birth of the baby.

Types of Placental Abruption

Revealed

Following separation of the placenta, the blood escapes from the placental site, separates the membranes from the uterine wall and drains through the vagina.

Concealed

The blood collects behind the separated placenta or between the membranes and decidua. The collected blood is prevented from coming out of the cervix by the presenting part, which presses on the lower segment. Sometimes it is retained behind the placenta and forced into the myometrium where it infiltrates between the muscle fibers of the uterus, resulting in a condition known as couvelaire uterus.

Mixed

In this type, some portion of the blood collects inside (concealed) and a portion is expelled out (revealed). Usually one type predominates the other.

Causes

The exact cause is unknown, but several factors have been considered as causes:
❖ Spasm of the uterine vessels followed by flooding into the choriodecidual space
❖ Malnutrition
❖ Folic acid deficiency
❖ Traction of short cord
❖ Trauma from external cephalic version.

Abruptio placentae is seen associated with the following conditions:
❖ Multiparity, 5th pregnancy and over
❖ Major congenital malformations
❖ Abruption in previous pregnancy
❖ Pregnancy induced hypertension.

Grading of Placental Abruption

Grade 1
❖ Mild separation of the placenta
❖ Slight vaginal bleeding and some uterine irritability are present. Maternal blood pressure is unaffected. Fibrinogen level is unaffected. The fetal heart rate is normal.

Grade 2
❖ Moderate separation of the placenta
❖ External bleeding is mild-to-moderate. The uterus is irritable. Tetanic contractions may be present. Maternal blood pressure may be normal. The fetal heart rate shows signs of distress. The maternal fibrinogen level is decreased.

Grade 3

❖ Severe separation of the placenta
❖ The bleeding may be severe and may be concealed. Uterine contractions are titanic and painful. Maternal hypotension may be present. The fibrinogen level is greatly reduced with resultant coagulation problems.

Signs and Symptoms

❖ Small to moderate amount of bright or dark red vaginal bleeding *bleeding.*
❖ Acute abdominal pain associated with vaginal bleeding → *severe & constant pain.*
❖ Uterine tenderness and high uterine tonicity often described as "board-like" abdomen
❖ Increase in the size of the uterus, particularly if the bleeding is concealed
❖ Failure of the uterus to relax between contractions
❖ Fetal heart sounds absent with concealed or mixed type
❖ Urine output usually diminished.

Diagnosis

❖ Ultrasonography to visualize the location of the placenta and presence of clot or hematoma
❖ Coagulation profile to rule out disseminated intravascular coagulation
  – Clotting time
  – Bleeding time
  – Fibrinogen level
  – Platelet count
  – Prothrombin and partial prothrombin time
  – Fibrin degradation products.
❖ Renal function tests.

Management

❖ Fluid and blood replacement
❖ Vaginal delivery if bleeding is minimal, the mother's condition is stable, the labor is progressing and the presenting part is in the pelvis. Labor may have to be augmented (induced) if it is not progressing well.
❖ Cesarean delivery if hemorrhage is severe, fetal heart tones are present, the presenting part is not in the pelvis, the cervix is closed or if it is anticipated that birth is not imminent.

If the fetus is dead, a cesarean section is performed only if the bleeding is life-threatening. A cesarean hysterectomy may be necessary if the bleeding cannot be controlled.

Possible Complications

❖ Severe shock may cause renal failure with first hematuria, then oliguria or anuria due to necrosis of the nephrons.
❖ Coagulation defect if not treated successfully can lead to catastrophic bleeding due to disseminated intravascular coagulation.
❖ Heavy blood loss and shock can cause pituitary necrosis leading to Sheehan's disease.
❖ Postpartum hemorrhage may occur as a result of the couvelaire uterus and disseminated intravascular coagulation.

Nursing Care

❖ All maternal and fetal vital signs should be monitored frequently and recorded carefully.
❖ The amount and nature of bleeding to be assessed and recorded.
❖ Contraction pattern and cervical status to be monitored if the woman is in active labor.
❖ Urinary output and skin color should be observed and recorded.
❖ The woman should be grouped and crossmatched for packed red blood cells.
❖ If the pain is extreme, an analgesic such as morphine is given, as pain can exacerbate shock, which must be avoided.
❖ An intravenous line must be set up with a 16-gauge intracatheter to administer plasma expander and blood. Blood is collected for investigations.
❖ A central venous line is usually inserted in order to monitor the central venous pressure two hourly or more frequently.
❖ Physical comfort and emotional support must be provided. The woman must be assisted to rest in left lateral position, which relieves occlusion of vena cava and compression of aorta by the gravid uterus.
❖ Fundal height and abdominal girth are to be measured hourly. An increase indicates continued bleeding behind the placenta.

❖ If the fetus is alive, the fetal heart rate should be monitored continuously and oxygen to be administered to relieve hypoxia. Once the woman's condition is stabilized cesarean section may be indicated.

❖ Observation must be made for any developing complication such as hypotension, hypovolemia, shock and DIC.

SUMMARY OF NURSING PROCESS

Assessment

Assess for the following clinical manifestations:

1. Scant or profuse vaginal bleeding.
2. Uterine irritability, tenderness and rigidity.
3. Abdominal pain that is intermittent or continuous.
4. Signs of maternal shock—hypotension, rapid pulse, dyspnoea.
5. Violent fetal activity followed by inactivity.
6. FHR—slow to absent.
7. Late deceleration noted in monitor strip.
8. May have blood stained amniotic fluid (port-wine stained).

Analysis /Nursing Diagnosis

1. Risk for fetal injury.
2. Risk for infection.
3. Ineffective airway clearance.
4. Actual/risk for aspiration.
5. Anxiety.
6. Anticipatory grieving.
7. Altered family processes.
8. Actual/risk for altered parenting.
9. Health seeking behavior.

Planning

1. Promote safe care environment.
2. Monitor for presence of pre-existing conditions.
3. Assess maternal-fetal status and initiate emergency care.
4. Provide encouragement and support.
5. Administer measures to treat shock and blood loss.

Implementation

1. Monitor maternal and fetal vital signs.
2. Treat shock symptoms.

❖ Assess vital signs every 5 to 15 minutes
❖ Administer oxygen by face mask at 7 to 10 L/min
❖ Increase IV flow rate
❖ Administer blood
❖ Monitor urinary output
❖ Monitor FHR continuously.

3. Observe for signs and systems of coagulation problems.
4. Measure abdominal girth.
5. Remain with woman.
6. Monitor labor pattern continuously if allowed to progress or prepare for cesarean section.

Evaluation

Ensure that:

1. The woman and her spouse understand the treatment plan.
2. The physiological status of the woman and the fetus remains within normal limits.
3. The woman and her spouse verbalizes, decrease of anxiety and feelings of support.
4. The woman remains normotensive.
5. The hemoglobin and hematocrit levels are within normal limits.

DISSEMINATED INTRAVASCULAR COAGULATION (DIC)

This is a condition of inappropriate coagulation within the blood vessels, which leads to the consumption of clotting factors. As a result clotting fails to occur at the bleeding site.

Etiology

DIC always occurs as a response to another disease process, it is never a primary disease. The response triggers widespread clotting with the formation of microthrombi throughout the circulation. Clotting factors get used up. The DIC triggers fibrinolysis and production of Fibrin degradation products. FDPs reduce the efficiency of normal clotting. A paradoxical feedback system is thus set up in which clotting is the primary problem, but hemorrhage is the predominant clinical finding.

When DIC occurs during or after delivery, the reduced level of clotting factors and the presence of FDPs prevent normal hemostasis at the placental site. FDPs inhibit myometrial action and prevent the uterine muscle from constricting the blood vessels in the normal way. Torrential bleeding may be the outcome. The lost blood may be observed to remain uncoagulated for several minutes and even when clotting does occur, the clot is unstable.

Microthrombi may cause circulatory obstruction in the small blood vessels. The effects of this vary from cyanosis of fingers and toes to cerebrovascular accidents and failure of organs such as the liver and kidneys.

Obstetric Conditions which may Precipitate DIC

Placental Abruption

In placental abruption, due to the damage of tissue at the placental site large quantities of thromboplastins are released into the circulation, which may cause DIC. If the placenta is delivered, as soon as possible after the abruption the risk of DIC is reduced.

Intrauterine Fetal Death

If a dead fetus is retained in uterus for more than 3 or 4 weeks, thromboplastins are released from the dead fetal tissue. These enter the maternal circulation and deplete clotting factors. If fetal death occurs and labor does not follow spontaneously, it should be induced. If fetal death is known to have occurred some time previously, clotting studies should be performed prior to induction of labor and if DIC is diagnosed, appropriate management must be instituted.

Amniotic Fluid Embolism

Thromboplastin in the amniotic fluid is responsible for setting off the cascade of clotting. If death does not occur from maternal collapse, DIC may develop.

Intrauterine Infection

The causes of infection in obstetric patients include septic abortion, chorioamnionitis, placenta accreta and endometrial infection before or after delivery. In such conditions, DIC is caused by endotoxins entering the circulation and damaging the blood vessels. Therefore, while treating the DIC, the infection itself must be treated aggressively with antibiotics. If the woman develops hemolytic septicemia, the bacteria in the blood-stream may destroy any blood administered. In postpartum infection, any retained products must be evacuated from the uterus.

Pre-eclampsia and Eclampsia

The factors which precipitate DIC in these patients is unclear, FDPs are seen increased in the serum and urine, which indicates fibrinolysis is taking place.

Management

In patients suspected of having DIC, blood investigations, such as blood grouping and cross-matching, clotting studies, platelets, fibrinogen and FDPs are done. Treatment involves the replacement of blood cells and clotting factors. Fresh frozen plasma and platelet concentrates are usually given. Whole blood may also be given.

Nursing Care

The midwife should be aware of the conditions in her patients, which may cause DIC. Her observation should include looking for signs of defective clotting and the nature of clot formation during the third stage of labor. Oozing from a venepuncture site or bleeding from the mucous membrane of the mother's mouth and nose during the third and fourth stage of labor must be noted and reported.

DIC is a frightening situation and an obstetric emergency. The nurse must be quick to recognize the signs and to take necessary action. She has to maintain her own calmness and clarity of thinking to deal with the situation. The patient, spouse and family need help to deal with the situation. Frequent and accurate observations must be made to monitor the mother's condition. This includes vital signs, fluid balance, and other parameters to assess the patient's general condition. The death of the mother is a real possibility and if the midwife finds herself in such a situation, supporting the bereaved family will be an important responsibility.

DISORDERS OF THE AMNIOTIC FLUID

Amniotic fluid normally increases in amount throughout pregnancy from a few milliliters to a liter at 38th week. The fluid is not static; the water and solutes in it are changed every few hours. There are two chief abnormalities of amniotic fluid—Ployhydramnios and oligohydramnios.

Polyhydramnios (Hydramnios)

Polyhydramnios is an excessive amount of amniotic fluid, which exceeds 1,500 ml. It occurs in 0.9 percent of pregnancies.

Causes

There is a higher incidence of polyhydramnios in women with the following conditions:

❖ Multiple pregnancy, especially with monozygotic twins
❖ Diabetes mellitus
❖ Erythroblastosis
❖ Fetal malformations, especially of the gastrointestinal tract and the central nervous system, e.g. anencephaly, meningomyelocele
❖ Esophageal atresia
❖ Chorioangioma, a rare tumor of the placenta.

Chronic polyhydramnios is gradual in onset, usually from about 30th week of pregnancy. This is the most common type.

Acute polyhydramnios is very rare. It occurs at about 20th week and comes on very suddenly. The uterus reaches the xiphisternum in about 3 or 4 days. It is often associated with monozygotic twins and or severe fetal abnormalities.

Signs and Symptoms

The signs and symptoms of polyhydramnios include the following:

❖ Uterine enlargement, abdominal girth and fundal height are far beyond that expected for gestational age

❖ Tenseness of the uterine wall making it difficult or impossible to
  – Auscultate fetal heart tones
  – Palpate the fetal outline and large and small parts.
❖ Elicitation of uterine fluid thrill (Fluid thrill may be elicited by placing a hand on one side of the abdomen and tapping the other side with the fingers).
❖ Mechanical problems such as:
  – Severe dyspnea
  – Lower extremity and vulvar edema
  – Pressure pains in the back, abdomen and thighs
  – Nausea and vomiting.
❖ Frequent change in fetal lie (unstable lie).
❖ Auscultation of the fetal heart is difficult because the quantity of fluid allows the fetus to move away from the stethoscope.

In women, suspected of having polyhydramnios, the following work-up are done to confirm the diagnosis:

❖ An ultrasound scanning (sonogram) to confirm the diagnosis and identify any coexisting conditions or complications
❖ Screening for diabetes
❖ Screening for ABO/Rh disease.

Complications

❖ Maternal ureteric obstruction
❖ Increased fetal mobility leading to unstable lie and malpresentation
❖ Cord presentation and prolapse
❖ Premature rupture of the membranes
❖ Placental abruption when the membranes rupture
❖ Premature labor
❖ Increased incidence of cesarean section
❖ Postpartum hemorrhage
❖ Raised perinatal mortality rate.

Management

Mild asymptomatic polyhdramnios is managed expectantly. The woman is not admitted. She is advised to get adequate rest. She should be advised that if she suspects that membranes have ruptured, immediate admission would be necessary.

For a woman with symptomatic polyhydramnios admission to a hospital is required. Care

Talipes — one or both feet can not stand with the sole of the foot flat on the ground.

CHAPTER 27: DISORDERS OF PREGNANCY

293

will depend on the condition of the woman and fetus, the cause and degree of hydramnios and the stage of pregnancy. Upright position will help to relieve dyspnea. Antacids may be prescribed to relieve heartburn and nausea. If the discomfort from the swollen abdomen is severe, amniocentesis or amnioreduction may be considered. Up to 500 ml of amniotic fluid may be removed to provide temporary relief. Fluid will accumulate again and there is risk of introducing infection with this procedure. Labor will be induced if the symptoms become worse or gross abnormality is diagnosed. For induction, the fetal lie must be corrected if it is not longitudinal. Membranes will be ruptured cautiously, allowing the amniotic fluid to drain out very slowly in order to avoid altering the lie and to prevent cord prolapse or placental abruption. Labor will be usually normal, but postpartum hemorrhage is a possibility. The baby will need to be examined for abnormalities.

Oligohydramnios

Oligohydramnios is an abnormally small amount of amniotic fluid. At term it may be 300 to 500 ml but the amount vary and it can be even less.

Causes

There is a higher incidence of oligohydramnios in women with the following conditions:

* Congenital anomalies, e.g. renal agenesis (absence of kidneys), Potter's syndrome (pulmonary hypoplasia in addition to renal agenesis)
* Early rupture of fetal membranes (24–26 weeks)
* Post mature pregnancy
* Intrauterine growth retardation due to placental insufficiency. Reduction in placental function causes inadequate perfusion of fetal organs including the kidneys. The decrease in fetal urine formation leads to oligohydramnios, as the major component of amniotic fluid is fetal urine.

Complications

Oligohydramnios may lead to the following further complications:
* Limb deformities, e.g. Talipes (club foot)

* A squashed looking face, flattening of the nose and micrognathia (small jaw)
* Dry, leathery skin.

Clinical Signs and Symptoms

These are because the amniotic fluid volume is below what is normally found for the particular gestational age.
* The uterus appears smaller than expected for the period of gestation
* Reduced fetal movements compared to previous normal pregnancies
* The uterus is small and compact and fetal parts are easily felt
* The fetus is not ballotable
* Auscultation is normal.

Amniotic fluid volume detection is done by ultrasonography.

Management

The woman will be admitted to the hospital. If ultrasound scan demonstrates renal agenesis, the baby will not survive. If agenesis is not present, placental function tests are performed. Where fetal anomalies are not considered lethal, amnioinfusion with normal saline or Ringer's lactate may be performed in order to prevent compression deformities and hypoplastic lung disease.

In women with oligohydramnios, labor may intervene or it may be induced because of the possibility of placental insufficiency. Epidural anesthesia may be indicated because uterine contractions are often unusually painful. Continuous fetal heart monitoring is essential because of the possibility of cord compression or placental insufficiency and resultant hypoxia. Constriction rings are a possibility owing to the small amount of amniotic fluid. In rare cases, the membranes may adhere to the fetus. Aspiration of amniotic fluid, which is more concentrated with meconium, may be an added danger to an asphyxiated baby when born.

SUMMARY OF NURSING PROCESS

Assessment

Assess for the following:
1. Ballottement results in fluid waves.
2. Fundal height excessive for gestation.

3. Fetus difficult to outline with palpation.
4. Supine hypotension.
5. Fetal abnormalities of central nervous system or GI tract.
6. Easy fatigability.

Analysis/Nursing Diagnosis

1. Risk for fetal injury.
2. Impaired physical mobility.
3. Actual/risk for fluid volume deficit.
4. Anxiety.
5. Anticipatory grieving.
6. Altered family process.
7. Actual/risk for altered parenting.
8. Health seeking behaviors.

Planning

1. Promote maternal comfort.
2. Promote maternal-fetal wellbeing.
3. Provide opportunities for counseling and support.
4. Provide education for selfcare measures in increasing comfort.

Implementation

1. Facilitate testing: amniocentesis, sonogram.
2. Assess FHR.
3. Anticipate premature labor and postpartum hemorrhage caused by over distention of the uterine muscle.

4. Instruct and explain:
   Nature of problem
   a. Need to obtain immediate medical attention for problems
   b. Need to observe for pre-eclampsia.

Evaluation

Ensure that the expectant mother
1. Verbalizes increased comfort.
2. Progresses to uneventful birth, as does her baby.
3. Verbalizes support.
4. Verbalizes self-care measures.

BIBLIOGRAPHY

1. Beare PG. Davis's NCLEX-RN Review, 3rd edn. Philadelphia; FA Davis Company, 2001.
2. Crafter H. Problems of Pregnancy, In: Myles Textbook for Midwives 13th edn. Edinburgh; Churchill Livingstone, 1999.
3. Dutta DC. Textbook of Obstetrics 5th edn. Calcutta; New Central Book Company, 2001.
4. Knuppet RA, Drukker JE. High Risk Pregnancy: A Team Approach: Phildelphia; WB Saunders, 1993.
5. Nicholas FN, Zwelling E. Maternal Newborn Nursing: Theory and Practice. Philadelphia; WB Saunders Co. 1997.
6. Varney Helen. Nurse-Midwifery, 2nd edn. Boston; Jones-Barlett Publishers, 1996.

28

Hypertensive Disorders of Pregnancy

Learning Objectives

Upon completion of this chapter, the learner should be able to:

❖ List the classifications of hypertensive disorders in pregnancy including the differentiating characteristics
❖ Describe the signs, symptoms and potential complications of hypertensive disorders
❖ Describe the management of different hypertensive disorders
❖ Outline the nursing care and support for clients with hypertensive disorders.

Hypertension is one of the common disorders of pregnancy and contributes significantly to the maternal and perinatal morbidity and mortality. Hypertension may appear for the first time during pregnancy as a direct result of the gravid state or as a sign of underlying pathology, which may be pre-existing.

Classification of Hypertension in Pregnancy

A. Pregnancy induced hypertension (PIH):
   1. With proteinuria and/or edema
      ❖ Pre-eclampsia
      ❖ Eclampsia.
   2. Without gross edema or proteinuria
      ❖ Gestational hypertension.
B. Chronic hypertension in pregnancy. Pregnancy is unrelated to the hypertensive state:
   1. Essential hypertension
   2. Renovascular hypertension
   3. Pheochromocytoma
   4. Coarctation of aorta
   5. Thyrotoxicosis
   6. Connective tissue disease—systemic lupus erythematosus.

C. Hypertension worsened by pregnancy:
   1. Superimposed pre-eclampsia
   2. Superimposed eclampsia.

PREGNANCY INDUCED HYPERTENSION

The hypertension develops as a direct result of the gravid state. The woman does not have a history of previous hypertension or evidence of it. The clinical types of PIH are:
❖ Pre-eclampsia
❖ Eclampsia and
❖ Gestational hypertension.

PRE-ECLAMPSIA

Definition

Pre-eclampsia is a multisystem disorder of unknown etiology characterized by development of hypertension to the extent of 140/90 mm Hg or more with proteinuria induced by pregnancy after the 20th week in a previously normotensive and nonproteinuric woman (International Society for Study of Hypertension in Pregnancy, 1988).

Incidence

About 5 to 8 percent of all pregnancies are complicated by hypertension and of these pre-eclampsia accounts for 80 percent (Llewellyn Jones, 1990). It occurs more frequently in young primigravidae and in mothers over 35 years of age. It is known to be associated with hydatidiform mole, multiple pregnancy and maternal diabetes.

Etiology

The exact nature of the primary event causing pregnancy-induced hypertension is not known.

The following are thought to be the possibilities:

1. There is a relative or absolute deficiency of vasodilator prostaglandin (PGI$_2$), synthesized in vascular endothelium and increased synthesis of thromboxane (TXA$_2$), a potent vasoconstrictor in platelets.
2. There is increased vascular sensitivity to the pressor agent angiotension-II. The sensitizing substances are yet to be explored.
3. Nitric oxide, which normally relaxes vascular smooth muscle, inhibits platelet aggregation and prevents intervillous thrombosis, is found deficient in preeclamptic clients. Hence, preeclampsia is characterized by complex endothelial cell dysfunction (Dutta, 2001).
4. In pre-eclampsia, trophoblastic invasion of the spiral arteries is thought to be inhibited by some immunological mechanism (Roberts and Redman, 1993).

The cause of excessive accumulation of fluids in the extracellular spaces is not clear. Excessive retention of sodium in the edematous state is probably due to the increased aldosterone out of activation of corticosterone by angiotensin-II. Diminished renal blood flow, decreased glomerular filtration rate and increased tubular reabsorption are responsible for retention of sodium.

The probable events that contribute to proteinuria are spasm of the afferent glomerular arterioles, anoxic damage to the endothelium of the glomerular tuft, increased capillary permeability and increased leakage of proteins. Tubular reabsorption is simultaneously depressed.

Pathophysiology

The pathological changes that occur in the various organs in severe preeclampsia and eclampsia are well documented.

* Uteroplacental bed: There is increased evidence of premature aging of the placenta. Areas of occasional acute infarcts are visible on the maternal surface of the placenta.
* There is acute atherosis of spiral arteries with obliteration of the lumen. Intervillous circulation is impaired to the extent of about one-third, secondary to changes in the maternal blood vessels. This results in placental changes, which are responsible for fetal jeopardy.
* In the kidneys, there is reduced blood flow and glomerular filtration rate and impaired tubular reabsorption or secretary functions.
* In the blood vessels, there is intense vasospasm. Circulation in the vaso vasorum is impaired leading to damage of the vascular walls including the endothelial integrity.
* Hemorrhagic necrosis occurs in the liver due to thrombosis of the arteriols. Hepatic insufficiency seldom occurs because of the reserve capacity and regenerative ability of the liver.

Clinical Classification of Pre-eclampsia

The clinical classification of pre-eclampsia is principally dependent on the level of blood pressure for management purpose.

Mild pre-eclampsia is diagnosed when there is sustained rise of blood pressure of more than 140/90 mm Hg but less than 160 systolic or 110 diastolic without significant proteinuria on two occasions six hours apart.

Severe pre-eclampsia is diagnosed when the blood pressure exceeds 160/100 mm Hg, when there is an increase in the proteinuria (75 gm per day) and where edema is marked. The woman may complain of frontal headaches, visual disturbances and upper abdominal pain with or without vomiting (imminent eclampsia). Reduced platelet count (less than 100,000), elevated liver enzymes, retinal hemorrhages or papilledema, pulmonary edema and intrauterine growth retardation of the fetus are also seen.

Clinical Features

* Pre-eclampsia frequently occurs in primigravidae (70%).
* It is often associated with obstetrical-medical complications, such as multiple pregnancy, polyhydramnios, preexisting hypertension, diabetes, etc.
* The clinical manifestations usually appear after the 20th week.
* The onset is usually insidious and the symptoms run a slow course. On rare occa-

sions, however, the onset becomes acute and follows a rapid course.

❖ Edema is seen in approximately 80 percent of women with preeclampsia. It may appear rather sudden and be associated with a rapid weight gain. Clinical edema may be mild or severe in nature and the severity is related to the worsening of the preeclampsia. The edema pits on pressure and may be found in the following anatomical areas—the face, hands, lower abdomen, vulva, sacral area, pretibial region, ankles and feet.

❖ Elevated blood pressure: More than 140/90 mm Hg in mild cases and above 160/110 mm Hg in severe preeclampsia.

Alarming Symptoms and Signs

The following symptoms and signs may be evident either singly or in combination. These are usually associated with acute onset of the syndrome.

❖ Headache over the occipital or frontal region

❖ Disturbed sleep

❖ Diminished urinary output (less than 500 ml in 24 hours)

❖ Epigastric pain associated with vomiting, at times coffee colored due to hemorrhagic gastritis or subcapsular hemorrhage in the liver

❖ Blurring or dimness of vision or at times complete blindness (vision is usually regained 4 to 6 hours following delivery)

❖ A rapid gain in weight of more than 2.5 kg (5 lbs) a month or more than 500 gm (1 lb) a week in the later months of pregnancy

❖ Visible edema over the ankles on rising from the bed in the morning. Sudden and generalized edema may indicate imminent eclampsia.

❖ Scanty liquor or growth retardation of the fetus.

Preeclampsia is principally a syndrome of signs and when symptoms appear it is usually late.

Effects on the Fetus

❖ Reduced placental function can result in low birth weight.

❖ There is an increased incidence of hypoxia in both the antenatal and intrapartum period.

❖ Placental abruption, if minor, will contribute to fetal hypoxia, if major, intrauterine death will occur.

❖ Early delivery, if the disease worsens, or if abruption occurs, which will produce a preterm baby requiring resuscitation.

Complications

Immediate

During pregnancy:

❖ Eclampsia 2 percent (more in acute cases)

❖ Placental abruption and intrauterine fetal death

❖ Oliguria and anuria

❖ Dimness of vision and blindness

❖ Preterm labor

❖ HELLP syndrome (Hemolytic anemia, Elevated Liver enzymes, Low Platelet count).

During labor:

❖ Eclampsia

❖ Postpartum hemorrhage—may be related with coagulation failure.

Puerperium:

❖ Eclampsia (usually occurs within 48 hours)

❖ Shock (related to reduced sodium and chloride)

❖ Sepsis (due to increased incidence of induction and operative delivery and low vitality).

Remote complications

❖ Residual hypertension: The hypertension may persist even after 6 months following delivery in about 50 percent of cases.

❖ Recurrent preeclampsia: There is 25 percent chance of preeclampsia to recur in subsequent pregnancies.

Preventive Measures

Preeclampsia is not a very preventable disease. However, some specific "high-risk" factors leading to preeclampsia may be identified in individuals. These are:

❖ Primigravida especially young and elderly

❖ Poor nutrition

- ❖ Low level of education
- ❖ Presence of complicating factors like pre-existing hypertension, twins, polyhydramnios, clinical or latent diabetes and nephritis
- ❖ History of preeclampsia or hypertension in the family or in previous pregnancy
- ❖ Abnormal weight gain
- ❖ Rising serum uric acid level.

The following regime is enforced in such patients in an attempt to prevent or to detect early manifestations of preeclampsia:

- ❖ Regular antenatal check-up at frequent intervals from the beginning of pregnancy to detect at the earliest, the rapid gain in weight or a tendency of rising blood pressure especially the diastolic pressure.
- ❖ Advice to take adequate rest in bed on her left side at least for two hours in the afternoon from the 20th week of pregnancy onwards.
- ❖ Low dose aspirin (60 mg) daily, beginning early in pregnancy to potentially high-risk women. It selectively reduces platelet thromboxane production.
- ❖ Calcium supplementation (2 gm per day) reduces the risk of preeclampsia.
- ❖ Antioxidants, vitamin C and E from 16 to 22 weeks onwards.
- ❖ Well balanced diet rich in protein.

Management and Nurse's Role

As the etiology of preeclampsia remains unclear the management is mostly empirical and symptomatic. Objectives of care are to:

- ❖ Provide rest and a tranquil environment
- ❖ Monitor the condition
- ❖ Prevent eclampsia and other complications
- ❖ Deliver a healthy baby in optimal time with minimum maternal morbidity.

Rest

The woman should be in bed preferably in left lateral position as much as possible to lessen the effects of vena caval compression. Rest is to be continued until all the preeclamptic manifestations subside. When proteinuria develops in addition to hypertension, the risks to the mother and fetus are considerably increased. Admission to the hospital is required at this stage to monitor and evaluate the maternal and fetal condition.

Rest increases the renal blood flow causing increased diuresis, increases the uterine blood flow causing improved placental perfusion and reduces the blood pressure.

Diet

As for any pregnant woman, a diet rich in protein, fiber and vitamins is recommended. Salt is neither restricted nor forced. Omission of salty food and extra salt in the dish is desirable. Fluids need not be restricted. Total calorie may be approximately 1,600 per day with about 100 gm proteins. There is some evidence to suggest that prophylactic fish oil in pregnancy may act as an antiplatelet agent, thereby preventing hypertension and proteinuric pre-eclampsia (Redman and Roberts, 1993). Calcium supplementation is also thought to be helpful as low serum calcium level is associated with hypertension.

Antihypertensive Therapy

Blood pressure usually comes down with adequate rest and sedatives. Antihypertensives have limited value in controlling the rise of blood pressure due to preeclampsia. They are used to prevent increase in blood pressure and the development of severe preeclampsia, especially when the diastolic pressure is over 110 mm Hg and when associated with proteinuria. The common oral drugs used are either methyldopa (aldomet) 0.5 to 2 gm/day or an adrenoreceptor antagonist (a and b blocker)—labetalol 200 mg six to eight hourly. If blood pressure is not under control, nifedipine, a calcium channel blocker 10 to 20 mg twice a day or hydralazine 25 mg twice daily are added.

Sedatives

Mild sedatives are given to reduce the emotional factor that contributes to elevation of blood pressure. Phenobarbitone 60 mg or diazepam 5 mg at bedtime or more frequently are given.

Laxative

If the woman is constipated, a mild laxative like milk of magnesia 4 teaspoons at bedtime may be given.

Abdominal Examination

Abdominal examination is to be carried-out daily for women admitted to the hospital. Any discomfort or tenderness must be recorded and reported to the physician immediately as this may be indicative of placental abruption. Upper abdominal pain is highly significant and indicative of the HELLP syndrome (Hemolysis, Elevated Liver enzymes and Low Platelet count).

Fetal Assessment

Assessment of the fetal wellbeing must be done by the use of kick charts, cardiotocograph monitoring and serial ultrasound scans.

Assessment of Treatment

The effect of treatment should be evaluated by maintaining records of:
- Blood pressure four times a day
- Status of edema and daily weight
- Fluid intake and urinary output
- Urine examination of protein daily
- Blood values of hematocrit, platelet count, uric acid, creatinine and liver function test once a week
- Ophthalmoscopic examination on admission and later as needed.

Favorable Signs

In favorable cases, there is fall of blood pressure and weight with subsidence of edema. Urinary output increases with diminishing protein-uria.

Treatment

The definitive treatment for preeclampsia is termination of pregnancy. The aim of treatment is to continue the pregnancy if possible, without affecting the maternal prognosis until the fetus becomes mature enough to survive in the extra-uterine environment. Thus, the duration of treatment depends on (1) severity of pre-eclampsia, (2) duration of pregnancy, and (3) response to treatment.

For those women who respond to treatment, if pregnancy is far from term the treatment is continued with weekly assessment. If the pregnancy is near term, the woman is kept in the hospital until completion of 37th week. Thereafter, a decision is taken either to terminate the pregnancy or to wait for spontaneous onset of labor by the due date.

For women whose blood pressure remains high, if the pregnancy is beyond 37 completed weeks, termination is considered. If less than 38 weeks, expectant treatment may be continued with careful monitoring of maternal and fetal wellbeing.

For those women who do not respond to treatment or develop additional symptoms, such as headache, epigastric pain and oliguria, termination of pregnancy is to be done irrespective of the period of gestation. Such patients may need prophylactic anticonvulsant therapy with magnesium sulphate. Methods of termination are (1) induction and (2) cesarean section.

Indications for Induction

- Aggravation of preeclamptic symptoms in spite of medical treatment
- Persistence of hypertension in spite of medical treatment with pregnancy reaching 38 weeks or more
- Acute fulminating pre-eclampsia irrespective of the period of gestation
- Tendency of pregnancy to overrun the expected date
- Recurrent preeclampsia with previous history of intrauterine fetal death.

If the cervix is ripe, surgical induction with low rupture of the membranes is the method of choice. Oxytocin infusion may be added to accelerate the process in selected cases. If the cervix is unripe and the termination is not urgent, intracervical prostaglandin gel (PGE_2) may be inserted to make the cervix ripe when low rupture of membranes can be performed. In severe pre-eclampsia, sedatives and antihypertensives are used during induction.

Indications for Cesarean Section

- Urgent termination is indicated but the cervix is unfavorable (unripe and closed) for surgical induction

❖ Severe preeclampsia with a tendency to prolong the induction delivery interval

❖ Associated complicating factors, such as elderly primigravida, contracted pelvis, malpresentation, etc.

Management of Labor

First Stage

The midwife should remain with the mother throughout the course of labor. Blood pressure tends to rise during labor and convulsions (intrapartum eclampsia) may occur. It is essential to document blood pressure and urinary output. Fluid balance should be monitored carefully. The patient should be in bed and sedatives (injection Pethidine) should be given at intervals. Marked deviations should be noted and medical assistance sought. The mother should be made as comfortable as possible by providing general nursing care.

Vital signs: Blood pressure and pulse are measured half hourly. Measurement of the mean arterial pressure (MAP) is recommended because of the hemodynamic changes in eclampsia. Respiratory rate and level of consciousness must be assessed periodically. Examination of the optic fundi can give an indication of cerebral edema. Cerebral irritability can be assessed by the degree of hyperreflexia or the presence of clonus.

Fluid balance: Intravenous fluids are administered using infusion pumps and the recommended infusion rate is 85 ml/h. Because of the reduced intravascular compartment in preeclampsia, poorly controlled fluid balance can result in circulatory overload, pulmonary edema, adult respiratory distress syndrome and ultimately death. A urinary catheter is inserted and urine output is measured hourly. A quantity about 30 ml/h reflects adequate perfusion. Urinalysis to detect the presence of protein, ketones and glucose is done four hourly.

Pain relief: Epidural analgesia may procure the best pain relief and reduce the blood pressure. If cesarean section should be done, epidural anesthesia is the best.

Fetal condition: The fetal heart rate should be monitored continuously and deviations from the normal must be reported and acted on.

Second Stage

When the second stage commences, the obstetrician and pediatrician should be notified. The midwife will continue to care for the mother. Duration of the second stage is usually shortened by the application of a forceps or ventouse. Depending on the blood pressure reading, the woman is sedated immediately following delivery of the baby with intramuscular morphine to prevent postpartum eclampsia. Usually blood pressure drops after delivery.

Third Stage

Ergometrine and syntometrine should not normally be used as they can cause peripheral vasoconstriction and increase blood pressure. In the presence of severe hemorrhage, Methergine intramuscularly or Syntocinon in the drip may be given.

Puerperium

The maternal condition should continue to be monitored at least every four hours for the next 48 hours, the period during which convulsions usually occur. Tab. Phenobarbitone 60 mg in repeated doses can produce effective sedation. Hypotensive drugs may be prescribed if the diastolic pressure is raised beyond 100 mm Hg. The woman is kept in the hospital, until the blood pressure reaches a safe level and proteinuria disappears.

Signs of Impending Eclampsia

The following signs and symptoms will alert the midwife to the onset of eclampsia:

❖ A sharp rise in blood pressure

❖ Diminished urinary output, which is due to acute vasospasm

❖ Increase in proteinuria

❖ Headache, which is usually severe, persistent and frontal in location

❖ Drowsiness or confusion due to cerebral edema

* Visual disturbances such as blurring of vision or flashing lights due to retinal edema
* Epigastric pain due to liver edema and impairment of liver function
* Nausea and vomiting.

The midwife should be alert to any of these and summon medical help immediately.

Acute Fulminant Pre-eclampsia

This is a clinical entity where the onset of pre-eclamptic manifestations is acute, occurring a new or there is rapid deterioration in an established case of pre-eclampsia over a short period. There is a constant threat of either convulsion or coma. All the features of pre-eclampsia generalized edema, raised blood pressure and proteinuria are intensified. Alarming symptoms such as headache, epigastric pain, visual disturbances, etc are evident either singly or in combination.

Treatment

Prophylactic anticonvulsant therapy with Magnesium sulphate is instituted immediately in dose and schedule as outlined in the treatment of eclampsia. Blood pressure is to be stabilized by antihypertensive drugs given parenterally (Aldomet, Labetalol or Hydralazine). Response to treatment should be carefully watched by noting the blood pressure, urinary output, proteinuria and hematological parameters at regular intervals.

Obstetric Management

In cases with pregnancy beyond 37th completed week or where the condition fails to improve within reasonable period (6–8 hours), delivery should be considered irrespective of the period gestation. Termination is done depending on the Bishops score, either by low rupture of the membranes aided by oxytocin infusion or by cesarean section.

HELLP Syndrome

The syndrome of hemolysis (H) elevated liver enzymes (EL) and low platelet count (LP) is a rare complication of PIH. The condition was first described by Weinstein in 1982. It is generally thought to represent a variant of the preeclampsia-eclampsia syndrome. This syndrome is manifested by nausea, vomiting, epigastric or right upper quadrant pain along with biochemical and hematological changes. It is observed in 10 to 15 percent of those with preeclampsia and eclampsia. Treatment is immediate delivery and management as that for acute fulminant preeclampsia.

Pregnancies complicated by HELLP syndrome have been associated with both poor maternal and poor fetal outcome. Serious maternal morbidity includes: Disseminated intravascular coagulation, acute renal failure, pulmonary edema, subcapsular liver hematoma and retinal detachment (Sibai et al, 1993). Infants whose mothers have the syndrome are often small for gestational age and at risk for perinatal asphyxia. The affected low birth weight babies have relatively high incidences of leukopenia, neutropenia and thrombocytopenia (Harms et al, 1995).

Diagnosis

The variety of signs and symptoms makes diagnosis difficult. Hypertension and proteinuria may be absent or slightly elevated. Upper abdominal pain is a common manifestation of the disorder, which should be investigated. Occasionally, the presence of this syndrome is associated with hypoglycemia leading to coma, severe hyponatremia and cortical blindness. Laboratory findings may show the following:

Hemolysis
* Abnormal blood picture
* Increased bilirubin (> 20 μmol/L)
* Increased lactic dehydrogenase (LDH > 600 IU/L)

Elevated Liver Enzymes
* Increased serum glutamic oxaloacetic transaminase (SGOT)/aspartate aminotransferase (AST) > 72 IU/L
* Increased lactic dehydrogenase (LDH) >600 IU/L.

Low Platelets
* Platelet count < 100,000/μL.

Complications

Subcapsular hemorrhage of the liver is a rare but potentially fatal complication of the HELLP syndrome. The condition usually presents with severe epigastric pain that may persist for several hours and in addition, the woman may complain of neck and shoulder pain.

Treatment

Women with HELLP syndrome should be admitted to a hospital with facilities for intensive care. In pregnancies less than 34 weeks' gestation, conservative treatment is given using plasma volume expanders and vasodilators.

In term pregnancies and where there is a deteriorating maternal or fetal condition, immediate delivery is recommended.

ECLAMPSIA

Pre-eclampsia when complicated with convulsion and/or coma is called eclampsia. The term eclampsia is derived from a Greek word meaning "like a flash of lightning". It may occur quite abruptly, without any warning manifestations. In majority (over 80%), the disease is preceded by features of severe pre-eclampsia. Thus, it may occur in women with pre-eclampsia or in women who have pre-eclampsia superimposed on essential hypertension or chronic nephritis.

Incidence

The incidence varies widely from country to country and even between different zones in the same country. In the developed countries, its prevalence is estimated to be around one in two thousand deliveries. In the developing countries, particularly in the rural areas, it contributes significantly to the maternal deaths. The hospital incidence in India ranges from one in five hundred to one in thirty. It is more common in primigravidae (75%), five times more common in twins than in singleton pregnancies and occurs between the 36th week and term in more than 50 percent (Dutta, 2001).

Pathophysiology

Since eclampsia is a severe form of pre-eclampsia, the histopathological and biochemical changes are similar although intensified than those of preeclampsia.

Onset of Convulsions

Convulsions occur more frequently beyond 36th week. On rare occasions, convulsion may occur in early months as in hydatidiform mole.

❖ *Antepartum (50%):* Fits occur before the onset of labor. More often, labor starts soon after and at times, it is impossible to differentiate it from intrapartum fits

❖ *Intrapartum (30%):* Fits occur for the first time during labor.

❖ *Postpartum (20%):* Fits occur for the first time in puerperium, usually within 48 hours of delivery.

Except on rare occasions, an eclamptic patient always shows previous manifestations of acute fulminating preeclampsia called premonitory symptoms.

Eclamptic Convulsions

The convulsions are epileptiform and consist of four stages:

Premonitory Stage

The patient becomes unconscious. There is twitching of the muscles of the face, tongue and limbs. Eyeballs roll or are turned to one side and become fixed. This stage lasts for about 30 seconds.

Tonic Stage

The whole body goes into a tonic spasm—The trunk opisthotonus, limbs are fixed and hands clenched. Respiration ceases and the tongue protrudes between the teeth. Cyanosis appears. Eyeballs become fixed. This lasts for about 30 seconds.

Clonic Stage

All the voluntary muscles undergo alternate contraction and relaxation. The twitchings start in the face and then involve one side of the extremities and ultimately the whole body is involved in the convulsion. Biting of the tongue occurs, breathing becomes stertorous and blood stained frothy secretions fill the mouth. Cyanosis gradually disappears. This stage lasts for 1-4 minutes.

Stage of Coma

Following the convulsion, the patient passes on to the stage of coma. It may last for a brief period or may persist until another convulsion. At times, the patient appears to be in a confused state following the fit and fails to remember the happenings. Rarely coma occurs without convulsion.

The fits usually are multiple, recurring at varying intervals. When it occurs in quick succession, it is called *status eclampticus*. Following convulsions, the temperature usually rises; pulse and respiration rates, and the blood pressure are also increased. The urinary output is markedly diminished, proteinuria is pronounced and the serum uric acid is raised.

Management

The patient, if at home or in the peripheral health centers, should be shifted urgently to the referral hospitals. The patient must be heavily sedated before moving her to the hospital. The aims of immediate management in the hospital are to:

❖ Clear and maintain the airway
❖ Prevent hypoxia
❖ Prevent injury
❖ Arrest convulsions
❖ Effect delivery in 6 to 8 hours.

The midwife must remain with the mother constantly. In the first instance, all effort is devoted to the preservation of the mother's life.

1. The patient should be placed in a railed cot in an isolated room, protected from noxious stimuli, which might provoke further fits. The patient is to be positioned in semiprone position in order to facilitate drainage of saliva and vomit. Side lying position helps to minimize vena caval compression. If the patient is unconscious, the position should be changed at intervals to prevent hypostatic pneumonia and bedsore. Airway is maintained and oxygen administered to prevent severe hypoxia.

2. Detailed history is to be taken from the relatives relevant to the diagnosis of eclampsia—Duration of pregnancy, number of fits and the medications administered outside.

3. After the patient is properly sedated, thorough but quick general, abdominal and vaginal examinations are done. A self-retaining catheter is introduced and the urine is tested for protein. Continuous drainage is established for measurement of the urinary output, periodic urinary analysis and for prevention of soiling of the bed due to incontinence, likely to occur during fits.

4. Vital signs check (pulse, respiration and blood pressure) is to be done half hourly and recorded. Progress of labor and fetal heart rate must be monitored. Urinary output is to be noted hourly.

5. Fluid balance: Crystalloid solution (Ringer's lactate) is started as a first choice. Total fluids should not exceed the previous 24 hours urinary output plus 1,000 ml (insensible loss through lungs and skin). Normally it should not exceed two liters in 24 hours. In preeclampsia and eclampsia, although there is hypovolemia, the tissues are over loaded.

6. Anticonvulsant therapy is given to control the fit and to prevent its recurrence. Magnesium sulphate is the drug of choice. It reduces motor end plate sensitivity to acetylcholine and thereby reduces neuromuscular irritability. Magnesium sulphate induces cerebral vasodilation, dilates uterine arteries and inhibits platelet activation. It has no detrimental effects on the neonate within therapeutic level.

Administration of Magnesium Sulfate
The regimens given below may vary between hospitals.

Prichard Regimen
Loading dose: 4 gm IV over 3 to 4 min. (20 ml of 20% solution), and then 10 gm deep IM.

Maintenance dose: 5 gm IM in alternate buttock 4 hourly (10 ml of 50% solution).

Zuspan Regimen
Loading dose: 4 gm IV over 5 to 10 min
Maintenance dose: 2 gm per hour IV infusion.

Sibai Regimen
Loading dose: 6 gm IV over 20 min
Maintenance dose: 2 gm per hour IV infusion.

Repeat injections are given only if the knee jerks are present, urine output exceeds 30 ml/hour and the respiration rate is more than 12 per minute. The therapeutic level of serum magnesium is 4 to 7 mEq/L. Magnesium sulfate is continued for 24 hours after the last seizure. For recurrence of fits, further 2 gm IV bolus is given over 5 minutes in the above regimens.

Magnesium sulfate is now the recommended drug of choice for routine anticonvulsant management of women with eclampsia rather than diazepam or phenytoin (Robson and Duley, 1996). Magnesium sulfate is superior to all other drugs because it does not depress maternal or fetal respiration within the therapeutic level. The mother remains conscious and hence cooperation in childbirth and nursing are easier. Complications of deep sedation and immobilization are avoided.

High levels of the drug can be toxic and therefore the patellar reflex and respiratory rate or oxygen saturation levels (pulse oxymetry) should be measured hourly. In women with oliguria, regular monitoring of serum magnesium level is necessary. Calcium gluconate is the antidote for magnesium toxicity and should be readily available.

7. Antihypertensives and diuretics: In spite of anticonvulsant and sedative regimen, if blood pressure remains more than 160/110 mm Hg, antihypertensive drugs are administered. Hydralazine 5 mg is given intravenously slowly and repeated after 20 minutes with 10 mg if there is no response. The blood pressure should be monitored every 5 minutes. Hydralazine is repeated whenever the diastolic pressure rises to 110 mm Hg. Alternatively, labetalol is given by slow intravenous route 20 mg per hour, for smooth control of blood pressure. Presence of pulmonary edema requires diuretics. In such cases, frusemide is administered in doses of 20 to 40 mg intravenously and repeated at intervals.

The Role of the Midwife

❖ The woman should be placed in a sound protected room to minimize auditory stimulation
❖ Eye pads to be applied to minimize optic stimulation
❖ The room should be well lighted so as not to miss development of cyanosis
❖ Bed railings to be padded in order to minimize physical injury during convulsion
❖ Patient to be placed in semi-prone position and the position to be changed every two hours if the patient is heavily sedated or in deep coma to avoid hypostatic pneumonia and bedsores
❖ Keep Foley's catheter in the urinary bladder and chart urinary output every hour
❖ Minimal handling and stimulation in order to reduce the risk of occurrence of another convulsion
❖ Maintain an intravenous line patent, preferably in a central vein
❖ Keep a tracheotomy tray available
❖ Apply a thromboelastic stocking to prevent deep vein thrombosis.

Management during a Fit

❖ In the premonitory state, a mouth gag is to be placed in between the teeth to prevent tongue bite and should be removed after the clonic phase is over
❖ The air passage is to be cleared off the mucus with a mucus sucker after convulsion
❖ The patient's head is to be turned to one side and the pillow taken off. Raising the foot end of the bed facilitates postural drainage of the upper respiratory tract
❖ Oxygen is to be given until cyanosis subsides.

The parameters to monitor are—a return to normal blood pressure, an increase in urinary output, a reduction in edema and a return to normal laboratory indices.

Complications of Eclampsia

❖ Injuries—Tongue bite, injuries due to falling out of bed
❖ Cardiovascular—Vasospasm, pulmonary embolism
❖ Renal—Oliguria, renal failure
❖ Hematological—Hypovolemia, hemoconcentration, thrombocytopenia, disseminated intravascular coagulation
❖ Neurological—Cerebral edema, cerebral hemorrhage
❖ Hepatic—Subcapsular hematoma, hepatic necrosis
❖ Respiratory—Pneumonia (aspiration, hypostatic or infective).
❖ Sensory—Disturbed vision due to retinal edema or detachment (usually reversible).
❖ Puerperal—Sepsis, psychosis
❖ Fetal—Placental abruption, intrauterine growth retardation, fetal distress, intrauterine death.

Mortality

Maternal mortality is very high in India and varies from 2 to 30 percent and more in rural hospitals. Causes for maternal death are: (1) Cardiac failure, (2) Pulmonary edema, (3) Aspiration and/or septic pneumonia, (4) Cerebral hemorrhage, (5) Anuria, (6) Pulmonary embolism, (7) Postpartum shock and (8) Puerperal sepsis.

Perinatal mortality is very high to the extent of about 30 to 50 percent. The causes are: (1) Prematurity, (2) Intrauterine asphyxia due to placental insufficiency, (3) Effects of drugs used to control convulsions and, (4) Trauma during operative delivery.

Prevention

In majority of cases, eclampsia is preceded by a severe preeclampsia. Hence, the prevention of eclampsia rests on early detection and effective institutional management with judicious termination of pregnancy. However, eclampsia can occur bypassing the preeclamptic state and as such, it is not always a preventable condition.

Adequate sedation and or prophylactic anticonvulsant therapy soon after delivery of the baby in pre-eclampsia and meticulous observation for 24 to 48 hours are definite steps to prevent postpartum eclampsia.

Future Management

There is no indication that pregnancy-induced hypertension causes later hypertensive disease, but it can leave an inherent disposition towards hypertension. Women with a history of pre-eclampsia before 32 weeks' gestation have a 5 percent risk of recurrence by this gestational age and 15 percent risk of recurrence overall.

Usually the blood pressure returns to normal within several weeks but the proteinuria may persist for a longer period. Six months after delivery, the obstetrician will examine the mother and if all is well, she will be advised to seek medical advice as soon as a subsequent pregnancy occurs.

SUMMARY OF NURSING PROCESS

Assessment

Assess for the following clinical manifestations of preeclampsia and eclampsia:
1. Edema
   ❖ Mild to moderate in preeclampsia
   ❖ Severe in face, hands and pretibial area in eclampsia.
2. Proteinuria
   ❖ Trace, 1+ to 2+ in preeclampsia
   ❖ Copious, 3+ to 4+ in eclampsia.
3. Weight gain
   ❖ 0.75 to 1.0 kg/week in preeclampsia
   ❖ Sudden large increase in eclampsia.
4. Blood pressure
   ❖ 140/90 to 160/110 mm Hg in preeclampsia
   ❖ Above 160/110 mm Hg in eclampsia.
5. Other symptoms
   ❖ Headache, blurred vision, epigastric pain and oliguria
   ❖ Tonic-clonic seizures, cyanosis and fetal distress in eclampsia.
6. Age and parity
   Occur more frequently in young primiparous women and multiparous women over 35 years.

7. Predisposing factors include:
   ❖ Inadequate protein intake
   ❖ Multiple pregnancies
   ❖ Hydatidiform mole
   ❖ Chronic renal and vascular disease.

Analysis/Nursing Diagnosis

1. Risk for fetal injury
2. Risk for infection
3. Ineffective airway clearance
4. Actual/risk for aspiration
5. Anxiety
6. Anticipatory grieving
7. Altered family processes
8. Actual/risk for altered parenting
9. Health seeking behavior.

Planning

1. Prevent progression of PIH to convulsions
2. Monitor maternal and fetal wellbeing
3. Provide counseling and support
4. Provide teaching related to diet, rest parental care and self-care activities.

Implementation

1. Facilitate early prenatal care
2. Assess physical parameters
   ❖ Blood pressure
   ❖ Weight
   ❖ Urine for protein
   ❖ Edema of face, hands and pretibial area
   ❖ Check reflexes for hyperreflexia.
3. Provide diet instructions
   ❖ Avoid added salt and high protein diet
   ❖ Maintain adequate fluid intake
   ❖ Ensure protein intake 1 gm/kg/day
   ❖ Maintain good prenatal nutrition.
4. Instruct regarding medications
   ❖ Antihypertensive drugs
   ❖ Sedatives.
5. Facilitate hospitalization, if required
6. Promote bed rest, rest on left side and quiet environment
7. Prevent convulsions
   ❖ Administer magnesium sulphate as prescribed
   ❖ Obtain $MgSO_4$ blood levels every 4 to 6 hours
   ❖ Monitor fetal heart rate

❖ Assess urine output, proteinuria, vital signs, reflexes and respiratory effort hourly
❖ Administer calcium gluconate for $MgSO_4$ overdose/toxicity
❖ Prepare for labor induction or cesarean birth
❖ Continue $MgSO_4$ for 24 hours after delivery.

Evaluation

Ensure that the expectant woman:
1. Complies with treatment regimen and does not develop eclampsia
2. Progresses to labor without further complications
3. Verbalizes support and increased coping ability
4. Verbalizes self-care measures.

GESTATIONAL HYPERTENSION

Gestational hypertension is a sustained rise of blood pressure to 140/90 mm Hg or more on at least two occasions, 4 or more hours apart beyond the 20th week of pregnancy or during the first 24 hours after delivery in a previously normotensive woman. It is associated with a much higher incidence of essential hypertension in later life than preeclampsia. Both are like the two phases of the same disorder. Essential features of this condition are:
❖ Absence of any evidence for the underlying cause of hypertension
❖ Unassociated with other evidences of preeclampsia such as edema or proteinuria
❖ The blood pressure returns to normal within 10 days following delivery.

The hypertension may be a stress response. Perinatal mortality remains unaffected. These patients are more likely to develop hypertension with the use of oral contraceptives or in subsequent pregnancies.

CHRONIC HYPERTENSION IN PREGNANCY

Chronic hypertensive disease is defined as the presence of hypertension of any cause before the 20th week of pregnancy in the absence of hydatidiform mole or is present long after delivery.

Chronic hypertension has two possible causes:

❖ It may be a long-term problem, present before the beginning of pregnancy, for example essential hypertension

❖ It may be secondary to existing medical problems such as
  – Renal disease
  – Systemic lupus erythematosus
  – Coarctation of the aorta
  – Cushing's syndrome
  – Pheochromocytoma (a rare tumor of the adrenal medulla).

Diagnosis

Consistent blood pressure recordings of 140/90 mm Hg or more on two occasions more than 24 hours apart during the first 20 weeks of pregnancy suggest that the hypertension is a chronic problem and unrelated to pregnancy. Women with chronic hypertension tend to be older, parous and have a family or personal history of hypertension. Serial blood pressure recordings should be made in order to determine the true pattern as even normotensive women show occasional peaks. Physical examination may reveal the long-term effects of hypertension, such as retinopathy, ischemic heart disease and renal damage.

Complications

The perinatal outcome in mild chronic hypertension is good. However, the perinatal morbidity and mortality are increased in those women who develop severe chronic hypertension or superimposed preeclampsia. Other complications are independent of pregnancy and include renal failure and cerebral hemorrhage. In 1 to 2 percent of cases, hypertensive encephalopathy may develop if the blood pressure suddenly rises above 250/150 mm Hg (Sibai, 1996).

ESSENTIAL HYPERTENSION IN PREGNANCY

Apart from the specific hypertensive disorder in pregnancy (PIH), essential hypertension is the commonest hypertensive state in pregnancy. Its incidence varies from 1 to 3 percent.

Diagnosis

The diagnostic criteria of essential hypertension are:

1. Rise of blood pressure to the extent of 140/90 mm Hg or more during pregnancy prior to the 20th week.
2. Persistence of blood pressure even after 3 months following delivery.
3. Common in multiparae and elderly women.
4. Presence of prepregnant hypertension and often family history.
5. Presence of hypertensive retinopathy.

Effects of Pregnancy on the Disease

1. There may be a midpregnancy fall of blood pressure in about 50 percent. However, the blood pressure tends to rise in the last trimester, which may or may not reach its previous level.
2. In about 50 percent, the blood pressure tends to rise progressively as pregnancy advances.
3. In about 20 percent, it is superimposed by preeclampsia.
4. Rarely, malignant hypertension supervenes.
5. In about 30 percent, there is permanent deterioration of the hypertension following delivery.

Risks to Mother and Fetus

In the milder form, the maternal risk remains unaltered but in the severe form or when superimposed by preeclampsia, the maternal risk is much increased. The babies are likely to be growth retarded due to chronic placental insufficiency. Perinatal loss is about 10 percent in the milder form with blood pressure less than 160/100 mm Hg. When the blood pressure exceeds 160/100 mm Hg, the perinatal loss doubles and when complicated by preeclampsia, it trebles (Dutta, 2001).

Management

In mild cases with blood pressure less than 160/100 mm Hg, adequate rest, low salt diet and a sedative (phenobarbitone 60 mg 1 to 3 times daily) are given. Weekly or more frequent check ups are needed up to 28 weeks and thereafter weekly.

In severe cases or in cases of superimposed preeclampsia, the patient should be hospitalized and placed in the treatment protocol as described under preeclampsia. Antihypertensive drugs are given only when the blood pressure is raised beyond 160/100 mm Hg because the diminished blood pressure may reduce the placental perfusion, which may be detrimental to the fetus. In cases where these drugs have been used before pregnancy, care is taken to adjust the dose during pregnancy, especially during midpregnancy, when the blood pressure tends to fall.

Spontaneous labor at term is awaited in mild cases. In severe or complicated cases, termination is done after 38 weeks by low rupture of membranes with or without oxytocin drip or by cesarean section. Prostaglandin gel (PGE_2) is used to make the cervix favorable before low rupture of membranes. Labor is managed in a manner similar to that of preeclampsia.

SUMMARY OF NURSING PROCESS FOR PREGNANT WOMEN WITH HYPERTENSION

Assessment

Assess for the following clinical manifestations.
1. Blood pressure elevation to 140/90 mm Hg if no pre-existing hypertension.
2. More frequent in older multiparae.

Planning

1. Monitor blood pressure on routine basis.
2. Promotion of maternal-fetal wellbeing.
3. Provide counseling and support.
4. Provide education for self-care.

Analysis/Nursing Diagnosis

1. Risk for fetal injury.
2. Risk for infection.
3. Ineffective airway clearance.
4. Actual/risk for aspiration.
5. Anxiety.
6. Anticipatory grieving.
7. Altered family processes.
8. Actual/risk for altered parenting.
9. Health seeking behavior.

Implementation

1. Assess blood pressure every 2 weeks for the first two trimesters, then weekly until delivery.
2. Assess weight, test urine for protein, indicating preeclampsia.
3. Administer and instruct regarding drug therapy antihypertensives.
4. Instruct regarding nature and progress of disease.
5. Encourage frequent rest periods.
6. Counsel to avoid undue stress.
7. Provide diet instructions
   - No added salt in diet
   - High protein
   - Maintain fluid intake
   - Routine prenatal nutrition.
8. Anticipate early vaginal or cesarean delivery.

Evaluation

Ensure that the expectant woman:
1. Remains normotensive.
2. Progresses to delivery with no further complications.
3. Verbalizes support.
4. Verbalizes knowledge of self-care measures, treatment regimen, balanced activity and rest, and information regarding medication.

BIBLIOGRAPHY

1. Chesley LC. Hypertensive Disorders in Pregnancy. New York: Appleton-Century Crofts 1978.
2. Chesley LC. Hypertensive Disorders in Pregnancy. Journal of Nurse-Midwifery 1985;30(2): 99-104l.
3. Duley L. Magnesium sulphate regimens for women with eclampsia. British Journal of Obstetrics and Gynecology 1996;103:103-5.
4. Dutta DC. Textbook of Obstetrics 5th edn. Calcutta: New Central Book Company 2001.
5. Harms K, Rath W, Herting E. Maternal hemolysis, elevated liver enzymes, low platelet count and neonatal outcome. American Journal of Perinatology 1995;12(1):1-6.
6. Hendricks CH, Brenner WE. Toxemia of Pregnancy: Relationship between fetal weight, fetal survival and maternal state. American Journal of Obstetrics and Gynecology 1971;109:225.

7. Llwellyn Jones D. Fundamentals of Obstetrics and Gynecology, Volume 1. Obstetrics, London: Faber and Faber 1990.

8. Lloyd C Lewis VM. Hypertensive disorders of pregnancy. In: Bennett R, Brown L. Myles (Eds). Textbook for Midwives 13th edn. Edinburgh: Churchill Livingstone 1999.

9. Redman CWG. Eclampsia still kills. British Medical Journal 296(6631):1209-10.

10. Roberts JM Redman CWG. Preeclampsia: More than pregnancy induced hypertension. Lancet June 5, 1993;341.

11. Robson SC. Magnesium sulfate: The time of reckoning. British Journal of Obstetrics and Gynecology February 1996;103.

12. Sibai BM. The HELLP Syndrome: Much ado about nothing? American Journal of Obstetrics and Gynecology 1990;162(2):311-6.

29

Medical Disorders Associated with Pregnancy

Learning Objectives

Upon completing this chapter, the learner will be able to:

❖ Outline the common medical disorders
❖ Describe the effects of different disorders on the woman and her fetus or the newborn
❖ Outline the management of women with different medical conditions during pregnancy and labor
❖ Describe the midwifery care and support required by the client and her family during pregnancy, labor and the postnatal period.

Pregnancy may be complicated by a variety of disorders and conditions that can profoundly affect the woman and her fetus. The disorders, which predate pregnancy, are important because of the way in which pregnancy affects them or the treatment for the disorders affects the pregnancy. Physical, social and psychological problems requiring nursing diagnosis and interventions are usually present.

CARDIAC DISEASE

The overall incidence of cardiac disease in pregnancy is falling in both the developed and developing parts of the world. It is less than one percent in hospital deliveries. The commonest cardiac lesion is of rheumatic origin followed by the congenital disorders. Adequate treatment for rheumatic fever with appropriate antibiotics with the advancement in cardiac surgery to rectify the congenital cardiac lesions, are responsible for the change in profile over the past two decades.

Rheumatic valvular lesion predominantly includes mitral stenosis. Predominant con-genital lesions include patent ductus arteriosus, aterial or ventricular septal defect, pulmonary stenosis, coarctation of aorta and Fallot's tetra-logy. Rare causes are hypertensive, syphilitic or coronary heart disease.

To manage pregnancy effectively in a woman with heart disease, the normal compen-satory changes in the cardiovascular system that occur during pregnancy must be under-stood. These normal responses are only detri-mental to the mother and fetus if heart disease is present (Nolan, 1990).

Changes in Cardiovascular Dynamics during Pregnancy and their Effects on Heart Lesion

In normal pregnancy, the cardiovascular dynamics alter in order to meet the increased demands of the fetoplacental unit. This increases the workload of the heart quite signi-ficantly. The major cardiac changes are:

❖ An increase in cardiac output by 30 to 50 percent
❖ An increase in blood volume by 20 to 40 percent
❖ A rise in stroke volume by 20 to 40 percent in early pregnancy
❖ A fall in the blood pressure in the second trimester.

These changes commence in early preg-nancy and gradually reach a maximum by the 30th week and maintained until term. Estrogens and prostaglandins are thought to be the mediators of the alterations in hemo-dynamics during pregnancy (deSwiet, 1995). A normal heart has enough reserve power so that the extra load can be tackled. A damaged heart with poor reserve may suffer cardiac failure eventually. Cardiac failure occurs during pregnancy around 30 weeks, during labor and mostly soon following delivery. Additional factors responsible for deterioration of function of the damaged heart are: (1) Advancing age, (2) Left ventricular hypertrophy, (3) Appearance of risk factors such as infection, anemia, pre-eclampsia excessive weight gain and multiple pregnancies, which further increase the cardiac load, (4) History of previous heart failure and, (5) Inadequate supervision.

Gradings

Depending upon the cardiac response to physical activity, heart diseases are graded according to the classification of the New York Heart Association.

Grade I
- Uncomplicated
  - Patients with cardiac disease but no limitation of physical activity

Grade II
- Slightly compromised
  - Patients with cardiac disease with slight limitation of physical activity. The patients are comfortable at rest but ordinary physical activity causes discomfort.

Grade III
- Markedly compromised
  - Patients with cardiac disease with marked limitation of activity. They are comfortable at rest, but discomfort occurs with less than ordinary activity.

Grade IV
- Severely compromised
  - Patients have discomfort even at rest (Benson, 1990).

Rheumatic Heart Disease

Valvular lesions predominate in rheumatic heart disease and constitute approximately 50 percent of all heart diseases seen in pregnancy (Nolan, 1990).

Mitral and Aortic Valve Incompetence

Pregnancy can be helpful in this case as it lowers the pressure in the arterial system, encouraging blood to flow the right way through the valves. There is however, a risk of endocarditis (Landon and Samuels, 1996).

Mitral Stenosis

As the demand for cardiac output rises in pregnancy, pressure in the left atrium rises. This may lead to back pressure in the pulmonary system and pulmonary edema. The left atrium being unable to cope with the demands made upon it begins to fibrillate and heart failure may occur (deSwiet, 1995).

Congenital Heart Disease

The most common congenital defects, which may remain uncorrected during the child-bearing years, are:
- Atrial septal defect
- Patent ductus arteriosus
- Ventricular septal defect.

All of these are openings, which allow communication between the right and left sides of the heart or, in the case of patent ductus arteriosus between the pulmonary artery and the aorta. Problems arise when pulmonary vascular resistance rises, as it does in pre-eclampsia, and blood flows from right to the left instead of passing through the lungs, leading to cyanosis. This may also happen in the third stage of labor when there is a sudden return of blood to the heart (Landon and Samuels, 1996).

Risk to Mother and Fetus

Structural defects of the heart whether congenital or acquired, predispose the women to bacterial endocarditis and thromboemboli. Expert attention from obstetricians and cardiologists is needed for them.

In Rheumatic Heart Disease (RHD), the maternal mortality is low and pregnancy does not affect long-term survival. The fetal outcome in RHD is usually good and little different from that in women who do not have heart disease. Maternal mortality is most likely in those conditions where pulmonary blood flow cannot be increased as in Eisenmenger's syndrome.

During pregnancy, fetuses of women with heart disease are generally growth retarded and fetal loss may be high. There is also increased incidence of congenital heart disease in children born to mothers who have CHD themselves.

Antenatal Care

Diagnosis

Diagnosis of cardiac disease in some women may only be made during antenatal visits. Breathlessness, fatigue, swollen ankles and palpitations may all be attributable to the normal changes associated with pregnancy, but if they were present before the pregnancy began, the woman must be referred to a cardiologist. Diagnosis will be made with the aid of the clinical picture, radiography, electrocardiography (ECG) and echocardiography.

Assessment

Where there is no cardiac lesion, no further follow-up will be required. Women who have mild lesions with no hemodynamic effect may continue the pregnancy, although prophylactic antibiotic cover in labor is recommended (de-Swiet, 1995). For those with a significant lesion with real or potential hemodynamic implications, the future of pregnancy needs to be considered and careful counseling given. If termination of pregnancy is decided upon, it is preferable that this should be done in the first trimester, as termination after 16 weeks' gestation is no safer than later delivery.

General Management

Principles

1. Early diagnosis and functional grading.
2. Detection and institution of effective therapy for cardiac failure.
3. Prevention and control of additional complications such as pulmonary hypertension.
4. Mandatory hospital delivery.

Preconception Care and Advice

Women who know that they have heart disease must seek advice from both cardiologist and an obstetrician before becoming pregnant so that the risks of her condition can be discussed. In some cases preconception surgery such as initial valvotomy may be advised (Shabetai, 1988). The woman should be helped to control obesity and choose a diet, which will prevent anemia in order to minimize risk. It is advisable that family size should be limited, as the risks increase with each pregnancy. Contraceptive advice is therefore an important aspect of management.

Place of Therapeutic Termination

Considering high maternal deaths, cases of primary pulmonary hypertension, Eisenmenger's syndrome and pulmonary veno-occlusive diseases are absolute indications for termination of pregnancy. The termination should be done within 12 weeks by suction evacuation or by conventional dilatation and evacuation.

Management

The aim of management is to maintain or improve the physical and psychological well-being of mother and fetus. This involves keeping a steady hemodynamic state and preventing complications. The major maternal complications are:

❖ Bacterial endocarditis
❖ Thromboemboli
❖ Cyanosis and
❖ Heart failure.

The risk factors for heart failure include:

❖ Infections, particularly urinary tract infection
❖ Hypertension
❖ Anemia
❖ Multiple pregnancy
❖ Obesity and
❖ Smoking.

The following advices are given to the women:

❖ Adequate rest—The women should have 10 hours rest in bed at night and 2 hours in the afternoon.
❖ Avoid undue strain and excitement—To limit the activities short of breathlessness.
❖ Avoid caffeine, alcohol, betamimetic drugs and high calorie or spicy diet—The diet should contain low salt, less carbohydrate, caffeine, alcohol and fat but more protein.
❖ Anemia is to be corrected by appropriate therapy.
❖ Cold and infections are to be avoided as they might precipitate heart failure. Intramuscular injections of penidure 12 LA (benzathine penicillin) may be given at intervals of 4 weeks throughout pregnancy

and puerperium to prevent recurrence of rheumatic fever (Dutta, 2001).

❖ Adequate dental care and care for such other potential sources of infection—Dental extraction if necessary, should be carried out with antibiotic cover to eliminate sources of sepsis and reduce the risk of endocarditis (Shabetai, 1988).

Hospitalization

Elective admission is recommended for:

Grade I: At least two weeks prior the expected date of delivery

Grade II: At 28th week especially in case of unfavorable social surroundings

Grade III and IV: As soon as pregnancy is diagnosed, the woman should be kept in the hospital throughout pregnancy.

Intrapartum Care

The First Stage of Labor

The least stressful labor for a woman with cardiac disease will be spontaneous in onset and vaginal delivery. In addition to the obstetrician, the cardiologist, anesthetist and pediatrician must be informed when the woman goes into labor.

❖ The woman should be confined to bed and be placed in lateral recumbent position to minimize aortocaval pressure by the gravid uterus

❖ Oxygen and resuscitation equipment must be ready and functioning. Oxygen to be administered at 5-6 L/min as and when required

❖ In the majority, analgesia is best given by epidural anesthesia

❖ Intravenous fluids should be given cautiously. As a rule, the quantity of infused fluid should not be more than 75 ml/hour to prevent pulmonary edema

❖ Observation of pulse and respiratory rate should be made every 15 minutes. If the pulse rate exceeds 110 per minute between uterine contractions, rapid digitalization is done by intravenous digoxin 0.5 mg

❖ Cardiac monitoring (ECG) and pulse oxymetry are done to detect arrhythmias and hypoxemia early. Deviations such as breathlessness and tachycardia should be reported immediately

❖ Prophylactic antibiotics are given during labor and for 48 hours after delivery, as these women are at increased risk from endocarditis (deSwiet, 1995). The recommended regimens include intravenous ampicillin 2 gm and gentamicin 1.5 mg/kg (not to exceed 80 mg), at the onset, followed by repeat doses at 8 hours interval.

Women with heart disease usually have quite rapid, uncomplicated labors. The midwife should help the woman to use the techniques that she has learned for coping with stress, as she is likely to be very anxious. The mother will need encouragement to a position in which she is comfortable (lateral) and must be informed that supine position may result in marked hypotension and maternal and fetal distress. Positions such as the lithotomy position in which the feet are higher than the trunk are best avoided because of the risk of acute heart failure resulting from the sudden increase of venous return to the heart.

The place of induction: Labor is not usually induced for uncomplicated heart disease. It is only considered safe if the benefits outweigh the disadvantages. If it is necessary to induce labor, the use of prostaglandins is advocated, but with caution as they are potent vasodilators and cause a marked rise in cardiac output (Willis et al, 1987).

ergometrin → vasoconstrict

The Second Stage of Labor

This should be short and without undue exertion on the part of the mother. Prolonged pushing withheld breath such as the Valsalva maneuver may be dangerous for a woman with heart disease. It raises the intrathoracic pressure, pushes blood out of the thorax and impedes venous return, with the result that cardiac output falls. Midwives need to suggest to the woman that she avoids holding her breath and follows her natural desire to push, giving several short pushes during each contraction. In this way, she will also avoid facial petechiae and subconjunctival hemorrhages. Any tendency to delay in the second stage of labor is to be curtailed by forceps or ventouse under pudental and/or perineal block anesthesia. Ventouse is preferred to forceps as it can be applied without putting the woman in lithotomy position. Some obstetricians advocate delivery in the left lateral position.

The Third Stage of Labor

 Conventional management is to be followed. No ergot containing preparations should be used for the third stage of labor as it causes a tonic contraction, which returns 300 to 500 ml of blood to the venous system. If the blood loss is excess, syntocinon may be used as it has less effect on blood vessels than ergometrine. If the woman is in heart failure, oxytocics should be avoided. If syntocinon is required, it is to be given by infusion accompanied by intravenous frusemide to prevent pulmonary edema (deSwiet, 1995).

The Place of Cesarean Section

In general, there is no indication of cesarean section for heart disease. However, in coarctation of aorta, elective cesarean section is indicated to prevent rupture of the aorta or cerebral aneurysm. The anesthesia should be epidural (preferred) or general.

The Puerperium

During the first 48 hours following delivery, the heart must cope with the extra blood from the uterine circulation and it is important to monitor the woman's condition closely during this time.

❖ She should be in absolute bedrest in a position comfortable to her. Intramuscular injection of morphine is given following delivery. Oxygen is administered either continuously or intermittently as required.
❖ Pulse and respirations are recorded hourly and temperature four hourly.
❖ Puerperal fever of any origin should be dealt with seriously by appropriate antibiotic therapy.

❖ Breastfeeding is not contraindicated unless the woman is in heart failure. The baby needs to be examined carefully for any sign of hereditary heart disease.
❖ The woman should be kept in the hospital for at least two weeks. In the first week, she should be confined to bed and allowed to move her limbs and to have breathing exercises. After a week, if everything is normal, she may be allowed to be out of bed.
❖ The woman may need advice to choose a suitable method of contraception. Steroidal preparations are contraindicated as it may precipitate thromboembolic phenomenon. Intrauterine device is contraindicated due to the risk of infection, which may lead to endocarditis. Barrier method of contraception (condom) is the best recommendation. Sterilization if chosen with the completion of the family, is usually delayed for 2 to 3 months after delivery. If the heart is not well compensated, the husband is advised for vasectomy.
❖ On her return home, the woman may need extra help in the house and may need to arrange for it.

SUMMARY OF NURSING PROCESS

Assessment

Assess for the following clinical manifestations:
1. Pedal edema, progressive generalized edema.
2. Dyspnea on exertion.
3. Moist cough.
4. Tachycardia, irregular pulse.
5. Increasing fatigue.
6. Cyanosis of lips and nail beds.
7. Heart murmurs.
8. Severe/persistent fungal infections (Candida, etc.).
9. Frustration as activity level is reduced.
10. Anxiety associated with fear of fetal and maternal demise.

Analysis/Nursing Diagnosis
1. Risk for fetal injury
2. Risk for infection

3. Ineffective airway clearance
4. Actual/risk for aspiration
5. Anxiety
6. Anticipatory grieving
7. Altered family processes
8. Actual/risk for altered parenting
9. Health seeking behavior

Planning

1. Protection from infection.
2. Promotion of graded activity with periods of rest.
3. Promotion of client acceptance of need for activity restriction.
4. Promotion and maintenance of health.
5. Education for self-care.

Implementation

If no symptoms with physical activity:
1. Additional evening rest.
2. Early treatment of infections.

If comfortable at rest and with symptoms during ordinary physical activity:
1. Avoid strenuous activity.
2. Administer prophylactic digitalis, diuretics and antibiotics.
3. Encourage frequent rest periods.
4. Anticipate forceps assisted vaginal delivery.

If comfortable at rest with symptoms during less than ordinary activity:
1. Reduce physical activity.
2. Avoid emotional stress.
3. Administer digitalis, diuretics and penicillin.
4. Facilitate early hospitalization and delivery.
5. Anticipate recommendation of early therapeutic abortion.

If symptoms present at rest:
1. Anticipate recommendation of early therapeutic abortion (50% mortality associated with delivery).
2. Administer penicillin, digitalis, diuretics and rotating tourniquets.
3. Prepare for vaginal delivery.

Evaluation

Ensure that the woman:
1. Remains free of infection.
2. Follows activity and rest recommendations.
3. Monitors her physical response to activity.
4. Participates in selfcare activities.

RESPIRATORY DISORDERS

Pulmonary Tuberculosis

The incidence of tuberculosis with pregnancy ranges between 1 to 2 percent amongst the hospital deliveries in the tropics, being confined predominantly to the underprivileged sectors of society. Incidence of tuberculosis is rising worldwide with the increasing prevalence of HIV patients (Dutta, 2001).

Effects on the Woman

The onset of tuberculosis is often insidious, producing night sweats, weight loss, anorexia, coughing, purulent sputum, hemoptysis, low-grade fever and malaise. The overall effect of this is to debilitate the woman, making her less able to cope with pregnancy and her existing family.

The disease may be pre-existing or the diagnosis may be made for the first time during pregnancy. The disease may be found in the quiescent or active phase. If the patient remains under medical supervision with adequate care and treatment during pregnancy, no deleterious effect may be seen on the course of the disease, nor has the disease any adverse effect on the course of pregnancy. In active disease, fetus can be affected by transplacental route or by aspiration of amniotic fluid. Neonatal infection is mainly by postpartum maternal contact.

Management

The woman will be under the care of an obstetrician and chest physician during her pregnancy. If the disease is in the inactive or quiescent phase, periodic chest X-rays must be taken after 12 weeks and repeated at 3 monthly intervals during pregnancy and one after a month following delivery.

If the disease is in the active phase, anti-tubercular therapy is to be started and continued for at least six months following delivery or until the disease is arrested. Initial treatment includes isoniazid 300 mg per day with rifampicin 600 mg per day, both given orally for 9 months. Ethambutol 15 mg/kg/day orally is added if isoniazid resistance is suspected. Pyridoxine 50 mg per day is given routinely.

None of the drugs used is teratogenic in human. *Streptomycin* is ototoxic and is avoided. Rest, both physical and emotional and hospitalization in advanced cases is necessary.

Antenatal Care

Antenatal care is to be carried out rigidly to minimize complications like anemia or pre-eclampsia. The woman should be admitted at least two weeks prior to the expected date of delivery. If the woman is infectious, she should be in a single room. Help of a social worker will be required if she has financial and domestic difficulties. Dietary counseling to improve the nutritional status will be required.

Intrapartum Care

Problems in labor stem from fatigue and reduced lung function. Hence, the woman is kept in bed and nourishment maintained to avoid fatigue. For sedation, pethidine 75 to 100 mg may be given intramuscularly. Episiotomies and forceps or ventouse delivery are advocated to reduce the strain of the second stage. Blood loss in the third stage should be minimized by giving prophylactic methergine 0.2 mg intravenously following the delivery of the anterior shoulder.

Postnatal Care

Adequate rest and good sleep are to be assured. Antituberculous therapy is to be repeated after one month of delivery. The baby is to be vaccinated with isoniazid resistant BCG whilst being protected from the disease by the use of prophylactic isoniazid syrup 20 mg/kg/day for 3 months. The vaccine becomes effective in 3 to 6 weeks as shown by a positive Mantoux test. If the mother has an active lesion or any of the baby's family is infected, the baby is to be separated until the baby becomes Mantoux positive.

Breastfeeding is not contraindicated with inactive or quiescent tuberculosis, if she wishes. In active lesion, however, not only is breastfeeding contraindicated but also the baby is to be separated promptly from the mother following delivery. However, if the mother has been on effective chemotherapy for at least two weeks, there is no need to isolate the baby. Mothers taking antitubercular therapy should be encouraged to breastfeed since the infant will receive a maximum of 20 percent of the normal infant dose by this route (Snider, 1984).

Caring for the baby at home makes great demands on the woman. Midwives should advice the woman and her spouse to arrange for extra help if possible. They must be explained that poor nutrition, stress and overtiredness will encourage a recurrence of active disease.

Contraception

Pregnancy is to be avoided until the disease has been quiescent for at least two years. When choosing a method of contraception, the woman needs to be aware that rifampicin reduces the effectiveness of oral contraception. Puerperal sterilization should be seriously considered, if the family is completed. Long-term medical follow-up is necessary in order to provide adequate help.

DIABETES MELLITUS

Carbohydrate Metabolism in Pregnancy

The fetus obtains glucose from its mother via the placenta by a process of facilitated diffusion (Smith, 1995). From 10th week of pregnancy, there is a progressive fall in the maternal fasting glucose level. During the third trimester, the mother begins to utilize fat stores, which were laid down during the first two trimesters. This results in a rise in free fatty acids and glycerol in the blood stream and the woman will become ketotic more easily (deSwiet, 1995).

The fetoplacental unit alters the mothers' carbohydrate metabolism in order to make glucose more readily available. The placenta manufactures human placental lactogen (HPL), which produces a resistance to insulin in the maternal tissues. These result in blood glucose levels, which are higher after meals and remain raised for longer than in the nonpregnant state. Estrogen and progesterone contribute to these changes and at the end of pregnancy cortisol levels rise, which also leads to rise in blood glucose.

More insulin is produced, sometimes two or three times as much as in the nonpregnant state (Oates and Beischer, 1987). The extra demands on the pancreatic beta cells can precipitate glucose intolerance or overt diabetes in women whose capacity for producing insulin was only just adequate prior to pregnancy. If a mother was already diabetic before pregnancy, her insulin needs will be increased (Landon, 1996).

Glycosuria in Pregnancy

During each antenatal visit, urine is examined as a routine for the presence of glucose. Repeat and random samples taken on one or more occasions throughout pregnancy reveal glycosuria in about 5 to 50 percent cases. Significant disturbances in carbohydrate metabolism occur in about one percent of pregnancies and the incidence of overt diabetes is about one in three hundred pregnancies (Dutta, 2001).

Causes of Glycosuria in Pregnancy

* *Renal glycosuria:* During pregnancy, renal threshold is diminished due to the combined effect of increased glomerular filtration and impaired tubular reabsorption of glucose. It is present more commonly in mid-pregnancy. If glucose tolerance test is done, glucose leaks out into the urine even though the blood sugar level is well below 180 mg per ml (normal renal threshold). No treatment is required and the condition disappears after delivery.

* *Increased glomerular filtration rate*: The glomerular filtration rate rises during pregnancy and glucose passes through the proximal convoluted tubule faster than it can be reabsorbed.

* *Impaired glucose tolerance*: During pregnancy there is accelerated absorption of glucose from the alimentary tract and delayed utilization of glucose to form liver glycogen due to anti-insulin activity. These indicate that pregnancy has a diabetogenic effect which results in glycosuria in small but distinct group of cases especially in later months.

* *Renal tubular damage:* This interferes with glucose reabsorption and may be revealed for the first time during pregnancy.

Glycosuria in pregnancy is not diagnostic of diabetes nor it can be used as a monitor of diabetes in the pregnant woman. Two episodes, however, are regarded as an indication for a glucose tolerance test (Jowett and Nichol, 1986). Glycosuria occurring any time during pregnancy with a positive family history of diabetes or past history of having a baby weighing 4 kg or more should be similarly investigated.

Gestational Diabetes

The term includes cases with abnormal carbohydrate tolerance with onset or first detected during the present pregnancy. The entity does not present until late in the second or during the third trimester. Women who are at special risk of developing gestational diabetes may be identified when the history reveals one or more of the following:

* Diabetes in a first degree relative (parents or sibling)
* Recurrent abortion
* Unexplained stillbirth
* Congenital abnormality
* A baby whose birth weight was 4 kg or more at 40 weeks
* Previous gestational diabetes or impaired glucose tolerance
* Persistent glycosuria
* Age over 30
* Obesity.

The progressive increase in insulin demand during pregnancy can make latent diabetes appear. This may resolve after the pregnancy.

Detection of Diabetes in Pregnancy

Women considered to be at risk of gestational diabetes undergo a glucose tolerance test. This will indicate whether they have normal or impaired glucose tolerance, or have developed diabetes. Before proceeding to a full glucose tolerance test, a fasting blood sample may be examined for glucose.

The methods employed for glucose tolerance tests vary slightly but the aim is always to assess the baby's response to a glucose load. The woman is asked to fast for a period time. The fasting blood glucose level is estimated and the woman is given a measured amount of glucose in the form of a drink such as Lucozade 265 ml, which provides 75 mg glucose. Blood samples are obtained at intervals for glucose estimation and the results compared with a normal range. The blood glucose level will rise initially but should return to normal within a given length of time. It would be considered abnormal if, between 28 and 34 weeks of pregnancy, glucose levels in two out of four venous samples exceeded the following:

- Fasting   90 mg
- One hour after ingestion of
  75 gm of glucose   165 mg
- Two hours after ingestion of
  75 gm of glucose   145 mg
- Three hours after ingestion of
  75 gm glucose.   125 mg

Effects of Diabetes on Pregnancy

When diabetes is well controlled, its effect on pregnancy is minimal. If the control is inadequate, there may be complications.

- Fertility is reduced and should conception occur, there is increased risk of spontaneous abortion and stillbirth.
- Increased incidence of macrosomia and birth trauma
- Perinatal mortality rate among infants of diabetic mothers is markedly increased
- More prone to urinary tract infections and a greater susceptibility to *Candida albicans*
- The incidence of preeclampsia and poly-hydramnios is increased.

Effect of Pregnancy on Diabetes

In the early stages of pregnancy, diabetic control may be complicated by nausea and vomiting. As the fetus grows, the mother needs more carbohydrate and ketosis is induced more easily, particularly in later stages of pregnancy. The diabetic, who is controlled by diet may become dependent on insulin. Women who have had diabetes since childhood and already have nephropathy or retinopathy must be monitored carefully for signs of any deterioration of their condition (deSwiet, 1995).

Effects on the Fetus

The effect of uncontrolled diabetes on pregnancy is due to disturbed maternal metabolism. Severe maternal ketosis can cause *intrauterine death*. Fetal blood glucose is similar to that of the mother and it is thought that congenital abnormality is caused by fetal hyperglycemia during the first trimester of pregnancy. No particular congenital abnormality is typical but the rare combination of sacral agenesis and neurological defects are most often seen in babies of diabetic mothers. Neural tubes defects are twice as common amongst babies of diabetic mothers and defects in the kidney and heart are seen (Hollingsworth and Resnik, 1988).

Glycosylated hemoglobin (hemoglobin bound to glucose) releases oxygen poorly to the fetus and this may lead to *intrauterine growth retardation*. A compensatory fetal polycythemia develops and may result in neonatal jaundice when the excess red cells are broken down (Roberton, 1992).

This is exacerbated by the relative immaturity of liver enzymes in these babies. In poorly controlled diabetes, the fetus responds to the extra glucose by producing more insulin, which increases its body fat and muscle mass resulting in *macrosomia*. Birth weight and body mass are both greater and the kidneys and adrenal cortex are larger. The head circumference and brain size are normal.

Neonatal complications include hypoglycemia, respiratory distress syndrome, hyperbilirubinemia, polycythemia, hypocalcemia, hypomagnesemia and cardiomyopathy.

Overt Diabetes   ↑ RBC

A woman with abnormal glucose tolerance test with or without symptoms and a raised fasting blood glucose level is called an overt diabetic. The condition may be pre-existing or detected for the first time during present pregnancy. Diagnosis can be presumptive if (a) the fasting plasma glucose exceeds 105 mg percent (b) the peak level exceeds 180 mg percent and (c) the two hour value exceeds 140 mg percent in glucose tolerance test.

Classification of Pregnant Diabetics

Group A   Gestational diabetes
Group B   Overt diabetes without vasculopathy
Group C   Diabetes with vasculopathy (retino-
           pathy and/or nephropathy)

Fetal and maternal outcome of diabetic pregnancy depends on the severity of the disease and its duration.

Management

Preconceptional Counseling

Pregnancy may lead to a deterioration of the diabetes and hence the woman must be carefully examined for the presence of renal, cardiovascular or retinal changes before becoming pregnant. The woman will need to continue using some form of contraception while improving control of her diabetes. Good control of diabetes is to be achieved before the onset of pregnancy. Appropriate advice about diet and insulin is to be given. Chances of having a diabetic child is about one percent when only the mother is diabetic, rising to 20 percent if both parents are diabetic.

Principles of Management

❖ Careful antenatal supervision and control of diabetes, to maintain the glucose level as near to physiological level as possible
❖ To find out the optimum time and method of delivery
❖ To make arrangements for the care of the newborn.

Antenatal Care

Antenatal supervision should be at monthly intervals up to 20th week and thereafter at two weeks intervals up to 30th week. Simultaneous consultation with a team consisting of physician, pediatrician and dietician is ideal. The *daily calorie requirement* is about 30 to 35 kcal per kg of body weight and an additional 200 kcal for the need of the fetus. Fat may be reduced if the woman is obese. Fiber containing food items are increased and a four-meal regimen with a bedtime snack is usually advised. Oral hypoglycemic agents are changed to insulin.

Frequent blood glucose estimation is required. Estimation of *glycosylated hemoglobin* should be done at the end of first trimester and three monthly thereafter. *Sonographic evaluation* is extremely helpful, not only to diagnose varieties of congenital malformations of the fetus but also to detect fetal macrosomia or growth retardation. *Assessment of the fetal well-being* is to be made from 32nd week onwards.

The midwife should alert the woman of her predisposition to urinary tract and vaginal infections so that she will seek treatment as soon as possible if symptoms develop. It is important to teach the woman about maintenance of hygiene. Examination of maternal weight and of her abdomen will help the midwife to detect polyhydramnios. In addition, the woman must be examined for any sign of diabetic complications.

Hospitalization

In uncomplicated cases, the woman is admitted in hospital at 34th to 36th week. Early hospitalization facilitates:
❖ Stabilization of diabetes
❖ Minimizes the incidence of preeclampsia, polyhydramnios and preterm labor
❖ Selection of the appropriate time for termination of pregnancy.

Termination of Pregnancy

Majority of intrauterine deaths of the fetus occur in the last two weeks of pregnancy. Hence, termination is done after 37 completed weeks. Early termination may have to be done for fetal jeopardy. Assessment of fetal lung maturity must be done beforehand and facilities of an equipped neonatal care unit should be available.

Management of Labor and Delivery

Induction of labor is done in the presence of following indications:
❖ Multiparae with good obstetric history
❖ Young primigravidae without any obstetric abnormality
❖ Presence of congenital malformation of the fetus.

Induction is done by low rupture of membranes and simultaneous oxytocin drip.

Cesarean section is indicated in the following conditions:
❖ Elderly primigravidae

- Multigravidae with bad obstetric history
- Diabetes difficult to control
- Obstetric complications like preeclampsia, polyhydramnios, and malpresentation
- Presence of large baby.

About 50 percent diabetic women are delivered by cesarean section. Spontaneous onset of labor at term and vaginal delivery are awaited in the following conditions:

- Young primigravidae or multiparae with good obstetric history
- Diabetes well controlled either by diet, insulin, or both or without any obstetrical complications.

During labor, control of blood glucose is achieved through administration of IV dextrose and soluble insulin with hourly estimation of blood glucose. Epidural analgesia is preferable than strong sedatives or analgesics as they might depress the fetal respiratory center.

The midwife should monitor fetal condition throughout labor using electronic fetal monitoring. A pediatrician should be present during delivery, especially if labor has been induced, as a baby with premature lungs may require resuscitation. Polyhydramnios increases the risk of malpresentation, cord prolapse and uterine inertia during labor. Birth asphyxia is more common in both macrosomic and growth retarded babies. The large baby is prone to birth injuries. Shoulder dystocia a possible hazard. Prophylactic ergometrine is given intravenously with the delivery of anterior shoulder to minimize blood loss. The cord should be clamped immediately after delivery to avoid hypervolemia. The placenta is usually large, the cord is thick and there is increased incidence of a single umbilical artery.

Postnatal Care

Carbohydrate metabolism returns to normal very quickly after delivery of the placenta and insulin requirements will fall rapidly. The woman can resume her prepregnancy regimen. A diabetic mother who is breastfeeding should be encouraged to increase her carbohydrate intake by 50 mg a day because of the increased nutritional demands. Insulin requirements are determined according to preprandial blood glucose estimation. Although a small amount of insulin may enter breast milk, these are destroyed in the baby's stomach.

The diabetic women are more prone to infection and delayed healing. Antibiotics are given prophylactically to minimize infection. The midwife will need to advise her to change her perineal pads frequently in order to keep any wound clean and dry.

Care of the Baby

A neonatologist should be present at the time of delivery. The baby should preferably be kept in an intensive neonatal care unit and observed closely for at least 48 hours, to detect and treat any complication likely to arise.

- Asphyxia is anticipated and to be treated effectively.
- Birth injuries and congenital abnormalities can be present and must be looked for.
- Hypoglycemia may occur and to prevent this the babies should be fed soon after delivery. Monitoring of neonatal blood glucose needs to be done according to the protocol. If the baby is lethargic or premature and breastfeeding is a problem, 10 percent glucose may be given orally as the first feeding and continued with breastfeeding every 3–4 hours.
- All babies should receive 1 mg vitamin K intramuscularly.
- The destruction of red cells and the relative immaturity of the liver predispose the baby to jaundice (Roberton, 1992).

Contraception

Barrier method of contraception is ideal for spacing of births. Low dose combined oral pills, containing third generation progestins, are effective and have minimal effect on carbohydrate metabolism. The IUCD increases the risk of pelvic infection. Tubal ligation should be seriously considered following second live birth, under local anesthesia in the puerperium.

SUMMARY OF NURSING PROCESS

Assessment

Assess for the following clinical manifestations:
1. Hyperemesis during early pregnancy.
2. Glycosuria, ketonuria.

3. Elevated blood glucose, glucose tolerance test.
4. Polydipsia, polyphagia, polyuria.
5. Rapid weight gain.
6. Previous large babies weighing 3,500 gm or more.

Analysis/Nursing Diagnosis

1. Risk for fetal injury
2. Risk for infection
3. Ineffective airway clearance
4. Actual/risk for aspiration
5. Anxiety
6. Anticipatory grieving
7. Altered family processes
8. Actual/risk for altered parenting
9. Health seeking behavior.

Planning

1. Regular tests for glucose levels.
2. Glycosuria, ketonuria.
3. Observing for signs of hypoglycemia and hyperglycemia.
4. Provision of counseling and support.
5. Teaching regarding disease and care activities.

Implementation

1. Obtain accurate obstetric and diet history.
2. Assess health status and report to physician regarding
   a. Hydramnios
   b. Large size fetus
   c. Fetal heart rate
   d. Weight, blood pressure.
3. Provide instructions regarding blood glucose control
   a. Blood tests
   b. Insulin injections
   c. Avoidance of oral hypoglycemics
   d. Management of hypoglycemia.
4. Encourage regular exercise for weight and blood sugar control.
5. Provide diet instructions:
   a. Prescribed diet (2200–2400 kcal/day)
   b. Avoid calorie restrictions
   c. Eat at regularly scheduled times (3 meals and 2 to 4 snacks daily)
   d. Observe for hypoglycemia.
6. Monitor for urinary and vaginal tract infections.
7. Prepare for delivery:
   ❖ Vaginal delivery is preferable to cesarean delivery.
8. Observe for the following complications:
   a. Hydramnios
   b. Preeclampsia and eclampsia
   c. Stillbirth
   d. Neonatal respiratory distress syndrome (RDS), congenital anomalies, hyperbilirubinemia and hypoglycemia
   e. Postpartum hemorrhage, infection.
9. Encourage breastfeeding because breastfeeding decreases insulin requirements.
10. Provide postpartum contraceptive information.
    a. Avoid oral contraceptives as it may increase the risk of deep vein thrombosis (DVT).
    b. Encourage barrier contraceptives.

Evaluation

Ensure that the pregnant woman:
1. Remains normoglycemic
2. Shows no signs or symptoms of hypoglycemia
3. Verbalizes support
4. Verbalizes understanding of the disease and the implications of diabetes on pregnancy.

THYROID DYSFUNCTION IN PREGNANCY

Thyroid disease is common in women of reproductive age. The incidence of thyroid disease associated with pregnancy is varied. Hyperthyroidism occurs in about two per 1,000 pregnancies and hypothyroidism about nine per 1,000 (Girling, 1996). Thyroid disease in pregnancy can have potential adverse effects on the fetus; the fetal morbidity and mortality rates in untreated women can be as high as 50 percent (Sugrue and Drury, 1980).

HYPERTHYROIDISM

The disease should be suspected on any woman who fails to gain weight satisfactorily despite a good appetite. Other symptoms include exophthalmos, eyelid lag and persistent tachycardia. Clinical diagnosis is difficult as the physiological signs and symptoms pregnant women normally exhibit, such as heat intolerance, palpitations, and mood lability may mask this condition. Hyperthyroidism when poorly controlled is associated with an increase in preterm delivery, low birth weight and fetal death (Mestman, 1980). Thyroid autoimmunity is related to abortion and chromosomal abnormality with increased fetal loss. Thyroid stimulating immunoglobulins can cross the placenta and produce neonatal thyrotoxicosis with increased neonatal death.

Diagnosis

Clinical diagnosis is confirmed by measuring free T_4 and T_3 levels along with TSH. Radioactive iodine uptake and scans should not be done during pregnancy as it will cross the placenta and damage the fetal thyroid gland permanently.

Treatment

The main form of treatment for hyperthyroidism is by means of antithyroid drugs (Carbimazole, methimazole and Propylthiouracil). Carbimazole is given orally with a daily dose of 20 to 60 mg and maintained at this dose until the woman becomes euthyroid. Then it is progressively reduced to maintenance of between 5 to 15 mg daily. Propylthiouracil is given at a daily dose of 300 to 450 mg and continued until the patient becomes euthyroid—the maintenance dose being 50 to 150 mg daily. Both the drugs may cause fetal goiter and hypothyroidism. Methimazole has been linked to a scalp defect—aplasia cutis of the neonate. Patients having marked tachycardia or arrhythmias should also have proponolol (β blocking agent). The drugs are not contraindicated during breastfeeding provided the dose is kept relatively low and close monitoring of the neonatal thyroid functions is carried out. Propylthiouracil is the drug of choice as it crosses into the breast milk to a lesser extent. Cord blood should be taken for TSH and free T_4 at the time of delivery to detect neonatal hyperthyroidism.

Preconceptional Counseling

Considering the hazards during pregnancy, preconceptional counseling is important.

Adequate treatment should be initiated to bring down the thyroid function profile to normal. Radioactive iodine therapy should not be given to women wanting pregnancy within one year. If pregnancy occurs inadvertently, termination should be done. Oral pill is to be withheld because of accelerated metabolism and disturbed liver function.

HYPOTHYROIDISM

Primary hypothyroidism in pregnancy is mostly related to thyroid autoimmunity. Myxedema rarely presents in pregnancy because they tend to be infertile. It is important to diagnose the condition because of the increased rate of fetal loss and reduced IQ in these children. Complications of pregnancy like preeclampsia and anemia are high.

Diagnosis

Diagnosis may be extremely difficult. Symptoms manifest as excessive weight gain despite poor appetite, cold intolerance, and a roughening of the skin. Thyroid function measurement is taken and if low, the woman is commenced on thyroxine. Therapy is started with levothyroxine, which is titrated to normalize thyroid function. The assessment is done on a monthly basis.

Antenatal Care

Women with pre-existing hypothyroidism will require monitoring of their thyroid function during pregnancy and their medication adjusted as necessary. Hypothyroid pregnant women tend to gain weight easily and the midwife needs to observe this closely for any deviation from the expected weight gain (Smith, 1990). Constipation may also be a problem because it is exacerbated by both hypothyroidism and pregnancy. Dietary advice such as increasing fiber content and fluid intake may help alleviate the problem.

Postnatal Care

After delivery, the neonate's thyroid status should be checked to identify whether there is any neonatal hypothyroidism present. There is no contraindication to breastfeeding, but the dose of thyroxine may need adjustment because of the maternal weight loss following delivery.

Postpartum Thyroiditis

About 10 to 15 percent of women develop this condition due to autoimmune thyroid disease. This is a transient disorder that occurs during the first year after parturition (Bishnoi and Sachmechi, 1996). The condition is characterized initially by symptoms of mild hyperthyroidism and may mimic postpartum psychosis (Walfish and Chan, 1985). Recovery is usually spontaneous in most women but the disorder tends to occur with subsequent pregnancies. About two-thirds will ultimately become euthyroid and the remaining one-third will become hypothyroid (Dutta, 2001).

ANEMIA IN PREGNANCY

Anemia is the most common hematological disorder that may occur in pregnancy. It is a reduction in the oxygen carrying capacity of the blood, which may be due to:

❖ A reduced number of red blood cells
❖ A low concentration of hemoglobin, or
❖ A combination of both.

According to the standard laid down by WHO, anemia in pregnancy is present when the hemoglobin concentration in the peripheral blood is 11 gm/100 ml or less. However, because of prevailing socioeconomic deprivation in the developing countries, the level is brought down to 10 gm/100 ml. The incidence of anemia in pregnancy ranges from 40 to 80 percent in the tropics compared to 10 to 20 percent in the developed countries (Dutta, 2001).

Classification of Anemia

Anemia may be classified in various ways. A simplified classification is given below:
❖ Physiological anemia
❖ Pathological anemia
  – Iron deficiency
  – Folic acid deficiency
  – Vitamin B_{12} deficiency
  – Protein deficiency.

❖ Hemorrhagic anemia
  – Acute—Following bleeding in early months of pregnancy or APH
  – Chronic—Hookworm infestation, bleeding piles, etc.
❖ Hemolytic anemia
  – Familial—Congenital acholuric jaundice, sickle cell anemia, etc.
  – Acquired—Malaria, severe infection, etc.
❖ Bone marrow insufficiency—Hypoplasia or aplasia due to radiation, drugs or severe infection
❖ Hemoglobinopathies.

The common types of anemia, which are of concern in obstetric practice, are the deficiency anemia and hemorrhagic anemia.

Physiological Anemia of Pregnancy

During pregnancy, maternal plasma volume gradually expands by 50 percent, an increase of approximately 1,200 ml by term. Most of the rise takes place before 32nd to 34th week's gestation and thereafter there is relatively little change (Letsky, 1987). The total increase in red blood cells is 25 percent, approximately 300 ml that occurs later in pregnancy. This relative hemodilution produces a fall in hemoglobin concentration, thus presenting a picture of iron deficiency anemia. However, it has been found that these changes are a physiological alteration of pregnancy necessary for the development of the fetus. Normal changes occurring in the blood are summarized in Table 29.1.

Erythropoiesis

In adults, erythropoiesis is confined to the bone marrow. Red cells are formed through stages of pronormoblasts → normoblasts → reticulocytes → mature nonnucleated erythrocytes. The average life-span of red cells is about 120 days after which the RBCs degenerate and the hemoglobin are broken down into hemosiderin and bile pigment. For proper erythropoiesis, adequate nutrients are needed. These are minerals, vitamins, proteins and hormones. Inadequate reserve, or increased demand or deficient supply of any of the constituents interferes with the normal erythropoiesis.

Table 29.1 Normal blood values in nonpregnant and pregnant states

	Nonpregnant state	Second half of pregnancy
Hemoglobin (Hbg)	14.8/100 ml	11–14 gm/100 ml
Red blood cells	5 million/Cu mm	4–4.5 m/mm^3
Packed cell volume (PCV)	39–42%	32–36%
Mean corpuscular volume (MCV)	75–100 Cubic micron (μm^3)	75–95 μm^3
Mean corpuscular hemoglobin (MCH)	27–32 micromicron (picogram—pg)	26–31 pg
Mean corpuscular hemoglobin concentration (MCHC)	32–36% (g/dl)	30–35 g/dl
Serum iron	60–120 µg/100 ml	65–75 µg/100 ml
Serum ferritin	20–30 mg/L (mean)	15 µg/L (mean)

Source: Dutta DC. Text Book of Obstetrics, 5th edn. New Central Book Company, Calcutta, 2001

* *Minerals*: Iron is an essential element in the synthesis of hemoglobin. Traces of copper and cobalt are also required in the synthesis
* *Vitamins*: The specific vitamins that are required in the maturation process are vitamin B$_{12}$ folic acid and vitamin C
* *Proteins*: The proteins supply the amino acid for the synthesis of globin
* *Erythropoietin:* The hormone is probably responsible for increase in red cells in the bone marrow. Increased secretion of erythropoietin is brought about mostly by placental lactogen and by progesterone. Erythropoietin is produced by the kidneys (90%) and liver (10%).

Causes of Increased Prevalence of Anemia in the Tropics

Iron deficiency anemia is very much prevalent in the tropics particularly among women of childbearing age, especially in the under-privileged sector. The causes for it are:
* Faulty dietetic habit—The diet rich in carbo-hydrate reduces the absorption of iron even when there is no deficiency of iron the diet.
* Faulty absorption mechanism—Because of the high prevalence of infestation, there is intestinal hurry, which reduces the iron absorption. Hypochlorhydria, often associated with malnutrition also hinders absorption.
* Iron loss—(a) More iron is lost through sweat to the extent of 15 mg per month. (b) Repeated pregnancies at short intervals along with a prolonged period of lactation

puts a serious strain on the iron reserve. It has been estimated that a normal healthy woman with adequate diet takes about two years to replenish about 1,000 mg of iron lost during childbirth and lactation. (c) Excessive blood loss during menstruation, which is left untreated. (d) Hookworm infestation with consequent blood depletion to the extent of 0.5 to 2 mg of iron daily. (e) Chronic blood loss due to bleeding piles and dysentery also cause iron deficiency anemia (Dutta, 2001).

Iron Requirements in Pregnancy

During pregnancy approximately 1,500 mg iron is needed for:
* The increase in maternal hemoglobin (400–500 mg)
* The fetus and placenta (300–400 mg)
* Replacement of daily loss through urine, stools and skin (250 mg)
* Replacement of blood lost at delivery (200 mg).
* Lactation (1 mg/day).

The woman who has sufficient iron reserve and is on a balanced diet is unlikely to develop anemia during pregnancy in spite of an increased demand of iron. But if the iron reserve is inadequate or absent, development of anemia is possible due to the following factors:
* Increased requirements of iron
* Disturbed metabolism—Depressed erythro-poietic function of the bone marrow.
* Prepregnancy health status—Pre-existing anemic state

- Excess demand—(a) Multiple pregnancy increases the iron demand by two-folds. (b) Rapid recurring pregnancy (within 2 years). (c) Teenage pregnancy—The demand of iron accompanies the natural growth. At the age of 17, the additional demand is estimated to be about 270 mg during the course of pregnancy, the requirement is however, brought down to nil at the age of 21.

Routine Screening for Anemia

Pregnant women are usually screened at their first antenatal visit and thereafter at monthly intervals from the 28th week. Some physicians prescribe iron supplements for all pregnant women while others give it to those at risk of anemia or are anemic already. Many physicians avoid giving iron during the first trimester of pregnancy owing to the gastrointestinal side effects. It may be more appropriate to administer prophylactic iron therapy in the third trimester of pregnancy. During this time the maternal iron store become depleted due to increasing fetal demand. Indications for prophylactic iron therapy include:

- Previous anemia
- Dietary conditions
- Chronic blood loss
- Low hemoglobin on booking
- Close family spacing.

Oral iron preparations given prophylactically consist of one of the iron salts, either alone or in combination with folic acid.

IRON DEFICIENCY ANEMIA

About 95 percent of pregnant women with anemia have the iron deficiency type. A pregnant woman is said to be anemic if her hemoglobin is less than 10 gm percent.

Causes

- Reduced intake or absorption of iron—This includes dietary deficiency and gastrointestinal disturbances such as morning sickness
- Excess demand such as multiple pregnancy, frequent or numerous pregnancies (more than four), chronic inflammation particularly of the urinary tract

- Blood loss from menorrhagia before conception, bleeding hemorrhoids, antepartum or postpartum hemorrhage and hookworm
- Decreased absorption due to decreased gastric acidity and dietary imbalance causing formation of insoluble salts of iron.

Signs and Symptoms

- Pallor of mucous membranes
- Lassitude and feeling of weakness
- Giddiness
- Tachycardia and palpitations
- Dyspnea
- Anorexia and indigestion
- Swelling of the legs.

Effects of Anemia on the Mother

- Reduced resistance to infection caused by impaired cell-mediated immunity
- Reduced ability to withstand postpartum hemorrhage
- Strain of even an uncomplicated labor may cause cardiac failure
- Predisposition to pregnancy induced hypertension and preterm labor due to associated malnutrition
- Reduced enjoyment of pregnancy and motherhood owing to fatigue
- Potential threat to life—Even a minor traumatic delivery without bleeding may produce shock or a minor hypoxia during anesthesia may be become lethal.

Effects of Anemia on the Fetus/Baby

- Increased risk of intrauterine hypoxia and growth retardation
- Prematurity
- Low birth weight
- Anemia a few months after birth due to poor stores
- Increased risk of perinatal morbidity and mortality.

Investigations

The patient having a hemoglobin level below 10 gm% should be subjected to a full hematological work up to ascertain the degree of anemia, the type of anemia and the cause of anemia.

By the time Hb falls, the iron store will already be depleted. The serum iron level demonstrates lack of iron, which will be usually below 30 µg/100 ml. Total iron binding capacity is elevated beyond 400 µg/100 ml. Serum ferritin level will be below 10 µg/100 ml. Midstream urine should be tested to exclude urinary tract infection, which will affect erythropoiesis. Stool examination should be done as a routine in the tropics to detect helminthic (particularly hookworm) infestation.

Prevention of Iron Deficiency Anemia

The midwife can help to identify women at risk of anemia by taking accurate history of medical, obstetric and social history. This may reveal a pre-existing problem or a lifestyle, which puts her at risk of anemia. It may also suggest that the woman is suffering from the effects of anemia.

She will be able to provide explanations appropriate to the particular woman taking into account her health and sociocultural preferences. Women need to be taught about the sources of iron, and ways in which absorption can be increased. Iron intake is closely linked with calorie intake; 2,000 kcal per day will contain approximately 12 to 14 mg of iron, sufficient to cover the recommended daily amount of 113 mg for pregnant woman (Torrance, 1992).

Management

In the tropics, majority of cases with iron deficiency anemia in pregnancy have a low socioeconomic status. The anemia is either pre-existing or is aggravated during pregnancy.

Prophylaxis

❖ *Avoidance of frequent childbirths*: A minimum interval between pregnancies, should be at least two years, to replenish the lost iron during childbirth and lactation. This can be achieved by proper family planning guidance.
❖ *Supplementary iron therapy*: After the woman becomes free of the nausea of pregnancy, daily administration of 200 mg of ferrous sulfate along with 1 mg of folic acid is a quite effective prophylactic procedure. Routine supplementation with iron and folic acid is not necessary when the hemoglobin level is high (> 13 mg/dl).
❖ *Dietary advice*: A balanced diet, rich in iron and protein, which is affordable by the woman and easily digestible, should be recommended.
❖ *Adequate treatments to eradicate illnesses likely to cause anemia*: These are hookworm infestation, dysentery, bleeding piles, malaria and urinary tract infections.
❖ *Early detection of falling hemoglobin level*: Hemoglobin level should be estimated at the first antenatal visit, at 28th and finally at 36th week.

Curative Management

Treatment of severe anemia must be preceded by an accurate diagnosis of the cause and type. Women having hemoglobin level of 7.5 mg% (ideally anyone with Hb less than 10 mg%) and those with associated obstetrical-medical complications even with moderate degree of anemia should be hospitalized. Following therapeutic measures are to be instituted.
❖ *Diet:* A balanced diet, which is rich in protein, iron and vitamins
❖ Appropriate antibiotic therapy to eradicate even a minimal septic focus
❖ Effective therapy to cure the disease contributing to the cause of anemia
❖ Iron therapy to raise the hemoglobin level and to restore the iron reserve at least in part, if possible, before the woman goes into labor.

This may be oral iron or parenteral iron depending on the severity of anemia, duration of pregnancy and associated complicating factors.

Oral Iron

The daily dose of iron for treating anemia is between 120 and 180 gm in divided doses. Iron is best absorbed in the ferrous form and ferrous sulphate 200 mg tablets or ferrous gluconate 300 mg tablets are generally used.

Side Effects of Oral Iron

Intolerance: This may be evidenced by epigastric pain, vomiting and diarrhea or constipation. To avoid intolerance, it is preferable to start the therapy with a smaller dose and then to increase the dose to a maximum of three tablets a day. These discomforts may be reduced by taking the iron after meals. Some women find one form of iron salts more tolerable than another does.

❖ The woman should be warned that her stools may turn black but that does not mean that iron is not being absorbed.

Parenteral Iron

Parenteral iron is indicated for women who have intolerance to oral iron and those with severe anemia in advanced pregnancy (last 8–10 weeks of pregnancy). Parenteral iron is contraindicated for women who have liver or renal disorders.

Intramuscular iron is given in the form of Iron dextran (imferon), which contains 50 mg of elemental iron in one milliliter, and one ampoule contains 2 ml. Injections should not be given in conjunction with oral iron as this enhances toxic effects such as headache, dizziness, nausea and vomiting. The injection should be given deep into the muscle to prevent staining of the skin, formation of abscess and fat necrosis.

After an initial test dose of 1 ml, the injections are to be given daily or on alternate days in doses of 2 ml intramuscularly. The injection is to be given in the buttock using the 'Z' track technique (pulling the skin and subcutaneous tissue to one side before inserting the needle).

Blood transfusion is used rarely to treat severe iron deficiency anemia. It may be used to raise the Hb level quickly if delivery is imminent (beyond 36 weeks). With transfusion, improvement is seen in 3 to 4 days.

Precautions to be taken for blood transfusion include:

❖ The blood to be transfused must be fresh (collected within 24 hours) and properly grouped

❖ Only packed cells are transfused and the quantity should be between 80 to 100 ml at a time

❖ The drip should be about 10 drops per minute and transfusion should not be repeated within 24 hours

❖ Prior to the transfusion patient is to be sedated with 60 mg phenobarbitone

❖ An antihistamine (phenergan 25 mg%) and a diuretic (frusemide 20 mg) are given

❖ Very close monitoring of vital signs and lung sounds.

Complications of transfusion are premature labor and cardiac failure. Features of transfusion reaction, if occur, are exaggerated.

Management during Labor

First Stage

The following are the special precautions to be taken when an anemic patient goes into labor:

❖ The patient should be in bed and should lie in a position comfortable to her

❖ Light analgesics are preferred for pain relief

❖ Oxygen administration to increase the oxygenation of maternal blood and thus diminish the risk of fetal hypoxia

❖ Strict asepsis to minimize the risk of puerperal infection.

Second Stage

Usually there is no problem. Intravenous methergine 0.2 mg should be given following the delivery of anterior shoulder.

Third Stage

Very vigilant observation is required during the third stage. Significant amount of blood loss should be replenished by fresh packed cell transfusion after taking the precautions outlined earlier. The volume of transfusion should not be more than the amount lost (to avoid overloading the heart).

Puerperium

❖ The patient should be on bed rest

❖ Any sign of infection should be promptly detected and treated

❖ Predelivery antianemic therapy should be continued until the patient restores her normal clinical and hematological status. Hematinics should be continued for at least three months following delivery. The anemic state usually improves following delivery

❖ Dietary advice outlined earlier must be reinforced

❖ Patient and family members must be counseled for help at home for baby care and other household chores.

FOLIC ACID DEFICIENCY ANEMIA (MEGALOBLASTIC ANEMIA)

Folic acid is needed for the increased cell growth of mother and fetus, but there is a physiological decrease in serum folate levels in pregnancy. Anemia is more likely to be found towards the end of pregnancy when the fetus is growing rapidly. In India, megaloblastic anemia is usually due to a deficiency of folic acid.

Causes

❖ Increased demands

❖ Increase in maternal tissue and red blood cell volume

❖ Reduced dietary intake

❖ Reduced absorption

❖ Interference with utilization; drugs such as anticonvulsants, sulphonamides and alcohol are folate antagonists

❖ Infections: They reduce the life-span of RBCs and increase cell production requiring more folic acid

❖ Decreased storage related to vitamin C deficiency and liver disease.

Clinical Features and Diagnosis

❖ The signs and symptoms are varied and may be mistaken as "minor disorders of pregnancy" such as pallor, lethargy, weight loss, depression, nausea and vomiting, glossitis, gingivitis and diarrhea

❖ Examination of the red cell indices will reveal that the red cells are reduced in number but enlarged in size (macrocytes)

❖ Peripheral blood smears show deficiency of iron and folic acid

❖ Examination of the bone marrow shows both megaloblasts and normoblasts

❖ MCV is either normal or raised.

The condition is generally diagnosed in the third trimester or puerperium. The patients are usually multiparas and in the middle or later years of reproductive life.

Effects of Megaloblastic Anemia

Deficiency of folic acid may cause placental abruption (abruptio placentae), neutral tube defects and congenital cardiac septal defects.

Management

Folic acid is administered orally in a dose of 5 mg eight hourly. If time is short, treatment may be given with 30 mg intramuscularly for 3 days or 90 mg intravenously in 250 ml of normal saline, to be followed by oral therapy. This is usually well tolerated with no side effects. Women must be taught about correct selection and preparation of foods, which are high in folic acid. Folic acid is found in leafy green vegetables such as spinach and broccoli, but is destroyed easily by prolonged boiling or steaming. Other sources include peanuts, chic peas, bananas and citrus fruits.

VITAMIN B$_{12}$ DEFICIENCY

Deficiency of vitamin B$_{12}$ also produces a megaloblastic anemia. vitamin B$_{12}$ levels fall during pregnancy, but anemia is rare because the body draws on its stores. Deficiency is most likely in vegetarians who eat no animal products at all and vitamin B$_{12}$ supplements must be taken during pregnancy. Folic acid should not be given in case of vitamin B$_{12}$ deficiency as it can hasten subacute degeneration of the spinal cord (Letsky, 1987).

HEMOGLOBINOPATHIES

Hemoglobinopathies are inherited specific biochemical disorders where the hemoglobin is abnormal. Hemoglobin consists of a group of four molecules, each of which has a hem unit and a protein chain. The position of the amino acids in the protein chain determines the type of hemoglobin produced. Adult hemoglobin (HbA) has two alpha and two beta chains while the fetal hemoglobin (HbF) has two alpha and two gamma chains. By six months 96 percent of a baby's Hb is HbA.

The type of protein is genetically determined. Defective genes lead to the formation of abnormal hemoglobin. Two common varieties are seen. *Sickle cell disease* is an inherited structural abnormality involving primarily the beta chain of HbA. *Thalassemia* is an inherited defect in the synthesis and production of globin in otherwise normal HbA. Homozygous and heterozygous forms occur. In *homozygous*, the abnormal globin chain is inherited from each parent and in *heterozygous*, the abnormal globin chain is inherited only from one parent. The later groups are not anemic but are carriers of the defect.

SICKLE CELL DISORDERS

The sickle cell hemoglobinopathies are hereditary disorders in which defectives genes produce abnormal hemoglobin beta chains; the resulting Hb is called HbS. In sickle cell anemia (Hbss), abnormal genes have been inherited from both parents whereas in sickle cell trait (HbAs) only one abnormal gene has been inherited. Sickle cell disorders are found most commonly in people of African or West Indian origin.

Sickle Cell Trait

HbS comprises 38 to 45 percent of hemoglobin, the rest being HbA, HbA_2 and HbF. The individuals are usually asymptomatic. There is no anemia even under the stress of pregnancy. Hematuria and urinary infection are common.

If the husband is also a carrier, there is 25 percent chance that the infant will be homozygous sickle cell disease and 50 percent chance for sickle cell trait.

Sickle Cell Disease

Homozygous sickle cell disease (HbSS) is a genetically inherited disease and transmitted equally by males and females. Sickle cells have an increased fragility and shortened lifespan of 17 days resulting in chronic hemolytic anemia and causing episodes of ischemia and pain; these are known as sickle cell crises.

Diagnosis

❖ Identification by sickling test
❖ Persistent reticulocytosis
❖ High fasting serum iron level
❖ Identification of the type of hemoglobinopathy by electrophoresis.

Effects on Pregnancy

Women with sickle cell anemia are subfertile, but those who do become pregnant may suffer the following:

❖ Increased incidence of abortion, prematurity, intrauterine growth retardation and fetal loss
❖ Perinatal mortality is high
❖ Incidence of preeclampsia, postpartum hemorrhage and infection is increased
❖ Increased maternal morbidity due to infection, cerebrovascular accident and sickle cell crises
❖ Maternal death is increased up to 25 percent due to pulmonary infarction, congestive heart failure and embolism.

Effects of Pregnancy on the Disease

There is chance of sickle cell crisis, which usually occurs in the last trimester. Two types of crises are generally seen: (1) hemolytic crisis (2) painful crisis.

Hemolytic crisis is due to hemolysis with rapidly developing anemia along with jaundice. There is associated leukocytosis and fever.

Painful crisis occurs due to vascular occlusion of the various organs by capillary thrombosis resulting in infarction. Abdominal pain, vomiting, chest pain, hemoptysis or hematuria occurs depending upon the site of vascular occlusion.

Precipitating factors include psychological stress, cold climate and extreme temperature changes, strenuous physical exertion and fatigue, respiratory disease, infection and pregnancy. When subjected to low oxygen tension, HbS contracts, damaging the cell and causing it to assume a sickle shape. Damaged cells block capillaries and the resulting infarction leads to pain, affecting particularly the bones, joints and abdominal organs. Emboli may be thrown off into the circulation, which may threaten life.

Management

Preconceptional counseling: As these conditions are inherited and in the homozygous form can be fatal, screening of the population at risk should be carried-out. Blood is examined by electrophoresis, which detects the different types of hemoglobin. Prospective parents, who are known to have or carry genes for abnormal hemoglobin, need genetic counseling in order to help them make an informed decision before deciding on a pregnancy. If both parents are carriers there is a 25 percent chances that the fetus will be homozygous. Prenatal identification of the homozygous state of the disorder is an indication for early termination of pregnancy (Dutta, 2001).

During Pregnancy

* Careful antenatal supervision
* Prophylactic folic acid 5 mg PO daily
* Iron supplementation in proven cases of deficiency
* Regular blood transfusion at 6 weeks intervals to keep the hematocrit values above 25 percent and HbS concentration under 50 percent
* Hospitalization for any infection or appearance of unusual symptoms:
  - *Treatment* involves rest, rehydration, treatment of infection, pain relief, oxygen therapy and blood transfusion
* Air travel is best avoided.

During Labor

* During labor, the midwife must ensure that the woman is kept well hydrated with intravenous fluids
* Prophylactic antibiotics, effective analgesia preferably epidural and oxygen therapy are needed
* The fetus should be monitored closely for signs of distress.

Postnatal Care

* Antibiotic cover is continued throughout the postnatal period for prevention of puerperal sepsis.

* Neonatal testing of all babies at risk must be done by testing the cord blood.
* Sickle test must be done for the babies at the age of 3 to 4 months and those with positive results must be followed-up by the hematologist. In order to prevent the high incidence of infant mortality from sickle cell anemia, early diagnosis combined with prophylaxis against infection, parental education and adequate follow-up are recommended (Streetly et al, 1993).

THALASSEMIA SYNDROMES

The thalassemia syndromes are commonly found genetic disorders of the blood. The basic defect is a reduced rate of hemoglobin chain synthesis. This leads to ineffective erythropoiesis and increased hemolysis with resultant inadequate hemoglobin content. The syndromes are of two types—The alpha and beta thalassemia depending on the globin chain synthesis affected. Alpha and beta thalassemia exist in both homozygous (major) and heterozygous (minor) states.

Alpha Thalassemia Major

This condition is more commonly found in South-east Asia. The child inherits abnormal genes from both parents. Rapid cell breakdown produces a severe anemia, which is incompatible with extrauterine life.

Beta Thalassemia Major

The defective genes result in severe hemoglobin deficiency, which may result in cardiac failure and death in early childhood. The use of frequent blood transfusion increases the possibility of survival. However, there is progressive hepatosplenomegaly, impaired growth, anemia, intercurrent infection and congestive cardiac failure. Chances of survival beyond teens are uncommon.

Alpha and Beta Thalassemia Minor

The heterozygous condition is the more common form of thalassemia and produces an anemia, which is more similar to iron deficiency in which the Hb, MCV and MCH are lowered. Serum iron and total iron binding capacity are normal or elevated because red cells are broken down more rapidly than normal and iron is stored for future use. Serum bilirubin may be raised to about 2 to 3 mg%.

The diagnosis is often late when the patient fails to respond to oral iron therapy to correct anemia. There is chance for hepatic and cardiac hemosiderosis from iron overload. The reproductive performance of thalassemia minor is usually normal. They require oral iron and folate supplementation during pregnancy. If hemoglobin is low, blood transfusion is better. Parenteral iron therapy should never be given (Letsky, 1987).

Renal Problems in Pregnancy

ASYMPTOMATIC BACTERIURIA

Asymptomatic bacteriuria occurs in 2 to 10 per cent of pregnant women owing to the physiological changes in the urinary tract during pregnancy. A diagnosis of ASB is defined as bacteriuria with more than 100,000 organisms per milliliter of urine from a clean voided urine (Duff, 1984). It is important that the midwife obtains, from the antenatal mother, proper history of any previous urinary tract infection in order to make a positive prediction.

The consequences of this condition in pregnancy represent a significant risk to both mother and fetus. Twenty-five percent of these women are likely to develop acute pyelonephritis, usually in third trimester, if left untreated. The incidence of anemia and hypertension is stated high. There is increased incidence of premature and growth retarded babies.

The penicillins and cephalosporins are the drugs of choice for initial treatment and are administered for 7 to 14 days. A urine sample should be obtained for culture one week after therapy is discontinued and thereafter at regular intervals throughout the pregnancy to ensure that reinfection has not occurred.

ACUTE PYELONEPHRITIS

Acute pyelonephritis occurs in 1 to 2 percent of all pregnancies. The causative organism is often *Escherichia coli* (*E. coli*). Bacteriuria in early pregnancy is a predisposing factor. The onset is acute and usually appears beyond the 16th week. The involvement is bilateral but if unilateral, it is most frequently on the right side.

Manifestations

Acute aching pain over the loins, often radiating to the groin
- Fever (often high) with chills and rigor
- Anorexia, nausea and vomiting
- Frequency of micturition and/or dysuria
- Flushed face and dry tongue (dehydration)
- Urine may appear cloudy.

Investigations

- Examination of midstream urine may show evidence of:
  - Acid reaction
  - Fishy smell
  - High specific gravity
  - Presence of slight proteins
  - Plenty of pus cells and RBCs
- Urine culture and sensitivity
- Blood tests may show high leukocytosis, raised blood urea nitrogen and creatinine depending on the extent of damage of the renal parenchyma.

Effects on Pregnancy

There may be increased fetal loss due to abortion and intrauterine fetal death caused by hyperpyrexia and low birth weight babies

Treatment

Preventive: Screening of susceptible women (having history of previous urinary tract infection) at the first antenatal visit to detect significant bacteriuria.

If it is found positive, a course of nitrofurantoin 50 mg thrice daily or ampicillin 250 mg six hourly for two weeks is given. The urine should be tested at intervals of four weeks. The woman should be advised to pass urine frequently.

Curative

Admission to the hospital is usual. Adequate rest, easily digestible diet and plenty of fluids are given. In case of persistent vomiting, intravenous fluid therapy is started. A clean-catch midstream urine is sent for culture and sensitivity test, and pending report, antimicrobial therapy is started. If the woman is febrile, intravenous cephadrine 1 gm every 6 hours is administered. Once the temperature subsides, oral cephadrine is started with 500 mg every 6 hours. Nitrofurantoin 100 mg thrice daily orally is the alternative. The therapy should be given for at least 10 days. After the therapy is stopped, if at least three urine cultures over the next 10 days are reported as sterile, the disease is considered cured.

Intravenous fluids may also be required to correct dehydration and an accurate record of fluid balance must be kept. During the early stages of illness, the woman will be confined to bed and the midwife should take steps to prevent complications of immobility, such as deep vein thrombosis and constipation. The midwife must monitor uterine activity, as there is a risk of labor commencing when the temperature rises. It may be necessary to reduce the temperature by tepid sponging and antipyretics. The temperature and pulse should be recorded four hourly.

The mother may be in considerable pain which may be eased by the use of hot water bag to her back and buscopan 20 mg. Antiemetics may be given to counteract nausea. Careful follow-up throughout pregnancy and especially in puerperium is mandatory. Relapses are common in puerperium (10%). The urine should be examined at monthly intervals including culture. Women should be encouraged to pass urine frequently. Any sign suggestive of urinary tract infection should be treated vigorously.

CHRONIC RENAL DISEASE

Chronic pyelonephritis may be a process from the beginning or may develop as sequelae of an incompletely treated and followed-up case of acute or recurrent mild pyelonephritis. Asymptomatic bacteriuria may prove to be a resting stage in the process of development of chronic pyelonephritis. A pregnant woman with pre-existing renal disease is considered to be at risk of pre-eclampsia and intrauterine growth retardation. Preterm birth and perinatal mortality are increased. The woman's own condition is likely to deteriorate. Hospital delivery is essential.

During pregnancy, proteinuria tends to increase. Damage to the kidney tubules causes an activation of the renin-angiotensin system, leading to salt and water retention and a consequent rise in blood pressure. Production of erythropoietin may be reduced, leading to anemia. The presence of chronic infection predisposes the mother to superimposed acute infection. The outcome of pregnancy depends on the degree of renal dysfunction, the blood pressure and episodes of infection. Termination of pregnancy or early induction of labor may be offered if the renal condition deteriorates severely.

Examples of Pre-existing Renal Diseases

❖ Polycystic kidney disease
❖ Glomerular nephritis
❖ Chronic pyelonephritis
❖ Renal calculi and nephrotic syndrome.

Chronic hypertension is a common sequel. Anemia may develop which become refractory to iron therapy and superimposed pre-eclampsia may aggravate the impaired renal function during pregnancy.

Management

The aim of management is to prevent deterioration in renal function. Renal function tests are performed at intervals throughout the pregnancy. The emergence and severity of hypertension, and preeclampsia are monitored by recording blood pressure and estimating urea, creatinine clearance and total protein excretion levels. Admission to hospital is advised if there is evidence of fetal compromise, if renal function deteriorates and proteinuria increases or if blood pressure rises. In severe cases, renal dialysis may be required.

Autoimmune Diseases

SYSTEMIC LUPUS ERYTHEMATOSUS (SLE)

Systemic lupus erythematosus is an autoimmune disease, which upsets the normal immunity of a person. It is characterized by the production of autoantibodies, which are antibodies, synthesized by an individual against a component of her own body. It is first diagnosed during pregnancy in 10 to 30 percent of cases.

SLE, which is a multisystem disease, is characterized by exacerbations (flares) and remissions but has no typical disease pattern, which often makes diagnosis difficult (Sala, 1993). It may manifest as polyarthritis, myalgia, skin rash, alopecia, pleurisy, dyspnea, pericarditis, proteinuria or anemia. Fertility rates are normal, therefore, pregnancy becomes a common management problem in these women.

Effects of Pregnancy on SLE

Long-term prognosis remains unaffected. There is chance of flare up, especially during first half and in puerperium. Deaths occur in puerperium due to pulmonary hemorrhage and lupus pneumonia.

Effects on Pregnancy

There is increased risk of first trimester abortion, lupus nephritis, recurrent deep vein thrombosis, PIH, IUGR, prematurity and stillbirths. Neonatal lupus syndrome occurs due to crossing of maternal lupus antibodies to the fetus causing hemolytic anemia, leucopenia and thrombocytopenia. Isolated congenital heart block is seen in about one-third of cases (Dutta, 2001).

Investigation

Antinuclear antibodies are the standard screening test for the disease.

Management

Preconception counseling is extremely important since conception during a period of quiescence is most likely to result in a live birth. The frequency of antenatal visits is dependent on the severity of the disease and should include full hematological and immunological investigations.

Control and treatment of SLE is mainly dependent on drugs starting with analgesics, such as paracetamol and progressing to corticosteroids, immunosuppressives and cytotoxic agents in severe cases. Drug therapy is individualized and dependent upon the disease activity and organs involved. Low dose aspirin 80 mg daily is prescribed usually. It is important that the woman is made aware of the risks to herself and her baby, if SLE is left untreated, as often women are reluctant to take drugs in pregnancy.

Intrapartum Care

The timing of delivery depends upon the severity of the disease and whether there are any complications such as preeclampsia or renal involvement. Delivery should otherwise be at term. SLE patients are at risk of infection and hence, the midwife should ensure that careful hand washing and strict aseptic technique are adhered to as well as limiting the number of vaginal examinations. Observations of vital signs need to be frequent along with measurement of fluid intake and output and assessment of urinary protein. Continuous fetal monitoring and fetal blood gas estimation are recommended. Vaginal delivery is aimed for where possible. However, because of associated problems, many fetuses are delivered by planned cesarean section. Women on long-term corticosteroid therapy should have parenteral steroid cover in labor and for 24 hours post-natally.

Postnatal Care

Following delivery of the baby, the midwife needs to encourage the woman to rest as much as possible in order to prevent exacerbation of her SLE which is likely to occur during stressful times. Close monitoring of vital signs should continue for 24 to 48 hours following delivery. Breastfeeding is generally safe if the mother is receiving nonsteroid antiinflammatory drugs or low-dose steroids. Salicylates, antimalarial and immunosuppressive agents need to be avoided (deSwiet, 1995). The newborn should have a careful clinical examination and undergo appropriate serological evaluation by a pediatrician in the postnatal period. The choice of contraceptives for the woman with SLE is limited to barrier methods and the midwife must educate the woman and her spouse in their proper use. Intrauterine device may predispose to infection, oral contraceptives may induce exacerbation of the disease, and hence both are contraindicated.

IDIOPATHIC THROMBOCYTOPENIC PURPURA (ITP)

ITP is the most common tissue or organ specific autoimmune disease in women of childbearing age and accounts for 2 to 4 percent of pregnant women. This condition causes increased platelet destruction by immune processes, which may arise following viral infection or an allergic response to drugs (Allison, 1989). If the platelet count falls below 50,000/mm³ the condition may manifest as bleeding from mucous surfaces and episodes such as epistaxis, multiple small bruises, petechiae in the skin, postpartum hemorrhage or bleeding from abdominal or perineal incisions.

Diagnosis

Diagnosis may be made following a routine full blood count of $< 100 \times 10^9/\mu L$, or when the woman presents with repeated episodes of bleeding in pregnancy.

Effects of ITP on Pregnancy and the Fetus

Postpartum hemorrhage is the major risk, which is directly related to the maternal platelet count. Maternal mortality and morbidity are now rare. The perinatal mortality can be as high as 15 percent in extreme cases. Complications to the fetus include gastrointestinal bleeding, hemopericardium, intraventricular hemorrhage and severe cutaneous manifestations of bleeding. Profound thrombocytopenia may develop in infants due to transplacental passage of IgG antibodies. In babies, it is a transient condition lasting between one week and four months of life.

Antenatal Care

Management of this condition during pregnancy is to be supervised by a hematologist and involves monitoring and maintaining the maternal platelet count at an acceptable level. Corticosteroid therapy is the initial treatment of choice, which will increase the maternal platelet count. If this fails, a high dose of immunoglobulin can be given intravenously.

Intrapartum Care

The objective is to plan for a vaginal delivery, avoiding an episiotomy and ensuring good control of the third stage of labor. Intravenous ergometrine is used prophylactically. A pediatrician should be present at delivery and an immediate cord platelet count is taken. Treatment may be required if the platelet count is $< 50 \times 10^9/l$ ($< 50 \times 100,000/\mu L$) or when the woman presents with repeated episodes of bleeding in pregnancy.

Postnatal Care

Following delivery, the midwife should inspect the genital tract to identify and control any bleeding sites. Strict attention to aseptic technique and careful repair of any tissue trauma is important. Breastfeeding is encouraged unless there are adverse complications. Discussion with the woman and her spouse regarding the risks of future pregnancies is important, and they should be advised that platelet levels need to be within normal limits prior to future conceptions.

Epilepsy in Pregnancy

The effect of pregnancy on epilepsy is unclear. Frequency of convulsions is unchanged in about 50 percent and is increased in some. Increased plasma clearance of anticonvulsant drugs during pregnancy has been observed and estrogens are thought to activate the seizure foci (Dutta, 2001). The adverse effects on the mother are third trimester bleeding and megaloblastic anemia, which may be related to anticonvulsant induced folate deficiency.

Birth defects are increased by twofold. Malformations include cleft lip and/or palate, mental retardation, cardiac abnormalities, limb defects and hypoplacia of the terminal phalanges. There is chance of neonatal hemorrhage which is related to anticonvulsant induced vitamin K dependent coagulopathy. The risk of developing epilepsy to the offspring of an epileptic mother is fourfold. Preconception counseling includes:

❖ Initiation of monotherapy, if possible and
❖ Administration of folic acid 1 mg daily.

Management

The dose of the chosen drug should be kept as low as possible and to be monitored regularly from the serum level. The commonly used drugs are:

❖ Phenobarbitone 60 to 180 mg daily in 2 to 3 divided doses
❖ Phenytoin 150 to 300 mg daily in two divided doses
❖ Carbamazepine 0.8 to 1.2 gm daily in divided doses.

The fits are controlled by intravenous diazepam 10 to 20 mg. Folic acid 1 mg must be continued throughout pregnancy. There is decrease in free level of most of the anticonvulsants in pregnancy. This is due to reduced absorption and at the same time increased hepatic metabolism and renal clearance. Vitamin K 10 mg daily must be given orally in the last two weeks. Termination of pregnancy may be considered in consultation with a neurologist. Seizure precautions and care will be required during the postpartum period.

There is no contraindication for breast-feeding. The infant may be drowsy. By 4 to 6 weeks postpartum, the anticonvulsant dose must be adjusted and brought to the pre-pregnant level. Steroidal contraceptives are to be avoided due to enzyme induction.

BIBLIOGRAPHY

1. Allison JV, et al. Lecture Notes on Human Physiology, 2nd edn. Oxford: Blackwell Scientific Publications. 1989.
2. Becks GP, Burrows GN. 'Thyroid disease and pregnancy'. Medical Clinics of North America. 1991;75(1):121-50.
3. Benson B. Handbook of Obstetrics and Gynecology. California: Lange Medical Publications. 1990.
4. Bishoni A, Sachmechi I. Thyroid disease during pregnancy. American Family Physician 1996; 53(1):215-20.
5. Carpenter MW. Testing for gestational diabetes. In: Reace et al. Diabetes Mellitus in Pregnancy, 2nd edn. New York: Churchill Livingstone, 1995.
6. deSwiet M. Medical Disorders in Obstetric Practice 3rd edn. Oxford: Blackwell Scientific Publications. 1995.
7. Duff P Maternal and Perinatal Infections. In: Gabbe SG, et al. Obstetrics: Normal and Problem Pregnancies, 3rd edn. New York: Churchill Livingstone. 1996.
8. Dutta DC. Textbook of Obstetrics, 5th edn. Calcutta: New Central Book Company. 2001.
9. Girling J. Thyroid disease in pregnancy. Maternal and Child Health. 1996;21(9):202-5.
10. Hollingsworth DR, Resnik R. Medical Counseling before Pregnancy. New York: Churchill Livingstone, 1988.
11. Jowett NI, Nichol SG. Gestational diabetes: are right women being screened. Midwifery. 1986; 2(2):98-100.
12. London MB, Samuels P. Cardiac and Pulmonary Disease. In: Gabbe SG, et al. Obstetrics: Normal and Problem Pregnancies, 3rd edn. New York: Churchill Livingstone 1996.
13. Lloyd C, Lewis VM. Common medical disorders associated with pregnancy. In: Myles Textbook for Midwives 13th edn. Edinburgh: Churchill Livingstone 1999.
14. Letsky EA. Anemia in obstetrics. In: Studd J (Ed.). Progress in Obstetrics and Gynecology. New York: Churchill Livingstone. 1987.
15. Mestman JH, et al. Thyroid disorders of pregnancy, endocrinology and metabolism. Clinics of North America. 1995;24:41-71.
16. Nolan J. Heart disease in pregnancy. British Journal of Hospital Medicine. 1990;39(1):50-3.
17. Oates JN, Beischer NA. Gestational diabetes. In: Studd J (Eds). Progress in Obstetrics and Gynecology. Edinburgh: Churchill Livingstone 1987.
18. Roberton NRC. A Manual of Normal Neonatal Care. London: Edward Arnold 1992.
19. Smith JE. Pregnancy complicated by thyroid disease. Journal of Nurse-Midwifery. 1990; 35(3):42-149.
20. Park K. Park's Textbook of Preventive and Social Medicine, (16th edn). Jabalpur: M/s Banarasidas Banot Publishers. 2000.
21. Sala DJ. Effects of SLE on pregnancy and neonate. Journal of Perinatal and Neonatal Nursing. 1993;7(3):34-48.
22. Shabetai R. Congenital or acquired heart disease. In: Hollingsworth D (Ed) et al. Medical Counseling before Pregnancy. New York: Churchill Livingstone 1988.
23. Snider DE. Should women taking antituberculosis drugs breastfeed? Archives of Internal Medicine. 1984;144:589-90.
24. Streetly A, Dick M Layton M. Sickle cell disease: The case of coordinated information. British Medical Journal. 1993;306:1491-2.
25. Sugrue D, Drury MI. Hyperthyroidism complicating pregnancy. British Journal of Obstetrics and Gynecology. 1980;87:970-5.
26. Torrance C. Absorption and functions of iron. Nursing Standards. 1992;6(19):25-28.
27. Walfish PG, Chan JY. Postpartum hyperthyroidism. Clinics in Endocrinological Metabolism. 1985;14:417-20.
28. Wills DC, et al. Cardiac output response to prostaglandin E_2 induced abortion in the second trimester. American Journal of Obstetrics and Gynecology. 1987;56:170-3.

30

Multiple Pregnancy

Learning Objectives

Upon completing this chapter, the learner will be able to:

❖ Describe the types of multiple pregnancies and the genesis of different varieties
❖ Describe the diagnosis and management of twin pregnancy and labor
❖ Describe the care of mother and babies after birth
❖ Explain the problems specific to babies of multiple births and the fetal abnormalities unique to the process of multiplication
❖ Explain the special needs of parents and nurses' role in management.

Multiple pregnancies are the development of more than one fetus at the same time in the gravid uterus. Simultaneous development of two fetuses is termed twins, which is the commonest. Although rare, simultaneously three fetuses (triplets), four fetuses (quadriplets), five fetuses (quintuplets) or six fetuses (sextuplets) may also develop.

INCIDENCE

The incidence varies widely. In the world, it varies from 5.6 to 46 per 1,000 births. It is highest in Nigeria, being 1 in 20 and lowest in far eastern countries, being 1 in 200 pregnancies. In India, the incidence is about 1 in 80. While the incidence of monozygotic twins remains constant throughout the globe, being 1 in 250, it is the dizygotic twins, which are responsible for the wide variation of the incidence. Since the 1980s, there has been a rise in the incidence due to the increased use of various kinds of treatments for infertility involving ovulation induction.

The number of triplets has more than trebled in the last 12 years due to the rise in infertility treatments such as *in vitro* fertilization (IVF) and ovulatory stimulating drugs like clomiphene citrate and gonadotropins (Bennett and Brown, 2000).

TWIN PREGNANCY

Simultaneous development of two fetuses in the uterus is the commonest variety of multiple pregnancies.

Varieties of Twins

1. Binovular twins—It is the most common (two-thirds) and results from the fertilization of two ova.
2. Uniovular twins (one-third) results from the fertilization of a single ovum.

Genesis of Twins

Binovular twins are also referred to as fraternal or dizygotic twins. They result from the fertilization of two ova, most likely ruptured from two different Graafian follicles, usually of the same or one from each ovary, by two sperms during a single ovarian cycle. Their subsequent implantation and development differ little from those of single fertilized ovum. The babies bear only fraternal resemblance to each other (that of brothers and sisters from different births). Approximately one-third of the binovular twins may be boy pairs, one-third girl pairs and one-third boy-girl pairs.

Uniovular twins are also termed as identical or monozygotic twins. They develop from one ovum and one spermatozoon and the twinning occurs at different periods after fertilization. The time at which the separation occurs is probably after the formation of the inner cell mass (between 4th-8th day). Thus, two embryos will develop enclosed by a single chorion, having single placenta and two separate amniotic sacs (monochorionic-diamniotic). These twins will be of the same sex and have the same genes, blood groups and physical features such as eye and hair color, ear shapes and palm creases. However, they may be of different sizes and sometimes have different personalities.

Etiology

The cause of twinning is not known. Prevalence of binovular twins is related to:

- ❖ *Race*: The frequency is highest amongst Negroes, lowest amongst Mongols and intermediate amongst Caucasians.
- ❖ *Heredity*: There is hereditary predisposition likely to be more transmitted through the female.
- ❖ *Advancing age of the mother*: Twinning increases with maternal age, peak being between 30 and 35 years.
- ❖ *Influence of parity*: The incidence increases with parity, especially from fifth gravida onwards.
- ❖ *Iatrogenic*: Drugs used for induction of ovulation may produce multiple fetuses to the extent of 20 to 40 percent following gonadotrophin therapy and to a lesser extent (5-6%) following clomiphene citrate.

Rare Forms

- ❖ *Superfecundation*: It is the fertilization of two different ova released in the same cycle, by separate acts of coitus within a short period of time.
- ❖ *Superfetation*: It is the fertilization of two ova released in different menstrual cycles. The nidation and development of one fetus over another fetus is theoretically possible until the decidual space is obliterated by 12 weeks of pregnancy.
- ❖ *Fetus papyraceous or compressus*: It is a state, which occurs if one of the fetuses dies

early. The dead fetus is flattened and compressed between the membranes of the living fetus and the uterine wall. It may occur in both varieties but is more common in uniovular twins and is discovered at delivery or earlier by sonography.

- ❖ *Fetus acardiacus*: It occurs only in uniovular twins. Part of the fetus remains amorphous and becomes parasitic without a heart.
- ❖ *Vanishing twin*: Occasional death of one twin and continuation of pregnancy with the surviving one. The dead fetus (if within 14 weeks) simply vanishes by resorption.

Determination of Zygosity

Determination of zygosity means determining whether or not the twins are identical.

Examination of Placenta and Membranes

Binovular twins

1. There are two placentae, either completely separated or more commonly fused at the margin appearing to be one (9 out of 10). There is no anastomosis between the two fetal vessels.
2. Each fetus is surrounded by a separate amnion and chorion.
3. The intervening membranes consist of four layers—2 amnions, 2 chorions.

Uniovular twins

1. The placenta is single. There is varying degree of free anastomosis between the two fetal vessels.
2. Each fetus is surrounded by a separate amnionic sac with the chorionic layer common to both (diamniotic, monochorionic).
3. The intervening membranes consist of two layers of amnion only (Figs 30.1A and B).

Sex

- ❖ Uniovular twins are always of the same sex
- ❖ Binovular twins may be of same sex or may differ.

Genetic Features (Dominant Blood Group)

If the fetuses are of the same sex and have the same genetic features (blood group), monozygosity is likely.

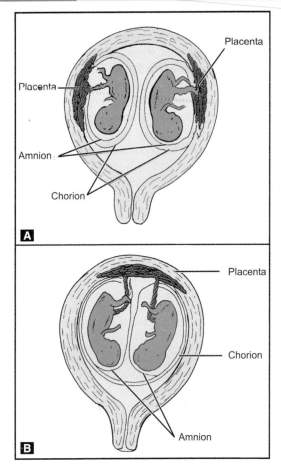

Figs 30.1A and B: Twin placentae: (A) Placenta of binovular (dizygotic) twins; (B) Placenta of uniovular (monozygotic) twins

Diagnosis of Twin Pregnancy

History

1. History of ovulation inducing drugs especially gonadotrophins for infertility.
2. Family history of multiple pregnancy (more often in the maternal side).

Symptoms

Minor ailments of normal pregnancy are often exaggerated. Some of the symptoms are related to the abnormal enlargement of the uterus.

1. Increased nausea and vomiting in early months.
2. Cardiorespiratory embarrassment in the later months such as palpitation or shortness of breath.
3. Tendency of swelling of the legs, varicose veins and hemorrhoids is greater.

4. Unusual rate of abdominal enlargement and excessive fetal movements may be noticed by an experienced parous mother.

General Examination

1. Prevalence of anemia is more than in singleton pregnancy.
2. Unusual weight gain, not explained by pre-eclampsia or obesity.
3. Evidence of pre-eclampsia (in about 25%).

Abdominal Examination

Inspection: (1) The size of the uterus may be larger than expected for the period of gestation, particularly after the 20th week. (2) The uterus broad or round (barrel shape) and fetal movements may be seen over a wide area. (3) Fresh striae gravidarum may be apparent. Polyhydramnios is common.

Palpation

1. On palpation, the fundal height may be greater than expected for the period of gestation (evident from midpregnancy onwards).
2. The presence of two fetal poles (head or breech) in the fundus of the uterus.
3. Palpation of multiple fetal limbs.
4. The girth of the abdomen at the level of umbilicus is more than the normal average at term (100 cm).
5. Lateral palpation may reveal two fetal backs or limbs on both sides. Pelvic palpation may give findings similar to those on fundal palpation although one fetus may lie behind the other and make detection difficult. Location of three poles in total is diagnostic of at least two fetuses.

Auscultation

Simultaneous hearing of two distinct fetal heart sounds, located at separate spots with a silent area in between by two observers, gives a certain clue in the diagnosis of twins, provided the difference in the heart rates is at least 10 beats per minute

Investigations

❖ *Ultrasound examination:* Two gestational sacs can be detected as early as 10th week of pregnancy. Considering that one fetus may vanish; repeat sonar is done in second trimester. Detection of two fetal heads and their measurement of biparietal diameters can be made by the 14th week. For assessment of placentation, sonar is done between 16th to 24th week. Zygosity could be determined by identifying the intervening layers. For assessment of IUGR, it should be repeatedly done at 4 weeks interval from the second half of pregnancy.

❖ *Radiography*: It is done less often these days. Two fetal heads and spines could be seen on X-ray.

Duration of Pregnancy

A multiple pregnancy tends to be shorter than a single pregnancy. The average gestation for twins is 37 weeks, triplets 34 weeks and quadruplets 33 weeks.

Effects of Pregnancy

Maternal

During pregnancy:

❖ *Exacerbation of minor disorders*: Nausea and vomiting occurs with increased frequency and severity. Heartburn may be more persistent and troublesome than in singleton pregnancy.

❖ *Anemia*: Iron deficiency and folic acid deficiency anemia are common in twin pregnancies. This is because of increased iron and folate requirements by the two fetuses. Deficiency of folic acid (after 28th week) leads to increased incidence of megaloblastic anemia.

❖ Pre-eclampsia (25%) is increased three times over singleton pregnancy. Over distension of the uterus may be the possible explanation.

❖ Antepartum hemorrhage may occur with slightly increased frequency. The increased incidence of placenta previa is due to the bigger size of the placenta encroaching on to the lower segment. Separation of the normally situated placenta may occur due to increased incidence of PIH, sudden escape of liquor following rupture of the membranes of the hydramniotic sac, deficiency of folic acid and following delivery of the first baby due to sudden shrinkage of the uterine wall adjacent to the placental attachment.

❖ Malpresentation is quite common in twins compared to singleton pregnancies. Malpresentation is more common in the second baby.

❖ Preterm labor (30%) frequently occurs and the mean gestational period for twins is 37 weeks. Over distention of the uterus, hydramnios and premature rupture of the membranes are responsible for preterm labor.

❖ Mechanical distress such as palpitation, dyspnea, varicosities and hemorrhoids may be increased. Increased weight and size of the uterus and impaired venous return from the lower limbs contribute to these discomforts. Backache and indigestion are common.

During labor:

❖ Early rupture of membranes and cord prolapse are likely to be increased due to increased prevalence of malpresentation. Cord prolapse is five times more common than in singleton pregnancy.

❖ Increased operative interference due to high prevalence of malpresentation.

❖ Bleeding following the birth of the first baby, may at times, be alarming and is due to separation of the placenta following reduction of placental site.

❖ Postpartum hemorrhage may occur due to atony of the uterine muscle due to overdistension of the uterus, longer time taken by the big placenta to separate, the bigger surface of the placenta exposing more uterine sinuses and implantation of a part of the placenta in the lower segment.

During puerperium:

❖ There is increased incidence of subinvolution because of bigger size of the uterus

❖ Chances of infection are more because of operative interference, pre-existing anemia and blood loss during delivery

Effects on Fetus

- Miscarriage rate is increased.
- Premature births are increased (80%) and the babies suffer from the hazards of prematurity.
- Growth problems (25%). Weight difference of 25 percent or more may be seen. This may be due to twin-twin transfusion syndrome or intrauterine anomalies occurring in one fetus.
- Intrauterine death of one fetus. This is increased in uniovular twin pregnancies. If a loss occurs early in gestation (before 14th week), the affected fetus simply vanishes by resorption. If the death occurs in the second trimester, a fetus papyraceous may form. If death occurs late in pregnancy, there may be death of the other fetus or it may complicate the mother with DIC. The deaths are due to cord compression, competition for nourishment or congenital malformation.
- Fetal anomalies are increased twofolds over the singleton pregnancy, more in uniovular twins. They are in the form of anencephaly, hydrocephalus, cardiac anomalies or Down syndrome.
- Asphyxia and stillbirth are more common due to increased prevalence of pre-eclampsia, malpresentation, placental abruption and increased operative interferences. The second baby is more at risk.

Antenatal Management

Early management of twin pregnancy is extremely important in order to prepare the parents by giving them the specialist support and advice they will need. This will help the mother to take additional care not only for her own benefit but also for the fetuses.

Advice

- *Diet*: Increased dietary supplement is needed for increased energy supply to the extent of 300 kcal per day, over and above that needed in a single gestation. The increased demand for protein must be met.
- Increased rest at home and early cessation of work is advised to prevent preterm labor and other complications.
- *Supplement therapy*: Additional iron, folic acid, vitamins and calcium are needed in multiple gestation.
- Interval of antenatal visit should be more frequent to detect at the earliest the evidence of anemia, pre-eclampsia or preterm labor.
- Fetal growth assessment must be done at every 2 to 3 weeks interval.
- *Preparation for breastfeeding*: Early in the antenatal period, the mother should be given as much information as possible about both breast and bottlefeeding. Mothers should be encouraged right from the beginning that breastfeeding will be possible for two or even three babies.

Hospitalization

Elective: In an uncomplicated twin pregnancy routine admission for bed rest is not essential. However, the woman may be admitted around the 32nd week if she prefers it. Bed rest improves uteroplacental circulation. This results in increased birth weight of babies, decreased frequency of pre-eclampsia, decreased frequency of preterm labor and lowered perinatal mortality.

Emergency: Development of complicating factors necessitates urgent admission irrespective of the period of gestation.

Management During Labor

The higher the number of fetuses the mother is carrying, the earlier labor is likely to start. Term for twins is usually considered 37th week rather than 40 and approximately 30 percent of twins are born preterm, that is before 37th week. As the twin pregnancy is considered a 'high-risk', the woman should be admitted in an equipped hospital preferably having an intensive neonatal care unit.

During the first stage of labor:
- The woman should be kept in bed and the enema withheld to prevent early rupture of membranes.
- Use of analgesics is limited as the babies are small and rapid delivery may occur. Epidural analgesia is preferred as it

facilitates manipulation of second fetus if it would become necessary.

- Careful fetal monitoring of both babies should be done; continuous monitoring using electronic fetal monitor is better.
- Vaginal examination should be done soon after the rupture of membranes to exclude cord prolapse.
- An intravenous line with Ringer's solution should be set up for any urgent intravenous therapy, if required.
- One unit of compatible and cross-matched blood should be made readily available.
- Neonatologist should be present at the time of delivery.
- If fetal distress occurs during labor, delivery will need to be expedited, usually by cesarean section.
- If uterine activity is poor, the use of intravenous syntocinon may be required once the membranes have been ruptured.
- Artificial rupture of membranes may be sufficient to stimulate good uterine contractions, but may need to be used in conjunction with IV syntocinon.
- Throughout labor, the mother will require emotional as well as physical support from the midwife.

Management of Delivery

The onset of second stage of labor should be confirmed by vaginal examination. The obstetrician, pediatrician and anesthetist should be present for the delivery because of the risk of complications. The possibility of emergency cesarean section is always present and the operating room should be ready to receive the mother at a short notice. Monitoring of both fetal hearts should continue until delivery. The delivery of the first twin should be conducted in the same manner as in normal labor if it presents by vertex. Liberal episiotomy is given to prevent intracranial damage to the forecoming or after-coming head of the premature baby. When the first twin is born, the time of delivery and the sex are noted. The baby must be labeled as 'twin one' immediately.

After delivery of the first twin, abdominal palpation must be done to ascertain the lie, presentation and position of the second twin and to auscultate the fetal heart. A vaginal examination should be done to exclude cord prolapse, if any, and to note the status of the membranes. If the lie is not longitudinal, an attempt may be made to correct it by external cephalic version. If the presenting part is not engaged it should be pushed into the pelvis by fundal pressure before the second sac of membranes are ruptured. If uterine activity does not recommence, intravenous oxytocin may be used to stimulate it.

When the presenting part becomes visible, the mother should be encouraged to push with contractions to deliver the second twin. Delivery will proceed as normal if the presentation is vertex. Delivery of the second twin must be completed within 45 minutes of the first twin as long as there are no signs of fetal distress. If there is delay, the baby is delivered by ventouse or low forceps. If the baby presents by breech, breech extraction is done.

Methergine 0.2 mg is given intravenously with delivery of the anterior shoulder of the second baby. The baby is labeled as 'twin two' and the time of delivery and sex of the baby are noted. The risk of asphyxia is greater for the second baby and may require active resuscitation and transfer to the neonatal unit.

Management of the Third Stage

The placenta is to be delivered by cord traction applied to both cords simultaneously. It is important to deliver the placenta immediately as emptying the uterus enables bleeding to be controlled and postpartum hemorrhage prevented. Oxytocin drip is continued for at least one hour, following the delivery of the second baby. The woman should be carefully watched for about two hours following delivery. A blood loss of more than average is often replaced by blood transfusion.

The placenta(e) should be examined and the number of amniotic sacs, chorions and placentae are noted. The umbilical cords should be examined and the number of cord vessels and the presence of any abnormalities noted.

Indications for Cesarean Section

Associated Causes

- ❖ Contracted pelvis
- ❖ Placenta previa
- ❖ Severe pre-eclampsia
- ❖ Previous history of cesarean section
- ❖ Cord prolapse of the first baby
- ❖ Abnormal uterine contractions.

Fetal Causes

- ❖ Both babies or even the first baby in transverse lie
- ❖ Nonvertex twins with estimated weight 2000 gm or less
- ❖ Conjoined twins
- ❖ Collision of both heads at brim preventing engagement of either head.

Complications Associated with Multiple Pregnancy

The high perinatal mortality associated with pregnancies is largely due to complications of pregnancy, such as premature onset of labor, intrauterine growth retardation and complications of delivery. The management of multiple pregnancies is concerned with prevention, early detection and treatment of these complications.

Polyhydramnios

Acute polyhydramnios may occur as early as 18th to 20th week. It may be associated with fetal abnormality and more likely due to the feto-fetal transfusion syndrome (FFTS) also known as twin-to-twin transfusion syndrome (TTTS).

Fetofetal transfusion syndrome can be acute or chronic. The acute form usually occurs during labor in uniovular twins where one twin appears to bleed into the other through some kind of placental vascular anastomosis. Both fetuses may die of cardiac failure if not treated immediately.

Chronic fetofetal transfusion syndrome can occur in up to 35 percent of mono-chorionic twin pregnancies (Fisk, 1995). As a result the receptor twin becomes larger, polycythemic and hypervolemic (hydrops) at the expense of the donor twin which becomes smaller, anemic and hypovolemic. Difference

of hemoglobin concentration between the two, usually exceeds 5 gm% and estimated fetal discrepancy is 25 percent or more. The fetal and neonatal mortality is high but some infants may be saved by early diagnosis and prenatal treatment with either amnio-reduction (amniocentesis) or laser coagulation of communicating placental vessels.

The smaller twin generally has better outcome. The plethoric twin runs the risk of congestive cardiac failure and hydrops.

Fetal Abnormality

This is particularly associated with monozygotic twins.

- ❖ *Conjoined twins*: This extremely rare malformation of monozygotic twinning results from the incomplete division of the fertilized ovum. Delivery has to be by cesarean section. Separation of the babies is sometimes possible and will depend on how they are joined and which internal organs are involved.
- ❖ *Acardiac formation*: This occurs in about 1:30,000 deliveries. In acardia, one twin presents without a well-defined cardiac structure and is kept alive through placental anastomosis to the circulatory system of the viable fetus (Moore, et al. 1990).
- ❖ *Fetus in fetu*: In fetus in fetu, parts of a fetus may be lodged within another fetus. This can happen only in monozygotic twins.

Malpresentations

Although the uterus is large and distended, the fetuses are less mobile than may be supposed. They restrict each other's movements, which may result in malpresentations. After delivery of the first twin, the presentation of the second twin may change.

Premature Rupture of Membranes

Malpresentations due to polyhydramnios may predispose to premature rupture of the membranes.

Prolapse of the Cord

This too is associated with malpresentations and polyhydramnios and is more likely if there is a poorly fitting presenting part. The second twin is particularly at risk of cord prolapse.

Prolonged Labor

Malpresentations are a poor stimulus to good uterine action and distended uterus is likely to lead to poor uterine activity and consequently prolonged labor.

Monoamniotic Twins

Approximately one percent of twins share the same amniotic sac. These twins risk cord entanglement with occlusion of the blood supply to one or both fetuses.

Locked Twins (Figs 30.2A and B)

This is a rare but serious complication of twin pregnancy. There are of two types. One occurs when the first twin presents by breech and the second by vertex, the other occurs when both are vertex. In both instances, the head of the second twin prevents the continued descend of the first. Interlocking occurs as the after-coming head of the first baby is locked with the forecoming head of the second baby.

With two vertex twins, the heads get locked at the pelvic brim preventing engagement of either of the head. Cesarean section is necessary in these cases for fetal interest. Occasionally, with interlocked twins of the first type decapitation of the first baby, if already dead, is done. The decapitated head is pushed up, followed by delivery of the second baby and lastly, delivery of the decapitated head. This saves one baby.

Figs 30.2A and B: Locked twins: (A) 1st twin breech, 2nd twin vertex; (B) Both twins vertex

Delay in the Birth of the Second Twin

After the birth of the first twin, uterine activity should commence within five minutes. Delivery of the second twin is usually completed within 45 minutes of the first birth. Delay may occur at times due to poor uterine action because of malpresentation. The risks of such delay are intrauterine hypoxia, birth asphyxia following premature separation of the placenta and sepsis as a result of ascending infection from the first umbilical cord, which lies outside the vulva.

The midwife may need to "rub-up" a contraction and to put the first twin to the breast to stimulate uterine activity. If there appears to be an obstruction, cesarean section may be necessary. If there is no obstruction *syntocinon* infusion may be commenced and forceps delivery commenced.

Premature Expulsion of the Placenta

The placenta may be expelled before delivery of the second twin. In dizygotic twins with separate placenta, one may be delivered separately. In monozygotic twins, the shared placenta may be expelled and the risks of severe asphyxia and death of the second twin are then very high. Hemorrhage is also likely if one twin is retained *in utero,* as this prevents adequate retraction of the placental site.

Postpartum Hemorrhage

Poor uterine tone because of over distension or hypotonic activity is likely to lead to post-partum hemorrhage.

Undiagnosed Twins

The possibility of an undiagnosed second baby should be considered if the uterus appears larger than expected after the delivery of the first baby or if the baby is surprisingly smaller than expected. This is unlikely with ultrasound scanning facility. If an oxytocic drug has been given after delivery of the anterior shoulder of the first baby, the second baby is in great danger and delivery should be expedited. The baby will require active resuscitation because of severe asphyxia.

Management of Postnatal Period

Care of the Babies

Immediate care after delivery involves ensuring that both babies have clear airway. Maintenance of body temperature is vital particularly if the newborns are small and use of overhead heater on the resuscitaire will help if available. Proper drying and wrapping with warm baby-blankets are important. Identification of the infants should be clear and parents must be given the opportunity to check the identity bracelets and cuddle their babies. The infants may have to be admitted directly to the neonatal unit from the labor ward and later transferred to the postnatal ward to be with the mother.

Both babies may be breastfed either simultaneously or separately. The mother may choose to feed the babies artificially. She may need help with the chosen method in the initial days. If the babies are small for dates or preterm, they may have to be fed with expressed breast milk or 'topped-up' after a breastfeed. At feeding time, the midwife must be with the mother to offer support and advice on positioning and fixing the babies as well as encouraging her to feed two babies. Using pillows to support the weight of the babies, the mother should be assisted to assume comfortable position for feeding. She might need the help of another person in the initial days whether the babies are breastfed or bottlefed.

If the infants are of low birth weight, they are more susceptible to infection and hence the mother should be encouraged to wash her hands before handling her babies and particularly after changing their nappies.

Care of the Mother

Involution of the uterus will be slower because of its increased bulk. 'After pains' may be troublesome and analgesics must be given when she needs. If the mother is breastfeeding, a high-protein, high-calorie diet is required. She may feel hungry between meals and must be encouraged to keep snacks for such times.

In order to improve the muscle tone of the abdomen and pelvic floor, she must be instructed in postnatal exercises and encouraged to carry them out regularly. Teaching parenting skills will be important, as she will need to gain confidence in managing two babies.

One or both babies may sometimes remain in the nursery for few days. Mothers in such situations need assistance with visiting the babies, feeding and bonding. Postnatal depression has been shown to be slightly higher in twin mothers (Thorpe et al, 1991). Stress, isolation and exhaustion are all significant precipitants of depression and mothers of twins are more bound to be vulnerable.

Triplets and Higher Order Births

Triplets may develop from fertilization of a single ovum or two or even three ova; similarly with quadruplets and quintuplets. Female fetuses usually outnumber the male ones. The diagnosis is often accidental following sonography, radiography or during births. Clinical course and complications are intensified compared to twins. Perinatal loss is markedly increased due to prematurity. Preterm delivery is common (50%) and usually occurs by 22nd to 34th week. Discordance of fetal growth is more common than in twins. Perinatal loss is related to low birth weight.

The mode of delivery for triplets or more is nearly always by cesarean section. The midwives must be prepared to receive several small babies within a very short time span. The special dangers associated with these births are asphyxia, intracranial injury and perinatal death.

All mothers of triplets or more must arrange for extra practical help well before the babies are born. The emotional stress and anxiety of the birth, having babies in the neonatal unit, and worries or practical and financial help will all seem overwhelming if no previous arrangements have been made.

Disability and Bereavement

Perinatal mortality and long-term morbidity are both more common among multiple births than singletons. The perinatal mortality rate for twins is about four times that of singletons and triplets 12 times.

The grief of parents, following the death of one of a multiple set, should not be underestimated. They often have conflicting emotions as they will feel and need to grieve for the child who has died, whilst wanting to rejoice at the birth of the healthy twin. They may need help in relating to the surviving baby. When one or more of a multiple set is disabled, often the healthy child needs special attention. As the healthy baby grows up, he/she may feel guilt for the disability of the other one, or feel resentful for the attention the other one needs or even the loss of twinship. Any of these may lead to emotional and behavioral problems if not addressed early on.

Embryo Reduction/Selective Reduction

This is the reduction of an apparently higher order multiple pregnancy down to two or even one embryo so the chances of survival are much higher.

This may be offered to parents who have conceived triplets or more, whether spontaneously or because of infertility treatment. The procedure is usually carried-out between the 10th and 12th week of pregnancy. It is done by inserting a needle under ultrasound guidance via the vagina or more commonly, through the abdominal wall into the fetal thorax. Potassium chloride or saline is used. All embryos remain in the uterus until delivery. Usually the pregnancy is reduced to two embryos, but in some cases to three or even one. Parents who are offered this treatment must be offered counseling, which should include:

- The advantages and disadvantages of reducing pregnancy
- The risks of continuing with a higher multiple pregnancy
- The risks of embryo reduction
- The effects on the surviving children
- How parents may feel afterwards
- Help for the parents to reach the right decision for them
- The offer of support if and when required.

Selective Fetocide

This may be offered to parents with a multiple pregnancy, where one of the babies has a serious abnormality. The affected fetus is injected as described in embryo reduction, so allowing the healthy fetus to grow and develop normally. Counseling must be offered to the parents as for embryo reduction. The full impact of the procedure and their bereavement will not often be felt until the birth of their remaining baby/babies many weeks later. At the time of delivery, the parents must be offered appropriate care and understanding in their bereavement.

BIBLIOGRAPHY

1. Davies Margie. Multiple Pregnancy, In: Myles (Ed). Textbook for Midwives, 13th edn. Edinburgh; Churchill Livingstone, 1999.
2. Dutta DC. Textbook of Obstetrics, 5th edn. Calcutta; New Central Book Company, 2001.
3. Fisk N. Scientific basis of fetofetal transfusion syndrome and its treatment. In: Whittle M, et al (Eds). Multiple Pregnancy. London; RCOG Press, 1995.
4. Moore TR, Gale S. Perinatal outcome of forty-nine pregnancies complicated by acardiac twinning. American Journal of Obstetrics and Gynecology. 1990;163:907-12.
5. Parulekar SV. Textbook for Midwives 2nd edn. Bombay; Vora Medical Publications, 1998.
6. Thorpe K, et al. Comparisons of prevalence of depression in mothers of twins and mothers of singletons. British Medical Journal 1991;302: 875-78.

31 Preterm Labor, Premature Rupture of Membranes and Intrauterine Fetal Death

> **Learning Objectives**
>
> Upon completing this chapter, the learner will be able to:
> - Describe the factors that contribute to premature labor
> - Describe the management of women during the different stages of preterm labor
> - Discuss the immediate care of preterm neonates
> - Describe the diagnosis and management of preterm rupture of membranes in different stages of pregnancy
> - Describe the diagnosis, management and care of women who have intrauterine fetal death.

PRETERM LABOR

Definition

Preterm labor is defined as labor occurring before 37th completed week of pregnancy counting from the first day of the last menstrual period. The lower limit of gestation is not uniformly defined. In the developed countries it has been brought down to 20 weeks, whereas in the developing countries, it is 28 weeks (Dutta, 2001).

Causes of Preterm Labor

In more than 50 percent of cases, the cause of preterm onset of labor is not known. The following are however, related with increased incidence of preterm labor.

History

- Previous history of induced or spontaneous abortion or preterm delivery
- Asymptomatic bacteriuria or recurrent urinary tract infection

- Smoking habits
- Low socioeconomic and nutritional status.

Complications in Previous Pregnancy

Maternal
- Pregnancy complications such as pre-eclampsia, antepartum hemorrhage, premature rupture of membranes and polyhydramnios.
- Medical and surgical illnesses like acute fever, acute pyelonephritis, diarrhea, acute appendicitis, toxoplasmosis and abdominal operation
- Chronic diseases such as hypertension, diabetes, decompensated heart lesion, severe anemia
- Genital tract infections such as bacterial vaginosis, beta hemolytic *Streptococcus*, *Chlamydia*, *Mycoplasma*.

Fetal
- Multiple pregnancy, congenital malformations, intrauterine death.

Placental
- Infarction, thrombosis, placenta previa or abruption

Idiopathic (Majority)
- Premature effacement of the cervix with a hyperirritable uterus and early engagement of the head. It is presumed that there is premature activation of the same system involved in initiating labor at term.

Presentation of the Woman

- Regular uterine contractions with or without pain (at least one in every ten minutes)
- Dilatation (> 2 cm) and effacement (90%) of the cervix

❖ Pelvic pressure, backache and/or vaginal discharge.

Management of Preterm Labor

The objectives of management are:
❖ To minimize the risk of perinatal mortality and morbidity
❖ To preserve maternal health.

Management Approaches

1. To prevent preterm onset of labor if possible.
2. To arrest preterm labor if not contra-indicated.
3. Appropriate management of labor.
4. Effective neonatal care.

Prevention

In about 50 percent of cases, the cause remains unknown. For the remaining group, decision has to be taken whether to allow the pregnancy to continue or not. The risk of delivery of a low birth weight baby has to be weighed against the risks to the unborn or to the mother if pregnancy continues.

Preventive Measures

❖ Identification of risk factors from the history and employing measures for rectification such as adequate rest, nutritional supplement, avoidance of smoking and encirclage operation, if required.
❖ Premature effacement of cervix: The women are to be put to bed rest and tocolytic agents may be administered.
❖ Selective continuation of complicated pregnancies such as twins, polyhydramnios, placenta previa, pre-eclampsia, etc. with rest and appropriate therapy. These patients are to be admitted in the hospital for close observation.
❖ Confirming the gestational age before induction.

Investigations

❖ Full blood count
❖ Urine for routine analysis, culture and sensitivity
❖ Endocervical swab for any causative organism
❖ Ultrasonography for fetal wellbeing, cervical length and placental location

❖ Serum electrolytes and glucose levels when tocolytic agents are to be used.

To Arrest Preterm Labor

Attempts to arrest preterm labor may be taken in about 10 to 20 percent of women where the fetus is not compromised, the maternal condition remains good and membranes are intact. The following regime may be instituted in an attempt to arrest premature labor.
❖ Adequate rest in bed. The woman is to lie preferably in left lateral position
❖ Adequate sedation is ensured with diazepam 5 mg PO or phenobarbitone 30 to 60 mg PO twice or thrice daily
❖ Adequate hydration is maintained
❖ Antibiotics are given if infection is evident or culture report suggests
❖ Tocolytic agents are administered to inhibit uterine contractions. Tocolytic agents can be used as short-term (1–3 days) or long-term therapy.

Short-term Therapy

Short-term therapy is used (1) To delay delivery for at least 24 hours, for glucocorticoid therapy to mother to enhance fetal lung maturation, if premature labor starts before 34th week. (2) To enable transfer of the woman with the baby *in utero* to a unit more able to manage a preterm neonate.

Long-term Therapy

Long-term therapy is instituted if pregnancy is to be prolonged for at least one week following established onset of labor prior to 34th week.

Glucocorticoid Therapy

Maternal administration of glucocorticoids is advocated where the pregnancy is less than 34 weeks. This helps in fetal lung maturation so that the incidence of respiratory distress syndrome can be minimized. Either betamethasone (Betnesol) 12 mg IM every 12 hours for two doses or dexamethazone (Decadrone) 8 mg IM every 12 hours three doses is given. If the delivery is delayed for more than seven days after the injection, treatment must be repeated.

Management of Preterm Labor

Labor is judged to have started when the woman experiences regular, painful uterine contractions accompanied by either show, rupture of membranes or complete effacement of the cervix. The principles in the management of preterm labor are: (1) To prevent asphyxia, which makes the neonate more susceptible to RDS (2) To prevent birth trauma.

First Stage

❖ The woman is put to bed to prevent early rupture of membranes
❖ Oxygen is given by mask to ensure adequate fetal oxygenation
❖ Strong sedatives or acceleration of labor is to be avoided. Epidural analgesia is the choice
❖ Progress of labor should be monitored clinically or (preferably) by electronic monitoring
❖ In case of delay or anticipating a tedious traumatic vaginal delivery, it is better to deliver by cesarean section.

Second Stage

❖ The birth should be gentle and slow to avoid rapid compression and decompression of fetal head
❖ Liberal episiotomies should be done under local anesthesia, especially in primigravidae to minimize head compression
❖ Tendency to delay must be curtailed by low forceps
❖ The cord must be clamped immediately at birth to prevent the development of hypervolemia and hyperbilirubinemia
❖ To place the baby in the intensive neonatal care unit under the care of a neonatologist. Preterm fetuses before 34th week presented by breech, are generally delivered by cesarean section.

Immediate Management of the Preterm Baby Following Birth

❖ The cord is to be clamped quickly to prevent hypervolemia and development of hyperbilirubinemia
❖ The cord length should be about 10 to 12 cm in case exchange transfusion will be required due to hyperbilirubinemia
❖ The air passage should be cleared of mucus promptly and gently. The stomach contents are also to be sucked out
❖ Adequate oxygenation must be provided.
❖ The baby should be wrapped in a sterile warm blanket or towel or laid in the warmer with the head slightly lowered (Temperature 36.5° to 37.5°C)
❖ Vitamin K_1 mg to be injected intramuscularly to prevent hemorrhagic manifestations
❖ Bathing is not appropriate for the preterm baby

Preterm babies are functionally immature and need special care for their survival.

Support for the Mother

The attendance of a support person throughout labor is crucial. This is usually the midwife who will monitor the maternal and fetal wellbeing as well as provide psychological support. An individual approach to care and instructions during labor will be required. It is quite important to communicate with the woman effectively, evaluate whether labor is progressing as expected and listen to her requests. Once the baby is born, the mother will be anxious about the baby's condition and appropriate communication must be maintained. The mother must be given the opportunity to see the baby prior to transfer to the nursery.

PREMATURE RUPTURE OF MEMBRANES (PROM)

(Syn. Prelabor Rupture of Membranes)

Definition

Spontaneous rupture of membranes any time beyond 28th week of pregnancy and before the onset of spontaneous uterine activity resulting in cervical dilation is called prelabor rupture of membranes (PROM). When rupture of membranes occurs beyond 37th week but before the onset of labor, it is called term PROM and when it occurs before 37 completed weeks, it is called preterm PROM, (PPROM).

Incidence

Prelabor rupture of membranes occurs in approximately 10 percent of all pregnancies.

Causes

In majority, the causes are not known. Possible causes are:

- Increased friability of membranes
- Decreased tensile strength of the membranes
- Polyhydramnios
- Cervical incompetence
- Multiple pregnancy
- Infection; chorioamnionitis, urinary tract infection and lower genital tract infection.

Manifestations

The only manifestation is the escape of watery discharge per vagina either in the form of a gush or slow leak.

Confirmation of diagnosis is done by employing the following methods.

- Speculum examination to inspect the liquor escaping out through the cervix
- Examination of the fluid collected from the posterior fornix (vaginal pool) for (a) detection of pH by litmus or Nitrazine paper. The pH becomes 6 to 6.2 (Normal vaginal pH during pregnancy is 4.5 to 5.5, whereas that of liquor amnü is 7 to 7.5). (b) To note the characteristic ferning pattern when a smeared slide is examined under microscope.

Risks of PROM

The implications are less serious when the rupture occurs near term than earlier in pregnancy.

- In term PROM, labor starts in 80 to 90 percent of cases within 24 hours. PROM is one of the important causes of preterm labor and prematurity
- Chances of ascending infection are more if labor fails to start within 24 hours. Liquor gets infected (chorioamnionitis) which may be followed by fetal and maternal systemic infection
- Increased incidence of cord prolapse, especially when associated with malpresentation

- Continuous escape of liquor for long duration may lead to dry labor
- Fetal pulmonary hypoplacia, especially in preterm PROM when associated with oligohydramnios
- Primary antepartum hemorrhage. Ultrasonography is done to assess the fetal wellbeing.

Management

If PROM is suspected, the woman is admitted to the labor room.

- Careful history is taken
- A sterile speculum examination is done to check the pooling of liquor in the posterior fornix, to note the state of the cervix and to detect any cord prolapse
- Patient is put to bed rest and sterile vulval pad is applied to look for leakage
- A digital vaginal examination should be avoided to reduce the risk of avoiding infection
- Fetal heart rate is checked to assess the fetal condition (an infected fetus may have a tachycardia)
- Maternal pulse, temperature, uterine tenderness and any offensively smelling discharge are observed and noted.

Once the diagnosis is confirmed, management depends on—(1) Gestational age of the fetus, (2) Whether the woman is in labor or not, (3) Any evidence of sepsis, and (4) Prospect of fetal survival if delivery occurs.

Term PROM: If the pregnancy is 38 weeks, the woman is not in labor and there is no evidence of fetal distress, she is observed in the hospital. Generally, in 90 percent of cases, spontaneous labor starts in 24 hours. If labor does not start in 24 hours, induction of labor is commenced with oxytocin. Cesarean section is performed for obstetric reasons (noncephalic presentations).

Preterm PROM: If the pregnancy is less than 34 weeks, the fetus appears to be uncompromised, and APH and labor have been excluded, she will be managed expectantly for fetal maturity.

If the gestational age is 34 weeks or more, spontaneous labor is awaited for 24 to 48 hours. If labor does not commence, induction with oxytocin is instituted. For presentations other than cephalic, cesarean section is chosen. On rare occasions, the leak seals spontaneously (especially if it is hind water leak) and the pregnancy continues.

If the membranes rupture before 24 weeks of gestation, the outlook is not good; the fetus is likely to succumb either to the problems caused by oligohydramnios or to those caused by preterm birth. Prophylactic antibiotics are given to minimize maternal and perinatal risks of infection. Oral ampicillin 500 mg is given six hourly for three days. Infection is evident by maternal tachycardia, rise in temperature, uterine tenderness, leukocytosis, and bacterial growth from vaginal swab. Intravenous ampicillin, or cephadrine along with metronidazole is administered in case of chorioamnionitis.

Psychological consideration of the woman and her spouse must be considered vital, as it is an extremely disturbing situation for them. Understanding care, adequate explanations and support from caregivers are required as the decisions for management are taken and executed.

INTRAUTERINE FETAL DEATH (IUD)

Intrauterine fetal death (IUD) includes antepartum deaths occurring beyond 28th week of gestation and usually results in the delivery of a macerated fetus.

Etiology

Fetal deaths during pregnancy are related to a number of maternal and/or fetal complications, which produce either chronic or acute placental insufficiency. However, in about 20 to 30 percent of cases, the cause remains unknown.

Pregnancy Complications

* *Pre-eclampsia*: Spasm of the uteroplacental vessels leads to reduction of placental blood flow and placental insufficiency.
* *Antepartum hemorrhage*: Both placenta previa and abruptio placentae can cause fetal

death by producing acute placental insufficiency. Abruptio placentae will cause more deaths than placenta previa with identical area of separation because of frequent association with pre-eclampsia.

Pre-existing Medical Diseases and Acute Illnesses during Pregnancy

* *Chronic hypertension*: It produces chronic placental insufficiency and is usually less lethal, unless pre-eclampsia supervenes
* *Diabetes*: Long-standing diabetes with atherosclerotic changes in the pelvic blood vessels may lead to chronic placental insufficiency and death of fetus. Associated pre-eclampsia, polyhydramnios, congenital malformation and maternal ketosis are some of the factors responsible
* *Chronic nephritis*: Continuation of pregnancy beyond the period of viability is rare and fetal death occurs due to massive placental infarction
* *Syphilis*: Though rare now a days, it produces fetal deaths by the spirochaete affecting the placenta and the fetus
* *Hyperpyrexia (malaria):* Acute fever of the mother over 39.4°C can kill the fetus directly
* Severe anemia may cause fetal death in some cases through maternal anoxemia
* Other rare causes include: Hepatitis (viral), toxoplasmosis, malaria, poliomyelitis, mumps, etc.

Fetal Causes

* *Congenital malformation*: A fetus with gross congenital malformations, incompatible with extrauterine independent existence is more vulnerable to die *in utero.*
* *Rh-incompatibility*: Excessive hemolysis of fetal blood by antibodies formed in the mother produces fetal anemia, anoxia and heart failure.
* *Postmaturity*: Unexpected death may occur during pregnancy due to placental insufficiency, however, the risk is more during labor.

Iatrogenic

❖ *External version*: It may result in a true knot of the cord or entanglement of the cord round the neck or limbs of the fetus.

❖ Quinine group of drugs if administered in higher than therapeutic doses.

Idiopathic

❖ In about 20 to 30 percent cases, the cause remains undetermined and is attributed to placental insufficiency .

Sometimes intrauterine fetal deaths recur in subsequent pregnancies.

Signs and Symptoms

Repeated examinations are often required to confirm the diagnosis.

❖ Absence of fetal movements, which were previously experienced by the woman.

❖ Retrogression of the breast changes that occur during pregnancy.

❖ Gradual retrogression of the height of the uterus so that it becomes smaller than the period of amenorrhea.

❖ Uterine tone is diminished and the uterus feels flaccid. Braxton-Hicks contractions are not easily felt.

❖ Fetal movements are not felt during palpation.

❖ Fetal heart sounds, which were audible before, is absent. Doppler effect of ultrasound is a better alternative to ordinary stethoscope.

❖ Eggshell crackling feel of fetal head, if elicited is more indicative of the diagnosis.

Investigations

❖ Sonography: Evidences of fetal death are lack of fetal movement (including cardiac) during a ten-minute period of careful observation, oligohydramnios and collapsed cranial bones.

❖ Straight X-ray abdomen may reveal the following features in varying degree either singly or in combination.

  ❖ Spalding sign: The irregular overlapping of the cranial bones one on another due to liquefaction of the brain matter and softening of the ligamentous structures supporting the vault. It usually appears seven days after death

❖ Hyperflexion of the spine and in some cases hyperflexion of the neck are seen

❖ Crowding of the ribs shadow with loss of normal parallelism

❖ Appearance of gas shadow (Robert's sign) in the chambers of the heart and great vessels may be seen as early as 12 hours after death.

Complications

1. *Extreme psychological upset of the woman*: She will need enormous amount of support to deal with the problem.

2. *Infection*: As long as the membranes remain intact, infection is unlikely but once the membranes rupture, infection, especially by gas forming organisms like *clostridium welchii* may occur.

3. *Blood coagulation disorders*: If the fetus is retained for more than four weeks (as occurs in 10 to 20 percent cases), there is possibility of defibrination from silent Disseminated Intravascular Coagulopathy (DIC). It is due to gradual absorption of thromboplastin, liberated from the dead placenta and decidua into the maternal circulation.

4. *During labor*: Uterine inertia, retained placenta and postpartum hemorrhage.

Prevention

While IUD cannot be totally prevented, prenatal care and monitoring can help to reduce the incidence.

❖ Regular antenatal care to prevent and detect early, the conditions that contribute to IUD and instituting effective therapy

❖ Screening the "at-risk mothers" for fetal wellbeing and to terminate the pregnancy at the earliest evidences of fetal compromise.

Management

Expectant Management (Noninterference)

In about 80 percent of cases, spontaneous expulsion occurs within 2 weeks of fetal death.

The woman may remain at home with the advice to come to the hospital for delivery. If spontaneous expulsion fails to occur within two weeks, the woman is to be admitted. Fibrinogen estimation is done every week and a falling fibrinogen level, approaching 150 mg percentage, should be arrested by infusion of heparin. The woman and her family are likely to be upset psychologically and should be assured of safety of noninterference.

Interference

Indications of interference are:
- ❖ Manifestations of uterine infection
- ❖ Falling fibrinogen level
- ❖ Tendency of prolongation of pregnancy beyond two weeks.

Early termination is now preferred as reliable diagnosis could be made with ultrasonography and prostaglandins are available for effective induction.

Termination of pregnancy is done by medical induction. Vaginal administration of *prostaglandin* (PGE$_2$) gel in the posterior fornix is used effectively where the cervix is unfavorable. The procedure may be repeated after 6 to 8 hours. The procedure may be supplemented with oxytocin infusion.

Oxytocin infusion is widely practiced and effective in cases where the cervix is favorable. To begin with 5 to 10 units of oxytocin in 500 ml of ringers solution is administered through intravenous drip. Consecutive two bottles may be administered at a time. In case of failure, a higher dose is administered on the following day. 20 units of oxytocin in 500 ml of Ringers solution are run at 30 drops per minute (80 mU/minute). The strength of the drip may be increased to 40 units after the first bottle, if contractions fail to start. More than two bottles should not be administered at one time because of the risk of antidiuretic effect. If the uterus still does not respond, the procedure is repeated after vaginal administration of prostaglandins.

Cesarean section is done only for those with major placenta previa, transverse lie or two or more previous cesarean sections.

Bereavement Management

The mother who has given birth to a dead baby suffers a great deal of emotional burden. This may be compounded by the process of maceration having changed the baby's appearance. The midwife should provide all the support and sympathy to the bereaved couple. Lactation is usually suppressed with bromocriptine (parlodel) 2.5 mg twice daily for 10 days. Counseling for future pregnancies is to be done at the time of postpartum check-up after six weeks.

BIBLIOGRAPHY

1. Dutta DC. Textbook of Obstetrics 5th edn. Calcutta: New Central Book Company, 2001.
2. Gunn GC, Mishell DR. Premature rupture of the fetal membranes. American Journal of Obstetrics and Gynecology 1970;106:268-79.
3. Hameed C, et al. Silent Chorioamnionitis as a cause of preterm labor refractory to tocolytic therapy. American Journal of Obstetrics and Gynecology 1984;149(7):726-30.
4. Kappy KA, et al. Premature rupture of the membranes: A conservative approach. American Journal of Obstetrics and Gynecology 1979; 134(6):655-61.

32

Post-term Pregnancy, Induction of Labor, Prolonged Labor and Disorders of Uterine Action

Learning Objectives

Upon completing this chapter, the learner will be able to:
* Discuss the diagnosis and management of post-term pregnancy
* Review the indications for induction of labor and the various methods used
* Describe how uterine dysfunction may result in a prolonged labor or a precipitate labor
* Discuss the serious complications of obstructed labor, which may result in morbidity or mortality of mother or baby or both
* Describe the role of the midwife in the care and management of such situations.

POST-TERM PREGNANCY

(Syn: Prolonged Pregnancy)

Post-term pregnancy is defined as one that exceeds 294 days calculating from the first day of the last menstrual period. The pregnancy continues beyond two weeks of the expected date of delivery. The terms prolonged pregnancy and post-term pregnancy, are used synonymously and relate to the duration of pregnancy. Postmaturity and postmature are terms that relate to the neonate and refer to features and conditions of the baby.

Incidence

The incidence of post-term pregnancy averages about 10 percent.

Etiology

The exact cause of the prolonged pregnancy is not clear, but certain factors are seen related.

* *Hereditary factors:* The condition often runs in family and often manifests in consecutive pregnancies in the same individual
* High standards of living with sedentary habits often tend to prolong the pregnancy
* Elderly primigravidae or elderly multiparae are more likely to have prolonged pregnancy
* Anencephaly without polyhydramnios.

Diagnosis

Menstrual history: If the woman is sure about her date with previous history of regular cycles, it is a reliable diagnostic aid in the calculation of the period of gestation. However, in cases of pregnancy occurring during lactational amenorrhea or soon following withdrawal of the pill, difficulty arises. In such cases previously documented antenatal records of first visit may help.

Clinical Findings

Clinical findings, which are evident when an otherwise uncomplicated pregnancy overrun the expected date by two weeks are:
* *Weight loss:* Regular periodic weight checking shows stationary or even falling weight.
* *Girth of the abdomen:* Normally, the girth of the abdomen at the level of umbilicus increases steadily up to the completion of 38th week and then remains steady up to term. Thereafter, the girth gradually diminishes because of diminishing liquor.
* *History of false pain:* Appearance of false pain followed by a subsidence with continuation of pregnancy is suggestive. The false pain is presumed to coincide with the expected date.

❖ *Abdominal palpation*: As liquor amnii diminishes there may be changes in the height of the fundus, size of the fetus and hardness of the skull bones. The uterus "full of fetus" is a feature usually associated with post-term pregnancy.

❖ *Internal examination*: Feeling of hard bones either through the cervix or through the fornix usually suggests maturity.

❖ *Ultrasound scan*: In early pregnancy, this can be used to assess the duration of pregnancy and fetal age. Measurements taken in the first or second trimesters have been found to be accurate within five days in 95 percent cases (Neilson, 1990). Crown-rump length (CRL), biparietal diameter (BPD) and femur length (FL) are the measurements of choice for assessment of fetal age. Composite biometry is of more value in the assessment of maturity of the fetus.

❖ *Straight X-ray abdomen*: Overall fetal shadow, thickness and density of the skull bone shadow, appearance and density of the ossification centers in the upper end of the tibia and lower end of the femur are taken together to assess the maturity.

Clinical Presentation for Retrospective Diagnosis

In addition to the increased length of gestation at which the baby is delivered, the following criteria have been used to establish the diagnosis of post-term pregnancy retrospectively, i.e. after the birth of the baby.

❖ *General appearance*: Baby looks thin and old. There is absence of vernix caseosa. Body and the cord are stained with greenish-yellow color. Head is hard without much evidence of moulding. Nails are protruding beyond the nail beds.

❖ *Liquor amnii*: Scanty and may be saffron colored with meconium.

❖ *Placenta*: There is evidence of aging of the placenta manifested by excessive infarction and calcification.

❖ *Cord*: There is diminished quantity of Wharton's jelly, which may precipitate cord compression.

❖ *Macrosomia*: Birth weight of 4 kg or more occurs in about 10 percent cases.

Dangers of Post-term Pregnancy

During Pregnancy

There is chance for fetal hypoxia due to placental insufficiency, as the pregnancy overruns the expected date. Placental aging leads to diminished placental function with resultant fetal hypoxia. The hypoxic state may be aggravated by such associated factors as elderly women, hypertensive disorders in pregnancy and history of bleeding during pregnancy.

During Labor

There is increased incidence of asphyxia and intracranial damage due to:

❖ Aggravation of pre-existing hypoxia leading to increased fetal distress

❖ Increased incidence of difficult labor due to big size baby, nonmoulding of the head due to hardening of the skull bones and occasional shoulder dystocia

❖ Increased incidence of operative delivery

❖ Cord compression related to scanty liquor amnii and less Wharton's jelly in the cord.

Following Birth

❖ Meconium aspiration syndrome and atlectasis as the result of intrauterine anoxia and consequent inhalation of meconium containing liquor amnii

❖ Low Apgar scores

❖ Hypoglycemia and polycythemia occur in growth retarded post-term babies

All these factors lead to increased perinatal loss, the magnitude of which is doubled at 43rd week and tripled at 44th week compared to that delivered at term.

There is increased maternal morbidity related to hazards of induction, instrumental and operative delivery.

Management of Post-term Pregnancy

The management of post-term pregnancy takes into account, the increased risk to the fetus as pregnancy lengthens. Two forms of care are generally offered, expectant management with fetal surveillance or elective induction of labor before 42nd week of gestation. Both aim to diminish the jeopardy to the fetus.

Expectant Management

❖ *Biophysical profile*: Ultrasound assessment of fetal breathing, fetal movement, fetal tone, reactivity of the heart rate and amniotic fluid volume could be used to predict fetal wellbeing in a high-risk pregnancy.

❖ *Cardiotocography or nonstress testing*: Fetal heart rate is monitored weekly and the monitor strip is assessed for the presence of reactivity and whether the baseline rate is within the normal range.

❖ *Amniotic fluid measurement*: Measurements are taken in several perpendicular planes to make the diagnosis of oligohydramnios. Intervention is indicated if the amniotic fluid volume falls below 30 mm (Crowley et al, 1984).

Elective Induction

The active approach to post-term pregnancy or one approaching the upper limits of term is for the mother to have labor induced. It is done between 10 to 14 days and a little earlier in primigravidae.

If the cervix is favorable (ripe), induction is done by stripping the membranes by low rupture of the membranes. If the liquor is found clear, oxytocin infusion is added to make it more effective. Careful fetal monitoring is mandatory. If the liquor amnii is thickly meconium stained, suggestive of chronic placental insufficiently, cesarean section is performed.

If the cervix is unripe, it is made favorable by vaginal administration of prostaglandins (PGE$_2$ gel). This is followed by low rupture of membranes. Oxytocin infusion is added when required.

When postmaturity is associated with complicating factors like contracted pelvis, post-cesarean pregnancy, malpresentation, elderly primigravidae, etc. an elective cesarean section is done.

Associated complications of pregnancy, that are likely to produce placental insufficiency, such as pre-eclampsia, history of bleeding during pregnancy, diabetes and Rh-negative pregnancy should not be allowed to go beyond the expected date and termination to be done either by induction or cesarean section as appropriate.

Care during Labor

Whether spontaneous or induced, the labor may be prolonged because of a big baby and poor moulding of the head. More analgesia is required for pain relief. Possibility of shoulder dystocia is present. Careful fetal monitoring must be done with available gadgets. If fetal distress appears, prompt delivery either by cesarean section or by forceps is to be done. Psychological care and measures to prevent maternal exhaustion must be taken.

INDUCTION OF LABOR

Induction of labor is the stimulation of uterine contractions before the onset of spontaneous labor. It is an obstetric intervention that should be used when elective birth will be beneficial to mother and baby. The purpose of induction is to effect the birth of the baby. Successful induction depends on adequate contractions, which are effective in bringing about progressive dilatation of the cervix. The procedure is more likely to be successful when the cervix is ripe, that is, it has undergone structural changes to produce softening, dilatation and effacement.

Indications for Induction

Induction is indicated when the benefits to the mother or the fetus outweigh those of continuing the pregnancy and it is associated with the following maternal, fetal or combined factors.

Maternal Indications

❖ *Prolonged or post-term pregnancy*: This is the main indication for induction of labor.

❖ *Previous history of unexplained intrauterine death*: Timely intervention provides an opportunity to avert the repetition of the disaster.

- *Medical problems*: Women with concurrent renal, respiratory or cardiac disease may require induction of labor
- Intrauterine death of the fetus
- Chronic polyhydramnios with maternal distress
- *Congenital malformation of the fetus*: For psychological reasons and to minimize the complications, termination is preferable to continuation of pregnancy. However, the pregnancy should be continued until such time when the induction is more likely to be successful.

Fetal Indications

- Chronic placental insufficiency leading to growth retardation of the fetus
- Rh-isoimmunization
- Unstable lie—after correcting into longitudinal lie
- Diabetes mellitus
- Postmaturity.

Combined Indications

Continuation of pregnancy may adversely affect both the mother and the baby
- Pre-eclampsia and eclampsia
- Minor degree of placenta previa
- *Abruptio placentae*: Early termination saves the mother from untoward complications like blood coagulation disorders and anuria. The baby can also be saved
- Premature rupture of membranes
- Chronic hypertension.

Contraindications to Induction of Labor

1. Contracted pelvis and cephalopelvic disproportion.
2. Persistent malpresentation—transverse or compound presentations.
3. Pregnancy with previous cesarean section.
4. Elderly primigravida especially associated with obstetric or medical complicating factors.
5. High-risk pregnancy with compromised fetus.
6. Cord presentation or cord prolapse.
7. Placenta previa.
8. Pelvic tumor.

In these circumstances, if delivery is imperative, it should be effected by cesarean section.

Dangers of Induction

Apart from the inherent hazards of the methods employed, the following are the dangers of induction. The hazards are however, to be weighed against the possible risks of continuation of pregnancy to the mother and/or the fetus due to the complication for which induction is contemplated.

Maternal

1. Psychological upset, more so when there is failure for which cesarean section is contemplated.
2. Tendency of prolonged labor due to abnormal uterine action.
3. Increased need of analgesia during labor.
4. Increased operative interference.
5. Increased morbidity.

Fetal

1. Iatrogenic prematurity.
2. Hypoxia due to disordered uterine action, prolonged labor and operative interference.

Methods of Ripening of the Cervix

The cervix is normally two centimeters long, firm and closed throughout pregnancy. Its shape is tubular with a rigid structure designed to retain the fetus within the uterus until term. Maturation of the cervix is the result of physiological processes that soften, efface and dilate the cervix prior to the onset of labor. This begins as much as 5 to 6 weeks prior to labor.

The ripeness of the cervix can be effectively achieved by employing the following methods:
1. Prostaglandin (PGE_2) used either in the form of gel 500 µg intracervical or 1 to 2 mg in the posterior fornix or in the form of a pessary 3 mg in the posterior fornix. The application may have to be repeated after 6 to 8 hours. Loosening of the cervical collagen fibers occurs following its application. Labor will start in 30 to 50 percent of cases.

2. Stripping of the membranes: It is possible if one finger can be introduced through the cervix. In order to carry-out the procedure, a vaginal examination with some cervical stretching is needed.
3. Oxytocin infusion may be used with some success. However, on occasion, labor starts following the use of any of the method.

Assessment of the Cervix

In order to decide on the method of induction, assessment of the cervix is required. A pre-induction score using the Bishop's score is done (Table 32.1). Key elements in the assessment are dilatation, effacement, position, consistency and station of the presenting part (Bishop, 1964). Five different features are considered and each is awarded a score of between zero and three. When a score of six or over is reached, the prognosis for induction is good.

Methods of Induction

❖ Medical
❖ Surgical
❖ Combined.

Medical Induction

1. Oxytocin induction
2. Prostaglandin induction.

Indications for medical induction
❖ Intrauterine death of fetus
❖ Premature rupture of membranes
❖ Along with surgical induction, to shorten the induction—delivery interval
❖ In cases of failure of surgical induction.

Drugs used:
1. Oxytocin
2. Prostglandins.

Oxytocin Induction

The synthetic preparation (syntocinon) is widely used as intravenous infusion; diluted in isotonic solution, such as normal saline. The infusion should be controlled through a pump to enable accurate assessment of volume and rate. Manual counting of the drops per minute may be followed carefully. The rate of infusion must be titrated against the assessment of strength and frequency of uterine contractions. As labor becomes established, the uterus becomes more sensitive to oxytocin and the infusion rate may need to be reduced as labor progresses. The midwife should aim to administer the lowest dose required to maintain, well-spaced uterine contractions, typically occurring every three minutes, lasting for 45 to 50 seconds. The objective of oxytocin administration is not only to initiate effective contraction but also to maintain the normal pattern of uterine activity until delivery and at least 30 to 60 minutes beyond that.

Calculation of the infusion dose
The infusion is expressed (recorded) in terms of milliunits per minute. This can give an accurate idea about the exact amount adminis-tered per minute irrespective of the concentra-tion of the solution (Table 32.2).

In majority of cases, a dose of less than 16 milliunits per minute (two units in 500 ml of Ringer's solution with drop rate of 60 per minute) is sufficient. Conditions where fluid

| Table 32.1 | Bishop's preinduction cervical scoring system |

Factors	0	Score		
		1	2	3
Cervix				
Dilatation (cm)	Closed	1–2	3–4	5+
Cervical length (cm)	> 2	1 or 2	< 1	Fully taken up
Consistency	Firm	Medium	Soft	–
Position	Posterior	Midline	Anterior	–
Head				
Station	(-3)	(-2)	-1. 0	+1, +2
Total score = 13		Favorable score = 6–13		Unfavorable score = 0–5

Table 32.2	Calculation of the dose of oxytocin delivered in milliunits (mU)		
Units of oxytocin mixed in 500 ml Ringer's solution or Normal saline	Drops per minute (15 drops = 1 ml)		
(1 unit = 1,000 milliunits (mU)	15	30	60
	Milliunits/Min		
1	2	4	8
2	4	8	16
3	16	32	64

Notes
1 unit (1000 mU) of oxytocin in 500 ml IV solution
@ 15 drops/min gives 2 mU/min
@ 30 drops/min gives 4 mU/min
@ 60 drops/min gives 8 mU/min

overload is to be avoided infusion with high concentration and reduced drop rate is used. The interval for escalating the drop rate is 15 to 30 minutes. The total dose required for initiating labor ranges from 600 to 12,000 milliunits with an average of 4,000 milliunits.

Observations during oxytocin induction
* ❖ The mother should never be left alone when the oxytocin infusion is running
* ❖ Rate of flow of the infusion should be maintained accurately, especially when the drip is regulated by counting the drops per minute
* ❖ Response to uterine contraction should be meticulously observed in the absence of an electronic monitoring device. The number of contractions in 10 minutes and the tonus of the uterus in between contractions (using finger tip palpation) should be noted
* ❖ Fetal heart rate should be noted every 15 minutes
* ❖ Continuous electronic fetal monitoring is ideal, especially for high-risk cases. Cardiotocographic equipment can record FHR and uterine contractions simultaneously
* ❖ Maternal condition: Pulse rate and blood pressure are to be checked hourly. The amount of urine should be noted when larger doses are administered (in excess of 20 mU/minute). Any untoward symptoms like precordial pain or uneasiness should be detected promptly
* ❖ Progress of labor: Progressive descent of the head and the rate of cervical dilatation are to be noted. The color of the liquor to be inspected periodically.

Indications for stopping the infusion
1. Nature of uterine contractions
   a. Abnormal uterine contractions occurring frequently (every two minutes or less) or lasting more than 60 seconds.
   b. Increased tonus (tension) in between contractions.
2. Evidences of fetal distress.
3. Appearance of untoward maternal symptoms.

Side effects of oxytocin
1. Hyperstimulation of the uterus: Oxytocin exposes the mother and fetus to the risk of hyperstimulation of the uterus, which could cause fetal hypoxia and uterine rupture. Hyperstimulation may cause the uterus to contract continuously for several minutes (contractions lasting longer than 60 seconds and more frequently than every two minutes). The relaxation between contractions is inadequate. If this occurs, the midwife should turn off the infusion and inform the obstetrician. The uterus recovers from the hyperstimulation rapidly as the infusion is discontinued. Oxytocin should not be given as a bolus injection during labor because of the risk of hyperstimulation.
2. Prolonged use may contribute to uterine atony postpartum.
3. Water retention and water intoxication can occur with prolonged use, due to its antidiuretic effect.

Effectiveness: The drug is effective in most of the cases either with single or repeat infusions. However, oxytocin is less effective in cases of intrauterine death, elderly primigravidae or early gestational period with unfavorable cervix.

Induction Using Prostaglandins

Prostaglandin is most commonly administered by the intravaginal route. Prostaglandin E_2 preparations are available in gel or pessary form and they are inserted close to the cervix, i.e. posterior fornix of the vagina. The usual dose is 1 to 3 mg, which may be repeated after 6 to 8 hours if necessary. Prostaglandin E_2, when administered to the cervix is absorbed, resulting in changes, which can be assessed on vaginal examination using the Bishop's score. Prostaglandin E$_1$ (Misoprostol), 50 mg intravaginal is also used and found more effective for induction of labor.

Prostaglandin produces frequent, but low intensity, contractions of the uterus. These may not be felt by all women and they wear off after 3 to 4 hours. Labor will result in 30 to 50 percent of cases (MacKenzie, 1990). Fetal heart rate and uterine contractions should be monitored continuously for 30 to 60 minutes thereafter. The mother should remain recumbent or resting for one hour.

Advantages
1. Effective method in intrauterine death or in cases with unfavorable cervix
2. No antidiuretic effect.

Drawbacks
1. More systemic side effects when used orally or intravenously, but vaginal administration has minimal side effects.
2. The adverse uterine effect (hyper-stimulation) if occurs, usually lasts for a longer period compared to oxytocin.
3. Systemic side effects include pyrexia, diarrhea and vomiting.

Surgical Induction of Labor

Methods
1. Artificial rupture of membranes (ARMs)
2. Stripping of the membranes.

Artificial Rupture of Membranes or Amniotomy
Amniotomy is performed to induce labor when the cervix is favorable or during labor to augment contractions. A well-fitting presenting part is essential, to prevent cord prolapse. ARM may also be done to visualize the color of the liquor or to attach a fetal scalp electrode for continuous electronic monitoring of the fetal heart rate.

Rupture of the membranes allows the presenting part to descend, with improved application to the cervical os. This increased stimulation results in stronger contractions, as levels of prostaglandins rise. Reduction of amniotic fluid volume causes the onset of labor.

Amniotomy may be used on its own or in association with oxytocin and may be either low rupture, involving rupture of the forewaters, or less commonly, high rupture which requires the hindwaters to be ruptured.

Hazards of ARM
❖ Intrauterine infection, particularly iatrogenic from digital or instrumental contamination
❖ Chance of umbilical cord prolapse: The chance is minimized in cases with an engaged head
❖ Bleeding from the following sources.
  – Fetal vessels in the membranes (vasa previa)
  – The friable vessels in the cervix
  – A low lying placental site (placenta previa)
  – Liquor amnii embolism.

Immediate beneficial effects of ARM
❖ Lowering of the blood pressure in preeclampsia and eclampsia
❖ Relief of maternal distress in polyhydramnios
❖ Control of bleeding in APH
❖ Release of tension in abruptio placentae thereby minimizing uterorenal reflex.

Low Rupture of Membranes (LRMs)
This method of amniotomy is widely practiced with high degree of success. The membranes below the presenting part overlying the internal os are ruptured using a Kocher's artery forceps to drain some amount of amniotic fluid.

Contraindication
Chronic polyhydramnios: The gush of amniotic fluid is difficult to control and sudden decompression may precipitate early separation of the placenta and accidental hemorrhage.

Observations
As the membranes rupture, the following are to be noted:
❖ Color of amniotic fluid
❖ Status of the cervix
❖ Station of the head
❖ Presence or absence of cord prolapse
❖ Quality of FHR.

Hazards

Same as mentioned for ARM.

High Rupture of Membranes (HRMs)

It is a procedure where the puncture of the hindwaters above the presenting part is made with a special instrument—Drew-Smythe catheter.

This method is almost obsolete now. It was used in chronic hydramnios associated with congenital malformations of the fetus or with floating head, where regulated escape of liquor amnii facilitates settling down of the presenting part. Slow decompression also prevents premature placental separation.

Conditions to be fulfilled

❖ Cervix should be at least one finger dilated
❖ Vertex must be presenting
❖ Forewaters must be present.

Contraindications

❖ Antepartum hemorrhage
❖ Severe pre-eclampsia or eclampsia.

Hazards

❖ Injury to the placenta
❖ Accidental injury to the uterine wall
❖ Injury to the fetal parts specially to the eye
❖ Accidental low rupture of membranes
❖ Displacement of the presenting part
❖ Intra-amniotic infection
❖ Longer induction—delivery interval compared to LRM.

While forewaters preservation is maintained and chance of cord prolapse is minimized with HRM, the LRM is widely practiced, as it is a more effective method of surgical induction.

Stripping the Membranes

Stripping the membranes off its attachment from the lower uterine segment is used as an effective procedure for induction provided the cervical score is favorable. It is used as a preliminary step prior to rupture of membranes. Prostaglandins are rapidly produced as the fetal membranes are detached from the decidua. Stretching and ripening of the cervix or at times initiation of labor results.

In order to carry-out the procedure a vaginal examination with some cervical stretching is needed. This provides additional stimulus for prostaglandin release. This method is employed as an alternative to medical induction in post-term pregnancy.

Combined Method

The combined medical and surgical methods are commonly used to increase the efficacy of induction by reducing the induction delivery interval. The oxytocin infusion is started either prior to or following rupture of membranes depending mainly upon the state of the cervix and head-brim relation. With the head engaged, it is preferable to induce with prostaglandin gel or to start oxytocin infusion followed by ARM.

Advantages of Combined Methods

1. More effective than any single method.
2. Shortens the induction delivery interval and thereby minimizes the risk of infection and lessens the period of observation.

PROLONGED LABOR

The labor is said as prolonged when the combined duration of the first and second stage is more than the arbitrary time limit of 18 hours. The prolongation includes prolonged cervical dilatation in the first stage and/or inadequate descend of the presenting part during the first and second stage of labor.

A latent phase that exceeds 20 hours in primigravidae and 14 hours in multiparae is abnormal. The causes include—unripe cervix, malposition and presentation, cephalopelvic disportion and premature administration of excessive sedation.

Causes of Prolonged Labor

Anyone or combination of the basic elements in labor could be responsible to create the situation.

First Stage

Failure to dilate the cervix.

❖ Fault in power includes—abnormal uterine contraction, such as uterine inertia or in coordinate uterine action

❖ Fault in the passage includes—contracted pelvis, cervical dystocia, pelvic tumor or even full bladder

❖ Fault in the passenger includes—malposition and malpresentation, congenital anomalies of the fetus, such as hydrocephalus

❖ Others—injudicious early administration of sedatives and analgesics before the actual active labor begins.

Second Stage

Sluggish or nondescend of the presenting part due to:

❖ Fault in the power
  – Uterine inertia
  – Inability to bear down
  – Epidural analgesia
  – Constriction ring.

❖ Fault in the passage
  – Contracted pelvis and disproportion
  – Undue resistance of the pelvic floor or perineum due to spasm or old scarring
  – Soft tissue pelvic tumor.

❖ Fault in the passenger
  – Malposition
  – Malpresentation
  – Big baby
  – Congenital malformation of the baby.

Diagnosis

Prolonged labor is a manifestation of an abnormality, the cause of which should be detected by a thorough abdominal and vaginal examination supplemented by partographic analysis of labor. Intranatal radiography is useful in determining the fetal station and position as well as pelvic shape and size.

First Stage Labor

If the first stage of labor lasts more than an arbitrary period of 12 hours or if the cervical dilatation arrests more than two hours, it is considered as abnormal.

Rate of cervical dilatation is sluggish to less than one cm/hr in nullipara and less than 1.5 cm/hr in multipara. There may be slow descending of the head (Normal one cm/hr in primi and 2 cm/hr in multi).

The first stage of labor is divided into a latent and an active phase. During latent phase, the uterus contracts regularly and the mother experiences discomfort and pain. The cervix effaces and dilatation occurs. The duration of latent phase varies according to each individual and with parity. The average duration of latent phase in nulliparous women is 8.6 hours.

The active phase is distinguished by an increased rate of dilatation of cervix; with descend of the presenting part. A prolonged active phase is caused by a combination of factors including the cervix, the uterus, the fetus and the mother's pelvis.

Second Stage

The second stage is considered prolonged if it lasts for more than two hours in primigravida and one hour in multipara. The diagnostic features are: (1) Sluggish or nondescend of the presenting part even after full dilatation of the cervix (failure of the head to descend within one hour is called arrest). (2) Variable degrees of moulding and caput formation in cephalic presentation.

Dangers of Prolonged Labor

Fetal

The fetal risk is increased due to the combined effect of:

1. Hypoxia due to diminished uteroplacental circulation specially after rupture of the membranes.
2. Intrauterine infection.
3. Intracranial stress or hemorrhage following prolonged stay in the perineum and/or increased moulding of the head.
4. Increased operative delivery.

All these result in increased perinatal loss due to asphyxia, intracranial hemorrhage and neonatal sepsis.

Maternal

There is increased incidence of:

1. Maternal distress.
2. Postpartum hemorrhage.
3. Trauma to the genital tract—concealed (undue stretching the perineal muscles

which may cause prolapse of uterus at a later stage), or revealed such as cervical tear, rupture of uterus.

4. Increased operative delivery.
5. Puerperal sepsis.
6. Subinvolution.

Management

The management of a mother experiencing a prolonged labor, will be the responsibility of the obstetric team. Midwives must seek medical advice on recognizing any aberration from normal.

1. When progress is slow, attempts should be made to determine the cause before deciding on management. An expectant management for inefficient uterine action is to *encourage ambulation* to produce a return to normal activity. Flynn, et al (1978) found that there was a reduced need for oxytocics to improve contractions when mobility was encouraged.

2. The upright position for the laboring mother improves the application of the presenting part on to the cervix and triggers the neuro-endocrine reflex. This would make the contractions less painful although stronger and more efficient than when remaining recumbent (Caldeyro-Barcia, 1979). Upright position or one where the woman adopts a forward-leaning posture, are helpful in encouraging an anterior rotation of the occiput.

3. When poor progress of labor is due to hypotonic, inefficient contractions, oxytocin increases the strength and frequency of the contractions. Cephalopelvic disproportion should be excluded before attempts are made to speed up the contractions. Correction of ineffective uterine contractions includes *amniotomy, amniotomy and administration of oxytocin or administration of oxytocin* in the presence of the previously ruptured membranes. When labor is induced or augmented with oxytocin, the midwife must be vigilant and aware of the risk of hyperstimulation of the uterus.

4. *Comfort and analgesia*: Adequate analgesia should be offered to the mother. Where

labor is prolonged intramuscular injection of pethidine or an epidural block affords complete pain relief in most cases. They should be helped to adopt the most comfortable position. General hygiene is important, especially where the membranes have been ruptured. Soiled pads and linen should be changed as necessary.

5. *Observations*: All observations are to be recorded on the partogram. Infection may develop where there has been prolonged rupture of membranes. Temperature should be taken four hourly. Vaginal swabs may be taken and broad-spectrum antibiotics commenced when infection is suspected. Pulse and blood pressure are recorded hourly or more frequently as the woman's condition requires.

6. *Fluid balance:* An accurate record should be kept. The woman should be encouraged to empty her bladder two hourly. If she is unable to void, a catheter should be inserted, as a full bladder may affect the uterine action in labor. Recording output is important when oxytocin is administered because of its antidiuretic effect. Fluid overload can occur which causes hyponatremia, affecting mother and baby.

7. *Assessment of progress*: Vaginal examination is carried out usually every four hours. Progress is noted by increasing dilatation along with the consistency of the cervix and application of the cervix to the presenting part. The degree of moulding should be noted, and any increase over successive examinations reported. Descend of the presenting part must be assessed by noting the station of the presenting part on vaginal examination. The color of the amniotic fluid needs to be noted and if meconium is present, this should be reported.

8. *Fetal wellbeing*: Fetal heart rate must be monitored carefully by frequent auscultation or continuously, using electronic fetal monitor. Fetal blood sampling may be used to support a decision to continue with labor or intervene.

The presence of meconium-stained liquor and an abnormal fetal heart tracing is suggestive of fetal hypoxia. A pediatrician should be present at the birth and precautions to be taken to prevent aspiration of meconium. If the mother is in labor at home, it may be necessary to transfer her to a hospital with facilities for operative delivery and care of the neonate.

Prolonged Second Stage of Labor

A lengthy second stage may result from ineffective contractions, poor maternal effort and loss of, or absence of, a desire to push caused by epidural analgesia. A full bladder or a full rectum can also impede progress. A large fetus, malpresentation or malposition may account for delay and an assisted birth may be necessary.

A reduced pelvic outlet in association with an occipitoposterior position may result in deep transverse arrest.

Management of a Prolonged Second Stage

A vaginal examination should be carried out to confirm position, attitude and station of the presenting part. The fetal heart should be auscultated after every contraction or electronic monitoring used.

In the presence of inefficient uterine contractions, an infusion of oxytocin should be commenced. The usual observations for the use of oxytocin are to be followed. Mothers with related factors, such as preeclampsia or prematurity, management of the second stage, will be assessed constantly.

Options for Delivery

Delivery may be expedited where the conditions alter or mother or fetus becomes distressed. Ventouse or forceps will be used where the pelvic outlet is adequate and vaginal birth can be safely carried out. Cesarean section may be necessary where there is evidence of cephalopelvic disproportion.

Maternal Distress

The following are the evidences of maternal distress:
- Anxious look with sunken eyes
- Dry tongue

- Acetone smell in mouth
- Rising pulse rate of 100 per minute or more
- Hot, dry vagina often with offensive discharge
- Scanty, high colored urine with presence of acetone.

DISORDERS OF UTERINE ACTION

Precipitate Labor (Over-efficient Uterine Action)

A labor is called precipitate when the combined duration of the first and second stage is less than two hours. It is common in multiparae and may be repetitive. Rapid expulsion is due to the combined effect of hyperactive uterine contractions associated with diminished soft tissue resistance.

Maternal Risks

- Extensive laceration of the cervix, vagina and perineum (to the extent of complete perineal tear)
- Postpartum hemorrhage
- Inversion of uterus
- Infection.

Fetal Risks

- Intracranial stress and hemorrhage because of rapid expulsion without time for moulding of the head
- The baby may sustain serious injuries if delivery occurs in standing position due to bleeding from the torn cord and direct hit on the skull.

Management

The woman with previous history of precipitate labor should be hospitalized prior to labor. The uterine contractions may be suppressed by administering ether during contractions. Delivery of the head should be controlled. Episiotomies should be done liberally. Elective induction of labor by low rupture of membranes and careful conduction of controlled delivery may be done.

Cervical Dystocia

Cervical dystocia is one where despite effective contractions the cervix (external os) fails to dilate, although it may efface. Cervical dystocia may be primary or secondary. The primary type of dystocia occurs predominantly during the first birth. The nondilatation may be due to the presence of excessive fibrous tissue or spasm of circular muscle fibers surrounding the os. The secondary cervical dystocia results usually from the effect of scarring or rigidity of cervix from the effect of previous operation or disease.

The cervix becomes very much thinned out and well applied to the head. Initially, the uterine contractions remain good but ultimately become ineffective. On occasion, edema of the anterior lip may occur and delivery may be accomplished by avulsion (tearing away) of the anterior lip or annular detachment of the cervix.

Management

In the presence of associated complications, where vaginal delivery is found unsafe, cesarean section is performed.

If the head is sufficiently low down with only a thick rim of cervix left behind, the rim may be pushed up manually during contraction or traction given by Ventouse. In others, where the cervix is very much thinned out, but only half dilated a Duhrssen's incision at 2 and 10 o'clock positions may be given followed by Ventouse or forceps application (Dutta, 2001).

Generalized Tonic Contraction (Uterine Tetany)

In this condition, pronounced retraction occurs involving whole of the uterus up to the level of internal os. There is no physiological differentiation of the active upper segment and the passive lower segment of the uterus. The uterine contraction ceases after a period and the whole uterus undergoes a sort of tonic muscular spasm holding the fetus inside.

Causes

- ❖ Failure to overcome the obstruction by powerful contractions of the uterus
- ❖ Irritability caused by repeated unsuccessful attempts at artificial delivery
- ❖ Injudicious administration of oxytocics, especially following intramuscular administration of oxytocin.

Clinical Manifestations

- ❖ The woman is in prolonged labor with severe and continuous pain
- ❖ Evidences of dehydration and ketoacidosis
- ❖ On abdominal examination:
  - The uterus is somewhat smaller in size
  - Tense and tender
  - Fetal parts are not well defined
  - Fetal heart sound not audible on auscultation.
- ❖ On vaginal examination:
  - Jammed head with big caput
  - Dry and edematous vagina.

Treatment

- ❖ Deep sedation by intramuscular morphine 15 mg or pethidine drip
- ❖ Correction of dehydration and ketoacidosis by administering Ringer's solution in rapid infusion
- ❖ Administration of antibiotics
- ❖ *Active management*: After a period of rest, the abnormal uterine action may subside when spontaneous delivery is possible, if there is no obstruction. In the presence of obstruction, however, operative procedure may be required to deliver the fetus.

Tonic Uterine Contraction and Retraction (Bandl's Ring)

This type of uterine contraction is predominantly due to obstructed labor. There is gradual increase in intensity, duration and frequency of uterine contraction. The relaxation phase becomes less and less, ultimately a state of tonic contraction results. Retraction, however, continues.

The lower segment elongates and becomes progressively thinner to accommodate the fetus driven from the upper segment. *A circular groove encircling the uterus is formed between the active upper segment and the distended lower segment, called pathological retraction ring or Bandl's ring.* In normal labor a ridge forms between the upper and lower segments, which is termed as the *retraction ring*. In obstructed labor, this phenomenon becomes exaggerated and is visible above the symphysis pubis as Bandl's ring (Figs 32.1A to C). Due to

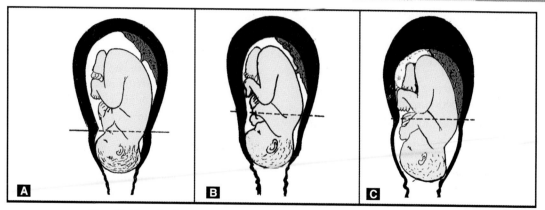

Figs 32.1A to C: Pathogenesis of retraction ring (Bandl's ring): (A) Normal labor; (B) Early obstruction; (C) Late obstruction

pronounced retraction, there is marked reduction of blood flow to the placenta, leading to fetal jeopardy and even death.

In primigravidae, further retraction may cease in response to obstruction and labor may come to a standstill as a state of exhaustion. Contractions may recommence after a short period of rest with renewed vigor. In multiparae, retraction continues with progressive circumferential dilatation and thinning of the lower segment. There is progressive rise of the Bandl's ring, moving nearer and nearer to the umbilicus and ultimately, the lower segment ruptures.

Clinical Features

- Patient is in agony from continuous pain and discomfort.
- Features of exhaustion and ketoacidosis.
- On abdominal palpation
  - Upper segment is hard, uniformly convex and tender, lower segment is distended and tender
  - The pathological retraction ring is placed obliquely between the umbilicus and symphysis pubis and rises upwards as time passes
  - Fetal parts may not be well defined
  - FHS is usually absent.
- Pelvic examination reveals
  - Dry, hot vagina
  - Fully dilated cervix
  - Membranes absent.

Prevention

It is a preventable condition. The abnormality either in the passage (bony or soft tissue) or in the passenger (malpresentation or malformation of the fetus) can be detected during antenatal or early intranatal period and appropriate treatment solves the problem.

Management

- Morphine 15 mg is given intramuscularly
- IV 5 percent dextrose and Ringer's solution to correct fluid volume deficit and ketoacidosis
- Vaginal delivery followed by exploration of the uterus to exclude rupture of the uterus
- Cesarean section is rarely indicated.

Constriction Ring
(Syn: Contraction Ring)

It is one form of incoordinate uterine action where there is localized spastic contraction of a ring of circular muscle fibers of the uterus. It is usually situated at the junction of the upper and lower segment around a constricted part of the fetus usually around the neck in cephalic presentation. It may appear in any stage of labor and is usually reversible.

Its occurrence is associated with injudicious administration of oxytocics, premature rupture of membranes and premature attempts at instrumental delivery.

Diagnosis

Diagnosis is difficult. Failure of the presenting part to advance even during effective contructions with the cervix lying loose is suspicious. It is revealed during:

- Cesarean section in the first stage
- During forceps application in the second stage.
- During manual removal of placenta in the third stage.

It is then referred to as *hour glass contraction*. The labor is prone to be delayed. Maternal condition is not much affected but the fetus may be in danger because of the hypertonic state.

Management

- *First stage*: The diagnosis is made during cesarean section. The ring may have to be cut vertically to deliver the baby.
- *Second stage*: Diagnosed when correct application of forceps fails to deliver the baby. Conformation is done by palpating the ring after removing the forceps. If the baby is in good condition, cesarean section is done even at this stage. If the baby is dead, forceps may be reapplied after relaxing the uterus by administering adrenaline subcutaneous and amyle nitrate by inhalation alternatively. If these fail to relax the uterus in five minutes, general anesthesia is given to complete the forceps delivery.
- *Third stage*: The diagnosis is made during attempted manual removal of the placenta. Deepening the anesthesia is usually effective. Alternatively, adrenaline or amyle nitrate may be administered.

Obstructed Labor

Obstructed labor is one where in spite of good uterine contractions, the progressive descend of the presenting part is arrested due to mechanical obstruction. This may result either from the faults in the fetus or in the birth canal or both.

Incidence is about 1 to 2 percent in the developing countries.

Causes

- Fault in the passage:
  1. Contracted pelvis and cephalopelvic disproportion are the common causes.
  2. *Soft tissue obstructions*: These include cervical dystocia, cervical or broad ligament fibroid and impacted ovarian tumor.
- Fault in the passenger:
  1. Brow presentation
  2. Congenital malformations, such as hydrocephalus, fetal ascitis, conjoined twins.
  3. Big baby associated with deflexed head and accipito-posterior position
  4. Impacted mentoposterior
  5. Compound presentation
  6. Locked twins.

Signs of Obstructed Labor

The presenting part does not enter the pelvic brim despite good contractions. The midwife should exclude reasons, such as full bladder, loaded rectum, or excessive liquor volume as factors contributing to the failure in descent.

As the presenting part does not descend, cervical dilatation is slow. The cervix hangs loosely like 'an empty sleeve' as the presenting part is not applied to it. Early rupture of membranes or formation of a large elongated sac of forewaters is seen.

Late Signs

Clinical signs include pyrexia and a rapid pulse rate. Urinary output is poor and hematuria may be present. Profound fetal bradycardia or fetal demise may follow.

The uterus becomes moulded round the fetus and it fails to relax properly between contractions. Uterus goes into tonic contraction. A visible retraction ring or Bandl's ring may be seen above the symphysis pubis. This is similar in appearance to a full bladder. Uterine exhaustion, in which contractions may cease for a while before recommencing with renewed vigor, may occur in primigravida.

Vagina may feel hot and dry. The presenting part is high and feels wedged and immovable. There is excessive moulding of the fetal skull and a large caput succedaneum present. Little urine is obtained on catheterization of the bladder.

Effects on Mother

1. Exhaustion due to constant agonizing pain and anxiety.
2. Dehydration due to increased muscle activity.
3. Metabolic acidosis due to accumulation of lactic acid produced by the contractile uterine and voluntary muscles.
4. Intrauterine infection may follow prolonged rupture of membranes.
5. Injury to the genital tract including rupture of uterus due to thinning of the lower uterine segment, which may be spontaneous in multiparae or may be traumatic following instrumental delivery.
6. Postpartum hemorrhage and shock due to the effects of traumatic delivery and blood loss or because of dehydration and ketoacidosis.
7. *Bladder injury due to trauma*: The base of the bladder and urethra, which may be nipped in between the presenting part and symphysis pubis, may undergo pressure necrosis. The devitalized tissue may become infected and later on slough off resulting in the development of vesicovaginal fistula.
8. Remote effects are variable degrees of vaginal atresia, rectovaginal fistula and secondary amenorrhea.

All these lead to increased maternal morbidity and mortality.

Effects on the Fetus

1. Asphyxia results from tonic uterine contraction, which interferes with uteroplacental circulation or due to cord prolapse, especially in shoulder presentation, leading to permanent brain damage.
2. Acidosis as the result of maternal acidosis.
3. Intracranial hemorrhage due to super-moulding of the head or due to traumatic delivery.
4. Ascending infection can cause neonatal pneumonia.

All these effects lead to increased perinatal loss.

Management of Obstructed Labor

Management includes prevention of obstructed labor in the first instance. Risk factors such as history of prolonged labor and difficult births must be noted in the antenatal period. Malpresentations or signs of cephalopelvic disproportion must be identified by abdominal examination and after confirmation, elective cesarean section may be advocated.

During labor, careful assessment of the progress will help to detect lack of descend before labor becomes obstructed. Correlation of findings from abdominal examination and vaginal examination helps to confirm descend of the presenting part through the pelvis. This is aided by observation of both maternal and fetal condition, and assessment of the length, strength and frequency of contractions. If the midwife suspects that labor is obstructed, she must seek appropriate medical aid immediately.

Measures of Management

1. Sedate the woman with pethidine 75 to 100 mg.
2. Correct dehydration and ketoacidosis by rapid infusions of appropriate solution.
3. Parenteral antibiotics are administered to overcome any infection that may be present.
4. Accurate record of observations of maternal and fetal conditions.

Obstetric Management

If obstructed labor is recognized in the first stage of labor, as when the head is extended to brow presentation, cesarean section is done. In the second stage of labor, failure to progress and descend may be caused by deep transverse arrest. If obstruction cannot be overcome by rotation and assisted birth;

cesarean section should be performed as soon as possible.

If the mother is laboring at home, she must be transferred to a hospital with facilities for immediate cesarean and resuscitation of the neonate. If the labor is obstructed and the fetus has died, this will still be the mode of delivery, as vaginal birth cannot be achieved. Following the birth of the baby and prior to repair of the uterus and abdomen, exploration of the uterus is done to exclude uterine rupture or tear.

The fetus is likely to be delivered in a shocked and asphyxiated condition and facilities for resuscitation and expert care should be available. The pediatrician should be present at birth and the parents need to be informed that the baby may need special care after birth.

BIBLIOGRAPHY

1. Caldeyro Barcia R. "The influence of maternal position on time of spontaneous rupture of membranes, progress of labor and fetal head compression". Birth and Family Journal 1979;6(1):7-15.
2. Crowley P, et al. "The value of ultrasound measurement of amniotic fluid volume in the management of prolonged pregnancies". British Journal of Obstetrics and Gynecology 1984;91: 444-8.
3. Dutta DC. Textbook of Obstetrics, 5th edn. Calcutta: New Central Book Company, 2001.
4. Flynn AM, Kelly J. "Ambulation in labor". British Medical Journal 1978;2:591-3.
5. Mackenzie IA. The therapeutic role of prostaglandins in obstetrics, In: Studd J (Ed). Progress in Obstetrics and Gynecology, Churchill Livingstone, Edinburgh, Volume 8;1990.
6. Shiers CV. Prolonged pregnancy and disorders of uterine action, In: Myles Textbook for Midwives, 13th edn. Edinburgh: Churchill Livingstone, 1999.

33

Malpositions and Malpresentations

The midwife must know, how to manage certain deviations from normal and obstetric complications until they are resolved or until the physician arrives. Occasionally she is confronted with these deviations from normal because a patient arrives in second stage with no prenatal care or record, or because of an emergency. Theoretically and ideally, all of these deviations from normal and complications should have been diagnosed and anticipated before delivery and before their occurrence. Situational circumstances with women in India, however, dictate that this will not always be the case. The conditions included in this chapter are:
* Occipito-posterior position
* Face presentation
* Brow presentation
* Breech presentation
* Shoulder presentation
* Compound presentation
* Shoulder dystocia
* Unstable lie.

OCCIPITO-POSTERIOR POSITION

Occipito-posterior position is a malposition of the head and occurs in about 13 percent of all head positions. The presenting part is the vertex and the denominator is the occiput. ROP is three times as common as LOP.

Postulated Causes of Occipito-posterior Positions

* Pendulous abdomen, common in multiparous women
* Anthropoid pelvic brim
* Android pelvic brim. The transverse diameter of the brim being nearer the sacrum encourages the biparietal diameter to accommodate posteriorly
* A flat sacrum with a poorly flexed head leads to further deflexion and occiput posterior position
* The placenta on the anterior uterine wall tends to encourage the fetus to flex round it.

Palpation

The fetal back is found to one side in early labor before descend of head. Fetal head is in the posterior position in early labor with descend of head. The limbs are to the front and give a hollowing above the head. This is particularly notable after rupture of membranes.

Auscultation

The fetal heart is heard best in the flank but descends to just above the pubis as the head rotates and descends.

Vaginal Examination

The membranes tend to rupture early, often before labor is well established. If the membranes are intact, they may protrude through the cervix. The head is deflexed so the anterior fontanelle is readily felt in the anterior part of the pelvis near the iliopectineal eminance. The sagittal suture is directed towards the right sacroiliac joint (in ROP). The posterior fontanelle is not readily felt till the head is in the lower pelvic cavity.

Course of Labor

Occipito-posterior position may lead to disorganized labor especially in the primigravida. Initially the contractions are sustained and irregular, accompanied by marked backache. Analgesia may be required to ease the discomfort. Engagement of the head is encouraged if the woman lies on the side, which the fetus faces. Walking about after rest also helps.

Labor tends to be long and contractions become more normal as labor progresses. Retention of urine is common in occiput-posterior labor and catheterization may be required.

The woman may feel the need to bear down before the second stage is reached, probably due to pressure on the sacrum and rectum. Dilatation must be confirmed before she is encouraged to bear down.

Mechanisms of Labor in Occipito-posterior Position

In the occiput-posterior position, the head engages in the right oblique diameter for the ROP and in the left oblique diameter for the LOP. The engaging transverse diameter is biparietal (9.5 cm) and the anteroposterior diameter is either suboccipitofrontal (10 cm) or occipitofrontal (11.5 cm).

Possible Courses of Labor

Long Arc Rotation

In favorable circumstances, with increasing flexion the occiput reaches the pelvic floor and rotates 3/8th of a circle (135°) forward (a long-arc rotation) to an occiput anterior position. Mechanisms will then continue as in an anterior position (ROA or LOA). In about 90 percent, delivery occurs in thin manner.

Posterior Rotation of the Occiput

With severe deflexion, posterior rotation of the occiput of 1/8th of a circle (45°) occurs as sinciput reaches the pelvic floor and rotates posteriorly. With posterior rotation the possible outcomes are (1) *Face to pubis delivery* with a spacious gynecoid pelvis, (2) *Persistent occipito-posterior position* in which the occiput goes into the hollow of the sacrum.

Short Arc Rotation

In unfavorable circumstances as with an android or athropoid pelvis and weak uterine contractions deflexion of the head persists. The occipit reaches the pelvic floor and rotates 1/8th of a circle (45°) anteriorly and the sagittal suture comes to lie in the transverse diameter of the pelvis. Further rotation is unlikely and the condition ends up as *deep transverse arrest.*

Nonrotation of the Occiput

As the fetal head descends, deflexion continues. There is nonrotation of the occiput resulting in an *oblique posterior arrest.*

Mechanism of Labor in Right Occipito-posterior Position (ROP)

- ❖ The lie is longitudinal
- ❖ The attitude of the head is deflexed
- ❖ The presentation is vertex
- ❖ The position is right occipito-posterior
- ❖ The presenting part is the middle or anterior area of the left parietal bone
- ❖ The occipitofrontal diameter 11.5 cm lies in the right oblique diameter of the pelvic brim
- ❖ The occiput points to the right sacroiliac joint and the sinciput to the left ileopectineal eminence.

Positional Movements

1. *Engagement:* Takes place in the right oblique diameter of the pelvis.
2. *Flexion:* Descent occurs with increasing flexion, the occiput becomes the leading part.
3. *Internal rotation of the head:* The occiput reaches the pelvic floor first and rotates

forwards 3/8th of a circle (135°) along the right side of the pelvis to lie under the symphysis pubis. The shoulders turn 2/8th of a circle (90°) and reach the right oblique diameter (long internal rotation).

4. *Crowning*: The occiput impinges beneath the symphysis pubis and the head is crowned.
5. *Extension*: The head (sinciput, face and chin) is born by extension.
6. *Restitution*: The occiput turns 1/8th of a circle (45°) to the right and the head re-aligns itself with the shoulders.
7. *Internal rotation of the shoulders*: The anterior shoulder rotates 1/8th of a circle (45°) to the right.
8. *External rotation of the head*: At the time of internal rotation of the shoulders, the occuped turns a further 1/8th of a circle (45°) to the right.
9. *Lateral flexion*: The anterior shoulder escapes under the symphysis pubis. Posterior shoulder sweeps the perineum and the body is born by lateral flexion. After the long internal rotation of 135°, further mechanisms continue as in a ROA delivery.

Mechanism of Labor with Posterior Rotation of the Occiput

With a spacious gynecoid pelvis, the baby may be born from a persistent occipito-posterior position as *face-to-pubis* (Fig. 33.1).
1. Engagement takes place in the right oblique diameter of the pelvis.
2. Flexion: With increasing flexion, the occiput becomes the leading part.
3. Internal rotation: The occiput turns 1/8th of a circle (45°) backwards and the sagittal

suture comes to lie in the anteroposterior diameter of the mother's pelvis.
4. Crowning: Further descend occurs until the root of the nose impinges under the symphysis pubis.
5. Birth of the baby's head is by a double mechanism of flexion and extension. The sinciput impinges beneath the symphysis pubis and becomes the pivotal point for delivery of head. The head stays in flexion as the occiput distends the perineum and is born to the nape of the neck. The remainder of the head is then born by extension as the head falls back towards the rectum with the face looking upward.
6. Restitution: The head moves 1/8th of a circle to the right.
7. External rotation of further 1/8th of a circle to the right.
8. Birth of a shoulders and body by lateral flexion.

FACE PRESENTATION

When the attitude of the head is one of extension, the occiput of the fetus will be in contact with its spine and the face will present.

The incidence is about 1:500 and the majority develops during labor from vertex presentations with the occiput posterior; this is termed as secondary face presentation. Less commonly, the face presents before labor; this is termed as primary face presentation. There are six positions in a face presentation (Figs 33.2A to F); the denominator is the mentum and the presenting diameters are the submento-bregmatic (9.5 cm) and the bitemporal (8.2 cm).

Causes

❖ *Contracted pelvis:* In the flat pelvis, the head enters in the transverse diameter of the brim, the head becomes extended and a face presentation develops. In an android pelvis, the occiput does not descend, the head becomes extended and face presentation results.
❖ *Polyhydramnios:* If the vertex is presenting and the membranes rupture spontaneously, the resulting rush of fluid may cause the head to extend as it sinks into the lower uterine segment.

Fig. 33.1: Face-to-pubis delivery, occipitofrontal diameter emerges out of the introitus

Figs 33.2A to F: Six positions of face presentation: (A) Right mentoposterior; (B) Left mentoposterier; (C) Right mentolateral; (D) Left mentolateral; (E) Right mentoanterior; and (F) Left mentoanterior

❖ *Congenital abnormality:* An anencephalic fetus in cephalic presentation ends up as face presentation, because the vertex is absent. Face is thrust forward. In very rare instances, a tumor of the fetal neck may cause extension of the head.

Diagnosis of Face Presentation

Antenatal diagnosis is rare because face presentation develops during labor in the majority of cases. A known anencephalic fetus in a cephalic presentation may be presumed to be a face presentation. Palpation in the intrapartal period may reveal the following:
❖ Occiput may feel prominent with a groove between head and back
❖ The limbs may be palpated on the side opposite to the occiput
❖ Fetal heart is best heard through the chest on the same side as the limbs.

In a mentoposterior position, fetal heart is difficult to hear because the fetal chest is in contact with the maternal pelvis. Many babies with face presentation begin labor either in brow presentation or with a hyperextended head and convert to a face during descend.

On vaginal examination, the fetal part is high. It may feel soft and irregular (lumpy) similar to a breech. When the cervix is fully dilated, orbital ridge, eyes, nose and mouth may be felt. Confusion between the anus and mouth could arise. The hard gums are diagnostic and the fetus may even suck the examining finger as it approaches the mouth.

Mechanisms of Labor

❖ The lie is longitudinal
❖ The attitude is one of extension of head and back
❖ The presentation is face
❖ The position is one of the following:
   LMA, LMP, LMT
   RMA, RMP, RMT
❖ The denominator is mentum
❖ The presenting part is the left malar bone.

Engagement

Engagement takes place when the submentobregmatic diameter has passed through the pelvic inlet. (About 70% of all face presentations engage as either mentum anterior or mentum transverse varieties. The remaining 30 percent engages as a posterior variety).

Extension

Descend takes place with increasing extension. The mentum (chin) becomes the leading part because the head is extended.

Descent Occurs Throughout

Internal rotation of the head occurs when the chin reaches the pelvic floor and rotates.
a. Rotation of the chin anteriorly:
   ❖ 45° (1/8th of a circle) for RMA and LMA to MA
   ❖ 90° (2/8th of a circle) for RMT and LMT to MA
   ❖ 135° (3/8th of a circle) for RMP and LMP to MA.

Submento-bregmatic diameter at outlet

A **B**

Figs 33.3A and B: Birth of head in mentoanterior position: (A) Chin escapes under symphysis pubis; (B) Head is born by a movement of flection

b. Rotation of the chin posteriorly
   ❖ 45° (1/8th of a circle) for RMP and LMP to MP.

Mentum Anterior Position

In mentum anterior position, birth of the head is by double mechanism of extension and flexion. Extension is maintained until the chin is born by escaping beneath the symphysis pubis. The submento area beneath the chin impinges beneath the symphysis pubis and becomes the pivotal point for the delivery of the rest of the head by flexion (Figs 33.3A and B). The remaining head is born sequentially starting with the sinciput, vertex and occiput as the head flexes.

If the chin rotates posteriorly into a mentum posterior position, the mechanisms of labor cease at this point because the baby cannot deliver vaginally from this position—*persistent mentoposterior position*. This is because the length of the neck of the fetus is only about half as long as the length of the sacrum. Therefore, it is not possible for the chin to escape from the vaginal floor over the perineum, thereby allowing the remainder of the head to be born by flexion. This condition must be recognized before impaction of the head takes place with its extremely poor prognosis for the baby. Delivery must be effected by immediate cesarean section.

Restitution

Restitution takes place when the chin turns 45° (1/8th of a circle) in the direction from whence the head rotated during internal rotation. For example, if the rotation was from

an RMT to an MA, the restitution is 45° to an RMA (to the woman's right) position.

Internal Rotation of the Shoulders

The shoulders enter the pelvis in the oblique diameter and the anterior shoulder reaches the pelvic floor first and rotates forwards 45° (1/8th of a circle) along the left side of the pelvis in the RMA position and along the right side in LMA position.

External Rotation of the Head

This occurs simultaneously. The chin moves further 45° (1/8th of a circle) in the same direction as restitution.

Birth of the Shoulders and Body by Lateral Flexion

The anterior shoulder escapes under the symphysis pubis, the posterior shoulder sweeps the perineum and the body is born by a movement of lateral flexion.

Midwifery Management of a Face Presentation

1. Recognition of the face presentation and notification of the physician of the malpresentation.
2. A fetal scalp electrode must not be applied, and care should be taken not to infect or injure the eyes during vaginal examination.
3. Close monitoring of the mechanism of labor or internal rotation and immediately informing the physician if rotation is to a direct mentum posterior position.
4. Immediately following rupture of membranes, a vaginal examination should be performed to exclude cord prolapse, as such an occurrence is more likely because the face is an ill-fitting presenting part.
5. For delivery of the head:
   a. Application of pressure on the fetal brow may be necessary to maintain extension until chin is born. This is done by pressing on the posterior end of the perineal body as the vulvovaginal orifice distends. The gloved hand must be

protected from contamination from the return by covering it with a sterile towel.

b. Exertion of head control, thereby allowing the gradual flexion and birth of the remainder of the head.

6. Request that the pediatrician to attend the delivery. If there is extensive edema of the neck, nose and mouth, respiratory function may be compromised.

7. Reassuring the parents, family and significant others that the position of the head and neck of the baby (neck extended, head fallen backwards) and the extensive swelling of the features of the face normally disappear in a few days and show noticeable improvement in a day or two.

Possible Complications

Obstructed Labor

Because the face, unlike the vertex does not mould, a minor degree of pelvic contraction may result in obstructed labor. In a persistent mentoposterior position, the face becomes impacted and cesarean section is necessary.

Cord Prolapse

A prolapsed cord is more common when the membranes rupture because the face is an ill-fitting presenting part. The midwife should always perform a vaginal examination when the membranes rupture in order to detect such an occurrence.

Facial Bruising

The baby's face is always bruised and swollen at birth with edematous eyelids and lips. The head is elongated and the baby will initially lie with his head extended.

Cerebral Hemorrhage

The lack of molding of the facial bones can lead to intracranial hemorrhage caused by excessive compression of the fetal skull or by rearward compression in the typical molding of the fetal skull found in this presentation (Fig. 33.4).

Maternal Trauma

Extensive perineal laceration may occur at the time of delivery due to the large submento-vertical and biparietal diameters distending the vagina and perineum. There is an increased incidence of operative delivery, either forceps or cesarean section, both of which increase maternal morbidity.

BROW PRESENTATION

In the brow presentation, the fetal head is primarily extended with the frontal bone lying at the pelvic brim. The presenting part is bounded by the anterior fontanel and the orbital ridges. The presenting diameter is mento-vertical (13.5 cm) (Fig. 33.5), which exceeds all diameters in an average-size pelvis. The incidence of this presentation is 1 in 1000 deliveries.

Causes

Causes are the same as for a face presentation.

Diagnosis

Brow presentation is not usually detected before the onset of labor.

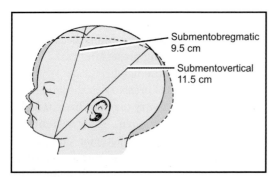

Fig. 33.4: Molding in a face presentation (dotted line)

Submentobregmatic 9.5 cm
Submentovertical 11.5 cm

Fig. 33.5: Molding in a brow presentation (dotted line)

Mentovertical 13.5 cm

Abdominal Palpation

The head is high, appears unduly large, and does not descend into the pelvis in spite of good uterine contractions.

Vaginal Examination

The presenting part may be high and difficult to reach. The anterior fontanel may be felt on one side of the pelvis and the orbital ridges on the other. A large caput succedaneum may mask these landmarks if the woman has been in labor of sometime.

Management

The obstetrician must be informed immediately if brow presentation is suspected. Obstructed labor usually results unless cesarean section is done immediately. In extremely rare cases vaginal delivery may be possible with a large pelvis and small a baby though the midwife should never expect such a favorable outcome.

If there is no fetal distress, the physician may allow labor to continue for a short while in case further extension of the head converts the brow presentation to a face presentation. Occasionally spontaneous flexion may occur, resulting in a vertex presentation.

BREECH PRESENTATION

In a breech presentation, the fetus lies longitudinally with the buttocks in the lower pole of the uterus. The presenting diameter is the bitrochanteric—10 cm (measured at the level of the hip joint) and the denominator the sacrum. This presentation occurs in approximately 3 percent pregnancies at term.

Positions of Breech Presentation

There are six positions for a breech presentation. These are illustrated in Figures 33.6A to F.

Types of Breech Presentation (Figs 33.7A to D)

Breech with Extended Legs (Frank Breech)

The breech presents with the hips flexed and legs extended on abdomen. Seventy percent of breech presentations are of this type. It is

Figs 33.6A to F: Six positions in breech presentation: (A) Right sacroposterior; (B) Left sacroposterior; (C) Right sacrolateral; (D) Left sacrolateral; (E) Right sacroanterior and (F) Left sacroanterior

Figs 33.7A to D: Types of breech presentation: (A) Frank breech; (B) Complete breech; (C) Footing presentation; (D) Knee presentation

particularly common in primigravidae whose good uterine muscle tone inhibits flexion of the legs and free turning of the fetus.

Complete Breech

The fetal attitude is one of complete flexion, hips and knees are both flexed and the feet tucked in behind the buttocks.

Footling Breech

One or both feet present because neither hips nor knees are fully flexed. The feet are lower than the buttocks, which distinguish this presentation from the complete breech.

Knee Presentation

One or both hips are extended, with the knees flexed. This is very rare.

Antenatal Diagnosis

On palpation, the lie is longitudinal with a soft presentation, which more easily felt during Pawlik's grip. The head can be felt in the fundus as a round hard mass, which may be made to move independently of the back by balloting it with one or both hands. If the legs are extended, the feet may prevent such nodding. When the breech is anterior, and the fetus well flexed, it may be difficult to locate the head, but a combined grip of upper and lower poles may aid diagnosis. The woman may complain of discomfort under her ribs, especially at night, due to pressure of the head on the diaphragm.

Auscultation

When the fetus has not passed through the pelvic brim, the fetal heart is heard above the umbilicus. When the legs are extended, the breech descends into the pelvis easily. The fetal heart is then heard at a lower level.

An ultrasound examination may be used to confirm a breech presentation. X-ray examination may be used for the purpose of diagnosis and pelvimetry.

Diagnosis during Labor

Breech presentation may be diagnosed by abdominal palpation on admission in labor.

On vaginal examination, the breech feels soft and irregular with no sutures palpable. The anus may be felt and fresh meconium on the examining finger is usually diagnostic. If the legs are extended, the external genitalia are very evident, but it must be remembered that these become edematous.

If a foot is felt, the midwife should differentiate it from the hand by noting that the toes are all of the same length and the big toe cannot be opposed to other toes. The foot is at right angles to the leg and the heel has no equivalent in the hand.

Presentation may be confirmed by ultrasound scan or X-ray.

External Cephalic Version

External cephalic version (ECV) is the use of external manipulation on the mother's abdomen to convert a breech to a cephalic presentation.

It has been demonstrated that the ECV can reduce the number of babies presenting by the breech at term by two-thirds and therefore reduce the cesarean section rate for breech presentations (Hofmyer, 1997).

Turning the fetus from a breech to a cephalic presentation before 37th week of gestation does not reduce the incidence of breech birth or rate of cesarean section as it is likely to turn itself back spontaneously (Zhang et al, 1993).

Method

An ultrasound scan is performed to localize the placenta and to confirm the position and presentation of the fetus. A 30 minute cardiotocograph (fetal heart monitoring) is performed to establish that the fetus is not distressed at the start of the procedure and maternal pulse and blood pressure are recorded.

The woman is asked to empty her bladder. The midwife then assists the woman to a comfortable supine position. The foot of the bed may be elevated to help free the breech from the pelvic brim. The abdomen is dusted with talcum powder to prevent pinching of the mother's skin during the procedure. The ECV may be uncomfortable for the mother, but may not be painful. The breech is displaced from the pelvic brim and iliac fossa. With one hand on each pole, the obstetrician makes the fetus perform a forward somersault. If this is not successful, then a backward somersault is attempted.

If the fetus does not turn easily, then the procedure is abandoned, but may be tried again after few days. The fetal heart should be auscultated after the procedure or a cardiotocogram performed.

Version may be performed immediately prior to the onset of labor. If the woman is Rh-negative, an injection of anti-D immunoglobulin is given as prophylaxis against isoimmunization caused by any placental separation.

Complications

1. Knotting of the umbilical cord should be suspected if bradycardia occurs and persists. The fetus is immediately turned back to a breech presentation. The woman is admitted for observation and, if necessary, cesarean section performed.
2. Separation of the placenta: Pain or vaginal bleeding during and after the procedure must be reported and taken care of.
3. Rupture of the membranes: If this occurs, the cord may prolapse because neither the head nor the breech is engaged.

Contraindications

1. Pre-eclampsia or hypertension because of the increased risk of placental abruption
2. Multiple pregnancy
3. Oligohydramnios
4. Ruptured membranes
5. A hydrocephalic fetus
6. Any condition, which would require delivery by cesarean section.

Assessment for Vaginal Delivery

The capacity of the pelvis to accommodate the fetal head must be assessed before the buttocks are delivered and the head attempts to enter the brim. The fetal size in relation to maternal pelvis must also be assessed by an ultrasound examination to avoid fetal hypoxia as the head enters the pelvic brim after the buttocks are delivered.

Mechanism of Labor for Left Sacroanterior Position

1. Lie is longitudinal
2. Attitude is one of complete flexion
3. Presentation is breech
4. Position is left sacroanterior
5. Denominator is the sacrum
6. Presenting part is the left (anterior) buttock
7. Bitrochanteric diameter 10 cm, enters the pelvis in the left oblique diameter of the brim
8. Sacrum points to the left iliopectineal eminence.

   ❖ Descend takes place initially with increasing compaction, owing to increased flexion of the limbs. Descend then occurs throughout.

   ❖ Engagement of the hips takes place in an LSA position with the sacrum in the left anterior portion of the mother's pelvis and the bitrochanteric diameter in the left oblique diameter of the mother's pelvis.

   ❖ *Internal rotation of the buttocks*: The anterior buttock reaches the pelvic floor first and rotates forwards 45° (1/8th of a circle) along the right side of the pelvis to lie underneath the symphysis pubis. The bitrochanteric diameter is now in the anteroposterior diameter of the outlet.

   ❖ *Birth of the buttocks by lateral flexion*: The anterior buttock escapes under the symphysis pubis, the posterior buttock sweeps over the perineum and the buttocks are born by a movement of lateral flexion.

   ❖ *Restitution of the buttocks*: The anterior buttock turns slightly to the mother's right side.

   ❖ *Internal rotation of the shoulders*: The shoulders enter the pelvis in the same left oblique diameter. The anterior shoulder rotates 45° (1/8th of a circle) along the right side of the pelvis and escapes under the symphysis pubis.

❖ *External rotation of the buttocks*: With the internal rotation of the shoulders, the delivered body also rotates and the sacrum returns to an LST position from an LSA position.

❖ *Birth of the shoulders takes place by lateral flexion*: When born spontaneously, the anterior shoulder impinges beneath the symphysis pubis and serves as the pivotal point for the lateral flexion necessary for the delivery of the posterior shoulder via the curve of Carus. Birth of the anterior shoulder then follows as the body straightens out.

❖ *Internal rotation of the head*: The head enters the pelvis with the sagittal suture in the transverse diameter of the brim. The occiput rotates forwards along the left side and the suboccipital region (nape of the neck) impinges on the under surface of the symphysis pubis.

External rotation of the body takes place simultaneously. The body turns so that the back of the baby is upward and the baby is facing down.

❖ *Birth of the head by flexion*: The chin, face and sinciput sweep over the perineum and the head is born in a flexed attitude.

Types of Breech Delivery

1. *Spontaneous breech delivery*: The delivery occurs with little assistance from the attendant.
2. *Assisted breech delivery*: The buttocks are born spontaneously, but some assistance is provided for delivery of extended legs or arms and the head.
3. *Breech extraction*: This is a manipulative delivery performed by an obstetrician to hasten delivery in an emergency, such as the fetal distress.

Management of Delivery

Before the actual delivery begins, the following should have taken place:
1. Complete dilatation of the cervix.
2. Elimination of any question about the adequacy of the pelvis.

3. Emptying of the bladder.
4. Adequate explanation to mother for effective pushing effort.
5. Readiness for a full-scale newborn resuscitation effort.
6. Positioning so, there is plenty of room for lateral flexion and downward traction, that is lithotomy position.
7. Notification and presence or immediate availability of the consulting physician, anesthesiologist and pediatrician.

When the buttocks are distending the perineum, the woman is placed in the lithotomy position and the vulva is swabbed and draped with sterile towels. The bladder is usually catheterized at this stage. An epidural anesthesia, pudendal block or local infiltration is carried out by the physician.

❖ The woman is encouraged to push with the contractions and the buttocks are delivered spontaneously.

❖ If the legs are flexed, the feet disengage at the vulva and the baby is born as far as the umbilicus.

❖ A loop of cord is gently pulled down to avoid traction on the umbilicus. If the cord is being nipped behind the pubic bone, it should be moved to one side.

❖ Feel for the elbows, which are usually on the chest. If so, the arms will escape with the next contraction. If the arms are not felt, they are extended. There is no need for facilitation of the progress of the mechanisms of labor until the baby is born up to the umbilicus. After that, the remainder of the baby is to be born in 3 to 5 minutes to avoid any anoxia with resulting possible brain damage. Traction exerted on the baby prior to birth up to the umbilicus may cause—(1) the arms to fly up in a reflex action, thereby extending them above, over or behind the head and causing later difficulties in the delivery and/or (2) the head to deflex, which may cause problems with delivery of the head.

❖ Place a warm towel around the baby from just below the umbilicus down. This would keep the baby warm as well as give a non-

Fig. 33.8: Correct grasp of baby on the hips in Lovset maneuver

slippery hold on the baby, which is essential to exert traction.

Delivery of the Shoulders

The uterine contractions and the weight of the baby will bring the shoulders down on to the pelvic floor where they rotate into the antero-posterior diameter of the outlet.

❖ The obstetrician now grasps the baby by the hips with thumbs on either sacroiliac region and fingers on the corresponding iliac crest (Fig. 33.8).

❖ The baby is then tilted towards the maternal sacrum in order to free the anterior shoulder

❖ When the anterior shoulder has escaped, the buttocks are lifted towards the mother's abdomen to enable the posterior shoulder and arm to pass over the perineum.

If the arm has become extended, it is delivered first by inserting the fingers of the hand in vagina (the hand other than the one holding the baby's feet) to reach the elbow and sweeping it across the baby's chest downwards to delivery.

In order to do this the feet of the baby is grasped in one hand with the index finger between the legs and the middle finger and thumbs each encircling a leg (Fig. 33.9).

Care must be taken in holding the baby at an angle so that the head will enter the pelvis in the transverse diameter. The back must remain lateral until this has happened.

Delivery of the Head

When the back has been turned, the infant is allowed to hang from the vulva without support

Fig. 33.9: Delivery of the posterior shoulder in a breech presentation

for 1 to 2 minutes. The baby's weight brings the head on to the pelvic floor on which the occiput rotates forwards. The sagittal suture is now in the anteroposterior diameter of the outlet. Gradually, the neck elongates, the hairline appears and the suboccipital region can be felt. Controlled delivery of the head is vital to avoid any sudden change in intracranial pressure and subsequent cerebral hemorrhage.

Methods of Delivering the Aftercoming Head

Forceps Delivery

The obstetrician usually applies forceps to the aftercoming head to achieve a controlled delivery.

Burns Marshall Method

The obstetrician grasps the baby's ankles from behind with forefinger between the two. The baby is kept on the stretch with sufficient traction to prevent his neck from bending backwards. The occipital region and not the neck should pivot under the apex of the pubic arch. The feet are taken up through an arc of 180° until the mouth and nose are free at the vulva. The right hand may guard the perineum in order to prevent sudden escape of the head.

An assistant may now clear the airway and the baby will breath. The mother should be asked to take deliberate, regular breaths, which allow the vault of the skull to escape gradually, taking 2 or 3 minutes.

Mauriceau-Smellie-Veit Maneuver
(Jaw flexion and shoulder traction)

This method is used when there is delay in descend of the head because of extension (excessive shoulder traction is avoided as it may cause Erb's palsy).

The baby is laid astride the right arm with the palm supporting the chest. Two fingers are inserted well back into the mouth to pull the jaw downwards and flex the head (two fingers may be placed on the malar bones and the middle finger in the mouth, if they can be accommodated). Two fingers of the left hand are hooked over the shoulders with the middle finger pushing up the occiput to aid flexion. Traction is applied to draw the head out of the vagina and, when the suboccipital region appears, the body is lifted to assist the head to pivot around the symphysis pubis. Once the face is free, the airway may be cleared and the vault delivered slowly (Fig. 33.10).

Delivery of Extended Legs

The baby can be born with his legs extended (Frank breech) and assistance is usually required. When the popliteal fossae appear at the vulva, two fingers are placed along the length of one thigh with the fingertips in the fossa. The leg is swept to the side of the abdomen (abducting the hip) and the knee is flexed by the pressure on its under-surface. As this movement is continued, the lower part of the leg will emerge from the vagina. This process should be repeated in order to deliver the second leg.

Complications of Breech Presentation

Apart from the difficulties already mentioned, other complications can arise, most of which affect the fetus.

1. *Impacted breech*: Labor becomes obstructed when the fetus is disproportionately large for the size of the maternal pelvis.
2. *Cord prolapse*: This is common in a flexed (complete) or footling breech, as these have ill-fitting presenting parts.
3. *Birth injury*: Superficial tissue damage. Edema and bruising of the baby's genitalia may be caused by pressure on the cervix. In a footling breech a prolapsed foot, which lies in the vagina or at the vulva for a long time, may become edematous and discolored.
4. Fracture of humerus, clavicle, femur, or dislocation of shoulder or hip caused during delivery of extended arms or legs.
5. Erb's palsy caused by the brachial plexus being damaged by the twisting of the neck.
6. *Trauma to the internal organs*: A ruptured liver or spleen may be produced by grasping the abdomen.
7. *Damage to the adrenals*: This also happens by grasping the abdomen. Adrenalin release can cause shock.
8. Spinal cord damage or fracture of the spine caused by bending the body backwards over the symphysis pubis while delivering the head.
9. Intracranial hemorrhage caused by rapid delivery of the head, which has had no opportunity to mould. Hypoxia may also cause intracranial hemorrhage.
10. *Fetal hypoxia*: This may be due to cord prolapse or cord compression or to premature separation of the placenta.
11. *Premature separation of the placenta*: Retraction of the uterus takes place while the head is still in the vagina and the placenta begins to separate. Excessive delay in the delivery of the head may cause severe hypoxia in the fetus.

Fig. 33.10: Delivery of head after flexing the head (Mauriceau-Smellie-Veit grip)

Figs 33.11A and B: Shoulder presentations:
(A) Dorsoanterior; (B) Dorsoposterior

12. *Maternal trauma*: The maternal complications of breech delivery are the same as found in other operative vaginal deliveries.

SHOULDER PRESENTATION (FIGS 33.11A AND B)

When the fetus lies with its long axis across the long axis of the uterus (transverse) the shoulder is most likely to present. Occasionally the lie is oblique but this does not persist, as the uterine contractions during labor make it either longitudinal or transverse.

Shoulder presentation occurs in approximately 1 in 300 pregnancies. Only 17 percent of these remain as transverse at the onset of labor. The head lies on one side of the abdomen, with the breech at a slightly higher level on the other. The fetal back may be anterior or posterior.

Maternal Causes

Lax Abdominal and Uterine Muscles

This is the most common cause and is found in multigravidae, particularly those of high parity.

Uterine Abnormality

A bicornuate or subseptate uterus may result in a transverse lie. More rarely, a cervical or low uterine fibroid may cause transverse lie.

Contracted Pelvis

This may prevent the head from entering the pelvic brim.

Fetal Causes

Preterm Pregnancy

The amount of amniotic fluid in relation to the fetus is greater, allowing the fetus more mobility than at term.

Multiple Pregnancies

There is a possibility of polyhydramnios but the presence of more than one fetus reduces the room for maneuver when amounts of liquor are normal. It is the second twin, which more commonly adopts this lie after delivery of the first fetus.

Polyhydramnios

The distended uterus is globular and the fetus can move freely in the excessive liquor.

Macerated Fetus

Lack of muscle tone causes the fetus to slump down into the lower pole of the uterus.

Placenta Previa

This may prevent the head from entering the pelvic brim.

Diagnosis

Antenatal

On abdominal palpation, the uterus appears broad; and the fundal height is less than expected for the period of gestation. On pelvic and fundal palpation, neither head nor breech is felt. The mobile head is found at one side of the abdomen and the breech at a slightly higher level at the other. Ultrasound examination may confirm the lie and presentation.

Intrapartum

The findings on abdominal palpation are as above when the membranes are intact. After the membranes have ruptured, the irregular outline of the uterus is more marked. If the uterus is contracting strongly and becomes moulded around the fetus, palpation is very difficult. The shoulder is wedged into the pelvis.

Vaginal examination should not be performed without first excluding placenta previa. The membranes usually rupture early because of the ill-fitting presenting part with a high risk of cord prolapse.

If the labor has been in progress for some time, the shoulder may be felt as a soft mass and ribs with their grid-iron pattern. With further progress of labor, an arm may prolapse, and this should be differentiated from a leg by checking the characteristics and differences.

Possible Outcome

There is no mechanism of labor for a shoulder presentation. Delivery must be by cesarean section to avoid obstructed labor and subsequent uterine rupture.

Management in the Antenatal Period

In the antenatal period, if placenta previa or contracted pelvis is detected as a cause, an elective cesarean section is required. Once such causes are excluded, an external version may be attempted. If this fails, or if the lie changes to transverse after an external version, the woman is admitted in the hospital until delivery because of the risk of cord prolapse, if the membranes rupture.

Management in the Intrapartum Period

If transverse lie is detected early in labor, when the membranes are still intact, the physician may attempt an external version followed by a controlled rupture of membranes. If the membranes have ruptured spontaneously a vaginal examination must be performed immediately to detect possible cord prolapse.

Immediate cesarean section is performed:
* If the cord prolapses
* When the membranes have already ruptured
* When external version is unsuccessful
* When labor has already been in progress for some hours.

Complications

* Prolapse of cord when the membranes rupture
* Prolapse of arm when the shoulder has become impacted
* Obstructed labor and rupture of uterus
* Fetal death.

Management

Immediate cesarean section under general anesthesia, regardless of whether the fetus is alive or dead

Fig. 33.12: Compound presentation

COMPOUND PRESENTATION (FIG. 33.12)

Compound presentation is one in which a hand or occasionally a foot, lies alongside the head. On rare occasions, head, hand and a foot are felt in the vagina. This is a serious situation, which may occur with a dead fetus.

Compound presentation tends to occur with a small fetus or a roomy pelvis. If diagnosed during the second stage of labor, the midwife should try to hold the hand back to allow delivery of the head.

SHOULDER DYSTOCIA

Shoulder dystocia by definition, is difficulty in the birth (or delivery) of the shoulders. In practice, this refers to cephalic presentations in which the shoulders have become impacted. Shoulder dystocia occurs when one shoulder (usually the anterior) or both shoulders (rarely) impact above the pelvic brim. The problem occurs if the shoulders attempt to enter the true pelvis with the bisacromial diameter in the anteroposterior diameter of the pelvic brim, instead of in either the left or right oblique diameter of the pelvic brim, which is the normal method of entry during the normal mechanism of labor (the oblique diameter is larger than the anteroposterior diameter).

Incidence

The incidence of shoulder dystocia is not accurately known. It is reported as varying from 0.37 to 1.1 percent (Bahar, 1996).

Risk Factors

The possibility of shoulder dystocia should be anticipated anytime when any of the following conditions exist:

- Maternal diabetes (fetal Macrosomia)
- Obstetric history of large babies (over 4,000 gm)
- Family history of large siblings
- Maternal obesity (over 90 kg)
- Large fetus (fetal macrosomia, over 4,000 gm)
- Any estimated fetal weight 500 gm or more greater than the woman's largest previous baby
- Maternal age over 35 years
- High parity.

Warning Signs and Diagnosis

The delivery of the head with or without forceps may have been quite easy, but more commonly the head may have advanced slowly and the chin may have had difficulty sweeping over the perineum. Once the head is delivered, it may look as if it is trying to return to the vagina. It is caused by shoulder traction and is called the *turtle sign*.

Shoulder dystocia is diagnosed when the maneuvers normally used by the midwife fails to accomplish delivery (Resnik, 1980). It is important for the midwife to know how to manage this situation because, even with anticipation, diagnosis cannot be made until after the head is born. This gives little time to resolve the problem before the baby is either damaged or dead.

Management

The following steps should be taken in sequence to manage the emergency of shoulder dystocia.
1. Stay calm and ensure mother's cooperation.
2. Request that an obstetrician, an anesthetist and a neonatologist be called *stat*.
3. Request readiness of a full-scale newborn resuscitation effort.
4. Request readiness to manage an immediate postpartum hemorrhage.

The obstetrician may try the following maneuvers to dislodge the shoulders and deliver the baby.

1. Check the position of the shoulders and rotate them into one of the oblique diameters of the pelvis. Instruct the mother not to push. Rotation is accomplished by placing all of the fingers of one hand on one side of the baby's chest and all of the fingers of the other hand on the baby's back on the opposite side and pressing with the amount of force necessary to move the baby. It is necessary that the entire hand is used and not just two finger for maximum strength. Under no circumstances, the baby's head should be moved as this would result in injury to the brachial or cervical nerve plexus or fracture of the cervical vertebrae.
2. Downward and outward pressure is applied on the sides of the baby's head while another person applies suprapubic pressure.

    Suprapubic pressure is most effective if the person applying it stands on a footstool in order to get greater force behind the downward push. In mild dystocia, the baby may be delivered with this step.

    Under no circumstances, allow the fundal pressure to be applied erroneously. This will only further impact the shoulders, waste time, possibly cause injury to the fetus and possibly rupture the uterus with disastrous sequelae to both mother and baby.

If the baby is not delivered:
3. Cut or enlarge the episiotomy. A deep mediolateral episiotomy will allow more room for manipulation.
4. Catheterize the woman to empty her bladder.
5. Place the woman in an exaggerated lithotomy position.
6. Do a vaginal examination to rule out causes of shoulder dystocia (after the head is born) other than impacted shoulders. This requires the insertion of the entire hand as far as it can be in. Other causes to be ruled out at this stage are:
    - Short umbilical cord (relative or absolute).
    - Enlargement of the thorax or abdomen of the fetus might be caused by tumors or severe edema.
    - Locked twins.

❖ Conjoined twins
❖ Bandl's retraction ring.

7. If the dystocia is diagnosed as resulting from shoulder dystocia, attempt is made again to deliver the baby by the application of suprapubic pressure while the obstetrician uses firm downward and outward pressure on the side of the baby's head. The baby may be delivered after this step if the condition was a moderate shoulder dystocia.

Other Manipulative Procedures

McRobert's maneuver: Maneuver involves helping the woman to lie flat and to bring her knees up to her chest as far as possible. This will rotate the angle of the symphysis pubis superiorly and use the weight of the mother's legs to create gentle pressure on her abdomen releasing the impaction of the anterior shoulder (Gonik et al, 1989). This maneuver is associated with the lowest level of morbidity and requires least force to accomplish delivery.

Suprapubic pressure: Suprapubic pressure should be exerted on the side of the fetal back and towards the fetal chest. This may help to adduct the shoulders and push the anterior shoulder away from the symphysis pubis.

Rubin's maneuver: This maneuver (Rubin, 1964) requires the midwife/obstetrician to identify the posterior shoulder on vaginal examination, then to push the posterior shoulder in the direction of the fetal chest, thus rotating the anterior shoulder away from the symphysis pubis. By adducting the shoulders, this maneuver reduces the 12 cm bisacromial diameter.

Wood's maneuver: (Woods, 1943) requires the obstetrician to insert her/his hand into the vagina and identify the fetal chest. Then, by exerting pressure on to the posterior fetal shoulder, rotation is achieved. This maneuver abducts the shoulders, rotates them into a more favorable diameter and enables the completion of the delivery.

Zavanelli maneuver: If the maneuvers, described above, have not been successful, the obstetrician may consider the Zavanelli maneuver (Sandberg, 1985) as a last hope for delivery of a live infant.

This requires the reversal of the mechanisms of delivery so far and reinsertion of the fetal head into the vagina. Delivery is then completed by cesarean section.

Complications following Shoulder Dystocia

Maternal Complications
❖ Hemorrhage
❖ Rupture of uterus.

Fetal Complications
❖ Neonatal asphyxia
❖ Erb's palsy from brachial plexus injury
❖ Neonatal death.

UNSTABLE LIE

An unstable lie is a condition in which, at any time after 36 completed weeks of pregnancy, the fetal lie is oblique or transverse, and the presentation changes from one examination to another.

Causes

Any condition in late pregnancy that increases the mobility of the fetus or prevents the head from entering the pelvic brim, may cause this.
❖ Lax uterine muscles in multigravidae
❖ Contracted pelvis
❖ Polyhydramnios.

Management

The woman is admitted to the hospital to avoid unsupervised onset of labor with a transverse lie.

After hospitalization, the lie may stabilize. If it does not, labor may be induced after 38th week of gestation, provided there is no placenta previa. The woman's bladder and rectum are emptied and an external cephalic version is done if the fetus is in a malpresentation. When the fetus is in a vertex presentation, labor is induced with an oxytocin infusion. Fetal presentation is checked in every five minutes.

Once regular contractions are established, a vaginal examination is done to rule out cord presentation. The membranes are then stripped and a high rupture of membranes is done, removing as much of amniotic fluid as possible so that the head enters the pelvis. Oxytocin infusion is continued and the woman is encouraged to empty her bladder frequently. Forewaters is not ruptured until the head is deeply engaged and labor is well advanced. Labor is regarded as a trial.

BIBLIOGRAPHY

1. Bahar AM. Risk factors and fetal outcome in cases of shoulder dystocia compared with normal deliveries of a similar birth weight. British Journal of Obstetrics and Gynecology. 1996;103:868-72.
2. Bennett RV, Brown LK. Myles Textbook for Midwives, 13th edn. Churchill Livingstone, 1999.
3. Coates T, Shiers CV. Midwifery and Obstetric emergencies, In: Myles Textbook for Nurses 13th edn. Edinburgh; Churchill Livingstone, 1999.
4. Dutta DC. Textbook of Obstetrics 5th edn. Calcutta; New Central Book Company, 2001.
5. Hofmyer GJ. Breech presentation and abnormal lie in late pregnancy, In: Chalmers I (Eds), et al. Effective Care in Pregnancy and Childbirth. Oxford; Oxford University Press 1997.
6. Resnik R. Management of shoulder girdle dystocia, Clinical Obstetrics and Gynecology. 1980;23(2):559-64.
7. Rubin A. Management of shoulder dystocia. Journal of the American Medical Association. 1964;189:835
8. Sandberg EC. The Zavanelli Maneuver: A potentially revolutionary method for resolution of shoulder dystocia. American Journal of Obstetrics and Gynecology 1985;152:479-87.
9. Woods CE. A principle of physics applied to shoulder delivery. American Journal of Obstetrics and Gynecology. 1993;45:797-805.
10. Zhang J, et al. Efficacy of external cephalic version: A review, Obstetrics and Gynecology 1993;82(2): 306-12.

34

Obstetric Operations

DILATATION AND EVACUATION

The procedure consists of dilatation of the cervix and evacuation of the products of conception from the uterine cavity. It may be done as a one-stage operation of dilatation and evacuation in the same sitting or a two-stage operation in which the first phase is slow dilatation of the cervix and the second phase is rapid dilatation of the cervix and evacuation.

One-Stage Operation

Indications

❖ Incomplete abortion (commonest)
❖ Inevitable abortion
❖ Medical termination of pregnancy (6–8 weeks).
❖ Hydatidiform mole in the process of expulsion.

Preparation for the Operation

Local preparation, perineal care and catheterization are done once the decision is made for evacuation. The woman and her spouse are given adequate explanation and psychological support.

Procedure

The procedure is done under general anesthesia. Internal examination is done by the obstetrician to note the size and position of the uterus and the state of dilatation of the cervix.

If the cervix is not sufficiently dilated to admit one finger, it is dilated up to the desired extend by the graduated metal dilators. The products are removed by an ovum forceps. The uterine cavity is then curetted gently by a blunt curette. Injection methergine 0.2 mg is administered intravenously during the procedure.

The uterus is massaged bimanually and when it is found firm and the bleeding is minimal, the vagina and perineum are cleaned and the woman sent back to her bed.

Two-Stage Operation

Indications

❖ First trimester abortion
❖ Missed abortion (8–10 weeks uterus)
❖ Hydatidiform mole with unfavorable cervix (long, firm and closed os).

Procedure

First phase (Figs 34.1A to C)
It consists of introduction of laminaria tents in to the cervical canal to effect its slow dilatation or introduction of intravaginal prostaglandin E_2 gel 2 mg or pessary 3 mg in to the posterior fornix at least 12 hours beforehand.

Figs 34.1A to C: Laminaria tents: (A) Prior to introduction; (B) Swollen while kept in the cervical canal; (C) Held by tent-introducing forceps

Prior to insertion of the tent, the woman is asked to empty her bladder, the tent of appropriate size is selected and the threads attached to one end are tied to the roller gauze.

Steps

1. Internal examination is done to note the size and position of the uterus and state of the cervix.
2. A vaginal speculum is introduced. The anterior lip of the cervix is grasped by an Allis forceps to steady the cervix.
3. The cervical canal may have to be dilated, especially in primigravidae, by one or two metal dilators to facilitate the introduction of tents.
4. The tents are introduced one after the other, holding it by tent introducing forceps. The tents are introduced for at least 4 cm (1.5″) so that the tips are placed beyond the internal os.
5. The upper vagina is packed with roller gauze to prevent the displacement of tents.
6. The patient is returned and preferably confined to bed.
7. Prophylactic antibiotic is usually administered. No anesthesia is required for the procedure.

Second phase

It consists of further dilation of the cervix by graduated metal dilators followed by evacuation of the uterus. The woman is brought to the operating room usually after 12 hours. Preparation of the patient for the procedure is same as for the one stage evacuation. The operation may be performed under local paracervical block or under general anesthesia.

Steps of the Evacuation Procedure

1. The posterior vaginal speculum is introduced after removing the vaginal packing. The tents are removed with a sponge holding forceps. The vagina and cervix are swabbed with an antiseptic solution and the speculum is removed.
2. Vaginal examination is done to note the size and position of uterus and the state of dilatation of the cervix.
3. A retaining speculum (Auvard's speculum) is introduced and the anterior lips of the cervix are held by an Allis forceps to steady it. A uterine sound is introduced in to the uterine cavity to ascertain the length of the cavity and position of the uterus.
4. The cervix is dilated with the graduated metal dilators up to the desired extent to facilitate introduction of the ovum forceps.
5. The products of conception are removed by introducing the ovum forceps. Intravenous methergine 0.2 mg is given during this stage to minimize blood loss.
6. The uterine cavity is thoroughly curetted by a flushing (blunt) curette.
7. The speculum and Allis forceps are removed and the uterus massaged bimanually. After confirming a well-contracted uterus with minimal bleeding, the vulva is cleaned and a perineal pad is placed.
8. Intramuscular methergine is repeated postoperatively and prophylactic antibiotic may be given.

Dangers of Dilatation and Evacuation Operation

Immediate Dangers

❖ Hemorrhage due incomplete evacuation or atonic uterus
❖ Injury such as cervical laceration or uterine perforation
❖ Shock due to excessive blood loss, uterine perforation or anesthetic complications
❖ Increased morbidity.

Late Dangers

❖ Pelvic inflammation
❖ Infertility

❖ Cervical incompetence
❖ Uterine adhesions.

FORCEPS DELIVERY

Forceps delivery is a means of extracting the fetus with the aid of obstetric forceps when it is inadvisable or impossible for the mother to complete the delivery by her own efforts. Forceps are also used to assist the delivery of the after coming head of the breech and on occasion to withdraw the head up and out of the pelvis at cesarean section.

Ever since the invention of obstetric forceps around 1,600 AD by the Chamberlen family, many designs were invented and modified. Forceps deliveries were formerly classified by the level of the head at the time the forceps were applied, i.e. high-cavity, mid-cavity and low-cavity. Low-cavity forceps is the one frequently performed, as cesarean section is usually preferred to the more traumatic high and mid-cavity operations.

Low-cavity forceps can be divided into *rotational* and *nonrotational*. Rotational forceps delivery refers to a maneuver of the fetal head from a malposition into a more favorable position with the aid of specially designed forceps usually Kielland's examples of nonrotational forceps are:

❖ Wrigley's forceps and Simpson's forceps (low cavity)
❖ Neville-Barne's and Haig Ferguson's forceps (high and midcavity forceps).

Basic Construction of the Forceps (Fig. 34.2)

Obstetric forceps consist of two separate blades, each with a handle. Each blade is marked 'L' (left) or 'R' (right). They are inserted separately on either side of the fetal head and locked together by English or Smellie lock (rotational forceps have a sliding lock). The blades are spoon shaped to accommodate the fetal head and fenestrated to minimize trauma and for lightness. The spoon shape of the blade is called the *cephalic curve*. When the blades are articulated it holds the fetal head. The blades are attached to the handle at an angle, which corresponds to the curve of Carus (curve on the axis of birth canal). This is termed as the *pelvic curve* of the blade. When the blades are

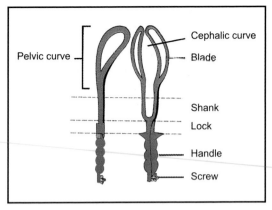

Fig. 34.2: Different parts of a long-curved obstetric forceps

correctly placed on the fetal head, the handles will be neatly aligned.

Types of Obstetric Forceps Currently Used

Only three varieties are commonly used in present day obstetrics (Figs 34.3A to C). They are:

❖ Long-curved forceps with or without axis traction device
❖ Short-curved forceps
❖ Kielland's forceps.

Long-Curved Obstetric Forceps

The long curved obstetric forceps is relatively heavy and is about 87 cm (15^2) long. In India Das's variety (named after Sir Kedar Nath Das) is commonly used. It is comparatively lighter and slightly shorter than its western counterpart, and is quiet suited for the comparatively small pelvis and small baby of Indian women (Dutta, 2001).

Its *measurements* are: Length 37 cm, distance between the tips 2.5 cm and widest diameter between the blades 9 cm. Blades are named left or right in relation to the maternal pelvis in which they lie when applied. Each blade consists of the following parts: (1) Blade, (2) Shank, (3) Lock, (4) Handle with or without screw.

The blades are fenestrated which facilitate a good grip of the fetal head. There is usually a slot in the lower part of the fenestrum of the blades to allow the upper end of the axis traction rod to be fitted.

Figs 34.3A to C: Different types of obstetric forceps; (A) Short-cured forceps; (B) Axis traction forceps and (C) Kielland's forceps

Blade: It has two curves. The 'pelvic curve' is designed to fit the curve on the axis of the birth canal (curve of Carus). The front of the forceps is the concave side of the 'pelvic curve'. The 'cephalic curve' on the flat surface, which when articulated, grasps the fetal head without compression.

Shank: It is the part between the blade and the lock, and usually measures 6.25 cm (2 ½"). It increases the length of the instrument and thereby, facilitates locking of the blades outside the vulva. When the blades are articulated, the shanks are not apposed together.

Lock: The common method of articulation consists of a socket system located on the shank at its junction with the handle (English lock).

Handle: The handles are apposed when the blades are articulated. It measures 12.5 cm (5"). A screw may be attached usually at the end (or at the base) of one blade, commonly left, to keep the blades in position.

Axis traction device: It can be applied with advantage in midforceps operation, especially

following manual rotation of the head. It provides traction in the correct axis of the pelvic curve and as such, less force is necessary to deliver the head. It consists of traction rods and traction handle.

Short-Curved Forceps (Wrigley's Forceps)

The instrument is lighter, shorter and stubby-handled. It is short due to reduction in the length of the shanks and handles. It has a marked cephalic curve with a slight pelvic curve. The instrument is used for very low forceps deliveries for the after coming head of a breech delivery or at cesarean section.

Kielland's Forceps

It is a long, almost straight (very slight pelvic curve) obstetric forceps without any axis traction device. It has a sliding lock. Kielland's forceps is used when the head is in an occipitolateral or occipitoposterior position. After the blades are applied, the head is rotated to an occipitoanterior position. It facilitates grasping and correction of asynclikic head because of its sliding lock.

In the hands of an expert, it is a useful and preferred instrument. It can be used in an unrotated vertex or face presentation. Grasping and correction of an asynclitic head is facilitated because of its sliding lock.

The blades are named anterior and posterior. The anterior blade is to be inserted first. Application of the blade is done either by wandering method or direct method. Wandering method is usually applied in deep transverse arrest. Anterior blade is introduced laterally over the baby's face. Then it is gently moved around the face to be placed over the anterior parietal bone. Posterior blade is introduced between the head and the sacrum. Rotation of the head can be achieved at the same level or at a lower level after pulling the head down. Epidural anesthesia is generally preferred for this procedure.

Limitations

Because of the complexity in the technique of its application, there are chances of injuries to the vagina or perineum. Deep mediolateral episiotomy is mandatory.

unless can't insert forcep blades

needs to fullfill......

Classification According to the Level of the Fetal Head at which the Forceps are Applied

1. *High forceps operation*: The application of forceps on a fetal head where the biparietal diameter has not yet passed the pelvic brim (nonengaged head). Cesarean section is preferred to this type of forceps application.

above the +2 station

2. *Mid forceps operation*: Refers to the application of the forceps where the biparietal diameter has passed the brim of the pelvis but not passed the level of ischial spines.

+2 station

3. *Low forceps operation*: Refers to the application of the forceps where the biparietal diameter has passed the level of ischial spines.

among the (+3-+4) station

4. *Outlet forceps*: The forceps are applied on the fetal head lying on the perineum and is visible at the introitus in between contractions. The sagittal suture should lie in the anteroposterior diameter of the outlet. In the present day practice 90 percent of forceps applications are the low forceps categories. All outlet forceps are low forceps, but not all low forceps are outlet forceps.

Indications of Forceps Operation

Delay in the second stage due to uterine inertia. If the head is on the perineum for 20 to 30 minutes without advancement, forceps application may be decided.

❖ Maternal indications
  – Maternal distress
  – Pre-eclampsia, eclampsia
  – Vaginal birth after cesarean section (VBAC)
  – Heart disease
  – Failure to bear down during the second stage of labor due to regional blocks, paraplegia or psychiatric disturbance.
❖ Fetal indications
  – Appearance of fetal distress in the second stage
  – Cord prolapse
  – After-coming-head of breech → *(breech delivery 2b© head delivery 2626 2y 2826.)*
  – Low birth weight baby
  – Postmaturity. *(After 42 weeks)*

Prerequisites for Forceps Delivery

There are certain conditions which must exist before forceps delivery can be performed.

❖ The cervix must be fully dilated and effaced
❖ Membranes must be ruptured
❖ Presentation and position must be suitable to apply the blades correctly to the sides of the head. (Sagittal suture in anteroposterior diameter of pelvic outlet)
❖ The head must be engaged with no parts of the head palpable abdominally
❖ No appreciable cephalopelvic disproportion
❖ The bladder must be emptied
❖ Presence of good uterine contractions as a safeguard to postpartum hemorrhage.

Preparation of the Woman

The woman should be prepared in advance for the possibility of a forceps delivery if this looks likely. Full explanation of the procedure and the need for it must be given to the woman.

Once the decision has been made, adequate and appropriate analgesia must be offered. When analgesia has been instituted and the obstetrician is ready to proceed, the woman's legs are placed in lithotomy position. Both legs must be placed simultaneously to avoid strain on the woman's back and hips.

The woman should be tilted towards the left at an angle of 15° by the use of a pillow or a rubber wedge under the mattress to prevent aortocaval occlusion.

Preparations must also be done for the baby including equipment for resuscitation. In some hospitals a pediatrician will also be present.

—large episiotomy.

Procedure of Low Forceps Operation

❖ The woman's vulval area is thoroughly cleaned and draped with sterile towels using aseptic technique. The bladder is emptied using a straight catheter
❖ A vaginal examination is performed by the obstetrician to confirm the station and exact position of the fetal head
❖ A pudendal block, supplemented by perineal and labial infiltration with 1 percent lignocaine hydrochloride, is given to produce effective local anesthesia
❖ An episiotomy may be done prior to introduction of the blades or during traction when the perineum becomes bulged and thinned out by the advanced head

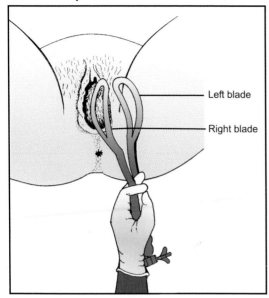

Fig. 34.4: Identification of the forceps blades

- The forceps are identified as left or right by assembling them briefly before proceeding (Fig. 34.4)
- The left blade is passed gently between the perineum and fetal head with the first two fingers of the operator's right hand lying alongside the fetal head protecting the maternal tissue. The tip of the forceps blade slides lightly over the head, in to the hollow of the sacrum and is then 'wandered' to the left side of the pelvis where it should sit alongside the head
- The procedure is repeated with the right blade until it sits on the right of the pelvis. It should then be easy to lock the two blades and there should be little or no gap between the handles. A significant gap suggests that the forceps are wrongly positioned and they should be reapplied after carefully checking the position of head
- During the application stage of the forceps, the woman should be given full support and attention by the midwife
- The fetal heart rate is to be monitored throughout
- As soon as the operator is ready and the uterus contracts, the woman is encouraged to push. To supplement her efforts the obstetrician exerts steady, downward

traction on the forceps. Traction is released between contractions. Intermittent traction is continued in a downward and backward direction until the head comes to the perineum. The pull is then directed horizontally straight towards the operator until the head is almost crowned. The direction of pull is gradually changed towards the mother's abdomen to deliver the head by extension (Figs 34.5A to D)
- The blades are removed one after the other, the right one first
- Following the birth of the head, usual procedures are to be followed as in normal delivery. Intravenous methergine 0.2 mg is to be administered with the delivery of the anterior shoulder. Episiotomy is repaired as quickly as possible and the woman made comfortable.

Manual Rotation of the Fetal Head Followed by Midforceps Operation

Some obstetricians prefer to rotate the fetal head manually in cases of occipitoposterior position, as this is likely to be less traumatic than instrumental rotation. The exact position of the fetal head must be determined. The obstetrician grasps the head usually by sinciput and rotates it, encouraging flexion.

The commonly used forceps is the long-curved one with or without axis traction device. Kielland's forceps is useful in the hands of an expert.

General anesthesia is preferable. The blades are introduced as in the low forceps operation. An assistant is required to hold the left handle after its introduction. If axis traction rod is used, this must be already attached to the blade. During introduction of the right blade, the traction rod must be held forwards otherwise it will prevent locking of the blades.

The direction of the pull is first downwards and backwards, then horizontal or straight and finally upward and forward. With axis traction device, the traction handle is to be attached to the traction rods. During traction, the traction rods should remain parallel to the shanks. When the base of the occiput comes under the

After forcep 'dilivery Uss-brain for baby to identify bleeding.

Figs 34.5A to D: Steps of forceps application: (A) Introduction of the left blade; (B) Introduction of the right blade; (C) Traction of the head and (D) Change of the grip in the final stage

symphysis pubis, the traction rods are to be removed.

Difficulties in Forceps Operation

The difficulties are mainly due to faulty assessment before the operative delivery is undertaken. However, there is hardly any difficulty with low forceps operation.

Difficulties in the application of blades are caused by incompletely dilated cervix and unrotated or nonengaged head. Difficulty in locking are caused by:
1. Application on unrotated head.
2. Improper insertion of the blade (not for enough in).
3. Failure to depress the handle against the perineum.
4. Entanglement of the cord or fetal parts inside the blades.

Causes of Failure

The causes of failure to deliver with traction are:
1. Undiagnosed occipitoposterior position
2. Faulty cephalic application
3. Wrong direction of traction
4. Mild pelvic contraction or
5. Constriction ring.

Complications of Forceps Operation

The hazards of the forceps operation are mostly related to the faulty technique and to the indications for which the forceps are applied.

In the Mother

Immediate
- Injury
  - Extension of the episiotomy towards rectum or upwards up to the vault of vagina

  - Vaginal lacerations
  - Cervical tear especially when applied through an incompletely dilated cervix
  - Bruising and trauma to the urethra
- Postpartum hemorrhage due to trauma, or atonic uterus related to prolonged labor or effect of anesthesia
- Shock due to blood loss, prolonged labor and dehydration *(damage)*
- Sepsis due to devitalization of local tissues and improper asepsis.

Late complications
- Chronic low backache due to tension imposed on softened ligaments of lumbosacral or sacroiliac joints during lithotomy position ?
- Genital prolapse or stress incontinence.

In the Infant   *Mx:- Pelvic Muscle Exercise.*

Immediate
- Asphyxia due to intracranial stress out of prolonged compression
- Intracranial hemorrhage due to malapplication of the blades
- Cephalhematoma
- Facial palsy due to damage to facial nerve
- Abrasions on the soft tissues of the face and forehead by the forceps blade, severe bruising will cause marked jaundice
- Tentorial tear from compression of the fetal head by the forceps.

Prophylactic Forceps (Elective)

It refers to forceps delivery only to shorten the second stage of labor when maternal and/or

→ hemorrhage between Skull & periosteum (fibrous membrane of cover the bones)

fetal complications are anticipated. The indications are:

❖ Eclampsia
❖ Heart disease
❖ Previous history of cesarean section
❖ Postmaturity
❖ Low birth weight baby
❖ Patients under epidural anesthesia
❖ To curtail the painful second stage.

Prophylactic forceps application is done only after the criteria of low forceps are fulfilled.

Trial Forceps

It is a tentative attempt of forceps delivery in a case of suspected midpelvic contraction with a preamble declaration of abandoning it in favor of cesarean section, if moderate traction fails to overcome the resistance. The procedure is conducted in an operating room keeping everything ready for cesarean section. If moderate traction leads to progressive descend of the fetal head, the delivery is completed vaginally, if not, cesarean section is done immediately.

Failed Forceps

When a deliberate attempt in vaginal delivery with forceps has failed to expedite the process, it is called failed forceps. It is predominantly due to lack of obstetric skill with poor clinical judgment. Failure in the operative delivery may be due to improper application or failure of descend of the head even with forcible contraction.

Cause for Failed Forceps

❖ Incompletely dilated cervix
❖ Unrotated occipitoposterior position
❖ Undiagnosed brow or hydrocephalus or fetal ascites
❖ Constriction ring
❖ Large baby with the shoulders impacted at the brim.

Management

❖ Assess the effect on mother and fetus
❖ Start IV infusion with 5 percent dextrose if one is not already in place
❖ Administer parenteral antibiotic
❖ Exclude rupture of uterus and plan for other modes of delivery
❖ The woman should be shifted to an equipped hospital.

VACUUM EXTRACTION (VENTOUSE DELIVERY)

Ventouse is an instrumental device designed to assist delivery by creating a vacuum between it and the fetal scalp.

Equipment (Fig. 34.6)

The ventouse or vacuum extractor consists of the following basic components:
1. Suction cup (4 sizes—30, 40, 50 and 60 mm)
2. A vacuum pump
3. Traction rod device.

Various modifications of the earlier instrument, introduced in 1956 by Mulstorm, are now

Fig. 34.6: Ventouse or vacuum extractor

available. Modern vacuum extractors use an electrical pump, which has sensitive controls. The vacuum is built-up steadily and is maintained efficiently, so that the cup is less likely to come off.

A metal or silastic (firm rubber) cup is applied to the fetal head; a vacuum is created inside this cup, which is connected to the pump by rubber tubing and traction is then applied. Inside the rubber tubing is a metal chain designed to take the strain of traction, with a metal handle to give the operator a good grip.

Indications

* Deep transverse arrest with adequate pelvis
* Delay in descend of the high head in case of the second baby of twins
* Malpositions: Occipitolateral and occipitoposterior
* Delay in the second stage of labor or late first stage
* As an alternative to forceps operation except in:
  - Face presentation and after-coming-head of breech
  - Fetal distress or prematurity.
* Maternal exhaustion.

Advantages of Ventouse Over Forceps

* It can be used in unrotated or malrotated occipitoposterior position of the head
* It can be applied even through an incompletely dilated cervix
* It is not a space-occupying device like the forceps blades
* Lesser traction force is needed (10 kg)
* It can be used safely even when the head remains at a high level in second baby of twins
* It is comfortable and injuries to the mother are less
* Requires less technical skill for the operator.

Advantages of Forceps Over Ventouse

* Forceps operation can quickly expedite the delivery in case of fetal distress, where ventouse will be unsuitable as it takes longer time

* Forceps is safe for a premature baby. The fetal head remains inside the protective cage
* It can be employed in anterior face or in after-coming head of breech
* In suspected pelvic contraction, where moderate traction is required, ventouse will be ineffective.

Contraindications for Ventouse

* Fetal distress, where urgent delivery is needed
* Face presentation
* Prematurity, chance of scalp avulsion or subaponeurotic hemorrhage is more
* Fetal bleeding disorder.

Conditions to be Fulfilled

* There should not be any bony resistance below the head
* The head of a singleton baby should be engaged
* Cervix should be at least 6 cm dilated.

Procedure (Fig. 34.7)

The prerequisites are as for forceps delivery. The operator must be completely familiar with the technique appropriate to the particular cup design. The woman is positioned and prepared as for forceps delivery. The position of the fetal head is determined and an appropriate size and type of cup selected. Pudental block or perineal infiltration with one percent lignocaine is done. The instrument is assembled and the vacuum is tested prior to its application.

Step-1: Application of the Cup

The cup is introduced after retraction of the perineum with two fingers of the hand. The cup is placed against the fetal head nearer to

Fig. 34.7: Application of vacuum extractor

the occiput with the "knob" of the cup pointing towards the occiput. This will facilitate flexion of the head.

A vacuum of 0.2 kg/cm² is induced by hand pump slowly, taking at least two minutes. A check is made with fingers round the cup to ensure that no cervical or vaginal tissue is trapped inside the cup. The pressure is gradually raised at the rate of 0.1 kg/cm² per minute until the effective vacuum of 0.8 kg/cm² is reached in about 10 minutes time. The scalp is sucked into the cup and an artificial caput succedaneum (chignon) is produced. The chignon usually disappears within few hours.

Step-2: Traction

Traction is exerted using one hand in the direction of the curve of Carus. Traction must be at right angles to the cup and synchronous with the uterine contractions while applying traction, fingers of the other hand are to be placed against the cup to note the correct angle of traction, rotation and advancement of the head. Ventouse delivery may take slightly longer than forceps delivery. However, if there is no advancement during four successive uterine contractions, it should be abandoned. On no account, traction should exceed thirty minutes.

As soon as the head is delivered, the vacuum is reduced by opening the screw—release valve and the cup is then detached. The delivery is then completed in the normal manner. Silicon rubber cups (Silc cups) are currently used as they are soft and can be smoothly applied over the contour of the fetal head. They could be folded and introduced into the vagina before being placed over the fetal head.

Silicone Rubber Cup/Silastic Rubber Cup (Fig. 34.8)

The silicone rubber cup can be used in place of the metal cup of malstrom vacuum extractor. The cup is used when the mother is cooperative, the baby is average sized and there is minimal caput.

The silicone rubber cup is used in the following manner: it is folded and gently

Fig. 34.8: Silicone rubber cup/silastic rubber cup

inserted into the vagina with one hand from above downwards while the other hand parts the labia. A gentle twist may help it to unfold into place in the vagina and thereafter it is essentially not maneuverable being larger in diameter than the metal cup and having a relatively inflexible handle.

With the pressure at 0.2 kg/cm², a check is made to ensure that no maternal tissue is caught under the cup and then the pressure is raised to 0.6 to 0.8 kg/cm² depending on the size of the baby/weeks of gestation. Gentle to moderate traction along the pelvic axis for the duration of next 2 to 3 contractions should deliver the head.

One hand should rest on the bell of the cup while the other applies traction. The hand on the cup detects any early detachment and also indicates whether the head moves downwards with each pull. The fingers on the head can promote flexion of the head.

Complications

Fetal

❖ Sloughing of the scalp
❖ Cephalhematoma
❖ Cerebral trauma, such as tentorial tear
❖ Chignon: This is an area of edema and bruising where the cup was applied, all babies delivered by ventouse will have a chignon. These normally subside uneventfully, but may occasionally become infected.

Maternal

Trauma to the mother is rare. Injuries may occur due to inclusion of the soft tissues such as the cervix or vaginal wall inside the cup.

Failure

An attempted vacuum extraction may be unsuccessful. Exerting too much traction will result in the cup coming off. The cup is likely to come off in unskilled or impatient hands.

CESAREAN SECTION

It is an operative procedure whereby the fetuses after the end of 28th week, are delivered through an incision on the abdominal and uterine walls. The first operation performed on a woman is referred to as a primary Cesarean Section. When the operation is performed in subsequent pregnancies, it is called repeat cesarean section.

Incidence

The incidence of Cesarean Section is steadily rising. During the last decade there has been two-to-three-fold rise in the incidence from the initial rate of about 10 percent. Factors responsible are—Increased safety of the operation due to improved anesthesia, availability of blood transfusion and antibiotics. Increased awareness of fetal well-being and identification of risk factors have caused reduction of difficult operative or manipulative vaginal deliveries. Obstetricians as well as women choose not to take even slightest risk of abnormal labor.

Indications for Cesarean Section

Elective Cesarean Section

The term, elective, indicates that the decision to deliver the baby by Cesarean Section has been made during the pregnancy and before the onset of labor. While some indications are absolute, others will depend on a combination of factors. Absolute (definite) indications include:

- Cephalopelvic disproportion
- Major degrees of placenta previa
- Multiple pregnancy with three or more fetuses
- Advanced carcinoma of cervix
- Pelvic tumors such as cervical fibroid

In all these cases, there is possibility of insuperable obstruction for vaginal delivery and Cesarean Section may have to be performed even if the fetus is dead. Relative (possible) indications include:

- Malpresentation
  - Persistent transverse lie, brow or mento-posterior
  - Big breech or average breech with associated complicating factors.
- Pregnancy induced hypertension
  - Acute fulminating pre-eclampsia
  - Eclampsia with uncontrolled fits and the woman is not in labor.
- Medical gynecological conditions
  - Chronic hypertension, chronic nephritis
  - Diabetes: Uncontrolled with previous history of fetal wastage
  - Heart disease: Uncorrected coarctation of aorta or organic heart lesions.
- Previous scar following classical cesarean section or hysterotomy
- Antepartum hemorrhage
- Bad obstetric history: History of recurrent fetal wastage.

If the indication for Cesarean Section pertains specifically to one pregnancy, such as placenta previa, vaginal delivery may be expected on subsequent occasions. However, certain conditions, such as cephalopelvic disproportion due to contracted pelvis, will recur and a uterus that has been scarred twice or more, carries a greater risk of uterine rupture and require repeat cesarean operation.

Emergency Cesarean Section

This is performed when adverse conditions develop during labor.

- Cord prolapse
- Uterine rupture (acute) or scar dehiscence
- Cephalopelvic disproportion diagnosed in labor
- Fulminating pregnancy: Induced hypertension
- Eclampsia
- Failure to progress in the first or second stage of labor
- Fetal distress, if delivery is not imminent. Fetal distress in the first stage is more likely in previously compromised baby of IUGR, hypertensive disorder, postmaturity or in hypertonus state following oxytocin induced or augmented labor and incoordinate uterine action
- Abnormal uterine contractions: Prolongation of labor due to incoordinate uterine action.

Contraindications

In the absence of maternal interest, the following are the contraindications for Cesarean section:

- ❖ Dead fetus
- ❖ Baby, too premature to survive outside the uterus
- ❖ Presence of blood coagulation disorders.

Types of Operations

Lower Segment Cesarean Section (LSCS)

In this operation, the extraction of the baby is done through an incision made in the lower segment through a transperitoneal approach. The lower segment of the uterus forms after about 32 weeks' gestation and is less muscular than the upper segment of the uterus. In a lower segment cesarean section, a transverse incision is made in the lower segment; this heals faster and successfully than an incision in the upper segment of the uterus. There is less muscle and more fibrous tissue in the lower segment, which reduces the risk of rupture in a subsequent pregnancy. It is the only method practiced in present day obstetrics and unless specified, cesarean section means lower segment operation. It is commonly performed through a transverse incision on the abdomen, the *pfannenstiel* or *bikini line* incision.

Classical Cesarean Section

In this operation, the baby is extracted through an incision made in the upper segment of the uterus. Its indications in the present day practice are very much limited and is rarely performed.

Indications

- ❖ Gestation of less than 32 weeks before the lower segment has formed
- ❖ Placenta previa, which is situated anteriorly, in order to avoid incision of the placenta
- ❖ Hour-glass constriction
- ❖ Lower segment approach is difficult due to dense adhesions from previous operation or severely contracted pelvis (osteomalacic or rachitic) with pendulous abdomen
- ❖ Lower segment approach is risky due to big fibroid in the lower segment, or carcinoma cervix
- ❖ Postmortem section: Contemplating to have a live baby
- ❖ A classical section is always performed through a midline incision.

Preparation of the Mother

Psychological Preparation

Different women require differing levels of information. Some women welcome Cesarean Section as a means of escaping the rigorous contractions of labor; others feel disappointed that they have not had the experience of a normal delivery and the accompanying enjoyment.

Some women need detailed explanations and reassurance. Women who have elective Cesarean Section may be given the information in stages. If the possibility of Cesarean Section arises during labor, the midwife should begin to prepare the woman for this eventuality. The woman and her spouse should be kept informed of the events and progress during labor as well as assured of assistance.

Physical Preparation

- ❖ Intravenous infusion is started if one has not already been established
- ❖ Abdomen is prepared as for laparotomy
- ❖ A nonparticulate antacid (0.3 molar sodium citrate 30 ml) is given orally before transferring the woman to operating room. It is given to neutralize the existing gastric acid
- ❖ If the Cesarean Section is an elective procedure, ranitidine (H_2 blocker) 150 mg is given orally the night before and repeated (50 mg IM or IV) one hour before surgery to raise the gastric pH
- ❖ Metoclopramide (Reglan) 10 mg IV is given to increase the tone of the lower esophageal sphincter as well as to reduce the stomach contents. It is administered about 3 minutes of preoxygenation in the operating room
- ❖ The stomach should be emptied, if necessary by a stomach tube (emergency procedure)

❖ Bladder must be emptied by passing a catheter before or after induction of anesthesia and left in place
❖ Bowel preparation is done the evening before (two glycerin suppositories) for elective Cesarean Section clients
❖ The woman is dressed in clean operation gown and any valuables are either placed in safekeeping or given to the family. Any rings or bracelets, which cannot be removed, are covered with adhesive strapping
❖ Premedicative sedatives must not be given.

Anesthesia

A method, which is considered safe by the anesthetist, is employed. General, epidural or spinal anesthesia may be used.

Position

The woman is placed in dorsal position. In susceptible cases, to minimize any adverse effects of venacaval compression, a 15° tilt to her left using sand bags until delivery of baby is beneficial.

Incision on the Abdomen

A low transverse incision is made about two fingers breadth above the symphysis pubis (modified pfannenstiel) or above the symphysis pubis (pfannenstiel or bikini line incision). Some obstetricians make a vertical infraumbilical or paramedian incision, which extends from about 2.5 cm below the umbilicus to the upper border of the symphysis pubis. The anatomic layers incised are:
❖ Fat
❖ Rectal sheath
❖ Muscle (rectus abdominis)
❖ Abdominal peritoneum
❖ Uterine muscle.
The surgeon usually incises the rectus sheath by a scalpel, but divides the rectus muscle digitally, splitting it transversely. This method minimizes blood loss. Alternatively, the incision may be extended on either side using a pair of curved scissors to make it a curved incision of about 10 cm (4″) in length, the concavity directed upwards.

Delivery of the Head

The uterine cavity is then opened, the membranes are ruptured and the amniotic fluid is aspirated. The head is delivered by hooking the head with the fingers, which are carefully inserted between the lower uterine flap and the head until the palm is placed below the head. As the head is drawn to the incision line, the assistant is to apply pressure on the fundus. Obstetric forceps (Wrigley's forceps) are often used to extract the head from the pelvis.

Delivery of the Trunk

As soon as the head is delivered, the mucus from the mouth, pharynx and nostrils is to be sucked out using rubber catheter attached to an electric sucker. When the baby is born, an oxytocic drug (methergine 0.2 mg) is administered before the placenta and membranes are delivered. The cord is cut between two clamps and the baby is given to the nurse.

Removal of the Placenta and Membranes

The placenta is extracted by traction on the cord with simultaneous pushing on the fundus towards the umbilicus (controlled cord traction). The placenta and membranes are removed intact.

Suturing of the Uterine Wound

The margins of the wound are picked up by Allis tissue forceps or Green Armitage hemostatic clamps. The uterine muscle is sutured in two layers using continuous running sutures, the second of which tends to align the cut edges of the pelvic peritoneum. Repair of the rectus sheath brings the rectus abdominis into alignment. The subcutaneous fat is sometimes sutured and finally the skin is closed with sutures or clips.

Postoperative Care

Immediate Care (4–6 Hours)

In the immediate recovery period, the blood pressure is recorded every 15 minutes. Temperature is recorded every two hours. The wound must be inspected every half hour to detect any blood loss. The lochia are also inspected and drainage should be small initially. Following general anesthesia, the woman is nursed in the left lateral or 'recovery' position until she is fully conscious, since the risks of airway obstruction or regurgitation and silent aspiration of stomach contents are still present. Analgesia is given as prescribed.

First 24 Hours

IV fluids (5% dextrose or Ringer's lactate) are continued. Blood transfusion is helpful in anemic mothers for speedy postoperative recovery. Injection methergine 0.2 mg may be repeated intramuscularly. Parenteral antibiotic is usually given for the first 48 hours. Analgesics in the form of pethidine 75 to 100 mg are administered as required. Ambulation is encouraged on the day following surgery and baby is brought to her.

After 24 Hours

The blood pressure, pulse and temperature are usually checked every four hours. Oral feeding is started with clear liquids and then advanced to light and regular diet. Intravenous (IV) fluids are continued for about 48 hours. Urinary catheter may be removed on the following day when the woman is able to get up to the toilet. The woman is helped to get out of bed as soon as possible and encouraged to become fully mobile.

The mother must be encouraged to rest as much as possible and needed help is to be given with care for the baby. This should preferably take place at the mother's bedside and should include support with breastfeeding.

The mother is usually discharged with the baby after the abdominal skin stitches are removed by the 4th or 5th day.

Complications of Cesarean Section

The complications are related either to the operation (inherent hazards) or to the indications for which the operation is done. Thus, the complications are more following emergency rather than elective operations.

❖ Postpartum hemorrhage related to uterine atony and rarely blood coagulation disorders

❖ Shock related to blood loss, it might occur when the operation is done following prolonged labor

❖ Anesthetic hazards—Mostly associated with emergency operations and related to aspiration of gastric contents

❖ Sepsis—The common sites of infection are urinary tract, abdominal wound, uterus, peritoneal cavity and lungs.

❖ Intestinal obstruction may be mechanical due to adhesions or bands, or paralytic following peritonitis.

❖ Thrombosis—Leg vein thrombosis and pulmonary embolism are likely following cesarean section.

❖ Wound complications, such as wound sepsis, hematoma, dehiscence and burst abdomen may happen.

Late complications include menstrual irregularities, chronic pelvic pain or backache. Remote surgical complications may be incision hernia and intestinal obstruction due to adhesions and bands.

The risk of scar rupture is a possible complication in future pregnancies. Babies born by cesarean section have increased risk of respiratory distress syndrome (RDS) compared to those delivered vaginally.

Cesarean Hysterectomy

Cesarean hysterectomy refers to an operation where cesarean section is followed by removal of the uterus. The common conditions are:

❖ Atonic uterus and uncontrolled postpartum hemorrhage

❖ Morbid adherent placenta

❖ Big fibroid

❖ Extensive lacerations due to extension of tears with broad ligament hematoma

❖ Grossly infected uterus

❖ Rupture of uterus with fetus inside.

DESTRUCTIVE OPERATIONS (EMBRYOTOMIES)

The destructive operations are designed to diminish the bulk of the fetus to facilitate easy delivery through the birth canal. It may occasionally be necessary to destroy the fetus

Figs 34.9A to C: Instruments for craniotomy: (A) Old-ham's perforator; (B) Craniodest; (C) Budin's connula

in the interest of saving the mother's life. There are four types of operations.

Craniotomy

It is an operation to make a perforation on the fetal head to evacuate the contents followed by extraction of the fetus. The various instruments used for craniotomy are shown in Figures 34.9A to C.

Indications

❖ Cephalic presentation producing obstructed labor with a dead fetus. This is the commonest indication of craniotomy in the referral hospitals of the developing countries

❖ Hydrocephalus even in a living fetus, this is applicable to the forecoming and after-coming head

❖ Interlocking heads of twins.

For the procedure to be done safely, the cervix must be fully dilated.

Sites of Perforation

Vertex: On the parietal bone, on either side of the sagittal suture

Face: Through the orbit or hard palate

Brow: Through the frontal bone

Suture is avoided to prevent collapse of the bone thereby preventing escape of brain matter.

Procedure

The obstetrician introduces two fingers (index and middle) into the vagina and the fingertips are placed on the proposed site of perforation. If the suture line cannot be defined because of a big caput, the perforation is done through the dependent part.

An assistant fixes the head suprapubically while the operator introduces the perforator with the blades closed, protecting the anterior vaginal wall and the bladder with the fingers in the vagina. When the tip reaches the site of perforation, the skull is perforated using rotating movements. After the skull is perforated, the instrument is advanced further and the handles are approximated so as to allow separation of the sharp blades which will extend the perforation. The blades are then apposed and brought out keeping the tip of blades still inside the cranium. The perforator is then rotated at right angles and the above step is repeated to make the perforated area look like a cross.

The instrument with the blades closed is again thrust beyond the guard, to churn the brain matter. After the brain matter is churned, the perforator is brought out under the guidance of two fingers still placed in the vagina.

Similar procedure could be performed using a sharp-pointed Mayo scissors. With the fingers, the brain matter is evacuated in order to make the skull collapse as much as possible.

When the skull is found sufficiently compressed, the extraction of the fetus is achieved either by using a cranioclast or by two giant vulsella. Traction is now exerted in the same direction as in forceps operation. After the delivery of the placenta, the vaginal canal and uterus are explored for evidence of any tear or rupture. Injection methergine is given and rest of the delivery is completed as in normal delivery.

Figs 34.10A to D: Special instruments for decapitation: (A) Giant vulsellum; (B) Hook with crochiet; (C) Embryotomy; (D) Decapitation hook with knife

In after-coming head of breech, the perforation is done through the occipital bone while the baby is being pulled forwards or backwards to fix the head during perforation. After the perforation, the brain matter is evacuated and the skull collapsed. Delivery is completed by traction on legs.

Decapitation

It is a destructive operation in which the fetal head is severed from the trunk and the delivery is completed with the extraction of the trunk and then of the decapitated head per vagina. Special instruments used fordecapitation are shown in Figures 34.10A to D.

Indications

❖ Neglected shoulder presentation with dead fetus where the neck is easily accessible
❖ Interlocking head of twins.

Procedure

If the fetal hand is not prolapsed, a hand is brought down. For this, a roller gauze is tied on

Fig. 34.11: Blond Heidler wire saw and Thimble with rim

the wrist and an assistant gives traction towards the side away from the fetal head to make the neck more accessible and fixed. Two fingers of the hand (index and middle) are then introduced into the vagina with the palmar surface downwards and the fingertips are placed on the superior surface of the neck. The decapitation hook with knife is introduced under the guidance of the fingers in the vagina, the knob pointing towards the fetal head. The hook is pushed above the neck and rotated about 90° to place the knife firmly against the neck.

By upward and downward movement of the hook with knife, the vertebral column is severed. The rest of the soft tissue may be severed by the same instrument or by an embryotomy scissors. The decapitated head is pushed up and the trunk is delivered by traction of the prolapsed arm.

The decapitated head is delivered by using the crochet (blunt hook) or forceps. Decapitation may be performed using a Blond Heidler wire (Fig. 34.11) saw and Thimble. The neck is severed by the wire saw after passing the wire loop around the fetal neck.

Eviceration

The operation consists of removal of thoracic and abdominal contents piecemeal through an opening on the thoracic or abdominal cavity at the most accessible site. The objective is to diminish the bulk of the fetus, which facilitates the extraction.

Indications

❖ Gross fetal malformations such as fetal ascitis or hugely distended bladder.
❖ Neglected shoulder presentation with dead fetus and neck is not easily accessible. The procedure is more feasible in a breech presentation. Embryotomy scissors are used for the procedure.

Cleidotomy

The operation consists of reduction of the width of the shoulder girdle by division of one or both the clavicles. The operation is done only in dead fetus with shoulder dystocia. The clavicles are divided by the embryotomy scissors or long straight scissors introduced under the guidance of two fingers of left hand placed inside the vagina.

Postoperative Care Following Destructive Operations

1. A self-retaining (Foly's) catheter is inserted following craniotomy and maintained for 3 to 5 days or until bladder tone is regained.

2. Intravenous drip is to be continued until dehydration is corrected. Blood transfusion may be given if required.

3. Antibiotic is given either parenterally or orally.

Complications

❖ Injury to the uterovaginal canal
❖ Postpartum hemorrhage: Atonic or traumatic
❖ Shock due to blood loss and/or dehydration
❖ Puerperal sepsis
❖ Subinvolution of uterus
❖ Injury to the adjacent viscera: Vesicovaginal fistula or rectovaginal fistula.

BIBLIOGRAPHY

1. Bevis Ruth. Obstetric anesthesia and operations. In: Myles (Ed). Textbook for Midwives, 13th edn. Edinburgh; Churchill Livingstone, 1999.
2. Depp R. Cesarean delivery and other surgical procedures. In: Gabbe SG, et al, (Eds). Obstetrics: normal and problem pregnancies, 2nd edn. Edinburgh; Churchill Livingstone, 1991.
3. Dutta DC. Textbook of Obstetrics, 5th edn. Calcutta; New Central Book Company, 2001.
4. Mac Donald R. Indications and contraindications for epidural blockade in obstetrics. In: Reynolds S (Ed). Epidural and Spinal Blockade in Obstetrics. London: Bailliere Tindall, 1990.

35

Obstetric Emergencies

Learning Objectives

Upon completing this chapter, the learner will be able to:

❖ Describe the emergency situations in midwifery including vasa previa, cord prolapse and shoulder dystocia with possible causes and actions to be taken

❖ Describe the conditions of uterine rupture

❖ Discuss the causes, detection and management of amniotic fluid embolism

❖ Discuss the different types of shock in obstetric clients and management

❖ Describe the procedure of basic life support.

VASA PREVIA

This term is used when a fetal blood vessel lies over the os in front of the presenting part. This usually occurs when fetal vessels from a velamentous insertion of the cord cross the area of the internal os to the placenta. However, vasa previa may also occur when there is a succenturiate placenta since the vascular connections to the succenturiate lobe are also unprotected vessels coursing between the chorion and amnion. With fetal descend and rupture of the membranes, the vessels are subject to compression and rupture with resulting exsanguination and anoxia of the fetus.

Vasa previa occurs in less than 0.2 percent of pregnancies. While extremely rare it should be thought of as a possibility, any time the midwife is not positive of what she feels presenting at the cervical os.

Diagnosis

❖ Vasa previa may sometimes be palpated on vaginal examination when the membranes are still intact. Pulsations felt may be synchronous with the fetal heart rate

❖ A speculum examination may be done to visualize the blood vessel

❖ It may also be visualized on ultrasound

❖ Fresh vaginal bleeding, which commences at the time of rupture of membranes, may be due to ruptured vasa previa.

Management

Immediate consultation with the physician is mandatory when the midwife believes the presenting part to be abnormal. The fetal heart rate should be monitored. If in the first stage of labor and the fetus is alive, an emergency cesarean section is carried out. If the mother is in the second stage of labor, delivery should be expedited and a vaginal birth may be achieved. The mode of delivery will be dependent on parity and fetal condition.

A pediatrician should be present at delivery and, if the baby is alive, hemoglobin estimation is necessary after resuscitation. The baby will require a blood transfusion, but the mortality rate is high with this emergency.

PRESENTATION AND PROLAPSE OF THE UMBILICAL CORD (FIGS 35.1A AND B)

There are three clinical types of abnormal descend of the umbilical cord by the side of the presenting part. All these are included under the heading cord prolapse.

❖ *Occult prolapse*: The cord lies alongside but not in front of the presenting part and is not felt by the fingers on internal examination

Figs 35.1A and B: Cord presentation and prolapse: (A) Cord presentation; (B) Cord prolapse

❖ *Cord presentation*: The cord is slipped down below the presenting part and lies in front of it in the intact bag of membranes
❖ *Cord prolapse*: The cord lies in front of the presenting part inside the vagina or outside the vulva following rupture of the membranes. *pulse feel in umbilical artery.

Incidence

The incidence of cord prolapse is about 1 in 300 deliveries. It occurs mostly in parous women especially in higher parities.

Predisposing Factors

These are same for both presentation and prolapse of cord. Any situation where the presenting part is neither well applied to the lower uterine segment nor well down in the pelvis may make it possible for a loop of cord to slip down in front of the presenting part. Such situations include:
❖ Malpresentations
❖ Prematurity
❖ Multiple pregnancy
❖ Polyhydramnios
❖ High head
❖ High parity.

Malpresentations

The commonest malpresentation associated with cord prolapse is transverse followed by breech, especially complete (legs flexed) or footling. This relates to the ill-fitting nature of the presenting part and the proximity of the umbilicus to the buttocks. In this situation, the degree of compression will be less than with a cephalic presentation, but there is still a danger

of asphyxia. Face and brow presentations are less common causes of cord prolapse.

Prematurity

The size of the fetus in relation to the pelvis and the uterus allows the cord to prolapse. Babies of very low birth weight, less than 1,500 gm, are particularly vulnerable.

Multiple Pregnancy

Malpresentation of the second twin is common in multiple pregnancy.

Polyhydramnios

The cord is liable to be swept down in a gush of liquor if the membranes rupture spontaneously. Controlled release of liquor with artificial rupture of membranes is sometimes performed to prevent this.

High Head

If the membranes rupture spontaneously when the fetal head is high, a loop of cord may pass between the uterine wall and the fetus resulting it lying in front of the presenting part.

Multiparity

The presenting part may not be engaged when the membranes rupture and malpresentation is more common.

Diagnosis

Occult Prolapse

This is difficult to diagnose. The possibility should be suspected if there is: (1) Persistence of variable deceleration of fetal heart rate pattern detected on continuous fetal monitoring in an otherwise normal delivery or (2) Persistent fetal souffle with irregular heart sounds.

Risk IUD r/t anoxia.
Fear e Anxiety r/t life threating to baby or mother.
CHAPTER 35: OBSTETRIC EMERGENCIES 405
Risk for Hypovolemia r/t blood loss.

Cord Presentation

The diagnosis of cord presentation is made by feeling the pulsation of the cord through the intact membranes. It is however, rarely detected but may also be associated with aberrations in fetal heart monitoring, such as decelerations.

Cord Prolapse

The cord is felt below or beside the presenting part on vaginal examination. A loop of cord may be visible at the vulva. The cord is more commonly felt in the vagina or in cases where the presenting part is high; it may be felt at the cervical os. Pulsation can be felt between contractions if the fetus is alive.

Risks to Mother and Fetus

Maternal

The maternal risks are incidental due to emergency operative delivery, which involves the risk of anesthesia, blood loss and infection.

Fetal

The fetus is at risk of anoxia due to acute placental insufficiency from the moment cord is prolapsed. The blood flow is occluded either due to mechanical compression by the presenting part against the incompletely dilated cervix or pelvic wall, or due to vasospasm of the umbilical vessels due to exposure to cold or irritation when exposed outside the vulva or as a result of handling. The danger is more in vertex presentation, especially when the prolapse is through the anterior segment of the pelvis or when the cervix is partially dilated.

Management of Cord Presentation

The aim is to preserve the membranes and to expedite the delivery.

❖ The midwife should discontinue vaginal examination in order to reduce the risk of rupturing the membranes
❖ Medical help should be summoned immediately
❖ Fetal heart should be auscultated as frequently as possible or obtained through continuous electronic monitoring

❖ Cesarean section is the most likely method of delivery
❖ During the time of preparing the woman for operative delivery, she is kept in exaggerated Sim's position to minimize cord compression.

Management of Cord Prolapse

Immediate Action

❖ When the diagnosis of cord prolapse is made, the midwife calls for urgent assistance
❖ The mother and her family must be given explanation about the findings and the emergency measures that will be needed
❖ If oxytocin infusion is in progress, it should be stopped
❖ If the baby is alive, the aim of immediate management is to minimize pressure on the cord until such time when the woman is prepared for assisted delivery or is transferred to an equipped hospital. For this, the gloved fingers are to be introduced into the vagina to lift the presenting part of the cord. The fingers should be placed inside the vagina until definitive treatment is instituted
❖ Postural treatment is given until the delivery of the baby, either vaginally or by cesarean section. The woman is placed in exaggerated elevated Sim's position with pillow under the hip. The foot end of the bed may be elevated. High Trendlenberg or knee-chest position, which has been traditionally mentioned, is very tiring and distressing to the woman
❖ If the cord lies outside the vagina, it should be replaced in to the vagina to minimize vasospasm due to irritation and to maintain the temperature
❖ If much of the cord is outside the vulva, it should be covered with sterile wet gauze, to prevent spasm of the umbilical vessels due to draughts.

Definitive Management

❖ Cesarean section is the ideal management when the baby is sufficiently mature enough to survive. Where the fetus is confirmed alive and delivery is not imminent, the birth must be expedited with the greatest possible speed to reduce the mortality and morbidity associated with this condition

❖ If immediate cesarean section is not possible or the baby is too premature, reposition of the cord may be an alternative. The cervix must be at least half dilated and the cord wrapped in a large piece of sterile roller gauze, is manually pushed above the presenting part under general anesthesia. This is followed by stimulation of uterine contraction with oxytocin drip, if necessary. When the cervix is about three-fourths dilated, ventouse traction may be applied to deliver the baby. This is possible only with vertex presentation and carries high fetal risks

❖ If the head is engaged, delivery is completed by forceps. With a breech engaged, a breech extraction is done

❖ If the fetus is confirmed dead, labor is allowed to proceed, awaiting spontaneous termination.

DYSTOCIA CAUSED BY FETAL ANOMALIES

Fetal Macrosomia (Generalized Fetal Enlargement)

Birth weight of more than 4 kg is considered overweight. The causes are hereditary, size of parents, particularly the mother, poorly controlled maternal diabetes and gestational diabetes, postmaturity and multiparity. Diagnostic evidence includes disproportionate increase in uterine size, feeling the fetus big and firm and sonographic evaluation of the dimensions of the head, thorax and abdomen.

Dangers of macrosomia are dystocia due to cephalopelvic disproportion and shoulder dystocia. Fetal risks include asphyxia, birth trauma and meconium aspiration syndrome leading to increased perinatal loss. Management includes selective preterm induction of labor and wider use of cesarean section.

Shoulder Dystocia

The term shoulder dystocia is used to describe failure of the shoulders to spontaneously traverse the pelvis after delivery of the head.

The anterior shoulder becomes trapped behind or on the symphysis pubis, whilst the posterior shoulder may be in the hollow of the sacrum or high above the sacral promontory.

Shoulder dystocia is not a common emergency. The incidence varies between 0.37 to 1.1 (Bahar, 1996). Risk factors, diagnosis and management are explained in Chapter 33.

Hydrocephalus

Excessive accumulation of cerebrospinal fluid in the ventricles with consequent thinning of the brain tissue and enlargement of the cranium occurs in about 1 in 2,000 deliveries. It is associated with other congenital malformations in one-third of cases. Recurrence rate is about 5 percent and breech presentation occurs in about 25 percent cases.

Diagnosis

Minor degree may escape attention in the antenatal period but the severe degree presents with the following features.

❖ The head is felt larger, globular and softer than the normal head

❖ The head is high-up and impossible to push down into the pelvis

❖ The sensation felt is comparable to that obtained when a ping-pong ball is squeezed

❖ Fetal heart sound is situated high-up above the umbilicus

❖ X-ray will reveal:
  – Cranial shadow as globular rather than normal ovoid
  – Fontanels and sutures are wide
  – Vault bones may show irregular thinning.

❖ Sonography may show dilatation of the lateral ventricles and thinning of the cerebral cortex

❖ Internal examination during labor reveals:
  – Gaping sutures and fontanels and
  – Crackling sensation on pressing the head.

In breech presentation, however, the diagnosis is not made until the after-coming head is arrested at the brim.

Management

The pregnancy is continued until a stage when induction can be performed, usually beyond

36th week. Induction is done by rupture of membranes and oxytocin when the cervix is 3 to 4 cm dilated; decompression of the head is done using a sharp pointed scissors or a perforator.

In breech presentation, the arrested head is decompressed by perforating the sub-occipital region. Exploration of the uterus is done after delivery of the head. If an open spina bifida is present, a uterine dressing forceps or a Drew-Smythe catheter is passed through the opening into the ventricle to drain the fluid.

Outcome

Fetal outlook is extremely poor. The fetus either is delivered stillborn or dies in the neonatal period. Babies, which survive, may be mentally defective. Maternal prognosis is favorable in diagnosed cases. In undiagnosed cases, obstructed labor with its consequences may occur. Rupture of membranes occurs even before the cervix is fully dilated because of too much distension of the lower segment by the head.

Neural Tube Defects

Anencephaly and spina bifida comprise 95 percent of neural tube defects and the remaining 5 percent is encephalocele. It is more common in lower socioeconomic group.

Anencephaly

The incidence of anencephaly is about 1 in 1,000 births. The anomaly develops from deficient development of the vault of the skull and brain tissue, but the facial portion is normal. The pituitary gland is often absent or hypoplastic.

About 70 percent of anencephalic fetuses are females. It is more prevalent in first birth and in young and elderly mothers.

Diagnosis

In the first half of pregnancy, the diagnosis is made by detecting elevated alfa-fetoprotein in amniotic fluid and confirmed by sonography. In the later half of pregnancy, the diagnosis is difficult, especially when associated with hydramnios. On internal examination, face presentation is diagnosed and confirmed by sonography or X-ray.

Complications

❖ Hydramnios
❖ Malpresentation—Face and breech
❖ Premature labor—Specially when associated with hydramnios
❖ Tendency of postmaturity
❖ Shoulder dystocia
❖ Obstructed labor—If the head and neck try to engage together because of short neck.

Management

If confirmed before, in the antenatal period, termination of pregnancy is to be done. During labor if shoulder dystocia occurs, it should be managed by cleidotomy.

Prevention

Prepregnancy counseling is essential for future pregnancies. Folic acid supplementation beginning one month before conception to about 12 weeks conception has reduced the incidence of NTD significantly (Dutta, 2001).

Enlargement of Fetal Abdomen

Enlargement of fetal abdomen sufficient to produce dystocia, may be due to ascites, distended bladder or enlargement of kidney by a tumor or an umbilical hernia.

Antenatal diagnosis may be made accidentally by X-ray or by sonography. Fetal appearance on X-ray resembles "Buddah position". The diagnosis is usually made when there is difficulty in the delivery of the trunk following birth of the head. Confirmation is done by introducing the hand and palpating the hugely distended abdomen. Decompression of the abdomen is done by simple puncture with a trocar, which is soon followed by spontaneous delivery.

Conjoined Twins

The varieties of incomplete twinning result in the development of conjoined twins. The condition is extremely rare and often causes surprise dystocia.

AMNIOTIC FLUID EMBOLISM

This condition occurs when amniotic fluid enters the maternal circulation through a tear in the membranes or placenta. The body responds in two phases—The initial phase is one of vasospasm causing hypoxia, hypotension and cardiovascular collapse. The second phase is the development of left ventricular failure, with hemorrhage and coagulation disorder followed by pulmonary edema. Mortality and morbidity are very high.

The presence of thromboplastin rich liquor amnii in the maternal circulation blocks the pulmonary arteries and triggers the complex coagulation mechanism leading to DIC. There will be severe clotting defect with profuse bleeding per vagina or through the venepuncture sites due to consumption of coagulation factors.

Predisposing Factors

Amniotic fluid embolism can occur at any stage in gestation. It is mostly associated with labor, though cases in early pregnancy and postpartum have been reported (Bennett and Brown, 1999).

❖ Transfer of amniotic fluid from the uterus to the maternal circulation can be insidiously associated with a tear in the membranes
❖ Amniotic fluid under pressure may enter maternal circulation in the first phase of hypoxia during hypertonic uterine activity
❖ Procedures such as insertion of an intrauterine catheter and artificial rupture of membranes are associated with the condition
❖ In cases of placental abruption, the placental bed is disrupted, and the barrier between the maternal circulation and amniotic sac may be breached
❖ It can occur during a cesarean section or termination of pregnancy or in association with ruptured uterus
❖ Trauma may occur during intrauterine manipulation such as internal podalic version

The condition is difficult to predict and equally difficult to prevent.

Clinical Features

❖ Sudden onset of maternal respiratory distress: The woman becomes severely dyspnic and cyanosed
❖ There is maternal hypotension and uterine hypertonia
❖ Fetal distress in response to hypoxia caused by hypertonia
❖ Cardiopulmonary arrest follows quickly in minutes
❖ Many mothers present with convulsions immediately preceding the collapse (Clark, 1990).

Emergency Management

Any one of the above symptoms is indicative of an acute emergency. The mother may be in a state of collapse and resuscitation must be started at once. Specific management of the condition is life support and high levels of oxygen are required. Mothers who survive may suffer neurological impairment.

Complications

Disseminated intravascular coagulation (DIC) is likely to occur within 30 minutes of the initial collapse.

Acute renal failure occurs due to heavy bleeding and the prolonged hypovolemic hypotension. Transfer to an intensive therapy unit for specialized care is indicated.

Effect on the Fetus

Perinatal mortality and morbidity are high, where amniotic fluid embolism occurs before the birth of the baby. Delay in the time from initial maternal collapse to delivery needs to be minimal if fetal death is to be avoided.

SHOCK

Shock is defined as a state of circulatory inadequacy with poor tissue perfusion resulting in generalized cellular hypoxia leading to dysfunction of organs and cells.

Shock can be acute but prompt treatment results in recovery with little detrimental effect on the mother. However, inadequate treatment or failure to initiate effective treatment can result in chronic multisystem organ failure, which may be fatal.

Classification of Shock

Based on the basic pathophysiology of shock and its clinical correlation, shock may be classified as follows:

Hypovolemic Shock

The result of a reduction in intravascular volume.

❖ *Hemorrhagic shock*: Associated with post-partum or postabortal hemorrhage, ectopic pregnancy, placenta previa, abruptio-placentae, rupture of uterus and obstetric surgery
❖ *Fluid loss shock*: Associated with excessive diarrhea, vomiting, diuresis or too rapid removal of amniotic fluid
❖ *Supine hypotensive syndrome*: Associated with compression of inferior vena cava by pregnant uterus
❖ *Shock associated with disseminated intra-vascular coagulation*: Intrauterine dead fetus syndrome and amniotic fluid embolism.

Cardiogenic Shock

Impaired ability of the heart to pump blood.

❖ Failure of the left ventricular ejection in cardiac arrest and myocardial infarction
❖ Failure of left ventricular filling associated with cardiac tamponade and pulmonary embolism.

Neurogenic Shock

❖ *Chemical injury*: Associated with aspiration of gastrointestinal contents during general anesthesia, especially in caesarean section (Mendelson's syndrome)
❖ *Drug induced*: Associated with spinal an-esthesia.

Septic Shock (Endotoxic Shock)

Associated typically with septic abortion, chorioamnionitis, pyelonephritis and rarely postpartum endometritis. This type of shock

may be hypovolemic but has primary cardio-genic and cellular components also. In this section, hypovolemic shock and septic shock are discussed as either of which may occur because of child bearing.

Hypovolemic Shock

The body reacts to the loss of circulating fluid in stages as follows:

❖ *Initial stage*: The reduction in fluid or blood decreases the venous return to the heart. The ventricles of the heart are inadequately filled, causing a reduction in stroke volume and cardiac output. As cardiac output and venous return fall, the blood pressure is reduced. The drop in blood pressure decreases the supply of oxygen to the tissues and cell function is affected
❖ *Compensatory stage*: The drop in cardiac output produces a response from the sympathetic nervous system through the activation of receptors in the aorta and carotid arteries. Blood is redistributed to the vital organs. Vessels in the gastro-intestinal tract, kidneys, skin and lungs constrict. The response is seen by the skin becoming pale and cool. Peristalsis slows, urinary output is reduced and exchange of gas in the lungs is impaired. The heart rate increases in an attempt to improve cardiac output and blood pressure. Pupils of the eyes dilate. The sweat glands are stimulated and the skin becomes moist and clammy.

  Adrenaline and aldosterone from adrenal glands and antidiuretic hormone from posterior pituitary gland are secreted causing vasoconstriction, an increased cardiac output and a decrease in urinary output. Venous return to the heart will increase but, unless the fluid loss is replaced, this will not be sustained.
❖ *Progressive stage*: This stage leads to multisystem failure. Compensatory mecha-nisms begin to fail, with vital organs lacking adequate perfusion. Volume depletion causes further fall in blood pressure and cardiac output. The coronary arteries suffer lack of supply. Peripheral circulation is poor, with weak or absent pulses.
❖ *Late stage:* (Irreversible).

❖ Hypotension continues and cannot be reversed by replacement of fluid because of stagnation of blood at the microvascular level. Color of skin becomes ashen gray. Metabolic acidosis starts and for elimination of accumulated carbon dioxide, the respiratory rate becomes rapid. Imperceptible low volume pulse, oliguria and mental confusion occur. Multisystem failure and cell destruction are irreparable. Treatment of any kind is practically useless in this phase. Death ensues (Dutta, 2001).

Management

Urgent resuscitation is needed to prevent the mother's condition from deteriorating and causing irreversible damage. The priorities are to:

1. *Maintain the airway*: If the mother is severely collapsed, she should be turned on to her side and oxygen administered at a rate of 6 to 8 liters per minute. If she is unconscious, endotracheal intubation may be necessary.
2. *Replace fluids:* (Infusion and transfusion): Blood should be taken for cross matching prior to commencing intravenous fluids. A plasma expander or fresh frozen plasma is given until whole blood is available.
3. *Avoid warmth*: Constriction of the peripheral blood supply occurs in response to the shock and keeping the mother warm may interfere with this response, causing further deterioration in her condition.
4. *Control of hemorrhage*: Specific surgical and medical treatment for control of hemorrhage should start along with the general management of shock.

Clinical Observations for the Mother in Shock (Monitoring)

❖ Assess the level of consciousness. Signs of restlessness and confusion are to be noted
❖ Monitor blood pressure every 30 minutes or continuously
❖ Cardiac rhythm may be monitored continuously
❖ Assess skin color and temperature hourly

❖ Assess central venous pressure and fluid balance for adequacy of circulating volume
❖ Watch for occurrence of any further bleeding.

Detailed observation charts are to be maintained and the mother may be transferred to a critical care unit.

Septic Shock

There is an overwhelming infection, commonly from gram-negative organisms such as *Escherichia coli*, *Proteus* or *Pseudomonas pyocyaneus*. These organisms are common pathogens in the female genital tract and have endotoxins present in their cells. Endotoxins release components that trigger body's immune response. Septic shock can less commonly be caused by gram-positive bacteria or by multiple organisms.

The placental site is the main point of entry for an infection associated with pregnancy and childbirth. This may occur following septic abortion, prolonged rupture of membranes, obstetric trauma or in the presence of retained placental tissue.

The body's primary response to infection is alteration in the peripheral circulation. Cells damaged by the infecting organisms release histamine and enzymes that contribute to vasodilatation and increased permeability of the capillaries. Mediators are also reduced that have the opposite action of vasoconstriction. The overall response, however, is one of vasodilatation, which reduces the systemic vascular resistance.

Clinical Signs of Septic Shock

❖ In the initial phase, there is marked flushing of the face and the skin feels warm
❖ Temperature rise varies between 101°F to 105° F
❖ Tachycardia, tachypnea and rigors occur
❖ Hemorrhage may be present which either could be due to the events of childbearing or because of disseminated intravascular coagulation
❖ As vasodilatation continues, hypotension leads to kidney damage with reduced glomerular filtration and acute tubular necrosis and oliguria

- If the shock condition does not improve, the patient passes clinically to the stage of "irreversible shock". She remains cold and clammy with ashen-gray cyanotic appearance
- Anuria, cardiac or respiratory distress and coma may supervene
- Disseminated intravascular coagulation is also a feature of septic shock
- Multisystem organ failure will result as an effect of the continued hypotension and myocardial depression. Failure of the liver, brain and respiratory systems follows, and death results.

Management of Septic Shock

Management is based on preventing further deterioration by restoring circulatory volume and eradication of the infection. A full infection screening should be carried out including a high vaginal swab, midstream urine and blood cultures. Retained products of conception if detected on ultrasound should be removed.

Measures of management include intravenous administration of antibiotics, intravenous fluids, adjustment of acid-based balance, steroids, prevention and treatment of intravascular coagulation and toxic myocarditis, administration of oxygen and elimination of the source of infection.

- Antibiotics: Broad-spectrum antibiotics are given to start with and after confirming the sensitivity, specific antibiotics are given intravenously
- Intravenous fluids and electrolytes: Septic shock associated hemorrhagic hypotension is treated with liberal infusion and blood transfusion. Oliguria with high specific gravity is an indication for liberal fluid administration, whereas a low specific gravity indicates fluid restriction. Impairment of renal function contraindicates administration of electrolytes
- Correction of acidosis: Bicarbonate is administered to correct metabolic acidosis
- Maintenance of blood pressure: Inotropic agents such as adrenaline, noradrenaline, dopamine and dobutamine are administered to increase the cardiac contractility.

Vasodilator drugs, such as sodium nitroprusside and nitroglycerine and diuretics are used in selected cases to reduce the after load and pulmonary edema
- Corticosteroids are given to exert an anti-endotoxin effect and to counteract anaerobic oxidative mechanism
- As a prophylactic measure for DIC, heparin may be given. Fresh frozen plasma or whole blood transfusion may be used
- In unresponsive septic shock following septic abortion or puerperal sepsis, hysterectomy may be done to eliminate the source of infection

The mother may require care and management in a critical or intensive care unit. The family should be kept informed of progress.

BASIC LIFE SUPPORT/CARDIOPULMONARY RESUSCITATION (CPR)

Basic life support refers to the maintenance of an airway and support for breathing, without any specialized equipment. The basic principles of BLS are: A—airway, B—breathing and C—circulation.

Steps of Basic Life Support

Airway

Determine Unresponsiveness
- If a mother is found collapsed, her level of consciousness is to be determined by gently shaking a shoulder and enquiring *are you alright.*

Call for Help
- If there is no response, assistance must be called for by ringing the emergency bell or asking another person *call for help.*

Position the Victim (Mother)
- The mother is then laid flat on her back, removing pillows. Once the body is supine, the victim's arms should be placed alongside the body. The surface under the mother must be firm and flat for effective maneuver.

Rescuer Position (Midwife)
- To perform basic life support, the midwife must stand at a suitable height at the victim's side near the chest or have the

victim on the floor and kneel at the side, at the level of the victim's shoulders.

Open Airway (Fig. 35.2A)
❖ The airway is cleared of any mucus or vomit and any dentures removed
❖ To open the airway, the chin is lifted up gently with one hand while pushing down on the forehead with the other to tilt the head back.

Determine Breathlessness (Fig. 35.2B)
❖ Once the airway is open, the chest is observed for signs of respiratory effort. For this the midwife places her ear close to the victim's mouth and:
   – Looks at the chest for movement
   – Listens for sounds of breathing
   – Feels for breath on her cheek.
If none of these signs is present, the victim is confirmed not breathing.

Breathing

Perform Rescue Breathing (Fig. 35.2C)
Rescue breathing is provided using the mouth-to-mouth technique.
❖ Using the thumb and index finger of the hand on the victim's forehead, the nose is pinched shut while the heel of the hand is kept in place to maintain the head tilt. The other hand is placed under the woman's chin to lift it up.
❖ Two full breaths are given while maintaining an airtight seal around the victim's mouth with the rescuer's mouth.

Circulation

Determine Pulselessness
❖ After giving the two full breaths, the woman's *carotid artery pulse is located* to see if the heart is beating. This is felt in the neck at the side of the mother's larynx using the hand that was supporting the chin
❖ If pulse cannot be palpated, artificial circulation is provided in addition to rescue breathing. A *precordial thumb* (short, sharp blow) is delivered on the center of the sternum using the fist. The blow should be

Figs 35.2A to C: Basic life support—rescue breathing: (A) Opening the airway; (B) Determining breathlessness; (C) Rescue breathing—mouth-to-mouth

from a height of about 15 cm. The fist is removed quickly and the *carotid pulse rechecked* to see whether the precordial thumb has been effective in restarting the heart
❖ If the precordial thumb is unsuccessful, the mother may be in cardiac arrest. External chest compressions are needed

Call for Assistance

If no one has reached for help and the rescuer (midwife) is alone, chest compression should be started.

External Chest Compressions
(Figs 35.3A and B)

❖ The woman's *xiphisternum* is located and hands placed on the lower half of the sternum with palms extended and fingers interlaced on top of one another. The heel of the lower hand is positioned on the lower two-thirds of the sternum. With the arms straight (the elbows locked into position directly over the hands), the rescuer leans on to the sternum depressing it 3.8 to 5 cm (1½-2 inches) with heals of the hands and releases it slowly at the same rate as compression. The chest should be allowed to return to its normal position between compressions without removing the hands from the victim's sternum. Relaxation and compression should be of equal duration.

Figs 35.3A and B: Basic life support—Determining breathlessness and external chest: (A) Determining breathlessness; (B) External chest compression

The rate of compressions should be 80 to 100 per minute. If the victim requires both *rescue breathing* and external chest compressions the proper ratio is 15 chest compressions to two breaths. If two persons are available, the rate is five compressions to two breaths (American Heart Association, 1986).

❖ Chest compressions and ventilation should be continued until help arrives and until those experienced in resuscitation are able to take over.

Summary of the Sequence of BLS

❖ Determine unresponsiveness
❖ Call for help
❖ Position the victim
❖ Rescuer position
❖ Open airway
❖ Determine breathlessness
❖ Perform rescue breathing
❖ Determine pulselessness
❖ Call for assistance
❖ Perform chest compressions.

BIBLIOGRAPHY

1. American Heart Association. Standards and guidelines for cardiopulmonary resuscitation and emergency cardiac care. The Journal of American Medical Association. 1986;255(21):2841-3044.
2. Bahar AM. Risk factors in fetal outcome in cases of shoulder dystocia compared with normal deliveries of a similar birth weight. British Journal of Obstetrics and Gynecology 1996;103: 868-72.
3. Clark Sl. New concepts of amniotic fluid embolism: A review, Obstetrical and Gynecological Survey. 1990;45(6):360-8.
4. Dutta DC. Textbook of Obstetrics, 5th edn. Calcutta; New Central Book Company 2001.
5. Gonik B, Allen SC. An alternate maneuver for management of shoulder dystocia. American Journal of Obstetrics and Gynecology 1983;145: 882-3.
6. Naef RW, Morrison JC. Guidelines for management of shoulder dystocia. Journal of perinatology, 1994;15(6):435-441.
7. Watson P, Besch N. Management of acute and sub-acute inversion of the uterus. Obstetrics and Gynecology 1980;55(1):12-6.

36

Complications of Third Stage of Labor

Learning Objectives

Upon completing this chapter, the learner will be able to:
- ❖ Describe the causes and management of postpartum hemorrhage
- ❖ Discuss the diagnosis and management of placenta accreta
- ❖ Describe the varieties and dangers of inversion of uterus
- ❖ Describe the measures to prevent inversion of uterus and management if the problem occurs.

Of all the stages of labor, third stage is the most crucial for the mother. Dangerous complications may appear unexpectedly in an otherwise uneventful first or second stage.

POSTPARTUM HEMORRHAGE

Definition

Postpartum hemorrhage is defined as excessive bleeding from the genital tract at any time following the baby's birth up to six weeks after delivery. A quantitative definition is related to the amount of blood loss in excess of 500 ml following birth of the baby.

While the quantitative definition may be useful for statistical purposes, the effect of the blood loss is more important rather than the amount of blood lost. Hence, the clinical definition states—"Any amount of bleeding from or into the genital tract following birth of the baby up to the end of the puerperium which adversely affects the general condition of the mother, evidenced by rise in pulse rate and falling blood pressure is called postpartum hemorrhage" (Dutta, 2001).

Incidence

The incidence varies widely because of lack of uniformity in the criteria used in definition. The incidence is about 1 percent amongst hospital deliveries.

Classification

Depending on the time of occurrence postpartum hemorrhage is classified as:
- ❖ Third stage hemorrhage—Bleeding that occurs before expulsion of placenta.
- ❖ Primary postpartum hemorrhage or true postpartum hemorrhage—Bleeding that occurs subsequent to expulsion of placenta and within 24 hours.
- ❖ Secondary postpartum hemorrhage—Bleeding occurs subsequent to the first 24 hours following birth up until the sixth week postpartum. This is also termed as delayed or late puerperal hemorrhage.

Postpartum hemorrhage is one of the most alarming and serious emergencies, which a midwife may face and is especially terrifying if it occurs immediately following a normal delivery. It may also prove a frightening experience for the mother. The midwife is often the first and may be the only professional person present when a hemorrhage occurs. Her prompt and competent action will be crucial in controlling blood loss and reducing the risk of maternal morbidity or even death.

Causes of Postpartum Hemorrhage

There are several causes for third stage bleeding and primary postpartum hemorrhage, which include atonic, traumatic and blood coagulopathy.

Atonic Uterus

Atonicity of the uterus is the most common cause (80%) of postpartum hemorrhage. This is a failure of the myometrium at the placental site to contract and retract, and to compress torn blood vessels and control blood loss by a living ligature action. When the placenta is attached, the volume of blood flow at the placental site is approximately 500 to 800 ml per minute. The following are the conditions, which often interfere with the retraction of the uterus as a whole and of the placental site in particular.

1. Incomplete separation of the placenta. If the placenta remains fully adhered to the uterine wall, it is unlikely to cause bleeding. However, once separation has begun, maternal vessels are torn. If placental tissue remains partially embedded in the spongy decidua, efficient contraction and retraction is interrupted.
2. Retained cotyledon, placental fragments or membranes will similarly impede efficient uterine action.
3. Precipitate labor—When the uterus has contracted vigorously and frequently resulting in duration of labor, that is less than one hour, then the uterine muscle may have insufficient opportunity to retract.
4. Prolonged labor—In a labor where the active phase lasts more than 12 hours, uterine inertia (sluggishness) may result due to muscle exhaustion.
5. Over distension of the uterus—In multiple pregnancy, polyhydramnios and large baby, the myometrium becomes excessively stretched and therefore less efficient.
6. Placenta previa—The placental site is partly or wholly in the lower segment where the thinner muscle layer contains few oblique fibers. This results in poor control of bleeding.
7. Placental abruption—Blood may have seeped between the muscle fibers, interfering with effective action. When severe, this results in a Couvelaire uterus.
8. General anesthesia—Anesthetic agents may cause a uterine relaxation, particularly in inhalational agents like halothane.
9. Mismanagement of the third stage of labor—"Fundus fiddling" or manipulation of the uterus may precipitate arrhythmic contractions, so that the placenta only partially separates and retraction is lost.
10. A full bladder—If the bladder is full, its proximity to the uterus in the abdomen, on completion of the second stage, may interfere with the uterine action.
11. Initiation or augmentation of delivery by oxytocin—Postdelivery uterine atonicity is likely to develop, as oxytocin will increase the power of contraction without improving the retraction power of the uterine muscle.
12. Constriction ring—Hour-glass constriction formed in the upper segment across the partially separated placenta or at the junction of upper and lower segments with the fully separated placenta trapped in the upper segment, may produce excessive bleeding.
13. Etiology unknown—A precipitating cause may never be discovered. Predisposing factors, which might increase the risk of atonic postpartum hemorrhage include:
    ❖ Previous history of postpartum hemorrhage or retained placenta—In such women there is a risk in subsequent pregnancies
    ❖ High parity—With each successive pregnancy, fibrous tissue replaces muscle fibers in the uterus, reducing its contractility and the blood vessels become more difficult to compress. Women who have had five or more deliveries, are at increased risk
    ❖ Fibroids—These benign tumors may impede efficient uterine action
    ❖ Anemia—Women who enter labor with reduced hemoglobin concentration (below 10 g/dl) may succumb more quickly.

Traumatic Hemorrhage in Third Stage

Causes

1. Perineal, vaginal and cervical tears
2. Lower segment tears

3. Uterine rupture
4. Vulval injuries.

If bleeding occurs despite a well-contracted uterus, it is almost certainly the consequence of trauma. Trauma to the genital tract usually occurs following operative delivery, though it may occur even after spontaneous delivery. Trauma involves usually the cervix, vagina, perineum (episiotomy wound and lacerations), paraurethral region and rarely rupture of the uterus. The bleeding is usually revealed, but can rarely be concealed (vulvo-vaginal or broad ligament hematoma).

In order to identify the source of bleeding, the mother is placed in lithotomy position under a good directional light. The external injuries are usually identified and torn vessels are clamped and ligated. A speculum is inserted to visualize internal trauma (vagina and cervix). Tissue or artery forceps may be used to obtain hemostasis prior to suturing under general anesthesia.

If bleeding persists when the uterus is well contracted and no evidence of trauma can be found, uterine rupture must be suspected. Following a laparotomy, this is repaired, but if bleeding remains uncontrolled, a hysterectomy may become inevitable.

Blood Coagulation Disorders

Causes

1. Disseminated intravascular coagulation.
2. Excessive fibrinolysis.
3. Inherited coagulation disorders.
4. Idiopathic thrombocytopenic purpura.

Postpartum hemorrhage may be the result of coagulation failure. The failure of the blood to clot may be due to diminished procoagulants (wash out phenomenon) or increased fibrinolytic activity. It can occur following severe pre-eclampsia, abruptio placentae, amniotic fluid embolism, HELLP syndrome, intrauterine death or sepsis.

Fresh blood is usually the best treatment, as this will contain platelets and the coagulation factors V and VIII. Fresh frozen plasma and fibrinogen may also be infused.

Signs of Postpartum Hemorrhage

1. Vaginal bleeding is visible outside, either as slow trickle or rarely a copious flow. Rarely, the bleeding is concealed either remaining inside the uterovesical canal, or in the surrounding tissue space resulting in hematoma.
2. Pallor.
3. Rising pulse rate.
4. Falling blood pressure.
5. Altered level of consciousness may become restless or drowsy.
6. Enlarged uterus, as it fills with blood or blood clot. It feels boggy on palpation, i.e. soft and distended lacking tone.
7. Maternal collapse.

The effect of blood loss depends on pre-delivery hemoglobin level, degree of pregnancy-induced hypervolemia and the speed at which blood loss occurs. Alteration of pulse and blood pressure appears only after substantial amount of blood loss and as such is a comparatively late manifestation. On occasion, blood loss is so rapid and brisk that death may occur with in a few minutes.

The state of the uterus, as felt per abdomen, gives a reliable clue as regards the cause of bleeding. In traumatic hemorrhage, the uterus is well contracted. In atonic hemorrhage, the uterus is flabby and becomes hard on massaging. However, both the atonic and traumatic may coexist.

Prophylaxis

Postpartum hemorrhage cannot always be prevented. However, the incidence and magnitude can be reduced substantially if following guidelines are followed.

Antenatal

❖ Improvement of the health status of women, especially to raise their hemoglobin level as near to normal as possible, so that they can withstand the blood loss
❖ Screening of high-risk women, such as those with twins, hydramnios, grand multipara, APH, history of previous third stage complications and severe anemia for delivery in a well equipped hospital

❖ Blood grouping and typing should be done for the high-risk mothers so that no time is lost during an emergency.

During Labor

Prevent prolonged labor and ketoacidosis by following good management practices:

❖ Prophylactic administration of oxytocic drugs for the third stage

❖ Baby should be pushed out by the retracted uterus and not be pulled out. One should take 2 to 3 minutes to deliver the trunk after the head is born

❖ Temptation of fiddling with or kneading the uterus, pulling the cord or Crede's expression of placenta to be avoided

❖ In all cases of induced or accelerated labor by oxytocin, the infusion should be continued for at least one hour after the delivery and prophylactic ergometrine should be given with the delivery of the anterior shoulder

❖ For any woman known to have placenta previa, two units of cross-matched blood should be kept available

❖ The woman should be observed for about two hours after the delivery and after being satisfied that the uterus is hard and contracted. The pulse and blood pressure should be within normal limits before transferring the woman to the ward/postpartum floor.

Management of Third Stage Bleeding

Three basic principles apply in the management of postpartum hemorrhage in the third stage.

❖ Call the obstetrician when the midwife thinks that the bleeding is more than expected

❖ Stop the bleeding by employing the following measures:
  – Rub up a contraction. The fundus is felt gently with the fingertips to assess its consistency. If it is soft and relaxed, the fundus is massaged with a smooth circular motion without applying undue pressure. When a contraction occurs, the hand is held still.

  – Give an oxytocic to sustain the contraction. Ergometrine 0.2 mg is given intravenously.

  – Empty the uterus. If the placenta is still inside, it should be delivered. If it has been born, any clots should be expelled by firm but gentle pressure on the abdomen.

❖ Resuscitate the mother.
  – Start a dextrose saline drip and arrange for blood transfusion if necessary.

  – The mother's legs may be lifted up in order to allow blood flow from them up to the central circulation (the foot of the bed should not be raised as this encourages pooling of blood in the uterus, which prevents the uterus contracting).

  – The bladder is to be catheterized in order to minimize trauma, should an operative procedure be necessary and to exclude a full bladder as a precipitating cause for further bleeding.

  – The woman may be sedated with morphine 10 to 15 mg intramuscularly. The placenta and membranes must be re-examined for completeness since retained fragments are often responsible for uterine atony.

Manual Removal of Placenta (Figs 36.1 and 36.2)

When the placenta remains undelivered even 30 minutes following the birth of the baby, it is considered a retained placenta requiring manual removal. The procedure is done by the physician under anesthesia. General anesthesia is used if the mother's condition permits. Epidural or spinal anesthesia offers an alternative depending on the situation.

Manual removal is performed with full aseptic precautions. The vulva and vagina are swabbed with antiseptic solution and sterile leggings are placed as in other vaginal operations. The bladder is catheterized.

With the left hand, the umbilical cord is held taut while the right hand is coned and inserted into the vagina and uterus following the direction of the cord. Once the placenta is

Fig. 36.1: Introduction of the hand into the uterus in a cone shaped manner

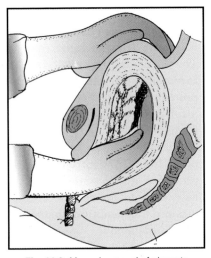

Fig. 36.2: Manual removal of placenta

located, the cord is released, so that the left hand may be used to support the fundus abdominally.

The operator will feel for a separated edge of the placenta. The fingers of the hand are extended and the border of the hand is gently eased between the placenta and the uterine wall with the palm facing the placenta. With a sideways slicing movement, the placenta is carefully detached. When the placenta is completely separated, it is extracted by traction of the cord by the left hand. The right hand is still inside the uterus for exploration of the cavity to be sure that nothing is left behind. The placenta should be checked immediately for completeness so that any further exploration, if needed, may be carried out immediately.

After the completion of manual removal, inspection of cervicovaginal canal is made to exclude any injury. Intravenous ergometrine 0.25 mg is given and the uterus is massaged to make it hard.

Difficulties

❖ Hour-glass contraction leading to difficulty in introducing the hand
❖ Morbid adherent placenta, which may cause difficulty in getting to the plane of cleavage of placental separation.

Complications

❖ Hemorrhage due to incomplete removal
❖ Injury to the uterus
❖ Shock
❖ Infection
❖ Inversion
❖ Subinvolution
❖ Thrombophlebitis
❖ Embolism.

Observation of the Mother Following Third Stage Hemorrhage

Once the bleeding is controlled:
❖ Total blood volume lost must be estimated as accurately as possible
❖ Maternal pulse and blood pressure are recorded quarter hourly and temperature taken four hourly
❖ The uterus should be palpated frequently to ensure that it remains well contracted and lochia lost must be observed
❖ Intravenous fluid replacement should be carefully calculated and administered to avoid circulatory overload. Monitoring the central venous pressure will provide an accurate assessment of the volume required, especially if blood loss has been severe
❖ Fluid intake and urinary output are recorded as indicators of renal function. The output should be measured on an hourly basis by the use of a self-retaining catheter
❖ The woman should remain in the labor ward until her condition is stable for close monitoring
❖ All records should be meticulously completed and signed as soon as possible
❖ Continued vigilance will be important for 24 to 48 hours

❖ Provision should be made for the woman to have a quiet period of recuperation.

MANAGEMENT OF PRIMARY POSTPARTUM HEMORRHAGE

Principles

❖ To diagnose the cause of bleeding—atonic or traumatic
❖ To take prompt and effective measures to control bleeding
❖ To correct hypovolemia.

Immediate Measures

The following immediate measures are taken by the attending physician when the amount of blood loss is more than a liter.

❖ Calls for additional help
❖ Puts in one or two large bore (16 gauge) intravenous cannula
❖ Sends blood for group and cross matching (if not done before) and requests for two units of blood
❖ Starts rapid infusion with normal saline (crystalloid) or plasma substitutes like hemaccel (colloids) to reexpand the vascular bed. Monitoring of pulse, blood pressure, fluids infused, urinary output, drugs given and central venous pressure (when cited) are important.

Management Steps

Step 1

❖ The first step is to feel the uterus for its consistency to determine the likely cause of bleeding. If the uterus is found atonic:
  – Massage the fundus to make it hard and express the blood clot
  – Methergine 0.2 mg is to be given intramuscularly
  – Empty the bladder if it is found full (by inserting a self-retaining catheter)
  – Examine the expelled placenta and membranes, if available, for evidence of missing cotyledons or pieces of membranes.

Step 2

❖ If the uterus fails to remain firm and relaxes again with more bleeding:

Fig. 36.3: Bimanual compression of the uterus

  – The uterus is to be explored under general anesthesia. Simultaneous inspection of the cervix, vagina and paraurethral region is done to exclude coexistent bleeding sites. Another dose of ergometrine is given. In refractory cases, 0.25 mg of 15 methyl PGF_2 is administered either intramuscularly or transabdominally into the myometrium to bring back the uterine tone. This may be repeated every 1 to 1.5 hours whenever necessary. If the uterus remains atonic, the next step is taken.

Step 3—Bimanual Compression (Fig. 36.3)

This is done to apply pressure to the placental site. The fingers of the right hand are inserted into the vagina like a cone; the hand is formed into a fist and placed into the anterior vaginally fornix, the elbow resting on the bed. The left hand is placed behind the uterus abdominally, the fingers pointing towards the cervix. The uterus is brought forward and compressed between the palm of the left hand and the first in the vagina. If bleeding persists, a clotting disorder must be excluded before exploration of the vagina and uterus.

During this period, the resuscitative measures are to be continued unless the general condition improves. With oxytocics and blood transfusion, most cases respond well. Uterine contraction and retraction regain and bleeding stops. However, in rare cases, when the uterus fails to contract, the following measures may be tried as an alternative to hysterectomy.

Step 4—Hot Intrauterine Douche

It is an effective method to stimulate the uterus to regain its tone. The temperature of the fluid should be about 108°F (47.8°C) and some antiseptic lotion are mixed in the douche. If the method fails, the next step may be tried.

Step 5—Tight Intrauterine Packing

Intrauterine packing is done under general anesthesia. A five-meter long and 8 cm wide strip of gauze is soaked in antiseptic cream is used. The gauze is placed high up and packed into the fundal area while the uterus is steadied by the external hand. Gradually, the rest of the uterine cavity is packed so that no empty space is left behind. A separate pack is used to fill the vagina. An abdominal binder is placed. The intrauterine packing exerts direct hemostatic pressure to the open uterine sinuses and stimulates uterine contraction. Antibiotic is given and the plug should be removed after 24 hours under morphine premedication. Intrauterine packing is useful in uncontrolled postpartum hemorrhage where other methods have failed and the patient is being prepared for transfer to a tertiary care center.

Last Step—Hysterectomy

If, in spite of the above measures, the uterus fails to contract and blood coagulopathy is excluded, hysterectomy may have to be performed.

Prognosis

Postpartum hemorrhage is one of the life-threatening emergencies in the third stage. It is responsible for maternal deaths in about 1 percent, especially in the developing countries (Dutta, 2001). Prevalence of malnutrition and anemia, inadequate antenatal care and lack of blood transfusion facilities are some of the important contributing factors. There is also increased morbidity. These include shock, puerperal sepsis, failing lactation, pulmonary embolism, thrombosis and thrombophlebitis.

Late sequelae include Sheehans syndrome (selective hypopituitarism) or rarely diabetes insipidus.

Breaking of the Cord

This is an occasional occurrence during completion of the third stage of labor. It is crucial to check that the uterus remains firm before further action is taken. If the placenta remains adherent, manual removal of the placenta is to be done by the obstetrician. If the placenta is palpable in the vagina, it is probable that separation has occurred. The mother may be encouraged to push with the next contraction and fundal pressure may be used. Great care must be taken not to exert undue pressure on the fundus. It may cause considerable pain and discomfort to the mother. If fundal pressure is performed without good uterine contraction, acute inversion may occur.

SECONDARY POSTPARTUM HEMORRHAGE

Secondary postpartum hemorrhage is bleeding from the genital tract more than 24 hours after delivery of the placenta and may occur up to six weeks after delivery. It is most likely to occur between 8th and 14th day after delivery.

Causes

❖ Retained bits of cotyledons, membranes, or a large uterine blood clot
❖ Separation of slough over a deep cervico-vaginal laceration
❖ Subinvolution of the placental site due to delayed healing process because of low-grade infection
❖ Secondary hemorrhage from cesarean section wound
❖ Withdrawal bleeding following estrogen therapy for suppression of lactation
❖ Other causes are chorion epithelioma, carcinoma cervix, placental polyp or fibroid polyp.

Clinical Features

❖ The lochia are heavier than normal and will consist of a bright red loss

- The lochia may be offensive if infection is a contributing factor
- Subinvolution of uterus and often a patulous os
- Pyrexia and tachycardia
- Varying degrees of anemia: Proportionate to the blood loss.

As this is an event most likely to occur at home, women should be alerted to the possible signs of postpartum hemorrhage prior to discharge from the postnatal ward.

Management

The principles of management are—(1) To assess the amount of loss and to replace the lost blood, (2) To find out the cause and to take appropriate steps to rectify it.

Supportive Therapy

- Resuscitative measures including blood transfusion, if the bleeding is heavy
- Ergometrine 0.5 mg intramuscularly, if the bleeding is uterine in origin
- Antibiotics as a routine.

Conservative Therapy

- Bed rest and observation for 24 hours, if the bleeding is mild.

Active Management

- Exploration of the uterus under general anesthesia, if retained bits of placenta or membranes is the cause
- Gentle curettage is done and the materials removed are to be sent for histopathological examination
- Ergometrine 0.5 mg is given intramuscularly.

Secondary bleeding following cesarean section may at times require laparotomy for applying hemostatic sutures. Rarely, ligation of internal iliac artery or hysterectomy may become necessary.

Nursing Considerations

- If the uterus is still palpable, massaging the uterus and expressing the clots may help
- The mother must be encouraged to empty her bladder

- All the pads and linen must be assessed for the volume of blood lost
- Vital signs and general condition must be monitored
- Hemoglobin estimation and iron treatment and teaching about iron rich foods
- Help to breastfeeding mothers to save the milk for the baby.

RETAINED PLACENTA

The placenta is said as retained when it is not expelled out even after 30 minutes of the birth of the baby.

Causes

There are three physiological phases involved in the normal expulsion of the placenta:
1. Separation through the spongy layer of the decidua.
2. Descend into the lower uterine segment and vagina.
3. Expulsion to outside.

Interference with any of these physiological processes results in its retention in the following manner:
- Placenta completely separated but retained. This is due to poor voluntary expulsive efforts specially following prolonged and exhaustive labor
- Simple adherent placenta due to uterine atonicity in case of grand multipara, over distention of uterus, prolonged labor, bigger placental surface area or uterine malformation. The commonest cause of retention of nonseparated placenta is atonic uterus
- Placenta becomes incarcerated following partial or complete separation due to construction ring (hour-glass contraction). This may be due to intravenous ergometrine given at the delivery of anterior shoulder, premature attempts to deliver the placenta before it is separated and unnecessary kneading or fiddling of the uterus
- Morbid adherent placenta—partial or rarely complete.

Signs of Retained Placenta

- Presence or absence of the features of placental separation depending on whether it is retained following separation or not

❖ Hour-glass contraction or the nature of adherence is diagnosed during manual removal.

Dangers

❖ Hemorrhage
❖ Shock due to blood loss, frequent attempts of abdominal manipulation to express the placenta out
❖ Puerperal sepsis
❖ Risk of its recurrence in subsequent pregnancies.

Management

❖ A separated placenta, that is retained, is expressed by controlled cord traction
❖ An unseparated retained placenta is removed manually under general anesthesia as described earlier. During manual removal, complications such as hour-glass contraction or morbid adherent placenta may be detected which are managed as follows:

Hour-glass contraction: The ring should be made to relax by (a) deepening the plane of anesthesia, (b) subcutaneous injection of 0.5 ml of one in 1,000 adrenaline hydrochloride or (c) inhalation of two amyl nitrate capsules of 5 minimum each.

If the ring is too tight and bleeding is absent, the operation is to be postponed. The woman is to be sedated with morphine 15 mg intramuscularly. After 4 to 6 hours of observation, manual removal is done.

If the ring is not too tight and bleeding is continuing, the ring is to be manually stretched by the cone-shaped hand, beginning at the upper border of the placenta in order to minimize bleeding.

Morbid adherent placenta: Diagnosis is made during attempted manual removal. On rare occasions, no cleavage between the placenta and the uterine wall is noted and a diagnosis of a total placenta accreta is made.

Complications Accompanying Retained Placenta and Management

❖ *Retained placenta with shock but not hemorrhage:* To treat the shock and when

the condition improves, manual removal is to be done, if not already separated
❖ *Retained placenta with hemorrhage:* Same management as outlined for third stage hemorrhage
❖ *Retained placenta with sepsis:* The woman is usually delivered outside and is admitted in the referral hospital after few hours or even days after delivery. Sepsis is a potential risk or may already be present. Intrauterine swabs are taken for culture and sensitivity test and broad spectrum antibiotic is given. Blood transfusion is usually required. On examination, if the placenta is found separated, it is expressed out. If found retained, manual removal is to be carried out as soon as the patient's general condition permits
❖ *Retained placenta with an episiotomy wound:* The bleeding points of the episiotomy wound are to be secured by artery forceps. A manual removal is done without delay followed by repair of episiotomy wound.

PLACENTA ACCRETA

Placenta accreta is an abnormal partial or total adherence of the placenta to the uterine wall. The placenta is directly adhered to the myometrium with either defective decidua or no decidua in between. When the chorionic villi extent further than contact with the myometrium and actually penetrate the uterine wall, the condition is called *placenta increta*. *Placenta percreta* occurs when the chorionic villi invade through the entire uterine wall to the serosa layer. These conditions are rare complications.

The probable cause is defective decidual formation. The condition is usually associated with placenta previa. It may also occur when the placenta is situated over injured sites as following cesarean section, dilatation and curettage operation, manual removal or myomectomy.

Diagnosis

❖ A partial placenta accreta is first seen as an acute third stage hemorrhage resulting from a partially separated placenta. Clinical diagnosis is made when the placenta's adherence is discovered during attempted manual removal of the retained placenta

❖ A complete placenta accreta has no signs and symptoms since there is no partial separation and, therefore, no hemorrhage. It is discovered during attempted manual removal of the retained placenta

❖ Definitive diagnosis of placenta accreta is made by microscopic examination. Pathological confirmation includes absence of decidua basalis, absence of fibrinoid layer and varying degrees of penetration of the villi in to the muscle bundles.

Placenta accreta is an obstetric disaster. Any suspicion that a retained placenta is due to placenta accreta requires that the midwife immediately place an urgent call for the physician. While waiting, the midwife must do all she can to maintain the woman and prepare her for immediate surgery.

Management

❖ In partial placenta accreta, where major separation is possible, the adherent area is separated manually leaving behind bits of placental tissue with the uterine wall. Oxytocin is administered for uterine contraction and intrauterine plugging to achieve hemostasis. If the uterus fails to contract, hysterectomy is done.

❖ In complete placenta accreta, hysterectomy is done in parous women. In women desiring to have another child, conservative management may be undertaken. This consists of cutting the umbilical cord as high as possible and leaving behind the placenta, which is expected to be autolysed in due course of time. Appropriate antibiotics are given.

Risks of placenta accreta include hemorrhage, shock, infection and rarely inversion of uterus.

INVERSION OF THE UTERUS

This is a rare but potentially life-threatening situation in which, the uterus is turned inside

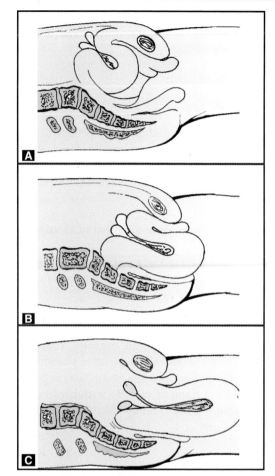

Figs 36.4A to C: Acute inversion of the uterus: (A) First degree; (B) Second degree; (C) Third degree

out partially or completely. The incidence is about 1 : 20,000 deliveries (Dutta, 2001). The obstetric inversion is usually an acute one and usually complete.

Classification of Inversion (Figs 36.4A to C)

❖ *First degree*: There is dimpling of the fundus, which remains above the level of the internal os

❖ *Second degree*: The uterus is inverted and the fundus passes through the cervix but lies inside the vagina

❖ *Third degree* (complete): The endometrium with or without the attached placenta is visible outside the vulva. The uterus, cervix and part of the vagina are inverted and visible.

Causes

The inversion may be spontaneous or more commonly induced.

Spontaneous (40%)

This is brought about by local atony of the placental site over the fundus associated with sharp rise of intra-abdominal pressure as in coughing, sneezing or bearing down effort. Fundal attachment of the placenta, short cord and placenta accreta are often associated.

Induced (60%)

This is due to mismanagement of third stage of labor.

*   Pulling the cord when the uterus is atonic specially when combined with fundal pressure
*   Crede's method of placental expression while the uterus is relaxed
*   Faulty technique in manual removal: Pulling the partially separated placenta, or firmly pressing on the atonic uterus by the external hand or rapidly withdrawing the internal hand thereby creating a negative pressure.

Dangers

*   Shock which is profound and mainly neurogenic in origin due to:
    *   Tension on the nerves from stretching of the infundibulopelvic ligament
    *   Pressure on the ovaries as they are dragged with the fundus
    *   Peritoneal irritation.
*   Hemorrhage, especially after detachment of the placenta
*   Pulmonary embolism
*   Infection and uterine sloughing, if left uncared.

Diagnosis (Signs and Symptoms)

*   Acute lower abdominal pain with bearing down sensation
*   Varying degree of shock
*   On abdominal examination:
    *   Dimpling or cupping of the fundal surface
    *   Fundus cannot be palpated.

*   Incomplete variety, a pear-shaped mass protrudes outside the vulva with the broad end pointing downwards and looking reddish-purple in color.

Management

Before Shock Develops

Immediate medical support must be summoned. Urgent manual replacement (even without anesthesia if not easily available) must be done as outlined below:

*   To push the fundus with the palm of the hand, along the direction of the vagina towards the posterior fornix
*   To apply counter support with the other hand placed on the abdomen
*   After replacement, the hand should remain inside the uterus until the uterus becomes contracted by parenteral oxytocis
*   The placenta is to be removed manually only after the uterus becomes contracted. A partially separated placenta may be removed prior to replacement to reduce the bulk, which facilitates replacement
*   Usual treatment of shock including blood transfusion should be arranged as and when required.

After Shock Develops

*   The treatment of shock should be instituted vigorously. Morphine 15 mg IM, dextrose saline drip and arrangements for blood transfusion to be made
*   To push the uterus inside the vagina if possible and to pack the vagina with antiseptic roller gauze
*   Foot end of the bed to be raised
*   Replacement of the uterus under general anesthesia to be done along with resuscitative measures.

If manual replacement fails, the method of hydrostatic replacement is instituted. This involves the instillation of warm saline through a douche nozzle. The pressure of the fluid builds up as several liters are run in to the vagina and restores the uterus to the normal position, while the operator seals off the introitus by one hand inserted into the vagina.

If the inversion cannot be manually replaced it may be due to the development of a cervical constriction ring. Drugs can be utilized to relax the constriction ring and facilitate the return of the uterus to its normal position.

Throughout the procedure, the woman and her husband and/or family should be kept informed of what is happening. Assessment of vital signs and level of consciousness is of great importance.

BIBLIOGRAPHY

1. Bonnar J, Mc Nicol GP. "Coagulation and fibrinolytic mechanisms during and after normal childbirth". British Medical Journal 1970;25:200-03.
2. Dutta DC. Textbook of Obstetrics 5th edn. Calcutta: New Central Book Company. 2001.
3. Levy V, Moore J. The midwife's management of the third stage of labor. Nursing times 1985;81(5):47-50.
4. McDonald S. Physiology and management of the third stage of labor. In: Bennett RV, Linda KB (Eds). Myles Textbook for Midwives, 13th Edn. Edinburgh: Churchill Livingstone. 1999.
5. Newton M, Mosey LM. Blood loss during and immediately after delivery. Obstetrics and Gynecology. 1961;17:9-18.

37

Injuries to the Birth Canal

Learning Objectives

Upon completing this chapter, the learner will be able to:

❖ Describe the causes of perineal lacerations and management including perineal repair
❖ Describe the perineal management at delivery and perineal care following delivery
❖ Discuss the causes, detection and management of women in the event of uterine rupture.

LACERATIONS OF PERINEUM

Injuries to the birth canal commonly occur during childbirth and contribute significantly to maternal morbidity. The maternal genital tract injuries occur in both natural and instrumental deliveries. Avoidance, early detection and effective management can minimize the morbidity and prevent gynecological problems in future life.

Injuries to Vulva

Lacerations of the vulval skin posteriorly and the paraurethral tear on the inner aspect of the labia minora are common sites. Paraurethral tears often bleed briskly as the labia are highly vascular. Prompt repair may be necessary to secure hemostasis.

Perineal Tears

The perineum may be torn due to several factors.
❖ Over stretching of the perineum due to large baby, face delivery, outlet contraction with narrow pubic arch, shoulder dystocia and forceps delivery
❖ Rapid stretching of the perineum due to rapid delivery of the head during uterine contraction, precipitate labor and delivery of the after coming head in breech
❖ Inelastic perineum as in rigid perineum in elderly primigravidae, scar in the perineum following previous operations, such as episiotomies or perineorrhaphy and vulval edema
❖ Unattended delivery and inability of the woman to stop bearing down.

Classification

Spontaneous tears are usually classified in degrees, which are related to the anatomical structures, which have been traumatized. The classification only serves as a guideline because it is often difficult to identify the structures precisely.

First Degree

Involves lacerations of the fourchette (lower end of the posterior vagina) only.

Second Degree

Involves the fourchette and the superficial perineal muscles, namely the bulbocavernosus and the transverse perineal muscles and in some cases the pubococcygeus.

Third Degree (Complete Tear)

Involves in addition to the above structures, the anal sphincter.

Fourth Degree (Central Tear)

The tear extends to the rectal mucosa.

Prevention

Conduct of second stage of delivery with due care in those with increased likelihood of laceration.

- Maintain flexion of the head until the occiput comes under the symphysis pubis so that lesser suboccipitofrontal (10 cm) diameter emerges out of the introitus
- Assure the woman not to bear down during contractions to avoid forcible delivery of the head
- Deliver the head in between contractions
- Perform timely episiotomies
- Take care during delivery of the shoulders.

Management

Tears must be repaired immediately following the delivery of the placenta in order to minimize blood loss and to reduce the chance of infection. In case of delay beyond 24 hours, the repair is to be withheld. Antiseptic dressing and antibiotics are given and the wound allowed to heal by granulation tissue or repaired after the infection is controlled. Complete tears (Third degree) that are delayed beyond 24 hours are repaired after 3 months.

Repair

The woman is placed in lithotomy position. A good source of light is essential. Vagina, vulva and perineal region are swabbed with antiseptic solution and the area is draped. Perineal infiltration is carried out by the physician with 1 percent lignocaine hydrochloride (10–20 ml). Infiltration is not required if the delivery is conducted under pudendal block or epidural anesthesia. In complete tear, general anesthesia may be administered.

In the first and second degree tears, the vaginal mucosa is sutured first. The first suture is placed at or just above apex of the tear. Thereafter, the vaginal walls are apposed by interrupted sutures with chromic catgut number '0' using curved, round body needle from above downwards until the fourchette is reached.

In third degree perineal tear, the rectal and anal mucosa are sutured first from above downwards with chromic catgut number '00' by interrupted stitches using curved atraumatic needle. Muscle walls and facia are then sutured by interrupted stitches using the same materials. The torn ends of the sphincter ani are then reconstituted with a figure of eight stitch using number '0' chromic catgut.

Repair of the perineal muscles is done in two layers by interrupted sutures using number '0' chromic catgut.

The perineal skin is apposed by interrupted sutures either with chromic catgut or nylon or silkworm gut using a cutting needle. The sutured area should be inspected in order to confirm hemostasis before the vaginal pack is removed. A vaginal examination is made to ensure that the introitus has not been narrowed. Upon completion, a rectal examination is done in order to ensure that no sutures have penetrated the rectal mucosa. Any such sutures if found must be removed to prevent fistula formation.

The area is cleaned and a sterile, sanitary pad placed over the vulva and perineum. The mother's legs are then removed gently and simultaneously from the lithotomy supports and she is made comfortable.

Aftercare

- The mother should be given explanation about the nature of trauma and repair and information given on whether or not the sutures will need to be removed
- A low residue diet is given from the second day onwards
- Stool softeners, such as mild milk of magnesia are given twice daily. If the woman does not pass stool and has discomfort, a small quantity enema (fleet enema or oil enema) is given
- Intestinal antiseptics, such as metronidazole are given for 5 to 7 days.

Vaginal Tears

Vaginal lacerations without involvement of the perineum or cervix sometimes occur. The most common site is the lower third of the vagina. The lower end of the vagina may be torn transversely from its junction with the perineum, leaving a deep cavity behind an intact perineum. Injuries of the upper and lower third of the vagina are rare. These are usually seen following instrumental or manipulative delivery. In such cases, the tears are extensive and often associated with active bleeding.

Management

A vaginal tear is sutured by interrupted or continuous sutures using chromic catgut number '0'. In case of extensive lacerations, in addition to sutures, hemostasis may be achieved by intravaginal plugging by roller gauze soaked with glycerine and acriflavine. The plug should be removed after 24 hours.

Colporrhexis

Rupture of the vault of the vagina is called colporrhexis. It may be primary where only the vault is involved or secondary when associated with cervical tear (more common). It is said to be complete when the peritoneum is opened up. The tear may be traumatic or spontaneous especially in multiparae.

Treatment is exploration and repair from below if the tear is limited to the vault and accessible part of the cervix. If however, the tear extends high up into the lower segment, laparotomy is to be done simultaneously with resuscitative measures.

Cervical Tears

Minor degrees of cervical tears often occur during first delivery. Major extensive tears requiring attention is also common. This is the commonest cause of traumatic postpartum hemorrhage.

Causes

* *Iatrogenic:* Attempted forceps delivery or breech extraction through an incompletely dilated cervix
* *Rigid cervix:* This may be congenital or due to scarring from previous operations on the cervix
* Strong uterine contractions as in precipitate labor
* Extremely vascular cervix as in placenta previa
* *Detachment of the cervix:* Annular detachment of the cervix may occur following prolonged labor in primary cervical dystocia
* Partial detachment may occur when the cervix is caught between the head and the pelvic wall
* Failure to remove a circlage suture
* Congenital elongation of the cervix or vaginouterine prolapse.

Signs of Cervical Tear

Excessive vaginal bleeding following delivery in the presence of a hard and contracted uterus is suggestive of cervical tear. Exploration of the uterovaginal canal under good light is essential to confirm the diagnosis and assess the tear.

Management

Minor tears require no treatment. Deep cervical tears associated with bleeding should be repaired soon after delivery of the placenta. The repair should be done under general anesthesia in lithotomy position with a good light.

PELVIC HEMATOMAS

Collections of blood anywhere in the area between the pelvic peritoneum and the peritoneal skin are called pelvic hematoma.

Anatomical Types

Depending upon the location of the hematoma, whether below or above the levator ani muscle, it is termed as:
* Infralevator hematoma
* Supralevator hematoma.

Infralevator Hematoma

Vulval hematoma is the commonest in this type.

Causes

* Trauma of spontaneous labor, prolonged labor and forceps operations resulting in rupture of paravaginal venous plexus
* Improper hemostasis during repair of vaginal or perineal tears or episiotomy wound
* Rough uterine massage for controlling postpartum hemorrhage may cause development of small hematomas in the supraperitoneal connective tissue and in the broad ligaments.

Manifestations

* Persistent, severe pain in the perineal region

- Rectal tenesmus or bearing down efforts when extension occurs to the ischio-rectal fossa
- Retention of urine
- Variable degrees of shock or collapse
- Tense swelling at the vulva which becomes dusky and purple in color and tender to touch
- Pallor, rapid pulse and low blood pressure
- A tender pelvic lump on palpation.

Treatment

A small hematoma (<5 cm) is treated conservatively with cold compress. When it is larger than 5 cm or increasing in size, it needs to be evacuated. The patient is given blood and narcotic analgesics for pain.

The hematoma is drained under general anesthesia and bleeding points are secured. The dead space is to be obliterated by deep mattress sutures and a closed suction drain may be kept for 24 hours. Prophylactic antibiotic is to be administered.

Supralevator Hematoma

Causes

- Extension of cervical laceration or primary vault rupture (colporrhexis)
- Lower uterine segment rupture
- Spontaneous rupture of paracervical venous plexus adjacent to the vault.

Diagnosis

- Unexplained shock with features of shock following delivery
- Abdominal examination reveals swelling above the inguinal ligament pushing the uterus to the opposite side
- Vaginal examination reveals occlusion of the vaginal canal by a bulge or a bogy swelling felt through the fornix
- Ultrasonography may show the exact localization of the hematoma.

Management

- Treatment of shock
- Exploratory laparotomy and drainage of the hematoma (blood clots are scooped out)

- The bleeding points, if seen, are to be secured and ligated
- Any injury to the uterus and/or cervix is repaired
- The broad ligament is drained extraperitoneally using corrugated rubber drain
- Bilateral internal iliac artery ligation may be required to control bleeding.

RUPTURE OF THE UTERUS

Rupture of the uterus is an uncommon injury and when it happens, it can be a catastrophic event, as it places the mother and fetus at high risk for morbidity and mortality.

Definition

A rupture is defined as an abrupt tearing of the uterus and can be complete or incomplete.

Classification of Rupture

Scar Rupture and Dehiscence

- In scar rupture disruption of the entire length of the scar occurs. With classical scars, rupture occurs late in pregnancy or early labor. Bleeding is slight unless the placenta is lying underneath. Rupture lower segment scars occur with obstructed labor. It is accompanied by a "tearing pain". Bleeding may not be heavy
- Dehiscence is disruption of part of the scar and not the entire length. It tends not to cause any bleeding and is without clinical significance.

Complete and Incomplete Rupture

- Complete uterine rupture extends through the entire wall and peritoneum with the entire contents spilling into the abdominal cavity
- An incomplete uterine rupture extends through the endometrium and myometrium without involving the peritoneum.

Spontaneous and Traumatic Rupture

- A spontaneous rupture is one that occurs during labor owing to a myometrium weakened by a previous scar

❖ A traumatic uterine rupture may be caused by trauma resulting from obstetric instruments, obstetric interventions or accidents such as fall or blow on the abdomen.

Risk Factors

❖ A tumultuous labor resulting from oxytocin induction when not controlled carefully
❖ Multiparity combined with use of oxytocin
❖ Obstructed labor such as with absolute CPD
❖ Accidents such as falling face downwards
❖ Trauma due to forceps, breech extraction or internal version late in labor
❖ Excessive fundal pressure
❖ Shoulder dystocia.

Signs and Symptoms

❖ Exquisite abdominal pain: When the rupture is complete, the woman experiences a transient relief from pain followed by cessation of contractions
❖ Vaginal bleeding
❖ Intra-abdominal bleeding, which may lead to rapid collapse. Blood may be confined retroperitoneally as a broad ligament hematoma
❖ Lack of progress in labor
❖ Shock from hemorrhage (hypovolemic shock)
❖ Alteration in shape of abdominal swelling. The uterus contracts and may be mistaken for a fetal head in the suprapubic region
❖ Palpation of fetal parts outside the uterine wall (superficial fetal parts): The fetus is wholly or partly extruded into the abdominal cavity and quickly dies whether or not the tear is complete or incomplete (complete when the peritoneum is also torn through)
❖ Rapid onset of fetal distress progressing to absence of fetal heart sounds
❖ Restlessness and anxiety
❖ An empty pelvis on vaginal examination.
  Dehiscence of a lower segment scar may cause virtually no bleeding or shock and is described as silent rupture. The injury is discovered only on section for delay in labor.

Management

❖ Emergency cesarean delivery with repair of the rupture, if the woman is undelivered and the symptoms are not severe

❖ Cesarean hysterectomy, if the tear is severe and cannot be repaired.

Nursing Care

❖ Continuous assessment of the woman who is predisposed to develop a rupture. In those with classical cesarean scar, the rupture is likely to occur even before labor begins
❖ Monitor the progress of labor carefully in order to facilitate early identification or abnormal symptoms
❖ Cautious use of oxytocin in women with uterine scar.

Once a Rupture is Diagnosed

❖ Monitor maternal and fetal vital signs and fluid status
❖ Administer oxygen for the benefit of both mother and fetus
❖ Urinary catheterization to be done and mother to be prepared for surgery
❖ Provide information to the woman and her family of the situation, interventions being planned and the prognosis
❖ Emotional support to the woman and her immediate family.

VISCERAL INJURIES

Injury to bladder may be due to:

Trauma
1. During instrumental vaginal delivery such as forceps delivery or destructive operations.
2. Abdominal operation, such as hysterectomy for rupture of uterus or repeat cesarean section.

Sloughing Fistula
This results from prolonged compression of the bladder between the fetal head and symphysis pubis in obstructed labor.

Clinical Manifestations

Traumatic
❖ Urine dribbles out following the operative surgery
❖ Blood stained urine following cesarean section or hysterectomy.

Sloughing Fistula

❖ Dribbling of urine occurs after varying interval following prolonged labor (5-7 days)

❖ Missing of a chunk of tissue seen on examination.

Management

Immediate repair is preferable for traumatic fistula, if the woman's general condition is good and facilities are available.

In unfavorable condition, a self-retaining catheter is introduced and kept for 10 to 14 days. Urinary antiseptics are given and bladder wash done daily. Spontaneous closure may occur and if it does not, repair is done after three months.

Injury to the Rectum

Rectal injury is rare because the middle third of the rectum is protected by the curved sacral hollow and the upper third is protected by the peritoneal lining. Prolonged compression of the rectum by the head in midpelvic contraction with a flat sacrum predisposes to ischemic necrosis of the anterior rectal wall and results in rectovaginal fistula. The repair in such cases should be postponed for at least three months.

Injury to the Urethra

Urethral injury may be traumatic resulting from instrumental delivery or during pubotomy. It may occur due to ischemic sloughing, the mechanism of which is similar to that of bladder necrosis. The principles of management are similar to those of bladder injury.

BIBLIOGRAPHY

1. Dutta DC. Textbook of Obstetrics, 5th edn. Calcutta: New Central Book Company, 2001.
2. Grant A. Repair of episiotomies and perineal tears. British Journal of Obstetrics and Gynecology, 1986;93:176-78.
3. Grant A. Repair of perineal trauma after childbirth. In: Chalmers I, Enkin M (Eds). Effective Care in Pregnancy and Childbirth. Oxford: Oxford University Press, 1989.
4. Harrison RF. Brennan M. "Is routine episiotomies necessary. British Medical Journal 1984;288:1971-5.
5. Hillan EM. Physiology and management of the second stage of labor, In: Myles Textbook for Midwives, 13th edn. Edinburgh: Churchill Livingstone, 1999.
6. Varney Helen. Nurse-Midwifery, 2nd edn. Boston: Jones and Barlett Publishers, 1999.

38

Complications of Puerperium

PUERPERAL PYREXIA

An elevation of temperature to 38°C (100.4°F) or more occurring on two separate occasions at 24 hours apart (excluding the first 24 hours) within the first 10 days following delivery is called puerperal pyrexia.

Causes

❖ Puerperal sepsis
❖ Urinary tract infection: Cystitis, pyelonephritis
❖ Breast infection
❖ Infection of laparotomy wound (cesarean section)
❖ Intercurrent infection: Acute bronchitis, pneumonia, influenza, acute appendicitis and enteric fever
❖ Thrombophlebitis
❖ Deep vein thrombosis
❖ Flaring up of tuberculosis

Puerperal sepsis is thought to be due to genital tract infection unless proved otherwise.

PUERPERAL SEPSIS

Definition

It is an infection of the genital tract, which occurs as a complication of delivery.

Conditions that Favor the Development of Sepsis

The vaginal flora in late pregnancy and during labor consists of the following organisms: *Doderleins bacillus, Candida albicans, Staphylococcus albus* or *aureus, Streptococcus, E. coli* and *Clostridium welchii* on occasion. These organisms remain dormant and are harmless during normal delivery, conducted in aseptic condition. However, the following conditions favor the development of sepsis in puerperal women:

❖ Damage to the cervicovaginal mucous membrane
❖ The open wound created by the cleavage of the decidua, which takes place when the placenta is separated (placental site)
❖ The blood clots at the placental site are an excellent media for the growth of bacteria.

Predisposing Factors of Puerperal Sepsis

Antepartum Factors

❖ Malnutrition and anemia
❖ Pre-eclampsia
❖ Premature rupture of membranes
❖ Chronic debilitating illness
❖ Sexual intercourse during late pregnancy.

Intrapartum Factors

❖ Introduction of organisms in to the upper genital tract during vaginal examinations especially after rupture of membranes' during manipulative delivery
❖ Dehydration and ketoacidosis during labor (prolonged labor)
❖ Traumatic operative delivery
❖ Hemorrhage antepartum or postpartum
❖ Retained bits of placental tissue or membranes
❖ Placental site lying close to vagina (placenta previa).

Organisms

The organisms responsible for puerperal sepsis are the following:

❖ Aerobic: *Staphylococcus pyogenes, E. coli, Klebsiella, Pseudomonas, Staphylococcus aureus, nonhemolytic Streptococcus*
❖ Anaerobic: Anaerobic *Streptococcus, Clostridium welchii, Clostridium tetani, Bacteroides.*

Mode of Infection

Puerperal sepsis is essentially a wound infection. Placental site (being a raw surface), lacerations of the genital tract or cesarean section wounds may be infected in the following ways.

❖ *Endogenous:* Organisms present in the genital tract before delivery become pathogenic
❖ *Autogenous:* Organisms present elsewhere in the body migrate to the genital organs either through bloodstream or by droplet infection or are conveyed to the site by the woman herself or her attendants. Common sites from where organisms are transferred include septic throat, feces and skin infection
❖ *Exogenous:* Infection is contracted from sources outside the client. The organisms are introduced by the attendants, usually from the respiratory tract of physicians or nurses. The infection may be dust borne or as droplet and may occur during vaginal examination or from contaminated linen.

Pathology

Puerperal infection is a wound infection. The primary sites of infection are perineum, vagina, cervix and uterus.

❖ *Perineum:* Lacerations of the perineum are likely to be infected. The wound edges become red and swollen. There may be collections of sanguinopurulent discharge or pus resulting in complete disruption of the wound
❖ *Vagina:* The vaginal lacerations are infected directly or by extension from the perineal infection. The mucosa is swollen and hyperemic, resulting in necrosis and sloughing
❖ *Cervix:* The cervical lacerations become the site of infection
❖ *Uterus:* The uterus is the most common site of infection. The decidua over the placental site is the common site to be infected first. The infection usually manifests between the third and sixth day of delivery. Uterine infection is termed as *endometritis.* In *putrid endometritis,* the decidua becomes infected and necrosed and sloughs off. The infection to the deeper myometrium is prevented by a zone of leukocytic barrier. The discharge becomes offensive

Invasion to the myometrium and spread to the distant sites may occur when the infection is severe by organisms like beta *hemolytic streptococci.*

Spread of infection to other sites may lead to the following:

❖ *Pelvic cellulites (parametritis):* Infection of the pelvic peritoneum and levator ani muscle
❖ *Salpingitis:* Infection of the fallopian tubes and ovaries with formation of tubo-ovarian mass
❖ *Peritonitis:* Localized pelvic abscess or generalized infection
❖ *Thrombophlebitis:* Ovarian vein of one side is usually involved. Uterine veins may also be involved
❖ *Septicemia and pyemia:* These may lead to endocarditis, pericarditis, renal abscess, lung abscess, meningitis or arthritis. These are rare these days with the advent of potent antibiotics.

Clinical Features

Local Infection

- Slight rise of temperature, generalized malaise or headache
- Redness and swelling of the local wound
- Pus formation and disruption of wound.

Uterine Infection

- Pyrexia of variable degrees and tachycardia
- Red, copious and offensive lochia
- Subinvoluted, tender and soft uterus.

With Severe Infection

- Fever with chills and rigor
- Rapid pulse
- Scanty, odorless lochia
- Involuted uterus.

Parametritis

- Sustained rise of temperature (7th to 10th day)
- Constant pelvic pain
- Tenderness on either side of the hypogastrium
- Unilateral, tender mass felt on vaginal examination
- Leukocytosis.

Pelvic Peritonitis

- Pyrexia with increased pulse rate
- Lower abdominal pain and tenderness
- On vaginal examination, tenderness of the fornix and with movement of the cervix
- Collection of pus in the pouch of Douglas.

General Peritonitis

- High fever with rapid pulse
- Vomiting
- Generalized abdominal pain
- Tender and distended abdomen.

Thrombophlebitis

- Swinging temperature with chills and rigor
- Features of pyemia according to the organs involved.

Septicemia

- High temperature associated with rigor
- Rapid pulse

- Headache, insomnia or mental confusion
- Positive blood culture
- Symptoms and signs of metastatic infection in the lungs, meninges or joints.

Investigations

1. Bacteriological study:
   - Smear
   - Culture and antibiotic sensitivity of purulent material
   - High vaginal and cervical swabs
   - Peritoneal fluid
   - Blood culture as appropriate.
2. Urine: Routine and microscopic examination
   - Culture if infection is suspected.
3. Complete blood count.
4. Ultrasonography: For diagnosis of pelvic masses, pelvic abscess, pelvic peritonitis, retained bits of placenta and/or membranes.
5. Other specific investigations as per clinical condition such as chest X-ray or blood for malaria parasites.

Prevention

Antenatal

- Improvement of general condition
- Treatment of septic focci
- Abstinence from sexual intercourse in the last two months
- Care about personal hygiene—bathing in dirty water to be avoided
- Avoiding contact with people having infection, such as cold, boils
- Avoiding unnecessary vaginal examinations and douches in the later months.

Intrapartum

- Staff (physicians and nurses) attending on labor clients should be free of infections
- Full surgical asepsis to be taken while conducting delivery
- Women having respiratory tract infection or skin infection should be admitted in single room or separate ward
- Membranes should be kept intact as long as possible and vaginal examination should be restricted to minimum
- Traumatic vaginal delivery and intrauterine manipulation should be preferably avoided. If required, should be done using

fresh (sterile) gloves with liberal use of strong antiseptic solutions

* Lacerations of the genital tract should be repaired promptly and meticulously with perfect hemostasis
* Excessive blood loss during delivery should be replaced promptly by transfusion to improve the general body resistance
* Prophylactic antibiotics must be administered in cases of premature rupture of membranes, prolonged labor or following traumatic delivery.

Postpartum

* Nurses to take aseptic precautions while dressing the perineal wound
* Restriction of visitors in the postpartum ward
* Mothers to be instructed to use sterile sanitary pads and to change them frequently
* Vulva and perineum to be washed/cleaned with mild antiseptic solution following urination and defecation
* Infected mothers and babies are to be isolated
* To keep the floor of the in-patient ward dust free by frequent mopping (wet swabbing).

Treatment

* The woman should be placed in a separate room/ward with adequate light and ventilation
* Complete rest is to be given in head high position, which helps in drainage of lochia and localization of infection to the pelvis if there is pelvic peritonitis
* Analgesics and sedatives are administered to enforce rest
* Broad-spectrum antibiotics are given intravenously until antibiotic sensitivity reports are available, followed by specific antibiotics
* Stool softeners are administered (milk of magnesia at bed-item) to keep the bowels open
* Anemia to be corrected by blood transfusion
* Infected wounds of perineum, vulva and vagina are laid open for drainage, cleaned and dressed with antiseptic preparations.

Surgical Treatment

* The stitches of the perineal wound may have to be removed to facilitate drainage of pus and relieve pain. After the infection is controlled, secondary sutures may be given later
* Infected retained products should be removed as early as possible under cover of antibiotics by digital exploration of the uterine cavity
* Pelvic abscess should be drained by colpotomy
* Abscess above the Poupart's ligaments should be incised and the pus drained.

NURSING PROCESS FOR MOTHERS WITH PUERPERAL SEPSIS

Assessment

Assess for the following clinical manifestations:

* Elevated temperature 38°C (101°F) or above with chills
* Foul smelling lochia
* Abdominal tenderness and pelvic pain
* Pain and burning on urination
* Tachycardia
* Increased WBC
* Presence of predisposing
  - Traumatic birth
  - Prolonged difficult labor
  - Dehydration
  - Excessive vaginal discharge
  - Pronged rupture of membranes
  - Anemia
  - Retained placental fragment
  - Hemorrhage.
* Mother frustrated due to extreme fatigue
* May appear uncooperative and uninterested.

Analysis/Nursing Diagnosis

* Risk for injury
* Knowledge deficit
* Interrupted breastfeeding
* Fluid deficit
* Impaired gas exchange
* Fear
* Body image disturbance
* Ineffective individual coping
* Self-care deficit

- ❖ Altered family process
- ❖ Risk for altered mother-baby attachment.

Planning

- ❖ Provide teaching regarding hygienic measures
- ❖ Administer treatment specific to infection
- ❖ Provide opportunities to express feelings
- ❖ Provide education for self-care.

Implementation

- ❖ Assess vital signs every 2 to 4 hours
- ❖ Obtain cultures, blood and urine samples
- ❖ Evaluate pain and lochia
- ❖ Provide routine postpartum care
- ❖ Use meticulous hand washing techniques
- ❖ Teach hand washing to mother
- ❖ Provide warm sitz baths and compresses or heat lamp
- ❖ Provide reassurance and support
- ❖ Isolate woman as indicated.

Evaluation

Ensure that woman:

- ❖ Demonstrates hand washing and verbalizes understanding of hygienic measures
- ❖ Continue ordered medications to full recovery
- ❖ Verbalizes feelings and increased ability to cope
- ❖ Verbalizes understanding of self-care measures to treat infection, prevent infection and increase comfort.

SUBINVOLUTION OF THE UTERUS

Subinvolution of the uterus is impaired and deficient involution of the uterus following delivery.

Causes of Subinvolution

Predisposing Factors

- ❖ Grand multiparity
- ❖ Over-distension of uterus as in twins and hydramnios
- ❖ Maternal ill health
- ❖ Cesarean section
- ❖ Prolapse of the uterus
- ❖ Uterine fibroids (leiomyomas)
- ❖ No sucking of the baby.

Aggravating Factors

- ❖ Retained products of conception
- ❖ Uterine sepsis
- ❖ Retention of lochia (lochiametra).

Clinical Features

- ❖ Excessive or prolonged discharge of lochia
- ❖ Irregular or excessive uterine bleeding
- ❖ Irregular cramp like pain
- ❖ Uterine height more than normal for the particular day of postpartum.

Subsequently the patient may suffer from conditions such as uterine prolapse or retroversion, which is the cause of subinvolution.

Management

Subinvolution is managed by treating the cause.

- ❖ Antibiotics for sepsis
- ❖ Exploration of the uterus for retained products
- ❖ Pessary in prolapse or retroversion.

BREAST COMPLICATIONS

The common breast complications in puerperium are breast engorgement, cracked and retracted nipple, mastitis, breast abscess and failing lactation.

Breast Engorgement

Breast engorgement may occur due to excessive production of milk, obstruction to outflow of milk or poor removal of milk by the baby. It usually manifests after the milk secretion starts (3rd or 4th postpartum day).

Symptoms

- ❖ Both breasts feel tender, tense and firm
- ❖ Nipples become edematous and flushed
- ❖ The veins over the breasts become engorged and prominent
- ❖ Generalized malaise and rise of temperature
- ❖ Painful breastfeeding.

Preventive Measures

- ❖ To initiate breastfeeding early and feeding at frequent intervals

❖ Exclusive breastfeeding on demand
❖ Feeding in correct position (sitting).

Management

❖ Support the breasts with a binder or brassiere
❖ Manual expression of any milk after each feeding and keeping the interval short between feeds
❖ Analgesics for pain
❖ The cause of poor sucking by the newborn should be corrected.

Cracked and Retracted Nipple

The nipple may become painful due to loss of surface epithelium with the formation of a raw area on the nipple or due to a fissure situated at the tip or the base of the nipple. These two conditions often co-exist, which are referred to as the cracked nipple.

Causes

❖ Inadequate hygiene resulting in the formation of a crust over the nipple
❖ Retracted nipple
❖ Vigorous sucking and an inadequate milk flow.

The woman experiences soreness and pain at the site of the fissure. The fissure may become infected. When infected, the infection may spread to the deeper tissue producing mastitis and hence, it should be treated vigorously.

Prophylaxis includes local cleanliness during pregnancy, and in the puerperium before and after each breastfeeding to prevent crust formation over the nipple.

Treatment

❖ Application of tincture of benzoin after the night feeding and the fissure is likely to be healed in 8 to 12 hours
❖ The nipple is to be kept dry and exposed to air
❖ Breast milk should be removed by manual expression or pump
❖ If infected, an antiseptic cream is applied locally
❖ If it fails to heal, breastfeeding from the affected breast is stopped for 24 hours.

Retracted Nipple

It is common in primigravidae. If left uncorrected, it may lead to difficulty in breastfeeding and predispose to cracked nipple. Manually pulling out the retracted nipple during the last two months of pregnancy is useful to rectify the defect. After delivery, the nipple is pulled out by the suction action of a disposable syringe. The procedure may have to be repeated for few days.

Acute Mastitis

There are two types of mastitis:
1. Infection follows a cracked nipple to involve the breast parenchymal tissues leading to cellulites. The lacteal system remains unaffected.
2. Infection reaches the lactiferous ducts leading to the development of primary mammary adenitis.

In either type, the responsible organism is predominantly *Staphylococcus aureus*. In superficial cellulites, the onset is acute during the first week of puerperium. In mammary adenitis, the onset is insidious and usually occurs near the end of the second week. The infection may occur even several weeks after the delivery.

Clinical Features

❖ Generalized malaise and headache
❖ Fever (102°F or over) with chills
❖ Severe pain and swelling in one quadrant of the breast with its apex at the nipple
❖ The overlying skin is hot and flushed and feels tense and tender.

If not treated adequately, it can lead to destruction of breast tissues with the formation of a breast abscess.

Treatment

❖ *Prophylactic:* Antenatal care to nipple, prevention of engorgement and isolation of the infected baby.
❖ Curative
   – Isolation of mother and baby
   – Suspension of breastfeeding on the affected side until the infection is controlled

– Manual expression of milk to relieve engorgement
– Suppression of lactation by bromocriptine (parlodel) 2.5 mg orally for 14 days
– Antibiotic therapy for at least ten days
– Analgesics and sedatives as required.

Breast Abscess

Features of breast abscess are flushed breasts, brawny edema, marked tenderness and swinging temperature. If an abscess is formed, it is to be drained under general anesthesia. The cavity is packed with gauze, which should be replaced after 24 hours, by a smaller pack. The procedure is continued until it heals up.

Failing Lactation

Causes

❖ Debilitating state of the mother
❖ Elderly primigravidae
❖ Failure to suckle the baby regularly
❖ Depression or anxiety state in the puerperium
❖ Reluctance or apprehension to nursing
❖ Premature baby, who is too weak to suck
❖ Ill development of breasts
❖ Painful breast lesion.

Treatment

Antenatal

❖ Education regarding the advantages of breastfeeding
❖ Correction of abnormalities like retracted nipple
❖ Maintenance of adequate breast hygiene especially in the last two months of pregnancy
❖ Improving the general health status of the mother.

Postnatal

❖ Encourage adequate fluid intake
❖ Nurse the baby regularly
❖ Treat painful lesions promptly
❖ Express residual milk after each feeding
❖ Drugs like thyroid extract or prolactin are useful.

VENOUS THROMBOSIS

Thrombosis of the leg veins and pelvic veins is one of the common and important complications in the puerperium. The prevalence is low in Asian and African countries compared to western countries.

Causes

❖ Stasis of blood in the pelvic and leg veins, as in cases where the woman has been on prolonged bed rest during pregnancy and following operative delivery
❖ Alteration in the blood constituents: Continuation of hypercoagulable state
❖ *Infection*: Pelvic cellulites, which causes inflammation of the venous wall to which a thrombus may be attached
❖ Traumas to the venous wall: Pelvic veins are traumatized during labor due to the pressure of the fetal head
❖ Other high-risk factors, such as advancing age, high parity, use of estrogen, obesity, anemia, and heart disease.

Types

The puerperal venous thrombosis is classified as:
❖ *Phlebothrombosis*: Superficial, deep
❖ Thrombophlebitis
   In *phlebothrombosis*, the initial event is intravascular thrombosis. In *thrombophlebitis*, the initial event is inflammation of the venous wall to which the thrombus is attached.

Superficial Vein Thrombosis

Superficial thrombosis usually occurs in preexisting varicose veins in the legs. It usually remains localized. On rare occasion, it may spread upwards to involve the long saphenous vein and thence to the femoral vein. Detachment of the thrombus if occurs leads to *pulmonary embolism*. The onset is within the first week. There is pain and tenderness on the affected area. There may be slight rise in temperature and pulse rate. The overlaying skin looks red due to reaction of the clot. The condition subsides within a week with obliteration of the vein.

Deep Vein Thrombosis (DVT)

Deep vein thrombosis may develop as a primary condition or the deep vein may be involved secondarily as an extension of superficial venous thrombosis. Occasionally superficial and deep vein thrombosis occurs simultaneously.

Symptoms include pain in the calf or sole, swelling in the leg and often slight rise of temperature and pulse rate between the 7th and 10th day of postpartum.

On *examination,* there is calf tenderness on deep pressure and a positive Homan's sign—pain in the calf on dorsiflexion of the foot and edema of the leg.

Investigations

❖ Doppler ultrasound to detect the changes in the velocity of blood flow in the femoral vein
❖ Phlebography to note the filling defect in the venous lumen
❖ Isotopic venography to detect radioactivity.

Management

In high-risk situations, the following preventive measures are to be adopted.
❖ Leg movement and exercises
❖ Elastic stockings
❖ Active breathing exercises
❖ Avoiding sitting with legs dangling down
❖ Intermittent calf muscle compression: pneumonic cuff, passive dorsiflexion
❖ Prophylactic anticoagulant therapy
❖ Avoiding the use of estrogens for suppression of lactation.
Management measures for the client with DVT include:
❖ Bed rest with the foot end raised above the heart level
❖ Analgesics to relieve pain in the affected area and sedatives to ensure sleep
❖ Antibiotics
❖ Heparin therapy—15,000 units IV followed by 10,000 units 4 to 6 hourly. Heparin is continued for 7 to 10 days or even longer. *Warfarin* orally is commonly used in addition to heparin and may be continued for 3 to 6 months as maintenance therapy

❖ Gentle movement in bed to be started when the pain subsides, in about a week
❖ Caval filter may be inserted if there is a free-floating thrombus detected by scan or phlebogram.

Thrombophlebitis

Postpartum thrombophlebitis originates in the thrombosed veins at the placental site by organisms such as *anerobic streptococci* or bacteroides (fragilis). When localized in the pelvis, it is called *pelvic thrombophlebitis*. There is no specific clinical feature for pelvic thrombophlebitis but it is suspected when pyrexia continues for more than a week in the absence of any other cause in postnatal mothers.

Extrapelvic spread may reach to the lungs or kidney (left). Retrograde extension to ileo-femoral vein produces the clinico-pathological condition of *phlegmacia alba dolens* or *white leg.*

Clinical Features of Phlegmacia Alba Dolens

❖ Usually develops in the second week of postpartum
❖ Mild fever prior to local manifestations and at times fever with chills
❖ Headache, malaise and rising pulse rate
❖ Affected leg is painful, swollen, white and cold
❖ Tenderness and induration along the course of the femoral vein
❖ Polymorphonuclear leukocytosis seen on blood count.

Prevention and Management

Preventive and curative measures are the same as those outlined for deep vein thrombosis.

PULMONARY EMBOLISM

Pulmonary embolism occurs when part of a clot breaks away from a vessel wall and enters the systemic circulation. It causes an obstruction once it reaches a vessel with a lumen smaller than it and usually a pulmonary artery.

While deep venous thrombosis in the leg or in the pelvis is most likely, the cause of pulmonary embolism in 80 to 90 percent, it occurs without any previous clinical manifestations of deep vein thrombosis. The predisposing factors are those already mentioned in venous thrombosis.

Signs and Symptoms of Small Pulmonary Emboli

The clinical features depend on the size of the embolus and on the preceding health status of the mother. The classic symptoms of small emboli are:

❖ Chest pain
❖ Dyspnea, coughing, slight hemoptysis
❖ Pyrexia
❖ Tachycardia.

Any of the above symptoms, however slight, must be reported to the physician immediately. The woman should be offered reassurance and oxygen, if required, until medical assistance is obtained.

Signs and Symptoms of Major Pulmonary Embolism

❖ Sudden acute chest pain
❖ Marked distress, shock or sudden collapse
❖ Dyspnea, cyanosis
❖ Pyrexia, tachycardia/bradycardia, hypotension
❖ Distension of jugular veins.

This constitutes an obstetric emergency. If a major pulmonary artery becomes blocked, sudden acute chest pain will occur immediately followed by respiratory collapse, cardiac failure and possibly death. Death usually occurs within a short time from shock and vagal inhibition.

Diagnostic Procedures

❖ X-ray of the chest
❖ Lung scan
❖ Pulmonary angiography.

Treatment and Management

❖ Resuscitation—cardiac massage, oxygen therapy and intravenous heparin
❖ IV fluid support

❖ Blood pressure to be maintained by dopamine or adrenaline
❖ Thrombolytic therapy with streptokinase
❖ Tachycardia is counteracted with digitalis
❖ Pain may be relieved by intravenous morphine.

If the woman does not respond to this therapy or if repeated attacks occur, surgical treatment like embolectomy, placement of caval filter or ligation of inferior vena cava and ovarian veins may have to be done. Surgical treatment is done following pulmonary angiography.

PSYCHOLOGICAL DISTURBANCES IN THE PUERPERIUM

The events of pregnancy, labor and delivery together with the peak experience of giving birth, all contribute to a mixture of emotional reactions in the mother during the first week of puerperium. There are three distinctive types of psychological disturbances seen in the puerperium—postpartum blues (baby blues), postpartum depression and puerperal psychosis.

Postpartum Blues (Baby Blues)

It is a mild, benign and transient mood change that begins within 3 to 4 days after delivery and peaks on the 4th to 5th day. It affects nearly 7 in 10 mothers (Donica.com).

The most common symptom is unprovoked weeping and spikes of elation. Other symptoms include irritability, anger, hostility, headache, feelings of unreality, exhaustion, sleep deprivation and restlessness. Baby blues generally disappear without medical intervention within two weeks. If the symptoms persist longer, another diagnosis may be identified.

Social interventions, such as a relative baby-sitting for few hours, so that the mother can get some sleep or assistance with household chores or providing instruction on newborn care can often help significantly. Women who have this condition are likely to have it recur with subsequent pregnancies.

Postpartum Depression

The onset of postpartum depression is gradual, developing after the second week. The condition may last for 3 to 6 months and in some cases, it will persist throughout the first year of the baby's life. Such depression is disabling for the mother. It causes much disruption of family life and mother-baby relationships.

Causes

Postnatal depression is a reactive illness provoked by demand overload. A specific etiology is not known, however, certain contributory factors identified are:

❖ Experiencing stress-inducing life events around the time of childbirth such as bereavement or relationship disharmony
❖ Low self-esteem, lack of support and stress associated with postnatal care
❖ Severe 'maternal blues' later developing to depression
❖ Demands of motherhood and loss of personal freedom.

Diagnosis

Symptoms of postpartum depression are similar to those of depression occurring at any other time. Characteristic symptoms include bouts of crying, sadness and emotional liability, guilt, loss of appetite or anorexia, profound sleep disturbances, poor concentration and memory, irritability and feelings of inadequacy to care for the newborn or other children.

In postpartum depression, there is the tendency to experience difficulty falling asleep, but once asleep, the woman will sleep for long periods. They often feel well in the morning but deteriorate as the day goes on. In most other depression, early waking is the pattern with symptoms more acute in the morning. The woman may feel constantly tired in spite of adequate periods of rest and may appear over anxious about her baby in spite of evidence that the baby is well and thriving.

Some women may not communicate or admit their feelings. They conceal their depression so well that the condition may not be diagnosed for months. Knowledge of the individual woman and awareness of her body language may help to identify potential risk.

Management

Early detection and initiation of appropriate treatment brings the best prognosis. If the midwife suspects a woman is depressed, this should be reported to the physician.

In less severe cases, treatment with mild sedation or antidepressants may be prescribed. Counseling is known to be helpful, particularly if initiated at an early stage (Holden, 1990). Involvement of the spouse and other family members may also be advantageous. When the depression is more advanced, admission to a hospital will be necessary. Untreated or undiagnosed depression can evolve into a psychotic illness.

Puerperal Psychosis

The onset of puerperal psychosis is usually rapid, occurring within the first few days of delivery and rarely beyond the first 2 to 3 weeks. The condition is more common in primiparous women and in those who have suffered previous psychosis. No defined cause has been identified.

Diagnosis

Puerperal psychosis may have an acute onset. The woman may appear to be experiencing normal emotional adaptive responses to childbirth and may exhibit symptoms similar to those of maternal blues which is a psychological phenomenon manifested as unexplainable sadness and frequent bouts of crying.

These become more profound with extreme mood swings during which feelings of guilt or anxiety may be expressed. The euphoria following childbirth is seen extended and exaggerated in puerperal psychosis. The onset of symptoms may be heralded by a time of acute restlessness and inability to sleep. Subsequently the behavior of the woman may become bizarre. She may do or say inappropriate things or react out of character. She may experience delusions or hallucinations and become detached from the reality of her situation. She may state that her baby is abnormal, believe it to be possessed and may avoid the baby.

There may be periods of normal behavior and at other times, she may appear depressed. She may experience suicidal impulses or desires to harm her baby.

Treatment

Because of extreme nature of the illness, medical help is required as a matter of emergency. The woman must be kept under constant observation until appropriate psychiatric help is obtained.

Heavy sedation is given at the time of onset. Early treatment with antipsychotic drugs under the care of a psychiatric team is usually instituted. Admission to a psychiatric unit and treatment with lithium and/or electro convulsive therapy is given. Psychosis may persist for 8 to 10 weeks even with prompt treatment, especially when the woman has a pre-existing history of schizophrenia or manicdepressive illness.

Prognosis

Whilst complete recovery is often achieved, it is possible that further episodes of illness will occur throughout the woman's life and there is an increased risk of recurrence in subsequent pregnancies.

Role of the Midwife

The community midwife should continue to visit both mother and baby to undertake the nonpsychiatric aspects of postnatal care. Family support also needs consideration. The midwife needs to offer advice and support to women during subsequent pregnancies and to alert the physician regarding psychiatric care when appropriate, in order to initiate prompt referral, should it become necessary.

The community midwife should be able to help the mother reestablish the mother-baby relationship and to rebuild self-esteem by encouraging care of the baby within a safe environment.

BIBLIOGRAPHY

1. Calhoun BC, Brost B. Emergency management of sudden puerperal fever. In: Martin J (Ed). Intrapartum and postpartum obstetric emergencies. Obstetrics and Gynecology Clinics of North America 1995; 22(2):357-67.
2. Dutta DC. Textbook of Obstetrics, 5th edn. Calcutta; New Central Book Company, 2001.
3. Hynes L. Physiology, complications and management of the puerperium, In: Myles Textbook for Midwives, 13th edn. Edinburgh; Churchill Livingstone, 1999.
4. Llewellyn Jones D. Infections of the genital tract, Fundamental of Obstetrics and Gynecology, 6th edn. London; Mosby. 1994.
5. McKenzie CAM, Vestal KW. High-Risk Perinatal Nursing, St Louis. St. Louis; WB Sounders, 1983.
6. Neeson JD. Clinical Manual of Maternity Nursing. Philadelphia; JB Lippincott, 1987.
7. Ridgway LE. Puerperal emergency: Vaginal vulvar hematomas. Obstetrics and Gynecology Clinics of North America 1995;22(2):275-82.
8. www.drdonnica.com, Postpartum Depression, article 154.

SECTION

8

The Normal Neonate

39

The Baby at Birth

Learning Objectives

Upon completing this chapter, the learner will be able to:

❖ Identify the physiological changes that must occur for the newborn at birth to adapt to extrauterine life
❖ Identify the normal characteristics of the newborn
❖ Describe the care of the baby during and immediately after birth
❖ Identify factors to be considered when the baby fails to establish respirations at birth and describe the goals and methods of neonatal resuscitation.

Fig. 39.1: A healthy newborn
(*For color version see Plate 2*)

The transition from intrauterine to extra-uterine life presents a number of challenges for the newborn. To leave the nurturing environment of the mother's womb, it must endure intense contractions of the uterus and pass through the birth canal or the mother's abdomen to the waiting world. Upon birth, the newborn's body must establish circulation, initiate respirations and maintain its own metabolism—All tasks previously managed by the mother through the placenta. Incredible and formidable as all these tasks are, most newborns sail through this transition smoothly. Yet, when difficulty is encountered, an astute midwife is often the first to note the changes and alert the pediatrician so that prompt intervention can begin (Fig. 39.1).

EXTRAUTERINE ADAPTATION

In order to care for newborns, the midwife requires knowledge of the transition from the fetus to the newborn. All the systems in the nondistressed full-term neonate are adequate to adapt to extrauterine life immediately after birth. This complex process of change and instability is known as the transitional period. The midwife must know, understand and be aware of, as well as assess the changes that take place as the neonate goes through its transitional period.

Respiratory Changes

The respiratory system is the most challenged in the change from intrauterine to extrauterine environment. Upon arrival into an atmospheric environment, there is an immediate demand on the neonate for respiration. The organ responsible for fetal respiration prior to delivery is the placenta. Upon delivery, the lungs change from a fluid-filled state to a system well prepared for and capable of respiration.

The phenomenon that occurs to stimulate the neonate to take the first breath is believed to be a combination of biochemical changes and a number of physical stimuli to which the neonate is subjected, such as cold, gravity, pain, light and noise, which cause excitation of the respiratory center. The first active breaths of air, once taken and sustained, set in motion a nearly inexorable chain of events that:

- ❖ Converts the fetal circulation to adult circulation
- ❖ Empties the lung of fluid
- ❖ Establishes the neonatal lung volume and the characteristics of pulmonary functions.

The primary concern at the time of delivery is the establishment of respiration. The prompt onset of breathing is essential to subsequent mental and physical development.

When the head is delivered, mucus drains from the nares and mouth. Many neonates gasp and even cry at this time. Therefore, suctioning the mouth and nares with a bulb syringe or mucus sucker to prevent aspiration of mucus or amniotic fluid may be necessary as soon as the head is accessible. More mucus will be noted as the body is compressed during delivery. This release of fluid allows air to be taken into the lungs.

Gentle rubbing of the neonates back, flicking the sole of the foot, or vigorous drying of the infant to reduce heat loss are sufficient aids in stimulation of respiration. If stimulation is too vigorous, such as slapping or exposure to extreme cold, it becomes distressful and tends to inhibit respirations.

Sustained regular respirations are established normally within 60 seconds of delivery and are accompanied by simultaneous changes occurring in the cardiovascular system.

Circulatory Changes

With the initiation of respiration, the fetal circulation undergoes changes that allow the newborn to sustain extrauterine existence. These begin with the clamping of the umbilical cord and the first breath taken by the newborn. Korones (1986) identifies five attributes of fetal circulation that must be altered for the infant to make the switch from the fetal to mature circulation.

- ❖ Closure of the ductus arteriosus
- ❖ Closure of the foramen ovale
- ❖ Closure of the ductus venosus
- ❖ Decreased pulmonary vascular resistance
- ❖ Increased aortic blood pressure.

These changes are initiated in the normal infant by the clamping of the cord and the first breath. This eliminates the placental supply of oxygen and forces the neonate to obtain oxygen from the lungs. This alters the path of blood flow and causes changes in blood volume, pressure, and chemical composition. The onset of respiration increases the arterial oxygen pressure (PO_2). This increase in oxygen causes a vasodilatation of pulmonary arterioles and an abrupt decrease in pulmonary resistance. The anatomic changes then follow.

A much larger amount of blood is pumped into the pulmonary arteries by the right ventricle and a smaller amount through the ductus arteriosus. The ductus arteriosus begins to atrophy and eventually is known as *ligamentum arteriosum.*

As the pulmonary circulation increases, more blood is returned from the lungs to the left atrium. Increase in pressure in the left atrium causes the foramen ovale to close. Placental circulation ceases to function when the umbilical cord is clamped. The ends of the hypogastric arteries atrophy and are known as the *hypogastric ligaments.*

The ductus venosus becomes occluded and is known as the *ligamentum venosus.* The umbilical vein becomes obliterated and is known as the *ligamentum teres.* These interdependent cardiopulmonary adaptations, which take place at birth, are essential to survival.

Other Systems

The newborn must begin to manufacture, breakdown and excrete substances on its own. Disorders of metabolism such as hypocalcemia or hypoglycemia may result if the newborn is not up to the challenge. The neurological system must begin the functions that protect and preserve life. The urinary system must be patent and excrete urine, and the gastrointestinal system must become functional.

Thermal Regulation

The neonate loses heat instantly at birth because of a large body surface area, especially the head, which comprises 25 percent of his size. Specific ways in which the neonate loses heat are:

* *Evaporation*: Whenever the skin becomes wet in a relatively dry room or incubator
* *Radiation*: When heat is transferred from the body to cooler objects in the environment (surfaces not in contact with the body)
* *Convection*:With the movement of cool air passing over the surface of the body (skin)
* *Conduction*: When heat is lost from the surface of the body to other objects in direct contact with the skin.

The newborn will attempt to conserve energy by peripheral vasoconstriction and adoption of a flexed posture. However, the neonate is capable of producing heat through both general and brown fat (adipose tissue) metabolism. Brown fat is located in the upper thorax, in the axillae and beneath the skin in the upper part of the back. This fat is different from white fat. If the neonate is cold, the autonomic nervous system triggers the brown fat deposits to release and metabolize the stored fat. The white fat or the ordinary adipose tissue, which acts as a reservoir for potential energy cannot be utilized as readily as brown fat. Brown fat is a limited resource, which is rapidly depleted during periods of cold stress.

The neonate uses up energy at the time of delivery. If the delivery room is cooler than the intrauterine temperature, the neonate will lose heat through evaporation, conduction, convection and radiation. Washing and placing the baby in an unwarmed crib causes further heat loss. Heat loss can be minimized by having the room where the baby is born warm, drying the neonate as soon as possible after delivery, wrapping the baby in a warm blanket and placing him/her in a warm crib next to the mother. Particular care must be taken to prevent heat loss from the head, which can represent 25 percent of a neonates surface area.

IMMEDIATE CARE OF THE BABY AT BIRTH

The immediate care of a newborn is based on the knowledge of the midwife of his transitional requirements and capabilities. Chances of heat loss by convection, radiation and evaporation are very high and hence appropriate preparations must be made for the provision of an optimal thermal environment in the delivery room. This would facilitate a successful transition to extrauterine life. Switching off the fan prior to delivery helps to minimize heat loss by convection. Closing the curtains in the room helps in reduction of radiant heat loss.

Initial Care

As the baby's head is born, excess mucus may be wiped gently from his/her mouth taking care not to touch the nares as it may cause reflex inhalation. The baby is to be handled gently, while he/she will be drawn up towards the mother's abdomen. The time of baby's birth and the sex are noted and recorded soon after the baby is expelled from his/her mother.

Clearing the Airway

In normal births this usually involves:
* Holding or placing the baby so that the head is lower than the body and is turned somewhat to the side for drainage
* Wiping of the baby's face and fluid from the nose and mouth
* Suctioning the nasal and oral passages with a soft rubber bulbsyringe or mucus sucker.

If necessary, the airway may be cleared with the aid of a mucus extractor or soft suction catheter attached to low pressure (10 cm of water) mechanical suction. It is important to aspirate the oropharynx prior to the nasopharynx so that when the baby gasps as his/her nasal passages are aspirated, mucus or other material is not drawn down into the respiratory tract.

Clamping and Cutting the Cord

Separation of the baby from the placenta is achieved by cutting the umbilical cord between two clamps, which should be applied approximately 8 to 10 cm from the umbilicus with enough space between them to allow easy cutting. Application of a gauze piece (4 × 4) over the cord while cutting it with scissors will avoid blood spraying the delivery field. There is no pain for either the baby or the mother at the site of the cutting of the umbilical cord.

The timing of clamping of the cord is not crucial unless asphyxia, prematurity, or Rhesus incompatibility is present. Some centers advocate delay of clamping until respirations are established and cord pulsation has ceased, thus ensuring that the infant receives placental transfusion of about 70 ml of blood. Leboyer (1976) advocated delayed cord clamping for an entirely different reason. He believed that this allowed the newly born baby to have two sources of oxygen during transition: (1) From the lungs and (2) From the placenta through the umbilical cord. Then, when the gradual transition from dependence on the placenta to dependence on the lungs is completed, as evidenced by cessation of cord pulsations, the umbilical cord is clamped and cut. The process is completed by approximately 4 to 5 minutes after birth.

There is also the view that the placental circulation so acquired may predispose to neonatal jaundice. Name bands are to be applied to the infant and mother before the cord is cut.

Identification

When babies are born in the hospital, it is essential that they are identifiable from one another. Name bands are used in most places for this purpose, usually one on the infants wrist and one on the ankle, each of which should indicate legibly the mother's name (family name), sex of the infant and date and time of birth. The midwife should ensure that the name bands are fastened securely and are neither too tight to excoriate the skin nor impede circulation or too loose risking loss. The identification bands should remain on the baby until his/her discharge from the hospital.

Evaluation of the Newborn at Birth

After the baby is seen making respiratory effort, the midwife can proceed to dry the infant in order to avoid evaporative heart loss, while attending also to the assessment procedure. At one minute after the baby's birth, she will assess the baby's general condition and will repeat this at five minutes. The factors assessed are—

Figs 39.2A and B: (A) Newborn with good muscle tone—Apgar score 2; (B) Newborn with poor muscle tone—Apgar score 0

Fig. 39.3: Achrocyanosis

heart rate, respiratory effort, muscle tone, reflex response to stimulus and color (Figs 39.2A and B and 39.3). A score of 0, 1 or 2 is awarded to each of the signs in accordance with the guidelines in Table 39.1. This scoring system, the Apgar score (Apgar, 1966) is recognized and used universally. Of the five signs, the heart rate and the respiratory rate are the most important.

The color of babies with pigmented skin is best assessed by inspecting the color of the mucus membrane. Of the five signs, color is least important and some centers have discontinued recording this part of the score making the maximum score eight rather than ten. Documentation of this modified system when used, requires to be specified in the baby's

Table 30.1	Apgar score			
Sign		Score		
	0	1		2
Heart rate	Absent	Less than 100 bpm		More than 100 bpm
Respiratory effort	Absent	Slow, irregular		Good or crying
Muscle tone	Limp	Some flexion of limbs		Active
Reflex response to stimulus	None	Minimal grimace		Cough or sneeze
Color	Blue, pale	Body pink, extremities blue		Completely pink

birth record, for example "Apgar minus color score = 7".

A normal infant in good condition at birth will achieve an Apgar score of 7 to 10. Medical aid should be sought if the score is less than seven. For an Apgar minus color scoring, a score of less than six requires medical aid.

Prevention of Heat Loss (Fig. 39.4)

It is important to keep the baby warm. This is initiated by wiping off and drying the baby, so that body heat is not lost. Subsequent actions vary but may include use of:

❖ Bodily contact with the mother
❖ Radiant warmer or 200 watt bulb
❖ Warmed blankets.

The wet towel must be removed before wrapping the baby in warm blankets. Skin-to-skin contact with the mother assists the baby to conserve heat. Covering the baby's head is of particular importance. The baby is to be shown to the mother and her significant others after he/she is wrapped well. After a period of rest in the warmer, basinet or in his/her mother's arms, preliminary care of the baby is to be continued.

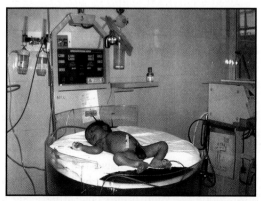

Fig. 39.4: Newborn in radiant warmer
(*For color version see Plate 2*)

Prior to transferring the baby to the ward with his/her mother, or to the nursery or leaving the mother's home in the case of home delivery, the midwife must carry-out a gross examination of the baby for any visible deformities or congenital defects. The initial cord clamp is to be replaced with disposable plastic clamp or cord ligatures approximately 2 to 3 cm from the umbilicus (skin edge) and the excess cord cut off.

Vitamin K 1 mg IM may be given as prophylaxis against bleeding disorders. Erythromycin or gentamycin eye ointment is applied as prophylaxis against gonococcal infection within one hour of birth.

NORMAL CHARACTERISTICS AND PHYSICAL FEATURES OF A HEALTHY NEWBORN

A healthy neonate born at term (between 38th to 42nd week) has an average birth weight (above 2,500 gm), cries immediately following birth, establishes independent rhythmic respiration and quickly adapts to the changed environment.

The weight is variable from country-to-country. In India, the weight varies from 2.7-3.1 kg with a mean of 2.9 kg. The length is 50 to 52 cm. Head circumference measures about 35 cm and the biparietal diameter measures about 9.5 cm.

Posture

The newborn assumes the attitude of its intrauterine life, i.e. extremities flexed and fists clenched. However, the extended attitude of the head in face presentation or legs in frank breech persists for few days more.

Skin

Slight peripheral skin cyanosis (achro-cyanosis), is common, but soon becomes pinkish with the establishment of cardiopulmonary function. Vernix caseosa covers the skin, particularly the back and creases. Lanugo is present over the face, back and extremities. Mongolian spots (benign bluish pigmentation) are present over the sacrum and they disappear by 4 years of age.

Head

Head is larger in relation to the rest of the body. Evidences of varying degrees of molding are present in vaginally delivered babies with cephalic presentation. Varying degrees of caput may be evident (Cephalhematoma is not present at birth).

Face

The face is comparatively smaller in relation the head. The eyes remain closed most of the times. The gums are smooth. The cartilages of the ears and nose are well formed and the cheeks are full.

Neck

The neck is short.

Trunk

The chest is barrel shaped. The circumference is less than that of the head. Breathing is abdominal. Heart rate is usually 120 to 140 per minute. Respiration rate is usually 30 to 60 per minute. Abdomen is usually soft and may be protuberant or flat. Bowel sounds are audible.

Genitalia

In the male, the foreskin will cover the glans, an orifice is present at the tip. The testes can usually be palpated in the scrotum. In the female, the labia minora and clitoris are covered by labia majora.

Extremities

Symmetrical and proportionate to the rest of the body.

Temperature

Normal body temperature for a neonate is 97.7° to 99.5° F or 36.5° to 37.5° C.

Urine

Small amount of urine of low specific gravity is passed.

Stool

Meconium may be passed soon after birth or within the first 24 hours.

Hematological Findings

The total blood volume is about 300 ml a few hours after birth. The average blood volume is estimated be 85 ml per kg body weight consisting of 41 ml of plasma and 44 ml of red blood cell mass.

The normal newborn's glucose levels are 50 to 60 mg per 100 ml, RBCs—6.8 millio/cu mm, and platelets 3,50,000/cu mm. Clotting power may be poor because of deficient vitamin K. Newborn reflexes are present at birth.

INITIAL ASSESSMENT OF THE NEWBORN

During the early hours of life, the newborn should receive a complete assessment. According to Phibbs (1982), there are three general goals when assessing the newborn:

❖ To detect significant medical problems so that they can be treated appropriately
❖ To protect the newborn from harmful processes such as chilling or nosocomial infections
❖ To promote good health by facilitating the normal adaptations to extrauterine life.

At delivery and before the initial assessment takes place, some obstetricians or midwives elect to place the apparently normal neonate on the mother's abdomen where she and the baby glimpse at each other for the first time. Others immediately hand the infant to the obstetric or neonatal nurse for assessment and care. In either case, after the mother has seen the infant the midwife places the baby on the baby bed in the delivery room, briefly examines it, suctions the mouth and nose if necessary, obtains footprints (if it is a requirement), applies identifying bands to the extremities, and cleans the baby superficially.

Much of the newborn's physical examination can be conducted without awakening him although the baby must be fully exposed at intervals for a complete and accurate examination. The neonate must be recovered as soon as possible after the examination to avoid chilling. Scrupulous handwashing is essential before touching the newborn to avoid transferring microorganisms. The infant must be examined systematically, but speedily beginning from the head followed by inspecting the whole body to detect any congenital abnormality. It is important to determine whether the newborn appears of normal size and development for the estimated gestational age. From there, many examiners take a head to toe or systems approach to the examination.

General Appearance

The overall appearance of the newborn must be noted. The following should be found in the normal baby:

- Body symmetrical and cylindrical in contour
- Head large in proportion to the rest of the body
- Small hips
- Narrow chest
- Protruding abdomen.

Measurements

Variations in measurements may occur, but relationships are consistent. The following are the average measurements:

- Head circumference— 35 cm
- Chest measurement— 32 cm
- Crown-rump length— 35 cm
- Crown-heal length— 51 cm

Activity

General body movements are symmetric and include sneezing, yawning, sucking, rooting, swallowing, grasping, responding to sound, blinking and crying. Variations in the infant's cry indicate the following:

- Persistent weak cry—The infant is sick
- Persistent, high-pitched cry—Possible intracranial injuries
- Persistent inconsolable cry—The infant is sick
- Cry stops when the baby is picked up— normal
- Any type of cry that is not normal must be reported to the pediatrician.

Color

Melanin pigmentation is present in varying degrees at birth. The color of the epidermis darkens with exposure to light in infants of dark-pigmented parents. If the infant is pink with bluish nail beds, palms, soles, and extremity, and color improves with activity, the infant is normal. However, if this coloring becomes worse with activity, watch for cyanosis around the mouth and fingernail beds. It may be due to intracranial hemorrhage, cardiac problems or central nervous system involvement.

Skin

The normal full term infant is covered with vernix caseosa. The skin has a velvet softness and elastic texture because of subcutaneous fat. Premature newborn's skin is thin, red, shiny due to lack of subcutaneous fat, and covered by plentiful lanugo and vernix caseosa. Postterm babies will have less vernix caseosa on the body and the skin may be wrinkled and peeling. Other observations to be made on the skin are:

1. Vascular nevi
   - *Stork's beak mark (Stork's bite) (Fig. 39.5):* Dilatation of capillary vessels and minute arteries; found at the nape of the neck and extending over the lower occipital area between the eyebrows, on upper eyelids and around the nose
   - *Strawberry mark (Fig. 39.6):* Bright red spot. It may be seen anywhere on the baby's body
   - *Port-wine stain (Fig. 39.7):* Smooth, flat, superficial angioma, varies in size from a few millimeters to an area that covers most of the face and neck.

Fig. 39.5: Stork beak mark

Fig. 39.8: Mongolian spots

Fig. 39.6: Strawberry mark

Fig. 39.7: Port-wine stain

Fig. 39.9: Forceps marks

2. *Pigmented nevi*: Moles from light brown to black.
3. *Mongolian spots (Fig. 39.8)*: Bluish or slate colored pigmentation over sacral area.
4. *Trauma*: Firm areas of indurations in subcutaneous tissue. The skin may be reddened or purplish, mainly caused by forceps injuries (Fig. 39.9).
5. Deep blue face with pink body is noticed following tight nuchal cord.

Head

The head is to be examined for the following:
1. Temporary asymmetry because of molding and overlapping of cranial bones should be noted.
2. Fontanelles:
   * Anterior—Diamond shaped
   * Posterior—Triangle shaped
   * Bulging fontanelles indicate intracranial pressure
   * Depressed fontanelles indicate dehydration.

3. Caput succedaneum: Swelling on the scalp resulting from pressure of the cervix.
4. Cephalhematoma: Subperiosteal bleeding. Does not cross suture lines, has hard edges around the soft center.

Eyes

The eyes should not be forced open for the examination. The following observations should be made:

❖ Puffy: Common after forceps delivery
❖ Minor drainage after eye prophylaxis drops is instilled
❖ Pupils react to light. Unequal size may be due to brachial plexus paralysis. Ptosis may also be present
❖ Opaqueness: Suggest cataract formation
❖ Almond-shaped eyes if present concomitantly with other signs, suggests Down syndrome
❖ Subconjunctival hemorrhage: Small patch or patches of red within the sclera
❖ Ptosis of the eyes or lids: May indicate nerve damage.

Nose

Newborns breathe through the nose. Any flaring of the nostrils may indicate respiratory distress.

Ears

The ears of the term infant are well formed. Preterm infants lack cartilage and their ears are very soft and flexible. Check the ears for the following:

❖ Presence of canal
❖ The awake infant reacts with a startle to a sudden noise
❖ Size and shape
❖ Deformed ear lobes with the upper margin of the pinna rolled down and thickened-in Down syndrome (trisomy 21)
❖ Low set ears: Autosomal chromosome abnormalities (trisomy 15 and 18).

Mouth

The following should be noted when examining the mouth.

❖ Cleft lip or palate
❖ Epstein pearls: Tiny cysts found on the palate at the junction of the hard and soft palate.

❖ Facial nerve paralysis: Asymmetry of the mouth when open, especially when crying.
❖ Natal teeth or macroglossia.
❖ Circumoral cyanosis: A bluish tinge of the lips in the first few hours of life.
❖ Pooling of saliva: First symptom of tracheo-esophageal fistula. First feeding must be observed.

Neck

Check the neck for the following:

❖ Head is freely movable
❖ Neck webbed on shoulders may indicate Down syndrome or Turner's syndrome
❖ Tightness of muscles on one side may indicate torticollis
❖ Brachial palsy or fractured clavicle—Reflexes absent on the side of fracture, arm remains extended when lying on back and immobilization of affected side.

Chest

The newborn has a barrel chest.

❖ Respiration: After the first period of activity, respirations should be quiet and free of adventitious sounds like rhales or ronchi; both sides of the chest should expand equally with inspiration. A grunding sound on expiration or a gasping, shrill sound on inspiration indicates respiratory distress. If the chest appears to be pulled back towards the spine on inspiration, retractions associated respiratory distress is indicated and the pediatrician should be notified immediately
❖ Heart: Normal heart rates are 120 to 160 beats per minute
❖ Clavicles should be palpated. One or both may be fractured during delivery
❖ Breasts: Supernumerary nipples—Extra nipples are relatively common, but glandular tissue does not usually accompany the nipples.

Abdomen

❖ Should look round and protruding
❖ Umbilical cord stump—Two arteries and one vein should be present. If three vessels are not found, congenital malformations should be investigated

- Masses—Umbilical or inguinal hernias or other abnormal masses are sometimes seen.
- Bowel sounds are generally active.

Genitalia

The genitals of the full-term newborn should appear to be normally formed.

Male
- The foreskin will cover the glans
- Urethral meatus should be at the tip. Deviations indicate hypopadias or epispadias
- The testes can usually be palpated in the scrotum.

Female
- Labia minora is prominent, but should be covered by labia majora
- Some vaginal discharge in response to maternal hormones is normal. In breech infants, the genitals may be edematous and discolored from passage through the vagina.

Back
Hold the infant prone and evaluate the spine. It should not have abnormal curvatures or lesions. Observe for the following:
- A dimple in the coccygeal-sacrococcygeal area may denote a pilonidal cyst, sinus opening or spina bifida
- Tufts of hair may indicate fistula.

Anus
Presence of a perforate anus must be verified. A soft rubber catheter is gently inserted in the rectum if no stools have been passed.

Upper Extremities

Note the proportion to the rest of the body, the symmetry and spontaneous movement of the arms and hands.

Arms
1. Arms should be of equal length when extended.
   - Infant should resist having arms extended.
2. Hands: Holds hands in fists and will normally grasp fingers or objects placed in their hands.
   - A single deep, sharp, transverse palmar crease (simian line) along with a flat and

stubby thumb and a short little finger is found in Down syndrome
- Fingers may show webbing (abnormal fusion of fingers), polydactylism (extra digits), or syndactylism (fewer digits)
- Nails: Fingernails are well developed in most instances, extending beyond fingertips. Long nails are present in post-term infants
- Skin tags may be seen occasionally.

Lower extremities
Check the legs for symmetry, range of motion and proportion to the rest of the body.
- Should be of equal length when extended.
- With knees flexed, legs should abduct to table in frog like position. Dislocated hip is suspected if abduction is asymmetrical and a hip click is present.
- If legs are persistently limb, it is indicative of spinal cord lesion.

Feet
Soles of the full-term neonate are normally wrinkled. Wrinkles may be absent in preterm infants.
- Acrocyanosis (blue discoloration of the hands and feet) is common immediately after birth
- Congenital malformations such as talipes equinovarus, talipes calcaneovalgus and bowing of legs must be noted
- Toes may show webbing, polydactylism or syndactylism
- The first and second *toes* are widely separated in Down syndrome.

Neurologic Examination

The normal newborn exhibits the following reflexes—The Moro or embracing reflex, the tonic neck reflex, the stepping reflex, the palmar grasp reflex and the rooting/sucking reflex. The newborn that appears jittery or exhibits jerky movements of the extremities may suffer from low blood sugar, disturbances of calcium metabolism or may, in fact, be having seizures.

Cardiovascular Examination

After quieting the baby with a pacifier or finger, auscultate the heart sounds and feel for pulses in the upper and lower extremities. Although cardiac murmurs are common as the newborn makes the transition from intrauterine to extra-uterine life, they should be documented and the pediatrician informed. Congenital heart defects may or may not be obvious in the first days of life.

Failure to Establish Respirations at Birth

Infants who fail to establish and sustain respirations within 60 seconds of birth require prompt and effective intervention. Knowledge of the predisposing factors and causes of hypoxia will be helpful for the nurse to be prepared for effective resuscitation of the newborn.

Intrauterine hypoxia occurs when there is inadequate perfusion of the placental site, reduction in placental function, impaired feto-placental circulation or inadequate hemoglobin. The fetus develops tachycardia followed by metabolic acidosis and bradycardia. The anal sphincter relaxes and the fetus may pass meconium into the liquor. Gasping breathing movements triggered by hypoxia may result in the aspiration of meconium stained liquor into the lungs. Auscultation of the fetal heart, use of cardiotocography and observation of meconium staining of liquor draining per vagina must alert the midwife to fetal distress.

Causes of Respiratory Depression in the Neonate

- ❖ Fetal hypoxia (described above)
- ❖ Obstruction of the baby's airway by mucus, blood, liquor or meconium
- ❖ Depression of the respiratory center due to the effects of drugs administered to the mother
- ❖ Mechanical dysfunction because of under-developed lungs, lack of surfactant and a soft pliable thoracic cage in premature infants
- ❖ Intranatal pneumonia developed when membranes have been ruptured for some-time
- ❖ Severe anemia caused by fetomaternal hemorrhage or Rhesus incompatibility, which diminishes oxygen carrying capacity of blood

- ❖ Major congenital abnormalities such as congenital heart defects, abnormalities of central nervous system or abnormalities in the respiratory tract.

Failure to establish respirations compounds hypoxia as previously described. It is necessary therefore to be able and be prepared to undertake specific resuscitative measures for any infant who had difficulty establishing respirations at birth.

RESUSCITATION OF THE NEWBORN

Rationale for Resuscitation

The goals of resuscitation are to establish and maintain a clear airway, to ensure effective circulation to correct acidosis and to prevent hypothermia, hypoglycemia and hemorrhage. Careful intrapartum assessment of the fetal heart rate can alert the midwife to the probable need for resuscitation. The fetus undergoing prolonged periods of asphyxia may make gasping attempts followed by apnea *in utero* (*primary apnea*). At birth, weaker gasps may be followed by a last gasp and *secondary period of apnea*. The heart rate falls dramatically and, without intervention, the infant dies. The infant born in secondary apnea cannot be revived with suctioning and tactile stimulation; ventilation and perhaps cardiac massage are required.

The asphyxiated infant has low oxygen levels, elevated carbon dioxide and lower blood pH (acidosis). This condition contributes to vasospasm of pulmonary arterioles and increased resistance to blood flow in the lungs after birth. The weak gasp of the asphyxiated newborn cannot overcome this resistance and establish adequate respirations. As the hypoxia continues, the heart rate slows and the myocardium contracts ineffectively. Blood pressure drops and systemic circulation slows, leading to organ damage.

Degrees of Resuscitation (Fig. 39.10)

Resuscitative requirements vary with the infant's condition at one minute of age.

- ❖ The baby with an Apgar score of 7 to 10 has a blood pH of 7.20 to 7.40. This baby has

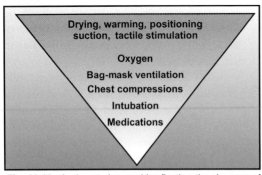

Fig. 39.10: An inverted pyramid reflecting the degrees of neonatal resuscitative efforts

minimal depression; and a normal transition period can be expected.

❖ Suction the oropharynx and then the nose to clear the airway and provide tactile stimulation (Flow chart 39.1).

❖ Dry the infant and provide warmth: Apply warm blankets to the baby on the mother's abdomen, or use radiant warmer (warmer may not be required in the tropics)

❖ Continue to observe transition closely.

Flow chart 39.1: Resuscitation of the newborn in the delivery room

Source: Textbook of Neonatal Resuscitation, © 1990 American Heart Association and the American Academy of Pediatrics, recommended by the National Neonatology Forum, India

❖ The baby with an Apgar score of 4 to 6 has a blood pH of 7.09 to 7.19 (moderate acidosis). This baby has moderate depression probably reflecting a period of primary apnea.
- Dry the infant
- Place infant under radiant heat source
- Suction the oropharynx and then the nose to clear the airway and provide tactile stimulation; give free-flow oxygen by facemask
- If infant is still apneic or has a heart rate below 100, begin positive pressure ventilation by facemask attached to an anesthesia bag or self-inflating bag with an oxygen reservoir; both give nearly 100 percent oxygen
- Continue free-flow oxygen after infant has established good respiratory effort.

❖ The infant with an Apgar score of 0 to 3 has a blood pH of 7.00 or below (severe acidosis). This baby has severe depression reflecting secondary apnea.
- Suction the infant to clear the airway
- Dry the infant
- Place infant in the work area under radiant heat source
- Begin positive pressure ventilation
- If positive pressure ventilation does not ensue with bag and mask, perform endotracheal intubation
- If heart rate is less than 60 after 30 seconds of adequate ventilation, begin cardiac massage. Continue massage until infant can sustain heart rate over 80 with ventilation alone.

Supplies and Equipment

Though the need for resuscitation can be anticipated in some situations, there are occasions when a baby is born in poor condition without forewarning. It is essential that resuscitation equipment is always available and in working order in the delivery room and nursery area in close proximity to oxygen and suction outlets. The equipment and medications should include those that will provide for adequate ventilation or resuscitation, thermoregulation, correction of hypoglycemia, fluids and electrolytes, plasma expanders and cardiac stimulants. The personnel in attendance at the delivery of a baby must be familiar with the equipment and resuscitation techniques. A list of essential equipment includes the following:

Suctioning Equipment

❖ Bulb syringe
❖ DeLee mucus trap with No. 10 Fr catheter or mechanical suction
❖ Suction catheters Nos. 6, 8 and 10
❖ Feeding tube No. 8 Fr and 20 ml syringe.

Bag and Mask Equipment

❖ Infant resuscitation bag with pressure release valve or pressure gauge with a reservoir capable of delivering 90 to 100 percent oxygen
❖ Facemasks with cushioned rims: Newborn and premature sizes
❖ Oral airways: Newborn and premature sizes
❖ Oxygen with flowmeter and tubing.

Intubation Equipment

❖ Laryngoscope with straight blades No. '0' (premature), No. '1' (newborn)
❖ Extra bulbs and batteries for laryngoscope
❖ Endotracheal tubes—sizes 2.5, 3.0, 3.5 and 4.0 mm internal diameter
❖ Stylet
❖ Scissors.

Medications

❖ Epinephrine 1:10,000 ampoules (1 ml ampoule of 1:1,000 available in India)
❖ Naloxone hydrochloride (neonatal narcan 0.02 mg/ml)
❖ Volume expander (one or more of these)
❖ 5 percent albumin solution
❖ Normal saline
❖ Ringer's lactate
❖ Sodium bicarbonate 4.2 percent (1 mEq/2ml) (7.5% strength available in India approximately 0.9 mEq/ml)
❖ Dextrose 10 percent concentration 250 ml
❖ Sterile water 30 ml
❖ Normal saline 30 ml.

Miscellaneous

- Radiant warmer
- Stethoscope
- Adhesive tapes
- Syringes 1 ml, 2 ml, 5 ml and 20 ml sizes
- Needles Nos. 21, 22 and 26
- Umbilical cord clamp
- Umbilical catheters 3.5 and 5 Fr. Sizes
- Umbilical artery catheterization tray
- Gloves.

Initial Steps

Preventing heat loss
- Place infant under a warmer
- Quickly dry off amniotic fluid
- Replace wet sheets with a dry one.

Positioning
- Place the baby on his back with head slightly down (15° tilt)
- Neck slightly extended

Suctioning
- Suction the mouth first and then nose
- Tactile stimulation
- If infant does not breathe immediately give tactile stimulation but only twice (Flick or tap the sole of foot twice or rub the back).

Evaluation
- After the above steps evaluate the baby's vital signs:
  - Respirations
  - Heart rate
  - Color.
- If respirations are normal, go on to evaluating heart rate
- If baby is apneic, begin positive pressure ventilation
- If heart rate is over 100 beats per minute, go on to evaluating color
- If less than 100 beats per minute, initiate positive pressure ventilation
- If infant is pink, no further action is necessary
- If there is central cyanosis, administer free flow oxygen (tip of the tube held ½″ from nares delivers approximately 90 percent oxygen).

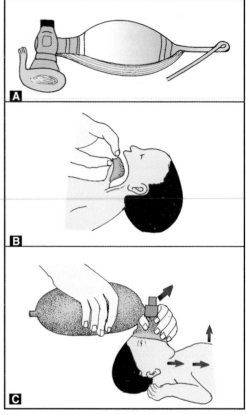

Figs 39.11A to C: Bag and mask ventilation: (A) Bag and mask for ventilation; (B) Correct position (sniffing position) of the baby's head for ventilating; (C) Bag squeezed to move the chest with each squeeze

Bag and Mask Ventilation/Positive Pressure Ventilation (Figs 39.11A to C)

Indications
- Infant apneic
- Heart rate less than 100 bpm

Procedure

The newborn should be on his back with neck slightly extended.

A tight seal to be formed over the infant's mouth and nose.

- Ventilate at the rate of 40 to 50 per minute with 20 to 25 cm, H_2O pressure
- Ventilate for 15 to 30 seconds and evaluate
- Have an assistant to evaluate, listen to the heart rate for 6 seconds and multiply by 10.

Evaluation

❖ Heart rate above 100/minute and sponta-neous respiration—Discontinue bagging
❖ Heart rate 60 to 100 per minute and increa-sing: continue ventilation
❖ Heart rate 60 to 100 per minute and not increasing: Continue ventilation
❖ Check whether chest is moving, adequately
❖ Heart rate below 80/minute—Start chest compressions
❖ Heart rate below 60 per minute—In addition to bagging and chest compressions, consider intubation and initiate medications.

Signs of Improvement

❖ Increasing heart rate
❖ Spontaneous respirations
❖ Improving color
Continue to provide free flow oxygen by facemask after respirations are established.
If the baby deteriorates, check the following:
❖ Placement of facemask for tight seal
❖ Head position and presence of secretions
❖ Pressure being used
❖ Presence of air in the stomach preventing chest expansion
❖ Oxygen being delivered (100% or not)
For bagging lasting for more than two minutes insert an orogastric tube to vent the stomach.

Chest Compressions

Chest compressions (Figs 39.12A and B) consist of rhythmic compressions of the sternum that compresses the heart against the spine, increases the intrathoracic pressure and circulates blood to the vital organs.

Chest compressions must always be accompanied by ventilation with 100 percent oxygen to assure that the circulating blood is well oxygenated.

Indications

❖ Heart rate less than 60 per minute after bagging with 100 percent oxygen for 15 to 30 seconds
❖ Heart rate 60 to 80 per minute and not increasing after bagging with 100 percent oxygen for 15 to 30 seconds.

Procedure

Site: Lower third of the sternum below an imaginary line between the two nipples.

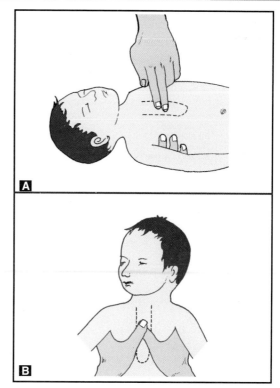

Figs 39.12A and B: External cardiac massage: (A) Two-finger technique; (B) Thumb technique

Depth: Depress the sternum to a depth of ½ to ¾ inch at a rate of 100 to 120 per minute.

Rate: 100 to 120 per minute. Coordinate heart compression with ventilation.

Discontinue when infant can maintain heart rate above 80 by ventilation alone.

Endotracheal Intubation

Indications

❖ Heart rate below 60 per minute in spite of bagging and chest compressions
❖ Presence of meconium in the amniotic fluid.

Procedure

❖ Place infant with head lightly extended with a rolled towel under the shoulder
❖ Introduce laryngoscope over the baby's tongue at the right corner of the mouth
❖ Advance 2 to 3 cm while rotating it to midline, until the epiglottis is seen. Elevation of the epiglottis by the tip of the laryngoscope reveals the vocal cords
❖ Suction secretions if needed

Table 39.2 Medications for neonatal resuscitation

Medication	Concentration	Preparation	Dosage/route	Total dose/infant			Rate/precautions
Epinephrine (Adrenalin)	1 : 10,000	1 ml	0.1-0.3 ml/kg IV or IT	*Weight* 1 kg 2 kg 3 kg 4 kg		*Total ml* 0.1-0.3 ml 0.2-0.6 ml 0.3-0.9 ml 0.4-1.2 ml	Give rapidly
Volume Expanders	Whole blood 5% Albumin Normal Saline Ringer's Lactate	40 ml	10 ml/kg IV	*Weight* 1 kg 2 kg 3 kg 4 kg		*Total ml* 10 ml 20 ml 30 ml 40 ml	Give over 5–10 minutes
Sodium Bicarbonate	0.5 mEq/ml (4.2% solution)	20 ml	2 mEq/kg IV	*Weight* 1kg 2 kg 3 kg 4 kg	*Total dose* 2 mEq 4 mEq 6 mEq 8 mEq	*Total ml* 4 ml 8 ml 12 ml 16 ml	Give slowly, over at least two min. Give only if infant being effectively ventilated
Naloxone (Narcan)	0.4 mg/ml	1 ml	0.25 ml/kg IV, IM, SQ, IT	*Weight* 1 kg 2 kg 3 kg 4 kg		*Total ml* 0.25 ml 0.50 ml 0.75 ml 1.00 ml	Give rapidly
	1.0 mg/ml	1 ml	0.1 ml/kg IV, IM, SQ, IT	*Weight* 1 kg 2 kg 3 kg 4 kg		*Total ml* 0.1 ml 0.2 ml 0.3 ml 0.4 ml	
Dopamine			Begin at 5 mcg/kg/min may increase to 20 mcg/kg/min (if necessary) IV	*Weight* 1 kg 2 kg 3 kg 4 kg		*Total mcg/min* 5-20 mcg/min 10-40 mcg/min 15-60 mcg/min 20-60 mcg/min	Give as a continuous infusion using an infusion pump. Monitor HR and BP closely. Seek consultation

IM—Intramuscular; IT—Intratracheal; IV—Intravenous; SQ—Subcutaneous
Source: Text Book of Neonatal Resuscitation, 1990 © American Heart Association, recommended by the National Neonatology Forum, India

- Pass the endotracheal tube a distance of 1.5 to 2 cm into the trachea, hold it firmly but gently in place and withdraw the laryngoscope slowly
- Attach the endotracheal tube to the adapter on the bag
- Ventilate with oxygen by bag. An assistant should check for adequate ventilation of both lungs with stethoscope.

Medications (Table 39.2)

Medications should be administered if, despite adequate ventilation with 100 percent oxygen and chest compressions, the heart rate remains 80 beats per minute. Medications used are Adrenalin (for hypotonia), Sodium bicarbonate (to correct acidosis), volume expanders (for hypovolemia) and Dopamine (for hypotension). Naloxone is given if needed to reverse the effects of maternal narcotics given in the perceding three hours. The dosages and routes of administration of drugs are detailed in Table 39.2.

BIBLIOGRAPHY

1. Apgar V. The newborn (Apgar) scoring system: Reflections and advice. Pediatric Clinics of North America 1966;13:599-619.
2. Arnold HW, et al. Transition to extrauterine life, American Journal of Nursing. 1975;65-77.
3. Dutta DC. Textbook of Obstetrics, 5th edn. Calcutta; New Central Book Company: 2001.
4. Karpen M, et al. Essentials of Maternal-Child Nursing, 2nd edn. Massachusetts; Western Schools Press, 1995.
5. Korones SB. High Risk Newborn Infants: The Basis for Intensive Nursing Care, 3rd edn. Mosby; St Louis, 1981.
6. Leboyer F. Birth Without Violence, Knopf; New York, 1976.
7. Michie MM. The baby at birth, In: Myles Textbook for Midwives, 13th edn. Edinburgh; Churchill Livingstone, 1999.
8. Moore ML. The Newborn and the Nurse. Philadelphia; Saunders 1972.
9. Phibbs RH. Evaluation of the newborn, In: Ruldoph AM, Hoffman J (Eds). Pediatrics, Norwalk, CT: Appleton-Century-Crofts.
10. Varney Helen. Nurse. Midwifery, 2nd edn. Boston; Jones and Barlett Publishers 1996.

40

Physiology, Screening, Daily Care and Observation of the Newborn

Learning Objectives

Upon completing this chapter, the learner will be able to:

❖ Describe the external features of the normal newborn baby
❖ Describe the functioning of the different body systems in relation to their stage of maturity
❖ Describe the behavior of the baby during the first weeks of life
❖ Describe the daily examination and observations of the newborn baby
❖ Discuss the role of the midwife in providing guidance and assistance to mothers in the care of their babies.

Extrauterine life presents a challenge to the newborn infant. The most important changes take place, are in the heart and lungs at birth. However, continued adaptations are necessary in the first week of life as the infant assumes independence from the maternal and placental nurturing, which he enjoyed before birth. The newborn remains dependent on his mother or caregiver for nutrition and protection, but is responsible for his own metabolism homeostasis and other functions essential to survival.

PHYSIOLOGY

Respiratory System

At birth, the respiratory system is developmentally incomplete, growth of new alveoli continuing for several years. Respiration rate is usually 30 to 60 per minute. The breathing is diaphragmatic, chest and abdomen rising and falling synchronously. Breathing pattern is erratic. Respirations are shallow and irregular,

being interspersed with brief 10 to 15 seconds of apnea. This is known as periodic breathing. The pattern of respiration alters during sleeping and waking states. Babies are obligatory nose breathers and do not convert automatically to mouth breathing when nasal obstruction occurs. Respiratory difficulties can occur because of neurological, metabolic, circulatory or thermoregulatory dysfunction as well as infection, airway obstruction or abnormalities of airway tract itself.

The baby has a lusty cry, which he uses to evoke a response from his attendants with a view to controlling his environment. The cry is normally loud and of medium pitch unless neurological damage, infection or hypothermia is present, when it may be high pitched or weak. Transient cyanosis may arise in the first few days when the baby is crying.

Cardiovascular System

The heart rate is rapid, 120 to 160 per minute and fluctuates in accordance with the baby's respiratory function and activity or sleep rate. Peripheral circulation is sluggish. This results in mild cyanosis of hands and feet and circumoral areas and in generalized mottling when the skin is exposed. Blood pressure fluctuates according to activity and ranges from 80 to 85/50 to 55 mm Hg in the first ten days of life.

The total circulating blood volume at birth is 80 ml/kg bodyweight. However, this may be raised if there is delay in clamping the umbilical cord at birth. The hemoglobin levels are high (18–20 gm/dl) of which 50 to 80 percent is fetal hemoglobin (Blackburn and Loper,

1992). Conversion from fetal to adult hemoglobin is completed in the first 1 to 2 years of life. Hemoglobin, red cell count and hematocrit levels decrease gradually during the first 2 to 3 months of life during which time erythropoiesis is suppressed. The white cell count is high initially and decreases rapidly (Perry, 1995).

Breakdown of excess red blood cells in the liver and spleen predisposes to jaundice in the first week. Because colonization of the intestine by the bacteria, which synthesize vitamin K, is delayed until feeding is established, vitamin K dependent clotting factors II (prothrombin), VII, IX and X are low. This inhibits blood clotting. During the first week platelet levels equal those of the adult but there is a reduced capacity for adhesion and aggregation (Blackburn and Lopper, 1992).

Thermal Regulation

Thermal control in the neonate remains poor for sometime. Owing to the immaturity of the hypothalamus, temperature regulation is inefficient and the infant remains vulnerable to hypothermia, particularly when exposed to cold or draughts, when wet, when unable to move about freely or when deprived of nutrition. As a baby, who is cold is unable to shiver; he will attempt to maintain his body heat by adopting flexed posture, increasing his respiratory rate and activity. He may also cry. These activities increase calorie consumption and may result in hypoglycemia, which in turn will compound the effects of hypothermia.

The infant's normal core temperature is 36 to 37°C. A healthy, clothed, term infant will maintain this body temperature satisfactorily if the environment is not cold, his nutrition is adequate and his movements are not restricted by tight swaddling. An unstable temperature may indicate infection.

Renal System

The kidneys are functionally immature at birth. Glomerular filtration rate is low and tubular resorption capabilities are limited. The infant is not able to concentrate or dilute urine very well in response to variations in fluid intake. The ability to excrete drugs is also limited and the baby's renal function is vulnerable to physiological stress.

The first urine is passed at birth or within the first 24 hours and thereafter with increasing frequency as fluid intake rises. The urine is dilute, straw colored and odorless. Cloudiness caused by mucus and urates may be present initially until fluid intake increases. Urine is voided by reflex emptying of the bladder. As the neonatal pelvis is small, the bladder becomes palpable abdominally when full.

Gastrointestinal System

The gastrointestinal tract of the neonate is structurally complete though functionally immature. The mucus membrane of the mouth is pink and moist. The teeth are buried in the gums and ptyalin secretion is low. Small epithelial pearls (Epstein's pearls) are sometimes present at the junction of the hard and soft palates. Sucking pads in the cheek give them a full appearance. Sucking and swallowing are coordinated.

The stomach has small capacity (15–30 ml) at birth, which increases rapidly in the first week of life. The cardiac sphincter is weak which give rise to regurgitation or posseting. Gastric emptying time is normally 2.5 to 3 hours. Enzymes are present though there is a deficiency of amylase and lipase, which diminishes the infant's ability to digest compound carbohydrates and fat.

When food enters the stomach, a gastrocolic reflex results in increased peristalsis, often accompanied by reflex emptying of the bowel. Bowel sounds are present within one hour of birth. Meconium present in the large intestine from 16th week's gestation, is passed within the first 24 hours of life and is totally excreted within 48 to 72 hours. This first stool is blackish green in color, is tenacious and contains bile, fatty acids, mucus and epithelial cells. From the third to fifth day, the stools undergo a transitional stage and are brownish-yellow in color. Once feeding is established, yellow feces are passed. The consistency and frequency of stools reflect the type of feeding. Breast milk results in loose, bright yellow and inoffensive acid stools. The baby may pass eight to ten stools a day. The stools of the bottle-fed infant are paler in color, semiformed, less acid and have a slightly sharp smell. The bottle-fed baby passes four to six stools a day and there is increased tendency to constipation.

Physiological immaturity of the liver results in low production of glucuronyl transferase for the conjugation of bilirubin. This together with a high level of red cell breakdown may result in a transient jaundice, which is manifest on the third to fifth day (physiological jaundice). Glycogen stores are rapidly depleted after birth and hence early feeding is required to maintain normal blood glucose levels. Feeding stimulates liver function and colonization of the gut, which assists in the formation of vitamin K.

Reproductive System

Spermatogenesis in boys does not occur until puberty but the total complement of primordial follicles containing primitive ova is present in the ovaries of girls at birth. In both sexes withdrawal of maternal estrogens results in breast engorgement, sometimes accompanied by secretion of 'milk' by the fourth or fifth day. Baby girls may develop pseudomenstruation for the same reason.

Musculoskeletal System

The muscles are complete, growth occurring by hypertrophy. The long bones are incompletely ossified to facilitate growth at the epiphyses. The bones of the vault of the skull also reveal lack of ossification. This is essential for growth of the brain and facilitating moulding during labor. Moulding is resolved within a few days of birth. The posterior fontanelle closes at 6 to 8 weeks. The anterior fontanelle remains open until 18 months of age, making assessment of hydration and intracranial pressure possible by palpation of fontanelle tension.

Immunological Adaptations

Neonates are susceptible to infections, particularly those gaining entry through the mucosa of the respiratory and gastrointestinal systems. Minor infections become generalized very easily.

The baby has some immunoglobulins at birth. There are three main immunoglobulins IgG, IgA and IgM, and of these only IgG is small enough to cross the placental barrier. It affords immunity to specific viral infections during the first few months of life.

IgM and IgA do not cross the placental barrier. Levels of IgM at term are 20 percent of those of the adult and takes two years to attain the adult levels. This relatively low level of IgM is thought to render the infant more susceptible to enteric infections. IgA levels are also very low and increase slowly. IgA protects against infection of the respiratory tract, gastrointestinal tract and eyes. Breast milk and especially colostrum provides the infant with passive immunity in the form of *Lactobacillus bifidus*, lactoferrin, lysozyme and secretary IgA.

The thymus gland, where lymphocytes are produced, is relatively large at birth and continues to grow until eight years of age (Michie in Bennett and Brown, 1999).

Neurological System

The nervous system is remarkably immature both anatomically and physiologically at birth. This results in predominantly brainstem and spinal reflex activity with minimal control by the cerebral cortex in the early months. After birth, brain growth is rapid, requiring constant and adequate supplies of oxygen and glucose. The immaturity of the brain renders it vulnerable to hypoxia, biochemical imbalance, infection and hemorrhage. Temperature instability and uncoordinated muscle movement reflect the incomplete development of brain.

The neonate is equipped with a wide range of reflex activities, the presence of which at varying ages provides indication of the normality and integrity of neurological and musculoskeletal systems.

Moro Reflex or Embracing Reflex (Fig. 40.1)

This reflex occurs in response to a sudden stimulus. Acceptable ways to elicit a Moro reflex include the following:
* Holding the baby at 45° angle and then permitting the head to drop 1 or 2 centimeters

Fig. 40.1: Moro reflex *(For color version see Plate 3)*

Fig. 40.2: Tonic neck reflex

❖ The examining table is struck near the head of the baby
❖ The table is jarred suddenly
❖ A loud noise or handclap is utilized.

The infant responds by abducting and extending his arms and fanning of fingers, sometimes accompanied by a tremor. The arms then flex and embrace the chest. A similar response may be seen in the legs, which, following extension, flex onto the abdomen. The reflex is symmetrical and is present for the first eight weeks of life. Absence of Moro reflex may indicate brain damage or immaturity. Persistence of the reflex beyond the age of six months is suggestive of mental retardation.

Tonic Neck Reflex (Fig. 40.2)

The infant is placed on his or her back and the head is turned to the side. The arm and leg on the same side extend and the opposite arm and leg flex; thus the infant assumes a fencing position. The head is turned to the opposite side and the same reaction should occur. The response may be present in the newborn for about 2 to 3 months. If it persists longer than this time, it usually indicates neurological dysfunction.

Palmar Reflex/ Grasp Reflex (Fig. 40.3A)

With the baby in supine and the head in midline, the finger of the examiner or a thin object such as a pencil is placed in the baby's hand. The newborn shows palmar reflex by wrapping the palm and the fingers around it. Normally, there should be flexion of all the infant's fingers around the examiner's finger.

When fingers of the examiner are plaed in both the hands, if the newborn holds so tightly

Fig. 40.3A: Palmar reflex *(For color version see Plate 3)*

Fig. 40.3B: Plantar reflex *(For color version see Plate 3)*

that they can be picked up and held by their grasp alone, this may present a hyperkinetic reaction. This reflex diminishes, weakens and disappears after three months. Complete absence of the reflex may be found in brain damage.

Plantar Reflex (Fig. 40.3B)

The examiner's thumb or a thin object such as a pencil is pressed against the ball of the infant's foot. There should be flexion of all toes.

Fig. 40.4: Stepping reflex *(For color version see Plate 3)*

The absence of this response is correlated with defects of the lower spinal cord. This reflex disappears in two to three years.

Walking/Stepping Reflex (Fig. 40.4)

The baby is held so that the sole of the foot touches a flat surface. This should stimulate a stepping or dancing movement with both legs. This reflex is present at birth and gradually disappears after three to four weeks.

Reflexes of the Eyes

❖ *Blink reflex*: A bright light is shone suddenly at the infant's eyes. Normally a quick closure of the eyes and a slight dorsal flexion of the head are elicited. With impaired light perception, this response is absent.

❖ *Corneal reflex:* When the eyes are open, the cornea is touched lightly with a piece of cotton, with care to avoid touching eyelids or lashes. Normally the eyes close. The absence of this response denotes lesions of the fifth cranial nerve.

Reflexes of the Mouth

❖ *Rooting reflex:* The corner of the baby's mouth, the upper lip and the lower lip are touched in turn with the finger (Fig. 40.5).

Fig. 40.5: Eliciting rooting reflex

Upon stimulation, the head turns toward the stimulated side, the mouth opens, the tongue moves to the point of stimulation and infant tries to suck on the stimulating object. Rooting reflex is elicited when the baby is alert. A baby whose hunger has been satisfied will turn away from the stimulation

❖ *Sucking and swallowing reflex*: If the examiner's index finger is placed in the infant's mouth, rhythmical sucking movements will be felt. Sucking is often less intense and less regular during the first three to four days. Poor sucking may be noted in apathetic or hyperactive babies and is the first indication of problems such as sepsis

❖ *Gag, Cough and Sneeze reflexes*: These protect the infant from airway obstruction.

❖ *Babinski's reflex*: The lateral aspect of the sole of the infant's foot is scratched, going from heel to toes. This must be more than pressure; if not, a plantar reflex instead of a Babinski's reflex will be elicited. The Babinski's reflex shows a dorsal flexion of the big toe. It is present in the newborn until ninth to tenth month. A poor response may be due to nervous system immaturity; absence of the response may be due to defects in the lower spinal cord

❖ *Traction response: Head lag*: When pulled upright by the wrists to a sitting position the head will lag initially, then right itself momentarily before falling forward on to the chest (Fig. 40.6)

❖ *Ventral suspension*: When held prone, suspended over the examiner's arm, the baby shortly holds his head level with his body and flexes his limbs (Fig. 40.7).

Fig. 40.6: Traction response / Head lag

Fig. 40.7: Ventral suspension

❖ *Incurvation of trunk / Peres reflex:* Hold the baby suspended ventrally and stroke the sides of spine alternately. The baby would turn his pelvis to the side stimulated. This response indicates general muscle tone as the baby is suspended. No response indicates Central Nervous System (CNS) deficit. The reflex disappears in one month.

Special Senses and Behavior Pattern

Vision

The structures necessary for vision are present and functional at birth although immature. The baby is sensitive to bright lights, which cause him to frown or blink. He demonstrates a preference for black and white patterns and the shape of human face. His focusing distance is about 15 to 20 centimeters, which allows him to see his mother's face when being nursed. He can track a moving object briefly within the first five days. His ability to establish eye contact with his mother helps to enhance bonding. By two weeks of age, he can differentiate his mother's face from that of a stranger.

Hearing

The baby turns his eyes towards sound. He is comforted by low-pitched sounds. High-pitched sounds make him agitated. A sudden sound elicits a startle or blink reflex. He prefers the sound of the human voice to other sounds. He can discriminate between voices and prefers his mother's. This too, promotes mother-baby interaction (De Casper and Fifer, 1987).

Smell and Taste

Babies prefer the smell of milk to that of other substances and show a preference for human milk. Within a few days, the baby can differentiate the smell of his mother's milk. He turns away from unpleasant smells. His preference for sweet taste is demonstrated by vigorous and strong sucking and a grimacing response to bitter, salty or sour substances (Blackburn and Loper, 1992).

Touch

Infants are acutely sensitive to touch, enjoys skin-to-skin contact, immersion in water, stroking, cuddling and rocking movements (Blackburn and Loper, 1992). A puff of air on his face induces an inspiration or gasp reflex. His curving response to touch and his gasp reflexes enhance his relationship with his mother. The baby withdraws from painful stimuli, bulges his brow and nasolabial furrow and may cry vigorously (Rushforth and Levene, 1994).

Sleeping and Waking

Following the initiation of respiration at birth, the baby remains alert and reactive for a period of approximately one hour, after which he relaxes and sleeps. The length of this first sleep varies from a few minutes to several hours. Subsequent sleeping and waking rhythms show marked variations and the baby takes some time to settle into his individual pattern. Initially, waking periods are related to hunger, but within a few weeks, the waking periods last longer and meet the need for social interaction.

Two Sleep States are Identifiable

Deep sleep in which the baby's eyes are closed, respirations are regular, no eye movements are present, response to stimuli is delayed and is quickly suppressed. Jerky movements may occur at intervals.

Light sleep in which eye movements could be observed through the closed eyelids. Respirations are irregular and sucking movements occur intermittently. Response to stimuli occurs more readily and may result in alteration of sleep state. Random movements are noted.

Awakening States

A wider range of awakening states is observed, ranging from drowsiness to crying.

Drowsy state: The baby's eyes may be open or closed with some fluttering of the eyelids. Smiling may occur. Limb movements are generally smooth, but are interspersed by startle responses.

Quiet alert state: Motor activity is minimal, the baby is alert to visual and auditory stimuli.

Active alert state: The baby is generally active and reactive to his environment.

Active crying state: The baby cries vigorously and may be difficult to console. Muscular activity is considerable.

The amount of time that the baby spends in which state varies and influences the way in which he responds to stimuli, whether visual, auditory or tactile (Brazelton, 1984).

Crying

Crying is the way in which the baby communicates discomfort and summons assistance. With experience, it is possible to differentiate the cry and identify the need, which may be hunger, thirst, pain general discomfort (for example, wanting a change of position or feeling too cold or too warm), boredom, loneliness or a desire for physical and social contact. The mother needs to learn how to comfort her baby. Rocking induces sleep, swaddling and upright position appear to be soothing (Downey and Bidder, 1990).

Growth and Development

Because of his physical limitations, the baby is dependent on his mother (or other care giver) for his continued growth, development and survival. These will progress satisfactorily only if he is in a safe environment, his nutritional needs are met, and his psychological development is promoted by appropriate stimulation and loving care. Abnormality of the baby's body systems, inadequate nutrition or emotional deprivation will compromise the baby's ability to grow and develop to his full potential. His relatively immature organ functions and his vulnerability to infection and hypothermia demand that his care must be designed to meet his needs and capabilities.

PHYSICAL EXAMINATION (SCREENING)

All newborn babies are routinely examined by a pediatrician within the first 24 hours of life and again prior to discharge home. Some of the examination duplicates what has been described earlier under initial assessment and hence only additional aspects are considered here. A general appraisal of the baby's color, overall appearance, muscular activity and response to handling are made throughout the examination.

Neurological assessment: The baby's reflex responses are elicited in order to establish normality of the nervous system. These are tested when the baby is in quiet alert state. Absent or weak responses may indicate immaturity, cerebral damage or abnormality.

Auscultation: The heart and lung sounds are auscultated. A heart murmur may be present for some days after birth.

Palpation: The abdominal organs, particularly the liver, spleen and kidneys are palpated, noting any enlargement. Femoral pulses are assessed ensuring that they are full and of equal strength.

Figs 40.8A and B: Assessing for Barlow's and Ortolani's signs: (A) Barlow's sign; (B) Ortolani's sign

Examination of hips: The hips are examined to detect developmental dysplasia. In order to examine the hips, the examiner places the baby on a firm flat surface at waist height.

a. *Barlow's test (Fig. 40.8A)*: This is used to detect hip instability. The examiner holds the baby's hips and knees at 90 degrees of flexion with the fingers over the greater trochanters. Backward pressure is applied while adducting the hips. The femoral head is felt slipping out of the acetabulum posteriolaterally when the test is positive.

b. *Ortolani's test (Fig. 40.8B)*: This sign is present when the hip is dislocated. The maneuver relocates the femoral head. With the examiners fingers on the baby's greater trochanters, the hips and knees are flexed to 90 degrees. The hips are then abducted while applying upward pressure over the greater trochanters. A positive sign is detected when a "click" is felt as the femoral head renters the acetabulum.

GESTATIONAL AGE ASSESSMENT

The American Academy of pediatrics recommended since 1967 that all newborns be classified by birth weight and gestational age, and the Dubowitz scoring system by Ballard et al (1991) remains the most popular method for determining gestational age. The examination provides a score of neuromuscular and physical maturity that can be mathematically projected onto a corresponding age, to reveal the gestational age, in weeks.

The ballard gestational age by maturity Rating consists of two scoring systems (Fig. 40.9). Physical maturity and neuromuscular maturity of six to seven characteristics each; scores from each system are added together and mathematically projected on the maturity rating scale to determine the gestational age by examination. The systems scored reflect the decreasing flexibility of muscles and joints in prematurity and the return to original positioning after movement indicative of a mature term infant. This examination is usually performed within the first 12 hours of life and is more accurate when done on term infants between 10 and 36 hours of life when the baby has had sufficient opportunity to rest following birth and when he is awake.

Gestational age and birth weight are considered jointly and marked on centile chart. The baby's birth weight is plotted against his gestational age. A baby whose weight lies between the 10th and 90th percentile this is described as appropriate for gestational age (AGA); if the birth weight is greater than 90th percentile this is described as large for gestational age (LGA) and a baby whose weight is below the 10th centile is described as being small for gestational age (SGA).

Assessment of Neuromuscular Maturity (Fig. 40.9)

The assessments are done in the following manner:

❖ *Posture:* Posture is the natural position that the newborn assumes on its back. It is observed with the infant quiet and in supine position.

NEUROMUSCULAR MATURITY

	–1	0	1	2	3	4	5
Posture							
Square window (wrist)	> 90°	90°	60°	45°	30°	0°	
Arm recoil		180°	180°	140°-180°	110°-140°	90°-110°	< 90°
Popliteal angle	180°	160°	140°	120°	100°	90°	< 90°
Scarf sign							
Heel to ear							

PHYSICAL MATURITY

Skin	Sticky, friable, transparent	Gelatinous, red, translucent	Smooth, pink, visible veins	Superficial peeling and/or rash few veins	Cracking pale areas, rare veins	Parchment deep cracking, no vessels	Leathery, cracked, wrinkled
Lanugo	None	Sparse	Abundant	Thinning	Bald areas	Mostly bald	
Plantar surface	Heet-toe 40-50 mm:–1 < 40 mm:–2	> 50 mm, no crease	Faint red marks	Anterior tranverse crease only	Creases anterior two-thirds	Creases over entire sole	
Breast	Imperceptible	Barley perceptible	Flat areola, no bud	Stippled areola, 1-2 mm bud	Raised areola, 3-4 mm bud	Full areola, 5-10 mm bud	
Eye/Ear	Lids fused loosely:–1 tightly:–2	Lids open, pinna flat, stays folded	Slightly curved pinna, soft, slow recoil	Well-curved pinna, soft but ready recoil	Pinna formed and firm instant recoil	Thick cartilage, ear stiff	
Genitals (male)	Scrotum flat, smooth	Scrotum empty, faint rugae	Testes in upper canal, rere rugae	Testes descending, few rugae	Testes down, good rugae	Testes pendulous, deep rugae	
Genitals (female)	Clitoris prominent, labia flat	Clitoris prominent, labia minora small	Clitris prominent, labia minora enlarged	Labia majora and minora equally prominent	Labia majora large, labia minora small	Labia majora cover clitoris and labia minora	

MATURITY RATING

Score	Weeks
–10	20
–5	22
0	24
5	26
10	28
15	30
20	32
25	34
30	36
35	38
40	40
45	42
50	44

Fig. 40.9: The new Ballard scale (NBS)

Source: From Ballard J New Ballard Scale, expended to include extremely premature infants. Journal of Pediatrics 1991;119:417. Reproduced by permission

Score: 0 Arms and legs extended.
1. Beginning of flexion of hips and knees, arms extended.
2. Stronger flexion of legs, arms extended.
3. Arms slightly flexed, legs flexed and abducted.
4. Full flexion of arms and legs.

❖ *Square window:* The examiner uses his or her thumb to gently press the infant's wrist and palm toward the infant's forearm. Either the angle that the wrist and the third and fourth fingers make against the forearm or the angle that the wrist and thumb make against the forearm is used for scoring.

❖ *Arm recoil:* With the infant in supine position both the forearms are flexed at chest level for 5 seconds, then fully extended by pulling on the hands, and then released. After release from extension, the amount of return to original position is observed and scored. The sign is fully positive (4) if the arms return briskly to full flexion. If the arms return to incomplete flexion or the response is sluggish, it is graded less (1 to 3). If they remain extended or only followed by random movements, the score is 0.

❖ *Popliteal angle:* This is the assessment of the angle created when the knee is extended. The infant is assessed in the supine position with the pelvis flat and the thigh of one leg resting on the abdomen while the knee is extended by exerting upward pressure on the heel of the leg with the examiner's right index finger behind the angle until resistance is met. The popliteal angle is measured.

❖ *Scarf sign:* In the supine position, the infant's hand is grasped between the thumb and first finger of the nurse's hand and, in one sweeping movement, the nurse attempts to place the hand on the opposite shoulder. Using a finger, the nurse marks on the infant's chest where the elbow of the infant falls and the scores in this category is made accordingly.
1. Elbow reaches opposite axillary line.
2. Elbow between midline and opposite axillary line.
3. Elbow reaches midline.
4. Elbow will not reach midline.

❖ *Heel to ear:* This maneuvre assesses hip flexibility in infants. With the baby in supine position, with the pelvis on a flat surface, one leg is gently extended and moved toward the infant's head on the corresponding side as near to the head as it will go without forcing it. When resistance is met, the visual distance between the ear on the infant's head and the great toe of the foot, along with leg position is scored (Grade according to diagram). Infants who experienced breech positioning or who are suspected of having developmental dysplasia of the hip may show a great amount of flexibility (Fig. 40.9).

Assessment of Physical Maturity

❖ *Skin:* Scoring in this category is based on palpation and visual inspection. Skin texture, transparency, relative thickness and flaking and peeling of the epidermis are noted. Transparency, defined as skin through which veins can be seen, is evident in premature (preterm) infants and disappears with increasing maturity. Flaking of skin and peeling with wrinkles occur in post-term infants.

❖ *Lanugo:* Lanugo is the fine hair seen mostly on the back and arms of premature infants. It eventually thins out in the lumbar region and disappears, leaving small traces on shoulders. Lanugo is lighter in colour and softer than body hair and curls at the end.

❖ *Palmar surface:* Creases on the soles of both feet are scored according to the extent to which the creases cover the soles. The best way to visualize the extent of plantar creases is to gently curl the infant's toes toward the heel, and determine the score.

❖ *Breast:* The amount of breast tissue is approximated by gently measuring the tissue present on the infant using a measuring tape in millimeters or by grasping the tissue between the examiner's thumb and forefinger. In addition, the bud and areola are inspected for size and stippling (shade of color). Lastly, the area of breast tissue is palpated to determine its elevation from the chest wall.

❖ *Eye and ear:* Eyelids should be open and should open easily in the mature infant. Ears are inspected for incurving of the pinna and palpated for a determination of the thickness of cartilage. The upper lobe recoil is performed bilaterally to validate the return to the posterior upright position when moved anteriorly and inferiorly.

❖ *Genitalia:* Both male and female genitalia are assessed with the infant in the supine position and the legs abducted. At about 35 weeks' gestational age, the testes descend into the scrotum. Deep creases gradually develop as crevices on the scrotum as the infant becomes more mature. Visualization of a pendulous scrotum occurs in the supine position with the lower extremities abducted. In this same position, female infants are assessed for the covering of the clitoris and the size of the labia majora. The distance between the edges of the labia majora and how much of the genitalia are covered can also be visualized and scored.

Once the scoring is complete on the Ballard Newborn Maturity Rating, the scores from both the neuromuscular and physical maturity categories are totaled. This score is compared mathematically to the gestational age (in weeks) through a simple proportionate formula that equates the score range with the gestational age in weeks and calculates the exact position of score within that range. An infant determined to be less than 37 weeks' gestational age is called preterm or premature. An infant whose score falls between 37 weeks and 42 weeks' gestational age is called term, and an infant that has scored beyond 42 weeks' gestation is called post-term.

DAILY CARE AND OBSERVATION OF THE NEWBORN

The daily assessment is important for identification of early problems. If the initial assessment supports that the infant is normal, the following should be done daily.

Vital Signs Check

* Respirations are to be regular, smooth and quiet, the rate about 40 per minute
* Temperature to be taken in the axilla, ear (tympanic membrane), or in the groin every 4 to 6 hours.

Weight

Weight is to be checked daily and evaluated according to birth weight. Weight loss is normal in the first few days but more than 10 percent body weight loss is abnormal. Most babies regain birth weight in 7 to 10 days, thereafter gaining weight at a rate of 150 to 200 gm per week.

General Changes in Color and Activity

Any cyanosis should be reported to the pediatrician immediately. Jaundice may be noted from the third day and is abnormal if it rises earlier, deepens or persists beyond the seventh day.

Feeding Status

The amount taken and difficulties, if any, are to be observed and recorded.

The Head

Assessment of the anterior fontanelle, which should be level, resolution of caput succedaneum and moulding and identification of any new swelling such a cephalhematoma to be done.

The Mouth

Should be clean and moist. Adherent white plaques indicate oral thrush infection (Fig. 40.10).

Fig. 40.10: Oral thrush

Umbilical Cord

The umbilical cord base is inspected and cleaned daily.

Elimination

The stools are observed and compared with expectations in relation to the baby's age and feeding method. Constipation, loose stools or sore buttocks may be observed and noted. The frequency of passing urine and stools in the past 24 hours should be noted.

Bath

Cleansing the skin may be done daily or as frequently as required, specially the face, skin flexures and napkin area, to prevent excoriation. A daily bath is recommended if the baby is at home. As the baby is undressed, his skin is inspected for rashes, septic spots or abrasions.

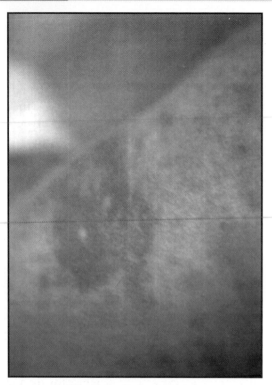

Fig. 40.11: Erythema toxicum

Skin rashes, such as erythema toxicum may alarm the mother, although it is of little significance (Fig. 40.11).

Parent-Infant Interaction

The baby is kept in a cot/crib by the bedside of the mother (rooming-in). This practice helps to establish the mother-baby relationship and to become conversant with the art of baby care when she goes home with the baby.

Vaccination and Immunization

BCG and Polio '0' dose are given during the early neonatal period where early protection is desirable.

BIBLIOGRAPHY

1. Ballard JL, Khoury JC, Wedig K, et al. New Ballard score expanded to include extremely premature infant. The Journal of Pediatrics 1991;119:417-23.
2. Blackburn ST, Loper DL. Maternal, Fetal and Neonatal Physiology: A clinical perspective, Philadelphia: WB Saunders; 1992.
3. Brazelton TB. Neonatal Behavioral Assessment Scale, 2nd edn. Spastics International Medical Publications, London: Blackwell Scientific, 1984.
4. Clausen, Flook, Ford. Maternity Nursing Today. New York: McGraw-Hill Book Co 1973.
5. De Casper A, Fifer W. Of human bonding: newborns prefer their mother's voices. In: Oates J, et al. Cognitive Development in Infancy. Hove; Lawrence Erlbaum Associates 1987.
6. Downey J, Bidder RT. Perinatal information on Infant Crying, Child: Care, Health and Development 1990;16(2):113-21.
7. Lynna LY, John EC. Maternity Nursing Care. New York; Thomson, Delmar Learning 2007.
8. Michie MM. The normal baby. In: Bennett RV, Linda KB (Eds). Myles Textbook for Midwives 13th Edn. Edinburgh: Churchill Livingstone, 1999.
9. Perry SE. The Newborn, In: Bobak IM, et al. Maternity Nursing (4th edn). St. Louis: Mosby, 1995.
10. Rushforth JA, Levene MI. Behavioral response to pain in healthy neonates. Archives of disease in childhood, 1994;70(3):F174.

41

Infant Feeding

Learning Objectives

Upon completing this chapter, the learner will be able to:
- ❖ Describe the structure and functions of the female breast
- ❖ Outline the properties and components of breast milk
- ❖ Describe the role of the midwife in ensuring successful breastfeeding
- ❖ Discuss the different causes of difficulty with breastfeeding
- ❖ Discuss the principles of bottle-feeding and the foods used.

THE BREASTS AND LACTATION

The breasts are secreting glands, composed of 15 to 24 *lobes,* separated from one another by fatty tissue. These lobes are divided into lobules, each lobule containing a certain number of *alveoli* and ducts. The alveoli contain *acini cells,* which produce milk and are surrounded by myoepithelial cells, which propel the milk out in to small ducts. These ducts connect, with larger ones called *lactiferous ducts.* One large duct leaves each lobe and widens to form a *lactiferous sinus* or *ampulla,* which acts as a temporary reservoir for milk. A *lactiferous tubule* from each sinus opens on the surface of the nipple (Fig. 41.1).

The nipple, which is composed of erectile tissue, is covered with epithelium, contains plain muscle fibers, and have sphincter-like action in controlling the flow of milk. Surrounding the nipple is an area of pigmented skin called the *areola,* which contains the montgomery's glands. These produce a sebum-like

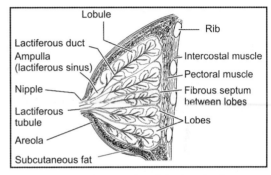

Fig. 41.1: A cross-section of the lactating breast

substance, which acts as a lubricant during pregnancy and throughout breastfeeding. Breasts, nipples and areolae are vary considerably in size from one woman to another.

The mechanism of milk production and ejection, called *let-down,* is determined hormonally. During pregnancy, estrogens and progesterone induce alveolar and ductal growth as well as stimulate the secretion of colostrum. Other hormones are also involved and they govern a complex sequence of events, which prepare the breasts for lactation. The production of milk is held in abeyance until after delivery, when the levels of placental hormones fall. Immediately after the delivery of the placenta, these hormones diminish, thereby activating the anterior lobe of the pituitary to release prolactin, which acts on the acini cells, stimulating them to produce milk. This process, which takes from 2 to 4 days, is enhanced by the sucking stimulus of the baby.

Prolactin is more important to the initiation of lactation than to its continuation. As lactation progresses, the prolactin response to suckling diminishes and milk removal (by the baby feeding or breast expression) becomes the driving force behind milk production. Oxytocin causes contraction of the myoepithelial cells as well as the uterine myometrical cells. In the early days of lactation, the let-down or milk ejection reflex is unconditioned and therefore likely to be inhibited by emotions. Later, it becomes a conditioned reflex responding to the baby's cry or other circumstances associated with the baby or feeding. Negative emotions such as fear, anger, anxiety and embarrassment as well as the presence of pain may inhibit the let-down reflex.

PROPERTIES AND COMPONENTS OF BREAST MILK

Breast milk is bluish-white in color and appears to be very watery. It is high in both lactose and fat, low in protein and phosphate. The composition is reversed in its precursor, colostrum, which is normally found in the alveoli during the later phase of pregnancy. Colostrum, a yellowish fluid, which is high in antibodies, is an excellent food for the baby during the 2 to 3 days before the milk comes in.

Human milk varies in its composition with the time of day, the stage of lactation and in response to maternal nutrition. It meets all the nutritional requirements of the new baby and has many other important properties as well.

Fat

Fat in breast milk provides the baby with more than 50 percent of his caloric requirements. The fat content is lowest in the morning and highest in the afternoon and the proportion increases during the course of the feed. It is utilized very rapidly because of the action of the enzyme lipase, which is present in the milk.

Lactose

Lactose in breast milk is converted into galactose and glucose by the action of the enzyme lactase and these sugars provide energy to the rapidly growing brain. Lactose enhances the absorption of calcium and promotes the growth of lactobacilli, which increase the intestinal acidity.

Protein

Protein in human milk is much less compared to any other mammalian milk, which makes it thinner. Human milk is whey dominant and forms soft, flocculent curds when acidified in the stomach. This provides a continuous flow of nutrients to the baby. Colostrum contains nearly three times the amount of protein that is present in mature milk and contains all the amino acids. It also contains secretary IgA and lactoferrin.

Fat-soluble Vitamins

Mature human milk contains vitamin A, D, E and K. For blood-clotting factors vitamin K is essential and the baby's gut flora synthesizes adequate amounts only after two weeks of birth. All babies are given vitamin K soon after birth to meet the need until colonization of the gut occurs.

Water-soluble Vitamins

All of the B vitamins are present at levels necessary for daily requirement. Vitamin C, which is required for collagen synthesis, is also present in adequate quantity if the mother eats a good diet.

Minerals and Trace Elements

Although the amounts of iron are less than those found in formula, the bioavailability of iron found in breast milk is very much higher; 70 percent of iron found in breast milk is absorbed whereas only 10 percent is absorbed from formula (Saarinen and Siimes, 1979). Babies who are fed on fresh cow's milk or formula need iron supplements to prevent anemia. Preterm babies do not have good iron stores and may need supplementation with oral iron. Human milk contains zinc, calcium, phosphorous, sodium and potassium in quantities lesser than in formula. However, the higher bioavailability of these minerals and trace elements ensure that the infant's needs are met.

Anti-infective Factors

Breast milk has the following anti-infective agents, which are protective for the newborn.

❖ Leukocytes (macrophages and neutrophils) that surround and destroy harmful bacteria by their phagocytic activity

❖ Secretary IgA and interferon produced by lymphocytes in human milk

❖ Immunoglobulins IgA, IgG, IgM and IgD are all found in breast milk. It 'paints' the intestinal epithelium and protects the mucosal surface against entry of pathogenic bacteria and enteroviruses

❖ Lysozyme, a general anti-infective agent

❖ Lactoferrin that prevents pathogenic *E. coli* from obtaining the iron they need for survival

❖ The bifidus factor promotes the growth of gram-positive bacilli in the gut flora particularly, *Lactobacillus bifidus*, which discourages the multiplication of pathogens.

MANAGEMENT OF BREASTFEEDING

Antenatal Preparation

The majority of women decide when they conceive that they want to breastfeed their babies. Some may not take a decision early. However, it is important to teach all pregnant women about the benefits of breastfeeding. Preparation for breastfeeding must begin when pregnancy starts altering the breasts and nipples. A comfortable brassiere that does not compress the breast, may be worn to support the increasing weight. Daily cleansing with water and a soft clean cloth followed by careful drying must be done. If nipples are inverted or flat, the procedure of nipple rolling must be explained to the mother. With lightly lubricated thumb and index finger, the mother will need to roll the nipple of each breast for approximately thirty seconds every day in the ninth month. If the mother understands how the milk is produced and how much her baby will benefit from breastfeeding, she may well be a success with feeding her baby.

Commencement of Breastfeeding

The first feed is a profoundly important experience for the mother and her baby. Unless individual circumstances indicate otherwise, the mother should have her baby with her immediately after delivery and breastfeeding should begin as soon as possible. The time of first feed, depend largely on the needs of the baby. Some babies demonstrate a need to feed almost as soon as they are born. Other babies show no interest until they are an hour or so old.

Whenever the first feed takes place, the quality of that experience is of utmost importance for the mother and baby. The early feedings might best consist of approximately 5 to 10 minutes suckling on each breast while the nipples are accustomed to it. This frequent suckling stimulates the production and let-down of lactation and reduces the potential severity of engorgement. Therefore, it is essential that there be no missed feedings, including those at night.

Preparation and Position of the Mother

The mother should be prepared for each feeding. She should be:

❖ In a comfortable position, this means any position that is comfortable for her and allows for proper positioning of her baby. This can be accomplished in a side lying, reclining or sitting position (Figs 41.2A to C). Generous use of pillows for support and comfort is most useful

❖ Without discomfort or pain. Her bladder should be empty. Any pain such as after birth-pains, episiotomy, or laceration repair pain should have received comfort measures prior to breastfeeding time

❖ Rested and relaxed

❖ Assured of available help as necessary

❖ Her hands should be washed and nipples cleansed with plain water.

Preparation and Position of the Baby

The baby's immediate preparation for breastfeeding is to have a clean, dry diaper and if necessary, to be swaddle wrapped. Swaddle wrapping (Figs 41.3A to D) when properly done, may be comforting rather than confining to babies because they feel held close and secure rather than bound. The wrapping is to be loose enough for freedom of motion of the legs. What

Fig. 41.2A: Feeding in side lying position (*For color version see Plate 3*)

Fig. 41.2B: Feeding in sitting position (*For color version see Plate 3*)

Fig. 41.2C: Sitting position with the baby in football hold (*For color version see Plate 4*)

has to be achieved is control of waving arms. For new mothers who will need this initially, it will be just a few feedings before they can cope without swaddle wrapping their baby.

Position the baby so that he or she will not be doubled up or have a twisted neck when sucking and that the head and body are supported. In bringing the baby and breast together, the following are helpful:

❖ Let the baby find the breast and grasp the nipple. Do not thrust the breast in the baby's face, as this is frightening to the baby

❖ Help the mother learn to hold her breast in such a way as to guide and control the breast and facilitate the baby's grasping of it

❖ Touch the baby's cheek with the nipple so the baby will turn towards the breast (use of the rooting reflex)

❖ Express a few drops of colostrum/milk so they are on the surface of the nipple. This provides the baby with instant gratification and reinforces learning (Fig. 41.4).

❖ As the baby grasps the nipple, the mother must make sure that the infant has enough of it for proper positioning in the mouth. The baby must grasp more than just the end of the mother's nipple. The baby must compress the lactiferous sinuses located beneath the areola with his gums when sucking in order to obtain colostrum or milk. The sequence

Figs 41.3A to D: Swaddle wrapping
(*For color version see Plate 4*)

Fig. 41.4: Initiating sucking with a drop of milk on nipple
(*For color version see Plate 4*)

Figs 41.5A and B: Technique of breastfeeding: (A) Baby
feels the nipple at his lips; (B) Nipple is sucked into the mouth

of movements of compression, sucking and swallowing is rhythmic and the mother can feel a steady pull.

❖ Once the baby's mouth is properly positioned well on to the areola, the mother releases her grasp of her breast. She now provides breathing space for the baby if needed by pressing with a finger on her breast where the baby's nose is. This may be needed during the learning period only (Figs 41.5 and 41.6).

Fig. 41.6: Baby's lips in contact with areola
(*For color version see Plate 5*)

Helping the Mother to Begin

During the early days of nursing, the mother should be instructed not to feed too long at any one feeding, as her nipples will become sore. It is recommended that she nurse from 3 to 5 minutes at every feeding during the first day, from 5 to 7 minutes during the second day, and from 7 to 10 minutes during the third day. In a week, she should be able to nurse 10 to 20 minutes on each side (the time it will probably take to empty it).

If the infant is crying hard when she wants to start breastfeeding, she should first calm the baby by holding him firmly and closely and by talking gently to him. An upset baby, who is put to breast, does not realize the nipple is in his mouth and will continue to cry loudly which may upset the mother and frustrate the baby. Once the baby is calm, he will be able to grasp the nipple and begin sucking.

The mother should nurse from both breasts at each feeding, alternating the side on which she begins. A suggestion to help the mother remember which side to start on at the next feeding is to have her put a safety pin in the bra strap on the side on which she will begin to nurse the next time. The baby should nurse on both sides because he sucks hardest on the first side and gets about 90 percent of the milk in that breast during the first 5 to 10 minutes of nursing. Using both breasts provides the necessary stimulus to keep up a sufficient amount of milk production in the breasts. This is especially important during the early weeks of nursing.

Feeding Behaviors

Babies usually will suck a bit; rest a bit (maintaining their hold on the nipple while they rest) and then suck some more. Some babies go to sleep once they get little food in their stomach and feel warm and comfortable next to the mother. The mother should be prepared for this, so she does not get upset. She can loosen the blankets around the baby, so that he is not quite so warm and drowsy during feeding. If this does not work, she may try any of the following—Rub the soles of the baby's feet, stroke his abdomen or change his position. The mother should also be prepared for the strong uterine contraction, she will feel when the baby first latches on to her breast.

Suction must be broken before trying to remove the baby from the breast. Pulling the baby off causes injury to the nipple. Suction is broken by slipping a finger into the corner of the baby's gums. Once the suction is broken, the baby is easily removed from the breast without injury to the nipple. The baby is then burped and put to the other breast (Figs 41.7 and 41.8).

Fig. 41.7: Breaking suction before removing the baby from breast *(For color version see Plate 5)*

Fig. 41.8: Burping the baby *(For color version see Plate 5)*

Lactation is established and maintained by a combination of the following:

❖ Starting breastfeeding as soon as possible after delivery
❖ Frequent feedings during the first few days, using both breasts
❖ No missed feedings or supplementary feedings
❖ Rotation of breasts as the starting and ending breasts to provide for complete emptying of both breasts
❖ Rested, relaxed and pain-free mother during feeding times
❖ Baby properly positioned on the breast.

The baby's neck should be slightly extended and the chin should be in contact with the breast. A generous portion of areola should be taken in by the lower jaw.

Timing and Frequency of Feeding

It is usual in the first day or two for the baby to have 6 to 8 hours gaps between good feeds. This is normal and provides an excellent opportunity for the mother to rest. As the milk volume increases, the feeds become more frequent and a little shorter. After the first few days, the baby will settle into his/her individual pattern of feeding frequency. This is described as "self-demand feeding" or "baby-led feeding" (i.e. feeding the baby when he or she is hungry). It is unusual for a healthy baby to feed less often than six times in 24 hours from the third day. If he demands fewer feeds, the reasons should be investigated. Individual mother-baby pairs develop their own unique pattern of feeding and, provided the baby is thriving, there is no need to change it.

Care of the Breasts

❖ Daily washing is all that is necessary for breast hygiene. The normal skin flora is beneficial to the baby. Using soap, alcohol or other drying agents can lead quickly to cracking of the nipples. Providing good support to breasts is important to avoid discomfort
❖ If the breasts become engorged, apply warmth to breasts, prior to each breastfeeding, to promote milk flow. This can be

Fig. 41.9: Applying warm towel to engorged breast
(For color version see Plate 5)

accomplished with warm washcloths or warm showers (Fig. 41.9).

❖ If there is areolar enlargement, manual expression of the milk to soften the area prior to nursing the baby will help the baby latch on to the nipple properly and easily
❖ Use manual expression of milk to empty the breasts after the baby has nursed, if they are still uncomfortably full and engorged after the feeding
❖ Ice bags may be applied to breasts between feedings to reduce swelling and pain
❖ If the nipples become tender:
   – Nurse on the less sore nipple first until there is let-down, then switch the baby to the sore nipple to empty that breast and meet the baby's sucking needs
   – Use a pacifier rather than the end of feedings on the nipples to meet the baby's sucking needs until the nipples are not sore
   – Breastfeed more frequently for shorter periods
   – Be sure the baby is properly positioned on the breast and change the baby's position, which will change the precise pressure points on the nipple; for example, shifting from an arm hold to football hold
   – Be sure to use a combination of exposure (of the breasts) to both air and heat after each breastfeeding, followed by application of nipple cream.
❖ Be sure to break the suction before removing the baby from the breast.

Benefits of Breastfeeding to the Mother

There are well-known and documented physiological benefits to the breastfeeding mother:

- ❖ Studies conducted on women of various cultures have shown that women who breastfeed have markedly decreased chance of developing breast cancer
- ❖ The incidence of thrombophlebitis is lower in breastfeeding mothers
- ❖ Postpartum uterine involution is more rapid in mothers who breastfeed. Therefore, delayed postpartum hemorrhage is also less common
- ❖ Lactation has been shown to suppress ovulation for about 75 days postpartum in almost 100 percent of women who do not supplement their infants with bottle. Thus, breastfeeding for a short time is a preferred contraceptive.

Benefits to the Baby

- ❖ Breast milk is of ideal composition for easy digestion with low osmotic load
- ❖ Colostrum and breast milk provide antibody protection (passive immunity) against several types of viruses
- ❖ Breastfed babies show a marked decrease in respiratory infections and gastroenteritis. Lysozyme, an enzyme present in breast milk destroys invasive organisms, especially *E coli*. Additional resistance to the gut from invading organisms is given by lactoferrin and bifidus factor and secretary IgA contained in breast milk
- ❖ Allergic disorders, such as infantile eczema, asthma and hay fever are much less common in breastfed babies
- ❖ Since the weight gain of a breastfed baby is less than that of a bottlefed one, obesity is less common
- ❖ Breastfeeding offers a psychological benefit by establishing healthy mother-baby relationship
- ❖ Breastmilk is readily available for the baby at the right temperature.

Volume of the Feed

Wellgrown infants are born with good glycogen reserve and high levels of antidiuretic hormone. Consequently, they do not need large volumes of milk or colostrum any sooner than they are made available physiologically. In the first 24 hours, the baby takes an average of 5 ml per feed; in the second 24 hours, this increases to 14 ml per feed (Moody et al, 1996).

The average requirement of milk is about 100 ml/kg/24 hours on the third day and is increased to 150 ml/kg/24 hours by the tenth day.

Difficulties in Breastfeeding and Management

At times, breastfeeding causes some problems.

Difficulties due to Mother

- ❖ *Inadequate supply of milk:* The mother who says she does not have enough milk for her baby probably is not nursing often enough. The nurse should instruct the mother that the oftener the baby nurses, the more milk she will have. The milk supply is directly related to the frequency of nursing—the more often the baby nurses, the more milk is produced
- ❖ *The baby who will not suck:* An infant who refuses to suck at the breast or who thrusts his tongue toward the roof of his mouth presents special problem. These babies will usually suck beautifully from a bottle nipple and therefore it is important not to supplement them with an artificial nipple. Expressed milk may be given by spoon or eyedropper. Milk can be dribbled down over the breast into the baby's mouth; which might help him to begin sucking from the breast
- ❖ *Breast ailments such as engorgement of breast, cracked nipple, depressed nipple and mastitis:* (Management of each condition is discussed earlier in this chapter) for mastitis, she should consult the physician. Once treatment has begun, she will be able to nurse the baby.
- ❖ *Anxiety and stress:* Anxiety, upset or emotional trauma influence milk ejection; therefore a mother who is not able to relax prior to nursing may find that her milk will not let-down. If possible, she should be

encouraged to lie down while nursing and concentrate on relaxing her baby. If lying down is not possible, she could sit down, put her feet up and perhaps read something. Her goal must be gearing her thoughts towards something other than the cause of upset

❖ *Blistered nipple:* A blistered nipple is usually an indication of improper sucking by the baby. It most often is caused by the infant grasping only the nipple and not the areolar area. These blisters may bleed when they are broken. Ultraviolet light and resting the nipple for 24 to 48 hours are preferred methods of treatment

❖ *Poor attachment of breast:* It leads to quick, shallow sucks instead of slow and deep. Areola remains outside the mouth. This causes nipple pain. Assistance and instructions from the midwife can improve the technique of breastfeeding. Proper placement of the nipple is on top of the baby's tongue with as much of the areolar space as possible in his mouth

❖ *Short nipples:* As the baby has to form a teat from both the breast and nipple, short nipples can cause problems and the mother should be reassured of this

❖ *Abnormally large nipples:* If the baby is small, his mouth may not be able to get beyond the nipple and on to the breast. Lactation could be initiated by expressing the milk. As the baby grows and the breast and nipple become more protractile, breast-feeding may become possible

❖ *Inverted and flat nipples:* Many babies are able to attach to the breast, even if the nipple is considered unfavorable. In difficult cases, it may be necessary to initiate lactation by expressing and delay attempting to attach the baby to the breast until lactation is established and the breasts have become soft and the breast tissue more protractile.

Difficulties due to Baby

❖ *Low birthweight baby:* The baby is too small or too feeble to suck. Tube feeding of expressed milk and artificial feeding are given until the baby becomes able to suck from breasts.

❖ *Temporary illness* such as cerebral irritation, respiratory tract infection, nasal obstruction due to congestion and lethargy due to jaundice or oral thrush may all lead to improper suckling. Due to lack of proper nipple stimulation and improper emptying, the milk may dry up. This must be recognized early and prevented

❖ *Over-distension of the stomach with swallowed air:* The problem can be prevented by burping the baby several times during feeding

❖ *Cleft palate:* The baby is unable to form a vacuum and thus form a teat out of the breast and nipple. Feeding expressed milk using special teat device can be done until the baby has had a surgical repair. Feeding with spoon can be another method.

Contraindications to Breastfeeding

❖ Drugs used for cancer, certain hormones and radioactive isotopes. When the mother uses any of these, breastfeeding should be suspended

❖ *HIV infection:* The human immunodeficiency virus may be transmitted in breast milk. In cases where artificial feeding is difficult, the mother may be counseled as regard the risks and benefits and helped to make an informed choice

❖ Chronic medical illness, such as decompensated organic heart lesion and pulmonary tuberculosis

❖ Puerperal psychosis

❖ Women receiving high doses of anti-epileptic, anticoagulant and antithyroid drugs

❖ Breastfeeding may be suspended when the mother is treated with metronidazole and chloramphenicol.

Underfeeding and Overfeeding

Normal progress of feeding is evidenced by: (1) General condition—happy baby, sleeps between feeds and at night, does not vomit and passes urine at least six times in 24 hours.

(2) Vigor which is manifested by movements of the limbs and cry, (3) Expected level of weight gain.

Features of Underfeeding

❖ Failure of the infant to gain weight as per schedule, evidenced from the weight curve
❖ Dissatisfied baby evidenced by cry in between feeds and at night
❖ Constipation
❖ Scanty, high colored urine

Management is to substitute the lesser amount of milk by artificial feed.

Features of Overfeeding

Overfeeding usually occurs at the end of first week. The features are:

❖ Vomiting soon after feeding
❖ Frequent, loose, bulky stools with undigested curds and fat
❖ Excoriation over the buttocks
❖ Variable weight curve—excess, stationary or at times falling.

Management is to put the baby to breast for shorter periods. It may be helpful to give little sterile water prior to each feed.

Suppression of Lactation

If a mother chooses not to breastfeed or if has a late miscarriage or stillbirth, lactation needs to be suppressed. The woman may experience discomfort for a day or two, but if unstimulated, the breasts will naturally cease to produce milk. In order to reduce discomfort the breasts must be supported with a breast binder. Suppression with hormones is effective but carry the risk of thrombosis.

Complementary and Supplementary Feeds

Complementary feeds are given after giving the baby breastfeeds. Complementary feeds may become necessary for babies who are small for dates, lethargic, jaundiced or difficult to attach. Mothers may be instructed to give their expressed milk by bottle.

Supplementary feeds are given in place of breastfeeds. This is justified only in cases where the mother has severe illness, because each breastfeed missed by the baby will interfere with the establishment of lactation and damage the mother's confidence.

The Babyfriendly Hospital Initiative

In 1992, United Nations International Children's Emergency Fund (UNICEF) and World Health Organization (WHO) launched the babyfriendly initiative amongst doctors, nurses, health workers and parents in hospitals and maternity centers to promote, protect and support breastfeeding. The objective is to reestablish the superiority of breastfeeding in order to protect the newborn's health by becoming baby friendly. In order to fulfill the initiative, the UNICEF and the WHO laid down ten steps to create the babyfriendly environment. These are:

❖ There must be a written breastfeeding policy
❖ All health care workers must be trained to implement this policy
❖ All pregnant women must be informed about the benefits of breastfeeding
❖ Mothers must be helped to initiate breastfeeding within half an hour of birth
❖ Mothers are shown the best way to breastfeed
❖ Unless medically indicated, the newborn should be given no food or drink other than breast milk
❖ To practice "roomingin" by allowing mothers and babies to remain together 24 hours a day
❖ To encourage demand of breastfeeding
❖ To encourage exclusive breastfeeding
❖ No artificial teats should be given to babies
❖ Breastfeeding support groups are to be established and mothers must be referred to them on discharge.

A babyfriendly hospital should also provide other preventive health cares, e.g. infant immunization, rehydration salts against diarrheal dehydration and child's growth and development surveillance (Dutta, 2001).

Artificial Feeding

When the infant is fed by any preparation other than human milk, it is called artificial feeding. As artificial feeding is commonly accomplished by using a bottle, it is often called as bottle-feeding.

Indications of Artificial Feeding

❖ Contraindications of breastfeeding either temporary or permanent (as mentioned earlier).
❖ Inadequate quantity of breast milk.
❖ Changing lifestyle of women (expressed breast milk may be an alternative).

FOOD USED

The kind of formula used varies. In general, boiled, diluted cow's milk, dried milk and milk formulas are commonly used. In some countries, goat's milk and buffalo's milk are used. Ready-to-use formulas in single use bottles are used in developed countries. However, there is no perfect substitute for breast milk.

Cow's Milk

Cow's milk when compared with human milk contains more protein and minerals and less lactose and about the same amount of fat (Table 41.1).

Qualitative Differences

Though, the quantitative differences, shown above, can be rectified, some of the qualitative differences are difficult to approximate. *Sugar* content in both human and cow's milk is in the form of lactose but as the concentration is higher in human milk, it is sweeter. *Fat proportion* in both milks is same, but the fat globules in the cow's milk are coarser and hence more difficult to digest than human milk. Protein of human milk contains two-thirds lactalbumin, which is soluble and easily digestible, and one-third caseinogen. The caseinogen content of the breast milk can be digested by the gastric juice with formation of flocculent curd (woolly), whereas in cow's milk, it is converted into heavy, tough casein curd causing indigestion. The sodium content of cow's milk is about four times higher than that of human milk, which may lead to hypernatremia and the resulting thirst causes baby to cry.

Modification of Cow's Milk

Quantitative changes in the constituents in the cow's milk can be done by dilution followed by addition. One part of milk is added to one part of water. This reduces the protein content to half while fat and sugar contents are reduced greatly. Sugar is added in the form of glucose or cane sugar to bring about readjustment in sugar content. Boiling changes the caseinogen and makes it easily digestible.

Preparation of a Feed

Preparation of a feed for the infant should preferably be done each time prior to feeding. A formula that can be used is to divide the weight of the baby in pounds by two, which gives the amount of feed in ounces; 1 ½ ounces should be water and the remainder cow's milk. One teaspoon of cane sugar is to be added.

Example of preparation of a feed for an infant weighing 8 lbs:

Amount of feed = Four ounces, which is made up of water 1 ½ ounces, milk 2 ½ ounces and cane sugar 1 teaspoon full.

The mixture is to be boiled in a clean saucepan to be followed by cooling before the baby is fed (Dutta, 2001).

Dried Milk

Three varieties of dried milk are commercially available. Full cream dried milk, half cream dried milk and humanized dried milk. If full strength is to be used, one level scoop measure is added

Table 41.1 Composition of human and cow's milk

	Sugar	Fat	Protein	Minerals	Water	Calories
Human	7	3.5	1.2	0.4	89	67
Cow's	4.5	3.5	3.4	0.8	88	67

to 30 ml (one ounce) of water. This gives the same composition and calorie value as that of cow's milk. When half strength is required, one level scoop measure is to be added to 60 ml.

Babies may be fed either by spoon from the bowl/cup or by feeding bottle. The cup and spoon are easy to clean. The feeding utensils (cup and spoon, or bottle and teat) should be cleaned prior to and after each feeding. The rubber teat and bottle should be boiled once a day (Dutta, 2001).

Preparation of the Mother for Artificial Feeding

❖ Mothers who choose to feed their babies artificially should be shown how to prepare a bottle feed safely. If the mother and baby are at home, this demonstration should take place in her house, using her own articles. If she is in the hospital, she may be shown there

❖ Clear instructions about the volumes of milk/powder, water and sugar must be given so that she understands accurate measurements

❖ Effective cleaning of utensils must be explained. For boiling, full immersion is essential and the contents of the pan must be boiled for at least five minutes

❖ Rinsing of the bowl and spoon or bottle prior to feeding must be done using recently boiled water

❖ The mother should try to stimulate breastfeeding conditions for the baby by holding him close, maintaining eye-to-eye contact

❖ The size of the hole in the teat should be of correct size. A useful test for the correct hole-size is to turn the bottle upside down; the feed should drip at a rate of about one drop per second

❖ Burping of the baby should be done in the middle and at the end of each feed

❖ Not more than twenty minutes should be spent for each feed

❖ The mother should be warned about the dangers of "bottle propping" and told that the baby must never be left unattended while feeding from a bottle.

Weaning from the Breast

It is the period during which the baby gets accustomed to food other than its mother's milk. This period extends from sixth months to one year. During this period, the baby's demand is more, breast milk cannot supply the necessary need, and as such, additional foods are required.

Breastfeeding should be stopped gradually. The mother may eliminate one breastfeeding a day and offer cup or bottlefeeding at that time. In a few days, the mother may eliminate another nursing and feed the baby twice by cup or bottle or additional food. She should continue in this manner until her milk has dried up. Weaning may be completed by ten months to one year.

Semisolid foods such as rice, dhal, boiled fish, boiled egg and fruits such as banana are incorporated in the tropical countries. Problems usually encountered during the weaning period are nutritional disturbances and weaning diarrhea due to altered composition of the food.

BIBLIOGRAPHY

1. Applebaum RM. The modern management of successful breastfeeding. Pediatric Clinics of North America 1970;17:203-05.
2. Clausen JP, et al. Maternity Nursing Today, New York; McGraw Hill, 1973.
3. Dutta DC. Textbook of Obstetrics, 5th edn. Calcutta; New Central Book Company, 2001.
4. Fisher C. Feeding, In: Bennett RV, Linda KB (Eds). Myles Textbook for Midwives 13th edn. Edinburgh; Churchill Livingstone, 1999.
5. Moody J, Britten J. Breastfeeding your baby. A National Childbirth Trust Guide. HMSO, London 1996.
6. Saarinen UM, Siimes MA. Iron absorption from breastmilk, cow's milk and Iron supplemented formula. Pediatric Research 1979;13:143-47.
7. Varney Helen. Nurse-Midwifery, 2nd edn. Boston; Jones-Barlett Publishers 1996.

42

The Low Birthweight Baby, the Preterm Baby and Intrauterine Growth Retarded Baby

Learning Objectives

Upon completing this chapter, the learner will be able to:
- ❖ Describe the different classes of low birthweight babies
- ❖ List the characteristics of low birthweight babies
- ❖ Discuss the appropriate care for these babies.

DEFINITION

The internationally accepted definition of a low birthweight (LBW) baby is one whose weight at birth is 2500 gm or less (WHO, 1977). Further classification within the low birthweight group include the very low birthweight (VLBW) baby weighing 1001-1500 gm and the extremely low birthweight (ELBW) baby who weighs 1000 gm or less.

In order to assess a low birthweight baby's needs or likely progress, in addition to the birthweight, an assessment of the gestational age is important. Because, infants born at term or post-term may weight less than 2500 gm and occasionally the baby of a diabetic mother may weigh much more than 2500 gm even before 37 weeks. When gestational age is considered, a *term infant* is one born after 37 completed weeks of gestation. A preterm infant is one born before 37 completed weeks of gestation.

A classification of low birthweight babies is done after correlating both the birthweight and gestational age (Fig. 42.1).

Centile charts have been devised on which the baby's birthweight is plotted against his gestational age. A baby whose weight lies

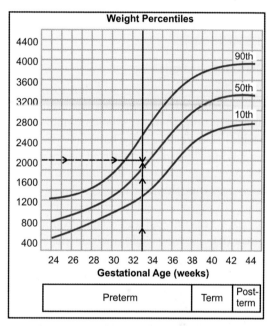

Fig. 42.1: Correlation of birthweight and gestational age in percentile

between the 10th and 90th centile is considered *appropriate for gestational age (AGA)*. The growth potential of this baby is normal. If birthweight is greater than the 90th percentile, this is described as a *large for gestational age (LGA)* and a baby whose weight is below the 10th percentile is described as being *small for gestational age (SGA)*. It follows that a baby born at term may be AGA, SGA or LGA; similarly, a preterm baby may be AGA, LGA or SGA.

INCIDENCE OF LOW BIRTHWEIGHT

The incidence of low birthweight is generally higher in those countries where the mean birthweight is low and as such varies from about 5 to 40 percent of live births. In India about a third of infants weigh less than 2500 gm (Dutta, 2001).

The factors influencing the low birthweight of the baby include short gestational period, Socioeconomic standard and nutritional and environmental factors. Ethnic background and genetic control are also significant.

SMALL FOR GESTATIONAL AGE TERM INFANT

Clinical Appearance

Typically, the body is long and thin with a disproportionately large head. The skin is often dry and peeling and there are abundant palmar and plantar skin creases. These babies are described as having the look of "worried old men". In behavior, they are active and indicate from an early age that they are hungry. These babies show an asymmetrical growth pattern. Their length is less affected and occipitofrontal head circumference may well be within the normal range for a term infant (Figs 42.2A and B).

A second group of SGA babies shows symmetrical growth retardation *in utero*. These are likely to be very normal babies whose size is compatible with ethnic and genetic expectations. Multiple gestation babies are frequently of this type—Symmetrically growth retarded.

A third group of babies with stunted growth *in utero* is by the teratogenic effects of infection, drug or alcohol abuse. In these babies, all three parameters, weight, length and occipitofrontal circumference are compromised. These babies are likely to present a variety of problems in the neonatal period.

Causes of Intrauterine Growth Retardation

These include maternal disease such as hypertensive disorders, which lead to poor placental perfusion, reduced availability of nutrients or placental transfer of substances, which have a teratogenic effect. Extremes of maternal age, socioeconomic factors, parity and the number of fetuses *in utero* may all affect the normal growth pattern.

Management at Birth

These babies are more susceptible to hypothermia. Extra care should therefore be taken to ensure that the baby is dried and wrapped in warm blankets soon after birth. All other aspects of management are same as for the normal baby.

Feeding

In order to meet the needs of a baby who has been starved *in utero*, early and frequent feeding must be instituted. These babies are hungry and mothers who choose to breastfeed may start as soon as possible. Breast milk from mothers of SGA babies has increased proteins and immunoglobulins for the first few days.

SGA babies have a higher metabolic rate and higher energy expenditure than AGA babies

Fig. 42.2A: Appearance of a SGA newborn
(*For color version see Plate 5*)

Fig. 42.2B: Appearance of a preterm newborn
(*For color version see Plate 5*)

and require more calories than AGA babies (Davies et al, 1996). Lack of subcutaneous fat and liver glycogen stores further compromise their nutritional reserves. For formula fed babies, feeds are therefore calculated at a rate of 9 ml/kg/day, increasing by 10 to 15 ml/kg/day. Blood glucose levels should be monitored at least six hourly for the first 48 hours. These babies loose minimal amounts of weight before gaining weight rapidly.

Temperature Control

Small for gestational age babies have relatively mature temperature control mechanism. However, due to lack of subcutaneous fat, they are more susceptible for hypothermia from fluctuations in environmental temperature.

The temperature should therefore be monitored regularly and maintained at optimum level.

Skin Care

Babies whose skin is dry, peeling or cracked require special attention. They must be kept clean and dry to prevent infection. An emollient may be applied to skin after bath.

THE PRETERM BABY

A baby born before 37 completed weeks of gestation calculating from the first day of last menstrual period is arbitrarily defined as a preterm baby. Babies born before 37 weeks (premature) usually weigh 2500 gm or less.

Less than 5 percent of preterm babies may weigh more than 2500 gm.

Incidence

The incidence of preterm babies is about 20 to 25 percent and constitutes two-thirds of low birthweight babies.

Causes of Prematurity

The causes of preterm birth remain unknown although several factors are considered to predispose to shortened pregnancy.

Multiple Pregnancy

Over distension of the uterus frequently results in spontaneous preterm labor especially when there are more than two babies.

Maternal Disease in Pregnancy

Pre-eclampsia, polyhydramnios or antepartum hemorrhage due to either placenta previa or placental abruption may prompt the decision to terminate the pregnancy early.

Previous Obstetric History

There is increased incidence of preterm labor in women who give history of previous induced or spontaneous abortion or preterm delivery.

Low Socioeconomic and Nutritional Status

Women in low socioeconomic group appear to have shorter gestation period though there may be other compounding factors such as maternal illness.

Uterine Anomalies

Uterine anomalies, such as cervical incompetence and malformation of uterus.

Infections

Infection's such as pyelonephritis, acute appendicitis or genital tract infections.

Chronic Diseases

Chronic diseases associated with pregnancy, such as hypertension, diabetes, severe anemia and decompensated heart lesions.

Fetal Causes

❖ Conditions where fetal well-being may be seriously compromised if pregnancy were continued, such as placental insufficiency and Rhesus disease

❖ Presence of congenital abnormalities possibly complicated by growth retardation.

Clinical Appearance

The weight is 2500 gm or less and length is usually less than 44 cm. Relative to his size the preterm baby has a big head, small thoracic area and large abdomen. The skull bones are soft, wide sutures and large fontanelles. Pinnae of ears are soft and flat. The eyes are kept closed.

The skin is thin, red, shiny, due to lack of subcutaneous fat, and covered by plentiful lanugo and vernix caseosa. Muscle tone is poor. Plantar creases are not visible before 34th week. The testicles are undescended; the labia minora are exposed because the labia majora are not in contact. The nails are not grown up to the fingertips.

Risks Associated with Prematurity

Asphyxia

The babies are likely to be asphyxiated because of anatomical and functional immaturity.

Hypothermia

A low birthweight baby has reduced subcutaneous as well as brown fat. Preterm babies often fail to maintain normal range of temperature.

Pulmonary Problems

The deficient lung surfactant in preterm babies born before 34th week predisposes to pulmonary problems such as respiratory distress syndrome (RDS) and atlectasis.

Cerebral Hemorrhage

The causes are soft skull bones, which allow dangerous degree of moulding, fragile capillaries and hypoprothrombinemia.

Infection

Protective passive immunity is usually acquired from the mother during the later months of pregnancy. As the protective immunoglobulins transferred from the mother is less, the incidence of infection is increased by 3 to 10 fold.

Jaundice

Physiological jaundice is exaggerated in preterm babies. Because of hepatic insufficiency, the bilirubin produced by the excessive hemolysis cannot be conjugated adequately for excretion as bile, leading to rise in unconjugated bilirubin, which is responsible for jaundice.

Anemia

Lack of stored iron, hypofunction of the bone marrow and excessive hemolysis all contribute to anemia.

Retrolental Fibroplacia (Retinopathy of Prematurity)

The cause is related to the liberal administration of high concentration of oxygen (above 40%) for a prolonged period (1–2 days) following birth. Blindness occurs usually within 6 months due to the formation of an opaque membrane behind the lens. Other factors like extreme prematurity, hypoxia, lactic acidosis, vitamin E deficiency and bright light have been implicated as causes of blindness (Dutta, 2001).

Care of the Preterm Baby at Birth

In the absence of problems during labor, the preterm baby will frequently establish respiration successfully and require no active resuscitation. It is important to be sure that optimum conditions surround his immediate care. Specific aspects of care are the following:

❖ The cord is to be clamped quickly to prevent hypervolemia and later development of hyperbilirubinemia
❖ Adequate oxygenation must be provided through mask in concentration not exceeding 35 percent
❖ The baby should be wrapped including head in a warm blanket or towel, and laid on the side with the head slightly lowered. Temperature must be maintained at 36.5 to 37.5°C
❖ The baby should be handled with extreme gentleness. Bathing is not appropriate for the preterm baby.

Preterm babies are functionally immature and "special care" is needed for their survival. Transfer to special baby care unit or neonatal intensive care unit may be needed in order to maintain their health status.

Principles of Care

❖ To maintain a relatively stable body temperature and adequate humidification
❖ To prevent or treat atlectasis
❖ To prevent infection
❖ To maintain adequate nutrition.

Body Temperature

Premature babies have difficulties maintaining temperature due to their:

❖ Large surface area to body mass ratio
❖ Lack of subcutaneous fat

Fig. 42.3: An Isolette/Incubator for care of preterm baby
(*For color version see Plate 6*)

❖ Lack of brown fat deposits—These are normally laid down after 36th week
❖ Comparatively thin skin with increase in transepidermal water loss and consequent heat loss from evaporation
❖ Lack of glycogen stores to use in heat generation by increasing metabolic rate
❖ Inability to reduce temperature by sweating.

In order to preserve and maintain thermal homeostasis, the preterm infant should be nursed in a neutrothermal environment. Failure to do so will cause an increase in metabolic rate, increase in oxygen requirements and may lead to respiratory difficulty.

Smaller babies are to be nursed in an incubator to maintain their temperature within normal limits. Alternatively, the baby can be managed under radiant warmer. The skin temperature should be maintained at 36 to 37°C with surrounding humidity at 50 percent (Fig. 42.3).

If it is not possible to maintain the temperature and humidity of the room, the baby should be kept in a warm crib or baby cot. Rubber hot water bottles, filled with hot (not boiling) water, may be used to warm the crib. Care should be taken to see that the bottles are stoppered and well-covered with clothings. The temperature of the crib should be maintained at 30°C (85°F).

Respiratory Support

Baby's air passages are to be cleared and oxygen administered with the baby in the incubator. Continuous oxygen monitoring by pulse oxymeter (90–92%) and periodic blood gas sampling are required.

Desirable levels are:
❖ PaO_2 55–65 mm Hg
❖ $PaCO_2$ 35–45 mm Hg
❖ pH 7.35–7.45.

Surfactant replacement therapy may be required for some babies.

Prevention of Infection

As the transfer of protective immunoglobulins from the mother to a preterm baby is less, the incidence of infection is increased 3 to 10 fold. The commonest types of infection are bronchopneumonia, meningitis and gastroenteritis. Great care should be taken to minimize risk factors. All caregivers should follow correct handwashing techniques. Use of bactericidal soaps or antiseptic solutions is recommended. Drying the hands properly is also important. While in the hospital, separate articles must be used for the baby and use of disposable articles must be encouraged to reduce the risk of nosocomial infection.

Nutritional Needs

Breast milk is the first choice of nutrition for all low birthweight babies. Colostrum, foremilk, hindmilk and preterm milk help faster growth of the body. Lucas et al (1994) have demonstrated that babies who were breastfed had a higher intelligence quotient (IQ) at the age of 5 and 8 years than their formula-fed counterparts (Halliday in Bennett and Brown, 1999). A further advantage of breast milk for the preterm baby is improved gastric emptying (Ewer et al, 1994).

The sucking swallowing reflex is developed by the preterm baby around 34th week's gestation, but the babies must be individually assessed. For babies who are able, direct feeding from the breast between 1 to 2 hours of birth eliminates hypoglycemia, lowers serum bilirubin and neurological sequelae. It should be remembered however, that a preterm baby may tire easily and not be able to sustain the effort long enough to obtain his necessary fluid requirements. In addition, the energy expended in sucking may leave insufficient calories to support growth and development. Hence, regular breastfeeding may be offered, if this does not overtire the baby. For smaller babies it is preferable to offer complementary and / or supplementary feeds from a cup or spoon. Those babies who are too immature to meet their nutritional needs by breastfeeding may still be put to the breast for short periods, as this will help establish lactation. If unable to put the baby directly to the breast, the mother may improve lactation by expressing milk.

Feeding intervals depend on the birthweight of the baby and range from hourly in extreme prematurity to three hourly feeds in babies born after 36th week.

Feeding Methods

The methods used for feeding depend on the size and vigor of the infant and his ability to suck and swallow. Thus, while comparatively bigger babies can be put to breast right from the beginning, smaller babies should be fed by any of the following methods:

- ❖ Tube feeding (Gavage)
- ❖ Dropper, bowl and spoon
- ❖ Bottle
- ❖ Intravenous.

Generally, babies weighing <1200 gm or less than 30 weeks gestational age are started on intravenous fluids first. Tube feeding is initiated after 2 to 3 days followed by spoonfeeding after 2 to 4 weeks and thereafter breastfeeding. Babies weighing 1200 to 1800 gm with gestational age 30 to 34 weeks may be started on tube feeding and gradually move on to spoon and breastfeeding. Whereas babies weighing over 1800 gm or above 34 weeks gestation may be started on breastfeeding straight away.

Tube Feeding or Gavage

Nasogastric or orogastric feeding may be given using a size 5 French gauge catheter (0.5 mm internal diameter). Preference for the oro- or nasogastric route may vary in institutions. An orogastric tube may be easier to pass but it is more likely to be dislodged. Hence, care should be taken to ensure that the tube is correctly positioned before instilling milk. The baby's position must be maintained in a head-up tilt. Measurement of the tube must be made from the root of the nose to the xiphisternum with the baby's head in a position of slight extension plus 2.5 cm. The tube must be aspirated and checked for the acidity of gastric aspirate prior to giving the milk. Expressed milk may be started with a small amount and is gradually built up. The ordered amount of fluid may be given by gravitation or by pressure.

Dropper or Spoonfeeding

This is used when the baby can swallow but fails to suck.

Bottlefeeding

It is used when the baby can suck and swallow but cannot manage to express the milk out from the breast.

Intravenous Fluid Therapy

Babies nursed within the incubator or under radiant warmer have increased fluid requirement due to the increased insensible water loss. Monitoring of fluid is done by measuring body weight, urine output, urine specific gravity and serum sodium.

Nature of Food

Breast milk expressed from the mother is ideal. If this is not available, diluted cow's milk in a proportion of 1:1 (milk: water) for the first month and 2:1 during the second month is an alternative substitute. One teaspoonful of glucose should be added to 50 ml of prepared milk for the first 10 days and thereafter reduced to one teaspoonful to 100 ml of formula. Premature infants require more calories than mature babies because of relatively greater loss of heat from the body surface. To meet the calorie requirements, the amount of milk given is progressively increased until the baby is receiving 200 ml per kg bodyweight. This may be achieved by two weeks. Because of small stomach capacity, weak cardiac sphincter and poor cough reflex, the feeds should be small and are to be given at shorter intervals. Thus, initially a much smaller volume is to be given.

All premature babies should receive additional supplement of vitamins and minerals, which should be started after two weeks (Dutta, 2000).

Skin Care

A newborn preterm baby is not bathed for the first few days. Depending on the gestational age of the baby, the epidermal layer of the skin may be more or less keratinized and therefore, afford variable protection against invading organisms. In the neonatal period, there is accelerated maturation of the epidermal layer of the preterm baby's skin (Blackburn and Loper, 1992). This process of keratinization may, however, be hampered if the baby is regularly immersed in a bath of water and toweled dry. Bathing will also alter the naturally low pH of the skin provided by normal skin flora, especially if alkaline or bactericidal soaps are used. Keeping the baby socially clean by removing milk or vomit debris and keeping the napkin area clean and dry will suffice.

Promotion of Growth and Development

Promotion of growth and development is one of the important objectives in caring for the low birthweight infant. One of the ways in which this can be done is by positioning the baby correctly. Encouraging the baby to adopt a flexed position will reduce heat loss and conserve energy. This can be achieved by using rolled blankets or sheets in the incubator to prevent the baby roaming around inside. Mother should be allowed to see her baby in the nursery. Stroking or caressing and interacting with the baby must be encouraged. They would then find it easier to pluck up courage to pick up and hold the baby. Macedo and Attree (1994) described that touching increases the production of growth hormone and strengthens the immune system. Parents may also enjoy the contact and feel that they are doing something possible and helpful for the baby. However, it should be remembered that each baby is an individual and some may be less responsive to this stimulation than others may. Close observation is necessary to pick up the behavioral cues that suggest the baby is unhappy.

Kangaroo Care

Placing the baby in skin-to-skin contact with his mother or father is called Kangaroo care. It was first described in Columbia (Whitelaw, 1990). The idea has since then spread to other parts of the world. This involves placing the naked baby (wearing only a napkin) against the mother's chest inside her blouse or dress. The baby's back may be covered with a blanket if necessary. Both mother and baby were found to enjoy the experience; the baby goes to quiet sleep, which is most beneficial for his growth and development (Halliday in Bennett and Brown, 1999).

Favorable Signs of Progress

Preterm babies, who thrive well, show the following favorable signs:
* Skin color remains pink all the time
* Smooth and regular breathing
* Increasing vigor evidenced by movements of limbs and cry
* Progressive gain in weight; Baby looses 1 to 1.5 percent of birthweight every day for the first 5 to 7 days. Thereafter, the baby gains birthweight by 10 to 14 days.

Preterm babies are discharged when they attain sufficient weight (approximately 2,000 gm in tropics), have good vigor and able to suckle the breast successfully (Dutta, 2001).

Advice to Mother on Discharge

Wherever possible, supervision of the baby to be continued at home by public health nurses or health visitors. The following advices are to be given to the mother:
* Feeding instructions, if formula feeding, all aspects of preparation of feeds and sterilizing of equipment
* Clothing, to prevent heat loss
* Bedding, to place the baby on his side to prevent aspiration and no pillows to be used in order to reduce the risk of suffocation

❖ Multivitamin and iron supplementation as prescribed
❖ Immunization and check-up.

INTRAUTERINE GROWTH RETARDATION (IUGR)

Intrauterine growth retardation is present in those babies whose birthweight is below the tenth percentile of average for the gestational age. Growth retardation can occur in preterm, term or post-term babies.

Other terms used are *Intrauterine growth restriction, Dysmaturity and Small for date.*

Incidence

Dysmaturity comprises about one-third of low birthweight babies. The incidence among term babies is about 5 percent and that among post-term babies is about 15 percent.

Types of IUGR Fetuses

Based on the clinical evaluation and ultrasound examination, the small fetuses are divided into two.
1. *Fetuses that are small and healthy*: The birthweight is less than tenth percentile for their gestational age. They have normal subcutaneous fat and usually have uneventful neonatal course.
2. *Fetuses whose growth is restricted by pathological processes (true IUGR).* Depending upon the relative size of their head, abdomen and femur, the fetuses are subdivided into (a) Symmetrical or Type I and (b) Asymmetrical or Type II.

The *symmetrical type* of growth retardation is most often caused by structural or chromosomal abnormalities or congenital infection (TORCH). The pathologic process is intrinsic to the fetus and involves all the organs including the head.

In the *asymmetrical type,* the fetus is affected in later months during the phase of cellular hypertrophy. The total cell mass remains the same but size is smaller than normal. Maternal disease alters the fetal size by reducing uteroplacental blood flow restricting the oxygen and nutrient transfer or by reducing the placental size.

Causes of Intrauterine Growth Retardation

Maternal
❖ Constitutional: Small women have small babies. Genetic and racial factors may be associated
❖ Maternal nutrition before and during pregnancy: As most of the fetal weight gain occurs beyond 24th week of pregnancy, malnutrition, anemia and hypertension in the second half of pregnancy play significant role in the reduction of the birthweight
❖ Low blood oxygen as in cyanotic disease
❖ Malabsorption syndrome
❖ Toxins: Alcohol, smoking, chronic renal failure, chronic urinary tract infection, etc.

Fetal
❖ Congenital anomalies either cardiovascular, renal or others
❖ Chromosomal abnormalities, such as trisomy 21, trisomy 18, trisomy 16, trisomy 13 and Turner's syndrome
❖ Accelerated fetal metabolism due to TORCH agents (toxoplasmosis, rubella, cytomegalovirus and herpes simplex)
❖ Multiple pregnancy.

Placental
Poor blood flow to the placental site, which leads to chronic placental insufficiency with inadequate substrate transfer. This occurs in conditions, such as preeclampsia, essential hypertension, chronic nephritis, organic heart disease, placental infarction, chronic placental abruption, circumvallate placenta, velamentous insertion of cord, etc.

Physical Features of the Baby at Birth
❖ Weight deficit at birth about 600 mg below the minimum percentile standard
❖ Length is unaffected
❖ Head circumference is relatively larger than the body
❖ Physical features show dry and wrinkled skin because of less subcutaneous fat, scaphoid abdomen, and thin meconium stained vernix caseosa and thin umbilical cord. Pinna of ears has cartilaginous ridges. Plantar creases are well defined

❖ The baby is alert, active and has normal cry. Eyes are open.

❖ Reflexes are normal.

Neonatal Complications

❖ Asphyxia (intrauterine and neonatal)

❖ Hypoglycemia due to shortage of glycogen reserve in the liver because of hypoxia

❖ Meconium aspiration pneumonia

❖ Hypothermia

❖ Pulmonary hemorrhage

❖ Polycythemia

❖ Necrotising enterocolitis (NEC) due to reduced intestinal blood flow

❖ Hyperviscosity syndrome.

Symmetrical growth retarded baby is likely to grow slowly after birth, whereas the asymmetrical baby is more likely to grow faster after birth. The fetuses, having retardation of growth evidenced before third trimester, are likely to have retarded neurological and intellectual development in infancy. The worst prognosis is for IUGR caused by congenital infection, congenital abnormalities and chromosomal defects.

When a small for gestational age fetus is suspected prenatally careful search is made to determine the presence of growth retardation with the help of sonography. If it is present, the type of IUGR and the possible causes are investigated. If a fetus is symmetrically growth retarded, tests are done to detect fetal anomalies including fetal blood sampling and karyotyping, to prevent unnecessary cesarean section for a malformed baby.

After exclusion of the possible structural and chromosomal abnormalities and congenital infections, the woman with growth retarded fetus is hospitalized. Termination of pregnancy is done after 38th week in an equipped hospital where intensive intranatal monitoring is possible and having facilities for intensive neonatal care. Precautions during labor are those required for preterm delivery. During labor, the woman should preferably be in left lateral position. Any slight evidence of hypoxia should be urgently dealt with by cesarean section in the first stage and forceps in the second stage.

Immediate Care of the Baby at Birth

A pediatrician should be available at the time of delivery. All precautions as outlined for premature delivery are to be taken. The baby should be placed preferably in the intensive neonatal care unit. All the protocols of management of preterm babies are to be followed. Special care is to be taken to prevent and treat hypoglycemia.

Early feeding within 1 to 2 hours is to be started with 5 to 10 ml of 10 percent glucose. The feeding is to be repeated at two hourly intervals. If the baby tolerates it, expressed milk or humanized milk may be given two hourly in small amounts for 48 hours (Dutta, 2001).

Blood glucose is checked using "dextrostix screening test" two hourly after birth and before each feeding for 48 hours. If the blood glucose level falls below 30 mg percentage, 10 percent glucose is to be given intravenously.

BIBLIOGRAPHY

1. Blackburn ST, Loper DL. Maternal, Fetal and Neonatal Physiology: A Clinical Perspective. Philadelphia: WB Saunders: 1992.
2. Davies PSW, et al. Total energy expenditure in small for gestational age infants. Archives of Disease in Childhood 1996;74:208-10.
3. Dutta DC. Textbook of Obstetrics, 5th edn. Calcutta: New Central Book Company, 2001.
4. Ewer AK, Durbin GM. Gastric emptying in preterm infants. Archives of Disease in Childhood. 1994;71:24-7.
5. Halliday AC. The healthy low birthweight baby, In: Bennett RV, Linda KB (Eds). Myles Textbook for Midwives, 13th edn. Edinburgh: Churchill Livingstone, 1997.
6. Hema KR, Johnson R. Management of growth-restricted fetus. The Obstetrician and Gynecologist 2000;2:13.
7. Kattwinkel, et al. Fetal evaluation and immediate newborn assessment. Virginia; Perinatal Continuing Education Program, 1995.
8. Lucas A, et al. A randomized multicenter study of human milk versus formula and later development in preterm infants. Archives of Diseases in Childhood, Fetal and Neonatal Education. 1994;70:141-6.
9. Whitelaw A. Kangaroo baby care: Just a nice experience or an important advance for preterm infants. Pediatrics 1990;85(4):604-5.

SECTION

9

The Ill Baby

43

Recognizing the Ill Baby

Learning Objectives

Upon completing this chapter, the learner will be able to:
- Assess and identify the ill neonate
- Provide an overview of the potential or presenting problems of the neonate
- Outline the needs of the family in the care of the newborn.

INTRODUCTION

The transition from intrauterine to extra-uterine life ordinarily proceeds smoothly and the majority of newborn babies are born normal and healthy. These babies require no intervention after delivery except to be dried and then to be given back to their mothers. However, even though the labor and delivery may have been uneventful, the baby still needs to be observed at this time to ensure that the respirations are normal, that there is good color, the body temperature is stable and that the baby is active and responsive.

The midwife must be able to recognize the signs and signals caused by illness, some of which may be subtle and nonspecific. The labor and delivery have an obvious effect on the well-being of the infant. Korones (1986) stated it well: "the events that follow birth have their origins in those that proceeded it". It is therefore critical that the nurse be aware of the mother's prenatal course and labor history to understand what has happened and prepare for what is to come.

ASSESSMENT OF GESTATIONAL AGE

Immediately following stabilization of respiration and temperature, the newborn should be examined for any gross congenital abnorma-lities or evidence of birth trauma. They should also have their weight and gestational age plotted on a standard growth chart. Infants can be classified as:
- Appropriate for gestational age (AGA): Between the 10th and 90th percentile
- Small for gestational age (SGA): Below the 10th percentile
- Large for gestational age (LGA): Above the 90th percentile
- *Preterm:* Born before 37th week of gestation.

This classification allows the midwife to assess infants who may require specialized care. Newborns, who are SGA, LGA or preterm, are at increased risk for respiratory distress, hypoglycemia, polycythemia and disturbed thermoregulation. In the recent years, it is increasingly being recognized that race, sex and maternal height have important effects on classification. Female babies have a lower neonatal mortality than males, blacks were found to have a higher survival rate than whites.

Decreasing morbidity and mortality is the goal of all those involved in the care of the newborn. Hence, early recognition of existing or potential problems is vital if the appropriate treatment is to be initiated as soon as possible. Reviewing the maternal health history is an essential starting point. Both prenatal and perinatal complications can affect the health of the neonate.

Maternal Conditions, which can affect the Newborn
- Pregnancy induced hypertension
- History of epilepsy
- Diabetes
- Substance abuse
- Sexually transmitted diseases

Factors Related to Labor and Delivery, which may have Effects on the Newborn

❖ Prolonged rupture of membranes
❖ Abnormal fetal heart rate pattern
❖ Meconium staining in amniotic fluid
❖ Difficult or rapid delivery
❖ Cesarean section and the reason for it.

Problems may become manifest in the newborn over a period of few hours as the baby adapts to living without placental support. The midwife needs to be able to recognize the warning signs and initiate prompt action if deterioration of the baby's condition is to be prevented.

WARNING SIGNS

Most of the information the midwife requires for the assessment of an infant's well-being comes from observation. The baby must be examined systematically commencing at the head and working gradually to the feet.

Pallor

The presence of underlying problems is often manifested in the skin. The presence of meconium on the skin, usually seen in the nail beds and around the umbilicus, is frequently associated with infants who have cardio-respiratory problems. A pale, mottled color of the skin is an indication of poor perfusion. The anemic infant's appearance is usually pale pink, white or in severe cases where there is vascular collapse, gray.

Cause of Anemia

Cause of anemia in the newborn period
❖ Hemolytic disease
❖ Twin-to-twin transfusion *in utero* (which causes one infant to be anemic and the other polycythemic)
❖ Maternal antepartum or intrapartum hemorrhage.

Causes of Pallor other than Anemia

❖ Hypothermia and hypocalcemia
❖ Shock
❖ Respiratory disorders
❖ Cardiac anomalies
❖ Sepsis.

Plethora

Plethoric babies are usually described as beetroot in color. Their color may indicate an excess of circulating red blood cells (polycythemia)—venous hematocrit greater than 70 percent. Newborn infants can become polycythemic if they are recipients of:
❖ Twin-to-twin transfusion *in utero*
❖ A large placental transfusion.

Contributing factors are delayed clamping of the umbilical cord, or holding the infant below the level of the placenta, thereby allowing blood to flow into the baby and giving a greater circulating blood volume (Bain in Bennett and Brown, 1999).

Other infants seen plethoric are:
❖ Small for gestational age (SGA) babies
❖ Infants of diabetic mothers (hypoglycemia)
❖ Those with Down syndrome.

Cyanosis

Central cyanosis is a serious condition. The mucous membranes are the most reliable indicators of central color in all babies. If the tongue and mucous membranes appear blue, this indicates low oxygen saturation levels in the blood, usually of respiratory or cardiac origin. Episodic central cyanotic attacks may be an indication that the infant is having convulsions. Peripheral cyanosis of the hands and feet is common during the first 24 hours of life and is a nonspecific sign of illness. Central cyanosis always demands urgent attention.

Jaundice

Early onset of jaundice (occurring in the skin and sclera within the first 12 hours of life) is abnormal and needs investigating. If a jaundiced baby is unduly lethargic, is a poor feeder, vomits or has unstable body temperature, this may indicate infection and steps should be taken to exclude this.

Other Factors that Affect the Appearance of the Skin

Preterm infants have thinner and redder skin compared to term infants. In post-term infants, the skin is often dry and cracked. The SGA infant may have folds of loose skin over joints due to the lack of subcutaneous fat. This can predispose the infant to hypoglycemia and hypothermia. If the infant is dehydrated, the skin may be pale, dry and cool to touch. Other signs of dehydration are—Pallor or mottled skin, sunken fontanelle or eyeball sockets and tachycardia.

Skin Rashes

Skin rashes are quite common in newborn babies and most are benign and self-limiting.

Milia are white or yellow papules seen over the chin, nose and forehead. These disappear spontaneously over the first few weeks of life.

Miliaria is clear vesicles on the face, scalp and perineum caused by retention of sweat in unopened sweat glands. The treatment is to nurse the infant in light clothes and to keep in cooler environment.

Petechiae or purpuric rash occur in neonatal thrombocytopenia. The petechial rash may appear over the whole body. There may also be prolonged bleeding from the umbilicus, puncture sites and into the gut. Thrombocytopenia may be found in infants with:

❖ Congenital infections
❖ Maternal idiopathic thrombocytopenia
❖ Severe Rhesus hemolytic disease.

Bruising can occur following breech extractions, forceps deliveries and ventouse extractions. The bleeding can lead to decrease in circulating blood volume predisposing the infant to anemia or hypotension.

Erythema toxicum or urticaria neonatorum: It is a rash that consists of white papules on an erythematous base and occurs in about 30 to 70 percent of infants. This condition is benign and can be confirmed by examination of smear of aspirate from a pustule, which will show numerous eosinophils (white blood cells indicative of allergic response).

Infectious Lesions

Oral thrush is a fungal infection of the mouth and throat. It is very common in neonates, especially if they have been on antibiotics. It presents as white patches seen over the tongue and mucous membranes and as a red rash on the perineum.

Herpes simplex virus: The infection usually occurs during delivery. Seventy percent of infected newborns will produce a rash, which appears as vesicles or pustules. It is a serious viral infection. Mortality depends on the severity of the illness.

Umbilical sepsis can be caused by a bacterial infection. Periumbilical redness or discharge may occur and antibiotic therapy is required to prevent an ascending infection.

Bullus impetigo is a condition, which makes the skin, look as though it has been scalded and is caused by streptococci or staphylococci. It presents a widespread tender erythema, followed by blisters, which break, leaving raw areas of skin. It is particularly noticeable around the napkin area but can also cause umbilical sepsis, breast abscess and conjunctivitis and in deep infections, there may be involvement of bones and joints (Bain in Bennett and Brown, 1999).

Pyoderma: Pustules are seen on the scalp, neck, groin and axillae. These are more common in summer. Spread of infection may lead to formation of abscess and septicemia. Hexachlorophene skin care is adequate in most cases. If the lesions are spreading, antibiotics are administered.

Conjunctivitis: Sticky eyes are common during the first two or three days after birth. Unilateral conjunctivitis is often due to chlamydia trachomatis. Purulent conjunctivitis is generally due to Gram-positive cocci. It is treated with antibiotic drops.

Respiratory System

Respiratory distress in the newborn can be a presentation of a number of clinical disorders and is the major cause of morbidity and mortality in the neonatal period.

It is important to observe the baby's breathing when he is at rest and when he is active. The midwife should always start by observing the skin color and then carry-out a respiratory inspection, taking into account whether the baby is making an extra effort or insufficient effort to breathe.

Breathing: Respiration should be counted by watching the lower chest and abdomen rise and fall for a full minute. The rate should be between 40 and 60 breaths per minute but will vary between levels of activity. The chest should expand symmetrically.

If the baby's respiratory rate is above 60 breaths per minute, this is described as *tachypnea*. An infant with tachypnea may be described as having respiratory distress and further observations should be made of the quality of respirations to identify if there is any inspiratory pulling in the chest wall above and below the sternum or between the ribs (retraction). If nasal flaring is also present, this may indicate that there has been a delay in the clearance of lung fluid or that a serious respiratory problem is developing.

Grunting, heard either with a stethoscope or audibly, is an abnormal expiratory sound. These infants require help with their breathing by either intubation or continuous positive airway pressure ventilation.

Apnea is cessation of breathing for 20 seconds or more. It is associated with pallor, bradycardia, cyanosis, oxygen desaturation or a change in the level of consciousness (Faranoff and Martin, 1987). The most common cause of apnea in preterm babies is pulmonary surfactant deficiency or immaturity of the central nervous system.

Other disorders that may produce apnea in the newborn are—Hypoxia, pneumonia, aspiration, pneumothorax, metabolic disorders (hypoglycemia, hypocalcemia, acidosis) and maternal drugs. Neurological problems such as intracranial hemorrhage, developmental disorders of the brain and congenital anomalies of the airway may also cause apnea. Apnea may be induced by stimulation of the posterior pharynx by suction catheter.

Body Temperature

Thermoregulation is a critical physiological function in the newborn that is closely related to the survival of the infant. "A neutral thermal environment is defined as the ambient air temperature at which oxygen consumption or heat production is minimal with body temperature in the normal range" (Bain in Bennett and Brown, 1999).

Normal Body Temperature Range for Term Infants
* Axillary—36.5 to 37°C
* Rectal (core temperature)—36.7 to 37.2°C (Mayfield et al, 1984).

Environments that are outside the neutral thermal environment, may result in the infant developing hypothermia or hyperthermia. Hypothermia is defined as a core temperature below 36°C. When the body temperature is below this level, the infant is at risk from cold stress. This can cause complications such as increased oxygen consumption, lactic acid production, apnea, decrease in coagulability and hypoglycemia. In preterm infants, cold stress may also cause a decrease in surfactant secretion and synthesis. The stress of hypothermia can be disastrous in babies compromised at birth as with:
* Severe asphyxia
* Extensive resuscitation
* Delayed drying at birth
* Respiratory distress
* Hypoglycemia
* Sepsis.
* Preterm or small gestational age (due to poor glucose stores, decreased tissue and little or no brown fat stores).

When the neonate is exposed to cold he will at first become very restless, then as his body temperature falls, he adopts a tightly flexed position to try to conserve heat. The sick or preterm infant will tend to lie supine in a frog-like position. The baby often looks pale or mottled and uninterested in feeding. Hypoglycemia is common in infants who develop hypothermia and this can cause them to have jittery movements of limbs.

Hyperthermia

Hyperthermia is an axillary temperature above 37.5°C. The usual cause of hyperthermia is overheating of the environment. It can also be a clinical sign of sepsis, brain injury or drug therapy. If the infant is too warm, he/she may become restless and may have bright red cheeks. The respiratory rate will be increased. Problems caused by hyperthermia are: hypernatremia, jaundice and recurrent apnea. Variability in body temperature may be the first and only sign that a baby is unwell.

Cardiovascular System

The normal heart rate for term infants is 120 to 160 bpm and for preterm infants 130 to 170 bpm. Heart rate persistently outside this range may suggest an underlying cardiac problem. Warning signs suggestive of congenital heart disease are:

- ❖ Cyanosis which is out of proportion to the degree of respiratory distress
- ❖ Persistent tachypnea
- ❖ Persistent tachycardia at rest
- ❖ Poor feeding: May become breathless and sweaty during the feed or after feeding; they may not complete their feeds and subsequently fail to thrive
- ❖ A sudden gain in weight leading to clinical signs of edema; usually noted as the baby having puffy feet or eyelids and swollen scrotum in males
- ❖ A very loud systolic murmur
- ❖ Evidence of cardiac enlargement on X-ray, persisting beyond 48 hours of life
- ❖ Enlargement of the liver.

Cardiovascular dysfunction should be suspected for infants who present with lethargy and restlessness during feeding. Problems that occur in neonatal cardiovascular functions are usually caused either by congenital defects or by failure of the transition from fetal to adult circulation. Persistent pulmonary hypertension of the newborn is seen in term or post-term infants who have a history of hypoxia or asphyxia at birth. Respiratory distress and cyanosis are seen before 12 hours of age. Infants who have congenital heart disease will be asymptomatic in the neonatal period. Infants who are breathless may have heart disease. The first indication of an underlying cardiac lesion may be the presence of a murmur, heard on routine examination. However, a soft localized systolic murmur with no evidence of any symptoms of cardiac disease is usually of no significance.

Central Nervous System

Assessment of an infant's neurological status is usually carried out when the baby is awake and not crying. Abnormal postures, which include neck retraction, frog-like postures, hyperextension or hyperflexion of limbs, jittery or abnormal involuntary movements, high pitched or weak cry could be indicative of neurologic impairment.

Neurological Disorders

Neurological disorders found at or soon after birth, may be either prenatal or perinatal in origin and include:

- ❖ Congenital abnormalities—Hydrocephaly, microcephaly, encephalocele, chromosomal anomalies
- ❖ Hypoxic or ischemic cerebral injuries
- ❖ Birth traumas, skull fractures, spinal cord and brachial plexus injuries, subdural and subarachnoid hemorrhage
- ❖ Infections passed on to the fetus (toxoplasmosis, rubella, cytomegalovirus, syphilis).

Neurological disorders that appear in the neonatal period need to be recognized promptly in order to minimize brain damage. They include:

- ❖ *Infection*: Meningitis, encephalitis, etc
- ❖ *Hypoxia*: Birth asphyxia, respiratory distress, apneic episodes
- ❖ *Metabolic*: Acidosis, hypoglycemia, hyponatremia, hypernatremia, hypothermia, hypocalcemia
- ❖ *Drug withdrawal*: Narcotics, barbiturates, general anesthesia
- ❖ Intracranial hemorrhage, intraventricular hemorrhage
- ❖ *Secondary bleeding*: Intracranial hemorrhage from thrombocytopenia or disseminated intravascular coagulation.

Manifestations of Neurological Disorders

- ❖ *Jitteriness:* The baby has tremors that are rapid movement of the extremities or fingers that are stopped when the limb is held or flexed. This is seen in infants who are affected by drug withdrawal or in infants with hypoglycemia.

❖ *Irritability*
❖ *Jerking activity:* Movement of one body part
❖ Seizures: These are often very subtle and easily missed. Common causes are asphyxia, metabolic disturbance, infection, intracranial hemorrhage and genetic defects
❖ Twitching
❖ *Hypotonia (floppiness):* Poor muscle tone or loss of body tension—As a result, the infant adopts an abnormal position. *Causes* of hypotonia are:
  – Maternal sedation
  – Birth asphyxia
  – Prematurity
  – Infection
  – Down syndrome
  – Metabolic problems, e.g. hypoglycemia, hyponatremia, inborn errors of metabolism
  – Spinal cord injuries
  – Hypothyroidism
  – Neuromuscular disorders.

Genitourinary System

Urinary infections in the newborn period are quite common, especially in males. The baby typically presents with lethargy, poor feeding, increasing jaundice and vomiting. Urine may be cloudy in appearance or smelly.

Renal problems may present as a failure to pass urine. The normal infant usually passes urine 4 to 10 hours after birth. Normal urine output for a term baby in the first day of life should be 2 to 4 ml/kg/hr. Urine output less than 1 ml/kg/hr (oliguria) should be investigated (Halliday et al, 1989).

Common Causes of Reduced Urinary Output

❖ Inadequate fluid intake
❖ Increased fluid loss due to hyperthermia related to the use of radiant heaters and phototherapy units
❖ Congenital abnormalities
❖ Infection
❖ Birth asphyxia

Gastrointestinal Tract

Gastrointestinal problems commonly seen in newborns are gastroschisis or omphalocele, esophageal atresia, malrotation of the gut, volvulus, meconium ileus, necrotising enterocolitis, imperforate anus, rectal fistulas and Hirshsprung's disease.

Omphalocele can be diagnosed prenatally by ultrasound, which provides time for parents to be prepared for the events that will follow birth. Esophageal atresia can be diagnosed when the mother presents with polyhydramnois, because the fetus is unable to swallow the amniotic fluid. Newborn usually presents with copious saliva, which causes gagging, choking, pallor or cyanosis. If not careful with feeding, the baby may aspirate the milk and develop severe respiratory arrest.

Vomiting and Diarrhea

Vomiting in the newborn can occur due to obstruction, malformations or structural damage anywhere below the stomach. Gastrointestinal disorders often present with vomiting, abdominal distension, a failure to pass stools, or diarrhea with or without blood in the stools. Vomiting can also occur due to overfeeding, infection or intestinal abnormalities. The midwife should distinguish between posseting that occurs with winding and overhandling after feeding, and vomiting due to overfeeding, infection or intestinal abnormalities. Early vomiting may be caused by the infant swallowing meconium or maternal blood at delivery. This can cause a gastritis, which will eventually settle.

The normal full-term infant usually passes about eight stools a day. Breastfed babies' stools are often looser and more frequent than those of bottle-fed and the color varies. The infant who has infection can often display signs of gastrointestinal problems, usually poor feeding, vomiting and/or diarrhea. Diarrhea caused by gastroenteritis is usually very watery and may sometimes resemble urine. Babies with bacterial or viral gastroenteritis must be isolated. Loose stools can also be a feature of infants being treated for hyperbilirubinemia with phototherapy.

Duodenal Atresia

This condition usually presents with bile-stained vomiting within 24 hours of birth. Abdominal distension is not usually present, but often visible peristalsis is seen over the stomach. Insertion of a nasogastric tube may reveal large amount of bile in the stomach and usually there is a history of polyhydramnios and a delay in passing meconium. The most common associated anomaly is Down syndrome, which occurs in nearly 30 percent of cases (Davis and Young, 1992).

Malrotation of the Gut

Malrotation may present as a mechanical bowel obstruction caused by the abnormal attachments (Ladd's bands). The infant usually has no problems in the first few days of life, then presents with bilious vomiting and abdominal distention.

Volvulus

Volvulus can occur in infants who have an incomplete rotation of the gut. Because of venous impairment and mucosal injury, there may be blood passed per rectum. Bilious vomiting also occurs. These infants are commonly very ill.

Meconium Ilius

Meconium ilius is usually seen in babies with cystic fibrosis. Meconium is usually not passed, but occasionally small pellet-like stools, pale in color may be passed. This must not be mistaken for a bowel movement. Vomiting occurs and gradually increases. Initially the vomitus may contain gastric secretions and feed, but later becomes bilious.

Necrotizing Enterocolitis (NEC)

NEC is an acquired disease of the small and large intestines caused by ischemia of the intestinal mucosa. It occurs more often in premature babies who have been asphyxiated at delivery or SGA babies who suffer polycythemia and hypothermia. Vomiting is the common manifestation. Gastric aspirate is large and bile stained. The abdomen becomes distended, stools are large and blood stained. Nonspecific signs include temperature elevation, unstable blood glucose, lethargy and poor peripheral circulation in the early stages. As the illness progresses, the infant becomes apneic and bradycardic and may require ventilating.

Imperforate Anus

This anomaly is seen in some babies. All infants should be checked for this at birth.

Rectal Fistulas

Presence of meconium in the urine is diagnostic of this condition. In female infants, meconium may be passed through the vagina.

Hirschsprung's Disease

This condition should be suspected in babies with delayed passage of meconium, i.e. beyond 24 hours of life. It is caused by an absence of ganglion cells in the distal rectum, colon and sometimes in the small intestine. An incomplete obstruction occurs above the affected segment. Abdominal distention and vomiting are present. The vomit becomes bile stained if meconium is not passed.

Metabolic Disorders

Metabolic disorders commonly seen are galactosemia and phenylketonuria. Infants present with vomiting, weight loss, jaundice and lethargy.

Nursing Management of the Hospitalized Newborn and the Family

Admission of a newborn into a neonatal unit interrupts the normal course of events that surrounds a birth. This can seriously damage the parent-infant bond. In the care of the baby, the midwife should try to normalize the environment of the neonatal unit as much as possible so that the neonate, who is separated from his mother and subjected to multiple caregivers, will have reduced stress. Specific measures to reduce stress for which she must pay special attention are minimizing handling of the baby and reducing noise levels. At the start of the shift, the midwife should determine the needs of the infant and carry-out the required care, all at one time, instead of repeatedly disturbing the baby. Lester and Tronick (1990) have stated that the best care for the sick infant is rest.

A lot of noise that occur in neonatal units are unnecessary and can be eliminated if thought is given. Staff may talk in normal speaking voice. Noise produced by banging of feeding bottles, closing of incubator doors or dropping items on the incubators are to be avoided. Day and night cycles should be recognized and lights should be dimmed at night-time and noise further reduced.

Involvement of Parents of the Hospitalized Baby

Following the delivery, if a baby is to be admitted to the neonatal unit, the parents should be allowed to touch or hold the baby, even if it is just for a few moments, before he is taken to the neonatal unit.

Parents should be encouraged to visit their baby in the neonatal unit as soon as they are able. They should be given explanation about the baby's condition and the equipment being used. Any questions the parents may have should be answered in a positive manner.

The premature infant may require a lengthy stay in a neonatal unit, in which case parenting roles may be difficult to establish owing to the physical condition of the baby who may be in a ventilator, being fed intravenously, or be under phototherapy light. All these may be barriers between the infant and the parents, which affect their confidence. Parents should be encouraged to communicate with the baby even if it has to be through the porthole window of the incubator.

As soon as the baby's condition and tolerance to handling permits, the parents should be encouraged to involve in the baby's care. This early involvement will strengthen their understanding of the baby belonging to them and increase their confidence in their ability to provide care. This is of fundamental importance to the general well-being of the baby. Encouraging the mother to breast or bottle-feed the baby in the nursery or to express the milk may make her feel she is contributing to her baby's care in a way that nobody else can.

Parents should be allowed to hold and cuddle their babies as soon as possible, based on the baby's condition. Skin-to-skin contact (Kangaroo care), where the baby is placed naked (apart from a nappy) between the mother's breasts has been shown to be most beneficial. It can improve oxygenation and breathing rates, have a calming effect and, in the infant, reduce stress levels; it may also increase breast milk supply and boost the mother's confidence (Whitewall et al, 1988).

Discharge planning should commence long before the baby is ready for home. Encouraging parents to participate in the care of their baby from the beginning enables them eventually to be the sole caregivers and resume total charge. Every mother should learn how to feed, bathe, dress and generally care for her child. If the baby has special needs related to feeding or observation, the mother/parents must be given needed training so that she will feel comfortable about caring for their baby before going home.

BIBLIOGRAPHY

1. Bain JE. Recognizing the ill baby, In: Bennett RV, Linda KB (Eds). Myles Textbook for Midwives 13th edn. Edinburgh: Churchill Livingstone, 1999.
2. Davis CF, Young DG. Gastroenterology, In: Roberton NRC. Textbook of Neonatology, 2nd edn. New York: Churchill Livingstone, 1992.
3. Dutta DC. Textbook of Obstetrics 5th edn. Calcutta: New Central Book Company, 2001.
4. Faranof AA, Martin JM. Neonatal Perinatal Medicine. St. Louis: Mosby, 1987.
5. Halliday HL, et al. Handbook of Neonatal Intensive Care. London: Bailliere Tindall, 1989.
6. Korones SB. High Risk Newborn Infants 4th edn. St Louis: Mosby, 1986.
7. Lester BM, Tronick EC. Guidelines for stimulation with preterm infants. Clinical Perinatology 1970; 17(1):15-17.
8. Mayfield SR, et al. Temperature measurements in term and preterm neonates. Journal of Pediatrics 1984;104:271-5.
9. Whitewall A, Sleath K. Skin-to-skin contact for very low birthweight babies and their mothers. Archives of Disease in Childhood 1988;63:1377-81.

44

Respiratory Problems of the Newborn

Learning Objectives

Upon completing this chapter, the learner will be able to:

- ❖ Review the anatomy and physiology of the respiratory system
- ❖ Describe the clinical signs of respiratory problems in the newborn
- ❖ Outline the causes of respiratory problems in the neonatal period
- ❖ Describe the management of common respiratory problems
- ❖ Describe the principles of caring for a baby with respiratory problems.

Respiratory problems are the most common cause of morbidity and mortality in the neonatal period. Problems can occur in term as well as in premature infants. The midwife; in managing labor and giving direct care to the newborn baby, is able to recognize the first signs of respiratory distress.

ANATOMY AND PHYSIOLOGY OF THE RESPIRATORY SYSTEM

The lungs *in utero* are nonfunctional as the placenta oxygenates the fetus and carries away waste products. They are bathed in fluid, which is expelled by pressure during the process of labor. Ultrasonographic studies have shown that some respiratory movements occur *in utero*. It has also been proved that such movements are essential for the normal growth of the lungs.

The basic requirements for initiation and maintenance of pulmonary respiration are:

- ❖ Intact neurological and respiratory apparatus
- ❖ Clear airway

- ❖ Adequate alveolar area and stable expanded alveoli
- ❖ Sufficient pulmonary perfusion
- ❖ Satisfactory lymphatic drainage
- ❖ Oxygen diffusion and dissociation capacity
- ❖ Carbonic anhydrase activity of blood.

With the completion of the second stage, the following events play a major role in the initiation of respiration:

- ❖ The clamping of the umbilical cord results in a fall in arterial oxygen and a slight rise in carbon dioxide tension. These factors taken together stimulate the respiratory center directly and via chemoreceptors in the carotid body
- ❖ Sensory impulses from changes in skin temperature and proprioreceptive impulses from joints directly stimulate the respiratory center
- ❖ With the inflation of the lungs, there is augmentation of respiratory effort

The first cry, gasp or breath (short inspiration followed by long expiration) establishes a functional residual capacity and brings about a huge increase in pulmonary perfusion and subsequent normal pattern of breathing. A negative intrathoracic pressure of 15 cm water is needed to establish regular respiration. This should also be sufficient to overcome the surface tension of 20 dynes per cm^2 at the fluid interface of alveolar epithelium. This is helped by pulmonary surfactant, which reduces it to 4 dynes per cm^2 (Dutta, 2001). With the first breath the lungs are inflated with air and the placenta is replaced as the organ of respiration. After birth, the baby develops additional conductive airways and alveoli. The lungs are not fully developed until the age of 8 years.

Differences in Anatomy and Physiology Between the Baby and Adult

The main differences are:

❖ The baby is an obligatory nose breather because of the high, anterior position of the larynx, which produces a direct airway to the lungs from the nasal cavity

❖ The narrowest part of the baby's airway is below the vocal cords at the level of the cricoid cartilage, which increases the risk of obstruction (in adults and older children the narrowest part of the airway is above the vocal cords)

❖ The infant's airways are smaller in diameter and become easily blocked by inflammation and secretions

❖ The infant has fewer alveoli for exchange of gases and to maintain air reserves (resting volume) in his lungs, making him more sensitive to hypoxia

❖ The muscles in the chest wall are weak and the ribs are more pliable than in the adult, providing less support to keep the lungs expanded

❖ The ribs are more horizontally placed, so that contraction of the diaphragm in breathing draws in the lower ribs. In addition, a baby's breathing movement is more diaphragmatic

❖ Because of the weaker chest muscles and pliable ribs, the baby is at great risk of respiratory fatigue than an adult

❖ The baby has a greater metabolic rate than an adult does. Oxygen consumption in the baby is 6 to 8 ml/kg/min compared to 3 to 4 ml/kg/min in adult (Livingston in Bennett and Brown, 1999).

CLINICAL SIGNS OF RESPIRATORY PROBLEMS

Common signs found in most respiratory problems are as follows:

❖ Increased work of breathing causing
  – Recession of intercostals and subcostal muscles and retraction of the sternum; the chest wall appears to be caving in

  – The chin appear to pull down the head to move up and down and the nostrils to flare as the baby tries to draw in as much air as possible, using accessory muscles in the upper body
  – Grunting caused by the baby breathing out against a partially closed glottis in an effort to keep as much air as possible in the lungs.

❖ Hypoxia causing pallor or cyanosis of the skin and mucous membrane

❖ Alteration in general appearance and behavior:
  – A tense worried appearance and distorted chest because of the increased work of breathing
  – The baby may be restless and unable to feed adequately because of breathing difficulties
  – The baby will become lethargic with more severe respiratory difficulties in struggling with the effort of breathing. An exhausted baby may become apneic

❖ *Tachypnea:* The respiratory rate will be increased (beyond 60 breaths per minute) in an effort to achieve adequate gaseous exchange.

CAUSES OF RESPIRATORY PROBLEMS

Breathing problems have many causes, which are not necessarily respiratory in origin. Causes include:

❖ Infection
❖ Aspiration
❖ Lung immaturity
❖ Transient tachypnea of the newborn
❖ Pneumothorax
❖ Central nervous system disorders
❖ Cardiovascular and circulatory problems
❖ Apnea of prematurity.

Infection

Generalized Infection

A baby having generalized infection may present with signs of respiratory distress. He may have a respiratory rate greater than 60 breaths per minute and be pale or cyanosed because of hypoxia.

Congenital or Acquired Pneumonia

A baby may be born with pneumonia that will present soon after birth. If the membranes have been ruptured for longer than 24 hours, the baby is at greater risk of developing pneumonia. In order to prevent serious neonatal infection the midwife needs to be vigilant for signs of sepsis in the mother, such as purulent vaginal discharge, maternal pyrexia or offensive smelling liquor. When maternal sepsis is suspected an intravenous antibiotic is administered to mother before delivery. When the membranes are ruptured for longer than 18 to 24 hours, the baby is screened for infection. If the baby shows signs of sepsis such as raised or suppressed white cell count, or the baby exhibits signs of infection, such as poor temperature control, poor feeding, respiratory signs, or hypoglycemia, then intravenous antibiotics may be prescribed. Organisms such as Group B streptococcus, which may be commensal to the mother's vagina, can cause congenital pneumonia and generalized septicemia. A baby with severe Group B streptococcal sepsis will be critically ill.

After birth, the baby is exposed to organisms in the environment, which can cause pneumonia. Common organisms that are commensal to the skin of adults, such as *staphylococcus epidermis*, can cause serious respiratory infection in the newborn.

Aspiration

At the time of delivery, it is possible for the baby to inhale any of the fluids that are present when he takes his first breath.

Meconium Aspiration

During labor, if there is fetal distress, hypoxia can stimulate peristalsis and relaxation of the anal sphincter and meconium is then released into the amniotic fluid. If the fetus becomes very distressed, he may start to make gasping movements *in utero* before birth, taking in surrounding amniotic fluid. If the amniotic fluid is heavily stained with thick meconium, this can cause the baby breathing difficulties after delivery. In delivering a mother with meconium stained liquor, arrangements must be made for immediate resuscitation of the baby. The person responsible for resuscitation will visualize the vocal cords using a laryngoscope; if meconium is present around the cords, meconium aspiration is unlikely. However, if meconium is present below the vocal cords, the baby will be intubated and the trachea suctioned to remove any inhaled meconium that is accessible. Because meconium is thick and tenacious, it blocks the airways. Meconium is alkaline and irritant to lung tissues, and can lead to a chemical pneumonitis.

Clinical presentation: Meconium aspiration syndrome is typically seen in term and post-term infants, particularly the intrauterine growth restricted group. A baby with meconium aspiration syndrome will present with signs of respiratory distress, which can range from mild to severe (clinical signs of respiratory problems). The chest may appear barrel shaped or hyperinflated. There may also be yellow-green staining of the skin and nail beds. A baby with severe meconium aspiration will need mechanical ventilation, intravenous antibiotics and chest physiotherapy to help clear the lungs.

Other Aspiration Problems

The baby inhales maternal blood or amniotic fluid at delivery, which can result in similar problems to meconium aspiration. In addition, a baby may inhale milk resulting in aspiration pneumonia. This may occur because of vomiting, or when there is a fistula between the airway and the esophagus.

Lung Immaturity

Respiratory Distress Syndrome (RDS)/Hyaline Membrane Disease

Respiratory distress syndrome occurs commonly in preterm neonates, babies of diabetic mothers and infants delivered by cesarean section or breech delivery. It is the commonest cause of respiratory disease and one of the most common causes of neonatal mortality. The pathologic finding is widespread atelectasis. A homogeneous eosinophilic membrane (hyaline membrane) is found plastering the alveolar ducts and terminal bronchioles. Hyaline membrane is made up of proteins that are exuded into the alveoli and airways of a baby with RDS. It is caused by deficiency of surfactant in the baby's lungs. Surfactant is made by cells in the alveolar walls. Its production slowly increases from 20th week's gestation, with a surge at 30th to 34th week and at term with the onset of labor.

A number of factors cause surfactant deficiency in the neonate, which include:

❖ Gross lowering of the surface tension reducing factor (lecithin)
❖ Hypoperfusion of the pulmonary vascular bed
❖ Alteration in the fibrinolytic mechanism within the lung.

In cases with deficient surfactant (lecithin), as in premature baby, the pressure needed to open up and expand the alveoli are very high and much beyond the ability of the baby. Hence, there is collapse of the lung (atlectasis) and the clinical manifestations of RDS appear.

Hypoxia reduces surfactant synthesis, which in preterm with low reserves of surfactant has more impact than in the healthy term baby. With maternal diabetes, it is thought that surfactant maturation is delayed, particularly when the prenatal control of diabetes has been poor. In elective cesarean section delivery, the stimulus of labor, which increases surfactant production, is absent.

The course of development of RDS:

Neonates

❖ Preterm
❖ Diabetic mother
❖ Cesarean section
❖ Breech delivery
❖ Hypothermic
❖ Hypovolemic

→ Deficient surfactant → Pulmonary atlectasis → Hypoxia and acidosis → Formation of hyaline membrane

The infant develops both respiratory and metabolic acidosis. pCO_2 may rise to even 80 mm Hg in a severe case.

Clinical Features

The clinical manifestations usually appear abruptly, 4 to 6 hours after birth.

❖ Recession of intercostal and subcostal muscles, and retraction of the sternum
❖ Tachypnea with a breathing rate greater than 60 per minute
❖ Expiratory grunt
❖ Cyanosis

On X-ray examination, the lung field has a white 'ground glass' (nontransparent glass) appearance as the alveoli are collapsed and not filled with air. The main airways, that are air-filled, stand out as dark areas. The severity ranges from mild transient distress to rapidly progressing fatal illness causing death within a few hours. The more premature and sick the baby is at the onset of RDS, the more complicated his recovery will be.

Prevention

❖ Administration of betamethasone (steroid) before preterm delivery, especially to women who go into labor before 34th week of gestation. Crowley, et al (1990) suggested the use of antenatal steroids to reduce the incidence of RDS by 50 percent and the mortality by 35 percent
❖ Administration of prophylactic artificial surfactant into the baby's lungs after delivery (Roberton, 1993)
❖ Assessment of lung maturity before premature induction of labor and to delay the induction as much as possible to avoid risk to the fetus
❖ Prevention of fetal hypoxia in diabetic mothers.

Management

The overall aim of managing the treatment of RDS is to support the baby's breathing and to maintain the baby in as good a condition as possible.

❖ The baby should be in the intensive neonatal care unit and nursed in a warm incubator with high humidity. Air passage is to be cleaned periodically through endotracheal suction. Minimum disturbance and handling are to be ensured
❖ Adequate warmed and humidified oxygen therapy in concentration of 35 to 40 percent under positive pressure is to be administered through endotracheal intubation to relieve hypoxia and acidosis.

- Prevention and treatment of infection
- Correction of hypovolemia with albumin or other colloid solution
- Correction of anemia and electrolyte imbalance, if any
- Frequent monitoring of pO_2, pCO_2, pH and base excess to detect metabolic and respiratory acidosis and rectification accordingly. Acidosis is corrected by intravenous administration of sodium bicarbonate
- Surfactant therapy to reduce surface tension and to stabilize the alveolar air-water interface; direct tracheal instillation is done
- Feeding: Intragastric feeding is the preferred method. If there is chance for vomiting and aspiration, intravenous administration of 10 percent glucose may be done through a catheter inserted in to the umbilical or peripheral vein.

Complications

Complications of hyaline membrane disease are:

- Intraventricular hemorrhage
- Bronchopulmonary displasia
- Pulmonary hemorrhage
- Pneumothorax
- Retrolental fibroplasia
- Neurological abnormalities.

About one-third of the babies with RDS die. Infants with mild affection may survive with prompt and effective management.

Transient Tachypnea of the Newborn

Transient tachypnea occurs mostly in term infants, although it can affect the preterm group as well. It is caused by the delayed clearing of lung fluid after birth (Roberton, 1993). It is more common in babies born by cesarean section. The baby with transient tachypnea of the newborn (TTN) will present with tachypnea (sometimes the respiratory rate will be over 100 breaths per minute), mild grunding and slight subcostal and intercostals recession. The baby may also be cyanosed. The baby with TTN is treated with oxygen therapy and may even require ventilation, if the condition is severe. Prophylactic antibiotic therapy is likely to be started, as it is difficult to differentiate the condition from serious infection. The baby's condition improves as the lung fluid clears, usually within 24 hours.

Pneumothorax

Pneumothorax may occur spontaneously after delivery or may result from overvigorous bag and mask ventilation.

Clinical Signs of Pneumothorax

- Pallor or cyanosis
- Difficulty in breathing
- An asymmetrical appearance to the chest
- The abdomen may appear distended as the pneumothorax can push the diaphragm down
- The breath sounds will not be equal on auscultation.

A diagnosis will be made by chest X-ray. Treatment may require the pneumothorax to be drained with a chest drain. If the pneumothorax is not severe, and the baby is not distressed, the baby may be treated with oxygen therapy and intravenous fluids until the air from the pneumothorax is reabsorbed.

Pneumothoraces are most common in babies who require mechanical ventilation. This type of air leak may also involve air trapped in the lung tissue and this is known as pulmonary interstitial emphysema.

Congenital Problems

Several congenital problems can cause respiratory difficulties. These may involve a mechanical obstruction of the respiratory tract, and an abnormality of development in the chest and its structures.

Upper Airway Problems

- *Choanal atresia:* Nasal obstruction allowing the baby to breath only through the mouth
- *Cleft palate*, which allows the tongue to fall to the back of the pharynx causing obstruction
- *Laryngeal obstruction*: Presence of cysts or laryngomalacia when the baby has a 'floppy larynx' causing laryngeal strider.

Lower Airway Problems

- *Tracheoesophageal* fistula, providing an abnormal passage between the trachea and esophagus

❖ *Hypoplastic lungs*: Lung tissue that has not developed adequately
❖ *Diaphragmatic hernia,* where the gut herniates up into the chest cavity through a defeat in the diaphragm.

Central Nervous System Disorders

The newborn may show signs of respiratory distress with problems affecting the central nervous system. The most common among them is hypoglycemia, which results in deprivation of energy to brain tissue, which can cause convulsions. Apnea may be the only outward sign of a convulsion in the neonate, as his neurological system is immature. Intracranial hemorrhage may also result in signs of respiratory distress. This is most common after perinatal asphyxia.

Cardiovascular and Circulatory Problems

Because of the changes in circulation at birth, certain cardiovascular problems will present with some respiratory signs in the neonatal period. Among the problems presenting at birth are those, which involve failure of the fetal circulation to change fully to the postnatal pattern and congenital malformation of the heart and major blood vessels.

Patent Ductus Arteriosus (PDA)

In PDA, the ductus arteriosus fails to close causing blood to be diverted from the lungs. In normal neonates, the ductus arteriosus is functionally closed by about 12 hours of age. Closure may be delayed by hypoxia, RDS and cyanotic heart disease. The ductus arteriosus secretes prostaglandins from cells in its walls, which encourage it to stay open *in utero*. In preterm babies, these cells remain active after delivery and encourage the duct to remain open.

Persistent Pulmonary Hypertension of the Newborn/Persistent Fetal Circulation

It can present in babies without apparent cause and in babies who have conditions such as RDS, polycythemia, hypoglycemia due to maternal gestational diabetes, postmaturity and meconium aspiration syndrome.

A baby with persistent pulmonary hypertension will present with signs of respiratory distress and cyanosis. The aim of treatment is to maintain the general condition of the baby until the pulmonary vascular resistance falls, allowing normal circulation to be established.

Structural Heart Defects

Congenital heart defects will present in the neonatal period with signs of respiratory distress and include:

❖ Transposition of the great arteries
❖ Atrial and ventricular septal defects
❖ Valve stenosis
❖ Hypoplastic heart
❖ Coarctation of aorta.

Some conditions such as *tetralogy of Fallot* are a combination of several defects. In addition, congenital heart disease is common in the presence of other congenital abnormalities such as Down syndrome.

Apnea of Prematurity

Apnea is a common problem found in babies of less than 34 weeks' gestation. It occurs because of immaturity of the respiratory center in the brain and respiratory fatigue. Cardiorespiratory monitoring and use of therapeutic respiratory stimulants help to prevent prolonged apnea. Physical stimulation of the baby, when he is apneic, may be sufficient stimulus to 'remind' him to breathe. Alternatively, if he does not respond to tactile stimulation, a bag and mask without oxygen may be used to ventilate him until he breathe spontaneously.

PRINCIPLES OF CARING FOR A BABY WITH RESPIRATORY PROBLEM

Objectives of caring for a baby with respiratory problems are to provide support to relieve the work of breathing and detect signs of deterioration. The principles, which are to be applied by the midwife caring for a baby with respiratory problems, are:

❖ Positioning
❖ Observation
❖ Oxygenation

- ❖ Nutrition and hydration
- ❖ Basic physical care needs
- ❖ Meeting the emotional and psychological needs of the baby and family.

Positioning

A baby with breathing difficulties will breathe more easily in the prone position or supported on either side in a symmetrically flexed position and with his head slightly elevated. The neonate is more likely to block his airway if the chin is too far upwards or downwards because his neck is short in comparison to that of the adult or older child.

He should be nursed on a soft sheet to give him tactile warmth and comfort. Newborn babies are not comfortable with the feel of wide-open spaces and need to feel secure. Rolled soft blankets or sheets can be kept on his sides to provide boundaries. Care must be taken that the support does not impede breathing. It is important to instruct mothers that the prone or supported side position is contraindicated at home because of the danger of suffocation and cot death.

Observation

A baby with any type of breathing difficulty needs to be closely monitored for signs of deterioration in his condition. A baby with noisy breathing due to secretions in the airway and no sign of respiratory distress is to be kept warm and fed early. The noisy breathing often settles as the secretions disperse.

A respiratory rate over 60 breaths per minute is indicative of respiratory distress. Color of the baby and the work of breathing should also be noted. Continuous cardiopulmonary monitoring should be used in a baby showing signs of respiratory distress because it allows for close monitoring without disturbing him/her. The baby is then able to rest, conserving energy for breathing.

Oxygenation

The baby with breathing difficulties is provided with oxygen according to his needs as assessed by his color, rate and work of breathing and

measurement of blood oxygenation. The need for oxygen is determined by the blood gas results and by the clinical assessment. Oxygen can be provided to babies by the following methods.

Ambient or Head Box Oxygen

Warmed and humidified oxygen can be provided either into an incubator or enclosed cot or by head box/hood (a clear Perspex dome, that is placed over the baby's head into which oxygen is delivered). It is essential that the concentration of oxygen be assessed accurately by means of an oxygen analyzer placed near the baby's head.

Nasal Cannula

This method can be used when the baby's condition improves and he can be nursed out of the incubator. Low flow oxygen can be delivered by this method. With the cannula, the baby can be handled more easily.

Mechanical Ventilation

When a baby is unable to support his own respiratory effort, intubation followed by mechanical ventilation is used. Neonatal ventilators, which are pressure controlled are generally used. This mode of ventilation allows the lungs to inflate and gaseous exchange to occur. Methods of ventilation commonly used are:

- ❖ Intermittent mandatory ventilation (IMV)
- ❖ Intermittent positive pressure ventilation (IPPV)
- ❖ Trigger ventilation
- ❖ Continuous positive airway pressure (CPAP)
- ❖ High frequency oscillation ventilation (HFOV).

HFOV is used in babies with severe respiratory disease. It is thought that the lower volumes of gas given at lower pressures, at rates of 400 to 1,000 or more breaths/minute, reduce trauma to vulnerable lung tissue (Clark, 1994).

Nutrition and Hydration

A baby who has breathing problem will be either unable to feed or find sucking difficult.

A full stomach will also impede breathing, and intestinal peristalsis slows down in a sick infant. Gastric tube feeding is given to meet the nutritional needs and hydration requirements if the baby's breathing difficulty is minimal and short-lived. However, most babies with breathing difficulties will initially require an intravenous infusion of 10 percent dextrose, calculated according to weight.

If the baby's respiratory problem is not predicted to be resolved in 48 hours and if total parenteral nutrition is available, it will be administered especially in low birthweight and intrauterine growth restricted babies. Milk feeding is introduced as early as possible, as it is the most natural form of feeding. A small volume, such as 0.5 to 1.0 ml/hour of expressed breast milk may be fed by gastric tube to even very sick and preterm babies in order to stimulate natural enzyme activity in the gut.

As the baby develops the ability to suck, more sucking feeds can be introduced and orogastric or nasogastric feeds may be reduced gradually. For a baby with respiratory problem, it is important to assess the hydration status by maintaining accurate intake and output record. Urine output may be assessed by weighing the nappies before and after the baby has worn them. Weight of the baby must be taken daily. Blood electrolytes are measured daily for infants on intravenous fluids.

Mothers who wish to breastfeed their babies need all possible support and encouragement to maintain the milk supply through the stressful period. It is the midwife's role to educate the mother to express and store her milk and to feed her baby as he progresses with his sucking ability.

Basic Physical Care Needs

Babies who are preterm and critically ill have reduced ability to maintain normal body temperature. Incubators, heated cots and added humidity are generally used to assist in the maintenance of temperature.

The baby with breathing difficulty, receiving assistance for maintenance of body temperature may not tolerate the handling required for activities such as nappy changing. Midwives must therefore practice minimal handling and coordination of activities where possible.

Meeting the Emotional and Psychological Needs of the Baby and Family

The baby in the neonatal (intensive care) unit with breathing difficulties is separated from the family and deprived of physical contact with the family. The machinery surrounding the baby imposes barriers to his family, especially the mother who must provide the physical comfort of contact.

The midwife caring for the baby must be aware of the impact of this separation and involve the mother in the care of the baby whenever possible. Activities such as touching, stroking and talking to the baby must be encouraged whenever the mother and/or father will be in the unit.

Parents need to be provided with consistent and accurate information about their baby's condition.

BIBLIOGRAPHY

1. Clark R. High frequency ventilation. Journal of Pediatrics. 1994;124:661-70.
2. Crowley P, Chalmers I, Keirse M. The effects of corticosteroid administration before preterm delivery. British Journal of Obstetrics Gynecology. 1990;97:11-25.
3. Dutta DC. Text Book of Obstetrics 5th edn. Calcutta: New Central Book Company, 2001.
4. Livingstone A. Respiratory problems, In: Bennett RV, Linda KB (Eds). Myles Textbook for Midwives, 13th edn. Edinburgh: Churchill Livingstone 1999.
5. Northway R, et al. Pulmonary disease following respiratory therapy for hyaline membrane disease. New England Journal of Medicine. 1967;276:357.
6. Roberton NRC. Disorders of the respiratory tract, In: Roberton NRC. A manual of Neonatal Intensive Care, 3rd edn. London: Edward Arnold 1993.

45

Birth Trauma, Hemorrhage and Convulsions

Learning Objectives

Upon completing this chapter, the learner will be able to:
* Describe the trauma, which may occur during birth to various structures
* Describe the major types of hemorrhage in the newborn due to trauma, hypoxia, coagulopathies and other causes
* Discuss convulsions in the newborn
* Outline the preventive strategies, which will reduce the incidence of complications
* Describe the measures for effective management
* Describe the interventions with parents.

Birth trauma remains an important cause of perinatal mortality and morbidity in countries where comprehensive antenatal and intranatal care is inadequate.

TRAUMA DURING BIRTH

Trauma or injury during birth occurs to:
* Skin and superficial tissues
* Muscles
* Nerves
* Bones.

Trauma to Skin

Damage to the skin is often iatrogenic and results from forceps blades, vacuum extractor cups, scalp electrodes and scalpels. Poorly applied forceps blades or vacuum extractor cups can result in abrasions of the scalp and bruising of the face. Scalp electrodes and fetal blood sampling techniques can cause puncture wounds. Occasionally, during incision of the uterus at cesarean section, laceration of the baby's skin can occur.

All of these injuries are detected during the physical examination of the baby after birth. Abrasions and lacerations should be kept clean and dry. If there is any indication of infection, medical advice should be sought and antibiotics may be required. Deeper lacerations may need closure with band-aid or suture material.

Trauma to Superficial Tissues

Trauma to soft tissue involves edematous swellings and/or bruising. During labor, the part of the fetus overlaying the cervical os can be subjected to pressure from a 'girdle of contact'. This leads to obstruction of the venous blood return resulting in congestion and edema. The edema usually consists of serum and blood (serosanguineous fluid).

Caput Succedaneum (Figs 45.1A to C)

It is the formation of a swelling due to stagnation of fluid in the layers of the scalp beneath the girdle of contact. In occipitoanterior position, a single caput succedaneum may be present. If the occiput rotates anteriorly in occiput posterior positions, a second caput succedaneum can develop. If there is delay in the second stage of labor, the perineum acts as another 'girdle of contact' to form a second caput suceedaneum. A false caput succedaneum can occur when a vacuum extractor cup is used. Because of its distinctive shape, the resulting edematous swelling is known as a 'chignon'.

Caput usually forms after rupture of the membranes and is present at birth. The swelling does not tend to enlarge and, if double, is unilateral. It is likely that the baby will experience some discomfort, therefore, gentleness

Figs 45.1A to C: Caput succedaneum: (A) Caput succedaneum; (B) Caput succedaneum resolved; (C) Cephalhematoma

when handling or dressing the baby is important. The caput succedaneum usually resolves by 36 hours of life with no longterm consequences.

Other Injuries

The cervical os may restrict venous blood return when the fetal presentation is one other than cephalic. If the face is the presenting part, it will become congested and bruised and the eyes and lips edematous. In a breech presentation, the fetus will develop bruising and edema to the genitalia.

This type of trauma is immediately apparent at birth. As it is very likely that the baby will experience pain, the midwife must take extreme care when handling or dressing the baby. With the swollen genitalia, excoriation of the overlying skin is likely and care should be taken to keep the area clean and dry to prevent infection.

Muscle Trauma

Injuries to muscle can occur when it is torn or when its blood supply is disrupted.

Torticollis

The sternomastoid muscle can be damaged during the birth of the anterior shoulder when the fetus presents by vertex or during rotation of the shoulders when the fetus is being born by the breech. The damage causes torticollis, which means a twisted neck. Torticollis presents as a small lump of approximately 2 cm diameter over the sternomastoid muscle on the affected side of the neck. The lump consists of blood and fibrous tissue and appears to be painless for the baby.

Stretching of the muscle can be achieved by laying the baby to sleep on the affected side and by using musclestretching exercises. The swelling will resolve over several weeks.

Nerve Trauma

Trauma occurs commonly to the facial nerve or the brachial nerve plexus.

Facial Nerve Palsy

Damage to the facial nerve usually results from its compression against the ramus of the mandible by a forceps blade, resulting in unilateral 'facial palsy'. A unilateral facial weakness is seen with the eyelid of the affected

Fig. 45.2: Facial palsy (Eye is open on the paralyzed side)

Fig. 45.3: Erb's palsy (Affected arm rotated inwardly)

side remaining open even during sleep and the mouth drawn over to the normal side on crying (Fig. 45.2). There may be difficulty with the early feedings, if the baby cannot form an effective seal on the nipple or teat. There is no specific treatment. As the eyelid remains open, the eyeball must be kept lubricated by instilling antibiotic eyedrops or ointment. Feeding difficulties are usually overcome by the baby's own adaptation. Spontaneous resolution of the condition usually occurs within 7 to 10 days.

Brachial Palsy

Trauma to the brachial plexus (group of nerves) usually results from stretching or effusion due to excessive lateral flexion, rotation or traction of the head and neck during a birth by breech or when shoulder dystocia occurs. Unilateral involvement is common. There are three main injuries: Erb's palsy, Klumpke's palsy, and total brachial plexus palsy.

(a) Erb's Palsy

This is the commonest type when the fifth and sixth cervical nerve roots are involved. The resulting paralysis causes the arm to lie on the side with extension of the elbow, pronation of the forearm and flexion of the wrist. The hand is partially closed and the arm is inwardly rotated (Fig. 45.3). This is commonly known as the 'waiter's tip' position. Moro reflex and biceps jerks are absent on the affected side. Treatment consists of the use of a splint to hold the arm abducted to a right angle and externally rotated; the forearm is flexed at

right angle and supinated and the hand is dorsiflexed. Massage and passive movements are advocated. Full recovery may take several weeks or even months. Severe injury may produce permanent damage.

(b) Klumpke's Palsy

This type of palsy is due to the affection of the lower cords of the plexus involving 7th and 8th cervical or even the first thoracic nerve root. The upper arm has normal movement but the lower arm, wrist and hand are affected. The arm is flexed at elbow, the wrist extended, the hand flaccid and the fingers flexed. Grasp reflex is absent. When the first thoracic nerve is involved; there may be homolateral ptosis with small pupil due to sympathetic nerve involvement. Treatment consists of splinting the arm with the forearm pronated and the fingers extended. Prognosis is good when the injury is due to stretching. If it is due to hemorrhage or tear, the deformity may be permanent.

(c) Total Brachial Plexus Palsy

There is damage to all the brachial plexus nerve roots. There is complete paralysis of the arm and hand with a lack of sensation and circulatory problems. If there is bilateral paralysis, spinal injury should be suspected. Investigations include X-ray or ultrasound examination of the clavicle, arm, chest and cervical spine and assessment of joints. Passive movements of joints and limb should be initiated under the direction of a physiotherapist.

Spontaneous recovery within days to weeks is expected. For babies who do not recover spontaneously within 4 to 6 months, surgical repair has been effective (Brucker et al, 1991).

Bone Trauma

Fractures are rare but the most commonly affected bones are the clavicle, humerus, femur, and those of the skull. With all fractures, a 'crack' may be heard during the birth.

Clavicle Fracture

This can occur if there is shoulder dystocia or during a birth by breech. The affected bone is usually the one, which is nearest the maternal symphysis pubis. During neonatal examination, it is possible to feel a distortion in the bone and crepitus or callus formation.

Humerus Fracture

Midshaft fracture can occur if there is shoulder dystocia or during a birth by breech when the extended arm is brought down and born. Considerable deformity will be evident on examination and the baby will be reluctant to move the arm.

Femur Fracture

Midshaft fractures can occur during a birth by the breech when the extended legs are brought down and born. Considerable deformity is evident on examination and the baby will be reluctant to move the leg owing to pain.

Treatment

In cases of suspected fractures, X-ray examination is done to confirm the diagnosis. Fractures of limbs are usually of green-stick type but may be complete. Fractures of the clavicle require no treatment. In fractures of the humerus, immobilization of the arm is achieved by placing a pad in the axilla and splinting the arm to the chest with a bandage. With fractures of the femur, immobilization of the leg is achieved by using a splint and bandage. Rapid reunion occurs with callus formation. Union of the clavicle occurs in 7 to 10 days, while the humerus and femur take 2 to 3 weeks. Deformity is rare even where the bone ends are not in good alignment.

Skull Fracture

These fractures, although rare can occur during prolonged or difficult instrumental births. They are usually linear although depressed fractures are possible. There may be no signs. Signs of associated complications such as intracranial hemorrhage, raised intracranial pressure, neurological disturbances, leakage of cerebrospinal fluid or seizures can sometimes lead to the detection of a fracture. A cephalhematoma may sometimes overlie the fracture leading to its detection.

X-ray examination can confirm the diagnosis. Linear fractures of the skull usually require no treatment. Depressed fractures may require surgical intervention. If there is a leakage of cerebrospinal fluid through the ear or nose, antibiotic therapy is indicated.

Dislocations

The common sites of dislocations of joints are shoulder, hip, jaw and fifth-sixth cervical vertebrae. Confirmation is done by radiology, and the help of an orthopedic surgeon should be sought.

Visceral Injuries

Liver, kidneys, adrenals or lungs are occasionally injured mainly during breech delivery. The commonest result of the injury is hemorrhage. Severe hemorrhage is fatal. In minor hemorrhage, the baby presents features of blood loss in addition to the disturbed function of the organ involved. Treatment is directed to correct the hypovolemia and anemia, and specific management to tackle the injured viscera.

HEMORRHAGE

Hemorrhage in the newborn can be due to trauma or hypoxia, or it can be related to coagulopathies and other causes. Blood volume in the term baby is approximately 80 to100 ml/kg and in the preterm baby 90 to 105 ml/kg body weight; therefore, even a small hemorrhage can be potentially fatal. Hemorrhage in the newborn can be classified according to the principal cause.

Hemorrhage due to Trauma

Cephalhematoma (Figs 45.4A and B)

It is an effusion of blood under the periosteum, which covers the skull bones. During a vaginal birth, if there is friction between the fetal skull and the bones of the maternal pelvis, such as in cephalopelvic disproportion or precipitate, the periosteum is torn from the bone, causing bleeding underneath. It may be caused by forceps delivery and may be associated with fracture of the skull bone. Because the skull bones are not fused in the newborn and as the periosteum is adherent to the edges of the skull bones, a cephalhematoma is confined to one bone.

However, more than one bone may be affected; therefore double or multiple hematomas may develop.

A cephalhematoma is never present at birth but gradually develops after 12 to 24 hours, grows larger over the subsequent few days and can persist for weeks. The swelling is circumscribed, soft, fluctuant and incompressible, and does not cross a suture line.

No treatment is necessary; the blood is absorbed and the swelling subsides in 6 to 8 weeks leaving an entirely normal skull. Procautions to prevent infection and avoidance of trauma are important.

Subaponeurotic Hemorrhage (Fig. 45.5)

This type of hemorrhage is rare. The epicranial aponeurosis under the scalp is pulled away from the periosteum of the skull bones and bleeding occurs between with resultant swelling. It can occasionally result from an otherwise normal birth but more often; it is associated with vacuum extraction.

The swelling is present at birth, increases in size and is a firm, fluctuant mass. It can cross suture lines and the swelling can extend into the subcutaneous tissue of neck and eyelids. Bruising may be present for days and sometimes weeks. The blood is reabsorbed and the swelling resolves over 2 to 3 weeks. Normally no treatment is required. If the hamorrhage is severe, the baby will show signs of shock. Supportive care including blood transfusion may be required. In rare cases, the hemorrhage is massive and the baby may die.

Subdural Hemorrhage

Normally, molding of the fetal skull bones and stretching of the underlying structures during birth is well tolerated by the fetus. When there

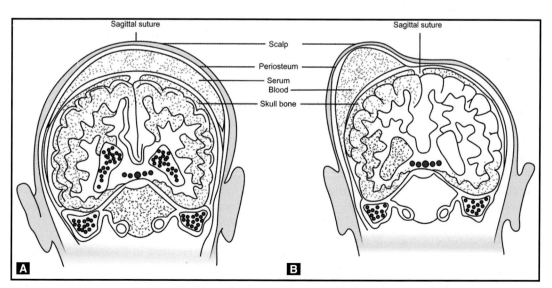

Figs 45.4A and B: (A) Caput succedaneum; (B) Cephalhematoma
(For color version see Plate 6)

Fig. 45.5: Subaponeurotic hemorrhage

is trauma to the fetal head involving excessive compression, abnormal stretching and eventually tearing of the dura can occur, leading to rupture of the venous sinuses and the development of a subdural hemorrhage. Predisposing traumatic circumstances include those in which the molding is rapid, abnormal or excessive such as precipitate or rapid birth, malpositions, malpresentations, cephalopelvic disproportion and undue compression during forceps maneuvers. A tentorial tear is the most common lesion and is most often experienced by term babies.

Slight hemorrhage produces hematoma, which may remain stationary or increase in size. Neurological symptoms may appear acutely or may have insidious onset, like vomiting, irritability and failure to gain weight. Hydrocephalus and mental retardation may be a late sequela.

Large subdural hemorrhage usually results from (1) Tear of the tentorium cerebelli thereby opening up the straight sinuses or rupture of the vein of Galen. (2) Injury to the superior *sagittal* sinus; the baby is likely to suffer severe asphyxia and be difficult to resuscitate or delivered stillborn. In lesser affection, the baby recovers from the respiratory depression. Gradually the features of cerebral irritation appear, such as frequent high pitch cry, neck retraction, incoordinate ocular movements, convulsion, vomiting and bulging of the anterior fontanelle.

Diagnosis is confirmed by cranial ultrasound scan. Supportive treatment is geared towards controlling the consequences of asphyxia and raised intracranial pressure. Subdural taps may be required to drain large collections of blood. This type of hemorrhage can be fatal.

Hemorrhage due to Hypoxia

Subarachnoid Hemorrhage

This hemorrhage occurs when small amounts of capillary or venous bleeding takes place in the subarachnoid space due to tear of some small veins running from the brain to one of the sinuses. Preterm babies, who suffer hypoxia and term babies who suffer traumatic births are vulnerable (McCulloch, 1993).

It often goes unnoticed, as many babies show no sign in the first week of life. After a week, the baby may show signs of twitching of the extremities, incoordinated eye movements and generalized convulsions. The baby becomes listless. Preterm babies may have apneic spells.

Diagnosis can be confirmed by computerized tomography scanning. If a lumbar puncture is performed, the cerebrospinal fluid will be uniformly bloodstained. Management involves the control of the consequences of asphyxia and the control of convulsions. Recovery is usually favorable.

Periventricular or Intraventricular Hemorrhage

This is the most common and serious of all intracranial hemorrhages. It affects infants of less than 32 weeks' (preterm) gestation and those weighing less than 1500 gm. Infants particularly at risk are those who experience hypoxia around the time of birth or in the early postnatal period. The mechanism of hemorrhage is due to intense congestion of the fragile coroidal plexus due to anoxia leading to rupture. The features of cerebral involvement appear abruptly and usually end fatally.

Prenatal administration of steroids to the mother to stimulate the maturation of surfactant followed by the administration of artificial surfactant postnatally to the preterm baby has reduced the incidence of intraventricular hemorrhage in the recent years (Jobe et al, 1993).

Hemorrhage Related to Coagulopathies

These hemorrhages occur because of temporary disruption in the baby's blood clotting abilities.

Hemorrhagic Disease of the Newborn

This is due to a temporary deficiency of the specific clotting factors, factor II (prothrombin), factor VII (proconvertin), factor IX (plasma thromboplastin component) and factor X (thrombokinase). These factors are proteins, which require vitamin K to convert them into active clotting factors.

The babies who are more susceptible to developing HDN are those suffering birth trauma, asphyxia, postnatal hypoxia and those who are preterm, of low birthweight or who are receiving antibiotic therapy. Babies who have been exclusively breastfed or who have been feeding poorly are also considered to be at risk. After the neonatal period, infants who have liver disease or cystic fibrosis are more likely to develop late HDN due to disruption of vitamin K absorption from the bowel. Manifestations of HDN are bleeding from the umbilicus; puncture sites, the nose and the skin as bruising.

Gastrointestinal bleeding is manifested as melena and hemetemesis. In early and late HDN, serious extracranial and intracranial bleeding can also occur. Diagnosis is confirmed if blood tests reveal prolonged prothrombin and partial thromboplastin times. The platelet count is normal.

With any form of HDN, the baby will require administration of vitamin K, 1 to 2 mg intramuscularly. In severe cases, when coagulation is grossly abnormal and there is active bleeding into vital structures, replacement of deficient clotting factors is essential and will involve transfusion of fresh frozen plasma and/or transfusion of the specific clotting factors. If circulatory collapse and severe anemia have occurred, a transfusion of red cell concentrate will be required in addition to fresh frozen plasma. Affected babies may also require other supportive therapy to assist in their recovery. Prophylactic administration of vitamin K, 1 mg intramuscularly to all babies, within the first hour after birth is an effective measure for preventing HDN.

Thrombocytopenia

Thrombocytopenia is a low count of circulating platelets, less than 100,000 per mm^3 and results from a decreased rate of formation of platelets or an increased rate of consumption. Babies who are at risk for developing thrombocytopenia are those:

❖ Who have severe congenital or acquired infection such as syphilis, cytomegalovirus, rubella, toxoplasmosis or bacterial infection
❖ Whose mother has idiopathic thrombocytopenia, systemic lupus erythematosus or thyrotoxicosis
❖ Whose mother takes thiazide diuretics
❖ Who have isoimmune thrombocytopenia
❖ Who have inherited thrombocytopenia.

In mild cases, localized petechial rash appear soon after birth. In a severe case, there is widespread and serious hemorrhage from multiple sites. Diagnosis is based on history, clinical examination and the presence of a reduced platelet count. It is differentiated from other hemorrhagic disorders because coagulation time, fibrin degradation products and red blood cell morphology are normal. In mild cases, no treatment is required, in severe cases where there is hemorrhage and very low platelet counts, a transfusion of platelet concentrate may be required.

Disseminated Intravascular Coagulation (DIC)

DIC is an acquired coagulation disorder, which is associated with the release of thromboplastin from damaged tissue, stimulating abnormal coagulation and fibrinolysis. The consequences include widespread deposition of fibrin in the microcirculation and excessive consumption of clotting factors and platelets.

DIC occurs secondary to other primary conditions. Maternal causes include preeclampsia, eclampsia and placental abruption. Fetal causes include severe fetal distress, the presence of a dead twin in the uterus and a traumatic birth. Neonatal causes include conditions resulting in hypoxia and acidosis, severe bacterial or viral infections, hypothermia, hypotension and thrombocytopenia. As the clotting factors and platelets are depleted and fibrinolysis is stimulated, the baby will develop a generalized purpuric rash and will bleed from multiple sites including pulmonary and intracranial hemorrhage. With the stimulation of the clotting cascade, multiple microthrombi appear in the circulation. These can occlude vessels, leading to organ and tissue ischemia and damage, particularly affecting the kidneys, resulting in hematuria and reduced urinary output. The baby will become anemic due to the hemorrhage and fragmentation of red cells.

Laboratory findings will show a low platelet count, low fibrinogen level, distorted and fragmented red blood cells, low hemoglobin and raised fibrin degradation products (FDPs) with a prolonged prothrombin time (PT) and partial thromboplastin time (PTT).

Treatment includes correction of the underlying cause, if possible, and full supportive care. In order to control the DIC, transfusions of fresh frozen plasma, cryoprecipitate, concentrated clotting factors and platelets are required. When the baby has anemia, transfusions of whole blood or red cell concentrate are required. Occasionally an exchange transfusion of fresh heparinized blood may be performed, removing FDPs while at the same time replacing the clotting factors (Greig in Bennett and Brown, 1999).

If treatment of the primary disorder and/or replacement of clotting factors do not lead to resolution, heparin may be administered to try to reduce fibrin deposition. The prognosis depends on the severity of the primary condition as well as of the DIC and the response to treatment.

Inherited Coagulation Factor Deficiencies

The X-linked recessive conditions such as hemophilia (factor VIII deficiency), rarely causes problems in the neonatal period but may present with excessive bleeding after birth trauma or surgical intervention, such as circumcision. Diagnosis is confirmed by a prolonged PTT and a normal PT with decreased levels of specific factors. Replacement transfusions are required.

An affected baby will require continuing follow-up by hematologists after discharge at home. Education, genetic counseling and support will be required for the family if they lack experience of the condition.

Hemorrhage Related to Other Causes

Umbilical Hemorrhage

This usually occurs because of poorly applied ligatures. Tampering with partially separated cords before they are ready to come off, can also cause bleeding. Cord hemorrhage is a potential cause of death. The use of plastic cord clamps has almost eliminated this type of hemorrhage. In places where plastic clamps are not used, care must be taken to tie the cord well using a reef knot. If umbilical bleeding does not stop after 15 or 20 minutes, a purse string suture should always be inserted.

Hematemesis and Melena

These signs are usually seen when the baby has swallowed maternal blood during delivery or from cracked nipples during breastfeeding. The diagnosis must be differentiated from hemolytic disease of the newborn, esophageal and gastric or duodenal ulceration and from other causes of melena such as intestinal duplications, hemangiomas within the gut, necrotising enterocolitis and anal fissure.

If the cause is swallowed blood, no specific treatment is required. If the cause is cracked nipples, appropriate treatment must be given to the mother.

Hematuria

Hematuria can be associated with coagulopathies, urinary tract infections and structural abnormalities of the urinary tract. Birth trauma may cause renal contusion and hematuria. Occasionally, after suprapubic aspiration of urine, mild hematuria may occur. Treatment of the primary cause usually resolves the hematuria.

Umbilical arterial and venous catheters, central venous lines, radial and femoral artery lines and peripheral venous infusion sites all carry potential danger of severe hemorrhage resulting from dislodgement of the catheter from the vessel or from accidental disconnection of the catheter from the infusion administering set.

Close observation and careful handling of these infants and their infusion lines are imperative to prevent these potentially fatal hemorrhages. If such a hemorrhage does occur, continuous pressure should be applied to the site or, especially for the umbilicus, it should be squeezed between the fingers until hemostasis occurs naturally or hemostatic sutures can be applied. A replacement transfusion of whole blood or packed red cells may be required (Greig in Bennett and Brown, 1999).

PREVENTION OF TRAUMA IN THE NEWBORN

Comprehensive antenatal and intranatal care is the key to success in the reduction of birth trauma and consequently in the reduction of perinatal mortality and neonatal morbidity.

Antenatal Period

Careful screening to identify babies likely to be traumatized during vaginal delivery in order to employ elective cesarean sections. Mothers with contracted pelvis, cephalopelvic disproportion, malpresentations like breech or transverse lie are to be included for cesarean section.

Intranatal Period

❖ Continuous fetal monitoring, if available, to detect early evidences of fetal distress
❖ Determination of pH by fetal blood sampling to detect early, any sign of distress in order to prevent traumatic fetal anoxia
❖ Careful cutting of the episiotomies after placing two fingers between the head and the stretched perineum to prevent injury to the scalp
❖ Undue stretching of the neck to be avoided to minimize injuries to the brachial plexus or sternomastoid muscle.

Preterm Delivery

❖ Avoidance of strong sedation
❖ Prevention of anoxia

❖ Liberal episiotomies and use of forceps to prevent intracranial compression
❖ Administration of vitamin K, 1 mg intramuscularly to prevent or minimize hemorrhage from the traumatized area.

Instrumental Delivery

❖ Difficult forceps to be withheld in preference to cesarean section
❖ Traction to forceps blades to be applied only after correct placement of blades (over the biparietal plane) is confirmed.

Vaginal Breech Delivery

❖ Proper selection of cases and utmost care and gentleness to be executed while conducting breech delivery
❖ Episiotomies to be given as a routine
❖ After-coming head to be delivered without haste and by forceps preferably
❖ Acute bending at neck to be prevented while applying forceps
❖ The trunk should not be pulled to one side too much (injury to the brachial plexus and sternomastoid muscle occur due to stretching)
❖ Care to be taken while performing different maneuvers to prevent fractures, dislocations and visceral injuries.

CONVULSIONS IN THE NEWBORN

A convulsion in the newborn is a sign of a neurological disturbance. Convulsions (seizures, fits) can present quite differently in a neonate than those of later infancy, childhood or adulthood due to the lack of development of neuronal contacts and myelination.

Manifestations

Neonatal convulsions are always visible manifestations of some underlying pathology. *It is manifested as abnormal sudden or repetitive movements of any part of the body.* Convulsive movements are to be differentiated from jitteriness or tremors in which the movements are rapid, rhythmic and equal which are often stimulated or made worse by disturbance and can be stopped by touching or flexing the affected limb. They are normal in an active, hungry baby and are usually of no consequences. *Convulsive movements tend to be slower, less equal, are not essentially stimulated by disturbance, cannot be stopped by restraint and are always pathological.*

Types of Neonatal Convulsions

Ballweg (1991) suggested that the type of movements a baby has could help classify the convulsions as either subtle, tonic, focal, clonic or myoclonic.

Subtle convulsions include movements such as blinking or fluttering of the eyelids, staring, clonic movements of the chin, horizontal or downward movement of eyes, sucking, drooling and sticking the tongue out, cycling movements of the tongue and apnea. Both term and preterm infants can experience subtle convulsions.

If the baby has *tonic convulsions*, there will be extension or flexion of limbs, altered patterns of breathing and maintenance of eye deviations. Tonic convulsions are more common in preterm babies.

Multifocal clonic convulsions are seen in term babies and the movements include random jerking movements of extremities. Term babies also experience *focal clonic convulsions,* which are localized, repetitive, clonic jerking movements. An extremity, a limb or a localized muscle group can be affected.

Myoclonic convulsions are the least common but affect both term and preterm babies. The movements are single or multiple flexion jerks of the feet, legs, hands or arms, which should not be confused with similar movements a sleeping baby can demonstrate.

During a convulsion, the baby may have tachycardia, hypertension, raised cerebral blood flow and raised intracranial pressure.

Causes of Convulsion in the Newborn

- Central nervous system causes
  - Intracranial hemorrhage
  - Intracerebral hemorrhage
  - Hypoxic-ischemic encephalopathy
  - Kernicterus.
- Metabolic
  - Hypo and hyperglycemia
  - Hypo and hypercalcemia
  - Hypo and hypernatremia
  - Hypomagnesemia
  - Inborn errors of metabolism.
- Infective
  - High fever
  - Meningitis
  - TORCH infection
  - Tetanus.
- Iatrogenic
  - Respiratory stimulants
  - Analeptic drugs
  - Drug toxicity, e.g. theophylline.
- Others
  - Cerebral malformations
  - Drug withdrawal.

Investigations

- Full blood count
- Blood, urine and CSF cultures
- Serum IgM and IgG specific TORCH titers.
- Biochemical estimation of glucose, calcium, magnesium, bilirubin and electrolytes
- Blood gas levels to detect acidosis and hypoxemia
- Ultrasonography and CT scan of the head to detect intraventricular and/or subarachnoid hemorrhage, or congenital malformations.

Management

Control of Convulsions

Immediate treatment of a convulsion includes getting the assistance of a pediatrician/neonatologist while ensuring that the baby has a clear airway and adequate ventilation either spontaneously or mechanically. It also includes turning the infant to the semiprone position with the head neither hyperflexed nor hyperextended. Gentle oral and nasal suctioning to remove any milk or mucus if required. If the baby is breathing but cyanosed, facial oxygen is to be given at a flow rate of 2 to 3 liters per minute. If apnea occurs and cyanosis persists, resuscitation may be required. The baby should be handled minimum. If the baby is nursed in an incubator without covering blankets yet dressed and well supported, observation and maintenance of neutral thermal environment can be achieved.

Intravenous administration of phenobarbitone 10 mg/kg body weight slowly over a period of 3 to 5 minutes is effective. A maintenance dose of 5 mg/kg bodyweight per day is administered intramuscularly for a period of four weeks or longer. In resistant cases IV phenytoin (Dilantin), 15 mg/kg at the rate of 0.5 mg/kg/minute, followed by maintenance dose of 5 mg/kg/day is administered.

Treatment of the Underlying Pathology

Hypoglycemia: Glucose infusion, 2 ml/kg of 10 percent glucose is given over a period of 2 to 3 minutes. Glucose infusion is continued at a rate of 6 to 8 mg/kg/minute. Blood glucose must be maintained at 40 to 60 mg/dl.

Hypomagnesemia: Magnesium sulphate 0.2 mEq/kg is given IV every six hours until magnesium level is normal.

Infection: Appropriate antibiotic therapy following septic work-up.

Hypocalcemia: Intravenous administration of 2 ml/kg of 10 percent calcium gluconate over 5 minutes. This is to be followed by oral calcium chloride 250 mg with each feed for few days.

Raised intracranial tension: 10 ml of 20 percent mannitol to be given intravenously over 30 to 60 minutes.

Observation and Recording

It is important that observations of a convulsion are documented, noting the type of movement, the areas affected, the length, any color change, any change in heart rate, respiratory rate or blood pressure and any immediate sequel.

The outcome for babies who have convulsions depends on the cause of the convulsion, the type of convulsion and the EEG tracing. Babies who have congenital malformations of the brain, hypoxic-ischemic encephalopathy or bacterial meningitis tend to have a higher mortality or a poor neurological outcome. Babies who have a late hypocalcemia, hyponatremia or primary subarachnoid hemorrhage are more likely to survive neurologically intact.

Babies, who experience subtle, generalized tonic and myoclonic convulsions tend to have a poorer neurological outcome than babies experiencing the other types of convulsions do. Abnormal EEG tracings generally indicate a poor prognosis (Ballweg, 1991; Blackburn, 1993).

Managing Parents

When their baby suffers trauma during birth, or hemorrhage or convulsions, parents are likely to be extremely shocked. Although the extent of parental contact with the baby will depend on the nature of the birth injury, all parents are entitled to be given honest and clear information about their baby's condition as soon as possible after detection. It is recommended that parents receive this type of bad news when they are together and from someone who is known to them (Richards and Reed, 1991). The neonatologist giving the information will need to give time for parents to clarify their questions. Follow up explanations by nursing personnel and encouragement for parental interactions are essential. Continuing supportive care will also be required for them to deal with the stressful situation.

BIBLIOGRAPHY

1. Ballweg DD. Neonatal Seizures: An overview, Neonatal Network 1991;10(1):15-21.
2. Blackburn ST. Assessment and management of neurological dysfunction. In: Kenner C (Eds), et al, Comprehensive Neonatal Nursing. Philadelphia; WB Saunders 1993.
3. Brucker J, et al. Brachial plexus birth injury, Journal Neuroscience Nursing 1991;23(6):374-80.
4. Dutta DC. Textbook of Obstetrics, 5th edn. Calcutta; New Central Book Company 2001.
5. Greig C. Trauma during birth, hemorrhage and convulsions. In: Bennett RV, Linda KB. Myles Textbook for Midwives, 13th edn. Edinburgh: Churchill Livingstone 1999.
6. Jobe AH, Mitchell BR. Beneficial effects of the combined use of prenatal corticosteroids and postnatal surfactant on perterm infants. American Journal of Obstetrics and Gynecology 1993;168: 508-13.
7. Mc Culloch M. Neurological disorders, In: Beachy P, Deacon J. Core Curriculum for Neonatal Intensive Care Nursing. Philadelphia;WB Saunders 1993.
8. Richards C, Reed J. Your baby has Down's syndrome. Nursing Times 1991;87(46):60-1.

46

Congenital Abnormalities

Learning Objectives

Upon completing this chapter, the learner will be able to:

❖ Describe and explain specific congenital abnormalities
❖ Explain the role of the midwife in the care of neonates with congenital problems
❖ Explain the possible psychological stress on staff and the measures to minimize stress.

A congenital abnormality is any defect in form, structure or function, present in a neonate.

The incidence of significant congenital malformations is about 2 to 5 percent at birth. A lower incidence of one in 500 is however, reported from the hospital statistics in India. In the western countries, major fetal abnormalities account for about 20 percent of perinatal deaths and many survivors are physically and/or mentally handicapped (Dutta, 2001).

CAUSES OF CONGENITAL ABNORMALITIES

Identifiable defects can be categorized as:
❖ Chromosome and gene abnormalities
❖ Teratogenic causes
❖ Multifactorial causes
❖ Unknown causes.

Chromosome Abnormalities

Each human cell carries a blueprint for reproduction in the form of 44 chromosomes (autosomes) and 2 sex chromosomes. Each chromosome comprises a number of genes. A fertilized zygote should have 22 autosomes and 1 sex chromosome from each parent. If a fault occurs in the formation of the gametes or following fertilization, an excess or deficit of chromosomal material will result. Each abnormal chromosomal pattern has a different clinical presentation. Common forms of chromosomal abnormalities are: Trisomy-21 (Down's syndrome), Trisomy-18 (Edward's syndrome) and Trisomy-13 (Patau syndrome).

Genetic Disorder (Mendelian Inheritance)

Genes are composed of deoxyribonucleic acid (DNA) and each is concerned with the transmission of one specific hereditary factor. Genetically inherited factors may be *dominant* or *recessive*. A dominant gene will produce its effect even if present in only one chromosome of a pair. An autosomal dominant condition can usually be traced through several generations. A recessive gene needs to be present in both chromosomes before producing its effect. Genetic disorders are classified as follows:

Teratogenic Causes

A teratogen is any agent that raises the incidence of congenital abnormality. The list of known and suspected teratogens is the following:

Prescription drugs
❖ Anticonvulsants
❖ Anticoagulants
❖ High concentrations of vitamin A (For acne treatment).

Drugs used in substance abuse
❖ Heroin
❖ Alcohol
❖ Nicotine.

Gene Disorders

Autosomal

Dominant
❖ Achondroplasia
❖ Osteogenesis imperfecta
❖ Adult polycystic kidney Disease
❖ Huntington's chorea
❖ Neurofibromatosis.

Recessive
❖ Cystic fibrosis
❖ Phenyle ketonuria
❖ Sickle cell anemia

X-linked disorders
❖ Hemophilia
❖ Duchenne muscular dystrophy
❖ Color blindness
❖ Fragile X-syndrome

Environmental factors
❖ Radiation
❖ Chemicals (Dioxins, pesticides).

Infective agents
❖ Rubella
❖ Cytomegalovirus
❖ Varicella
❖ Toxoplasma.

Maternal diseases
❖ Diabetes
❖ Epilepsy.

Several factors influence the effect(s) produced by any one teratogen such as gestational age of the embryo or fetus at the time of exposure, length of exposure and toxicity of the teratogen.

Multifactorial Causes

These are due to a genetic effect in addition to one or more teratogenic influences. These include neural tube defects, congenital heart defects, cleft palate and cleft lip.

Advancing maternal age increases the incidence of Down's syndrome (Mongolism) to the extent of one in 100 births at the age of 40. Increasing parity is associated with high incidence of malformation except anencephaly or spina bifida, which is common in first birth. Maternal malnutrition is associated with increased incidence of fetal malformations.

Unknown Causes

In spite of a growing body of knowledge, the specific cause of large number of abnormalities (80%) remains unspecified.

PRENATAL GENETIC COUNSELING

Genetic counseling is the screening procedure designed to identify the individual having a greater risk of producing an offspring with genetic abnormalities. Identification of the cases at risk is done by meticulous family and reproductive history as well as the possible effects of environmental factors. Birth of a congenitally malformed baby increases the chance of repetition to the extent of six-folds and that following two consecutive babies increases the chance to 70 percent as compared to a normal woman. The aim is to allow the woman and her spouse to make a unified decision regarding future management of pregnancy. The objectives are to provide information and assist the couple to adjust to the problem and thereby decrease the incidence of births of genetically defective babies.

Candidates for Screening

❖ Women over 35 years
❖ Family history of neural tube defects
❖ Previous baby born with neural tube defect
❖ Previous child with chromosomal anomaly
❖ One or both parents carriers of sex-linked autosomal traits
❖ A mentally retarded child with or without congenital anomaly
❖ History of recurrent abortion.

Risk Factors

Prenatal high-risk factors that are associated with multiple congenital anomalies are:

❖ Oligohydramnios
❖ Polyhydramnios
❖ Severe intrauterine growth restriction
❖ Decreased fetal activity
❖ Uncontrolled diabetes mellitus in the preconceptional period
❖ Contact with tertogens (infection with rubella or cytomegalo virus).

Detection

Improved prenatal screening and diagnostic techniques are now available for detection of abnormalities in early pregnancy which include:

❖ Maternal serum alpha-fetoprotein (MSAFP)
❖ Triple test: MSAFP, Unconjugated estriol (E$_3$) and HCG
❖ Amniocentesis
❖ Chorion villus biopsy
❖ High resolution ultrasonography
❖ Fetoscopy
❖ Embryobiopsy.

Termination of pregnancy is considered following early detection of genetic disorders, chromosomal abnormalities and structural abnormalities.

Management of at Risk Couples

Preconceptional counseling is an important step in the management so that the couple has adequate information before hand. Option of termination of pregnancy is offered if the fetus is affected with serious genetic, chromosomal or structural abnormality.

COMMON MALFORMATIONS AND SYNDROMES

Gastrointestinal Malformations

Most of the abnormalities affecting this system call for prompt surgical intervention, for example atresias, gastroschisis and exomphalos. If prenatal diagnosis has been made, the parents will be at least partially prepared. After the baby is delivered and prior to obtaining their consent for surgery, they should be permitted to hold the baby and the pediatric surgeon must provide adequate explanation.

Gastroschisis and Exomphalos

Gastroschisis is a paramedian defect of the abdominal wall with extrusion of bowel, which is not covered by peritoneum, thus making it very vulnerable to injury and infection. Surgical closure of the defect is usually possible.

Exomphalos or omphalocele is the bowel or other viscera protrude through the umbilicus. Very often these babies have other abnormalities such as heart defects, which could be a contraindication to surgery in the neonatal period. Closure of the defect may consequently be delayed as long as one or two years.

Immediate management of both the above conditions is to cover the herniated abdominal contents with warm sterile saline gauze or a sterile silastic bag. Stomach contents should be aspirated. Transfer of the baby to a surgical neonatal intensive care unit is then expedited.

Atresias

Esophageal Atresia

This occurs when there is incomplete canalization of the esophagus in early intrauterine development. It is commonly associated with tracheoesophageal fistula, which connects the trachea to the upper or lower esophagus or both. The commonest type of abnormality is where the upper esophagus terminates in a blind pouch and the lower esophagus connects to the trachea. This abnormality should be suspected in the presence of maternal polyhydramnios. At birth the baby has copious amounts of mucus coming from the mouth. An orogastric tube may travel less than 10 to 12 cm. Radiography will confirm the diagnosis.

The baby must be given no oral fluid. He should be transferred immediately to a pediatric surgical unit. It may be possible to anastomose the blind ends of the esophagus. If the distance is too large, a series of bouginages may be carried out in an attempt to stretch the ends of the esophagus, stimulate growth and thereby eventually facilitate repair by end-to-end anastomosis. Alternatively, a Teflon graft or transplant of a section of colonic tissue will be needed later. If the repair is delayed, a cervical esophagostomy may be performed to allow drainage of secretions. Meanwhile the baby will require to be fed via a gastrostomy tube.

Duodenal Atresia

If this has not already been diagnosed in the prenatal period, persistent vomiting within the first 24 to 36 hours of birth will be the first features encountered. The vomit will often contain bile unless the obstruction is proximal to the entrance of the common bile duct. Abdominal distension may not be present and the baby may pass meconium. A characteristic double bubble of gas may be seen on radiological examination. Treatment is by surgical repair. Outcome is good if the baby is otherwise healthy.

Rectal Atresia and Imperforate Anus

Imperforate anus is often obvious at birth on examination of the baby, but a rectal atresia might not become apparent until it is noted that the baby has not passed meconium. Where the first temperature is taken by rectal thermometer, the problem may be noted earlier. Both conditions require the baby to have surgical intervention.

Other possibilities that should be considered if a baby fails to pass meconium in the first 24 hours are *malrotation, cystic fibrosis and Hirschsprung's disease*.

Malrotation

This is a developmental abnormality, where incomplete rotation of the gut has taken place, giving rise to signs of obstruction. Surgical correction is necessary.

Cystic Fibrosis

This is an autosomal recessive condition. Majority of cases are not diagnosed until later in infancy or childhood when the child fails to thrive or have repeated chest infections. In this condition, the meconium is particularly viscous and causes intestinal obstruction. There is accompanying abdominal distension and bile-stained vomiting. Definite diagnosis will be by identifying a raised immunoreactive tripsin level. Treatment is supportive rather than curative and involves intravenous therapy and gastrografin enema to relieve obstruction, administration of pancreatin and chest physiotherapy.

Hirschsprung's Disease

In this disease, the bowel has an aganglionic section. The incidence is about 1 in 5,000 births. Due to the presence of the aganglionic section, peristalsis does not occur and the bowel therefore, becomes obstructed. The baby develops abdominal distension and bile-stained vomiting. Definite diagnosis is made by doing a colonic biopsy. Resection of the aganglionic section of the bowel and anastomosis is indicated.

Pyloric Stenosis

Pyloric stenosis arises from a genetic defect, which causes hypertrophy of the muscles of the pyloric sphincter. The characteristic clinical presentation is projectile vomiting usually around six weeks of age but it may occur earlier in some babies. Boy babies are usually affected and surgical repair is by Ramstedt's operation (Halliday in Bennet and Brown, 1999).

Cleft Lip and Cleft Palate

Cleft in the lip may occur as a single deformity or accompanied by cleft palate. The defect may be unilateral or bilateral. Clefts in the palate may affect hard palate, soft palate or both. Some defects will include alveolar margins and sometimes the uvula. The greatest problem with these babies initially is feeding. If the defect is limited to a unilateral cleft lip, the mother may be able to breastfeed the baby. Where there is the additional problem of cleft palate, feeding presents problems. Feeding with specially made teats or spoon will be required.

Middle ear infection is common in these babies and repeated infections could impede hearing and subsequent development of speech. Mothers should be encouraged to feed with expressed breast milk and assisted with the task of feeding, as it will require lot of patience.

Surgical repair of the cleft lip may be performed at the age of 3 to 4 months. Closure of the palate defect is often suggested at around the age of 12 to 15 months. The delay is to allow normal growth to take place, which may result in reducing the size of the defect, thus increasing the possibility of a more satisfactory repair.

Pierre Robin Syndrome

Pierre Robin syndrome is characterized by micrognathia (hypoplasia of the lower jaw), abnormal attachment of muscles controlling the tongue, which allows it to fall backward and occlude the airway, and a central cleft palate. Maintenance of a clear airway is paramount in the care of these babies. In order to achieve this, the baby will be nursed prone. Feeding is difficult and there is high risk for aspiration. Suction catheter and oxygen equipment should be ready to hand. The action of sucking may encourage development of the mandible. The baby may have to be kept in the hospital until the lower jaw has grown sufficiently.

ABNORMALITIES RELATING TO RESPIRATION

Any abnormality of the respiratory tract or accessory respiratory muscles is likely to hamper the process of successful transition from fetus to neonate.

Diaphragmatic Hernia

In this condition, there is a defect in the diaphragm, which allows herniation of abdominal contents into the thoracic cavity. The extent to which lung development is compromised as a result, depends on the size of the defect and the gestational age at which herniation first occurred. The condition may be suspected at birth if the baby is cyanosed and difficulty is experienced in resuscitation. Since the majority of such defects are left sided, heart sounds will be displaced. The abdomen may have a scafoid appearance. Chest X-ray will confirm the diagnosis. Immediate surgical repair of the defect is necessary. Prognosis relates to the degree of pulmonary hypoplasia. Coexistent abnormalities such as cardiac defects or chromosomal anomalies are usually seen.

Choanal Atresia

Choanal atresia is a unilateral or bilateral narrowing of the nasal passage(s) with a web of tissue or bone occluding the nasopharynx. Tachypnea and dyspnea are cardinal features particularly when a bilateral lesion is present. The baby's color will improve with crying. Maintaining a clear airway is obviously essential and an oral airway may have to be used to effect this. A unilateral defect may not be noticed until the baby feeds for the first time, when respiratory difficulty and cyanosis occur. Surgery will be required to remove the obstructing tissue. Occasionally choanal atresia is associated with other abnormalities.

Laryngeal Strider

This is a noise made by the baby usually on inspiration and exacerbated by crying. Most commonly, the cause is laryngomalacia due to laxity of the laryngeal cartilage. With strider, the baby is generally not in distress though it may sound distressing. Parents often require repeated reassuring. The condition may resolve over time, perhaps by two years. If however, there are other accompanying signs of dyspnea or feeding problems, further investigations would be necessary to rule out additional abnormalities.

CONGENITAL CARDIAC DEFECTS

Babies born with congenital defects comprise the second largest group of babies, born with abnormalities (Nixon and O'Donnel, 1992). The underlying mechanisms that produce cardiac defects are thought to be either abnormal cell migration or disordered intracardiac blood follow. Majority of the defects cannot be attributed to a single cause. About 10 percent of the defects occur due to chromosomal and genetic factors or caused by teratogens.

Detection of Cardiac Defects

An increasing number of problems are now being identified by ultrasound scanning. However, most defects are identified during the neonatal examination. Congenital cardiac anomalies of the newborn can be divided into two groups, cyanotic heart disease and acyanotic heart disease.

Cardiac Defects Presenting with Cyanosis

These defects include:

- ❖ Transposition of great arteries
- ❖ Total anomalous pulmonary venous drainage
- ❖ Tricuspid atresia
- ❖ Fallot's tetralogy
- ❖ Pulmonary atresia
- ❖ Univentricular heart.

The first signs that a cardiac defect is present are the persistence of central cyanosis, tachypnea and tachycardia. Administration of oxygen to these babies will be ineffective in improving their color. Chest X-ray should be performed to exclude anomalies of the respiratory tract, respiratory disease and diaphragmatic hernia. Echocardiography may be done to explore the precise nature of the defect.

Transposition of great arteries: This is a condition where the aorta arises from the right ventricle and the pulmonary artery from the left ventricle. Consequently, oxygenated blood circulates back through the lungs and deoxygenated blood back into the systemic circuit. Unless life saving intervention is instituted immediately, the baby will die. Prostaglandin infusion may be commenced to maintain patency of the ductus arteriosus, which may be followed by a Rashkind septostomy. This procedure involves creating an artificial septal defect to allow oxygenated blood to access the systemic circulation. Corrective surgery is then carried out later.

Some of the other defects do not initially present with marked cyanosis. These babies for a time may be considered healthy.

'Acyanotic' Cardiac Defects

Anomalies included in this group are:

- ❖ Left heart hypoplasia
- ❖ Coarctation of aorta
- ❖ Patent ductus arteriosus
- ❖ Atrial or ventricular septal defects.

These babies may manifest signs of cardiac failure such as tachypnea, tachycardia and cyanosis following the exertion of crying or feeding. Detailed examination may reveal heart murmurs and diminution or absence of femoral pulse.

Corrective surgery is sometimes possible for coarctation of aorta, depending on the extent of the stricture. Babies with hypoplastic heart disease have a poor prognosis. It is important that each baby is examined thoroughly before discharge from the hospital. It is equally important to realize, however, that not all heart murmurs heard at this time are significant. Parents must be instructed to seek medical advice for any change in the baby's behavior, such as breathlessness or cyanosis.

CENTRAL NERVOUS SYSTEM ABNORMALITIES

The number of babies born with abnormalities of the central nervous system has reduced due to the mothers taking folic acid supplements during the early months of pregnancy. Prenatal screening tests, such as measuring the alpha-fetoprotein levels and detailed ultrasound scanning has resulted in some parents choosing selective termination of pregnancies where severe neural tube defects are found.

Anencephaly

Anencephaly is characterized by the absence of the forebrain and vault of the skull. It is a condition which is incompatible with sustained life but occasionally such a baby is born alive. It is important for the midwife to wrap the baby (the head) carefully before showing to the mother. Parents may however, want to hold the baby and see the full extend of the abnormality. Though unpleasant, it may facilitate their grieving process and will help them to accept the reality of the situation.

Spina Bifida Aperta

This condition results from failure of fusion of the vertebral column. There are various forms of the spina bifida.

Meningocele (Fig. 46.1)

This is a saclike protrusion of either the cerebral or spinal meninges through a congenital

Fig. 46.1: Meningocele

defect in the skull or the vertebral column. It forms a hernial cyst that is filled with cerebrospinal fluid but does not contain neural tissue. The anomaly is designated as cranial meningocele or spinal meningocele depending on the site of the defect.

Meningomyelocele (Fig. 46.2)

It involves the spinal cord. This lesion may be enclosed or the meningocele may rupture and expose the neural tissue. Meningomyelocele usually gives rise to neural damage producing paralysis distal to the defect and impaired function of urinary bladder and bowel. The lumbosacral area is the most common site for these to present but they may appear at any point in the vertebral column.

When the defect is at the base of skull level, it is known as *encephalocele*. The added complication with encephalocele is that the sac may contain varying amounts of brain tissue. Normal progression of may be impeded by a large lesion of this type.

Immediate management involves covering open lesions with a nonadherent dressing. Babies with enclosed lesions should be handled with great care in order to preserve the integrity of the sac, reducing the risk of meningitis. Surgical closure is possible for meningocele (Halliday in Bennet and Brown, 1999).

Spina Bifida Occulta

Spina bifida occulta is the minor type of defect where the vertebra is bifid. There is usually no

Fig. 46.2: Meningomyelocele in the lumbosacral area

spinal cord involvement. A tuft of hair or sinus at the base of the spine may be noted on first examination of the baby. Ultrasound examination will confirm the diagnosis and rule out any associated spinal cord involvement.

Hydrocephalus

This is a condition, which arises from a blockage in the circulation and absorption of cerebrospinal fluid. The lateral ventricles increase in size and eventually compress the surrounding brain tissue. Hydrocephaly may either be present at birth or develop following surgical closure of a meningomyelocele. The risk of cerebral impairment may be minimized by the insertion of a ventriculoperitoneal shunt. As the baby grows, this will need to be replaced. Risks with the shunt devices are that the line blocks and the shunt becomes a portal for infection leading to meningitis. Signs of increased intracranial pressure to be watched for include:

- ❖ Large tense anterior fontanelle
- ❖ Splayed (spread out) skull bones
- ❖ Inappropriate increase in occipitofrontal circumference
- ❖ Sun-setting appearance to the eyes
- ❖ Irritability or abnormal movements.

Microcephaly

Microcephaly is the condition where the occipitofrontal circumference is more than two standard deviations below normal for gestational age. The disproportionately small head may be the result of intrauterine infection such as rubella, a feature of fetal alcohol syndrome, or part of a number of defects in some trisomic disorders. The baby will invariably be mentally impaired.

MUSCULOSKELETAL DEFORMITIES

These are vary from relatively minor anomalies such as an extra digit, to major deficits such as absence of a limb. *Polydactyly (super numerary digits)* (Fig. 46.3) occur either on the hands or on the feet. In fact, their occurrence on the hands is sufficiently frequent to make this the most common congenital anomaly of the upper extremity. In some families, it occurs as a hereditary trait. Most frequently, it appears as an accessory and often hypoplastic appendage, sometimes no more than a simple *skin tag* on the ulnar surface of the little finger. Alternatively, the thumb may be duplicated. Polydactyly is occasionally seen in conjunction with other congenital malformations.

With the exception of a simple *skin tag*, which may be ligated and allowed to slough, surgical intervention is almost invariably indicated. In cases that are more complex, the operation may be delayed until the age of two or three years, when phalangeal and meta-

Fig. 46.3: Polydactyly

Fig. 46.4: Syndactyly

carpel ossification centers are present and the anatomic status can be more precisely defined.

Syndactyly, (Fig. 46.4) second only in incidence to polydactyly as an abnormality of the upper extremity, is an abnormal fusion of the digits either partial or complete. It may consist of interdigital webbing of the skin only, or the bony structure, or both. Most often, it involves the third and fourth fingers or the second and third fingers. It is frequently a hereditary characteristic unaccompanied by any other abnormality. However, it can appear as a feature of a syndrome such as *Apert's syndrome*, which is a genetically inherited condition in which there is premature fusion of the sutures of the vault of the skull, cleft palate and complete syndactyly of both hands and feet.

Treatment is by surgical operation. Since premature intervention may lead to a poor result, surgery is best performed shortly before the child enters school.

Careful examination including separation and counting of the baby's fingers and toes during the physical examination is important in order not to miss anomalies such as polydactyly and syndactyly.

Limb Reduction Anomalies

Limb reduction anomalies comprise a wide range of possibilities. In some, either a hand or a foot will be completely missing while in others a normal hand or foot will be present at the end of a shortened limb. Thalidomide, an antiemetic, has been a proven teratogenic in this context.

Fig. 46.5: Talipes equinovarus

Fig. 46.6: Talipes calcaneovalgus

The child is not ill and will not be upset by the defect. However, the parents of a child with limb defect will grieve the loss of their perfect child. Children usually prove themselves most adaptable and able to cope.

Talipes Equinovarus (Fig. 46.5)

Talipes equinovarus is a common congenital anomaly, occurring once in 1,000 to 1,600 births and accounts for more than 95 percent clubfoot. It affects males twice commonly as females. In this condition, the foot is turned downward and inward so that the sole is directed medically. In some instances, the condition may be attributable to an unusual fetal posture—The foot (or feet) having been held in an abnormal position within the uterus. In such cases the position of comfort, which the foot assumes postnatally, will often indicate the origin of the deformity. If the foot can be passively placed in a normal position without force, correction will almost certainly take place spontaneously or with a conservative mode of treatment. Treatment should be started as early as possible.

When the condition is mild, it may be completely corrected within six to ten weeks. When force is required to place the foot in normal position, this indicates that shortening of the ligaments and tendon is present, are more involved and prolonged orthopedic treatment will be required.

Talipes Calcaneovalgus (Fig. 46.6)

Like talipes equinovarus, this deformity may stem from an abnormal intrauterine position. The foot is held in dorsiflexion and deviated laterally. Shortening of the soft tissues on the dorsum of the foot, limits the degree of plantar flexion and inversion.

Generally, the condition is positional and the only treatment required is regular passive stretching. Less frequently, correction by exercise and application of plaster cast is required. When the foot cannot be passively corrected, the causative structural abnormality should be sought and appropriate orthopedic treatment instituted.

Congenital Hip Dysplasia

Congenital dysplasia of the hip is a condition in which there is an abnormal development of the hip joint and related ligaments and soft tissues. The head of the femur may be in proper position although susceptible to dislocation by appropriate maneuvering. Alternatively, it may be either partially or totally dislocated. Characteristic clinical signs of hip abnormalities in the infant are asymmetry of the skin folds and creases on the dorsal surfaces, together with apparent shortening or lengthening of the affected leg. In congenital abduction contracture of the hip, for example, the skin folds of the thighs and popliteal creases are asymmetrical and the affected leg appears to be longer. In a dislocated hip where the head of the femur is displaced upward and laterally, the affected extremity appears shorter, and the inguinal crease is deeper and more cephalad on the affected side (Figs 46.7A and B).

The condition affects females 6 to 8 times as frequently as males and the left hip three times more than the right hip. In 25 percent of cases, the condition is bilateral. The fundamental cause of the defect is still controversial.

Fig. 46.7A: Normal gluteal and popliteal skin creases

Fig. 46.7B: Abnormal skin creases in congenital dislocation of right hip

Limitation of abduction, present at birth or developing within the first few weeks of life, is a cardinal sign of congenital subluxation (partial dislocation or displacement). Early evidence of the condition may be obtained by the Ortolani's maneuver. In this maneuver, the infants thighs are flexed to a right angle and fully abducted. The thigh under suspicion is then adducted while still in the flexed position and pressure is applied along the long axis of the femur in the direction of the posterior lip of the acetabulum. As dislocation occurs a click (the click of exit) is felt when the femoral head passes over the posterior lip. A similar click (the click of entry) is noted on reversal of the maneuver as the hip slips back into the joint. X-ray examination may help in the diagnosis.

In congenital dysplasia with dislocation, the femoral head is usually dislocated posteriorly and a reverse Ortolani's sign may be detected, i.e. a click of entry is felt on abduction and a click of exist on adduction. With lateral and upward displacement of the femoral head, there is an apparent shortening of the affected leg together with a 15 to 20° external rotation of the limb and limitation of passive abduction with the hip flex at 90°. The inguinal crease is deeper and more cephalad on the affected side and there is an asymmetry of the thigh. When the infant is placed in a prone position, the buttock on the affected side is wider and flatter than

normal. Radiographic examination should be used to confirm the diagnosis.

Early diagnosis is of vital importance in congenital hip displacia to prevent the development of persistent structural damage. Treatment is usually instituted as soon as the diagnosis is made. With early diagnosis, the sole therapy generally required is maintenance of the limb in a position of abduction and external rotation for 2 to 3 months. Application of double diapers help to keep the legs abducted. A splint or harness such as Pavlik harness may be applied to keep the legs in flexed and abducted position. Parents will require additional support in learning how to handle and care for their baby. Particular attention should be paid to skin care and checking for signs of chafing and excoriation.

Streeter's Dysplasia

Streeter's dysplasia is a rather infrequent condition in which constricting bands (streeter's bands) encircle one or more extremities. The constrictions are of varying depth and may appear on the digits, feet, hands or any part of the legs or arms. Somewhat more common on the legs than on the arms, their causation is unknown, although hereditary factors have been thought responsible in some instances. The bands vary considerably in depth, sometimes being deep enough to cause congenital amputation, and sometimes being so superficial that no treatment is required. Between these extremes, bands deep enough to interfere with circulation or lymphatic drainage call for surgical correction.

Achondroplasia

Achondroplasia is an autosomal dominant condition where the baby is generally small with a disproportionately large head and short limbs. These babies often develop marked lordosis. Cognitive development is not usually impaired.

ABNORMALITIES OF THE URINARY SYSTEM

At birth the first indication that there is an abnormality of the renal tract may be finding a single umbilical artery in the umbilical cord or alternatively recognizing the abnormal facies associated with Potter's syndrome (discussed later). Attention should be paid at the time of delivery to see if the baby passes urine. If no urine is passed within 24 hours or the baby is noted to be dribbling urine constantly, the pediatrician should be informed. Dribbling of urine is a sign of neural damage, which occurs with neural tube defects.

Polycystic Kidneys

It is likely that problems may arise in delivering this baby because of increase in abdominal girth. On abdominal examination, the kidneys will be palpable. Radiological or ultrasound examinations will be carried out to confirm the diagnosis. Renal failure is a likely outcome and the prognosis is poor. The condition has an autosomal recessive inheritance pattern.

Hypospadias and Epispadias

In *hypospadias*, the urethral meatus opens on to the undersurface of the penis. It can be at any point along the length of the penis and in some cases will open on to the perineum. This abnormality often coincides with another condition named *chordee* in which the penis is short and bent. Some of these babies may require surgical intervention in the neonatal period to release the chordee and enlarge the urethral meatus. In *epispadias* the urethral meatus opens on the upper (ventral) surface of the penis.

Cryptorchidism

If on examination of the baby after delivery, the scrotum is empty, the undescended testes may be found in the inguinal pouch. Sometimes the testis in this position can be manipulated into the scrotal pouch. Testes that are found too high in the inguinal canal to manipulate into the scrotum may be malformed. Cryptorchidism may be unilateral or bilateral. Parents should be encouraged to have their baby examined at regular intervals. If descend of the testes do not occur by the time the child has to go to school, orchidopexy will be required.

Ambiguous Genitalia

On some occasions the genitalia of a baby is such that it is difficult to determine the sex in order to give a definitive answer. Examination of the baby may reveal any of the following—a small hypoplastic penis, chordee, bifid scrotum, undescended testes or enlarged clitoris, incompletely separated or poorly differentiated labia. Most of these babies are found to be female.

One of the reasons for ambiguous genitalia is an autosomal recessive condition called *adrenal hyperplasia*. The adrenal gland is stimulated to overproduce androgens because of a deficiency of an enzyme called 21-hydroxylase. If aldosterone production is reduced, these babies will rapidly loose salt. Urea and electrolyte levels should be measured and appropriate fluid replacements given. Baby girls with this condition may require later cosmetic surgery. The condition is not always recognized in boys in the neonatal period.

Intersex

In this condition, the internal reproductive organs are at variance with the external appearance of the genitalia. Ultrasound examination will help identify the nature of internal reproductive organs. True *hermophroditism* is extremely rare. Following chromosomal studies to determine the genetic make up, hormone assays and consideration of the potential for cosmetic surgery, the decision of sex attribution is made. The difficulties of parents in accepting the condition and naming the baby are to be tackled with understanding. It is more common for a child of truly ambiguous gender to be raised as a girl.

COMMONLY OCCURRING SYNDROMES

Trisomy 21 or Down's Syndrome

It is a common malformation due to a chromosomal defect. The defect is due to the inclusion of an additional chromosome, trisomy 21, that is 47 instead of 46 chromosomes. In a small percentage (5%), especially in young mothers it occurs due to a translocation defect. There is transfer of a segment of one chromosome to a different chromosome.

The overall incidence is 1 in 600. The incidence rises with advancing age of the mother, reaching a peak of about 1 in 25 by the age of 45. The classic features of the syndrome were first described in 1866 by physician John Down. The commonly occurring features are as follows:

The head is round with flat occiput and a plump face, upward and outward slanting of the widely set eyes with epicanthic folds, short upper lip with small mouth and macroglossia. The baby's face resembles that of the Mongolian race. The hands are short and broad with a single palmar (simian) crease. There is increased association of congenital heart disease Ventricular Spetal Defect (VSD), hypothyroidism, omphalocele, cataract and intestinal atresia. The affected baby is often mentally retarded.

Expectation of life is reduced. Adult Mongol is likely to develop leukemia. Males are infertile. In females, puberty may be delayed and may be fertile. Diagnosis is established by chromosomal analysis (karyotyping) using bone marrow aspiration or leukocyte culture.

Parents who have a baby with Down's syndrome should be offered genetic counseling to establish the risk of recurrence. Apart from emotional support, the mother may need help with feeding the baby as the baby may have generalized hypotonia.

Trisomy 18 or Edward's Syndrome

This condition is found in about 1 in 5,000 births. An extra 18th chromosome is responsible for the characteristic features. The head is small with a flattened forehead, a receding chin and frequently a cleft palate. The ears are low-set and maldeveloped. The sternum tends to be short, the fingers often overlap each other and the feet have a characteristic rocker-bottom appearance. Malformations of the cardiovascular and gastrointestinal systems are common. The life span of these babies is short and the majority dies during their first year.

Trisomy 13 or Patau Syndrome

An extra copy of the 13th chromosome leads to multiple abnormalities. The affected infants are small and are microcephalic. Midline facial abnormalities are common and limb abnormalities are frequently seen. Brain, cardiac and renal abnormalities may coexist with this trisomy. These babies have a short life. Only 5 percent live beyond three years.

Potter Syndrome

The baby's face will have a flattened appearance, low-set ears, antimongoloid slant to the eyes with deep epicanthic folds, and a beaked nose. The babies are usually severely asphyxiated at birth because they have lung hypoplacia. They also have renal agenesis. It is a syndrome incompatible with sustained life.

Turner Syndrome (XO)

This is a monosomal condition, where only one sex chromosome exists—an X. The absent chromosome is indicated by 'O'. The baby is a girl with a short, webbed neck, widely spaced nipples and edematous feet. The genitalia tend to be underdeveloped and the internal reproductive organs do not mature. Congenital cardiac defects may be present.

The condition may not be diagnosed until puberty fails to occur. Mental development is usually normal.

Klinefelter Syndrome (XXY)

This is an abnormality—affecting boys. Normally it is not diagnosed until puberty fails to occur.

BIBLIOGRAPHY

1. Dutta DC. Textbook of Obstetrics, 5th edn. Calcutta: New Central Book Company 2001.
2. Halliday AC. Congenital abnormalities. In: Bennett RV, Linda KB (eds). Myles Textbook for Midwives, 13th edn. Philadelphia: JB Lippincott 1999.
3. May K, Mahlmeister L. Maternal and Neonatal Nursing, 3rd edn. Philadelphia:JB Lippincott 1994.
4. Nixon H, O'Donnell B. Essentials of Pediatric Surgery, 4th edn. Oxford: Butterworth Heinemann 1992.

47

Jaundice and Infections in the Newborn

Learning Objectives

Upon completing this chapter, the learner will be able to:

❖ Describe the process of bilirubin conjugation and underlying etiology of jaundice
❖ Describe the causes and management of physiological jaundice
❖ Explain the causes and consequences of pathological jaundice
❖ Explain the treatment of jaundice by photo-therapy and exchange transfusion
❖ Describe the infections that may be acquired by the neonate before, during or shortly after birth
❖ Discuss the role of the midwife in the prevention, assessment, diagnosis and treatment of neonatal infections.

JAUNDICE

Jaundice is the yellow discoloration of the skin caused by accumulation of excess of bilirubin in the tissues and serum. Neonatal jaundice becomes apparent at serum bilirubin concentrations of 5 to7 mg/dl. Jaundiced shoulders and trunk indicates a level of 8 to 10 mg/dl. Jaundice of the lower body appears at 10 to 12 mg/dl and jaundice of the entire body at 12 to 15 mg/dl.

Formation of Bilirubin

Bilirubin is formed mainly from the non-iron fraction of Hem of broken down hemoglobin. RBCs are removed from the circulation and broken down in the reticuloendothelial system. The hemoglobin in the red blood cells breaks down into its by products of globin, iron and hem. Globin is reused by the body to make proteins and iron is stored or reused for making new RBCs. Hem is rapidly bound to serum albumin and form unconjugated bilirubin-albumin complex (indirect bilirubin). The complex so formed is carried to the liver cells for conjugation by enzyme glucuronyl transferace to form water soluble (direct bilirubin). It is nontoxic and is excreted either in urine or feces.

Unconjugated bilirubin is fat-soluble, cannot be excreted easily either in bile or urine and can build-up in blood and be deposited in extravascular fatty and nerve tissues, e.g. under the skin and in the brain. Deposits under the skin lead to jaundice while deposits in the brain can cause bilirubin toxicity or kernicterus.

Excretion of Bilirubin

The conjugated or water-soluble bilirubin is excreted via the biliary system into the small intestine where it is converted into urobilinogen by intestinal bacteria. This urobilinogen is then oxidized to form orange-colored urobilin. Most of the conjugated bilirubin is excreted in the feces as stercobilinogen and a small amount is excreted in the urine.

Complications of Hyperbilirubinemia

*Kernicterus (Bilirubin toxicity):*Kernicterus is the most important complication, which can be fatal if not detected promptly and treated effectively. It is an encephalopathy that is caused by deposits of unconjugated bilirubin in the basal nuclei of the brain. The critical level of hyperbilirubinemia causing kernicterus varies from 15 to 20 mg percent, depending upon the maturity of the baby. Hypoxia, acidosis, hypoglycemia, hypothermia or sepsis enhances the pathogenesis so that the condition may develop even at a lower level of bilirubin. Excess level of conjugated bilirubin cannot produce kernicterus.

Clinical manifestations are lethargy, poor feeding, high-pitched cry and loss of moro reflex. Gradually severe illness is manifested by prostration, respiratory distress and finally opisthotonus, nystagmus, hyperpyrexia, convulsions and enlarged liver and spleen. The jaundice is intense along with anemia.

Prevention includes regular and periodic estimation of blood bilirubin level in susceptible babies. Exchange transfusion and phototherapy are used to effectively treat the condition.

TYPES OF JAUNDICE

Physiological Jaundice

More than 50 percent of full-term neonates and 80 percent of preterm neonates will have some physiological jaundice. There is regular rise of unconjugated bilirubin from 1.5 to 2.0 mg/dl in the cord blood serum to 5 to 7 mg/dl on the third day of life. In a full-term well baby, physiological jaundice never appears before 24 hours of age, never exceeds 12 to 13 mg/dl and usually fades by one week of age (Fig. 47.1).

Causes of Physiological Jaundice

❖ *Increased red cell break down*: The newborns' red blood cells have a shorter lifespan (100 days in term infants and 60 to 80 days in preterm infants as opposed to 120 days in adults).
❖ *Decreased albumin binding capacity*: The ability of neonates to actively transport

Fig. 47.1: Physiological jaundice

bilirubin to the liver for conjugation is reduced because of lower albumin concentration, or decreased albumin-binding capacity. Levels of unbound (free), unconjugated, fat-soluble bilirubin in the blood rise as the binding sites on albumin are used up.

❖ *Enzyme deficiency*: Newborn infants have low levels of Uride Diphospho Glucuronyl Transferance (UDP-GT) enzyme activity during the first 24 hours of life. UDP-GT is the major enzyme involved in bilirubin conjugation. Normal adult levels are not reached for 6 to 14 days.
❖ *Increased enterohepatic reabsorption*: Enterohepatic reabsorption of bilirubin is increased in neonates as they lack the normal enteric bacteria that break down bilirubin to urobilinogen.

Management

No specific treatment is generally required.
❖ *Adequate feeding*: Early, frequent feeding helps newborns deal with their increased bilirubin load. Demand feeding ensures adequate volume of colostrum and milk in the intestine. Effective feeding encourages bowel colonization with normal flora and increases bowel motility, which in turn helps in the production of enzymes needed for conjugation, and decreases enterohepatic reabsorption.
❖ Careful observation of newborns will help to distinguish between healthy babies with normal, physiological response (needing no active treatment) and those for whom serum bilirubin testing is required.
❖ In premature babies, rising bilirubin level to critical level require use of phototherapy or phenobarbitone administration.

Pathological Jaundice

Pathological jaundice usually appears within 24 hours of birth and is characterized by a rapid rise in serum bilirubin and prolonged jaundice.

Features of Pathological Jaundice

❖ Clinical jaundice appears within the first 24 hours of life

- Increase in bilirubin > 5 mg/dl per day
- Total bilirubin > 13 mg/dl
- Persistence of clinical jaundice for 7 to 10 days in full-term infants and two weeks in premature infants.

Cause of Pathological Jaundice

The underlying etiology of pathological jaundice is some interference with bilirubin production, conjugation, transport and excretion.

Increased production due to excessive red cell hemolysis
Conditions that can lead to increased hemolysis include:
- Hemolytic diseases of the newborn
  - Fetomaternal blood group incompatibilities—Rhesus and ABO incompatibility
  - Increased red cell fragility—Congenital sphirocytosis
  - Deficient red cell enzyme—Glucose-6-phosphate dehydrogenase (G_6-PD) deficiency.
- Neonatal sepsis, which can lead to increased hemoglobin break down
- Polycythemia, delayed cord clamping and infants of diabetic mothers
- Extravasated blood, such as in cephalhematoma and bruising.

Defective conjugation
- Diminished production of the enzyme glucuronyl transference
  - Immature liver cells as in premature babies
  - Dehydration, starvation, hypoxia and sepsis because oxygen and glucose are required for conjugation
  - Metabolic disorders such as galactosemia.

Transport and Excretion Failure
- Hepatic obstruction caused by congenital anomalies such as biliary atresia, bile plugs, or absence of common bile duct
- Excess conjugated bilirubin caused by infection, or idiopathic neonatal jaundice
- Umbilical cord sepsis leading to ascending thrembophlebitis, obstruction of biliary canaliculi and destruction of liver cells.

Management of Jaundice

For the management of jaundice, it is important to differentiate between healthy babies whose jaundice is a normal physiological response and those with an underlying serious illness or liver disease. More than 50 percent of full-term infants and 80 percent of preterm babies will have some physiological jaundice. About 7 in 500 babies have some form of liver disease.

Assessment and Diagnosis

In evaluating neonatal jaundice, it is important to determine whether the jaundice results from the physiological break down of bilirubin or the presence of another underlying factor and whether the infant is at risk for kernicterus. Assessment includes observation of risk factors.

Risk Factors

- Birth trauma or evident bruising
- Prematurity
- Family history of jaundiced siblings or hemolytic disease
- Ethnic predisposition to jaundice or inherited disease (incidence of pathological jaundice is more in Asian, African and Mediterranean male infants)
- Delayed feeding or meconium passage
- Jaundice within the first 24 hours suggests hemolysis
- Prolonged jaundice may indicate serious disease such as hypothyroidism or obstructive jaundice
- Extent of changes in skin and scleral color
- Presence of lethargy, decreased eagerness to feed, vomiting, irritability, a high-pitched cry, dark urine or light stools
- Presence of dehydration, starvation, hypothermia, acidosis, hypoxia.

Laboratory Evaluation

- Serum bilirubin to determine if the bilirubin is unconjugated or conjugated
- Direct Coombs' test to detect the presence of maternal antibodies on fetal RBCs
- Indirect Coomb's test to detect the presence of maternal antibodies in serum

❖ Hemoglobin/hematocrit estimation to assess any anemia

❖ Reticulocyte count (elevated with hemolysis when new RBCs are being formed)

❖ ABO blood group and Rhesus type for possible incompatibility

❖ Peripheral blood smear-red cell structure for abnormal cells

❖ White cell count to detect any infection

❖ Serum samples for specific immunoglobulins for the TORCH infections

❖ Glucose-6-phosphate dehydrogenase (G6PD) assay

❖ Urine for substances such as galactose (Percival in Bennet and Brown, 1999).

TREATMENT

A number of treatment strategies are available to reduce bilirubin levels. These include phototherapy, exchange transfusion and possibly drug treatments (Blackburn, 1995).

Phototherapy (Fig. 47.2)

Phototherapy can be used to prevent the concentration of unconjugated bilirubin in the blood from reaching levels where neurotoxicity may occur. During phototherapy the neonate's skin surface is exposed to high-intensity light, which photochemically converts fat-soluble, unconjugated bilirubin into water-soluble bilirubin, which can be excreted in bile and urine (McFadden, 1991).

Fig. 47.2: Baby undergoing phototherapy
(*For color version see Plate 7*)

Indications for Phototherapy

Phototherapy is started quickly, at lower bilirubin levels in infants:

❖ Who are smaller or preterm

❖ Who are sick particularly with hemolysis

❖ In whom jaundice appears within 12 to 24 hours

Bilirubin levels indicating phototherapy are:

❖ 17 to 22 mg/dl (280 to 365 mmol) for term infants who become jaundiced after 48 hours

❖ 8 to 10 mg/dl (140 to 165 mmol) for preterm infants > 1,500 gm

❖ 5 to 8 mg/dl (80 to 140 mmol) for preterm babies < 1,500 gm.

The serum bilirubin level at which phototherapy is discontinued varies. Declining serum bilirubin levels below 13 mg/dl (215 mmol) are generally accepted as necessary for stopping phototherapy.

Types of Phototherapy

Conventional systems: Fluorescent lamps are used to deliver high intensity light. The effectiveness depends on the wavelengths, the distance between the lights and the infant, and the amount of skin exposure. The infant usually is placed at a distance of about 45 to 60 cm from the phototherapy light with the skin exposed. The infants' testes/ovaries are covered with a nappy. Eyes are covered with eye shields or patches. Turning the neonate frequently ensures maximum skin exposure. Phototherapy treatment is generally continuous with interruption only for essential care, such as feeding or nappy changing. Intermittent therapy may be given for periods of 6 hours on and 6 hours off.

Fiberoptic light systems: Fiberoptic blankets or woven fiberoptic pads which deliver high intensity light with no ultraviolet or infrared radiation are wrapped around the infant under the clothing, thus ensuring that more skin is exposed to light. The pads can be used day and night with minimal supervision. They also reduce some of the side effects of phototherapy, e.g. increased insensible fluid loss. In addition, they eliminate the need for eye protection.

Fiberoptic phototherapy combined with the standard phototherapy is used to provide double phototherapy for optimum results. Fiberoptic mats were found more comfortable for infants and resulted in less restlessness (Costello et al, 1995).

Care of the Baby Undergoing Phototherapy

❖ *Observing any visible side effects:* These can include lethargy or irritability, decreased eagerness to feed, loose stools, hyperthermia, dehydration and fluid loss, skin rashes and skin burns, alterations in neurobehavioral organization, lack of usual sensory experiences including visual deprivation. Neonates may also experience hypocalcemia, low platelet counts, increased red cell osmotic fragility, bronze baby syndrome, riboflavin deficiency and DNA damage.

❖ *Eye care:* A potential side effect of phototherapy is the effect of the high-intensity light on the retina. The position of eye shields or patches is to be closely monitored to ensure that they are over the eyes, do not occlude the nose and that the headband is not tight. The infant is also observed for any eye discharge or weeping.

❖ *Estimation of bilirubin levels:* Bilirubin levels are usually estimated daily. The reduction in bilirubin levels appears to be greatest in the first 24 hours of phototherapy.

❖ *Skin care:* The skin is to be observed frequently for any rashes, dryness and excoriation, and cleaned with warm water when the midwife considers it necessary.

❖ *Temperature:* The infant is to be kept in a warm thermoneutral environment and observed for any hypo- or hyperthermia. If the infant is nursed in an incubator, servocontrol is usually used. Heat loss is to be minimized as far as possible.

❖ *Hydration:* Fluid intake and urine output are to be monitored (including the frequency, amount and color of urine and stool pattern). Good hydration is to be maintained with demand feeding, and if breastfeeding, the mother is to be encouraged to continue. Extra fluids may be required for severely ill or dehydrated infants. Intravenous fluids are not routinely required as they do not stimulate peristalsis or encourage meconium excretion.

❖ *Neurobehavioral status:* Infant's sleep and waking states, feeding behaviors, responsiveness, response to stress and interaction with parents and others are to be observed.

❖ *Sensory deprivation:* To reduce the effects of isolation when feeding, the eye patches are to be taken off and the infant is removed from the lights. Parents can be encouraged to hold, feed and care for their baby as much as possible.

❖ *Hypocalcemia:* Serum calcium level decreases in some babies and a level < 7 mg/dl is considered hypocalcemia in neonates. Symptoms include jitteriness, irritability, rash, loose stools, fever and dehydration and convulsions.

❖ *The needs of parents:* When the baby is undergoing phototherapy, parents will be in lot of distress due to anxiety about the baby's condition and the nature of treatment. The midwife has a particularly important role in providing information, support and reassurance. If the mother is breastfeeding, she may be encouraged to continue feeding as much as possible during her visit to the nursery.

Exchange Transfusion

Exchange transfusion is a life-saving procedure in severely affected hemolytic disease of the newborn. An exchange transfusion process removes bilirubin from the body and in cases of hemolytic disease, also replaces sensitized erythrocytes with blood that is compatible with the mother's and infant's serum (Sater, 1995).

Tan (1996) stated that phototherapy has largely replaced exchange transfusion when treating severe neonatal jaundice. Except in Rh incompatibility, exchange transfusion may now be seen as a second treatment of choice that is used only when phototherapy has failed. Exchange transfusion would certainly be considered when there is a risk of bilirubin toxicity or kernicterus.

Indications

Rh-positive with direct Coombs' test positive babies having:

- ❖ Cord blood hemoglobin less than 15 g percent
- ❖ Previous definite history of an affected baby due to hemolytic disease
- ❖ Birthweight less than 2,500 g
- ❖ Rapidly developing jaundice with unconjugated bilirubin above 5 mg percent.

Objectives

The objectives of exchange transfusion are to:

- ❖ Correct the anemia by replacing the Rh-positive sensitized red cells (normal or hemolysed) with compatible Rh-negative red cells
- ❖ Remove the circulating antibodies
- ❖ Eliminate the circulating bilirubin.

While about 80 to 90 percent of the fetal blood is exchanged during the procedure, transfusion of Rh-negative blood cannot alter the Rh factor of the baby's blood. The replacement temporarily helps to tide over the crisis from anemia and hyperbilirubinemia for about two weeks. Thereafter the baby produces his own Rh-positive blood.

Nature and Amount of Blood Transfused

- ❖ Blood for exchange should be Rh-negative, whole blood from unsensitized donors with the same ABO grouping to that of the baby or group 'O'. The blood should be cross-matched with the mother's serum. (It does not cause any harm if Rh-negative blood is transfused to an Rh-positive individual).
- ❖ The blood should be freshly collected.
- ❖ The amount is about 170 ml/kg bodyweight of the baby.

A number of risks are associated with exchange transfusion. These include risks from the transfused blood and from the procedure itself, e.g. acquired immune deficiency syndrome and hepatitis B from the use of blood products. Exchange transfusion also increases the risk of necrotising enterocolitis (Todd, 1995). Lack of experienced practitioners due to the infrequency of the procedure can also increase the morbidity and mortality.

Care of the Baby Undergoing Exchange Transfusion

The procedure is usually carried out in a neonatal intensive care unit with experienced neonatal nurses caring for the infant before, during and after the procedure. The transfusion is given by the umbilical vein. Removal of blood and replacement is conducted by removing approximately 10 to 15 ml at one time and replacing this with 10 ml, given slowly, taking at least one minute. This is usually continued until a total volume of 170 ml/kg of infant blood has been replaced.

For every 100 ml of blood transfused, one milliequivalent of sodium bicarbonate is given to combat metabolic acidosis and 1 ml of 10 percent calcium gluconate to prevent tetany due to transfusion of citrated blood. Bilirubin and hemoglobin levels are assessed prior to and after the exchange transfusion.

Following transfusion, the baby is placed under radiant warmer. The umbilicus is to be inspected frequently for any evidence of bleeding. Serum bilirubin is to be estimated six hours after transfusion and to be repeated as required. Blood glucose must be monitored four hourly to detect any hypoglycemia.

Complications

Immediate complications possible are:

- ❖ Cardiac failure due to raised venous pressure and overloading of the heart
- ❖ Air embolism
- ❖ Clotting and massive embolism
- ❖ Hyperkalemia
- ❖ Tetany
- ❖ Acidosis
- ❖ Sepsis
- ❖ Hypocalcemia
- ❖ Hypoglycemia
- ❖ Coagulopathies due to thrombocytopenia.

Delayed complications include:

- ❖ Necrotizing enterocolitis
- ❖ Extrahepatic portal hypertension due to thrombosis of portal vein.

Drug Therapy

Drugs are used as an adjuvant therapy.

- ❖ *Phenobarbitone 2 mg / kg* bodyweight is administered thrice daily intramuscularly for babies undergoing phototherapy. Phenobarbitone increases the glucuronyl transferase enzyme activity in the fetal and neonatal liver to conjugate the bilirubin, which hastens its clearance.

❖ *Antibiotics* are administered for 3 to 5 days (Dutta, 2001).

HEMOLYTIC DISEASES OF THE NEWBORN

Hemolytic diseases of the newborn include:
❖ Fetomaternal blood group incompatibilities
 – Rhesus incompatibility
 – ABO group incompatibility.
❖ Increased red cell fragility (Congenital sphirocytosis)
❖ Deficient red cell enzyme (Glucose-6 phosphate dehydrogenase).

Fetomaternal blood group incompatibilities are the commonest cause of hemolysis in the newborn. Hemolysis occurs when the fetus possesses an antigen (Rh or ABO), which the mother does not have and becomes exposed to that antigen. The maternal antibodies so produced, i.e. an immunoglobulin G (IgG), crosses the placental barrier to the fetus to produce hemolysis of the red blood cells by antigen-antibody reaction.

Rhesus Incompatibility

Rhesus or Rh (D) incompatibility can occur when a woman with Rh (D) negative blood type carries a baby with Rh (D) positive blood type. The antibodies produced in the maternal blood crosses the placenta and destroy the erythrocytes of the fetus. Usually sensitization occurs in the first pregnancy, and in subsequent pregnancies extensive destruction of fetal cells may occur.

Sensitization may also occur following such procedures as amniocentesis, abortion and external cephalic version or after antepartum hemorrhage. Antibodies once formed remain throughout life.

Effects on the Fetus

The effect on the fetus depends on the severity of the hemolysis.
❖ Congenital anemia—With lesser degrees of destruction

❖ Icterus gravis neonatorum—Babies are born without evidences of jaundice at birth, but develop it within the first 24 hours of life
❖ Erythroblastosis fetalis—Presence of increased number of immature RBCs
❖ Hydrops fetalis—Infants are born with edema and ascitis.

Management

When the bilirubin (unconjugated) level rises above 12 mg percent, the condition is called *Hyperbilirubinemia of the newborn*. The palms and soles of the infant are usually stained yellow at this level and treatment is required. Treatment strategies to reduce bilirubin levels include phototherapy, exchange transfusion and drug treatments.

ABO Incompatibility

ABO incompatibility occurs usually when the mother is blood group O and the body contains both anti-A and anti-B antibodies. The antibodies are usually IgM class and are too large to cross the placenta. However, some women produce antibodies of IgG class, which are smaller than IgM and can cross the placenta. Once in the fetal circulation, the IgG anti-A and anti-B antibodies attach to fetal red cells and destroy them.

ABO sensitization can occur from blood transfusion and blood leakage due to pregnancy. Both first and subsequent babies are at risk. In subsequent pregnancies, the problem may become more severe because previous exposure of the fetus to type O antigens strengthens the anti-A response. The management of ABO immunization depends on the severity of the hemolysis. In most such cases where the mother's blood type is O and the baby's A or B, the hemolysis is mild.

NEONATAL INFECTIONS

Infection is one of the leading causes of neonatal death in the developing countries. The neonates are more susceptible to infection because they lack in natural immunity and take some time for the acquired immunity to develop. Full immunocompetence requires both natural (innate) and acquired immune mechanisms.

Natural or Innate Immunity

This involves responses that do not require previous exposure to microorganisms. These include intact skin and mucous membranes and gastric acid and digestive enzymes that act as first line defense against infection in the neonate. Immediately after birth, the infant's bowel is not colonized with normal protective flora, and the skin is more easily irritated and damaged.

Acquired Immunity

Acquired or specific immune responses are responses that develop and improve with ongoing exposure to a pathogen or organism. Although the infant has some immune protection from the mother, largely he must actively acquire this immune response. Immunoglobulins are deficient at birth. Antibody levels are limited (transfer of IgG across the placenta occurs after 32nd week of gestation). Breastfeeding increases the infant's immune protection through the transmission of secretary IgA in breast milk. During the early weeks of life, the infant also has deficiencies in both the quantity and quality of neutrophils.

Preterm infants are particularly vulnerable to infection. They have less welldeveloped defense mechanism and are more likely to be exposed to invasive procedures that increase the risk of infection.

Modes of Acquiring Infection

- *Transplacental:* Maternal infections that can affect the fetus through transplacental route are predominantly the viruses. They are rubella, cytomegalovirus, herpes virus, HIV, chickenpox and hepatitis B virus. Other infections are syphilis, toxoplasmosis and tuberculosis.
- *From amniotic fluid:* Amnionitis following premature rupture of membranes can affect the baby following aspiration or ingestion of the infected amniotic fluid.

- *Intranatal*
  - Aspiration of infected liquor during labor in which early rupture of membranes and repeated internal examinations occur. This may lead to either congenital or neonatal pneumonia.
  - While the fetus is passing through the vagina, contamination of the eyes can occur with Gonococci leading to ophthalmia neonatorum. Contamination with Candida albicans can lead to oral thrush.
  - Improper asepsis while caring for the umbilical cord may lead to cord sepsis.
- *Postnatal*
  - Transmission of infection due to human contact as from infected mother, relatives or hospital staff
  - Cross infection from an infected baby in the nursery or postnatal unit
  - Infected utensils used for feeding or bathing—Clothing or air-borne.

Organisms in Newborn Infection

Soon after birth, the baby becomes colonized by bacteria derived from the mother, like *Staphylococcus* on the skin, *Streptococcus* in the respiratory tract and *E. coli* in the gastrointestinal tract. This colonization takes place uneventfully in most newborns, but in some, particularly those who have been harassed during labor and delivered following distress in prolonged difficult labor, instrumental delivery or delayed emergency cesarean section, the same organisms turn virulent and produce severe infection.

The onset of infection is most often quiet and insidious. Except when the lesion is visible externally, the evidences of internal organ involvement are rarely detected. Minor changes in the baby's behavior should be identified as early detection and treatment gives good response and prognosis.

Management of Infection in the Baby

The midwife's role in the management of fetal and neonatal infection includes prevention, assessment, diagnosis and treatment of infection.

Prevention

Midwives can play an important role in creating a safe environment that decreases the chances of infants acquiring infection after birth. They can do this by:

- Encouraging and assisting the mother with breastfeeding, thus increasing the infant's immune protection
- Ensuring careful and frequent hand washing by all caregivers to prevent the spread of infection
- Having the infant rooming-in with his/her mother
- Adequately spacing the baby cots, when the infants are in the nursery with other infants
- Always using individual equipment for each infant
- Avoiding any irritation or trauma to the infant's skin and mucous membranes, as intact skin provides a barrier against infection
- Discouraging visitors, who have infections or who have been exposed to communicable disease, from visiting the baby
- Isolating infected babies when necessary
- Observing for and appropriately treating any infection in the mother prior to the infant's birth
- Ensuring the appropriate administration of immunoglobulin and antibiotics to mother or baby, if required.

Protection of midwives and other caregivers is also vital. The underlying assumption of universal precautions is that every patient is presumed to be a potential source of bloodborne infections, e.g. hepatitis B, C and acquired immune deficiency syndrome. Therefore, universal precautions must be used when dealing with any substance or article that may be contaminated with blood. General infection control measures must also be used with respect to any other body fluids that may be a potential source of other infections (Percival in Bennett and Brown, 1999).

Assessment and Diagnosis

Prompt diagnosis and treatment of infection is critical in minimizing adverse or long-term effects for the neonate. Early signs of infection may be subtle and difficult to identify. Non-specific signs and symptoms can include temperature instability, lethargy, poor feeding, bradycardia or tachycardia and apnea. A maternal history of prolonged rupture of membranes, chorioamnionitis, pyrexia during birth, or offensive amniotic fluid increases the risk of infection for the baby. Laboratory evaluation may be dependent on the severity and type of signs and symptoms and may include:

- Complete blood cell count
- Testing of urine and stool for specific organisms
- Swabs from nose, throat and umbilicus
- Swabs from any skin rashes, pustules or vesicles
- Chest X-ray
- Lumbar puncture if central nervous system signs are present
- Testing of cord blood, amniotic fluid and placental tissue for specific organisms.

Treatment of Infection

The objectives of treatment essentially are the prevention of septicemia and septic shock and a reduction in the short and long-term effects of the infection.

- The baby is to be nursed in a warm thermo-neutral environment with the midwife observing for any temperature instability
- Maintenance of good hydration and the correction of electrolyte imbalance with demand of feeding and intravenous fluids, as required
- Systemic antibiotic or other drug therapy is always commenced as soon as possible as well as any local treatment of infection
- Monitoring of the infant's neurobehavioral status including sleep and wake states, feeding behaviors, responsiveness, response to stress and interaction with parents and other caregivers
- Any infant with septic shock is to be cared for in a neonatal intensive care unit as it is a life-threatening emergency.

The midwife has a particularly important role in providing information, support and reassurance to parents. Where possible, it is best to avoid separation of the mother and baby. If the baby requires, being in the nursery, parents could be encouraged to spend time with their baby. If the mother is breastfeeding she should be encouraged to continue or express the milk as appropriate and informed of the role of her milk in fighting infection.

INFECTIONS ACQUIRED BEFORE OR DURING BIRTH

Toxoplasmosis

Toxoplasmosis is a protozoal infection caused by *Toxoplasma gondii*. In adults infection is transmitted by encysted organism by eating infected raw or uncooked meat or through contact with infected cat and dog feces. It can also be acquired across the placenta. Transplacental infection to the fetus occurs during parasitemia.

Virulence of fetal infection is greatest, when maternal infection is acquired early in pregnancy. The affected baby may develop hydrocephalus, cerebral calcification, microcephaly and mental retardation. In less severe cases, infants may present with low birthweight, enlarged liver and spleen, jaundice and anemia. Infants born asymptomatic at birth can later develop retinal disease and neurological abnormalities, usually by the age of twenty. Maternal infection is rarely diagnosed clinically. On suspicion, serologic testing should be done for specific IgM antibody, which denotes acute infection. If current infection is confirmed amniocentesis and cordocentesis are done for detection of IgM antibody in the amniotic fluid and fetal blood. Ultrasonography is done at 20 to 22 weeks for ventricular dilatation.

If the fetus is infected and hydrocephalus is present, counseling for termination is done. If the fetus is infected but is otherwise normal, drug treatment is given to the mother. Pyrimethamine, sulphadiazine, folic acid and spiramycin are given orally. If infection occurs late in pregnancy, only spiramycin is given.

Prevention includes advising women about proper handwashing and washing of kitchen surfaces following contact with uncooked meat. Uncooked meat, unpasteurised milk and contact with cat and dog litter to be avoided.

Rubella

Rubella or German measles virus causes mild and insignificant illness in the mother, but can have serious consequences for the fetus. The virus is transmitted by respiratory droplet exposure. Fetal affection is by transplacental route throughout pregnancy. Risk of major anomalies is about 80 percent if infection occurs in the first 12 weeks of pregnancy. Early infection may result in spontaneous abortion. The mother may also be advised termination of pregnancy.

Surviving infants can have cardiac defects, hearing problems, cataracts and very significant developmental delays. Infants born with congenital rubella are highly infectious and should be isolated from other infants and pregnant women for up to one year after birth.

Active immunity can be conferred in non-immune individuals by giving rubella vaccine (live, attenuated, rubella virus) preferably during adolescence to girls. It is not recommended in pregnant women. When given during childbearing period, pregnancy should be prevented for three months.

Cytomegalovirus (CMV) Infection

Cytomegalovirus is the herpes class that is harbored in leukocytes and transmitted by saliva, semen, urine, cervical secretions and blood. Transmission may also occur by respiratory droplet or transplacental. Virus is excreted in urine and breast milk. Fetus is affected by transplacental route in about 30 to 40 percent of cases.

Infection in the mother may be primary or secondary. A primary infection in the mother during the first 20 weeks of pregnancy can result in spontaneous abortion, intrauterine growth retardation and premature birth of the infant. Infants with CMV may suffer from an enlarged liver and spleen, jaundice, developmental delay, blindness, epilepsy and hearing loss. Most congenitally infected babies are asymptomatic at birth with only 1 percent showing adverse clinical disease. However, they should be followed up for 5 to 7 years because of the possibility of long-term neurological problems. Infection can be confirmed by viral culture of urine and nasopharyngeal secretions. At this time, no specific antiviral treatment is effective against congenital CMV infection.

Herpes Simplex Virus (HSV)

Infection with herpes simplex virus (HSV) is associated with genital herpes in the mother. Neonatal infection is more likely with a primary maternal infection during pregnancy and results in high morbidity and mortality. The infection may be acquired through the placenta or from an infected birth canal. The risk of intrapartum infection is about 50 percent when the mother has primary genital herpes lesions at the time of birth. Prolonged rupture of the membranes and the use of scalp electrodes both increase the risk of neonatal infection. Therefore, when active maternal infection is present, the baby should be delivered by cesarean section.

Signs of neonatal infection can be non-specific at birth. A herpetic rash (blisters and a papular vesicular rash) is usually, but not always, seen by the end of the first week of life. Multiple organs may be affected, in particular the brain, liver and adrenal glands. Mortality can be as high as 80 percent.

Untreated survivors can have long-term neurological damage, in particular micro-cephaly, blindness and severe developmental delay. Encephalitis occurs in a high proportion of children.

The virus is present in vesicles, urine and CSF. An exposed infant should be isolated with the mother for care.

Acquired Immunodeficiency Syndrome (AIDS)

AIDS is caused by HIV (Human immuno deficiency virus), which is a group of retrovirus, HIV-1 and HIV-2. The virus specifically reduces CD-4 cells leading to immunodeficiency. As a result, the individual is susceptible to infections by opportunistic microorganisms and specific tumors. The incubation period is from two months to four years.

The main modes of transmission of HIV are sexual contact (Homosexual or heterosexual),

transplacental, exposure to infected blood or tissue fluids and through breastmilk. Increased incidence of abortion, prematurity, IUGR and perinatal mortality are seen in HIV positive women.

The vertical transmission to neonates is about 30 percent in seropositive mothers. The baby may be affected *in utero* through transplacental transfer, during delivery by conta-minated secretions and blood of the birth canal and through breastmilk in neonatal period. Women with AIDS are discouraged to become pregnant.

Varicella Zoster Virus

Varicella zoster virus does cross the placenta and may cause congenital or neonatal chicken-pox. Maternal mortality is high due to varicella pneumonia. In the neonate, infection can cause the milder symptoms associated with neonatal varicella or neonatal zoster. Maternal chicken-pox from four months' gestation up to almost the time of birth usually results in these milder forms of the disease. However, at different stages of pregnancy more severe infections can also occur.

Varicella zoster immune globulin (VZIG) should be given to exposed nonimmune mothers as it reduces the morbidity. VZIG should also be given to newborns exposed within five days of delivery. With maternal chickenpox during the first 20 weeks' gestation, up to 5 percent of infants will develop conge-nital varicella syndrome characterized by skin lesions, chorioretinitis and limb hypoplasia. About 24 percent will develop disseminated infection when the mother is infected from five days before to 2 days after delivery. This severe infection develops within days of birth and can result in disseminated skin lesions, viral pneumonia, liver problems, and death in 30 percent of cases.

Chlamydia

Chlamydia infection may be acquired by the infant during birth from a mother with chlamy-dial cervicitis. Infected infants may develop ophthalmia neonatorum and a small number may develop pneumonia.

Hepatitis B Virus

The most common source of neonatal infection with hepatitis B virus (HBV) is maternal blood during birth. The virus can be detected in any body secretion including breastmilk. Ninety percent of the infected infants will become carriers of the virus who are at risk of developing hepatocellular carcinoma in future. Infants with HBV positive mothers should be given hepatitis B immunoglobulin within 12 hours after birth. This is followed by administration of hepatitis vaccine during the first week, as part of an ongoing vaccination program. A booster dose is given at about 5 years of age.

Syphilis

This infection is caused by the spirochete treponema pallidum and is transmitted by sexual contact or by maternofetal transmission. The infant may contract the disease through the placenta or from the birth canal. There are 50 percent chances of a mother with primary or secondary syphilis infecting her fetus during pregnancy. When active lesions are present in the birth canal, a cesarean birth is recommended.

Infants with congenital syphilis may be asymptomatic at birth or present with serious abnormalities. Symptoms may include maculopapular rash, enlarged liver and spleen, jaundice, skin lesions, deformed nails, alopecia, chorioretinitis and pseudoparalysis. Late congenital syphilis can also involve the central nervous system, bones, teeth and skin. Intravenous or intramuscular antibiotic treatment is recommended immediately on diagnosis with the infant isolated for the first 24 hours.

Gonococcal Infections

Neonatal gonococcal infection is acquired during the birth process. It can cause a variety of symptoms including ophthalmia neonatorum, scalp abscesses, vaginitis, proctitis, oropharyngeal infections and systemic infections. These systemic infections can include pneumonia, sepsis, arthritis or rarely meningitis. Diagnosis is difficult. Early and appropriate antibiotic treatment of both mother and baby is important.

Ophthalmia Neonatorum

This is an inflammation of the conjunctiva during the first three days' life. The classical ophthalmia neonatorum caused by gonococcus is very rare these days. The most common cause for it is chlamydia trachomatis. The other causes include—Bacterial-staphylococcal, pseudomonal-pneumococcal, chemical silver nitrate and viral herpes simplex.

Infection occurs mostly during delivery by contaminated vaginal discharge. It is more likely in babies born by face and breech presentations. During neonatal period, there may be contamination from other sites of infection or by chemical. The clinical picture varies and the discharge may be watery, mucopurulent to frank purulent in one or both eyes. The eyelids may be sticky or markedly swollen. Cornea may be involved in severe cases.

The condition can be prevented by treating any suspicious vaginal discharge during the antenatal period and maintaining meticulous aseptic technique at birth. The newborn's closed eyelids should be thoroughly cleaned and dried. Sulphacentamide eyedrops or soframycin eyedrops are instilled into each eye for few days.

The discharge from the eyes is taken for gram stain smear and culture and sensitivity tests. Treatment depends on the specific etiology. For gonococcal infections, eyes are irrigated with sterile isotonic saline every one to two hours and topical gentamycin eyedrops are instilled four times a day for seven days. In severe cases, systemic benzyl penicillin 50,000 units/kg is given in two divided doses for seven days or Cefotaxime 100 mg/kg is given intravenously. For chlamydia, erythromycin suspension 40 mg/kg is given orally for 2 to 3 weeks with erythromycin eyedrops four times a day. For herpes simplex, systemic therapy with acyclovir 30 mg/kg for two weeks is given IV.

Candida Infections

Candida is a gram-positive yeast fungus. *Candida albicans* is responsible for most fungal infections including oral thrush in infants. Infection can affect the mouth (oral candidiasis), the skin (cutaneous candidiasis) and visceral organs (disseminated candidiasis).

Oral candidiasis or thrush presents as white patches on the gums, palate and tongue. It can also affect the skin around the mouth, perineum and anus. It can be acquired during birth or from caregivers' hands or feeding equipment. The fungus grows on the mucous membrane and produces milky white elevated patches resembling milk curd, which cannot be easily wiped off. Rarely, the infection may spread down to involve the gastrointestinal or respiratory tract. Removing the lesions is not recommended as this may leave raw areas. Nystatin (mycostatin) oral suspension dropped under the tongue four times a day is effective to treat the infection. Application of boroglycerine is soothing.

Cutaneous candidiasis presents as a moist papular or vesicular rash, usually in the region of the axilla, neck, perineum or umbilicus. The area is kept as dry as possible and topical nystatin applied. Oral nystatin is also used to reduce the yeast population.

Disseminated candidiasis is usually found only in preterm and ill newborns. Complications can include meningitis, endocarditis, pyelonephritis, pneumonia and osteomyelitis.

INFECTIONS ACQUIRED AFTER BIRTH

Skin Infections

Most neonatal skin infections are caused by *Staphylococcus aureus*. In newborn babies, the most likely skin lesions are septic spots or pustules, which may be either found as a solitary lesion or clustered in the umbilical and buttock areas. In a well neonate with limited lesions, regular cleansing with an antiseptic solution may be all that is required. Lesions that are more extensive require antibiotic treatment.

Pemphigus neonatorum is a serious form of skin infection in the newborn caused by *Staphylococcus aureus*. It can cause septicemia or pyemia. Superficial ulcers appear on any part of the skin; become pustules and then burst. They tend to appear in crops and are usually associated with systemic illness.

The baby is to be isolated. The blisters are pricked with a sterile needle and after removal of the dead skin; the area is to be smeared with antibiotic ointment. Systemic administration of gentamycin or cloxacillin is required in severe infections. *Pemphigus* may also be due to syphilis when the blisters appear on the palms, soles or trunk. Other features of syphilis are present. Antisyphilitic treatment is to be instituted.

Omphalitis

Omphalitis or infection of the umbilicus can include localized infection and an offensive discharge. Treatment includes regular cleansing, administration of an antibiotic powder and appropriate antibiotic therapy. Untreated infection can spread to the liver via the umbilical vein and cause hepatitis and septicemia.

Respiratory Infections

Nasopharyngitis and Rhinitis

These conditions though not severe, may be distressing for the infant. Babies with nasal pharyngitis may be isolated with their mothers to prevent the spread of the infection. Symptomatic treatment and antibiotics may be required.

Neonatal Pneumonia

Pneumonia is the most serious of neonatal respiratory infections. It may be acquired before, during or after birth. In newborns, pneumonia is life-threatening and early diagnosis is essential. Symptoms of general infection may be accompanied by nasal flaring, grunting, substernal and intercostal retraction and cyanosis. Blood evaluation and chest X-ray are done to diagnose pneumonia. Appropriate antibiotic therapy must be instituted promptly.

Gastrointestinal Infections

Gastroenteritis

Causative organisms include *Salmonella*, *Shigella*, and a pathogenic strain of *Escherichia coli.* Rotavirus is the most important cause of viral gastroenteritis in the newborn. Treatment depends upon the severity of symptoms. The correction of fluid and electrolyte imbalance is an urgent priority as vomiting and diarrhea can rapidly cause dehydration.

Infants with infective diarrhea are isolated and stool should be sent for culture and sensitivity prior to antibiotic therapy. Milk feeding is stopped and oral rehydration fluids are given in mild cases. In severe cases, parenteral therapy is required.

Necrotizing Enterocolitis

NEC is characterized by inflammation, ischemia and necrosis of the gastrointestinal tract. It is the most common and most lethal surgical abdominal emergency in the newborn.

Early symptoms can include temperature instability, lethargy, bradycardia, apnea, decreased appetite, vomiting, blood in the stool and abdominal distension. As the disease, progresses there may be severe abdominal distension and tenderness, grossly bloodied stools and presence of hepatic portal venous gas. Diagnosis is confirmed by X-ray showing pneumatosis intestinalis (submucosal or sub-serosal cysts filled with a gaseous mixture). In the late stages, perforation of the gut, peritonitis, septic shock and death can occur.

Possible risk factors for developing NEC include prematurity, low birthweight, enteral feeding, asphyxia, patent ductus arteriosus and bacterial infection. Treatment depends on the stage and severity of the disease. Nonsurgical treatment includes the prevention of shock, the correction of electrolyte imbalance and the administration of broad spectrum antibiotics. When surgical treatment is needed, the necrotic tissue is resected with the objective of preserving as much bowel as possible.

Urinary Infections

Urinary tract infections can occur because of bacterial invasion or congenital anomaly that obstructs urine flow. The causative organisms include *E. coli*, group B *Streptococcus* and other organisms. The signs and symptoms are usually those of an early nonspecific infection. Diagnosis is usually confirmed through laboratory evaluation of a urine sample. Specific treatment according to the organisms identified is instituted (Wright Lott, 1994).

Meningitis

Meningitis is inflammation of the membranes lining the brain and spinal column. The most common organisms causing neonatal meningitis are *E. coli*, group B streptococci and Listeria monocytogenes. Other types found include candidal meningitis and herpes meningitis.

Maternal infections and pyrexia at birth are often identified as the associated factor. In the early stages, the infant may have nonspecific signs of generalized infection. Specific signs of meningeal irritation may also be present, including irritability, raised intracranial pressure demonstrated by a bulging fontanelle, increasing lethargy, crying, tremors and twitching, severe vomiting, alterations in consciousness and diminished muscle tone. Infants may also present with hemiparesis, decreased pupillary reaction of the eye, decreased retinal reflex and an abnormal Moro reflex.

Diagnosis is usually confirmed by lumbar puncture and examination of CSF. Very ill babies will require intensive nursing care including intravenous fluids and antibiotic therapy. Early diagnosis and treatment offers better prognosis. About 30 to 50 percent of surviving infants suffer long-term neurological complications such as feeding problems and minimal brain damage (Adhikari, et al, 1995).

BIBLIOGRAPHY

1. Adhikari M, Coovadia YM, Singh D. Neonatal meningitis: Clinical and microbiological findings, Journal of Tropical Pediatrics 1995;41(2): 81-5.
2. Blackburn S. Hyperbilirubinemia and neonatal jaundice. Neonatal Network 1995;14(7):15-25.
3. Brown LP, et al. Incidence and pattern of jaundice in healthy breastfed infants during the first month of life. Nursing Research 1993;42(2):106-10.
4. Costello SA, et al. Bliblanket phototherapy system versus conventional phototherapy, Journal of Pediatric and Child Health 1995;31(1): 11-3.

5. Dutta DC. Textbook of Obstetrics, 5th edn. Calcutta; New Central Book Company, 2001.

6. Mc Fadden EA. The wallaby phototherapy ststem, a new approach to phototherapy. Journal of Pediatric Nursing 1991;6(3):206-8.

7. Percival P. Jaundice and infection, In: Bennett RV, and Linda KB (Eds). Myles Textbook for Midwives, 13th edn. Edinburgh;Churchill Livingstone, 1999.

8. Rubaltelli FF, Griffith PF. Management of neonatal hyperbilirubinemia and prevention of kernicterus, Practical therapeutics 1992;43(6): 864-72.

9. Sater K. Color me yellow. Caring for the new infant with hyperbilirubinemia and prevention of kernicterus. Journal of Intravenous Nursing, 1993;18(6):317-25.

10. Stephenson K. Neonatal jaundice. Physician Assistant 1996;20(4):19-38.

11. Tan KL. Phototherapy for neonatal jaundice. Acta Pediatrics. 1996;85(3):277-9.

12. Todd NA. Isovolemic exchange transfusion of the neonate. Neonatal Network 1995;14(6):75-7.

13. Wright Lott J, et al. Assessment and management of immunologic dysfunction. In: Kenner CA, et al (Edn). Comprehensive Neonatal Nursing. A Physiologic Perspective, Philadelphia;WB Saunders, 1994.

48

Metabolic and Endocrine Disorders in the Newborn

Learning Objectives

Upon completion of this chapter, the learner will be able to:
* Review the common disorders of metabolic and endocrine disorders
* Outline the screening methods available for the early detection of disorders
* Discuss the features, causes and management of diarrhea and vomiting in newborn
* Discuss the identification and management of babies with drugs or substance withdrawal.

INBORN ERRORS OF METABOLISM

Transient disorders of glucose and electrolyte balance are common in preterm and stressed neonates. Permanent disorders such as those caused by inborn errors of metabolism (IEM), may also present in the neonatal period. These disorders have the potential to cause brain damage, poor growth and development or even death. However, the occurrence of individual conditions is rare. As a group IEM contribute significantly to neonatal morbidity and mortality.

Common Features of IEM

Most inborn errors of metabolism are autosomal recessive inherited conditions. Certain conditions are more rare in different populations. In IEM, normal metabolism is disrupted by the absence or deficiency of an enzyme. Metabolites can then accumulate which are toxic to the body tissues, including the brain. *In utero*, the fetus is usually not affected as the placenta removes toxins. It is mostly after birth that the neonate will start to show signs of IEM.

Many of these signs can be nonspecific and could be attributed to other neonatal problems such as sepsis. The signs may become apparent within hours, days or weeks.

Possible Indicators of IEM

* History of previous unexplained neonatal death in the family, or parental consanguinity
* Failure of a sick neonate to respond to usual management
* History of a period of apparent health after birth, followed by adverse signs after the introduction of milk feeding
* Severe metabolic acidosis
* Diarrhea, vomiting and failure to thrive
* Apnea or respiratory distress secondary to neurological depression and/or severe metabolic acidosis
* Unusual odor from the baby's skin or urine, discoloration of urine, abnormally colored or offensive stool
* Prolonged or early jaundice.

Diagnosis of IEM

Antenatal diagnosis can be made by DNA analysis of fetal cells obtained at amniocentesis or chorionic villus biopsy. After birth, screening procedures done for neonates in developed countries ensures early diagnosis and prompt initiation of treatment.

One of the commonest screening procedures used is the Guthrie test in which blood dropped onto an absorbent filter paper is examined using microbiological techniques. Antibiotics may interfere with the microbiological methods used in this test. If a baby is on antibiotic therapy, or he is breastfeeding and his mother is taking antibiotics, this information is included in the Guthrie test card. Conditions screened for will vary in different conditions. However, in most developed countries, all newborn babies are screened for phenylketonuria and hypothyroidism.

Common investigations for IEM involve general tests such as:
- Blood glucose
- Blood gases
- Urine for ketones or reducing substances
- Metabolic tests for blood and urine
- Enzyme analysis of blood and urine.

PHENYLKETONURIA (PKU)

This is an autosomal recessive condition with an incidence of about one in ten thousand (Roberton, 1993). It is due to a deficiency of the enzyme phenylalanine hydroxylase, which converts phenylalanine (an amino acid) to tyrosine in the liver. Because of the failure of conversion, phenylalanine levels rise and although some will be excreted in the urine, most will be converted to phenylpyruvic acid. The raised level of phenylalanine in the blood is found within a few days of birth, after the baby has been subjected to dietary protein. The build-up of phenylpyruvic acid takes longer. It is toxic to the developing brain and without treatment mental retardation results.

Clinical Features

At birth, the baby looks and behaves normally. Signs usually appear after three months. These include vomiting, feeding difficulties, eczema, fair skin and hair, blue eyes and 'musty' (stale) smelling urine due to presence of phenylacetic acid.

Diagnosis
- Positive result on Guthrie test done on capillary blood drawn between 6th and 8th postnatal day
- Assessment of phenylalanine level in blood.

Management

Low phenylalanine diet is prescribed. Milk substitutes with iron supplements are usually given. After puberty, the child will be able to tolerate normal diet. Continued follow-up will be required. In females, a return to low phenylalanine diet is essential prior to conception and during pregnancy.

GALACTOCEMIA

Galactocemia is the most common disorder of carbohydrate metabolism to appear in the neonatal period. It is an autosomal recessive condition and can be screened for during the antenatal period and in the newborn period. The enzyme, which aids the conversion of galactose to glucose, is absent. Galactose and glucose are the component sugars present in the disaccharide lactose.

Clinical signs include vomiting, diarrhea, failure to gain weight, jaundice, lethargy and hypotonia. An affected baby may also present with septicemia secondary to damage to intestinal mucosa by high levels of galactose in the intestines. The diagnosis is confirmed by urine and blood enzyme assessment. Affected babies need to be fed lactose-free milk (Livingston in Bennett and Brown, 1999).

GLUCOSE-6-PHOSPHATE DEHYDROGENASE (G_6PD) DEFICIENCY

G_6PD is an inherited disorder of red blood cell metabolism. Hemolysis occurs, resulting in jaundice and anemia in the neonate. This condition is more prevalent in Asian, Middle Eastern and Mediterranean populations. Management includes treating the jaundice, correcting anemia and reducing the baby's exposure to oxidants, which can damage fragile red blood cells. Vitamin E is prescribed for its antioxidant properties.

CYSTIC FIBROSIS

This is an autosomal recessive condition, which causes dysfunction of secretary glands. Mucus secretions are thick and may block glands and ducts. The condition is more common in northern

European population. It may present in the neonatal period as meconium ileus. Delayed passage of meconium is usually present. Other signs are failure to thrive, prolonged jaundice, bulky pale stools and easy respiratory tract infections. Diagnosis in the newborn period is by measuring the serum immunoreactive trypsin. Treatment is aimed at preventing complications and optimizing growth and development. Parents will need genetic counseling and antenatal screening for future pregnancies (Livingston in Bennett and Brown, 1999).

ENDOCRINE DISORDERS

Endocrine disorders are rare in the newborn period. They are usually treatable, and if untreated can lead to significant morbidity. The most common disorders involve the thyroid gland, adrenal cortex and developing sexual organs.

Thyroid Problems

CONGENITAL HYPOTHYROIDISM

The incidence of congenital hypothyroidism is approximately 1 in 3,500 (Roberton, 1993). Often there is a strong family history of hypothyroidism. Some rare forms of hypothyroidism are autosomal recessive conditions. Hypothyroidism in the neonate can also be caused by the mother taking antithyroid drugs or by maternal treatment with radioactive iodides in pregnancy. Low circulating levels of thyroid hormones cause impaired intellectual and motor function.

Clinical Presentation

Depending on the amount of thyroid hormone produced, there are different degrees of hypothyroidism. Severe hypothyroidism has the following manifestations:

- Coarse facial expressions with a low hairline
- Wrinkled forehead and flat nasal bridge
- Short and thick neck
- Prolonged jaundice
- Constipation
- Lethargy
- Poor feeding
- Hypothermia.

Diagnosis and Treatment

Routine neonatal screening for hypothyroidism is done in many countries at the same time as the PKU screening. With this type of screening, diagnosis is often made before the baby shows signs and symptoms. A positive screening test will be followed up by radioimmune assays of the thyroid hormone T_4 or the thyroid stimulating hormone (TSH) before starting treatment with thyroxin replacement.

Prognosis is good if treatment is instituted quickly, but infants with complete absence of thyroid tissue will have a less favorable outcome. Genetic counseling should be offered to parents.

Acquired Metabolic Disorders

HYPOGLYCEMIA

This is the most common acquired metabolic disorder. The midwife's management of the neonate is important as any prolonged or recurrent hypoglycemia can result in mental retardation and permanent neurological, damage (Aynsley-Green and Soltesz, 1992).

In term infants, hypoglycemia occurs when blood glucose is 40 mg/dl, within the first three days of life. After the first three days of life 45 mg/dl signifies hypoglycemia. The fetus stores glucose as glycogen in the liver and muscles and as subcutaneous and body fat, and this occurs largely in the third trimester. After birth, the baby must make metabolic adjustments to maintain a normal blood sugar. To meet the baby's energy needs during the initial hours after birth, hepatic glycogen is released. After the first few hours, the neonate is able to use fatty acids as an alternative energy source.

Normal term babies who have not been stressed have adequate stores of glycogen to be able to meet their energy requirements, if they are kept warm and are able to feed.

Etiology
- Decreased stores
  - Prematurity
  - Intrauterine growth retardation
  - Starvation.

- ❖ Hyperinsulinism
  - – Infant of diabetic mother
  - – Erythroblastosis (Rhesus hemolytic disease)
  - – Islet cell hyperplasia or hyperfunction
  - – Beckwith-Weidemann syndrome
  - – Insulin producing tumors
  - – Inborn errors of metabolism
  - – Maternal tocolytic therapy with beta-sympathomimetic agents.
- ❖ Other causes
  - – Sepsis, shock
  - – Asphyxia
  - – Hypothermia
  - – Glycogen storage disease
  - – Galactocemia
  - – Adrenal insufficiency
  - – Abrupt stoppage of IV glucose 10 percent
  - – CNS hemorrhage
- ❖ Iatrogenic causes.
  - – Cessation of hypertonic glucose infusions
  - – Exchange transfusions.

Clinical Signs of Hypoglycemia

Many infants are asymptomatic, particularly the preterm. Common signs described are:
- ❖ Tremors and jittery movements
- ❖ Hypotonia
- ❖ Lethargy
- ❖ Poor feeding and refusal to suck
- ❖ Apnea and cyanosis
- ❖ Seizures
- ❖ Weak or high pitched cry.

Management of Hypoglycemia

It is important for the midwife to have the knowledge base to identify the infants who are at risk. Effective management of the baby's feeding and temperature control will help to prevent hypoglycemia. Blood glucose screening, using whole blood obtained by capillary heel stab, must be done.

Early oral or gavage feeding with 10 percent glucose water every two hours until blood glucose levels are stable and then wean to breast or formula.

Minimize calorie expenditures by minimizing stress and keeping the baby warm. The prognosis is good unless the hypoglycemia has been severe or has been prolonged over days.

HYPERGLYCEMIA

Blood glucose levels, greater than 130 mg percent in newborn, is considered as hyperglycemia. It is found most commonly in preterm infants. It is thought to be a result of the immature infant's inability to handle glucose. It can occur also as a response to infection, dehydration, intravenous glucose, stress and steroids used to treat bronchopulmonary dysplasia. Treatment is to reduce the concentration of administered dextrose infusions and give a continuous insulin infusion if necessary. Neonatal diabetes mellitus is a rare occurrence. The cause is thought to be immaturity of the pancreatic islets with a resultant insulin insufficiency. Treatment is with insulin until the condition resolves when the pancreas matures (Roberton, 1993).

ELECTROLYTE IMBALANCE

Electrolyte levels will become imbalanced in the neonate when the normal hydration is not maintained. The midwife needs to be aware of the factors that can cause fluid and electrolyte imbalance which include:
- ❖ Fluid loss through the skin, which is increased under radiant warmers and phototherapy
- ❖ Dehydration from inadequate feeding.
  Sick and premature infants are more at risk of electrolyte and fluid imbalance.

HYPERNATREMIA

Hypernatremia is the condition in which the serum sodium level is greater than 148 mEq/L (Roberton, 1993). It may be due to an excessive intake of sodium, from incorrectly made up feeds or a consequence of intravenous therapy and the administration of sodium bicarbonate. Excessive water loss from increased insensible water loss can also cause hypernatremia. The baby is usually dehydrated and may present with signs of cerebral irritation, which, if left untreated, can lead to intraventricular hemorrhage.

Management is to restore fluid and electrolyte balance and treat the underlying cause. It is important that the midwife ensures that a baby under phototherapy receives sufficient fluid to prevent dehydration.

HYPONATREMIA

Hyponatremia occurs when the serum sodium is less than 133 mEq/L (Roberton, 1993). It is the result of water retention or excessive water loss. Preterm babies are more at risk because of the immaturity of their kidneys, which allow a high sodium loss in the urine. The baby may be asymptomatic or present with signs of edema. If the sodium loss is acute, the baby may present with convulsions.

Management is to replace sodium either orally or intravenously, and correct the imbalance.

HYPOCALCEMIA

This is a condition where the serum calcium is less than 8.0 mg percent (Roberton, 1993). It occurs most commonly in low birthweight babies, infants of diabetic mothers, babies who have acquired exchange transfusion or in very sick babies. Other causes are deficiency of maternal and fetal vitamin D, renal failure and hypoparathyroidism in the infant.

Signs of hypocalcemia are irritability, rapid jerky limb movements or even convulsions. Management is to supplement the baby with either oral or intravenous calcium (Livingstone in Bennett and Brown, 1999).

HYPERCALCEMIA

Neonatal hypercalcemia is diagnosed when the serum calcium is over 11.0 mg percent (Roberton, 1993). This is rare in newborn babies. High calcium levels can lead to renal damage and pathological changes in the heart. It may be the result of over treatment with a calcium infusion or occur when there is insufficient phosphate in the baby's diet. It can also occur when the baby has abnormal vitamin D metabolism. Treatment will depend upon the underlying cause (Livingstone in Bennett and Brown, 1999).

DIARRHEA IN NEWBORN

Diarrhea is one of the serious problems in newborn. However, frequent passage of stools occurs in newborns, which should be differentiated from infective diarrhea or gastroenteritis.

Causes

Specific and nonspecific organisms such as *E. coli*, *Staphylococcus* or virus are usually responsible.

Clinical Features

True diarrhea of gastroenteritis is manifested by:
- ❖ Frequent watery stools
- ❖ Green stools due to unchanged bile
- ❖ Containing mucus and blood.

It is common in artificially fed babies because of problems in the quality of milk and maintaining asepsis of the utensils used. Associated features include:
- ❖ Colic and crying
- ❖ Evidences of dehydration such as:
  - – Dry, inelastic skin
  - – Sunken eyes
  - – Depressed anterior fontanelle
  - – Loss of weight and ultimately
  - – Circulatory collapse.

Dietetic Causes of Diarrhea (Noninfective)

- ❖ *Overfeeding*: Increased amount and/or frequent feeds lead to undue irritation of the gut and intestinal hurry causing diarrhea. The stool is bulky without any mucus. Maintenance of regularity and adjusting the amount of feeds cure the condition
- ❖ *Underfeeding*: It is called *hunger diarrhea*. There is frequent passage of small green stools. Increasing the quantity of the feeds by test feeding solves the problem
- ❖ *Excessive carbohydrate*: Produces flatulence, frequent frothy stools with excoriation of the buttocks. The reaction of the stool is acidic
- ❖ *Excessive fat (addition of cream)*: This may lead to vomiting and diarrhea with pale stool
- ❖ *Protein diarrhea*: This is associated with colic, vomiting and frequent bloody stools.

Treatment of Infective Diarrhea

The baby should be isolated and the stool should be sent for culture and sensitivity test prior to starting antibiotic therapy.

Mild diarrhea is managed as follows:

- Milk feeding is stopped.
- Oral rehydration solutions (ORS) are started. The WHO recommended ORS packet contains:
  - Glucose 20 gm,
  - Sodium chloride 3.5 gm,
  - Sodium citrate 2.9 gm and
  - Potassium chloride 1.5 gm.

The contents of a packet should be dissolved in one liter of drinking (potable) water and used within 24 hours.

- The total fluids should be at least 200 ml/kg bodyweight per day and should be given at 2 to 3 hourly intervals. If the baby fails to take the necessary amount by mouth, parenteral therapy is started
- After the diarrhea is controlled, breastfeeding is resumed. Alternatively, half-strength skimmed milk is given before the usual milk feeds are restored
- *Antibiotics*: If there is systemic infection with gastrointestinal manifestations, oral or parenteral antibiotics (colistin sulfate, ampicillin, amikacin or cefotaxime) are given.

Severe Diarrhea with Dehydration

- Dehydration should be corrected with intravenous fluids. Five percent dextrose in one-fifth saline or half-strength Hartmann's solution or Ringer lactate is administered. Once urine output is adequate, oral rehydration is started. Other treatment measures are same as for mild diarrhea.

VOMITING IN NEWBORN

Vomiting is one of the common manifestations in the neonates. Vomiting in neonates may either be trivial or manifestation of some graver pathology. Mucus vomiting tinged with blood is quite common soon after birth. It is due to irritation of the gastric mucosa by the swallowed materials during birth.

CAUSES OF VOMITING

- *Obstructive*: Vomiting may be a manifestation of congenital gastrointestinal tract obstruction. The conditions include esopha-geal atresia, cardiospasm, chalasia (continuous relaxation of esophageal-gastric sphincter), pyloric stenosis, duodenal atresia, diaphragmatic hernia or hiatus hernia, meconium ileus and imperforate anus (Dutta, 2001).
- *Intracranial injuries*: Raised intracranial tension due to hemorrhage or depressed skull bone fracture
- *Dietetic*: Overfeeding or qualitative change in the food constituents or excessive air swallowing
- *Milk allergy*: Allergy to cow's milk is manifested with mucus and blood in the vomitus. Recurrence of diarrhea after reintroducing cow's milk is very much suggestive
- *Infective*: Gastroenteritis, meningitis or septicemia.

Treatment

- Early diagnosis and correction of fluid imbalance   •
- Medical or surgical therapy as appropriate for the underlying pathology.

DRUG OR SUBSTANCE WITHDRAWAL

Drugs and substances that have been prescribed or abused in pregnancy can cause neonatal withdrawal symptoms. Among these are narcotics, alcohol, amphetamines, barbiturates, codeine, benzodiazepines, pentazocine, cocaine, lithium and tricyclic antidepressants. The drugs and substances abused vary according to current trends, availability and geographical location. Drug and substance abuse is associated with increased fetal and neonatal deaths, prematurity and intrauterine growth restriction. Pregnant users often have accompanying social, economic and housing problems. This group of women is also at more risk for sexually transmitted diseases such as chlamydia, gonorrhea, HIV and hepatitis B infection.

NEONATAL ABSTINENCE SYNDROME (NAS) OR WITHDRAWAL SIGNS

These are nonspecific and should be observed by the midwife when the mother presents with history of drug or substances use. The signs are:

❖ Tremor
❖ High-pitched cry
❖ Irritability
❖ Hyperactivity
❖ Sweating
❖ Pyrexia
❖ Sneezing
❖ Vomiting
❖ Disorganized suck
❖ Diarrhea
❖ Convulsions
❖ Respiratory distress.

In opiate misuse, the symptoms of withdrawal will generally appear within the first 24 to 48 hours of life. Barbiturate abstinence signs may not appear for two weeks and may go on for a period of several weeks or months.

Care of a baby undergoing withdrawal include the following aspects:

❖ Provision of a quiet environment with reduced light and noise stimulus
❖ Swaddling the baby to make him feel secure.
❖ Small frequent feeds for comfort and adequate nutrition
❖ Administration of phenobarbitone to control convulsions
❖ IV fluids, if oral feeding is not tolerated.

Treatment

Treatment will vary according to the drug of misuse and the severity of presenting signs. Narcotics such as morphine may be used until observable signs are controlled (Roberton, 1993). Chlorpromazine is also used until presenting symptoms are controlled.

Midwife's management of the baby and mother must include providing opportunities for parents to participate in the care of the baby and adequate explanation of the baby's behavior. Adequate follow-up arrangements, including community health and social services, must be ensured when planning discharge from the hospital.

FETAL ALCOHOL SYNDROME (FAS)

Fetal alcohol syndrome is characterized by intrauterine growth restriction, failure to thrive, developmental delay and dysmorphic (deformed) facial features. It is thought that ethanol (a component of alcohol) disrupts cell differentiation and growth in the fetus and impairs normal placental function.

Characteristics of Babies with FAS

❖ Small eyes with exaggerated epicanthic folds
❖ Poorly formed nasal bridge
❖ Fretfulness and difficulty to feed
❖ Associated abnormalities of the heart and musculoskeletal system, intestinal atresias, skin lesions and cleft palate
❖ The baby will also have delays in mental and motor development and may have learning and behavioral problems in later life.

Management

The midwife has an important role in the prevention and management of FAS by identifying women at risk and in giving effective antenatal education. In managing the baby suspected of having FAS, the midwife will need to monitor for signs of alcohol withdrawal. Follow-up care including community health and social services must be arranged prior to discharge from the hospital.

BIBLIOGRAPHY

1. Aynsley Green A, Soltesz G. Metabolic and endocrine disorders, Part 1. In: Roberton N. Textbook of Neonatology, 2nd edn. London; Churchill Livingstone, 1992.
2. Brown J, Philips CA, et al. Glucose testing in the neonate. Journal of Neonatal Nursing, 1997;3(3): 22-3.
3. Dutta DC. Textbook of Obstetrics, 5th edn. Calcutta; New Central Book Company, 2001.
4. Jones K. Fetal alcohol syndrome. Pediatric Review 1986;8(4):122.
5. Livingston A. Metabolic and endocrine disorders and drug withdrawal. In: Bennett RV, Linda KB (Eds). Myles Textbook for Midwives, 13th edn. Edinburgh; Churchill Livingstone, 1999.
6. Roberton NRC. A Manual of Neonatal Intensive Care, 3rd edn. Londonl; Edward Arnold, 1993.

Community
Midwifery

49

Preventive Obstetrics and Domiciliary Care in Maternity Nursing

Learning Objectives

Upon completing this chapter, the learner will be able to:
- Describe the concept of community midwifery
- Describe the role of the midwife and the scope of her practice during the antenatal, intrapartum and postpartum periods
- Review the skills a midwife requires for home birth.

The concept of home care combines obstetrical concerns with the concepts of primary health care. Such midwifery care takes into account the woman's and her family's personal and social circumstances, which influence the health and well-being of her and her baby.

Community midwifery is one of the functions of community health care. It aims to promote the well-being of mothers and babies and to support sound parenting and stable families. It is a component of the maternal and child health (MCH) program in India, which has its specific objectives for reduction of maternal, perinatal, infant and childhood mortality and morbidity and promotion of reproductive health.

ANTENATAL CARE

The aim of antenatal care is to achieve at the end of a pregnancy—a healthy mother and a healthy baby. Ideally, this care should begin soon after conception and continue throughout pregnancy.

Objectives of Antenatal Care

- Promote, protect and maintain the health of the mother during pregnancy

- Detect "high-risk" pregnancies and give the mothers special attention
- Foresee complications and prevent them.
- Remove anxiety and fear associated with delivery
- Reduce maternal and infant mortality and morbidity
- Teach mother, elements of childcare, nutrition, personal hygiene and environmental sanitation
- Sensitize the mother to the need for family planning.

Antenatal Visits

Ideally, the care should begin soon after conception and continue throughout pregnancy. A schedule to follow for the mother is to attend the antenatal clinic once a month during the first seven months, twice a month during the next two months and thereafter once a week if everything is normal. In India a large proportion of mothers are of low socioeconomic group for whom attendance at the antenatal clinic may mean loss of daily wages and hence a minimum of three visits are encouraged as below:

- First visit, as soon as the pregnancy is known or at 20th week
- Second visit, at 32nd week
- Third visit, at 36th week.

Further visits may be made if justified by the condition of the mother. At least one visit should be paid in the home of the mother.

Preventive Services for Mothers in the Prenatal Period

The first visit irrespective of when it occurs should include:

❖ Health history
❖ Physical examination
❖ Laboratory examination
  – Complete urine analysis
  – Stool examination
  – Complete blood count including Hbg estimation
  – Serological examination
  – Blood grouping and Rh determination
  – Chest X-ray, if needed
  – Gonorrhea test, if needed.

On subsequent visits:

❖ Physical examination including weight and blood pressure
❖ Laboratory tests including urine examination and hemoglobin estimation
❖ Iron and folic acid supplementation and medications as needed
❖ Immunization against tetanus
❖ Group or individual teaching on nutrition, self care, family planning, delivery and parenthood
❖ Home visiting by a female health worker or trained dai (trained traditional birth attendant)
❖ Referral services, when necessary.

Risk Approach

While continuing to provide appropriate care for all mothers, 'high risk' cases must be identified as early as possible and arrangements to be made for skilled care. These cases comprise the following:

❖ Elderly primigravida (30 years and above)
❖ Short statured primigravida
❖ Malpresentations, e.g. breech, transverse lie, etc.
❖ Antepartum hemorrhage, threatened abortion
❖ Pre-eclampsia and eclampsia
❖ Anemia
❖ Twins, hydramnios
❖ Previous stillbirth, intrauterine death, manual removal of placenta
❖ Elderly grand multipara
❖ Prolonged pregnancy (14 days beyond expected date of delivery)
❖ Previous cesarean or instrumental delivery

❖ Pregnancy associated with medical conditions, e.g. cardiovascular disease, kidney disease, diabetes, tuberculosis, liver disease, etc.

The purpose of risk approach is to provide maximum services to all pregnant women with attention to those who need them most. Maximum utilization of all resources, including human resources is involved in such care. Services of traditional birth attendants, community health workers and women's groups are utilized. The risk strategy is expected to lead to improvements in both the quality and coverage of healthcare at all levels, particularly at primary healthcare level.

Home Visits

Home visits are paid by the Female Health Worker or Public Health Nurse. If the delivery is planned at home, several visits are required. The home visit will provide opportunities to study the environmental and social conditions at home and to provide prenatal advice. In the home environment, the woman will have more confidence to make an informed decision about home birth.

Prenatal Advice

A major component of antenatal care is prenatal advice or education. The mother is more receptive to advice concerning herself and her baby at this time than any other time. The topics should cover not only the specific problems of pregnancy and childbirth but must also include family and child health care.

Diet

A balanced and adequate diet is of utmost importance during pregnancy and lactation to meet the increased needs of the mother, and to prevent nutritional stress. On an average a pregnant woman, gains about 12.5 kg of weight during pregnancy. Studies have indicated that Indian women of low-income group gain an average weight of 6.5 kg during pregnancy (ICMR Bulletin, Dec. 1977). Thus, pregnancy induces the need for calorie and nutritional requirements. If maternal stores of iron are poor as may happen after repeated pregnancies and if adequate iron is not available to the mother during pregnancy, it is possible that the fetus will lay down insufficient iron stores. Such a baby may show normal hemoglobin at birth but will lack the stores of iron necessary for rapid growth, and increase in blood volume and muscle mass in the first year of life.

Personal Hygiene

Advice regarding personal hygiene is equally important. The need to bathe every day and to wear clean clothes should be explained. About eight hours of sleep and at least two hours rest after midday meals should be advised. Constipation should be avoided by regular intake of green leafy vegetables, fruits and extra fluid. Purgatives such as castor oil to relieve constipation should be avoided. Light household work should be encouraged but manual physical labor during pregnancy may adversely affect the fetus.

Smoking should be cut down to a minimum, as heavy smoking by the mother can result in babies much smaller than average size due to placental insufficiency. The perinatal mortality amongst babies whose mothers smoked during pregnancy is between 10 to 40 percent higher than in nonsmokers. Mothers who are moderate to heavy drinkers (alcohol) become pregnant, have greater risk of pregnancy loss and if they do not abort, their babies may have various physical and mental problems. Heavy drinking has been associated with fetal alcohol syndrome (FAS), which includes intrauterine growth retardation and developmental delay. Advice should also be given about dental care and sexual behavior during pregnancy. Sexual intercourse should be restricted during the last trimester of pregnancy.

Drugs

The use of drugs that are not absolutely essential should be discouraged as certain drugs taken by the mother during pregnancy may affect the fetus adversely and cause fetal malformations. Some of the drugs known to cause damage include streptomycin that may cause eighth nerve damage and deafness in the fetus, iodide containing drugs that may cause

congenital goiter, corticosteroids that may impair fetal growth, sex hormones that produce virulism and tetracyclins that affect the growth of bones and enamel formation of teeth. A great deal of caution is required in the drug intake by pregnant women.

Radiation

Exposure to radiation is a positive danger to the developing fetus. The most common source of radiation is abdominal X-ray during pregnancy. Studies have shown that mortality rates from leukemia and other neoplasms were significantly greater among children exposed to intrauterine X-ray. Congenital malformations such as microcephaly are known to occur due to radiation. Hence, X-ray examination in pregnancy should be carried out only for definite indications.

Warning Signs

The mother should be given instructions that she should report immediately, any of the following warning signals: swelling of the feet, convulsions, headache, blurring of the vision, bleeding or discharge per vagina and any other unusual symptoms.

Childcare

Mothers attending antenatal clinics must be given mother craft education that consists of nutrition education, hygiene and childrearing, childbirth preparation and family planning information.

Specific Health Protection

Specific protection for pregnant women's health is an essential aspect of prenatal care. This is because 50 to 60 percent of women, belonging to low socioeconomic groups, are anemic in the last trimester of pregnancy. The major causative factors are iron and folic acid deficiencies. Anemia is known to be associated with high incidence of premature births, postpartum hemorrhage, puerperal sepsis and thromboembolic phenomena in the mother. The government of India has initiated a program in which 60 mg of elemental iron and

500 mcg of folic acid are being distributed daily to pregnant women through antenatal clinics, primary health centers and their subcenters.

Other Nutritional Deficiencies

Protection is required against other nutritional deficiencies that may occur during pregnancy such as protein, vitamin and mineral deficiencies. In some MCH centers fresh milk is supplied free of cost to all expectant and lactating mothers; where this is not possible skimmed milk is given. Vitamin A and D capsules are also supplied free of cost.

Tetanus Protection

If the mother was not immunized earlier, two doses of tetanus toxoid should be given, the first dose at 16th to 20th week and the second dose at 20th to 24th week of pregnancy. For a woman who has been immunized earlier, one booster dose will be sufficient. When such a booster dose is given, it will provide necessary cover for subsequent pregnancies for the next five years.

Syphilis

Syphilitic infection in the woman is transmissible to the fetus, especially when she is suffering from primary or secondary stages after the 6th month of pregnancy. Neurological damage with mental retardation is one of the most serious complications. Blood should be tested for syphilis (VDRL) at the first visit and late in pregnancy. Ten daily injections of procaine penicillin (600,000 units) are usually adequate to treat the infection.

German Measles

Rubella infection contracted during the first 16 weeks of pregnancy can cause major defects such as cataract, deafness and congenital heart diseases. Vaccination of all women of childbearing age, who are seronegative, is desirable. Before vaccinating, it is desirable that pregnancy is ruled out and effective contraception be maintained for eight weeks after vaccination because of possible risk to the fetus from the virus, should the mother become pregnant.

Rh Status

It is a routine procedure in antenatal clinics to test the blood for Rhesus type in early pregnancy. If the woman is Rh-negative and the husband is Rh-positive, she is kept under surveillance for determination of Rh-antibody levels during antenatal period. The blood is further examined at 28th week and 34th to 36th week of gestation for antibodies. Rh anti-D immunoglobulin should be given at 28th week of gestation so that sensitization during the first pregnancy can be prevented. If the baby is Rh-positive, the Rh anti-D immunoglobulin is given again within 72 hours of delivery. It should also be given after abortion. Postmaturity should be avoided. Whenever there is evidence of hemolytic process in fetus *in utero*, the mother should be shifted to an equipped center specialized to deal with Rh problems. The incidence of hemolytic disease due to Rh factor in India is estimated to be approximately one for every 400 to 500 live births (Park, 2000).

HIV Infections

HIV may pass from an infected mother to her fetus through the placenta or to her infant during delivery or by breastfeeding. About one-third of the children of HIV positive mothers become infected through this route. The risk of transmission is higher if the mother is newly infected or if she has already developed AIDS. Prenatal testing for HIV infection should be done as early in pregnancy as possible for pregnant women who are at risk (if they or their partners have multiple sexual partners, have sexually transmitted disease or use illicit injectable drugs). Universal confidential voluntary screening of pregnant women in high prevalence areas may allow infected women to choose therapeutic abortion, make an informed decision on breastfeeding or receive appropriate care.

Prenatal Genetic Screening

Screening for genetic abnormalities and for direct evidence of structural anomalies is performed in pregnancy in order to make the option of therapeutic abortion available when severe defects are detected. Typical examples are—screening for trisomy-21 and severe neural tube defects. Women aged 35 years and above, and those who already have an afflicted child are at high risk.

Mental Preparation

Mental preparation is as important as physical or material preparation. Sufficient time and opportunity must be given to expectant mothers to have free and frank talk on all aspects of pregnancy and delivery. The "mother craft" classes at the MCH centers help a great deal in removing their fears and in gaining confidence.

Family Planning

Family planning is related to every phase of the maternity cycle. Educational and motivational efforts must be initiated during the antenatal period. If the mother has had two or more children, she should be motivated for puerperal sterilization. The All India Postpartum Services (AIPS) are available to all expectant mothers in India.

INTRANATAL CARE

The need for effective intranatal care is paramount, even if the delivery is expected to be a normal one. Complications such as septicemia and tetanus neonatorum can occur from the use of improperly sterilized instruments. There must be emphasis on cleanliness, which includes clean hands and fingernails, a clean surface for delivery, clean cutting and care of the cord, and keeping birth canal clean by avoiding harmful practices. Hospitals and health centers should be equipped with midwifery kits, a regular supply of sterile gloves and drapes, towels, cleaning materials, soap and antiseptic solution as well as equipment for sterilizing instruments and supplies. Delivery kits (UNICEF) are available with the items needed for basic hygiene for delivery at home.

The objectives of good intranatal care are to achieve:

❖ Thorough asepsis
❖ Delivery with minimum injury to the newborn and mother
❖ Readiness to deal with complications such as prolonged labor, hemorrhage, convulsions, malpresentations, prolapse of the cord, etc.
❖ Care of the baby at delivery—resuscitation, care of the cord, care of the eyes, etc.

Domiciliary Care

Mothers with normal obstetric history may be advised to have their delivery in their own homes, provided the home conditions are satisfactory. In such cases, the delivery may be conducted by the Female Health Worker or Assistant Nurse Midwife or trained dai (trained traditional birth attendants). This is known as *domiciliary midwifery service.*

Domiciliary midwifery service continues to be a necessary mode of practice in India as a large portion of the population (74%) is in the rural areas where there may be no more than one physician per 20,000 to 30,000 populations. Domiciliary out-reach is a major component of intrapartum care.

Advantages of the Domiciliary Midwifery Service

❖ The mother delivers in the familiar surroundings of her home, which may remove her fear associated with delivery in a hospital
❖ The chances of cross infection are generally fewer than in the hospital/nursery
❖ The mother is able to keep an eye upon her children and domestic affairs
❖ The fear associated with hospitals is eliminated, which may tend to ease her mental tension
❖ The financial strain on the family is reduced, which would otherwise be a burden
❖ The load on hospital/health center facilities is reduced, so that other clients in greater need for urgent medical care, can be adequately treated.

Disadvantages of Domiciliary Midwifery

❖ The mother may have less medical and nursing supervision than in the hospital
❖ The mother may have less rest as she may resume domestic duties too soon
❖ Her diet and medications may be neglected
❖ Many homes in India are unsuitable for even a normal delivery
❖ Even though childbirth is a natural event, which should take place at home, not everything may be normal every time and hence extreme caution is essential in domiciliary midwifery.

A home delivery is contraindicated in certain home situations and when the mother and/or fetus present with *risk factors*. These include the following:

The Home
❖ Overcrowding
❖ Presence of infectious disease
❖ Poor (unsanitary) environmental conditions.

Maternal Factors
❖ Cephalopelvic disproportion
❖ Pregnancy induced hypertension
❖ Eclampsia
❖ Multiple pregnancy
❖ Hydramnios
❖ Antepartum hemorrhage
❖ Rh-isoimmunization
❖ Elderly primigravida
❖ Grand multipara
❖ Previous cesarean section, forceps delivery, postpartum hemorrhage
❖ Associated medical disorders.

Fetal Factors
❖ History of previous stillbirths or neonatal deaths
❖ Malpresentation
❖ Prematurity
❖ Intrauterine growth retardation.

Preparation for Home Delivery

The midwife/female health worker should assess the home conditions and provide necessary instructions. The mother must be told what she should prepare and provide for the event to take place at home.

All pregnant women must be instructed to make necessary preparations for delivery. They should be provided with a disposable delivery kit (DDK) from the health centre. In case the DDK is not available, they should be advised to buy a new razor blade and some thread themselves and keep them ready. The thread should be boiled for 20 minutes and sun dried before delivery. They should be advised to keep ready cotton cloth for themselves and for the newborn. It is important that these are clean to prevent infection. Clothes should be washed with soap and sun dried and kept away from dust.

All women who are pregnant must be informed about the nearest hospital so that they can be taken there immediately, if there is an emergency (MHFW, 1996).

The Room

In the week prior to delivery, the ceiling and walls should be dusted and the floor scrubbed. The mattresses should be beaten and exposed to sunlight for a day or two. The bed sheets should be washed and dried. Dirty surfaces should be wiped with a cloth wrung out of an antiseptic solution. The bed should be conveniently placed to have adequate light and access for health workers from both sides.

As the woman goes into labor, and the female health worker's arrival is awaited, the family should prepare the following:
❖ Boil two pots of water, one of which to be set to cool
❖ Bed linen and baby clothes to be kept ready
❖ A plastic sheet to be placed over the mattress to protect it from fluid and blood
❖ Arrangement to burn or deep bury the placenta.

Instruments, syringes and needles will have to be sterilized and brought from the hospital/health center along with the delivery kit. The management of labor and delivery is as in the hospital.

The Female Health Worker or Community Health Nurse, who is the pivot of domiciliary care, should be adequately prepared to recognize the 'danger signals' during labor and seek immediate help in transferring the mother to the nearest Primary Health Center or Hospital, should the need arises.

The Danger Signals

- Sluggish contractions or no contractions after rupture of membranes
- Good contractions for an hour after rupture of membranes, but no progress
- Prolapse of cord or hand
- Meconium stained liquor or a slow irregular or excessively fast fetal heart rate
- Excessive show or bleeding during labor
- A placenta which is not separated within half an hour after delivery of the baby
- Postpartum hemorrhage or collapse
- A temperature of 38°C or over, during labor.

There should be close liaison between domiciliary and institutional delivery service.

Equipments for Conducting Home Delivery

From Home for Mother

- Clean newspapers
- A large pot to boil articles
- Two shallow mud pots to use as bed pan and placenta receiver
- Clean sheets and linen
- A clean mat to spread on the floor or cot
- Clean rags.

For Baby

- Clothes for baby (old pieces washed with soap, dried by hanging in the sun and ironed with hot iron)
- A mild soap
- Small pieces of rags or cotton
- A cradle with firm bottom.

From the Bag and Midwifery Kit (As Suggested by UNICEF)

- Plastic apron
- Plastic sheet
- Two kidney trays
- Two bowls for lotion
- Two artery forceps
- Two thumb forceps
- Scissors
- Two to three packets of sterile gloves
- Syringe and needles
- Enema set
- Urethral catheter
- Mucus extractor (bulb syringe)
- Spring balance

- Thermometers (oral and rectal)
- Sterile cotton swabs and 4 × 4 gauze pieces
- Cord tie/cord clamp
- Dettol/any antiseptic solution
- Alcohol
- Eye drops/ointment for the baby
- Injection vitamin K for the baby
- Methergine (injection and tablets)
- Fetoscope
- Measuring tape
- Episiotomy scissors
- Suture items.

Other Items from the Health Center

- Prenatal record/card of the woman
- Notebook and pen.

Upon receiving the call for a home delivery, the midwife needs to:

- Collect information regarding the time of onset of labor and intensity of contractions
- Take out the woman's antenatal card or record
- Check the midwifery kit and public health bag and add any articles needed
- Leave information in the call register including name and address of the woman and the time of leaving.

Upon arrival in the home, further information regarding the onset of labor and other relevant data must be obtained. Monitoring the progress of labor, health of the mother and fetus and conducting the delivery are same as in a clinic or hospital setting.

About one percent of deliveries tend to be abnormal and four percent 'difficult', requiring the services of a physician. Institutional care may be sought for all difficult cases (Park, 2000).

The health status of the mother and baby must be stable before the midwife leaves the home. She must ensure that the woman's:

- Vagina and perineum are intact and does not have lacerations that require suturing in the health center
- Uterus is firm and contracted and bleeding is minimal
- Vital signs are stable and desirous of feeding and bonding with the baby.

An *initial assessment of the newborn* must be done to ensure that:

❖ The cord is tied or clamped securely
❖ The neonate's temperature and breathing are stable
❖ The neonate is able to feed from the mother's breasts
❖ There are no visible/identifiable congenital anomalies
❖ Injection vitamin K and prophylactic eye medication are administered.

Instructions regarding the continued care and observations of the mother and baby must be reviewed with the family. In the mother's antenatal card/record, the information about the management of labor and delivery are recorded including the medications used.

Articles used for the conduct of delivery must be cleaned and wrapped for transport to the health center for sterilization. Materials to be destroyed by burning, must be sorted and the family instructed about it. Before leaving the home, the midwife must leave with the family clear instructions as to where she can be contacted if any need arises.

POSTNATAL CARE

Care of the mother and the newborn after delivery is known as postnatal or postpartal care. The objectives of postpartal care are to:
❖ Prevent complications of the postpartal period
❖ Promote rapid restoration of the mother's health to optimum level
❖ Check the adequacy of breastfeeding
❖ Provide family planning instructions and services
❖ Provide basic health education to mother/family.

Following delivery, the mother and baby are visited daily for ten days. During each of these visits the midwife/FHW checks temperature, pulse and respirations of the mother, examines her breasts, checks the progress of normal involution of uterus, examines lochia for any abnormality, checks urine and bowels and advices on perineal toileting. The immediate postnatal complications such as puerperal sepsis, thrombophlebitis and secondary hemorrhage must be kept in mind. At the end of 6th week, the woman needs an examination by the physician in the health center to check-up involution of the uterus, which should be complete by then. Further visits should be done once a month during the first six months and thereafter once in 2 to 3 months until the end of one year. In rural areas, where only limited care is possible, efforts should be made by the FHW to give at least 3 to 6 postnatal visits. The common conditions found during the late postnatal period are subinvolution of uterus, prolapse of uterus and cervicitis. Postnatal examination offers an opportunity to detect and correct these defects. Anemia if present needs to be treated. Health education regarding affordable nutritious diet and postnatal exercises to restore the stretched abdominal and pelvic muscles must be provided to enable the mother have a normal postpartum period.

The psychological aspect of postnatal care needs to be addressed based on a needs assessment. New mothers may have timidity and fears due to ignorance and insecurity regarding the care of the baby. In order to endure the emotional stress of childbirth, she requires the support and companionship of her husband as well as encouragement and assistance of family. Fear and insecurity may be eliminated by proper prenatal instructions, postnatal enforcing, and supportive care.

Breastfeeding

Postnatal care includes helping the mother to establish successful breastfeeding. For many babies breast milk provides the main source of nourishment in the first year of life. When the standard of environmental sanitation is poor and education low, the content of feeding bottle is likely to be as nutritionally poor as it is bacteriologically dangerous. It is therefore very important to advise mothers to provide exclusive breastfeeding in the initial months. At the age of 4 to 5 months, breast milk should be supplemented by additional foods rich in protein and other nutrients (e.g. animal milk, soft-cooked mashed vegetables, fruits, etc). These supplementary foods should be introduced very gradually and in small amounts.

Family Planning

Every attempt should be made to motivate mothers when they attend postnatal clinics or during postnatal contacts to adopt a suitable method for spacing the next birth or for limiting the family size as appropriate. Postpartum tubal ligation is generally recommended on the 2nd day after delivery. Contraceptives that will not affect lactation, may be prescribed immediately following delivery after a physical examination.

Health Education

Health education during the postnatal period should cover the following areas:

- Hygiene—personal and environmental
- Feeding of infant
- Care of the umbilical cord/umbilical stump
- Bathing the baby
- Nutritious diet for the mother
- Pregnancy spacing

- Health check-up for mother and baby
- Birth registration

BIBLIOGRAPHY

1. Department of Family Planning, Ministry of Health, Government of India. Plan of Operation for All India Hospital (Postpartum) Family Planning Program, 1971.
2. Government of India, MCH. Division, National Child Survival and Safe Motherhood Program, 1971.
3. ICMR Bulletin, December 1977.
4. Ministry of Health and Family Welfare, Manual for Orientation of Auxiliary Nurse Midwives and Supervisors, Reproductive and Child health Approach, New Delhi, 1996.
5. Park K. Park's Textbook of Preventive and Social Medicine, 16th edn. Jabalpur: Banarasidas Bhanot Publishers, 2000.
6. Parulekar SV. Textbook for Midwives, 2nd edn. Mumbai: Vora Medical Publications, 1998.
7. WHO Health for All, Sr. No. 4.

50

Primary Health Care in India

Learning Objectives

Upon completing this chapter, the learner will be able to:

❖ Describe the organization of health care in the country
❖ Describe the role of trained dais
❖ Describe the place of female health workers in the health care system and outline their functions for implementing Maternal and Child Health (MCH) services
❖ Describe the job functions of the female health assistant in relation to MCH services
❖ Describe the program of Reproductive and Child Health (RCH) services.

The system of health care practiced in India presently includes treatment of illness, promotion of health and prevention of illness. Community participation is recognized as a major component. The stress is on the provision of these services to the people representing a shift from medical care to health care and from urban population to rural population.

LEVELS OF HEALTH CARE

In India, the complex of primary health centers and their subcenters through the agency of multipurpose health workers, village health guides/trained dais provide primary health care. Since India has opted for "Health for all by 2000 AD", the primary health care system has been recognized and strengthened to make the primary health care delivery system more effective (WHO Chronicle, 1977).

The health care service is organized at three levels, i.e. primary, secondary and tertiary.

These levels represent different types of care involving varying degrees of complexity.

Primary care level: It is the first level of contact of individuals, families and community with the national health system where primary health care (essential health care) is provided. As a level of care, it is close to the people, where most of their health problems can be dealt with and resolved. At this level, the health care will be most effective within the context of the needs and limitations of the area.

Secondary care level: The next higher level of care is the secondary (intermediate) health care level. At this level, problems that are more complex are dealt with. In India, this kind of care is generally provided in district hospitals and community health centers which also serve as the first referral level facility (WHO Chronicle, 1969).

Tertiary care level: The tertiary level is a more specialized level than secondary care level and requires specific facilities and attention of highly specialized health workers. This care is provided by the regional or central level institutions, e.g. Medical College Hospitals, All India Institutes, Regional Hospitals and Specialized Hospitals.

A fundamental and necessary function of the health care system is to provide a sound referral system. It must be a two-way exchange of information and returning patients to those who referred them for follow-up care (UNICEF-WHO Joint Committee on Health Policy, 1987). This will ensure continuity of care and inspire confidence of the consumer in the system.

Health Care at the Village Level

The Government of India evolved a national health policy based on primary health approach in 1983. Steps for implementing the national health policy were undertaken during the sixth (1980-1985) and seventh (1986-1990) five-year plans. One of schemes adopted to implement the policy was the training of local dais (traditional birth attendants) in the country to improve their knowledge in the elementary concepts of maternal and child health and sterilization (asepsis) besides obstetric skills. The dais were trained for 30 working days at the PHC, subcenters or MCH centers. During the training, the dais were to conduct two home deliveries under the guidance and supervision of the female health worker (FHW) or assistant nurse midwife (ANM). The emphasis during training was on asepsis so that home deliveries are conducted under safe hygienic conditions thereby reducing the maternal and infant mortality.

After successful completion of training, each dai was provided with a delivery kit and a certificate. These dais were also expected to play a vital role in propagating small family norm since they were more acceptable to the community. The national target was to train one local dai in each village.

Health Care at the Subcenters Level

The subcenters are the peripheral outposts of the health delivery system in rural areas. These were established on the basis of one subcenters for every 5,000 population in general and one for every 3,000 population in the hilly, tribal and backward areas. Each subcenter is manned by a male and a female multipurpose health worker. The functions of a subcenters are limited to mother and child health (MCH) care, family planning and immunization and imple-mentation of some aspects of national health programs such as Malaria Eradication Program.

Primary Health Centers Level

The primary health centers and its subcenters provide the infrastructure to provide health services to the rural population. The National Health Plan of 1983 proposed reorganization of primary health centers on the basis of one PHC for every 30,000 to 50,000 population in the plains and one PHC for every 20,000 population in hilly, backward and tribal areas for effective coverage.

In every community development block, there are one or more PHCs each of which covers 30,000 rural population with a 15 member of staff.

Community Health Centers

Community health centres were established by upgrading the primary health centers (established earlier), each community health center covering a population of 80,000 to 125,000 (one in each community development block), with 30 beds and specialists in surgery, medicine, obstetrics and gynecology and pediatrics with X-ray and laboratory facilities. A community health officer has been included in the 25 member staff in order to strengthen the preventive and promotive aspects of health care.

MATERNAL AND CHILD HEALTH (MCH) SERVICES

The maternal and child health and family planning programs were integrated in the fourth five-year plan. It is a method of delivering health care to special groups in the population, which are especially vulnerable to disease, disability or death.

The term "maternal and child health" refers to the promotive, preventive, curative and rehabilitative health care for mothers and children. It encompasses the health care aspects of obstetrics, pediatrics, family welfare, nutrition, child development and health education.

Objectives of MCH Services

The main objective of MCH services is lifelong health. The specific objectives are:
- ❖ Reduction of morbidity and mortality rates for mothers and children
- ❖ Promotion of reproductive health
- ❖ Promotion of physical and psychological development of the child within the family.

Components of MCH Services

The components of MCH services are:
- Maternal health
- Family planning
- Child health
- School health
- Handicapped children
- Care of children in special settings suit as day care centers.

The program includes all activities, which promote health and prevent or solve health problems of mothers and children, irrespective of whether they are carried out in health centers, or in the home by primary health care workers, traditional dais, or highly trained specialists. In the concept of "Health For All by the Year 2000", the National Health Policy suggested goals for MCH services with quantifiable targets for achievement.

Maternal Health Care

Antenatal care to women during pregnancy includes preventive services, risk approach, prenatal advice, specific health protection, mother-craft class for psychological preparation and family planning.

Intranatal care covers domiciliary midwifery, institutional care and rooming-in for the newborn. Postnatal care includes care of the mothers, management of postpartal complications, measures for restoration of optimum health, promotion of breastfeeding, family planning and basic health education.

Neonatal Care

Early neonatal care aims to assist the newborn in the process of adoption to the external environment which include:
- Establishment and maintenance of cardiopulmonary functions
- Maintenance of body temperature
- Avoiding infection
- Establishment of satisfactory feeding regimen
- Early detection and treatment of congenital and acquired disorders, especially infections.

Job Functions of the Female Health Worker for Implementing MCH Services

Under the multipurpose health worker scheme, a female health worker in the subcenters has the following functions:

Registration

- Registration of all pregnant women, married women in the reproductive period and children through systematic home visits and at clinics
- Maintenance of maternity records, register of antenatal cases, eligible couples register and children register
- Categorize the eligible couples according to the number of children and age of mothers.

Care at Home

During home visits, she will:
- Provide care to pregnant women especially, registered mothers, throughout the period of pregnancy
- Give advice on nutrition to expectant and nursing mothers
- Distribute iron and folic acid tablets to pregnant and nursing mothers, children and family planning adopters and vitamin A solution to children
- Immunize pregnant mothers with tetanus toxoid
- Refer women with abnormal pregnancies and medical or gynecological problems
- Conduct about 50 percent of total deliveries
- Supervise deliveries conducted by dais whenever called in
- Refer cases of difficult labor and newborns with abnormalities and help them to get institutional care and provide follow-up care to patients referred to or discharged from the hospital
- Provide at least three postdelivery visits for each delivery case and render advice regarding feeding of the newborn as well as diet and hygiene
- Spread the message of family planning to the couples; motivate them for family planning individually and in groups

❖ Distribute conventional contraceptives to the couples, provide facilities and help to prospective adopters in getting family planning services, if necessary by accompanying them or arranging dai to accompany them to hospital

❖ Provide follow-up services to family planning adopters, identify those who develop side effects and minor complaints and refer those cases that need attention by physicians, to the PHC/Hospital

❖ Assess the growth and development of the infant and take necessary action

❖ Administer DPT, polio, BCG and measles vaccination to all the infants in her area where facilities for these are available

❖ Provide treatments for minor ailments, provide first aid in case of emergencies and refer cases beyond her competence to PHC or nearest hospital

❖ Notify all the notifiable diseases, which she comes across during her visits

❖ Record and report all the births and deaths occurring in her area to the local birth and Death Registrar and to her supervisor

❖ Test urine for albumin and glucose during her home visits

❖ Identify clients who require help for medical termination of pregnancy, provide information on the availability of services and refer them to the nearest approved institution

❖ Provide health education on all health matters and healthful living.

At the Health Centers

❖ Arrange and help the Medical Officer and the Female Health Assistant in conducting MCH and FP clinics at the subcenters

❖ Conduct urine examination and estimate hemoglobin percentage

❖ Educate mothers individually and in groups in better family health including MCH and family planning, nutrition, immunization, hygiene and minor ailments.

In the Community

❖ Identify women leaders, help the female health assistant, and participate in the training of women leaders

❖ Set up women depot-holders for condom distribution and help the health assistant in training them

❖ Participate in *Mahila Mandal* meetings and utilize such gatherings for educating women in family welfare programs

❖ Utilize satisfied customers, village leaders, dais and others for promoting family welfare program.

Other Responsibilities

❖ Maintain the cleanliness of the centers

❖ Attend staff meetings at PHC and community development block

❖ List dais in her area and involve them in promoting family welfare work

❖ Help the female health assistant in the training program for dais

❖ Coordinate activities with health workers, particularly male health workers

❖ Prepare and maintain all registers, records, maps and charts for her area in the subcenters and submit the prescribed periodical reports in time to the health assistants as per standing orders and instructions (Park, 2001).

Specific Job Functions of the Female Health Assistant

The female health assistant will:

❖ Carry-out supervisory house visiting

❖ Guide the female health worker in establishing women depot-holders for distribution of conventional contraceptives

❖ Conduct MCH and family planning clinics and carry-out educational activities

❖ Organize and conduct training for dais and women leaders with the help of women health workers

❖ Visit each of the four subcenters at least once a week

❖ Respond to urgent calls from the health workers and trained dais and render necessary help

❖ Organize and utilize *Mahila Mandals* (women's groups), teachers, etc. in the family welfare programs

❖ Personally, motivate resistant cases for family planning

❖ Provide information on availability of services for medical termination of pregnancy and refer suitable cases to the approved institutions

❖ Supervise the immunization of all pregnant women and children from zero to five years.

REPRODUCTIVE AND CHILD HEALTH PROGRAM (RCH)

The population growth and health of women and children in India continued to be a major problem despite implementation of programmes such as Maternal and Child Health (MCH) and Child Survival and Safe Motherhood (CSSM) programs through reorganized health care systems.

In 1994, during the International Conference on Population Development (ICPD), held in Cairo, Egypt, a new approach to tackle the problem was recommended. Under this approach, it was decided that family planning services should be provided as a component of the comprehensive reproductive health care. The plan outlined in the program envisaged that men and women be well informed about and have access to safe and effective contraceptive methods, women will go through pregnancy and childbirth safely and that couples will be provided with the best chance of having a healthy infant.

India as one of the 180 participants in the ICPD conference agreed to adopt the "Reproductive Health Approach" to the population issues. The Government of India launched the RCH program in October 1997. The integrated package of services included in the program is:

❖ Services for mothers during pregnancy, childbirth and postnatal period including safe abortion services when required

❖ Services for children including newborn care, immunization, Vitamin A prophylaxis, Oral Rehydration Therapy (ORT) for diarrhea, management of Acute Respiratory Infections (ARI), anemia control, etc.

❖ Services for eligible couples through promotion of use of contraceptive methods as well as infertility services when required

❖ Prevention and management of Reproductive Tract Infections (RTI)

❖ Health services including counseling on family life and reproductive health for adolescents.

The approach adopted for rendering the services under the RCH program places special emphasis on client oriented, need-based, high quality, integrated services to the beneficiaries.

Specific Features of the RCH Approach

1. *Target-free program, based on community needs*: Instead of the centrally determined contraceptive specific targets, the workload of functionaries is estimated by using Community Need Assessment Approach (CNAA).

2. *Participatory planning*: The estimation of services required and its planning are to be actually undertaken with active involvement and consultation with community members including women's groups, panchayat institutions, members, etc.

3. *Quality of care and client satisfaction*: Special emphasis is placed on good quality of care. All care provided are to be of good quality and acceptable to the clients.

The organizers and planners of the program identified that well-trained and highly motivated health care personnel are an essential prerequisite for its successful implementation. In order to provide RCH services under the changed approach, service providers must have a desirable degree of technical competence, communication skill and managerial skills. Steps taken towards achieving this included:

❖ In service education for all health care personnel in order to orient them to the new approach

❖ Sensitizing all field functionaries at the most peripheral level through awareness generation training. The group included community leaders, members of *Mahila Mandals,* and *Panchayat* members. This was completed by December 2000

❖ Integrated skill, development training of various duration for all categories of health care personnel including physicians, nurses and paramedical workers at the Community Health Centres, Primary Health Centers and their subcenters.

Services included in the Program for Care of Mothers and Children

Essential Care for all Pregnant Women

- ❖ Registration by 12th to 16th week
- ❖ Antenatal check-up at least three times during pregnancy
- ❖ Tetanus toxoid to all women as early as possible during pregnancy with two doses at one-month interval. If already immunized during pregnancy, one dose to be given
- ❖ Iron and folic acid one tablet daily for 100 days to all pregnant women with clinical signs of anemia to receive two tablets daily for 100 days
- ❖ De-worming with mebendazole during 2nd/3rd trimester in areas where hookworm infestation is common
- ❖ Safe and clean delivery services
- ❖ Preparation of women for exclusive breast-feeding and timely weaning
- ❖ Postnatal care, including advises and services for limiting and spacing births.

Early Detection of Complications

- ❖ Clinical examination to detect anemia
- ❖ Referral and transportation to the nearest hospital of women with antepartum or postpartum hemorrhage
- ❖ Referral of all with a weight gain of more than 3 kg in a month or systolic blood pressure of 140 mm Hg or higher which arouse suspicion of pregnancy induced hypertension (preeclampsia/eclampsia)
- ❖ Referral of women with temperature of 39°C and above after delivery or after abortion for treatment in a hospital
- ❖ Transfer of women in labor for more than 12 hours to the nearest hospital where facilities for cesarean section are available.

Emergency Care for those who Need it

- ❖ Early identification of obstetric emergencies
- ❖ Initial management of emergencies and transfer to referral hospitals without delay using the fastest available mode of transport locally available
- ❖ While transporting, the patient should be made to lie on her left side and if she has fits, a roll of cloth should be placed between teeth to avoid tongue bite.

Care for Women in the Reproductive Age Group

- ❖ Counseling on
  - – Importance of girl child
  - – Optimal timing and spacing of birth
  - – Small family norms
  - – Use and choice of contraceptives
  - – Prevention of sexually transmitted diseases and reproductive tract infections.
- ❖ Information on availability of
  - – Medical termination of pregnancy services.
  - – IUD and sterilization services.
- ❖ Family planning services
  - – Condom distribution
  - – Oral contraceptive dispensing
  - – IUD services.
- ❖ Recognition and referral of clients with sexually transmitted diseases and reproductive tract infections.

Provision of Clean and Safe Delivery Practices at the Community Level

- ❖ Creation of awareness in the community on need for clean and safe deliveries
- ❖ Deliveries by trained personnel
- ❖ Provision of Disposable Delivery Kits (DDK) for all deliveries
- ❖ Promotion of institutional deliveries
- ❖ Identification and referral of high-risk cases at the community level by trained dais.

Newborn Care

- ❖ Weighing all newborns. Normal birth weight is 2500 gm and above (2500–2800 gm). Babies whose weight is between 2000 and 2500 gm would require special care. Such babies are to be covered well with clothes, kept close to the mother, breastfed well and not to be handled by too many people to prevent infections. Newborns weighing less than 2000 gm to be referred to a specialist for further examination and management.
- ❖ Resuscitation of asphyxiated babies— removal of means with a mucus sucker and mouth-to-mouth breathing, if required.

❖ Prevention of hypothermia—wiping dry, covering well with soft clean cloth or baby blanket
❖ Exclusive breastfeeding within one hour of delivery
❖ Referral of newborns who show signs of illness
❖ Advice to mother on essential newborn care, which includes:
  – Prevention of hypothermia and infections
  – Nutrition (breastfeeding)
  – Vitamin A prophylaxis
  – Detection of early signs of illness and management.

Immunization

❖ BCG: One dose at birth
❖ DPT: Three doses, beginning at 6th week at monthly interval
❖ Polio: '0' dose at birth for all institutional deliveries and three doses beginning at 6th week at monthly interval
❖ Measles: One dose at completion of 9 months
❖ Vitamin A: First dose (100,000 IU) with measles vaccination.

Children (1–3 Years)

Immunization

❖ DPT/OPV booster dose at 16th to 18th month
❖ Vitamin A
  – 2nd dose (200,000 IU) at 16th to 18th month along with DPT/OPV booster
  – 3rd to 5th dose (200,000 IU each) at 6 monthly intervals.

Children (3–5 Years)

❖ Iron and folic acid tablets (small) for children with signs of anemia
❖ Treatment for worm infestation with mebendazole.

Prevention of Deaths due to Diarrheal Diseases

❖ Correct management of all cases of diarrhea.
❖ Teach mothers:
  – To increase the volume of fluids (ORS) as soon as diarrhea starts
  – How to prepare ORS solution
  – To continue feeding the normal diet
  – To recognize when to seek help.

Prevention of Deaths due to Pneumonia

❖ Correct management of all cases of acute respiratory infections
❖ Referral of children with severe pneumonia or very severe illness.

BIBLIOGRAPHY

1. Menon MKK. Journal of Obstetrics and Gynecology in India 1969;15:113.
2. Ministry of Health and Family Welfare. Manual for Orientation for Auxiliary Nurse Midwives and Supervisors, Reproductive and Child Health Approach. New Delhi, 1996.
3. National Institute of Health and Family Welfare. Reproductive and Child Health, Module for Staff Nurses' (PHC/CHC), Integrated Skill Development Training, NIHEW, Munirka, New Delhi, 2001.
4. Park K. Park's Textbook of Preventive and Social Medicine, 16th edn. Jabalpur: M/s Banarasidas Bhanot Publishers, 2000.
5. UNICEF/WHO. Joint Committee on Health Policy 1987.
6. WHO Chronicle, 1977;32:231.
7. WHO Report of Training Courses on Organization of MCH Field Practice Programs, SEA/MCH, 1969.

SECTION

11

Special Topics

51

Pain Relief and Comfort in Labor

Learning Objectives

Upon completing this chapter, the learner will be able to:

❖ Identify the factors affecting perception of pain and individual reactions to it
❖ Identify the causes of pain during labor and delivery
❖ Discuss the effects of various pain relief methods on the well-being of the fetus
❖ Describe the advantages and disadvantages of the various methods of analgesia and anesthesia for use during labor and delivery
❖ Identify the nonpharmacological methods of pain relief that are effective for laboring women.

Most women expect and experience pain in labor and childbirth. Pain is a subjective experience, and it is whatever the woman says it is for her (Neeson, 1987; Martin, 1990). Labor pain is often described as the most intense ever experienced, and in many cases, it is the aspect of childbirth most feared by the expectant mother. Physical, psychological and cultural factors play an important role in the woman's response to childbirth, although the intensity of pain, experienced, varies a great deal from one woman to another.

Pain is managed in various ways, according to the following indicators; the frequency, duration and intensity of uterine contractions; the character of labor, the woman's emotional behavior, her response to pain; the dilatation of cervix, the condition of mother and fetus, the skill, attitude and experience of health care team, and the preferences of the woman and her family. Pain relief ranges from none or very mild sedation to regional anesthesia to heavy sedation and/or anesthetic medication. When considering any form of analgesia or anesthesia, the safety of the mother and fetus are paramount. Pain relief in labor presents unique problems. Sedatives and anesthesia cross the placenta and can cause respiratory distress in the fetus (Cunningham, MacDonald and Grant, 1989). Unlike its use in surgery, which is brief, obstetrical analgesia may be needed for as long as 12 hours. In addition, since labor begins without warning, the woman invariably has not had sufficient time to empty her gastric contents, leading to the threat of aspiration of vomitus. Therefore, the risks versus benefits of pain relief in labor must be carefully weighed prior to its administration. 'Comfort' in labor is not merely an emotional or physical relieving of malaise and pain. It is a complex process in which the midwife combines research-based knowledge and skills, with warmth, empathy and sensitivity in order to provide a birth environment, which is safe, caring and conducive to a satisfying birth experience (Page, 1995).

PERCEPTION OF PAIN

The way in which an individual perceives and reacts to pain is affected by many different factors (Moore, 1997).

❖ *Fear and anxiety*: This will heighten the individual's response to pain (Simkin, 1986). Fear of the unknown, fear of being left alone to cope with an experience such as labor and fear of failing to cope well will increase anxiety. A previous bad experience will also increase anxiety

❖ *Personality*: The woman who is naturally tense and anxious will cope less well with stress than one who is relaxed and confident

❖ *Fatigue*: The woman who is already fatigued by several hours of labor, perhaps preceded by a period when sleep was disturbed by the discomforts of late pregnancy, will be less able to tolerate pain

❖ *Cultural and social factors*: Some cultures expect fortitude in suffering while others encourage expression of feeling (Schott and Henley, 1996). The perception of pain may be altered if the woman has experienced pain and hardship previously

❖ *Expectations*: The woman who is realistic in her expectations of labor and about her likely response to it is probably the best equipped, as long as she feels confident that she will receive the help and support she needs and is assured that she will receive appropriate analgesia.

CAUSES OF PAIN

During the first stage of labor, pain occurs due to dilatation of the cervix, hypoxia of the uterine cells during contractions, stretching of the lower uterine segment and pressure on adjacent structures (Ladewig, London and Olds, 1990). Initially contractions are felt in the lower back, and then progress to the lower torso in the back and abdomen.

In the second stage of labor pain is due to hypoxia of the contracting uterine muscle cells, distension of the vagina and perineum, and pressure on adjacent structures.

During delivery, there is often a decrease in pain, although many women describe the sensations of stretching, splitting or burning. Most third-stage pain results from contractions and cervical dilatation as the placenta is expelled. After the third stage, anesthesia is needed primarily for episiotomy repair.

Analgesics and Anesthesia

In the recent years, with the family involvement in childbearing, the use of anesthesia and analgesia has diminished to some extent. Approaches to labor and delivery has been shifting from "always medicate" to "rarely medicate" in the western world. The practice of obstetrics now takes a middle of the road approach and the value of anesthesia and analgesia is in the process of re-evaluation (Karpen, Conrad and Chitwood, 1995).

Analgesics and their Fetal and Maternal Side Effects

When cervical dilatation and uterine contractions cause discomfort, a narcotic such as Demerol (meperidine) and a tranquilizer such as promethazine, usually are indicated (Cunningham, MacDonald and Gant, 1989). Administration is either by intramuscular (IM) or intravenous (IV) route. The advantage of the IM or subcutaneous injection is that this is the fastest route in regard to midwife time and observation. The disadvantages include the length of time it takes for the drug to cause relief of pain, the danger of the drug's crossing the placental barrier and affecting the fetus, and unequal absorption of the drug. The advantage of the IV route is prompt pain relief with predicable results and that small amounts can be given in equally divided doses. The disadvantage of IV administration is the possibility of a bolus, but if given in the correct manner this is not of concern.

Commonly used narcotic analgesics include the following:

❖ *Meperidine hydrochloride (Demerol)* is typically administered IV in 12.5 to 25 mg doses (with 50 mg maximum) and IM in 75 mg doses (with 100 mg maximum). Pain relief usually occurs within 10 minutes after IV administration. Maternal side effects include central nervous system depression, especially respiratory, nausea, vomiting and/or dry mouth, drowsiness, dizziness, flushing, transient hypotension, tachycardia, palpitation and convulsions. Fetal/newborn side effects include neonatal hypotonia and lethargy, interference of thermoregulatory response for up to 72 hours after delivery, neonatal respiratory depression, neurologic and behavioral alterations for up to 72 hours postdelivery and depressed attention and social responsiveness for the first six weeks of life

❖ *Meptazinol* has similar analgesic and sedative property as that of pethidine. It causes less respiratory depression of the newborn

❖ *Pentazocin (Fortwin)*: It is given intramuscularly in a dose of 30 to 40 mg. Its duration of action is shorter and causes some respiratory depression. It also causes some drug dependence

❖ *Butorphanol (Stadol)* is a synthetic narcotic agonist-antagonist analgesic. The typical dose is 2 mg IM every three to four hours. When given IV, lower doses are used. Its effects compare favorably to 40 to 60 mg of pethidine. Since it can cause respiratory depression, it is contraindicated in women with respiratory disease. Other side effects include sedation, nausea, dizziness, a clammy, sweaty sensation and a tendency to elevate cerebrospinal fluid pressure. Fetal side effects can include respiratory depression in the fetus. It must be used with great caution if premature delivery is expected. Nubain and Stadol must be used with extreme caution in women who are addicted to drugs, since narcotic antagonists can induce acute withdrawal symptoms in mother and fetus if the mother is addicted to heroin.

Patient Controlled Analgesia (PCA)

Narcotics can be administered by the mother herself from a pump at an intermittent demand rate through intravenous route. This offers better pain control than high doses given at long intervals by the midwife. Client satisfaction is high with this method. Drugs commonly used are Demerol (meperidine), and fentanyl.

Assessment and Intervention

Nursing intervention in pain relief should start with nonpharmacological methods, which will be discussed later in this chapter. For some women however, those methods will not bring adequate relief, and increasing discomfort will interfere with their ability to perform breathing techniques and maintain a sense of control.

Under these circumstances, pharmacological analgesics may be used to decrease discomfort, increase the woman's ability to relax, and reestablish her sense of control. However, since analgesics will affect the mother, the fetus and the contraction pattern, the midwife must first assess the woman's vital signs to determine that they are stable and must establish that the woman is willing to receive analgesia after being advised about its effects. She should understand the type of medication being administered, its route of administration, its expected effects, its implications for the fetus/neonate, and the safety measures required for its use. The fetus must also be assessed to determine that the FHR is between 120 and 160 beats per minute with no late or variable decelerations present; normal accelerations are present with fetal movement, the fetus is at term and there is no meconium staining.

Labor assessment includes a well-established contraction pattern, cervical dilation of 4 to 5 cm in nulliparas and 3 to 4 cm in multiparas, engagement of the fetal presenting part and progressive descend of the fetal presenting part with no complications existing.

When administering analgesic drugs, careful and continuous observation of maternal respirations and FHR are mandatory, with baseline FHR and maternal vital signs recorded on the monitor strip (if on continuous monitoring) both before and after administration. The physician's written order is checked and the drug is prepared and signed out on the narcotic sheet. The woman's arm band is checked/the woman correctly identified and she is again asked if she is allergic to any drug. The drug is administered by the route ordered, and the medication, time, dosage and site of administration are charted on the nurse's notes. Safety precautions include side rails and continuous observation for nausea and vomiting, to prevent aspiration. While receiving analgesia, the woman should preferably be in an individual birthing or labor room, with the environment free from sensory stimuli. She should be encouraged to empty her bladder before drug administration, and she should not be left alone.

ANESTHESIA

Regional

Regional anesthesia is the injection of local anesthetic agents that block the transmission of painful stimuli from the uterus, cervix, vagina and perineum to the thalamic pain centers in the brain. The methods most often used in labor are the pudendal block, the paracervical block, the peridural (lumbar, epidural and caudal) block, subarachnoid or saddle block (spinal for cesarean birth, low spinal for vaginal delivery) and local infiltration. These blocks are accomplished by means of a single injection or continuously, by means of an indwelling plastic catheter. Paracervical and peridural blocks are used in the first stage of labor. During the second stage, pudendal, peridural or subarachnoid blocks are used.

Pudendal Block

Pudendal block consists of a local anesthetic agent injected around the pudendal nerve, which causes perineal analgesia. Used late in second stage, just before spontaneous or low forceps delivery of the infant, it provides anesthesia for birth and for repair of the episiotomies. It does not alter maternal or fetal respirations or other body functions, and does not affect uterine contractions. However, it may affect the woman's bearing down reflex and may cause broad ligament hematoma.

Paracervical Block

Paracervical block is accomplished by injecting a local anesthetic transvaginally, adjacent to the outer rim of the cervix. It may be administered during the active phase of labor, achieving rapid and complete relief of uterine pain during cervical dilatation. It does not anesthetize the lower vagina or the perineum and it does not interfere with the bearing down reflex. However, it has several maternal disadvantages, including systemic toxic reaction and uterine vessel damage leading to severe hematoma. Fetal risks include bradycardia, acidosis and death. Because of these risks, electronic fetal monitoring is indicated. Paracervical blocks are used infrequently.

Peridural (Epidural) Anesthesia

Peridural (epidural) anesthesia, which can be used during the first or second stages of labor, consists of injecting an anesthetic agent into the extradural space. It does not penetrate the dura or the spinal cord, and may be administered into the caudal space within the sacrum or into the epidural space at the second, third or fourth lumbar interspace. It may be given by a single injection or by continuous injection over several hours. A small amount relieves the discomfort of uterine contractions, while a larger dose extends anesthesia to the vagina. An additional dose may be given to provide perineal anesthesia.

Its advantages are that it can be given during active labor, providing effective pain relief during uterine contractions and cervical dilatation. It also enhances the woman's rest, relaxation and ability to cope. However, it has several disadvantages; if given too early, it may slow labor, and may result in maternal hypotension and decrease in placental bloodflow. The second stage of labor may be lengthened, since the mother does not feel the bearing down sensation, thus possibly requiring a forceps delivery. It may interfere with the woman's ability to void and it may cause infection. In addition, the dura mater may be punctured, resulting in inadvertent spinal anesthesia. Epidural anesthesia is contraindicated when maternal hemorrhage is present or likely to occur, in the presence of local infection at the injection site, and when the woman has cardiac, pulmonary or central nervous system disease.

Spinal Anesthesia (Subarachnoid)

Spinal anesthesia (subarachnoid) involves the injection of a local anesthetic directly into the spinal fluid, providing anesthesia for vaginal or cesarean delivery. For vaginal delivery, it is given late in the second stage, when the fetal head is on the perineum. It has no effect on maternal or fetal respirations but may cause temporary hypotension and a postspinal maternal headache. A spinal block eliminates the bearing-down reflex, but proper patient preparation will usually allow for spontaneous delivery. If not, forceps are easily applied due to perineal relaxation. Its advantages are simplicity, rapidity of action, high success rate, and a low incidence of maternal and fetal side effects.

Contraindications include: Severe hypovolemia, central nervous system disease, infection at the puncture site, severe hypotension or hypertension, cephalopelvic disproportion, and fear of the procedure (Karpen, Conrad and Chitwood, 1995).

Advantages and Disadvantages of Regional Anesthesia

Regional anesthesia has become increasingly popular due to its compatibility with the goals of psychoprophylactic preparation for childbirth. Its many *advantages* include the following:

The area blocked is completely relieved from pain, depression of maternal vital signs is rare and aspiration of gastric contents is eliminated when no additional sedative is given, administration does not alter the course of labor, and the woman remains alert and able to participate in the birth.

The *disadvantages* of regional anesthesia include the high degree of skill required for its administration, the possibility of failure to adequately block pain, the side effects of some agents and the possibility of systemic toxic reactions which can range from mild symptoms to cardiovascular collapse. Mild reactions include palpitations, vertigo, tinnitus, apprehension, confusion, headache, and a metallic taste in the mouth. Moderate reactions include more intense degree of the above-mentioned mild symptoms plus nausea; vomiting, hypotension and muscle twitching that can lead to convulsions and loss of consciousness, coma, severe hyotension, bradycardia, respiratory depression, and cardiac arrest. Because of the possibility of adverse reactions, regional anesthetics should always be used with an intravenous line in place.

Nursing Considerations

Nursing considerations during the administration of regional anesthesia include the following:

* Support for the laboring woman, encouraging her participation in decision-making.
* Continuous monitoring of vital signs and fetal status.
* Adequate knowledge of medications, their proper dosages, possible complications, early signs and symptoms of complications and actions to initiate in the event of untoward reaction until the arrival of appropriate medical personnel.

Actions Specific to Blocks

* *Paracervical*: Assess maternal blood pressure, pulse and fetal heart rate, assure continuous FHR tracing, assess maternal bladder.
* *Epidural*: Initially assess maternal blood pressure and pulse and the fetal heart rate for baseline. An electronic fetal monitor must be used for continual tracing. Maternal blood pressure and pulse are assessed every two minutes during the first 15 minutes after the injection, and every 10 to 15 minutes until stable. Assess bladder at frequent intervals for distention after delivery. Delay ambulation until all motor control has returned. Assess for orthostatic hypotension.
* *Spinal*: Assess maternal vital signs and fetal heart rate for baseline. Assist with positioning during administration. Assess for uterine contractions and inform anesthesiologist. Place a wedge under patient's right hip to tip the uterus off the vena cava. Assess maternal blood pressure and pulse every 2 to 5 minutes until stable and continue to monitor contractions. Provide safety and prevent injury when moving the patient. Provide bed rest for 6 to 12 hours following delivery.
* *Pudendal*: Provide support and assess for development of hematoma.
* *Local infiltration*: Provide support and assess for perineal trama, such as swelling or bruising.

General Anesthesia

General anesthesia is inhalation anesthesia, which provides pain relief through the administration of a gaseous agent mixed with oxygen and inhaled until the client becomes unconscious. Its advantages are that it produces overall relaxation, which is useful in difficult forceps deliveries, breech and cesarean sections. The likelihood of convulsions in pre-eclamptic or eclamptic women is reduced when general anesthesia is administered and perhaps its greatest advantage is that it can be administered rapidly in emergencies when delivery must be immediate and pain relief is essential. However, its disadvantage is that delivery must occur within 5 to 7 minutes after administration, because inhalation anesthesia crosses the placenta quickly and can cause hypoxia and respiratory depression in the fetus. There is always risk of maternal aspiration of gastric contents, which can result in pulmonary complications and immediate postpartum recovery is more complicated due to the risks of nausea, vomiting, uterine atony and postpartum hemorrhage. With this type of anesthesia, the bearing-down reflex is stopped, and the mother cannot participate in the birth nor can she interact with the baby immediately following birth.

General anesthesia is used today because of previous complications or high-risk problems due to pregnancy. Women whose regional anesthesia is ineffective, those with pregnancy-induced hypertension, prolapsed cord; severe bleeding or fetal distress with a second twin may be candidates.

Contraindications for general anesthesia are fetal prematurity or distress, maternal upper respiratory infection, multiple births, and if the woman who has eaten before administration.

The patient receiving general anesthesia requires preoxygenation, IV fluid loading, and tracheal protection with cricoid pressure to prevent aspiration and a pelvic tilt for maximum uterine circulation to the fetus. The midwife attending the patient under general anesthesia must observe the fetal heart rate constantly, while monitoring maternal vital signs and checking for uterine bleeding. Although it may slow down uterine contractions, general anesthesia can also relax perineal musculature and cause rapid expulsion of the fetus, for which the midwife must be alert.

Types of General Anesthesia

Nitrous oxide (Entonox): The anesthetic, which is 40 percent nitrous oxide and 60 percent oxygen, is administered by facemask or inhaler. Its induction is fast and pleasant and it is non-irritating, nonexplosive and less disruptive of physiological functions than any other general anesthetic. Its main use is in the second stage of labor, as an induction agent or as a supplement to more potent general anesthesia.

Halothane (Fluothane): Not used as frequently as nitrous oxide, halothane nevertheless bears mention for obstetrical anesthesia. Its induction is rapid, predictable and safe, since it causes little or no nausea or vomiting. It provides moderate to good uterine relaxation, although it may cause respiratory depression as well as irritability of cardiac tissue, which can result in arrhythmia. It may also cause increased uterine contraction along with the risk of postpartum hemorrhage.

Methoxyflurane (Penthrane): Administered by inhaler for analgesia or in combination with other agents for anesthesia, methoxyflurane induction is pleasant but slower than with gas agents. Uterine contraction may result from its use and administration is restricted to low doses for short periods because of the risk of postpartum bleeding.

Thiopental sodium (Pentothal): This ultra short-acting barbiturate is given intravenously and it produces narcosis within 30 seconds. Induction and emergence are smooth and pleasant, with little nausea or vomiting. It is most frequently used for induction or as an adjuvant to more potent anesthetics.

Recovery

The recovery period from general anesthesia requires particular vigilance from the midwife. If the woman is conscious, her physiological and psychological well-being demand that she be with her baby and significant other. At the same time, the midwife must monitor temperature, blood pressure, pulse and respiration while watching for bleeding, checking uterine tone, and observing bladder filling. Vital signs and observations of the uterus, bladder and episiotomies or abdominal incision must be recorded every 15 minutes. The recovery period is generally of two hours.

Balanced Anesthesia

Today's trend is toward "balanced anesthesia" for both vaginal and cesarean births. This is achieved by giving several different agents by different routes, which increases effectiveness and safety. Because of the combined effect, smaller doses can be given of each agent than if given separately. For example, IV thiopental sodium may be given for sedation and induction, followed by halothane by facemask for analgesia and anesthesia.

NONPHARMACEUTICAL METHODS OF PAIN RELIEF

Gate Control Theory

According to the gate control theory, pain is the result of interactions between several specialized neural systems. This theory postulates that a mechanism in the dorsal horn of the spinal column serves as a valve (or gate) that can increase or decrease the flow of nerve impulses from the periphery to the central nervous system. The gate mechanism is influenced by the size of the fibers that transmit impulses and by the impulses that descend from the brain. Pain perception and response may activate the gate system and influence psychological processes, including experiences, attention and emotion. Therefore, according to the theory, the gates can either be opened or closed by central nervous system activities such as anxiety or excitement or through selective localized activity.

The gate control theory, as it applies to obstetrics, has vast implications. It suggests that pain can be controlled by tactile stimulation and can be modified by activities controlled by the central nervous system. These include back rub, sacral pressure, suggestion, distraction and conditioning. Abdominal effleurage, a specific type of cutaneous stimulation, is used before the transitional phase of labor. It consists of light abdominal stroking. It is used in the Lamaze method of childbirth preparation. It is particularly effective in relieving mild-to-moderate pain but is ineffectual for intense pain. The application of deep pressure over the sacrum is more effective for relieving back pain.

Other nonpharmaceutical methods of pain relief include acupuncture, acupressure, therapeutic touch, transcutaneous electrical nerve stimulation (TENS), bathing or showering, warmth and positioning.

Acupuncture

Acupuncture has been widely used in the orient for many years, and there is increasing evidence that it may be an effective tool during labor. In some cultures, women have pressed combs into the palms of their hands to reduce the pain of contractions. Similarly, acupuncture involves the insertion and rotation of needles on specific points of the body, which is thought to produce analgesia and sedation through the release of beta-endorphin. However, acupuncture is an invasive technique that may cause infection.

Acupressure

Also long used in the Orient, acupressure is thought to activate the release of endorphins in the body. It is defined as finger pressure or massage over "pain prevention (or acupressure) points", and is another form of touch therapy. Proponents of the gate control theory speculate that the acupressure's pain relieving qualities are based on blocking the gate at the level of the spinal cord.

This technique is now taught in many childbirth education classes in the developed countries.

Acupressure may be used to alleviate some of the common discomforts of pregnancy, such as dizziness, faintness, headache or sciatic nerve pain and leg cramps. In labor, acupressure is used as a part of pain control routine that includes relaxation, concentration and rhythmic breathing.

Contraindications to this technique include any site where there is red, swollen, broken or infected skin and selected points that should not be used during pregnancy because of the potential to induce labor.

Yoga and Meditation

These are claimed to have calming effect, assist the mother in becoming attuned to her body, and give a focus for distraction from pain and tension.

Therapeutic Touch

Throughout history, people have used touch (the ancient art of laying-on of hands) as a means of calming a person. Now, according to researchers, there is evidence of an actual transfer of energy taking place in some forms of touching, as evidenced in muscular relaxation. Therapeutic touch offers several advantages. No devices are required, no physician's order is needed, the technique is noninvasive, and it incurs no cost since the technique is incorporated into nursing care. Indeed, there has been extensive research by nurses into the background and application of therapeutic touch, which was originally, described by a nurse—Dolores Krieger. The technique has no religious base and requires only the conscious intent of the healer.

Therapeutic touch may offer a powerful means of enhancing relaxation, reducing anxiety, and controlling pain. It can be of help to couples increase their communication and alleviate the discomforts of pregnancy. During labor and birth, it is used along with breathing and other relaxation strategies; and in the early months of parenting, it is frequently used as a means of calming a crying baby, relaxing a distraught parent or helping a woman through "postpartum blues". Therapeutic touch can benefit not only the client, but also the healer through enhancing her sense of inner harmony, well-being and relaxation, enabling her to cope while healing. Touch is a means of making coping skills more powerful and effective.

Transcutaneous Electrical Nerve Stimulation (TENS)

This method of alleviating pain by electrical nerve stimulation generally require the services of a physiologist or other professional. Although TENS is widely used outside obstetrics, its use in labor is questionable. It may interfere with continuous electronic fetal monitoring, since it must be applied constantly to gain relief. Moreover, it is most effective only if introduced before crisis.

Bathing, Showering, Warmth

During the early stage of labor, bathing or showering may afford a measure of pain relief for the woman. No physician's order is needed for showering. Whichever method is employed, the midwife should remain in close attendance to avoid the possibility of accidents and hyperthermia. The midwife must also be alert to the mother's need for bodily warmth in cold climates and should provide blankets as needed or keep the room temperature at a comfortable level as appropriate.

POSITIONING

The midwife should encourage the laboring woman to assume whatever position she finds most comfortable. However, any position used during labor and delivery should facilitate the alignment of the presenting part to the axis of the pelvis, and should encourage the mother's effort towards accomplishing delivery.

Women may require help to find positions, which are comfortable for them. Leaning forward with the arms resting on a convenient windowsill, table or shelf during a contraction may help the woman cope with backache. A rocking chair provides a soothing, rhythmic distraction during contractions, the motion probably encourages release of endogenous opioids, and most rocking chairs give good support to the back. A reclining chair also gives good support, but a recumbent position should be avoided because of the risk of aortocaval occlusion. Birthing beds and chairs are designed specifically for women in labor and most are very versatile. Ideally, they are used for delivery only and the woman is encouraged to walk about and use alternative positions during the first stage of labor.

An alternative position may be described as any position other than recumbent, semirecumbent or sitting on the bed; the woman follows her natural instincts and finds a position and movements, such as pelvic rocking which feel right for her, making use of gravity to assist descend of the presenting part. An upright or kneeling position also allows maximum "give" of the pelvic girdle, whereas sitting causes pressure over the sacrum and coccyx. Any woman in normal labor may benefit from freer mobility.

During delivery, the upright position was considered normal in most societies until recent times, and only within the past two centuries has the recumbent (lithotomy) position been used, mainly for the convenience of the physician or midwife. Now some countries have accepted alternative positions based on the comfort of the laboring woman. These include sitting in a birthing chair, semi-Fowler's position, and left lateral Sims's position, squatting and sitting in a birthing bed.

In active birth, the woman participates fully in her labor, is very aware of all that is going on in her body and aims to respond to these events naturally. She will have to prepare herself during her pregnancy by exercising. She will not wish to have any form of medical intervention if this can be avoided.

HYGIENE AND COMFORT

The woman in labor will become very hot and will perspire profusely. If she is able, she will prefer a bath or shower. If the woman is not able to get up, she will appreciate frequent sponging, particularly of her face and neck with cold water. A clean, cool gown will be appreciated and a fan is comforting. Her mouth will feel much fresher if she can clean her mouth or have a mouthwash.

Care of the bladder and bowels is an important aspect of the mother's comfort. In helping the laboring woman to achieve pain relief, the midwife should focus on the body's natural resources and should emphasize supportive pain management techniques for labor and childbirth. The midwife must respect the woman's right to her feelings about pain medication and other aspects of labor and delivery. She must attempt to convey a realistic picture of the childbirth pain experience, assist the woman in her efforts to manage pain, and bolster her confidence, so that she can cope with the experience of childbirth.

BIBLIOGRAPHY

1. Bevis R. Pain relief and comfort in labor, In: Bennett RV, Linda KB. Myles Textbook for Midwives, 13th edn. Edinburgh: Churchill Livingstone; 1999.
2. Cunningham FG, MacDonald PC. Grant NF. Williams Obstetrics, 18th edn. London: Prentice Hall International; 1989.
3. Fairs PJ. Relieving Pain and Discomfort in Labor, The role of the Midwife, Nursing Times 1966; 62:599.
4. Field Peggy A. Relief of Pain in Labor, Canadian Nurse 1974;70:17-20.
5. Karpen M, et al. Essentials of Maternal-Child Nursing, 2nd edn. Western Schools Press, 1995.
6. Kemp S. The Diginity of Labor. Nursing Times 1970;66:1436.
7. Ladewig PW, et al. Essentials of Maternal-Newborn Nursing, New York: Addison-Wesley; 1990.
8. Martin E. Intrapartum Management Modules, Baltimore: Williams and Wilkins; 1990.
9. Moore S. Physiology of Pain, In: Moore S, Understanding Pain and its Relief in labor; Edinburgh: Churchill Livingstone; 1997.
10. Neeson JD. Clinical Manual of Maternity Nursing, Philadelphia: JB Lippincot; 1987.
11. Page L. Putting principles into practice, In: Page L, Effective Group Practice in Midwifery; Oxford: Blackwell Science; 1995.
12. Schott J, Henley A. Culture, Religion and Childbearing in a Multiracial Society; Oxford: Butterworth-Heinemann 1999.
13. Simkin P. Stress, Pain and Catecholamines in Labor, Part II, Birth 1986;13:234-40.
14. Thomton JA. The Relief of pain in Labor. Nursing Times 1961;16:1128.
15. Watson M. The Present Position of Pain Relief in Labor Part I, Nursing Mirror 1963;116:431-5.
16. Watson M. The present Position of Pain Relief in Labor Part II, Nursing Mirror 1963;116:447-52.

52

Childbirth Education and Preparation

Learning Objectives

Upon completing this chapter, the learner will be able to:

❖ State the goals of childbirth education and preparation
❖ Describe the different philosophical approaches to childbirth education
❖ Identify the role of the "coach" or support person
❖ Specify the responsibilities of the childbirth educator (midwife) in providing effective prenatal and parenting education.

Childbirth is one of the greatest events in every woman's life. Having had fantasies about pregnancy and motherhood, when confronted with the reality, many of them have doubt in their ability to cope with this great event in their lives. Influenced by family, friends and relatives, they get prepared in different ways as they approach the experience of childbirth. This preparation may be positive or negative, realistic or inaccurate.

At this time, the mother-to-be needs a lot of help for the realization and acceptance of childbirth as a normal physiological phenomenon. She needs to develop a healthy attitude towards pregnancy so that she might have a safe and emotionally satisfying experience of labor and a rapid recovery both mentally and physically in the puerperium. Realization of this need by the obstetricians led to the development of psychosomatic methods of preparation for childbirth.

NATURAL CHILDBIRTH APPROACH

Dr Grantley Dick Read originated the natural childbirth movement. He developed the method in 1933 in England. The basis of the program was the realization that childbirth was a normal physiological occurrence and as such should not be painful. He believed that the pain of labor and delivery was mental in origin. He attributed the cause of pain to culturally induced fear and anxiety. "The belief was that fear of labor and delivery was a learned response and fear created tension, which was responsible for the pain that occurred" (Chertock, 1961).

The physical exercise component of the Read's method was largely due to the work of Helen Heardman, a physiotherapist in England, who strongly supported Dr Read's contentions. She believed in the necessity of a healthy positive mental attitude in the prospective mother. She advocated a vigorous program of physical education in preparation for parturition. Thus, through the combined efforts of Dr Dick Read and Helen Heardman, education, psychological training, and physical exercise to enhance relaxation comprised the original natural childbirth program.

CHILDBIRTH PREPARATION PROGRAM

Childbirth education classes were developed for meeting women's pain-reduction needs during labor and delivery. Early contributors, such as Dick Read and Lamaze, formed the basis of today's childbirth education classes, which in addition to pain management is designed to help women cope with childbirth through active participation and increased decision-making. Childbirth education emphasizes making childbirth a more rewarding experience for the mother, her mate and her entire family.

GOALS OF EDUCATIONAL PROGRAMS

Antepartal education programs vary in content, leadership techniques and teaching methods (Ladewig, London and Olds, 1990). The ideal childbirth education program should help the woman/couple to cooperate through the "problem" of labor in a satisfactory manner to both. It should provide them with coping skills and impetus to practice what they have learned and it should encourage mutual participation. As the couple works toward assuming an active and independent role in the childbirth experience, they will learn to become more flexible and their potential for working together in future situations will be enhanced. Therefore, the objectives of childbirth education should include the following:

❖ Providing a supportive milieu
❖ Reducing anxiety
❖ Providing factual information
❖ Maintaining a focus on current concerns.

METHODS OF CHILDBIRTH PREPARATION

Read Method

This is a method of psychophysical preparation for childbirth designed by Dr Grantly Dick Read. It was the 'natural childbirth' program, a term coined by Dr Read. Dr Read held the view that childbirth is a normal, physiologic process and that the pain of labor and delivery is of psychogenic origin; the fear-tension-pain syndrome (fear causes tension which in turn causes pain). He countered women's fears with education about the physiologic process, encouraged a positive, welcoming attitude, corrected false information and led tours of the hospital before birth. In order to decrease tension, he developed a series of breathing exercises for use during the various stages of labor. To foster relaxation and optimal physical function in labor and in recovery after delivery, he incorporated a series of physical exercises to be performed regularly in classes and in practice at home during pregnancy. The woman is helped to manage labor and delivery using the Read method in the following way:

During the early and mid-first stage of labor, before cervical dilatation has reached 7 cm, contractions are 2 to 5 minutes apart and last for 30 to 40 seconds, the mother lies on her back with her knees bent. Abdominal breathing is used during contractions. Her hands are placed over her lower abdomen, fingers touching. She breaths slowly and deeply—in through her nose and out through her mouth. The abdominal wall rises with each inhalation, which she can feel with her hands. The rate of breathing is no more than six breaths in 30 seconds or 12 to 18 in one contraction.

During the late part of the first stage of labor, after 7 cm of cervical dilatation, the contractions are 1½ to 2 minutes apart and last for 40 to 60 seconds. Costal or diaphragmatic breathing is used during contractions. Her hands are placed on her sides over the ribs. She breaths in more shallowly feeling her ribs move sideways against her hands. Each breath is drawn in through her nose and exhaled through her mouth. The abdominal wall does not rise and fall with this kind of breathing. The rate of breathing is no more than six breaths in 30 seconds or 12 to 18 in one contraction.

At the end of first stage of labor, near full dilatation, contractions may be very strong occurring every 1½ to 2 minutes and lasting 60 to 90 seconds. The mother lies on her back with her knees bent. Panting respirations are used during contractions. The mother holds one of her hands on the sternum, which rises and falls as she pants lightly and rapidly through her mouth. Panting continues through the end of the first stage to full dilatation as the urge to push grows. Panting helps the woman to avoid pushing.

During the second expulsive stage of labor and after full dilatation of the cervix, the contractions occur every 1½ to 2 minutes, last for 60 to 90 seconds and are accompanied with an urge to bear down and push. The woman lies back with head and shoulders supported in a semisitting position. She is helped to draw her legs up, holding them with her hands behind the lower thighs, thighs on her abdomen and legs apart.

As each contraction begins, she raises her head, takes a deep breath, tucks her chin on her chest, blocks the escape of air from her lungs and bears down. During each contraction, she may need to blow the air out, refill her lungs and push again two or three times.

Throughout labor, the woman is helped to understand what is occurring and to participate and accept the experience in anticipation of the birth of the baby. Currently, many authorities that advocate the use of other aspects of the Read method strongly recommend that a woman in labor not lie on her back. Supine hypotension is frequently the result of this position, because the uterus can fall back occluding the vena cava and decreasing the volume of blood returned to the heart, thus reducing the volume of cardiac output. Maternal hypotension follows, resulting in decreased placental perfusion and an inadequate supply of oxygen to the fetus. Today, the woman using the Read method spends much of her labor lying on her side or in a semi-sitting position with her knees, back and head well supported.

Lamaze Method (Psychoprophylaxis)

A method of psychophysical preparation for childbirth was developed in the 1950s by a French obstetrician, Fernand Lamaze. It uses Pavlov's stimulus-response theory to decondition women in labor. His method of "painless childbirth" became popular in the 1960s and now it is one of the most frequently used methods of childbirth education in several countries. The classes consist of two components:

❖ Education to dispel fears, coupled with training to achieve relaxation of body musculature.
❖ Conditioning for labor, which is achieved through the development of consciously controlled activities that displace the pain sensations of contractions in the brain. Relaxation is achieved by means of breathing techniques for each stage of labor and by massage and counter pressure. Positioning is used as a means to assist in increasing maternal comfort and exercises to strengthen pelvic musculature are taught (Ladewig, London and Olds, 1990).

It requires classes, practice at home and coaching during labor and delivery, often by a trained coach called a "monitrice". The classes given during pregnancy, teach the:
❖ Physiology of pregnancy and childbirth
❖ Exercises to develop strength in the abdominal muscles and control of isolated muscles of the vagina and perineum
❖ Techniques of breathing and relaxation to promote control and relaxation during labor.

The woman is conditioned by repetition and practice to dissociate herself from the source of a stimulus by concentration on a focal point, by consciously relaxing all muscles and by breathing in a special manner at a particular rate, thereby training herself not to pay attention to the stimuli associated with labor.

Kind and Rate of Breathing Change with Advancing Stages of Labor

During the early part of the first stage of labor, when the cervix is dilated less than 5 cm and the contractions occur every 2 to 4 minutes lasting 40 to 60 seconds and are of mild to moderate strength, the mother does *slow chest breathing* during contractions. The abdominal wall does not move with respiration. She may perform an effleurage or rhythmic fingertip massage of her lower abdomen during the contractions. The rate of respiration is 10 or fewer breaths per minute increasing to 12 per minute as labor intensifies. A deep cleansing breath is taken before and after each contraction.

During the active part of the first stage of labor up to the transition to the second stage, the cervical dilatation is from 5 cm to nearly full dilation, the interval between contractions is 2 to 3 minutes and the duration of contraction is from 45 to 90 seconds. During this phase, the mother breathes *quietly and slowly in her chest*. The rate of her breathing varies with the strength of the contractions, increasing during a contraction to as fast as once a second at the peak slowing to once every six seconds as the uterus relaxes. She is coached to concentrate on the focal point and has selected to perform the effleurage of her abdomen to relax her perineal and vaginal muscles and to take a cleansing breath at the beginning and end of each contraction.

At the end of the first stage of labor, when the cervix is almost completely dilated and the contractions are strong, occurring every 1½ to 2 minutes and lasting 60 to 90 seconds, the mother begins to feel the urge to bear down and push during contractions. She avoids pushing before full dilatation by combining several *light, shallow breaths in the chest with short puffing exhalations* as the urge increases during contractions.

During the second stage of labor, the cervix is fully dilated and contractions are strong, frequent and expulsive. The mother's head and shoulders are supported on pillows. During contractions, she is helped to draw her legs back flexing the thighs against the abdomen, holding them behind the lower thigh with her hands. Her chin is tucked on her chest, the air is blocked from escaping from her lungs, her perineum is relaxed, and she bears down forcibly.

Depending on the strength of contraction, several pushes of 10 to 15 or more seconds may be possible during a contraction. As the head of the baby crowns, she is asked to *pant lightly* so that the head may be delivered slowly.

The advantages of the method include the need for little or no analgesia for pain relief and participation in the labor by the mother giving her a great sense of satisfaction at delivery. The father of the baby also benefits by participating in the birth of his baby.

Modified Lamaze Method

Childbirth educators have enhanced the Lamaze method by adding information on prenatal nutrition, infant feeding, cesarean birth and variations from the usual labor, discussions on sexuality and parenting and coping skills for the postpartum period (Table 52.1). The original Lamaze theory specified the presence of a female monitor (monitrice), now a father-husband coach is encouraged along with a medical attendant. The exercises have been modified to enhance comfort in pregnancy and birth. However, perhaps the most important modification involves a change in philosophy concerning the goals of expectant parents. The original Lamaze theory virtually demanded that in order to have a successful childbirth experience, the delivery was to be painless and without anesthetic. In many cases, the parturient that was unable to fulfill this goal was left with a feeling of inadequacy. Today childbirth educators encourage the couple to set their own goals, supplying them with the tools for accepting these goals while providing reassurance and information about other options for those who cannot achieve a pain-free and anesthetic-free delivery (Ladewig, London and Olds, 1990).

Bradley Method

A method of psychophysical preparation for childbirth developed by Dr Robert Bradley, involves education about physiology of childbirth, exercise and nutrition during pregnancy and techniques of breathing and relaxation for control and comfort during labor and delivery. The father is extensively involved in the classes and acts as the mother's "coach" during labor. Among the advantages of the method are its simplicity, the involvement of the father and the realistic approach to the efforts and discomforts of labor. This is also called the husband-coached childbirth.

Teaching Content

Childbirth preparation classes are designed to help the couple make informed decisions during the child bearing period and should contain information regarding changes in the woman and the development of the fetus. They are best conducted in chronological sequence, with both parents taught breathing and relaxation techniques, infant care and coping strategies.

First Trimester Classes

The content of the first trimester classes included the following—early gestational changes; self-care during pregnancy; fetal development and environmental dangers for the fetus; sexuality in pregnancy; birth settings; nutrition, rest and exercises;

Table 52.1   Content outline for Lamaze prepared childbirth classes

A. Theory of the Lamaze method.
B. Anatomy and physiology as they relate to:
   • Pregnancy
   • Labor and birth
   • The postpartum period (mother)
   • The newborn.
C. Emotional responses of expectant parents to:
   • Pregnancy experience
   • Childbirth experience
   • Early parenting experience (includes role changes).
D. Physical conditioning for childbirth:
   • Prenatal exercises
   • Posture/body mechanics
   • Guidelines for exercises.
E. Stages and phases of labor:
   • Overview
   • First stage
     – Latent phase
     – Active phase
     – Transition phase
   • Second stage
   • Third stage
   • Woman's physical responses
   • Woman's emotional responses
   • Coach's role.
F. Nonpharmacological Analgesia
   • Progressive relaxation
   • Touch relaxation
   • Imagery
   • Focusing techniques
   • Effleurage
   • Massage
   • Comfort measures (back rub, positioning etc.)
   • Support (role of the coach, hospital staff, physician or midwife).
G. Pharmacological analgesia and anesthesia
   • Types used (describe and explain)
   • How and when administered
   • Effects on mother and baby.

H. Breathing techniques
   • Respiratory theory and principles
   • Respiratory techniques
     – Slow paced
     – Modified paced
     – Patterned paced
   • Second stage expulsion
     – Physiologic techniques
     – Modified valsalva technique.
I. Birthing process
   • Vaginal birth
   • Cesarean birth
     – Indications
     – Procedure
     – Use of prepared childbirth techniques
     – Coach's role.
J. Variations in labor and birth
   • Amniotomy
   • Fetal monitoring
     – External
     – Internal
   • Induction and augmentation
   • Forceps and vacuum extraction
   • Episiotomies.
K. Hospital procedures
   • Admission
   • Labor and birth
   • Postpartum care (mother and baby)
   • Parent-infant interaction.
L. Other content
   • Nutrition
   • Infant feeding (breast or bottle)
   • Signs of premature labor (prevention of prematurity)
   • Grieving and loss of unexpected outcome
   • Postpartum "blues"
   • Family planning (contraception).

Source: Guidelines for developing a teaching plan, ASPO/Lamaze Teacher Certification Program for Childbirth Educators, Washington, DC, American Society for Psychoprophylaxis in Obstetrics, 1987.

relief measures for common discomforts of pregnancy and psychological changes in pregnancy. These classes should also highlight factors that place the woman at risk for preterm labor and discuss its signs and symptoms. The pros and cons of breastfeeding and bottlefeeding should be covered, since many women make their decisions regarding feeding before the third trimester.

breathing techniques and other measures that promote comfort and participation during the birth experience. Postpartum self-care should be taught, as well as early adjustment to parenthood and infant care including feeding, family nutrition, child health and safety, growth and development, infant stimulation and family development. A discussion of the car seat is important where applicable for child safety.

Second and Third Trimester Classes

Later classes should focus on preparation for labor, birth and early parenthood, stressing and allowing time for body conditioning, relaxation,

Refresher Courses

Refresher courses may be given for experienced mothers who have previously taken a course in prepared childbirth and who want to update their skills and knowledge. These classes may review the process of labor and delivery as well as methods of promoting comfort and participation during childbirth. They most often include a segment on sibling adjustment.

Cesarean Birth Preparation

With the increase in the proportion of cesarean deliveries, preparation for the possibility should be included in every childbirth education class. To help the couple avoid the feelings of anger, loss and grief that can occur with cesarean birth, it should be approached as a normal event, with the instructor stressing the similarities between it and vaginal birth. Information should be provided that will help a couple make personal choices and participate in the experience. The content should cover the details of a cesarean delivery and describe what the mother and father will feel as well as what they can do.

For the couple who know ahead of time that cesarean birth is planned (for instance, the handicapped woman or the woman with pelvic insufficiency) should receive more detailed cesarean preparation classes. The classes will also benefit those couples that anticipate a repeat cesarean birth. The instructor should stress that subsequent cesarean deliveries are often less painful than the first and for the woman whose first cesarean was preceded by a long or strenuous labor, there will be much less fatigue the second time around.

Prenatal Exercise Classes

A well conditioned body will perform better and more reliably under the stresses of labor than a body in poor physical condition (De Santo and Hassad, 1983). However, because of the body's changes during pregnancy, the pregnant woman must learn how to exercise safely and effectively to condition her body with minimum risk to herself and the fetus (Raff and Freisner, 1989). The goal of these exercises is to strengthen muscle tone in preparation for delivery and promote faster restoration of muscle tone after delivery.

The exercises taught include the pelvic tilt, abdominal exercises (tightening abdominal muscles in synchronization with respiration,

partial sit-ups, inner thigh exercises (done cross-legged in tailor position), and Kegel's exercises to strengthen the perineal muscles. An exercise prescription from the physician is encouraged. (For details on exercises, refer to Chapter 54).

EFFECTIVENESS OF PRENATAL EDUCATION

Prenatal education serves many purposes on many different levels. Although prepared childbirth does not preclude the use of medication when necessary, it allows for a decreased use of analgesics and anesthetics during labor, thereby lowering the probability of drug-related side effects to mother and baby (Raff and Freisner, 1989). It also intensifies the mother-father-child relationship by allowing for full participation in the birth process. It reduces fear, anxiety and pain by providing knowledge and understanding, helping to make the experience of parenthood one of joy. In sharing experience with other couples, lateral supports are strengthened, reducing the couples' feelings of isolation. The understanding gained concerning changes in the woman's body during pregnancy, labor and postpartum period provides a feeling of preparedness and calm. Added to this, are the benefits of increased circulation and respiratory exchange, a reduced perception of contractions as painful and increased confidence in the couple's ability to cope with the discomforts of labor.

As a counselor, teacher, professional and friend, the childbirth educator helps parents evaluate their feelings. Since pregnancy and childbirth are "normal crises of life", the educator helps parents gain internal as well as external resources for handling crises situations, which aids them in achieving a satisfactory and healthy adjustment. In the open and permissive classroom atmosphere, the educator encourages parents to examine their feelings and discuss how and why they react the way they do to situations. Through discussions and role-playing, the responsibility of learning to adjust is placed on the parents and the educator guides them through process of exploring their reactions and trying new ones. With the proper guidance, it becomes easier to choose appropriate responses in labor and cope with the stresses of the postpartum period.

ROLE OF COACH OR SUPPORT PERSON

Providing a supportive milieu is one of the most important functions of childbirth preparation programs. The childbirth coach, an integral member of the support team, goes to classes with the expectant mother, asks questions regarding issues of concern and uses the discipline of repetitive practice with the expectant mother to begin the process of conditioning (Ladewig, London and Olds, 1990). The coach's role is to help the mother use the techniques she has learned. During labor, the coach comforts and supports the woman with care-taking activities, such as soothing conversations, touching, staying close by giving back rubs, applying cool clothes to the face and forehead and maintaining eye contact. Using verbal clues, the couple practices together, the coach reinforces learned responses while encouraging and working with the laboring mother to achieve a satisfying birth experience. The coach is particularly important in helping the woman time her contractions, identifying the beginning of each one and breathing through it with her or encouraging and supporting her as she breathes.

ROLE OF THE CHILDBIRTH EDUCATOR

The childbirth educator has three responsibilities—assessment of parents, intervention and fulfillment of their educational needs (Raff and Freisner, 1989).

Assessment includes determining the accuracy and completeness of the parents' information regarding parenting, determining their misconceptions (if any) about the maternity role, determining their ability to understand information and instructions, assessing their motivation to learn and becoming familiar with any personal or cultural values that may influence their acceptance of information and their compliance with instructions.

Intervention may include conducting parents' classes, dispensing of literature (if any) appropriate to their level of understanding and educational level and individual counseling and teaching. Effectiveness of teaching is enhanced by:

- Choosing the time of optimum readiness for motivation to learn (for example, not teaching labor and delivery during the first trimester).
- Limiting the amount of new information given at one time.
- Summarizing and writing down points.
- Providing feedback mechanism to assess learning, such as asking clients to repeat the information, asking if they understand the material, and verifying their understanding by nonverbal clues; and providing an atmosphere where questions can be asked freely.

Educational Needs

- Anatomical and physiological changes in pregnancy
- The labor and delivery process
- Signs of labor, nutrition and signs of complications in pregnancy
- The rationale for early and regular prenatal care
- Safety precautions
- Hospital admission and daily routine procedures; hospital policies affecting mother-child interaction
- Planning and purchasing baby clothes and other materials
- Preparation for natural childbirth—exercises, hygiene and fetal development
- General health care and newborn care.

BIBLIOGRAPHY

1. Anderson KN, Anderson LE, Wanze WD. Mosby's Medical, Nursing and Allied Health Dictionary, 4th edn. Mosby, St. Louis, 1994.
2. Bing Elizabeth. Six Practical Lessons for an Easier Childbirth, New York, Bantom Books, 1967.
3. Chertock J. Psychosomatic methods of preparation for childbirth. American Journal of Obstetrics and Gynecology, 1967;98:698-707.
4. De Santo P, Hassid P. Evaluating Exercises, Childbirth Educator, American Baby, 1983.

5. Davis Clarence D, Morrone Frank A. An objective evaluation of a prenatal childbirth program. American Journal of Obstetrics and Gynecology, 1962;84: 1196-1201.

6. Dick Read G. Revelation of Childbirth: The Principles and Practice of Natural Childbirth, 2nd edn. London; William Heinemann, 1943.

7. Edwards Margo. Egostates and Stroking in Childbirth Experience, The Transactional Analysis Journal 1971;3-6.

8. Karpen M, et al. Essentials of Maternal-Child Nursing, 2nd edn. Western Schools Press, 1995.

9. Ladewig PW, London ML, Olds SB. Essentials of Maternal Newborn Nursing, New York: Addison-Wesley, 1990.

10. Raff B, Freisner A. Quick Reference to Maternity Nursing, Aspen Publishers, Rockville, 1989.

11. Read Dick Grantly. Childbirth Without Fear, New York: Harper and Row Publishers, 1972.

12. Sclare AB. Psychoprophylaxis in Obstetrics Nursing Times 1965;61:1373-4.

13. Yahia, Clement and Ulin. The theory and technique of psychoprophylactic preparation for childbirth American Journal of Obstetrics and Gynecology 1968;93:942-8.

53

Special Exercises for Pregnancy, Labor and Puerperium

Learning Objectives

Upon completing this chapter, the learner will be able to:

❖ Develop an insight into the postural and circulatory changes that may occur during pregnancy, which may lead to discomforts
❖ Discuss the measures for relaxation and relief of discomforts during pregnancy and labor
❖ Describe the posture for comfort in different positions in the prenatal period
❖ Describe the exercises that can be practiced during pregnancy
❖ Describe the exercises for relieving aches and pains following vaginal delivery and cesarean section.

Preparation for parenthood outlined in Chapter 52 includes information in physiology of pregnancy and childbirth as well as breathing and relaxation techniques, which the prospective parents can learn from a professional in a relaxed atmosphere. In such an atmosphere, prospective parents develop confidence to cope with pregnancy, labor and delivery. In this chapter, information related to postural and life-style changes and exercises for relief of discomforts during antenatal period, labor and postpartum period are explained.

POSTURAL CHANGES IN PREGNANCY

Accompanying the gradual weight gain in pregnancy and its centralizing distribution is the hormonal effect on ligamentous structures. These factors alter the posture of the pregnant women. The body's center of gravity moves forwards and when this is combined with stretching of weak abdominal muscles, it often leads to a subsequent hollowing of the lumbar spine with a rounding of the shoulders and poking chin. There is a tendency for back muscles to shorten and abdominal muscles to stretch, extra strain is placed on the ligaments and the result is backache, usually of sacroiliac or lumbar origin. Postural re-education, including correction of the 'pelvic tilt' should be taught. Advice relating to comfortable positions in sitting, standing, lying, general mobility and how to lift correctly must be given to avoid back pain.

POSTURE FOR COMFORT IN DIFFERENT POSITIONS

Sitting

The pregnant woman should choose a comfortable chair, which supports both back and thighs (Figs 53.1A and B). She should sit well back and if necessary, place a small cushion or folded towel behind the lumbar spine for additional comfort. The seat height should allow the feet to rest on the floor, or a small stool. If relaxing in an easy chair, the head can be supported and the legs elevated on stool.

Standing

The posture should be as tall as possible with both the abdomen and buttocks tucked in. Weight must be evenly distributed on both legs, to prevent undue strain on the pelvic ligaments and spread between the heels and the balls of the feet. A medium or low-healed shoes, which gives support, should be used; high heels should be avoided, as it will throw the balance

Figs 53.1A and B : Relaxation in sitting position

Figs 53.2A and B: Relaxation in lying position

of the pregnant woman too far forwards. Shoulders are to be down and relaxed to prevent thoracic aches.

Lying

Equal pressure on all parts of the body will lead to a good posture in lying with no undue strain on anyone area. Lying flat on the back should, be avoided as far as possible because of the danger of supine hypotension. Lying with two to three pillows to raise the head and shoulders, will avoid the risk. It may be more comfortable with an additional pillow under the thighs to reduce the tension behind the knees (Fig. 53.2A).

Side lying with pillows under the top arm and knee is usually a comfortable position in pregnancy (Fig. 53.2B).

Getting up from lying can be done by bending the knees, rolling on to one side, and then using the arms to push up into a sitting or kneeling position. This would avoid strain on both the back and the abdominal muscles.

Household Activities

Household tasks may be performed in a sitting position as much as possible. When activities are done in standing position, the working surface should be at the correct height to avoid the need to stoop and subsequent backache. For jobs at the floor level, kneeling position prevents lumbar strain (Figs 53.4A and B).

Lifting heavy objects should be avoided during pregnancy, if possible. If lifting is unavoidable, then the object must be held close to the body with the knees bent and the back kept straight (Fig. 53.3). This way the strain is taken by the thigh muscles and not those of the back. Twisting movements while lifting are dangerous and must not be performed.

Moderate exercises during pregnancy stimulates circulation, helps to keep joints flexible, creates good muscle tone and promotes a general scene of well-being (Jacobson et al, 1990). It has also been observed that women who exercise regularly during pregnancy have an improved course of pregnancy and compared to those who lead a sedentary lifestyle (Clapp, 1990).

Walking

Walking in the fresh air remains one of the most natural and simplest form of exercise and should be encouraged.

Fig. 53.3: Proper position for lifting

Figs 53.4A and B: Positions for changing baby's diaper: (A) Changing diaper in sitting position; (B) Changing diaper in standing position

Cycling

This is a good form of exercise, which allows for good mobility of the lower limbs with the bodyweight supported. Cycling when done should only be short distances and care must be taken to avoid steep areas. It is also advisable to stop before feeling tired.

Swimming

Swimming is another excellent exercise, as water relieves the effects of gravity on the body and muscles can be strengthened and flexibility of joints retained without undue fatigue. Light swimming with gentle supporting arm movements is often most comfortable. Strenuous strokes and diving should be avoided.

POSTURE FOR RELIEF OF ACHES AND PAINS

Back and Pelvic Pain

A good number of women experience backache at some stage of their pregnancy. Women who suffer backache can be helped by encouraging good posture and the practice of *pelvic tilting exercise* in standing, sitting and lying position. Sciatic-like pain may be relieved by lying on the side away from the discomfort, so that the affected leg is uppermost. Pillows should be placed to support the whole limb.

Cramp

Practicing foot and leg exercises can achieve prevention of cramp. To relieve sudden cramp in the calf muscles whilst in the sitting position, the woman should hold the knee straight and stretch the calf muscles by pulling the foot upwards (dorsiflexing) at the same time. Alternatively, standing firmly on the affected leg and striding forwards with the other leg will stretch the calf muscles and solve the problem.

Rib Discomfort

Discomfort around the rib cage can often be relieved by adopting a good posture or by specifically stretching one or both arms upwards, depending on which side the pain is present.

ANTENATAL EXERCISES

Muscles of good tone are more elastic and will regain their former length more efficiently and more quickly after being stretched than muscles of poor tone. Exercising the abdominal muscles antenatally will ensure a speedy return to normal postnatally, effective pushing in and the lessening of backache in pregnancy. The overstretched ligaments and weakened abdominal muscles during pregnancy can lead to chronic skeletal problems postnatally as well as backache antenatally. In order to prevent this and to maintain good abdominal tone, abdominal tightening and pelvic tilting exercises are to be taught.

Abdominal Tightening

The woman has to sit comfortably or kneel on all fours. Breathe in and out and then pull the lower part of the abdomen below the umbilicus while continuing to breathe normally. Hold upto ten seconds and repeat up to ten times.

This exercise strengthens the deep transverse abdominal muscles, which are the main postural support of the spine and will help to prevent backache in the future. When the woman masters this exercise, it can be practiced in any position whilst doing other activities.

Pelvic Floor Exercise (Kegel Exercise)

Sit, stand or half-lie with legs slightly apart. Close and draw up around the anal passage as though preventing a bowel action, then repeat front passages (vagina and urethra) as if to stop the flow of urine in midstream. Hold for as long as possible up to 10 seconds, breathing normally, then relax. Repeat up to ten times. All pregnant women should practice this exercise very regularly antenatally, particularly after emptying the bladder.

Foot and Leg Exercises

The circulation during pregnancy, particularly the venous return, is sluggish and this can lead to problems such as cramp, varicose veins and edema. To prevent these and to improve the circulation, the following simple exercises and advice will help.

Sit or half-lie with legs supported. Bend and stretch the ankles at least 12 times. Circle both feet at the ankle at least 20 times in each direction. Brace (hold tight) both knees for a count of four and then relax. Repeat 12 times.

These exercises should be performed before getting up from resting, last thing at night and several times during the day. Women should be discouraged from standing unnecessarily and encouraged to put their feet up whenever possible. Crossing the legs at the knee or ankle will impede circulation further. If varicose veins or edema is present, support tights or stockings may be worn before allowing the legs to drop over the edge of the bed.

Breathing Exercise

A few deeper breaths now and again can be done everyday. This will help the venous return and aid the oxygen supply to both pregnant woman and her fetus. Only three or four breaths are to be taken at a time. More deep breaths at one time can lead to hyperventilation.

POSITIONS FOR COMFORT DURING LABOR

Early First Stage of Labor

A woman in labor should be encouraged to keep mobile and active if there are no complications. She should be encouraged to try alternative positions of ease as alteration of position leads to productive uterine contractions (Roberts et al, 1983). When discomfort increases during contractions, the woman should be encouraged to stay relaxed and concentrate on rhythmical, easy breathing.

The following positions of ease may help during the early stages of labor and can be practiced in the antenatal period:

* Sitting against a table and relaxing forwards so that shoulders, arms and head are supported
* Standing, leaning backwards against the wall of the room
* Kneeling on the floor and leaning forwards against a chair
* Leaning forwards against a partner

❖ Sitting astride on armless chair with arms supported on the chair back and body relaxing backwards.

Pelvic rocking in any of these positions may be helpful. Deep massage of lower back or gentle stroking of the abdomen by the partner or coach sooths many women (Brayshaw in Bennett and Brown, 1999).

Later First Stage of Labor

As labor progresses, it becomes more difficult to find a comfortable position and frequent changes may be necessary. Some prepared women are content to sit back against pillows on the bed and concentrate on breathing and relaxation at this stage. If there is an urge to push, they must be encouraged to use an interrupted outward breath pattern that is two shorter breaths followed by a longer breath (Pant, pant, blow). This prevents the increase in intra-abdominal pressure. An alteration in position, such as the side lying, may take away some of the urge to push.

Second Stage of Labor

Position for second stage of labor will depend largely on the obstetric practice in the institution. In most places, women are delivered in supine position. However, alternative positions are possible, depending on the method of pain relief and obstetric factors. The positions that may be used include:
❖ Side lying
❖ Squatting on the bed
❖ Supported squatting with partner supporting from behind
❖ Sitting fairly upright against the back rest with knees bent and feet resting on the bed.
❖ Kneeling on all fours.

As the contraction starts, the mother is reminded to breathe in and out gently. When the urge to push becomes overwhelming, she will tuck in her chin and bear down, keeping the pelvic floor relaxed. Breath holding should not be encouraged because of the danger of fetal hypoxia in an already compromised baby (Caldeyro—Barcia, 1978). To prevent pushing

whilst the head is delivered, deep panting may be useful.

POSTNATAL EXERCISES

These should be started as soon after delivery as possible in order to improve circulation, strengthen pelvic floor and abdominal muscles and prevent transient and longterm problems (Brayshaw in Bennet and Brown, 1999).

Circulatory Exercises

Foot and leg exercises must be performed very frequently in the immediate postpartal period to improve circulation, reduce edema and prevent deep vein thrombosis. If edema is present, the foot of the bed may be raised slightly.

Pelvic Floor Exercises (Kegel Exercise)

The pelvic floor muscles have been under strain during pregnancy and stretched during delivery and it may be both difficult and painful to contract these muscles postnatally. Mothers should be encouraged to do the exercise (as explained in the antenatal section) as often as possible, in order to regain full bladder control, prevent uterine prolapse and ensure normal sexual satisfaction in future. The contraction should be held for ten seconds (to a count of six) and repeated up to ten times at any one session, breathing normally throughout.

The mother should continue to do this exercise for 2 to 3 months. After three months, if the mother is able to cough deep deeply with a full bladder without leaking urine (stress incontinuance), she may stop the exercise. If leaking occurs, she may to continue the exercise for the rest of her-life.

Abdominal Exercises

Abdominal muscles need to regain tone as soon as possible after delivery in order to protect the spine, prevent back problems and help the mother to regain her former figure. These include abdominal breathing, head and shoulder raising, leg raising, pelvic tilt, knee rolling, hip hitching and sit-ups.

Fig. 53.5: Abdominal breathing

Fig. 53.6: Head and shoulder raising exercise

Fig. 53.7: Leg raising exercise

Fig. 53.8: Pelvic tilt exercise

Abdominal Breathing

The mother is taught deep abdominal breathing to strengthen the diaphragm. This may be started on the first postpartum day. She is taught to take a deep breath, raising her abdominal wall and exhale slowly. To ensure that the exercise is being done correctly, place one hand on the chest and one on the abdomen. When inhaling, the hand on the abdomen should be raised and the hand on the chest should remain stationary. Repeat the exercise five times (Fig. 53.5).

Head and Shoulder Raising

On the second postpartum day, lie flat without pillow and raise head until the chin is touching the chest. On the third postpartum day raise both head and shoulders off of the bed and lower them slowly. Increase gradually until able to do ten times (Fig. 53.6).

Leg Raising

The exercise may be begun on the 7th postpartum day. Lying down on the floor with no pillows under the head, point toe and slowly raise one leg keeping the knee straight. Lower the leg slowly. Gradually increase to ten times each leg (Fig. 53.7).

Pelvic Tilting or Rocking

Lie flat on the floor with knees bent and feet flat. Inhale, and while exhaling, flatten the back hard against the floor so that there is no space between the back and the floor. While doing this, tighten abdominal muscles and the muscles of the buttocks. Inhale normally, hold breath for up to 10 seconds, and then relax. Repeat up to 10 times (Fig. 53.8).

Knee Rolling

This exercise will strengthen the oblique abdominal muscles and may be done only if there is no undue separation of the rectus muscles (diastasis of the rectus muscle). In back lying with knees bent, pull in the abdomen and roll both knees to one side as far as is comfortable, keeping shoulders flat. Return knees to and upright position and relax the abdomen. Pull in again and roll both knees to the other side. This exercise can be performed up to ten times.

Figs 53.9A and B: Hip hitching (up-drawing) exercise

Hip Hitching

Hip hitching or leg shortening is performed in back lying with one knee bent and the other knee straight. Slide the heel of the straight leg downwards thus lengthening the leg. Shorten the same leg by drawing the hip up towards the ribs on the same side. Repeat up to ten times, keeping the abdomen pulled in. Change to the opposite side and repeat (Figs 53.9A and B).

If the mother does these exercises faithfully and follows a sensible diet, she will most likely be able to regain her figure quickly (Clausen et al, 1973).

EXERCISES FOLLOWING CESAREAN SECTION

Foot and leg exercises as described earlier should be started as soon as possible, especially after epidural anesthesia, as distal circulation will be sluggish. These may be followed by not more than four deep breaths to ensure full expansion of the lungs and pumping action on the inferior vena cava. If a general anesthetic has been given, the mother may have extra secretions and needs to be taught how to clear them by coughing in a sitting position with the sutures supported by both hands and a pillow. Deep breathing and coughing will help loosen the secretions.

To ease backache and flatulence the *abdominal tightening, pelvic tilting* and *knee rolling* exercises can be practiced gently after 24 hours.

Mothers will progress to the pelvic floor exercises, head raising and hip hitching when they feel more comfortable, usually after 4 to 5 days if there is no undue separation of the rectus muscles. Pelvic floor exercises are still important following cesarean section even though the women in this group are less likely to suffer stress incontinence (Wilson, 1996).

Adequate rest is essential postnatally to allow the tissues to regain their normal function. After a cesarean section, the woman has not only given birth but has also undergone major surgery, yet she has to cope with her baby. The midwife must take every opportunity to remind relatives of the need to help with chores and the organization of rest periods for the mother.

Care of the Back Postnatally

It may take up to 6 months for the ligaments to completely resume their normal functions (Polden and Mantle, 1990). Therefore, it is vital that mothers receive advice on back care in relation to everyday activities during this period.

When feeding the baby, she should sit back in a chair, well supported, with the baby raised up on pillows to prevent a slouched forward position. Nappy changing and bathing of the baby are best carried out at waist level or with the mother kneeling at a coffee table height (*see* Figs 53.4A and B).

Lifting should be avoided if at all possible and the object should be as light as possible and kept close to the body. While lifting, the knees must be bent and back kept straight.

IMMEDIATE POSTNATAL PHYSICAL PROBLEMS

Diastasis Symphysis

This condition may be present in late pregnancy, occur during labor or appear after delivery (Fry, 1992). If the pain is severe, indicating complete separation of the pubic joint, complete bed rest with some support around the pubis is advised. The woman must be instructed to press her knees together when moving in bed. She should be encouraged to perform the abdominal tightening and pelvic tilting exercises plus circulatory exercises while she is resting. Mobilization of the woman may be allowed only when the acute pain has subsided. Therapeutic ultrasound, transcutaneous nerve stimulation or ice applications may be prescribed to relieve local pain.

Diastasis Recti

If the woman's rectus muscles are found more than two fingers width apart, the only exercises, which should be permitted, are abdominal tightening, pelvic tilting and head lifting. While performing head lifting, the woman should keep her hands crossed over the abdomen to support the muscles and draw them towards the midline.

Painful Perineum

This is a common problem and advice on positioning should be given plus analgesia and local pain-relieving measures, such as ice application. To avoid the possibility of local skin injury, ice should not be in direct contact with the skin. It may be crushed and placed inside a polythene bag or gauze and positioned against the painful area for no longer than 5 to 10 minutes. The woman will be most comfortable in side lying position and should be reminded not to sit on the ice pack, as the pressure would impede circulation. Alternatively, the perineum may be massaged for 5 to 10 minutes at a time by an ice cube, held in a disposable cloth or clean plastic bag. When the pain is less, pelvic floor exercises should be encouraged with the aim of increasing the local circulation.

Incontinence

Stress incontinence occurs in some women following delivery. Pelvic floor exercises will help to rehabilitate the pelvic floor, but the woman will usually require specific obstetric exercises prescribed by her physician.

Backache

Early postnatal backache is usually postural and can be relieved by warmth and pelvic tilting

exercises. Persistent and severe back pain if present, the woman will need physiotherapy.

Coccydynia

An acutely painful coccyx occasionally presents which may be incapacitating for a new mother. Placing pillow strategically may give some relief and alternative positions in feeding may be given. Specific physiotherapy or manipulation may be required for a displaced coccyx.

During pregnancy, labor and the puerperium, mothers should be influenced to incorporate a sensible approach to exercise. Relaxation, walking, cycling and other forms of exercises can be encouraged as part of a general lifestyle. Specific exercises for strengthening pelvic floor and abdominal muscles or relieving aches and pains such as cramps or backache, will be useful even beyond the months of childbearing.

BIBLIOGRAPHY

1. Brayshaw EM. Special exercises for pregnancy, labour and the puerperium, In: Bennett RV, Linda KB. Myles Textbook for Midwives, 13th edn. Edinburgh: Churchill Livingstone, 1979.
2. Caldeyro Barcia R. The influence of maternal position on labor and the influence of maternal bearing-down efforts in the second stage of labor on fetal well-being, In: Simkin PR. Kaleidoscope of Childbearing Preparation, Birth and Nurturing, Penny Press, Seattle, 1978.
3. Clapp J. The courses of labor after endurance exercise during pregnancy, American Journal of Obstetrics and Gynecology 1992;163(6):1799-1805.
4. Clausen JP, et al. Maternity Nursing Today, New York: McGraw Hill Book Company, 1973.
5. Fry D. Diastasis symphysis pubis, Journal of the Association of Chartered Physiotherapists in Obstetrics and Gynecology 1992;71:10-3.
6. Jacobson B, Smith A. The Nation's Health: A Strategy for the 1990s, London: Kings Fund, 1991.
7. Polden M, Mantle J. Physiotherapy in Obstetrics and Gynecology, London: Butterworth-Heinemann, 1990.
8. Roberts JE, et al. The effects of maternal position on uterine contractility and efficiency;Birth 1983;10:243-9.
9. Wilson PD. Obstetric practice and prevention of urinary incontinence, British Journal of Obstetrics and Gynecology 1996;103:154-61.

54

Drugs Used in Obstetrics

Learning Objectives

Upon completing this chapter, the learner will be able to
- Describe the use of oxytocic drugs and the nursing considerations related to each
- Describe the use of antihypertensive drugs for maternity clients
- Describe the use and nursing considerations for tocolytic agents
- Discuss the effects of maternal medications on fetus and breastfeeding infants.

Drugs commonly used for maternity clients, are described in this chapter. The midwife should have thorough knowledge of the indications, actions and side effects of these drugs as well as the nursing considerations related to each of them in order to plan and implement effective nursing process.

OXYTOCICS

Oxytocics are the drugs that have the power to excite contractions of the uterine muscles. Among a large number of drugs belonging to this group the ones that are important and extensively used are: oxytocin, ergot derivatives and prostaglandins.

Oxytocin

Oxytocin is an octapeptide synthesized in the hypothalamus and stored in the posterior pituitary.

Preparations

Synthetic oxytocin available for parenteral use include:
- Syntocinon 5 units/ml in ampoules of 1 ml.
- Pitocin 10 units/ml in ampoules of 0.5 ml
- Syntometrine: A combination of syntocinon 5 units and ergometrine 0.5 mg
- Oxytocin nasal solution 40 units/ml.

Actions
- Acts directly on myofibrils producing uterine contraction and stimulates milk ejection by the breasts.

Indications for Use

Pregnancy
- To induce abortion (inevitable, missed)
- To expedite expulsion of hydatidiform mole
- For oxytocin challenge test
- To stop bleeding following evacuation
- To induce labor.

Labor
- To augment labor
- In uterine inertia
- To prevent and treat postpartum hemorrhage.

Postpartum
- To initiate milk let-down in breast engorgement.

Contraindications

In late pregnancy
- Grand multipara
- Contracted pelvis
- History of cesarean section or hysterotomy
- Malpresentation.

During Labor
- All contraindications mentioned in pregnancy
- Obstructed labor
- Incoordinate uterine action.

Anytime

❖ Hypovolemic state
❖ Cardiac disease.

Adverse Effects

❖ Hypertonic uterine activity
❖ Fetal distress and fetal death
❖ Uterine rupture
❖ Hypotension
❖ Neonatal jaundice
❖ Water retention and water intoxication.

Dosage and Routes of Administration

❖ Controlled intravenous infusion (ten units of oxytocin in one liter of Ringers lactate or 5 percent dextrose in water)
❖ Nasal spray for milk let-down.

Nursing Considerations

Assess

❖ Intake and output ratio
❖ Uterine contractions and FHR
❖ Blood pressure, pulse and respiration

Administer

❖ By IV infusion
❖ After having crash cart (emergency trolley) available in the ward.

Evaluate

❖ Length and duration of contractions
❖ Notify physician of contractions lasting over one minute or absence of contractions.

Teach Client/Family

❖ To report increased blood loss, abdominal cramps or increased temperature.

Ergot Derivatives

Ergot alkaloids are either natural or semi-synthetic.

Preparations

❖ Ergometrine (Ergonovine) 0.25 mg or 0.5 mg ampoules and 0.5 to 1 mg tablets
❖ Methergine (Methyle-ergonovine) 0.2 mg ampoules and 0.5 to 1 mg tablets
❖ Syntometrine Ergometrine 0.5 mg + Syntocinon 5.0 units ampoules.

Ergometrine and methergine can be used parenterally or orally. As the drug produces titanic uterine contractions, it should only be used after delivery of the anterior shoulder or following delivery of the baby. It should not be used in induction of labor or abortion. Syntometrine should always be administered intramuscularly.

Mode of Action

❖ Ergometrine acts directly on the myometrium. It stimulates uterine contractions and decreases bleeding.

Indications

❖ *Therapeutic:* To stop the atonic uterine bleeding following delivery, abortion or expulsion of hydatidiform mole.
❖ *Prophylactic:* As a prophylaxis against excessive hemorrhage; it may be administered after the delivery of the anterior shoulder (active management of third stage), with crowning or following delivery of the baby.

Contraindications

❖ *Suspected plural pregnancy*: If given accidentally with the delivery of the first baby, the second twin is likely to be compromised by the titanic contractions of the uterus.
❖ *Organic cardiac disease*: It may cause sudden squeezing of blood out of the uterine circulation into the general circulation causing overloading of the right heart and precipitating failure.
❖ *Severe pre-eclampsia and eclampsia*: There may be sudden rise of blood pressure.
❖ *Rh-negative mother*: There is more chance of fetomaternal microtransfusion.

Note: For women with heart diseases or hypertension oxytocin is a better substitute.

Adverse Effects/Side Effects

❖ Because of its vasoconstrictive action, it may precipitate rise of blood pressure
❖ Prolonged use in puerperium may interfere with lactation by decreasing the concentration of prolactin
❖ Prolonged use may lead to gangrene of the toes due to its vasoconstrictive effect.

Nursing Considerations

Assess

❖ Blood pressure, pulse and respiration
❖ Watch for signs of hemorrhage.

Administer
- Orally or IM in deep muscle mass
- Have emergency cart readily available.

Evaluate
- Therapeutic effect: Decreased blood loss.

Teach Client/Family
- To report increased blood loss, abdominal cramps, headache, sweating, nausea, vomiting or dyspnea.

Prostaglandins (PGs)

Prostaglandins are synthesized from one of the essential fatty acids, arachidonic acid, which is widely distributed throughout the body. In the female, these are identified in the menstrual fluid, endometrium, decidua and amniotic membrane.

Preparations
- PGE_2—Prostin E_2 (dinoprostone)
- $PGF_2\alpha$—Prostin $F_2\alpha$ (dinoprost tromethamine)
- PGE_1—Misoprostol.

Actions

Both PGE_2 and $PGF_2\alpha$ have an oxytocic effect on the pregnant uterus. They also sensitize the myometrium to oxytocin. $PGF_2\alpha$ acts predominantly on the myometrium, while PGE_2 acts mainly on the cervix.

Indications
- For induction of abortion during second trimester and expulsion of hydatidiform mole
- For induction of labor in intra-uterine death of fetus
- In augmentation or acceleration of labor
- To stop bleeding from the open uterine sinuses as in refractory cases of atonic PPH
- Cervical priming.

Contraindications
- Hypersensitivity, uterine fibrosis, cervical stenosis, pelvic surgery, pelvic inflammatory disease, respiratory disease.

Side effects/adverse reactions
- Headache, dizziness, hypotension, leg cramps, joint swelling, blurred vision.

Dosage and Routes of Administration
- Tablets: Containing 0.5 mg Prostin E_2
- Vaginal suppository: Containing 20 mg PGE_2 or 50 mg $PGF_2\alpha$
- Vaginal pessary: Containing 3 mg PGE_2
- Injectable ampoules or vials of Prostin E_2, 1 mg/ml Prostin $F_2\alpha$, 5 mg/ml
- Misoprostol (PGE_1) 50 mg, given four hourly by oral, vaginal or rectal route for induction of labor.

Nursing Considerations

Assess
- Respiratory rate, rhythm and depth
- Vaginal discharge, itching or irritation indicative of infection.

Administer
- Antiemetic or antidiarrheal preparations prior to giving this drug
- High in vagina (if vaginal preparations are used)
- After warming the suppository by running warm water over package.

Evaluate
- For length and duration of contractions, notify physician of contractions lasting over one minute or absence of contractions
- Fever and chills.

Teach Client/Family
- To remain supine for 10 to 15 minutes after vaginal insertion.

ANTIHYPERTENSIVE DRUGS

Antihypertensive drugs are used in hypertensive disorders of pregnancy. The commonly used drugs are:
- Adrenergic inhibitors: Methyldopa
- Adrenergic blocking agents: Labetalol, propranolol
- Vasodilators: Hydralazine, Diazoxide, sodium nitroprusside
- Calcium channel blockers: Nifedipine.

Methyldopa

Preparations

❖ Aldomet, Dopamet.

Action

❖ Stimulates central α-adrenergic receptors or acts as false transmitter, resulting in reduction of arterial pressure.

Indication

❖ Hypertension.

Contraindications

❖ Active hepatic disease, congestive cardiac failure, blood dyscrasias, psychiatric disorders.

Side Effects/Adverse Reactions

❖ Nausea, vomiting, diarrhea, constipation
❖ Bradycardia, orthostatic hypotension, angina, weight gain
❖ Drowsiness, dizziness, headache, depression
❖ Leukopenia, thrombocytopenia Coombs' Test may be positive.

Dosage and Route of Administration

❖ Orally: 250 mg BID to 1 gm TID
❖ IV infusion: 250 to 500 mg.

Nursing Considerations

Assess
❖ Blood values: Neutrophils, platelets
❖ Renal studies: Protein, BUN, creatinine
❖ Liver function tests
❖ Blood pressure before beginning treatment and periodically thereafter.

Perform/Provide
❖ Storage of tablets in tight containers.

Evaluate
❖ Decrease in blood pressure (therapeutic response)
❖ Allergic reaction: Rash, fever, pruritis, urticaria
❖ Symptoms of congestive heart failure (edema, dyspnea, wet rales)
❖ Renal symptoms: Polyuria, oliguria, frequency.

Teach Client/Family
❖ To avoid hazardous activities
❖ Administer one hour before meals
❖ Not to discontinue drug abruptly or withdrawal symptoms may occur
❖ Not to use over the counter (OTC) medications (non-precription) for cough, cold or allergy, unless directed by physician
❖ Compliance with dosage schedule even if feeling better
❖ To rise slowly to sitting or standing position to minimize orthostatic hypotension
❖ Not to skip or stop drug unless directed by physician
❖ Notify physician of untoward signs and symptoms.

Labetalol

Preparations

❖ Trandate, Normodyne.

Action

❖ Nonselective β blocker.

Indication

❖ Hypertension.

Contraindications

❖ Hepatic disorders, sinus bradycardia, bronchial asthma.

Side Effects/Adverse Reactions

❖ Orthostatic hypotension, bradycardia, chest pain, ventricular dysrhythmias, drowsiness, headache, nightmares, lethargy, agranulocytosis, thrombocytopenia, sore throat, dry burning eyes.

Dosage and Routes of Administration

❖ Orally: 100 mg TID up to 800 mg daily
❖ IV infusion (Hypertensive crisis): 1 to 2 mg/min until desired effect.

Nursing Considerations

Assess
❖ Intake output and weight daily
❖ Blood pressure and pulse check q4h
❖ Apical or radial pulse before administration.

Administer
- ❖ PO, before food and h.s.
- ❖ IV, keep client recumbent for 3 hours.

Perform/Provide
- ❖ Storage in dry area at room temperature.

Evaluate
- ❖ Therapeutic response: Decreased BP after 1 to 2 weeks
- ❖ Edema in feet, legs daily
- ❖ Skin turgor and dryness of mucous membranes for hydration status.

Teach Client/Family
- ❖ Not to discontinue drug abruptly, taper over 2 weeks
- ❖ Not to use over the counter medications containing α-adrenergic stimulants, such as nasal decongestants and cold medications, unless directed by physician
- ❖ To report bradycardia, dizziness, confusion or depression
- ❖ To avoid alcohol, smoking and excess sodium intake
- ❖ Take medication at bedtime to prevent the effect of orthostatic hypotension
- ❖ Wear support hose to minimize effects of orthostatic hypotension.

Propranolol (Inderal)

Action
- ❖ β-adrenergic blocker: Decreases preload, afterload, which is responsible for decreasing left ventricular end diastolic pressure and systemic vascular resistance.

Indications
- ❖ Hypertension, prophylaxis of angina pain.

Contraindications
- ❖ Bronchial asthma, renal insufficiency, diabetes mellitus, cardiac failure.

Side Effects/Adverse Reactions
Maternal
- ❖ Severe hypotension, sodium retention, bradycardia, bronchospasm, cardiac failure.

Fetal
- ❖ Bradycardia and impaired fetal responses to hypoxia, IUGR with prolonged therapy, neonatal hypoglycemia.

Dosage and Routes of Administration
- ❖ Orally 80 to 240 mg in divided doses.

Nursing Considerations
Assess
- ❖ BP, pulse and respirations during therapy
- ❖ Weight daily and report excess weight gain
- ❖ Intake output ratio.

Administer
- ❖ Administer with 240 ml of water on empty stomach.

Evaluate
- ❖ Tolerance if taken for long period
- ❖ Headache, light-headedness, decreased BP.

Teach Client/Family
- ❖ There may be stinging sensation when the drug comes in contact with mucous membranes
- ❖ The drug may be taken before stressful activity exercise
- ❖ Client compliance with treatment regimen
- ❖ To make position changes slowly to prevent fainting.

Hydralazine

Preparations
- ❖ Apresoline, Hydralyn, Rolazine.

Action
- ❖ Vasodilates arteriolar smooth muscles by direct relaxation, reduction in blood pressure with reflex increase in cardiac function.

Indication
- ❖ Essential hypertension.

Contraindications
- ❖ Coronary artery disease, mitral *valvular* rheumatic heart disease.

Adverse Effects
Maternal
- ❖ Hypotension, tachycardia, arrhythmia, palpitation, acute rheumatoid state, muscle cramps, headache, dizziness, depression, anorexia, diarrhea, pruritis.

Dosage and Routes of Administration
- Orally—100 mg/day in 4 divided doses
- IV/IM bolus 20 to 40 mg q4-6h.

Nursing Considerations

Assess
- BP every 15 minutes initially for 2 hours then every hour for 2 hours, and then q4h, pulse q4h
- Blood studies: Electrolytes, CBC and serum glucose
- Intake: Output and weight daily.

Administer
- To patient in recumbent position, keep in that position for one hour after administration.

Evaluate
- Edema in feet and legs daily
- Skin and mucous membrane for hydration
- Rales, dyspnea, orthopnea
- Joint pain, tachycardia, palpitation, headache and nausea.

Teach Client/Family
- To take with food to increase bio-availability
- To notify physician if chest pain, severe fatigue, muscle or joint pain occurs.

Nifedipine

Preparations
- Adalat, procardia.

Action
- Calcium channel blocker
- Produces direct arteriolar vasodilatation by inhibition of inward calcium channels in vascular smooth muscles.

Indication
- Hypertension, angina pectoris.

Contraindications
- Simultaneous use of magnesium sulphate could be hazardous due to synergistic effect
- Second or third degree heart block.

Side Effects/Adverse Reactions
- Flushing, hypotension, palpitations, bradycardia, inhibition of labor, headache, fatigue, drowsiness, nausea, vomiting.

Dosage and Routes of Administration
- Orally—5 to 10 mg, tid.

Nursing Considerations

Assess
- Blood levels of the drug, therapeutic levels 0.025 to 0.1 µg/ml.

Administer
- Before meals and h.s.

Evaluate
- Therapeutic response, cardiac status, BP, pulse, respiration and ECG.

Teach Client/Family
- To limit caffeine consumption
- To avoid OTC drugs unless directed by the physician
- Stress patient compliance to all aspects of drug use.

Diazoxide

Preparation
- Hyperstat.

Action
- Vasodilator.

Indication
- Hypertensive crisis when urgent decrease of diastolic pressure is required.

Contraindications
- Diabetes, heart disease
- Diuretics should be used simultaneously.

Side Effects

Maternal
- Fluid and sodium retention
- Inhibition of uterine contraction
- Hyperglycemia

❖ Severe hypotension
❖ Palpitations.

Fetal
❖ Hypoxia.

Dosage and Routes of Administration

❖ IV—30 to 50 mg, may be repeated every 10 to 15 minutes or continuous infusion.

Nursing Considerations

Assess
❖ BP q5min for 2 hours, then q1hr for 2 hours and then q4h
❖ Pulse, jugular venous distention q4h
❖ Serum electrolytes, CBC, serum glucose
❖ Weight daily and intake output.

Administer
❖ To patient in recumbent position, keep in that position for one hour after administration.

Perform/Provide
Protection from light.

Evaluate
❖ Therapeutic response: Primarily decreased diastolic pressure
❖ Edema in feet and legs
❖ Hydration status
❖ Dyspnea and orthopnea
❖ Postural hypotension: Take BP sitting and standing.

Teach Patient/Family
❖ To limit caffeine consumption
❖ To report side effects if present
❖ To comply with the regimen.

Sodium Nitroprusside

Preparations

❖ Nipride, Nitropress

Action

❖ Peripheral vasodilator, directly relaxes arteriolar, venous smooth muscle, resulting in reduction of cardiac preload and afterload.

Indications

❖ Hypertensive crisis
❖ To decrease bleeding by creating hypotension during pregnancy.

Contraindications

❖ Should be used in critical care unit for short time
❖ Compensatory hypertension is possible.

Side Effects/Adverse Reactions

Maternal
❖ Nausea, vomiting, severe hypotension
❖ Restlessness, decreased reflexes, loss of consciousness.

Fetal
❖ Toxicity due to metabolites: Cyanide and thiocyanate.

Dosage and Route of Administration

❖ IV infusion 0.5 to 10 mg/kg/minute.

Nursing Considerations

Assess
❖ Serum electrolytes, BUN and creatinine
❖ Hepatic function (AST, ALT and alkaline phosphatase)
❖ BP and ECG
❖ Weight and intake output.

Administer
❖ Using an infusion pump only
❖ Wrap bottle with aluminum foil to protect from light.

Evaluate
❖ Therapeutic response: Decreased BP, absence of bleeding
❖ Edema: Feet and legs
❖ Hydration status.

DIURETICS

Diuretics are used in the following conditions during pregnancy.
❖ Pregnancy induced hypertension with massive edema
❖ Eclampsia with pulmonary edema

- Severe anemia in pregnancy with heart failure
- Prior to blood transfusion in severe anemia
- As an adjunct to certain antihypertensive drugs, such as hydralazine or diazoxide.

Common Preparations Used

Furosemide (Lasix)

Action

- *A loop diuretic:* Acts on loop of Henle by increasing excretion of sodium and chloride.

Dosage

40 mg tab, daily following breakfast for 5 days a week. In acute conditions, the drug is administered parenterally in doses of 40 to 120 mg daily.

Side Effects

Maternal
- Side effects include weakness, fatigue, muscle cramps, hypokalemia, hyponatremia, hypocalcemia, hypochloremic alkalosis and postural hypotension.

Fetal
- May occur due to decreased placental perfusion leading to fetal compromise. Thrombocytopenia and hyponatremia are other hazards.

Contraindications
- Hypersensitivity to sulphonamides, hypovolemia.

Interactions/Incompatibilities
- Increased toxicity—Lithium, skeletal muscle relaxants, and digitalis
- Decreased effects of antidiabetics
- Increased anticoagulant activity
- Increased action anticoagulants.

Nursing Considerations

Assess
- Weight, intake and output daily to determine fluid loss
- Respiration: Rate, depth and rhythm

- BP: Lying and standing
- Electrolytes: Sodium, chloride, potassium, BUN, blood sugar, CBC, serum creatinine, blood pH and ABGs
- Glucose in urine, if patient is diabetic.

Administer
- In AM to avoid interference with sleep.
- Potassium replacement, if serum potassium is less than 3.0
- With food, if nausea occurs, absorption may be decreased slightly.

Evaluate
- Improvement in edema of feet, legs and sacral area
- Signs of metabolic acidosis: Drowsiness, restlessness
- Signs of hypocalcemia, postural hypotension, malaise, fatigue, tachycardia and leg cramps
- Rashes and temperature elevation.

Teach Patient/Family
- To increase fluid intake 2 to 3 L/day unless contraindicated
- To rise slowly from lying or sitting position
- To report adverse reactions, such as muscle cramps, nausea, weakness or dizziness
- To take with food or milk
- To take early in day to prevent nocturia.

Hydrochlorothiazide

Preparations
- Esidrex, hydrodiuril, hydrozide.

Action
- Sulphonamide derivative
- Acts on distal tubule by increasing excretion of water, sodium, chloride and potassium.

Uses
- Edema, hypertension.

Dosage and Route
- PO, 25 to 100 mg/day.

Side Effects/Adverse Reactions
- Polyuria, glycosuria, frequency
- Nausea, vomiting, anorexia
- Rash, urticaria, fever
- Increased creatinine, decreased electrolytes.

Contraindications

❖ Hypersensitivity to thiazides or sulphonamides.

Nursing Considerations

Assess

❖ Weight, intake and output to determine fluid loss
❖ Rate, depth and rhythm of respiration
❖ BP: Lying and standing
❖ Electrolytes: Potassium, sodium and chloride
❖ BUN, blood sugar, CBC, serum creatinine, blood pH and ABGs
❖ Glucose in urine, if patient is diabetic.

Administer

❖ In AM to avoid interference with sleep
❖ Potassium replacement, if serum potassium is less than 3.0
❖ With food if nausea occurs.

Evaluate

❖ Improvement in edema
❖ Improvement in CVP
❖ Signs of metabolic acidosis, drowsiness and restlessness
❖ Signs of hypokalemia, postural hypotension, malaise, fatigue, tachycardia, leg cramps and weakness
❖ Rashes and temperature elevation.

Teach Patient/Family

❖ To increase fluid intake to 2 to 3 L/day unless contraindicated
❖ To notify physician of muscle weakness, cramps, nausea and dizziness
❖ Drug may be taken with food or milk
❖ To take early in day to avoid nocturia.

Spironolactone (Aldactone)

Mode of Action

❖ The drug antagonizes aldosterone by competitive inhibition in the distal tubules, thereby preventing the potassium excretion and decreasing the sodium reabsorption.

Dose

❖ Initially 25 mg PO may be increased to 100 mg in divided doses.

Advantages

❖ There is no potassium loss. It has some hypotensive action.

Nursing Considerations

Assess

❖ Weight, intake and output daily to determine fluid loss
❖ Blood pressure: Lying and standing as postural hypotension may occur
❖ Serum electrolytes (sodium, potassium, chloride), BUN, blood glucose, serum creatinine and CBC.

Administer

❖ In AM to avoid interference with sleep
❖ Potassium replacement, if serum potassium is less than 3.0
❖ With food: If nausea occurs.

Evaluate

❖ Improvement in edema: Feet, legs and scral area daily
❖ Signs of metabolic acidosis—drowsiness, restlessness
❖ Signs of hypokalemia: Postural hypotension, fatigue, tachycardia, leg cramps and weakness.

Teach Client/Family

❖ To increase fluid intake
❖ To rise slowly from lying or sitting position
❖ To take with food or milk for G1 symptoms
❖ To take early in day to prevent nocturia.

TOCOLYTIC AGENTS

These drugs can inhibit uterine contractions and used to prolong the pregnancy. In women who develop premature uterine contractions, in addition to putting them to absolute bed rest and sedating, tocolytic drugs are administered in an attempt to inhibit uterine contractions.

The commonly used drugs are: Isoxsuprine (duvadilan), ritodrine hydrochloride (yutopar) and magnesium sulfate.

Isoxsuprine (Duvadilan)

Action

❖ Acts directly on vascular smooth muscle, causes cardiac stimulation and uterine relaxation.

Dosage and Routes

Initial

IV drip 100 mg in 5 percent dextrose. Rate 0.2 µg per minute. To continue for at least two hours after the contractions cease.

Maintenance

❖ IM 10 mg six hourly for 24 hours, Tab 10 mg 6 to 8 hourly.

Side Effects

❖ Hypotension, tachycardia, nausea, vomiting, pulmonary edema, cardiac arrhythmias, adult respiratory distress syndrome, hyperglycemia, hypokalemia, lactic acidosis.

Contraindications

❖ Hypersensitivity, postpartum.

Nursing Considerations

Assess

❖ BP and pulse during treatment
❖ Take BP: Lying and standing—orthostatic hypotension is common
❖ Intensity and length of uterine contractions
❖ Fetal heart tones.

Administer

❖ With meals to reduce GI upset.

Perform/Provide

❖ Storage at room temperature.

Evaluate

Therapeutic response:

❖ Reduced uterine contractions
❖ Absence of preterm labor
❖ Increased pulse volume.

Teach Patient/Family

❖ To avoid hazardous activities until stabilized on medication. Dizziness may occur
❖ To make position changes slowly, or fainting may occur
❖ To notify physician if rash, palpitations or severe flushing develops.

Ritodrine Hydrochloride (Yutopar)

Action

❖ Uterine relaxant: Acts directly on vascular smooth muscle. Causes cardiac stimulation and uterine relaxation.

Dosage and Routes

Initial

❖ IV drip 100 mg in 5 percent dextrose. Rate, 0.1 mg per minute gradually increased by 0.05 mg per minute q10 min until desired response. To continue for at least 2 hours after the contractions cease.

Maintenance

❖ Tab 10 mg 6 to 8 hourly
❖ PO 10 mg given half hour before termination of IV, then 10 mg q2h x 24 hrs, then 10 to 20 mg q4h, not to exceed 120 mg/day.

Side Effects/Adverse Reactions

❖ Hyperglycemia, headache, restlessness, sweating, chills, and drowsiness
❖ Nausea, vomiting, anorexia and malaise
❖ Altered maternal and fetal heart tone and palpitations.

Contraindications

❖ Hypersensitivity, eclampsia, hypertension and dysrhythmias.

Nursing Considerations

Assess

❖ Maternal and fetal heart tones during infusion.
❖ Intensity and length of uterine contractions.
❖ Fluid intake to prevent fluid overload, discontinue if this occurs.

Administer

❖ Only clear solutions
❖ After dilution 150 mg in 500 ml D_5W or NS, give at 0.3 mg/ml
❖ Using infusion pumps or monitor carefully.

Perform/Provide

❖ Positioning of patient in left lateral recumbent position to decrease hypotension and increase renal blood flow.

Evaluate

Therapeutic response

❖ Decreased intensity
❖ Length of contraction
❖ Absence of preterm labor
❖ Decreased BP.

Teach Patient/Family

❖ To remain in bed during infusion.

ANTICONVULSANTS

The commonly used anticonvulsant is magnesium sulfate. Diazepam, phenytoin and phenobarbitone are also used.

Magnesium Sulfate

Action

❖ Decreases acetylcholine in motor nerve terminals, which is responsible for anticonvulsant properties, thereby reduces neuromuscular irritability. It also decreases intracranial edema and helps in diuresis. Its peripheral vasodilatation effect improves the uterine blood supply. Has depressant action on the uterine muscle and CNS.

Use

❖ It is a valuable drug lowering seizure threshold in women with pregnancy-induced hypertension. The drug is used in preterm labor to decrease uterine activity.

Dosage and Route

❖ For control of seizures, 20 ml of 20 percent solution IV slowly in 3 to 4 minutes; to be followed immediately by 10 ml of 50 percent solution IM, and continued 4 hourly till 24 hours postpartum. Repeat injections are given only if the knee jerks are present, urine output exceeds 100 ml in previous 4 hours and the respirations are more than 10/minute. The therapeutic level of serum magnesium is 4 to 7 mEq/L.
❖ 4 gm IV slowly over 10 min, followed by 2 gm/hr, and then 1 gm/hr in drip of 5 percent dextrose for tocolytic effect.

Side Effects

❖ *Maternal:* Severe CNS depression (respiratory depression and circulatory collapse), evidence of muscular paresis (diminished knee jerks).
❖ *Fetal:* Tachycardia, hypoglycemia.

Antidote

❖ Injection calcium gluconate 10 percent 10 ml IV.

Nursing Considerations

Assess
❖ Vital signs q 15 min after IV dose. Do not exceed 150 mg/min
❖ Monitor magnesium levels
❖ If using during labor, time contractions, determine intensity
❖ Urine output should remain 30 ml/hr or more, if less notify physician
❖ Uterine contractions when used as tocolytic agent
❖ Reflexes—Knee jerk, patellar reflex.

Administer
❖ Only after calcium gluconate is available for treating magnesium toxicity
❖ Using infusion pump or monitor carefully; IV at less then 150 mg/min; circulatory collapse may occur
❖ Only dilutions.

Perform/Provide
❖ Seizure precautions: Place client in single room with decreased stimuli, padded side rails
❖ Positioning of client in left lateral recumbent position to decrease hypotension and increase renal blood flow.

Evaluate
❖ Mental status, sensorium, memory
❖ Respiratory status: Respiratory depression, rate and rhythm. Hold drug if respirations are less than 12/min
❖ Hypermagnesemia: Depressed patellar reflex, flushing, confusion, weakness, flaccid paralysis, dyspnea
❖ Respiratory rate, rhythm and reflexes of newborn if drug was given within 24 hours prior to delivery
❖ Reflexes: Knee jerk and patellar reflex decrease with magnesium toxicity.
  Discontinue infusion if respirations are below 12/min, reflexes severely hypotonic, urine output below 30 ml/hr or in the event of mental confusion or lethargy or fetal distress.

Teach Client/Family
❖ On all aspects of the drug: Action, side effects and symptoms of hypermagnesemia
❖ To remain in bed during infusion.

Diazepam (Valium)

Action

Depresses subcortical levels of CNS, anticonvulsant, and antianxiety.

Dosage and Route of Administration

❖ PO, 2 to 10 mg tid—qid
❖ IV, 5 to 20 mg (bolus), 2 mg/min, may repeat q5—10min, not to exceed 60 mg, may repeat in 30 min if seizures reappear.

Side Effects

❖ *Mother:* Hypotension, dizziness, drowsiness, headache.
❖ *Fetus:* Respiratory depressant effect, which may last for even three weeks after birth. Hypotonea and thermoregulatory problems in newborn.

Nursing Considerations

Assess
❖ BP in lying and standing positions; if systolic pressure falls 20 mmHg, hold drug and inform physician
❖ Blood studies: CBC
❖ Hepatic studies.

Administer
❖ IV into large vein to decrease chances of extravasation.
❖ PO with milk or food to avoid GI symptoms.

Provide
❖ Assistance with ambulation during beginning therapy since drowsiness and dizziness may occur.
❖ Safety measures include side rails.

Evaluate
Therapeutic response:
❖ Mental status, sensorium, sleeping pattern
❖ Physical dependence, headache, nausea, vomiting

Teach Patient/Family
❖ That drug may be taken with food
❖ To avoid alcohol ingestion
❖ Not to discontinue medication abruptly
❖ To rise slowly as fainting may occur.

Phenytoin (Dilantin)

Action

❖ Inhibits spread of seizure activity in motor cortex.

Dosage and Route of Administration

❖ Eclampsia: 10 mg/kg IV at the rate not more than 50 mg/minute, followed 2 hours later by 5 mg/kg
❖ Epilepsy: 300 to 400 mg daily orally in divided doses.

Side Effects

Maternal
❖ Hypotension, cardiac arrhythmias and phlebitis at injection site.

Fetal
❖ Prolonged use by epileptic patients may cause craniofocal abnormalities, mental retardation, microcephaly and growth deficiency.

Nursing Considerations

❖ Blood studies: CBC, platelets every 2 weeks until stabilized
❖ Discontinue drug if neutrophils < 1600/mm^2.

Administer
❖ After diluting with normal saline, never water.

Evaluate
❖ Mental status, sensorium, affect, memory
❖ Respiratory depression
❖ Blood dyscrasias: Sore throat, bruising.

Teach Patient/Family
❖ All aspects of drug administration, when to notify physician.

Phenobarbitone (Luminal)

Action

❖ Decreases impulse transmission and increases seizure thresholds at cerebral cortex level.

Dose and Route of Administration

❖ 120 to 240 mg/day in divided doses.

Side Effects

Maternal

❖ Sedation, drowsiness, hangover headache, hallucinations.

Fetal

❖ Withdrawal syndrome.

Nursing Considerations

Assess

❖ Blood studies, liver function tests during longterm treatment
❖ Therapeutic level 15 to 40 mg/ml.

Evaluate

❖ Mental status, mood, senorium, affect and memory
❖ Respiratory depression
❖ Blood dyscrasias: Fever, sore throat bruising, rash.

Teach Patient/Family

❖ All aspects of drug administration and when to notify physician.

ANTICOAGULANTS

Heparin Sodium

Action

❖ Prevents conversion of fibrinogen to fibrin.

Indications

❖ Deep vein thrombosis, thromboembolism, disseminated intravascular coagulation, patients with prosthetic valves in the heart.

Dosage and Routes

❖ Administered parenterally; only 5,000 to 7,000 IU to be administered initially as IV push, followed by 2,500 units subcutaneously every 24 hours.

Side Effects

Leukopenia, thrombocytopenia, osteoporosis, hemorrhage, alopecia.

Nursing Considerations

Assess

❖ Blood studies: Hematocrit, platelets, occult blood in stools

❖ Partial prothrombin time
❖ Blood pressure: Signs of hypertension.

Administer

❖ At same time, each day to maintain steady blood levels
❖ Avoid all IM injections that may cause bleeding.

Evaluate

❖ Therapeutic response: Decrease of deep vein thrombosis
❖ Bleeding gums, petechiae, ecchymosis, black tarry stools, hematuria
❖ Fever, skin rash, urticaria.

Teach Patient/Family

❖ To avoid use of drugs unless prescribed by physician
❖ To use soft bristle toothbrush to avoid bleeding gums
❖ To comply with instructions
❖ To recognize and to sign of bleeding—gums, under skin, urine, stool.

Warfarin Sodium (Cumadin)

Action

❖ Interferes with blood clotting by indirect means—depresses hepatic synthesis of vitamin K—dependent coagulation factors (II, VII, IX, X).

Indications

❖ Deep vein thrombosis, pulmonary embolism.

Dosage and Route

❖ 10 to 15 mg orally daily for 2 days, followed by 2 to 10 mg at the same time each day depen-ding upon the prothrombin time.

Side Effects

Maternal

❖ Hemorrhage.

Fetal

❖ Skeletal and facial deformities, optic atrophy, microcephaly.

Nursing Considerations

Assess

❖ Blood studies: Hematocrit, platelets, occult blood in stools
❖ Prothrombin time
❖ BP: Watch for signs of hypertension.

Administer

❖ At same time, each day to maintain steady blood levels
❖ Alone—do not give with food
❖ Avoid all IM injections that may cause bleeding.

Perform/Provide

❖ Storage in tight container.

Evaluate

❖ Therapeutic response: Decrease of deep vein thrombosis
❖ Bleeding gums, petechiae, ecchymosis, black tarry stools, hematuria
❖ Fever, skin rash, urticaria.

Teach Patient/Family

❖ To avoid over the counter (OTC) preparations unless prescribed by physician
❖ Drug may be held during menstruation
❖ To use soft—bristle tooth brush
❖ Stress client compliance
❖ To report any sign of bleeding.

ANALGESICS

Pethidine (Meperidine)

It is synthetic narcotic analgesic agent, well absorbed by all routes of administration.

Action

❖ Inhibits ascending pain pathways in central nervous system, increases pain threshold and alters pain perception.

Indications

❖ Moderate to severe pain in labor, postoperative pain, abruptio placentae, pulmonary edema.

Dosage and Route of Administration

❖ Injectable preparation contains 50 mg/ml, can be administered SC, IM, IV. Its dose is 50 to 00 mg IM combined with promethazine 25 mg.

Contraindication

Pethidine should not be used intravenously within 2 hours and intramuscularly within 3 hours of the expected time of delivery of the baby, for fear of birth asphyxia. It should not be used in cases of preterm labor and when the respiratory reserve of the mother is reduced.

Side Effects/Adverse Reactions

Mother

❖ Drowsiness, dizziness, confusion, headache, sedation, euphoria, nausea and vomiting.

Fetus

❖ Respiratory depression, asphyxia.

Nursing Considerations

Assess

❖ Urinary Output: May cause urinary retention.

Administer

❖ With antiemetic (promethacin) to prevent nausea and vomiting
❖ When pain is beginning to return—Determine dosage interval by patient response.

Perform/Provide

❖ Storage in light: Resistant container at room temperature
❖ Assistance with ambulation
❖ Safety measures: Side rails, night light, call bell within easy reach.

Evaluate

❖ Therapeutic response: Decrease in pain
❖ CNS changes: Dizziness, drowsiness, euphoria
❖ Allergic reactions: Rash, urticaria
❖ Respiratory depression, notify physician if respirations are <12/minute.

Teach Patient/Family

❖ To report symptoms of CNS changes, allergic reactions.

Fentanyl

Fentanyl is a synthetic narcotic analgesic agent.

Action

❖ Inhibits ascending pain pathways in CNS, increases pain threshold and alters pain perception.

Indications

❖ Moderate to severe pain in labor, postoperative pain and as adjunct to general anesthetic

Dosage and Routes

❖ 0.05 to 0.1 mg IM q 1 to 2 hours prn. Available in injectable form, 0.05 mg/ml.

Contraindications

❖ Hypersensitivity to opiates.

Side Effects/Adverse Reactions

❖ Dizziness, delirium, euphoria, nausea, vomiting, muscle rigidity, blurred vision.

Nursing Considerations

Assess
❖ Vital signs
❖ Note muscle rigidity.

Administer
❖ By injection (IM-IV), give slowly to prevent rigidity
❖ Only with resuscitative equipment available.

Perform/Provide
❖ Storage in light resistant container at room temperature
❖ Coughing, turning and deep breathing for postoperative patients
❖ Safety measures: Side rails, night light, call bell within reach.

Evaluate
❖ CNS changes: Dizziness, drowsiness, hallucination, euphoria, LOC, pupil reaction
❖ Allergic reaction: Rash, urticaria
❖ Respiratory dysfunction: Respiratory depression: Notify physician if respirations are >12/min.

Teach Patient/Family
❖ To report any symptoms of CNS changes, allergic reactions.

Promethazine (Phenergan)

Promethazine is an antihistamine, H_1—receptor antagonist belonging to the phenothiazine group.

Action

❖ Decreases allergic response by blocking histamine, sedative and antiemetic.

Indications

❖ Treatment of vomiting in pregnancy
❖ Sedation during labor
❖ Pregnancy induced hypertension
❖ Combined with pethidine to prevent vomiting
❖ In Rh isoimmunization to decrease the production of antibodies
❖ Allergic reactions.

Dosage and Route of Administration

❖ Available for oral use as 12.5, 24 and 50 mg tablets and for parenteral use as 25 and 50 mg/ml solutions. The dose is 25 mg, 8 hourly orally and 25 mg intramuscularly, to be repeated as necessary.

Contraindications

❖ Acute asthma attack
❖ Lower respiratory tract disease.

Side Effects/Adverse Reactions

❖ Drowsiness, dizziness, poor coordination, fatigue, anxiety, confusion, neuritis, parasthesia.

Nursing Considerations

Assess
❖ Urinary output: Be alert for urinary retention, frequency, dysuria; drug should be discontinued if these occur.

Administer
❖ Coffee, tea and cola (caffeine) to decrease drowsiness
❖ With meals if GI symptoms occur when given orally
❖ Deep IM in large muscle; rotate site.

Perform/Provide

❖ Hard candy or gum, frequent rinsing of mouth for dryness

❖ Storge in light resistant container.

Evaluate

❖ Therapeutic response

❖ Respiratory status: Wheezing, chest tightness

❖ Cardiac status: Palpitation, hypotension, increased pulse.

Teach Patient/Family

❖ That drug may cause photosensitivity, to avoid prolonged sunlight

❖ To notify physician if confusion or hypotension occurs

❖ To avoid concurrent use of alcohol or other CNS depressants

❖ To avoid drinking or other hazardous activity, if drowsiness occurs.

EFFECTS OF MATERNAL MEDICATIONS ON FETUS AND BREASTFEEDING INFANTS

During early embryogenesis, the drugs taken by the mother reach the conceptus through the tubal or uterine secretions by diffusion. The harmful effect on the blastocyst is usually death. In case of survival, there is chance of congenital anomalies.

From 2nd to 12th week (period of organogenesis), drugs taken by the mother can cause serious damages. Gross congenital malformations and even death of the fetus may result, depending on the route, length of time and dose of exposure.

From the second trimester onwards, transfer of durgs takes place through the utero-placental circulation. The drug transfer across the placenta is increased due to the lowered serum albumin concentration, which results from hemodilution. As the albumin-binding capacity of the drugs is decreased, more free drug is available for placental transfer. In addition, the metabolism of the drugs may be hampered by the increase in plasma steroids. Increased utero-placental blood flow, increased placental surface area and decreased thickness of the placental membrane are the additional causes for increased drug transfer.

Fetotoxic or teratogenic drugs are prescribed only when the benefits outweigh the potential risks. Prior counseling is mandatory and minimum therapeutic dosage is used for shortest possible duration.

Maternal Medications with Established Teratogenic Properties and their Effects

❖ Cytotoxic drugs: Multiple fetal malformations and abortion

❖ Androgenic steroids, Hydroxy progesterone: Masculinization of the female offspring

❖ Lithium: Increased congenital malformations when used in the first trimester, neonatal goiter, hypotonia and cyanosis

❖ Diethyl stillbestrol: Vaginal stenosis, cervical hoods and uterine hypoplasia in female fetuses.

Possible Teratogens

❖ Antithyroid drugs: Goiter, mental retardation

❖ Oral antidiabetic drugs: Abnormalities in the eyes, central nervous system, skeletal system and neonatal hypoglycemia

❖ Vitamin D: Cardiopathies, hypercalcemia and mental retardation

❖ LSD (lysergic acid diethylamide): Chromosomal abnormality and stunted growth

❖ Anticonvulsants (- Phenytoin, valproate): Mental retardation, cardiac abnormalities, limb defects, neonatal bleeding, epilepsy.

Fetotoxic Drugs

❖ Aspirin: High doses in the last few weeks can cause premature closure of ductus arterious, persistent pulmonary hypertension and kernicterus in the newborn.

❖ Corticosteroids (prednisolone): Doses above 10 mg daily may produce fetal and neonatal adrenal suppression.

❖ Aminoglycosides (antibiotics, e.g. amikacin, streptomycin): Auditory or vestibular damage

❖ Chloramphenicol: Peripheral vascular collapse (gray baby syndrome)

❖ Tetracycline: Dental discoloration (yellowish) and deformity, inhibition of bony growth

❖ Long acting sulphonamides: Neonatal hemolysis, jaundice and kernicterus
❖ Nitrofurantoin (furadantin): Hemolysis in newborn with G_6 PD deficiency, if used at term
❖ Vitamin K (large doses): Hyperbilirubinemia and kernicterus
❖ Alcohol and smoking: Intrauterine growth retardation, pre-term labor, mental retardation.
❖ Narcotics: Depression of CNS—Apnea, bradycardia and hypothermia.
❖ Anesthetic agents: Convulsion, bradycardia, acidosis, hypoxia, hypertonia.
❖ Antihistamines: Tachycardia, vomiting, diarrhea.
❖ Anticoagulants: Optic atrophy, microcephaly, chondrodysplsia punctate.
❖ Diuretics: Fetal compromise due to diminished placental perfusion.
❖ Beta-blockers (antihypertensive drugs): IUGR, fetal bradycardia and impaired fetal responses to hypoxia.

Maternal Drug Intake and Breastfeeding

Maternal drug intake of nursing mothers have adverse effects on lactation and also on the baby as it may be present in the breast milk.

Milk concentration of some drugs such as iodides may even exceed those in the maternal plasma so that therapeutic doses in the mother may cause toxicity to the infant. Certain drugs in breastmilk may cause hypersensitivity in the infant when used in therapeutic doses. Transfer of drugs through breast milk depends on the following factors:
❖ Chemical properties
❖ Molecular weight
❖ Degree of protein binding
❖ Ionic dissociation
❖ Lipid solubility
❖ Tissue pH
❖ Drug concentration
❖ Exposure time.

Drugs that are non-ionized, of low molecular weight and lipid soluble compounds are usually excreted through breastmilk. Drugs identified as having effects on lactation and the neonate are listed below:
❖ Bromides: Rash, drowsiness and poor feeding.
❖ Iodides: Neonatal hypothyroidism.
❖ Chloramphenicol: Bone marrow toxicity.
❖ Oral pill (combined preparations): Suppression of lactation.
❖ Bromocriptine (parlodel): Suppression of lactation.
❖ Ergot: Suppression of lactation.
❖ Metronidazole (Flagyl): Anorexia, blood dyscrasias, irritability, weakness, neurotoxic disorders.
❖ Anticoagulants: Hemorrhagic tendency (warfarin appears safe in therapeutic doses).
❖ Isoniazid: Anti-DNA activity and hepatotoxicity.
❖ Antithyroid drugs and radioactive iodine: Hypothyroidism and goiter, agranulocytosis.
❖ Antimetabolites (methotraxate): Anti-DNA activity, immunosuppression.
❖ Diazepam, opiates, phenobarbitone: Sedation effect with poor sucking reflex.

Breastfeeding is discouraged for mothers on medications that are harmful for the infant.

BIBLIOGRAPHY

1. Clark JB, Queener SF, Karb VB. Pharmacological Basis of Nursing Practice, 4th edn. St. Louis, Mosby Year Book, 1994.
2. Drug Information 94, American Hospital Formalary Service, Bethesda, 1994.
3. Dutta DC. Textbook of Obstetrics, 5th edn. Calcutta: New Central Book Company, 2001.
4. Goodman A, et al. Goodman and Gilman's, The Pharmacological Basis of Therapeutics, 9th edn. New York: Pergamon Press, 1994.
5. McKenry LM. Salerno E. Mosby's Pharmacology in Nursing, 18th edn. St. Louis: Mosby Year Book, 1992.
6. Parulekar VS. Textbook for Midwives, 2nd edn. Calcutta: New Central Book Company, 2001.
7. Skidmore Linda. Mosby's Nursing Drug Reference. St. Louis: CV Mosby, 1996.

55

Vital Statistics in Obstetrics

Learning Objectives

Upon completing this chapter, the learner will be able to:

❖ Explain the vital events' registration system in the country and the place of it in health care

❖ Describe the maternal vital statistics, the magnitude of the problem and the measures to reduce the mortality and morbidity

❖ Describe the perinatal and neonatal mortality, the prevailing causes and the preventive measures for a faster decline of the rates

❖ Enumerate the role of midwives for record keeping.

Many of the advances in health services have come because of public health interventions. The ability to intervene in the health of populations is dependent upon development of appropriate tools for measuring health, illness and interventions. Only by standardizing communication on such issues as infant and maternal mortality can health managers hope to target high-risk populations with effective interventions.

Registration of Vital Events

Much importance is given to registration of vital events (e.g. births, deaths) in all countries, as it is the precursor of health statistics. If registration of vital events is complete and accurate, it can serve as reliable source of health information.

The United Nations defines vital events registration system as including "legal registration, statistical recording and reporting of the occurrence of, and collection, compilation, presentation, analysis and distribution of statistics pertaining to vital events, i.e. live births, deaths, fetal deaths, marriages, divorces, adoptions, legitimations, recognitions, annulments and legal separations" (WHO, 1981-Health for All, Sr, No 4).

India had Births, Deaths and Marriage Registration Act since 1873, but the Act provided only for voluntary registration. However, the registration system tended to be very unreliable, the data being grossly deficient in regard to accuracy, timeliness, completeness and coverage. The extent of under registration was high in several states because of illiteracy, ignorance, lack of concern and motivation. Reasons such as lack of uniformity in the collection, compilation and transmission of data and the working of multiple registration agencies contributed to the lack of adequacy and accuracy of the data.

In an effort to improve the civil registration system, the Government of India promulgated the Central Births and Deaths Registration Act in 1969. The Act came into force in 1970. The Act provides for compulsory registration of births and deaths throughout the country, and compilation of vital statistics in the states to ensure uniformity and comparability of data. The Act fixes the responsibility for reporting births and deaths while citizens (e.g. parents and relatives) are to report events occurring in their households, the heads of hospitals, nursing homes, hotels, jails or dharmashalas are to report events occurring in such institutions to the concerning Registrar. The time limit for registering the event of births is 14 days and that of deaths is 7 days. In case of default, a fine up to ₹ 50.00 can be imposed.

MATERNAL VITAL STATISTICS

The quality of health care delivery system of a country is reflected by its maternal and perinatal mortality rates. During the last 50 years, there has been marked reduction in the maternal and perinatal death rates in the developed countries and to some extent in the developing countries. Maintenance of accurate vital statistics, their critical analysis, and formulation of the preventive measures contributed to the reduction of deaths in advanced countries. Unregulated fertility, inadequate prenatal care and lack of trained birth attendants are mainly recognized as the factors responsible for high maternal and perinatal deaths in the developing countries.

MATERNAL MORTALITY

Maternal death is defined as death of a woman who is pregnant or within 42 days of the termination of pregnancy irrespective of the duration and the site of pregnancy from any cause related to or aggravated by the pregnancy or its management but not from accidental or incidental causes.

Maternal Mortality Rate

Maternal mortality rate measures the risk of women dying from 'puerperal causes' and is defined as:

$$\frac{\text{Total number of female deaths due to complications of pregnancy, childbirth or within 42 days of delivery from puerperal causes in an area during a given year}}{\text{Total number of live births in the same area and year}} \times 1,000$$

Ideally, the denominator should include all deliveries and abortions. However, the rate is expressed as a rate per 1,000 live births. In developed countries, MMR has declined significantly and because of this decline; they use the multiplying factor 100,000 instead of 1,000 to avoid fractions in calculating MMR.

It is estimated in a study carried out jointly by WHO and UNICEF that globally some 585,000 maternal deaths occur every year from pregnancy related causes. About 99 percent of these deaths occur in developing countries. For the year 1997, maternal mortality rate for India was estimated as 408 per 100,000 live births. The trend has not changed much in the last five years. The MMR in developed countries such as the USA, UK and Europe ranges from 5 to 8 per 100,000. The causes for the high maternal mortality in India is attributed to large number of deliveries conducted at home by untrained persons. In addition, lack of adequate referral facilities to provide emergency obstetric care for complicated cases also contribute to high maternal morbidity and mortality (Park, 2001).

Classification of Maternal Deaths

Direct Maternal Deaths (75%)

This is defined as deaths from complications of pregnancy, delivery or puerperium. Such conditions are abortion, ectopic pregnancy, pre-eclampsia, eclampsia, hemorrhage, chorioamnionitis, and puerperal sepsis and include any complications arising from their treatment, omissions, incorrect treatment or events resulting from any of the above.

Indirect Maternal Deaths (25%)

Indirect deaths often represent underlying medical conditions aggravated but not caused by the pregnancy. This would include conditions present before or developed during pregnancy. These are anemia, cardiac disease, diabetes, thyroid disease and connective tissue disease of which anemia is the most important single cause in the developing countries. Viral hepatitis when endemic, contributes significantly to maternal deaths.

Virtually all the direct maternal deaths demand intense scrutiny, because most can be shown to have been preventable under optimal circumstances. Indirect maternal deaths, however, simply may reflect the remarkable advances in medical care that allow these women to achieve reproductive age and, in some cases to voluntarily undertake pregnancy in the face of enormous disadvantages.

Nonobstetric or Unrelated Deaths

This rate measures deaths of pregnant or postpartum women that were neither caused by nor aggravated by the pregnancy and include those due to motor vehicle accidents, homicides, and infectious diseases such as malaria and typhoid.

Reproductive Mortality

This term is used currently to include direct maternal deaths and mortality resulting from the use of contraceptives.

Magnitude of the Problem

Maternal mortality statistics reveal an alarming picture in the developing countries. Out of an estimated 585,000 annual maternal deaths in the globe, 99 percent are distributed in the developing countries. There are more maternal deaths in India in the space of a week than there are in all Europe in a whole year (Dutta, 2001). In India, 148,000 women die every year because of pregnancy and childbirth, which is about one maternal death every four minutes. It is further estimated that for one maternal death, at least 15 more suffer from severe morbidities.

Factors Associated with Maternal Mortality

Age

The optimum reproductive efficiency appears to be between 20 and 25 years. In the young adolescent, pregnancy carries a higher risk due to pre-eclampsia, cephalopelvic disproportion, and uterine inertia. In women aged 35 years or over, the risk is 3 to 4 times higher.

Parity

The risk is slightly higher in primigravida and it is three times greater in Para 5 or above due to postpartum hemorrhage, malpresentations and rupture of uterus. The risk is lowest in the second pregnancy.

Socioeconomic Strata

Mortality rates are higher in women of low socioeconomic level as these women are likely to be less privileged in the areas of nutrition, education, housing and prenatal care.

Antenatal Care

Availability and acceptance of antenatal care is low among women of lower socioeconomic status and those who live in rural areas of the country.

Social Factors

Presence of social evils such as illiteracy, ignorance, prejudice, inadequate maternity services and underutilization of existing facilities, are responsible for increased number of avoidable maternal deaths.

Causes of Maternal Death

Hemorrhage

Hemorrhage is accounted for 20 to 25 percent of maternal deaths and is mostly due to postpartum hemorrhage, antepartum hemorrhage, abortion and ectopic gestation.

Sepsis

Deaths due to infections associated with labor and puerperium and unsafe abortions contribute to 20 to 25 percent of deaths.

Hypertensive Disorders in Pregnancy

About 5 to 15 percent of maternal deaths are attributed to preeclampsia and eclampsia and are mostly due to lack of antenatal care.

Anemia

About 40 percent of obstetric clients in the developing countries suffer from anemia and if it is severe, they may die from congestive cardiac failure during pregnancy or labor. Deaths among anemic women account for 15 to 20 percent.

Infective Hepatitis

This, when present in an epidemic form, results in a mortality rate of up to 20 to 25 percent in India. This risk of death is most in the last trimester with hepatic coma and coagulation failure leading to hemorrhage.

Thromboembolism

This accounts for about 2 to 5 percent of deaths in India. Deaths due to thrombophlebitis are higher (15–20%) in western countries.

Lack of Assistance of Trained Personnel

A large number of deliveries take place at home without the services of trained midwifery personnel. The risk of maternal death is higher for such women and is estimated to be 1 in 41 (Park, 2000).

Preventive Measures

High maternal mortality reflects not only an inadequacy of health care services for mothers but also a low standard of living and socio-economic status of the community. An attempt to lower maternal mortality rate (MMR) must take into consideration, the following measures.

- ❖ Early registration pregnancy
- ❖ At least three antenatal check-ups
- ❖ Improvement of nutritional status including correction of anemia
- ❖ Identification of high-risk cases and their referrals to appropriate referral hospitals
- ❖ Prevention of complications such as eclampsia, malpresentations, and ruptured uterus
- ❖ Treatment of medical conditions such as hypertension, diabetes and tuberculosis
- ❖ Antimalaria and tetanus prophylaxis
- ❖ Integration of domiciliary, rural and institutional deliveries with efficient referral system
- ❖ Institutional deliveries for women with bad obstetric history and risk factors
- ❖ Promotion of family planning to control the number of children to not more than two and spacing of births
- ❖ Identification of every maternal death and searching for its causes through regular maternal mortality review conferences
- ❖ To provide safe delivery services to all mothers by training the Traditional Birth Attendants (TBA), upgrading the health centers, making government vehicles available in emergencies and increasing the number of health care providers such as midwives, multipurpose health workers, health assistants and other ancillary personnel
- ❖ Frequent joint consultation amongst specialists in the management of medical disorders of pregnancy such as anemia, diabetes, hypertension and heart disease
- ❖ Periodic refresher courses for continuing education of all levels of health workers to highlight the preventive measures.

MATERNAL MORBIDITY

Maternal morbidity originates from any cause related to pregnancy or its management any time during antepartum, intrapartum and postpartum period usually up to 42 days after delivery. The parameters of maternal morbidity are:

- ❖ Temperature more than 100.4°F or 38°C and continuing for more than 24 hours
- ❖ Blood pressure more than 140/90 mmHg
- ❖ Recurrent vaginal bleeding
- ❖ Hemoglobin less than 10.5 gm percentage irrespective of gestational period
- ❖ Asymptomatic bacteriuria of pregnancy.

Classification

Direct Obstetric Morbidity

These include temporary conditions such as APH, PPH, eclampsia, obstructed labor, rupture of uterus, sepsis, ectopic pregnancy and molar pregnancy. Chronic or permanent causes of morbidity include VVF, RVF, uterine prolapse, secondary infertility and Sheehan's syndrome.

Indirect Morbidity

Indirect conditions of morbidity are exaggerated previously existing diseases like malaria, hepatitis, tuberculosis, anemia, etc. by changes in the various systems during pregnancy.

Reproductive Morbidity

It is a term used to include obstetric morbidity, gynecological morbidity and contraceptive morbidity.

PERINATAL MORTALITY

Perinatal mortality is defined as deaths among fetuses weighing over 1,000 gm at birth, that die before and during delivery or within the first 7 days of delivery (late fetal and early neonatal deaths weighing over 1,000 gm at birth). The perinatal mortality rate is expressed in terms of such deaths per 1,000 total births.

$$PMR = \frac{\text{Late fetal deaths (28 weeks gestation and more) + early neonatal deaths (first week) in one year}}{\text{Live births in the same year}} \times 1000$$

Perinatal mortality rate includes stillbirths and deaths within the first week of life. In India, stillbirths are seldom registered. Consequently, most studies on perinatal mortality in this country are hospital based. The PMR in India is reported to be 49.1 per 1,000 live births in rural areas and 32.7 per 1,000 live births in urban areas. Both rural and urban areas combined, the figure was 46.0 per 1,000 live births in 1991 (Park, 2000). In developed countries, the level has declined in the past decade to 15 to 20 per 1,000 total births due to improved obstetric and perinatal technologies.

Causes of Perinatal Mortality

About two-thirds of all perinatal deaths occur among infants with 2,500 gm weight. The causes involve one or more complications in the mother during pregnancy or labor, in the placenta, fetus or neonate.

The main causes of death are intrauterine and birth asphyxia, low birth weight, birth trauma and intrauterine or neonatal infections. The various causes of perinatal mortality may be grouped as follows:

Antenatal Causes

❖ *Maternal diseases:* Hypertension, cardiovascular diseases, diabetes, tuberculosis, anemia
❖ *Pelvic diseases:* Uterine myomas, endometriosis, ovarian tumors
❖ *Anatomical defects:* Uterine anomalies, incompetent cervix

❖ *Endocrine imbalance:* Inadequate uterine preparation
❖ Blood incompatibilities
❖ Malnutrition
❖ Toxemias of pregnancy
❖ Antepartum hemorrhage
❖ Congenital defects
❖ Advanced maternal age
❖ Preterm labor and preterm rupture of membranes.

Intranatal Causes

❖ Birth injuries
❖ Asphyxia
❖ Prolonged labor
❖ Obstetric complications: Dystocia, abnormal uterine action, malpresentation.

Postnatal Causes

❖ Prematurity
❖ Respiratory distress syndrome
❖ Respiratory and alimentary infections
❖ Congenital anomalies.

Measures for Reduction of Perinatal Mortality

Measures to reduce perinatal mortality rate are essential to accelerate the declining trend in neonatal and infant mortality rates. These are:

❖ Advice to women with medical problems to avoid pregnancy until health improves
❖ Birth spacing
❖ Tetanus toxoid immunization iron and folic acid supplements for anemia control
❖ Early treatment of maternal complications
❖ Institutional delivery for women at high risk
❖ Immediate referral and appropriate care of emergency obstetric complications
❖ Safe and clean delivery practices
❖ Essential newborn care
❖ Resuscitation of newborns without spontaneous cry at birth.

Preventive Measures

Many of the perinatal deaths are preventable with proper care and good organizational setup. The following measures may help in greatly reducing the perinatal mortality.

❖ Prepregnancy health care and counseling
❖ Genetic counseling to detect genetic, chromosomal or structural abnormalities
❖ Regular antenatal care, with advice regarding health, diet and rest
❖ Improvement of maternal nutrition
❖ Screening of high-risk mothers: Those of poor socioeconomic status, high parity, very young and those with multiple pregnancies for hospital delivery
❖ Careful monitoring during labor and avoidance of traumatic vaginal delivery
❖ Efficient neonatal service for preterm babies
❖ Health education to mothers about care of newborn
❖ Autopsy studies of perinatal deaths
❖ Continued study of perinatal mortality problems.

STILLBIRTHS

A stillbirth is a birth of a newborn after 28th completed week (weighing 1,000 gm or more) when the baby does not breathe or show any sign of life after delivery. Such deaths include antepartum deaths (macerated) and intrapartum deaths (fresh stillbirths).

Stillbirth rate is the number of such deaths per 1,000 total births (live and still) (Dutta, 2001).

Causes

Antepartum Deaths

❖ Pregnancy complications such as pre-eclampsia and antepartum hemorrhage
❖ Pre-existing medical diseases and acute illnesses during pregnancy such as chronic hypertension, diabetes, chronic nephritis, syphilis, hyperpyrexia (malaria), severe anemia and infections
❖ Fetal causes such as congenital malformations, Rh-incompatibility and post-maturity
❖ Iatrogenic as due to administration of quinine group of drugs and external version
❖ Placental insufficiency.

Intrapartum Deaths

The common causes are:
❖ Acute fetal distress
❖ Traumatic vaginal delivery leading to asphyxia or intracranial hemorrhage

❖ Asphyxia especially in premature babies
❖ Congenital malformations of the fetus.

NEONATAL MORTALITY

Neonatal deaths are deaths occurring during the neonatal period, commencing at birth and ending at 28 completed days after birth. Neonatal mortality rate is the number of neonatal deaths in a given year per 1,000 live births in that year. It is tabulated as:

$$NMR = \frac{\text{Number of deaths of babies under 28 days of age in a year}}{\text{Total live births in the same year}} \times 1000$$

Causes of Neonatal Deaths

About two-thirds of the neonatal deaths are related to prematurity and majority of the deaths occur within 48 hours of birth.
❖ Low birth weight
❖ Birth injury due to difficult labor
❖ Congenital anomalies
❖ Hemolytic disease of the newborn
❖ Conditions of placenta and cord
❖ Acute respiratory infections
❖ Tetanus
❖ Diarrheal diseases.

As the high concentration of neonatal deaths occur in the early neonatal period, there is need to improve the antenatal and postnatal services to mothers. Neonatal mortality is seen greater in boy babies throughout the world, because newborn boys biologically are more fragile (Park, 2001).

Neonatal mortality varies from 53 per 1,000 live births for the least developed countries to about 5 per 1,000 live births for the developed countries. In India, about 50 to 60 percent of infant deaths, occur within the neonatal period (first 28 days). Of these, more than half may die during the first week of birth, first 24 hours being the time of greatest risk. Neonatal mortality rate for the year 1995 was 50 per 1,000 live births.

INFANT MORTALITY RATE (IMR)

Infant mortality rate is defined as "the ratio of infant deaths registered in a given year to the number of live births registered in the same year; usually expressed as a rate per 1,000 live births (Hograh, 1978). It is given by the formula:

$$IMR = \frac{\text{Number of deaths of children less than one year of age in a year}}{\text{Number of live births in the same year}} \times 1000$$

During the past decades, there have been steady decline in infant mortality rate throughout the world and more so in the developed countries. By 1980s, most developed countries achieved rates below 10 per 1,000 live births. India had the goal of reducing the IMR of 72 in 1998 to 60 per 1,000 live births by the year 2000.

The decline in infant mortality has been attributed to:

❖ Improved obstetric and perinatal care; e.g. availability of oxygen, fetal monitoring during labor, improved techniques for induction of labor
❖ Improvement in the quality of life, i.e. economic and social progress
❖ Better control of communicable diseases, e.g. immunization and oral rehydration
❖ Advances in chemotherapy, antibiotics and insecticides
❖ Better nutrition especially emphasis on breastfeeding
❖ Family planning, e.g. birth spacing.

In India, the states, those have higher female literacy and improved primary health care have achieved lower infant mortality rates.

RECORD KEEPING

Records of activities and events related to vital statistics that occur in health care facilities, such as in hospitals and primary health centers must be maintained as accurate and complete as possible. Standard forms and acceptable formats are often available in the work place. Midwives functioning in different settings are required to keep detailed records, which must be made as contemporaneously as is reasonable.

Records commonly maintained by midwives include:

❖ Antenatal record for individual clients in which details of the pregnancy and treatments prescribed is entered
❖ Antenatal register with record of all women attending the clinic
❖ Birth register with details of childbirth, including mode of delivery, sex of the baby, birth weight, weight of placenta, Apgar score, etc
❖ Postnatal record contains details of childbirth, condition of the newborn, condition of the mother, etc
❖ Under-five record/card: A card for each baby with information such as serial weight and height, immunization, weaning and vitamin supplements given. These are entered until the child becomes 5-years-old
❖ Eligible couples register: Record of all couples in the reproductive age group and the mode of contraceptives used is maintained in the health centers.
❖ Register for recording contraceptives: Condom distribution, oral pill register, IUD register, and sterilization register for males and females.
❖ Morbidity registers for different categories of clients.
❖ Admission and discharge register.
❖ Outpatient treatment register: Names, diagnoses and treatments given to patients
❖ Referral register
❖ Stock register
❖ Contraceptive follow-up register
❖ Death register: Record of all deaths of mothers and babies including details such as full name, age address, age at the time of death, cause of death.

General Guidelines for Maintaining Records

1. All information must be entered in the proper place/particular column in the appropriate register or record.
2. Information must be entered as soon as possible to avoid incompleteness and inaccuracies.
3. All information to be written clearly and legibly for use by supervisors and others for statistical and related purposes.

4. All records must be arranged in order and safeguarded
5. Records should be treated as confidential material and away from handling by unauthorized persons.
6. All record should be kept safely for prescribed period of time, minimum period of five years in government institutions.

All the records written must be legible, accurate and complete with all the required details for effective tabulation and communication. The information may be used currently as well as retrospectively and hence, all records and reports must be preserved.

BIBLIOGRAPHY

1. Dutta DC. Textbook of Obstetrics, 5th edn. Calcutta: New Central Book Company, 2001.
2. Government of India, MCH Division, National Child Survival and Safe Motherhood Program, 1994.
3. Hogarh J. Glossarry of Health Care Terminology, Copenhagen: WHO, 1978.
4. National Institute of Health and Family Welfare, Reproductive and Childhealth Module for Staff Nurses' Integrated Skill Development Training, Munirka, New Delhi: NIHF, 2000.
5. Park K.r Park's Textbook of Preventive and Social Medicine, 16th edn. Jabalpur: Banarasidas Bhanot Publishers, 2000.
6. WHO, Health for All, Sr No 4, 1981.
7. WHO, World Health, 1981.

56

Perinatal Loss and Grief

Learning Objectives

Upon completing this chapter, the learner will be able to:
- Describe the grief situations in perinatal period
- Describe the nature of perinatal mourning
- Explain the phases of mourning
- Explain the help to be given to grieving parents
- Explain the care needed by care givers.

All expectant parents expect a healthy baby as the outcome of pregnancy. For most parents and families, healthy pregnancy, normal childbirth and healthy baby are the realities, but for a few others the reality is loss, grief and mourning. Caring for mothers who confront perinatal or neonatal loss are occasional yet important grief situations a midwife has to deal with. Providing assistance to cope with the loss through healthy grieving process is important for resumption of balance or homeostasis in the life of the bereaved person.

LOSS, GRIEF AND MOURNING

Loss

Loss is defined as the anticipated or actual removal of something or someone of value to a person. Perinatal losses include those, which involve loss the baby to abortion, miscarriage, stillbirth or having a baby but with loss of expectations of perfect baby image such as prematurity or congenital abnormalities.

Perinatal Grief

Perinatal grief is the emotional reactions to a significant loss related to childbearing that can occur from the pre-conception period through early infancy (Moore in Nicols and Zwelling, 1997).

Mourning

Mourning is the expression of sorrow with outward signs of grief, which include crying, fatigue, feeling of emptiness and a depressed mood. The process of mourning involves accepting the loss and experiencing the pain in response to the loss and redirecting the energy from grieving to reconstructing of one's life.

GRIEF SITUATIONS IN THE PERINATAL PERIOD

Feeling of loss and the need to grieve may occur at any time in the childbearing period.
- Grieving related to infertility occurs in those who have difficulty to conceive
- Spontaneous and induced abortions and ectopic pregnancies are losses in the first and early second trimesters
- Intrauterine fetal deaths, induced abortions, and premature births are losses in the late second and third trimester
- Stillbirths, neonatal deaths and birth of infants with congenital anomalies are losses in the immediate period after childbirth
- Birth of a baby of a sex different from that expected by the parents is a grief situation for some
- Mothers who choose elective abortion also mourn their infants
- Death of an infant in the neonatal nursery following the immediate period after birth is also included as perinatal loss.

THE NATURE OF PERINATAL LOSS AND GRIEF

Perinatal loss and grief are different from other types of grief in several respects.

Intense Feelings

For parents who experience an outcome of pregnancy different from their expectation and from the experience of most people they know, the feelings are intense. To them, a traumatic event has substituted for what was expected to be a joyful event.

Anticipatory Grief

When an intrauterine fetal anomaly or death is diagnosed before the onset of labor, there may be few hours or days of anticipation.

Emotional and Physical Stress

In some instances, perinatal loss follows a period of maternal illness. This leaves parents emotionally and physically strained.

Mourning in the Absence of a Visible Object or Baby

For losses in the first trimester, parents mourn in the absence of a visible object or baby.

Guilt and Anger

With abortions or miscarriages, they experience the loss of both the baby and the pregnancy, and guilt if they engaged or failed to engage in activities they think were related to the experience. When a seemingly perfect fetus is stillborn or extremely premature, there is also aggravated guilt and anger wondering if they did something wrong.

Loss of Relationship

A mother develops a unique and special relationship with her fetus during pregnancy that is different from her relationship to any other person. As a result when the baby is lost either before birth or after birth, her experience of loss is also different from that of any other loss.

Limited Memories

When a baby is lost to miscarriage, to stillbirth or to loss in the immediate period after birth, there are limited memories. For some, it may be an ultrasound image, a single photograph or remembering the feel of a fetal kick.

Social Support

Family and friends may not recognize the significance of the loss to the parents and may not, therefore, provide adequate support. The parents experiencing the loss may feel the need to be strong for each other. This often diminishes the ability of each to talk about their loss with others.

PHASES OF MOURNING (GRIEVING)

The stages grief through which a person is likely to have to work has been described by Kubler Ross (1970). These stages are not negotiated in a consistent, sequential order and there will be individual variations. Often a person moves back and forth through them eventually achieving resolution.

The stages of mourning include initial shock and disbelief, a phase of anxiety and searching, a phase of disorganization and a phase of resolution (reorganization). Each phase is characterized by physical symptoms, behaviors and feelings. Feelings such as anger or guilt may appear to be dissolved, only to reappear at a later time. Feelings, behaviors and physical symptoms may intensify at certain times and worn out at other times.

Period of Shock and Disbelief

Shock is always the initial response to loss. Responses associated with shock include disbelief, crying, wanting to escape and becoming numb or incoherent. The initial responses comprise a defense mechanism, which serves to protect the individual from the full impact of the loss in the period immediately after the loss. In this period, they may verbalize statements of denial and show apathy, inappropriate behavior, unexplained calm, impaired concentration, difficulty in decision-making and physical detachment. These feelings may last from several days to weeks. It is important for midwives to recognize that denial is a defense mechanism that serves a useful purpose of giving the person time to mobilize her coping recourses.

As decision-making is difficult at this stage, they will need help.

Phase of Anxiety and Searching

This is the second phase of mourning, which is commonly intense from the second to fourth or fifth month after a loss.

Phase of Disorganization

During this period, they find it difficult to accomplish their normal tasks. Physical symptoms such as body ache; restlessness, malaise and anorexia may be experienced. Feelings such as sadness, fertility, lowered self esteem, social withdrawal and preoccupation with the lost baby are some of the characteristics of this period.

Resolution or Reorganization

In this stage, the restoration of the capacity to interact with others and to plan for the future takes place. This process may be slow and vary with setbacks in different individuals. Although a mother is never likely to get over her loss, she will probably be able to eventually integrate it into her experience of life. This ultimate degree of resolution is recognizable in the person's ability to contemplate realistically the strengths and weaknesses of her lost relationship. Family relationships stabilize and the capacity to concentrate on activities and to interact with others is restored.

HELPING GRIEVING PARENTS

Nursing interventions to assist parents who face stillbirth or neonatal death and go through the mourning process requires several support strategies.

Immediate Support

Immediate support includes calling a support person such as a close friend, family or clergy and ensuring that the mother is not left alone.

Attitude and Empathy

The attitude and empathy of the staff are important in terms of how the process is remembered and perhaps resolved. Conveying an understanding that each fetus or infant is special and significant to the mother is important.

Validating the Loss

This includes understanding and accepting the family's feelings about their loss and encouraging the acceptance of the baby's existence.

❖ Be sensitive to the family's cultural values related to disposing the infant's body
❖ Encourage the father to share the grief of the mother and participate in her care
❖ Avoid rationalizing that she would have another baby and not to worry
❖ Provide opportunity to grieve and encourage to verbalizing their feelings
❖ Hold or touch the mother when she cries to convey a feeling of caring
❖ Give some momentos for the mother to keep such as a card with information of the baby, a lock of hair or certificate of life or death.

Making the Loss Real

❖ Prepare parents for what they will see if they choose to see and hold the dead baby. Give them some description like body temperature, color, size, bruises and deformities
❖ Stay with them unless they request time alone. Allow the parents to see and hold the dead baby if they wish
❖ Wrap the baby in a clean and warm blanket or sheet. The care taken with the baby demonstrates respect
❖ Refer to the baby by name if a name has been given. If no name, refer to the baby by the correct sex
❖ If the parents wish, take a photograph of the baby
❖ Encourage parents to have a burial or funeral for the baby
❖ Discuss medical findings and autopsy results (if done) in a frank and sensitive manner.

For Mothers who Grieve through the Miscarriage

❖ Convey an understanding that they mourn their fantasized baby
❖ Empathize the intense grieving they go through

❖ Provide privacy and support as they go through the process.

Death of an Infant in the Nursery

When a baby dies after surviving the immediate period of days or weeks, parents need special help.

❖ During the period between birth and death, encourage parents to spend as much time as possible with their baby
❖ Provide opportunities to hold the baby, touch the baby or care for the baby as appropriate
❖ Provide opportunity to be with the baby in the final period before death
❖ Immediately after death, be with the family or be available for support. The family should not be left to feel alone or abandoned.

CARING FOR THE CAREGIVER

The sense of loss and grief that accompanies perinatal loss are not limited to parents and family members. Nurses and other professionals grieve as well. Before nurses can be helpful to parents and families, they must recognize their own potential for grief. It is difficult for most nurses not to identify with young parents who grieve. Many nurses are in their own childbearing years and some may have experienced a perinatal loss themselves or may fear such a loss in the future. Shock and disbelief may be experienced for loses which occur suddenly. The inability to prevent the death may be perceived as a threat to selfesteem. They may try to cope with their anxiety by remaining detached. There may be feelings of anger at the baby, parents or other team members.

Nurses need opportunities to express their feelings and ask questions. They need acceptance of colleagues. An effective counseling service and team spirit will prevent staff burnout.

Record Keeping

Records regarding fetal demise, infant death or miscarriage are essential for accurate vital statistics of the country and for taking measure for preventing such occurrences in future when possible. Details of events and management is must, therefore be entered in all the relevant records and registers.

Continued Care

Ongoing support of the grieving mother/ parents will need to be provided by community health nurses or other health workers. The suppression of lactation may require particular attention during this period. If follow-up at home cannot be arranged, clear and detailed instructions will have to be given before the parents leaves the hospital. For a mother to go through a healthy grieving process and to come to terms with her loss, the care and attention given to her must be of the highest standard, empathetic and individualized.

NURSING PROCESS FOR THE CLIENT EXPERIENCING A LOSS

Assessment

Grief Behaviors

❖ Sleep disturbance
❖ Thoughts centered on loss
❖ Dependency
❖ Withdrawal
❖ Anger
❖ Guilt.

Support System

❖ Family members
❖ Friends
❖ Social and religious support.

Analysis/Nursing Diagnosis

❖ Ineffective individual/family coping
❖ Sleep pattern disturbance
❖ Altered thought process
❖ Impaired verbal communication
❖ Poor concentration
❖ Altered nutrition—Less than body requirements
❖ Altered family process
❖ Altered health maintenance.

Planning and Implementation Goals

Client/Family Will

❖ Discuss responses to loss
❖ Resume normal eating/sleeping patterns
❖ Resume activities of daily living (ADL) as they accept the loss
❖ Respond adaptively to the loss.

Interventions

❖ Encourage client/family to express feelings
❖ Accept negative feelings/defenses
❖ Employ empathic listening
❖ Educate the client and family of the grief stages and normalcy of their feelings and responses to the loss
❖ Refer client/family to support persons or groups.

Evaluation

Client/Family

❖ Express feeling
❖ Progress through mourning process
❖ Seek necessary support.

BIBLIOGRAPHY

1. Iles S. The loss of early pregnancy, In: Oats M.R., Psychological Aspects of Obstetrics and Gynecology, Bailliere. London: Tindall, 1989.
2. Kowalski K. "Perinatal loss and bereavement", In: Sonstegard L, Kowalski K, Jennings B, Women's health: Crisis and Illness in Childhearing, Orlando: Grune and Straffon, 1987.
3. Kubler-Ross E. On Death and Dying, London: Tavistock Publications, 1970.
4. Lewis E, Bourne S. Perinatal Death, In: Oates M, Psychological Aspects of Obstetrics and Gynecology, London, Bailliere Tindall, 1989.
5. Littlewood J. Aspects of Grief: Bereavement in Adult Life, Routledge, London: Tavistock Publications, 1992.
6. MaCaffery M. Nursing Management of the Patient with Pain, Philadelphia: Lippincott, 1979.
7. Nicholas FN, Zwelling E. Maternal Newborn Nursing: Theory and Practice, Philadelphia: WB Saunders Co, 1997.
8. O'Hare T, Creed F. "Life events and miscarriage", British Journal of Psychiatry 1995;167(6):799-05.
9. Redstad I, Nordin C, Steineck G. Psychological Complications after Stillbirth, British Medical Journal 1996;312(7045):1505-8.

57

Radiology and Ultrasonics in Obstetrics

Learning Objectives

Upon completing this chapter, the learner will be able to:

❖ Describe the use of radiology in obstetrics and list the hazards of radiation
❖ Enumerate the use of ultrasound in the present day obstetric practice
❖ Describe how ultrasound works and the different methods available for diagnostic purposes
❖ Explain the responsibilities of midwives regarding prenatal ultrasound screening.

RADIOLOGY IN OBSTETRICS

Radiology in obstetrics is used mainly to supplement and confirm findings, which have been made on clinical examination during pregnancy. Until recently, radiological examinations have been used extensively in obstetric clients. With the advent of Ultrasonography and Magnetic Resonance Imaging (MRI), the use of radiology is declining. Currently, radiological examinations are done on pregnant women only if the following principles are met:

❖ The benefits of radiation must outweigh the risks of the procedure
❖ Minimum radiation dose to be used
❖ Appropriate fetal shielding to be done
❖ First trimester should preferably be avoided
❖ Benefits and safety of ultrasonography must be considered as an alternative (Dutta, 2001).

Indications

Fetal

❖ Diagnosis of pregnancy: Fetal skeletal shadow is visible at 16th week of pregnancy.

❖ Diagnosis of hydatidiform mole: Negative fetal shadow beyond 16th-18th week
❖ Multiple pregnancy: To confirm the diagnosis, to note the lie of the fetus and to exclude malformations
❖ Hydramnios: To exclude multiple pregnancies and to diagnose congenital bone malformations such as open spina bifida or anencephaly
❖ Intrauterine death of the fetus: Overlapping of skull bones and hyper flexion of the spine may be present
❖ Diagnosis of congenital anomalies such as the extent of imperforate anus, intestinal obstruction, diaphragmatic hernia
❖ Diagnosis of limb defects such as Amelia (absence of limb), ectromelia (absence of a part of a limb), phocomelia (absence of proximal part of a limb) and mermaid (single lower limb)
❖ Fetal maturity: Evidenced by overall fetal shadow, thickness and density of ossification centers of the upper end of the tibia and lower end of the femur (usually after 38 weeks)
❖ Placental localization
❖ Pelvimetry in cases suspected to have pelvic contraction
❖ Secondary abdominal pregnancy
❖ Hydrops fetalis
❖ Amniography: Abnormalities such as atresia of gastrointestinal tract could be revealed
❖ Patients having cardio-pulmonary disease may require X-ray during pregnancy.

Radiation Hazards

The risk is primarily based on the estimated dose of radiation and period of gestation.

* Teratogenic effects: Irradiation of less than 5 rads is not associated with any defects. Higher doses can cause microcephaly, mental retardation, cataracts, retinal degeneration, cleft palate, hypoplasia of genitalia, etc.
* Oncogenecity: Fetal exposure in the first trimester is associated with an increased risk of malignancy.

Measures that Help to Reduce Radiation

* Avoiding as far as possible any radiological examination during pregnancy
* Use of minimum essential plates
* Use of high frequency X-rays
* Use of short exposure times
* Use of fast films
* Use of filters
* Use of screens when possible, e.g. shielding of the abdomen during chest radiography.

ULTRASONICS IN OBSTETRICS

The ultrasound is a sound wave beyond the audible range of frequency greater than 2 MHz (cycles per second). The commonly used frequency range in obstetrics is 3.5 to 5 MHz. SONAR stands for "Sound, Navigation and Ranging". In clinical practice, two main varieties of ultrasound (sound that is produced at a very high pitch) are used depending upon whether the reflected waves give audible or visual signals.

* The apparatus, which interprets the audible signals—doptone and sonicaid are easy to carry and simple to use even with batteries. It can detect fetal heartbeats as early as 10th week of gestation
* The apparatus for interpretation of visible signals—the sonar system, which is a much more sophisticated and bulky apparatus, is used in three forms:
  1. The A-scan, that gives a one-dimensional picture
  2. The B-scan, that gives a composite two-dimensional picture
  3. The real-time scanner that depicts movements—to display cardiac and breathing activity.

How Does Ultrasound Work?

Scanners are used to produce static pictures. The picture is built up as a single crystal transducer (a thin disk to which a wire is attached), which is moved backwards and forwards across the area scanned. When the transducer is placed on the body and as it encounters a structure, a fraction of that sound is reflected back. The echo is detected electronically and transmitted on to the screen as dots. The amount of sound from each organ varies according to the type of tissue encountered:

* Strong echoes give bright dots, e.g. bone
* Weaker echoes give various shades of gray according to their strength
* Fluid-filled areas cause no reflexion and give rise to a black image.

The real-time scanners are so called because it produces a moving picture on the screen as opposed to scanners that give static picture. The real-time scanner can have several types of transducers attached to it, which are interchangeable and are used according to the type of image needed and the part of the anatomy to be examined. Types of transducers in common use includes: *The linear array; the curved linear array; the sector and the vaginal probe*. Instead of a single crystal, all these types of transducers have many crystals that fire off electrical energy and collect the echoes very rapidly, thus producing the moving picture.

Use of Ultrasound in Obstetrics

Sonography is a noninvasive procedure and has been proved safe to the conceptus, even with repeated exposures at any stage of pregnancy (Dutta, 2001). Routine sonography in early months is used for:

* Diagnosis of pregnancy: Detects gestational ring at 5th week, fetal poles and gestational sac at 6th week, cardiac pulsation at 7th week and embryonic movements at 8th week of gestation.
* Detection of abnormal conceptus prior to clinical manifestations and fetal malformations.
* Accurate determination of gestational age is possible, which is helpful later in

pregnancy when IUGR is suspected. For this, crown-rump length (CRL) at 10 to 11 weeks gives the best predictive value.

❖ Diagnosis of twins can be made early in pregnancy for effective management.

❖ To diagnose unsuspected placenta previa: Because of the possibility of placental migration to the upper segment, repeat scanning should be performed later-around 34th week (Figs 57.1 and 57.2).

Selective sonography is done when indicated at any time during pregnancy for the following reasons:

❖ To determine the maturity of the fetus: Crown-rump length (CRL), biparietal diameter (BDP) and femur length (FL) are the measurements of choice for assessment of gestational age. Determination of the maturity is important in cases of:
   – Uncertain gestational age
   – Discrepancy between amenorrhea and uterine size
   – Prior to elective induction for post-maturity or elective cesarean section.

❖ Suspicion of fetal and/or placental abnormalities such as:
   – Suspected ectopic pregnancy
   – Blighted ovum (empty sac)
   – Incomplete abortion
   – Hydatidiform mole
   – Localization of placenta as in placenta previa
   – Abruptio placentae
   – Intrauterine growth retardation
   – Intrauterine death
   – Malpresentations such as breech, transverse or face
   – Structural defects such as neural tube defects, absent or abnormal limbs
   – Defects of gastrointestinal, and urinary system, and heart defects.

❖ Prior to invasive procedures such as chorion villus biopsy, amniocentesis, cordocentesis, fetoscopy and intrauterine fetal therapy

❖ As a part of antepartum or intrapartum fetal surveillance
   – Biophysical profile.

❖ Integrity of a previous cesarean scar—A weak scar or placental implantation over the scar can be detected.

Fig. 57.1: Image of a fetus in the second trimester

Fig. 57.2: Placenta previa: Longitudinal scan shows the placenta (P) lying just above the cervical os (O)

❖ Postpartum period:
   – Secondary PPH
   – Retained placental bits
   – Subinvolution due to fibromyoma.

❖ Neonatal head screening to diagnose:
   – Intraventricular hemorrhage
   – Hydrocephalus.

Transvaginal Ultrasonography (TVS)

This is usually done during the first trimester of pregnancy. As the transducer is closer to the object, the images are of enhanced quality.

A full bladder is not required. Transvaginal sonography is superior to transabdominal sonography in diagnosing placenta previa.

Doppler Ultrasound (Audible Signal)

Ultrasound transmitted into the body in a narrow beam is transferred back at the same frequency when the object is still. When moving, there is a change in frequency known as the Doppler shift. The frequency increases or decreases according to whether the movement is towards or away from the source of energy.

It is used for monitoring the fetal heart rate, which can be picked up as early as 10th week of gestation. Uterine and fetal blood flow can be assessed and the fetus at risk of compromise could be identified. Leg vein thrombosis can be diagnosed by noting the absence of hissing sound of blood flow through the veins.

Midwife's Responsibility Regarding Prenatal Screening

Midwives take care of pregnant women in different stages of their pregnancy. They often need to involve themselves in preparing and counseling women through the process. When giving information about the screening tests available or prescribed, it is important to include information regarding:

❖ Why the test is offered?
❖ What the test involves?
❖ When and how the results will be given?

In order to advise women regarding the tests that are available, the midwife needs to keep up-to-date with current technological advances.

Information given to women should also include how the woman needs to prepare herself, e.g. by attending with a full bladder for a scan.

The midwife needs to be available for women when ambiguous or screen positive results plunge them and their spouses into a period of anxiety as they try to make decisions regarding further tests and/or termination of the pregnancy.

BIBLIOGRAPHY

1. Chudleigh P, Pearce MJ. Obstetric Ultrasound, Edinburgh: Churchill Livingstone, 1983.
2. Dutta DC. Textbook of Obsterrics, 5th edn. Calcutta: New Central Book Company, 2001.
3. Lockwood MD, Benacerraf MD, Krinsdy A. A Sonographic Screening Method for Down's Syndrome, American Journal of Obstetrics and Gynecology, 1987;157:803-8.
4. Luck CA. Value of routine ultrasound at 19 weeks, British Medical Journal 1992;304:1474-8.
5. Proud J. Specialized Antenatal Investigations, In: Bennett RV, Linda KB, Myles. Textbook for Midwives, 13th edn. Edinburgh: Churchill Livingstone, 1999.

58

Legal and Ethical Aspects of Midwifery

Learning Objectives

Upon completion of this chapter, the learner will be able to:

❖ Identify the legal and ethical standards in the practice of maternal-newborn nursing
❖ Discuss the ethical principles involved in midwifery practice
❖ Describe the legal issues in midwifery practice
❖ Outline the patient's bill of rights and guidelines for legal protection.

While ethical and legal considerations are a component of all areas and specialties of nursing, some unique issues exist in maternal-newborn nursing. Many of these issues occur because two parties, tightly liked are involved–the mother and the fetus/newborn. Adequate knowledge of legal concepts and standards of care for practicing within legal boundaries is essential for all practitioners of nursing in general and midwifery in particular.

LAWS AND ETHICS

Ethics refers to the branch of philosophy that provides rules and principles that can be used for resolving ethical dilemmas.

Laws are rules that govern the behavior of individuals and represent the minimum standard of morality (Tschudin, 2003). Laws are written with the interests of society as the major consideration and ethics focus on the interests of an individual in the society. While laws are rules that are external to an individual and that members of a society must obey, ethics tend to be personal and involve values, beliefs and interpretations to guide behavior.

Standards of Practice

National standards provide an expectation of the delivery of care to clients. Regulations and policies at institutional levels provide for delivery of safe care. Educational programs of midwifery ensure that all new nurses/midwives can safely deliver care within the scope of usual midwifery practice.

State License or Registration

Practice of nursing and midwifery is regulated by state registration councils through license to practice. If a nurse/midwife moves to a different state, she must obtain registration in that state in order to practice there. The state license is meant to protect the consumers by ensuring that the midwife has appropriate education and can provide safe care.

Institutional Policies

Policies and regulations of an institution govern the nursing and midwifery care to clients seeking health care in that place.

Community Standards

A midwife's performance will be evaluated according to the availability of medical and nursing knowledge that would be used in the management of similar patients under similar circumstances by competent midwives, given the facilities, resources and options available.

Code of Ethics

The code of ethics published by "American College of Nurse-Midwives" (ACNM) serves as guidelines for practice of midwifery for all nurses.

❖ Nurse-midwifery exists for the good of women and their families. The goal is to safeguard this by practice in accordance with the philosophy and standards of ACNM for the practice of nurse-midwifery

❖ Nurse-midwives hold the belief that childbearing and parturition are normal life processes. When intervention is indicated, it is integrated into care in a way that preserves the dignity of the woman and her family

❖ Decisions regarding nurse-midwifery care require client participation in an on-going negotiation process in order to develop a safe plan of care. This process considers cultural diversity, individual autonomy and legal responsibilities

❖ Nurse-midwives share professional information with their clients that leads to informed consent participation. This sharing is done without coercion or deception

❖ Nurse-midwives practice competently. They consult and share when indicated by their professional scope of practice and personal limitations

❖ Nurse-midwives provide care without discrimination based on race, religion, lifestyle, sexual orientation, socioeconomic status or nature of health problem

❖ Nurse-midwives maintain confidentiality except when there is clear, serious and immediate danger or when mandated by law

❖ Nurse-midwives take appropriate action to protect clients from harm when endangered by incompetent and unethical practices

❖ Nurse-midwives interact respectfully with people with whom they work and practice

❖ Nurse-midwives participate in developing and improving the care of women and families through supporting the profession, research and education of nurse-midwifery students and nurse-midwives

❖ Nurse-midwives promote community, state and national efforts to ensure access to quality care and to meet the health needs of women and their families.

Ethical Principles that Guide Nursing Practice

Four major principles guide ethical thinking in nursing practice—*respect for autonomy, nonmaleficence, beneficence* and *justice*. These principles may be used in conjunction with theoretical perspectives as guidelines to help resolve ethical dilemmas.

❖ *Respect for autonomy:* It refers to individual independence in holding a particular view, making choices and taking action based on values and beliefs (Beauchamp and Childress, 2001). The concept of respect for autonomy recognizes the inherent worth of the individual and that a competent human being is qualified to make decisions in his/her own best interests. The concept of informed consent is firmly rooted in the principle of respect for autonomy.

❖ *Nonmaleficence:* It refers to the concept of preventing harm to others and is an important principle for nurses. Harm is the interference with mental or physical well-being of others (Beauchamp and Childress, 2001). Basic rules include not killing, not causing pain, not disabling, and not depriving of freedom. Nonmaleficence encompasses both harm and the risk of harm. The harm may be either intentional or nonintentional. Nurses have the obligation to exercise due care in professional practice so that unintentional harms do not occur. *Due care* is a legal and ethical standard of performance by which professionals abide. As professionals, nurses must possess sufficient knowledge and skills and render care that is cautious, diligent and thoughtful

❖ *Beneficence:* It means doing good and includes prevention of harm, removal of evil and promotion of good (Frankena, 1973). Nurses should have their goal to promote the welfare of clients in their care. These might include recommendations regarding diet, exercise, smoking and alcohol consumption

❖ *Justice:* It refers to how the benefits and burdens in the society are shared. Health care is a benefit that promotes the health and will-being of individuals in our society. All pregnant women should be treated equally in terms of access to care.

Legal Issues in Midwifery Practice

As in the practice of nursing in any medical specialty or health care facility, nurses practicing maternal-newborn nursing and gynecology nursing need also to be knowledgeable of the legal issues that may occur.

1. *Professional negligence:* Medical negligence is the legal error committed by medical personnel. In legal terms, this error is a *tort*. A tort is a civil wrong that injures a person. If a tort is intentional, it becomes a crime of *assault* or *battery*.

   Negligence is an unintentional tort—a form of malpractice. In order to prove that a negligent act or tort has occurred, four elements must be present.

   ❖ A duty must exist between the injured party and the professional accused of wrong doing

   ❖ A breach of duty must have occurred, i.e. the midwife must have practiced outside the standard of care of her profession

   ❖ The breach of duty must be the proximate cause of the claimed injury

   ❖ There must be damage or injury to the claimant that are recognized by law and compensable.

2. *Medication error:* Nurses are to administer medications correctly to patients. Administering wrong medicines, wrong doses, wrong routes or timing resulting in harm may be considered an act of malpractice.

3. *Failure of monitoring:* A nurse is responsible to monitor clients admitted with obstetric or gynecologic problems. Monitoring during intrapartum and postpartum period requires great care.

4. *Informed consent:* Based on a clients right to self-determination, informed consent demands that information regarding treatment procedures be given to clients and their consent obtained by concerned physician and nurses witness the patient's signing in the form. If she finds that a valid consent is missing, it must be reported on time.

5. *Nursing care of newborn:* Newborns require professional and specialized care. Failure of the neonatal nurse to meet her obligations can result in liability in employment or even a civil suit.

6. *Failure in assessing:* Failure in assessing and reporting changes in a client's condition for timely action can be considered a malpractice.

7. *Abortion:* Nurses assist in the performance of abortions under the act of medical termination of pregnancy (MTP) and take care of patients' following the procedure. They have the right to refuse to assist in the procedure if the abortion is illegal.

   Although most nurses assume that they will never be named in a law suit, it is true that a few are. Nurses these days take up employment in institutions of different levels in several countries of the world. Increasing awareness of health care and patients' rights in communities makes it imperative for health professionals to be more alert in delivering quality care that is ethically and morality right and to exercise adequate care not to give chance for legal issues.

A Patient's Bill of Rights

A patient's bill of rights was adopted by the American Hospital Association in 1973 and was later revised in 1992. This bill serves both care givers and recipients of care everywhere. The rights can be exercised on patient's behalf by a designated surrogate or proxy decision maker if the patient lacks decision-making capacity, legally incompetent or is a minor.

1. The patient has the right to considerate and respectful care.

2. The patient has the right to obtain from physician and other direct care givers relevant, correct and understandable information concerning diagnosis, treatment and prognosis. Patients have the right to know the identity of physicians, nurses and others involved in their care, as well as when those involved are students, residents or other trainees. The patient also has the right to know the immediate and long-term financial implications of treatment.

3. The patient has the right to make decisions about the plan of care, prior to and during the course of treatment and refuse a recommended treatment or plan of care to the extent permitted by law and hospital policy and to be informed of the medical consequences of this action.

4. The patient has the right to have an 'advance directive' such as a living will, health care proxy or durable power of attorney for health care concerning treatment or designating a surrogate decision maker with the expectation that the hospital will honor the intent of that directive to the extent permitted by law.

5. The patient has the right to every consideration of privacy. Case discussion, consultation, examination and treatment should be conducted so as to protect each patient's privacy.

6. The patient has the right to expect that all communications and records pertaining to his / her care will be treated as confidential by the hospital except in cases such as suspected abuse and public health hazards when reporting is required by law.

7. The patient has the right to review the records pertaining to his or her medical care and to have the information explained or interpreted as necessary.

8. The patient has the right to expect that when medically appropriate and legally permissible or when a patient has so requested, he may be transferred to another health care facility.

9. The patient has the right to ask and be informed of the existence of business relationship among the hospital, educational institutions and other health care agencies that may influence the patient's treatment and care.

10. The patient has the right to consent to or decline to participate in proposed research studies on human experimentation affecting care and treatment or requiring direct patient involvement and to have these studies fully explained prior to consent.

11. The patient has the right to expect reasonable continuity of care when appropriate and to be informed by physicians and caregivers of available and realistic patient care options when hospital care is no longer appropriate.

12. The patient has the right tot be informed of hospital policies and practices that relate to his care, treatment and responsibilities.

Nurses are responsible for determining their own actions and for supporting clients who are making their moral decisions or for whom decisions are made by others. Nurses can enhance their ethical practice and client advocacy by clarifying their own values, understanding the values of other healthcare professionals, and becoming familiar with nursing code of ethics. Client advocacy involves concern and actions on behalf of another person or organization in order to bring about change. Her functions of advocacy role are to inform, support and mediate for the patient.

Nurses need to know and apply legal aspects in their many different roles. Competent practice is a major legal safeguard for nurses.

Nurse-midwives and student midwives have specific legal obligations and responsibilities

| Table 58.1 | Practice guidelines for legal protection |

1. Function within the scope of your education, job description and nurse practice Act.

2. Follow the procedures and policies of the employing agency.

3. Build and maintain good rapport with clients.

4. Always check the identity of a client to make sure it is the right client.

5. Observe and monitor the client accurately, communicate and record significant changes in the client's condition to the physician.

6. Promptly and accurately document all assessments and care given.

7. Be alert when implementing nursing interventions and give each task your full attention and skill.

8. Perform procedures correctly and appropriately.

9. Make sure the right medications are given in the correct dose, by the right route, at the scheduled time and to the right client.

10. When delegating nursing responsibilities, make sure that the person who is delegated the task understands what to do and that the person had the required knowledge and skill.

11. Protect clients from injury.

12. Report all incidents involving clients.

13. Always check any order a client questions.

14. Know your own strengths and weaknesses. Ask for assistance and supervision in situations for which you are inadequately prepared.

15. Maintain your clinical competence. For students, this demands study and practice before caring for clients. For graduate nurses, it means continued study to maintain and update clinical knowledge and skills.

Source: Kozier, Erb, Berman & Burke "Fundamentals of Nursing, 2007.

to clients and employers. Nurses can be held liable for failure to carry out a task or procedure according to standards or for a harm or injury due to failure to follow the standard, which are considered unintentional torts. They can be held responsible for intentional torts such as assault and battery, false imprisonment or invasion of privacy. Practice guidelines for legal protection outlined in Table 58.1, if followed, provide good safeguard for nurses.

When a client is accidentally injured or involved in an unusual situation such as an obstetric emergency, the midwife's first responsibility is to take steps to protect the client and then to notify the physician.

BIBLIOGRAPHY

1. Beanchamp T, Childress J. Principles of Biomedical Ethics, 5th edn, New York; Oxford University Press 2001.
2. Fry S. The Ethics of Caring: can it survive in Nursing? Nursing Outlook 1988; 36(1):48.
3. Hall, JK. Nursing Ethics and Law. Philadelphia; WB Saunders, 1996.
4. Kozier B, Erb G, Berman A, Burke K. Fundamentals of Nursing, 7th edn, India. Dorling Kindersley Pvt Ltd, 2007.
5. Kumari N, Sharman S, Gupta P. Midwifery and Gynecological Nursing. India; S. Vikas & Company.
6. Littleton L, Engebretson J. Maternity Nursing Care; Thompson Delmar Learning, India, 2007.
7. Tschudin V. Ethics in Nursing, 3rd edn, Philadelphia, USA; WB Sounders, 2003.

59

National Population Policy and Family Welfare Programs

Learning Objectives

Upon completion of this chapter, the learner will be able to:

❖ Describe the present population status in India
❖ List the measures adopted since 1950 and the demographic achievements after half a century
❖ Describe the strategies and action plan of the National Population Policy (NPP)
❖ Describe the schemes under the National Family Welfare Programs (NFW) for maternal and child health.

India is currently the world's second largest country in population. India crossed the one billion mark in the year 2000; one year after the world population crossed the six billion threshold. India is currently home to about 1.21 billion people representing a full 17 percent of the earth's population. India's 2011 census showed that the country's population had grown by 181 million people in the prior decade.

Demographers expect India's population to surpass the population of China, currently the most populous country of the world by 2030. At that time, India is expected to have a population of more than 1.53 billion while China's population is forecast to be at its peak of 1.46 billion.

When India gained independence from the United Kingdom sixty four years ago, the country's population was a mere 350 million. Since 1947, the population of India has more than triple. In 1950, India's total fertility rate was approximately six children per women. Nonetheless since 1952, India has worked to control its population growth. In 1983, the country's National Health Policy was to have a replacement value of total fertility rate of 2.1 by the year 2000. That did not occur.

National Population Policy 2000

In the year 2000, the country established a new National Population Policy, to stem the growth of the country's population. One of the primary goals of the policy was to reduce the Total Fertility Rate (TFR) to 2.1 by 2010. One of the steps along the path towards the goal in 2010 was a total fertility rate of 2.6 by 2012.

India's demographic achievements half a century after formulating the national family welfare program are:

❖ Reduced crude birth rate (CBR) from 40.8 in 1951 to 26.4 in 1998
❖ Halved the infant mortality rate (IMR) from 146 per 1000 live births in 1951 to 72 per 1000 live births in 1998
❖ Quadrupled the couple protection rate (CPR) from 10.4 percent in 1971 to 44 percent in 1999
❖ Reduced crude death rate (CDR) from 25 in 1951 to 9 in 1998
❖ Added 25 years to life expectancy from 37 years to 62 years
❖ Achieved nearly universal awareness of the need for and methods of family planning
❖ Reduced total fertility rate from 6 in 1951 to 3.3 in 1997.

Stabilizing population is an essential requirement for promoting sustainable development with more equitable distribution.

However, it is as much a function of making reproductive health care accessible and affordable for all.

* Increasing the provision and outreach of primary and secondary education
* Extending basic amenities including sanitation, safe drinking water and housing
* Empowering women and enhancing their employment opportunities and providing transport and communication facilities.

The National Population Policy 2000 (NPP 2000) affirms the commitment of government towards voluntary and informed choice and consent of citizens while availing of reproductive health services and continuing of 'target free' approach in administering family planning services. The NPP 2000 provides a policy framework for advancing goals and prioritizing strategies during the next decade to meet the reproductive and child health needs of the people of India and to achieve net replacement levels by 2010.

Objective of NPP

The objective of the NPP 2000 was to address the unmet needs for contraception, health care infrastructure and health personnel and to provide integrated service delivery for basic reproductive and child health care. The medium-term objective was to bring the TFR to replacement level by 2010, through vigorous implementation of inter-sectoral operational strategies. The long-term objective was to achieve a stable population by 2045, at a level consistent with the requirements of sustainable economic growth, social development and environmental protection.

In order to achieve these objectives, the following targets were set:

* Address the unmet needs for basic reproductive and child health services, supplies and infrastructure
* Make school education up to age 14, free and mandatory and reduce drop outs at primary and secondary school levels to below 20 percent for boys and girls

* Reduce infant mortality rate (IMR) to below 30 per 1000 live births
* Reduce maternal mortality ratio to below 100 per 100,000 child births
* Achieve universal immunization of children against all vaccine preventable diseases
* Promote delayed marriage for girls, not earlier than 18 and preferably after 20 years
* Achieve 80 percent institutional deliveries and 100 percent deliveries by trained persons.
* Achieve universal access to information/counseling and services for fertility regulation and contraception with a wide basket of choices
* Achieve 100 percent registration of births, deaths, marriages and pregnancies
* Contain spread of Acquired Immuno-deficiency Syndrome (AIDS) and promote greater integration between the management of reproductive tract infections (RTI) and sexually transmitted infections (STI) and National AIDS control organization.
* Prevent and control communicable diseases. Integrate Indian Systems of Medicine (ISM) in the provision of reproductive and child health services, and in reaching out to households.
* Promote vigorously the small family norm to achieve replacement levels of total fertility rate (TFR).

Strategies of NPP 2000

* Decentralization of the plan and program implementation
* Convergence in services at delivery points
* Strengthening the measures for child survival
* Meeting the unmet needs for family welfare
* Special services to slum dwellers
* Attending to adolescents
* Increasing male participation.

Promotional Measures

* Providing fertility regulating information and services
* Furnishing family life/sex information
* Improving the status of women

- Improving the health and nutrition status
- Providing incentives and disincentives
- Improving research and evaluation
- Carrying out specific legal reforms to influence internal and international migration.

Legislation

As a motivational measure, in order to enable state governments to fearlessly and effectively pursue the agenda for population stabilization contained in the National Population Policy 2000, legislation was considered necessary. It was recommended that the 42nd constitutional Amendment that freezes till 2001, the number of seats to the Lok Sabha and Rajya Sabha based on the 1971 census be extended up to 2016.

The NPP 2000 is to be implemented and managed at Panchayat and Nagar palika levels in co-ordination with the concerned state/union territory administrations. This will require comprehensive and multi-sectoral co-ordination of planning and implementation between health and family welfare on the one hand along with schemes for education, nutrition, women and child development, safe drinking water, sanitation, rural roads, communication, transportation, housing, forestry development, environmental protection and urban development. Accordingly the following structures were recommended.

i. National commission on population: A national commission on population presided over by the Prime Minister, will have the Chief Ministers of all states and union territories and the central minister-in-charge of the department of family welfare and other concerned central ministers and departments.

ii. State and union territory commissions on population: Each state and union territory to have a state / UT Commission, presided over by the Chief Minister, on the analogy of the National Commission to oversee and review implementation of NPP 2000 in the state/UT.

iii. Coordination cell in the planning commission.

iv. Technology mission in the department of family welfare: This will be to provide technology support in respect of design and monitoring of projects and programs for reproductive and child health campaigns.

Action Plan of the NPP 2000

1. **Operational strategies**
   - Converge service delivery at village level
   - Utilize village self-help groups to organize and provide basic services for reproductive and child care, combined with the ongoing Integrated Child Development Scheme (ICDS)
   - Implement at village levels a one-stop integrated and coordinated service delivery package for basic health care, family planning and maternal and child health related services provided by the community for its members
   - At the village level, the anganwadi center may become the pivot of basic health care activities, contraceptive counseling and supply, nutrition education and supplementation as well as preschool activities.
   - Providing maternity services. The panchayat may appoint a competent and mature midwife and volunteers to assist her. Trained birth attendants, traditional dais and auxiliary nurse midwives at subcenters are to monitor and respond to maternal morbidity/emergencies at village level.

2. **Empowering women for improved health and nutrition**
   - Create an enabling environment for women and children to benefit from products and services disseminated under reproductive and child health program
   - Open more child care centers in rural areas and in urban slums, where a woman worker will have her children in responsible hands

- Pursue drinking water schemes for increasing access to potable water
- Give rewards and priority schemes for households who use energy saving devices such as solar cookers, making sanitation facilities or extending telephone facilities
- Improve district, subdistrict and Panchayat level health management with co-ordination and collaboration between district health officer and Panchayat for planning and implementing health care activities.
  - Encourage adequate transportation at village level, subcenter level, Zillah parishads, primary health centers and at community health centers, so that the women with complications can reach emergency care in time
  - Strengthen the capacity of primary health centers to provide basic emergency obstetric and neonatal health care
  - Involve professional agencies in developing and disseminating training modules for standard procedures in the management of obstetric and neonatal health care
  - Involve professional agencies in developing and disseminating training modules for standard procedures in the management of obstetric and neonatal health care
  - Improve supervision by developing guidance and supervision checklists
- Monitor performance of maternal and child health services at each level by using various monitoring systems
- Improve technical skills of maternal and child health care providers through in-service education and training
- Develop and implement health package for adolescents
- Expand the availability of safe abortion care
- Develop maternity hospitals, district hospitals and community health centers

to function as first referral units for complicated and life-threatening deliveries
- Formulate and enforce standards of clinical services in the public, private and NGO sectors
- Focus on distribution of nonclinical methods of contraception such as condoms and oral pills.

3. Improving child health and survival
- Support community activities from village level upwards to monitor early and adequate antenatal, natal and postnatal care. Focus attention on neonatal health care and nutrition
- Promote compulsory registration of births in coordination with ICDS program
- After birth of a child, provide counseling and advocacy about contraception to encourage adoption of a reversible or terminal method
- Improve capacity of health centers in basic midwifery services and essential neonatal care including management of sick neonates
- Sensitize and train health personnel in the integrated management of childhood illnesses
- Strengthen critical interventions aimed at bringing about reductions in maternal malnutrition, morbidity and mortality by ensuring availability of supplies and equipment at village levels and sub-centers
- Pursue rigorously the pulse polio campaign to eradicate polio
- Ensure 100 percent routine immunization for all vaccine preventable diseases
- Expand ICDS to include children between 6 and 9 years of age, especially to promote and ensure 100 percent school enrolment.

4. Meeting the unmet needs of family welfare services
- Address on priority, the different unmet needs in particular an increase in rural

infrastructure, deployment of sanctioned and appropriately trained health personnel, and provisioning of essential equipment and drugs

❖ Improve facilities for referral transportation at Panchayat, Zillah parishad and primary health centre levels.

5. **Uplifting the under-served population**
   Groups in urban slums, tribal communities, hill area population and displaced, and migrant populations.

   ❖ Integrate aggressive health education programs with health and medical care programs with emphasis an environmental health, personal hygiene and healthy habits, nutritional education and population education

   ❖ Streamline the referral systems and linkage between the primary, secondary and tertiary levels of health care in urban areas

   ❖ In tribal areas provide information and counseling in respect of infertility

   ❖ Health care providers in tribal and hilly areas to adopt a 'burden of disease' approach to meet the special needs of such communities

   ❖ Provide for adolescents the package of nutritional services under the ICDS program

   ❖ Enforce the Child Marriage Restraint Act, 1976, to reduce the incidence of teenage pregnancies

   ❖ Encourage increased participation of men in planned parenthood. Re-popularize vasectomies, in particular the no-scalpel vasectomy as a safe, simple, painless procedure, more convenient and acceptable for men.

6. **Utilizing diverse health care providers**

   ❖ At district and subdistrict levels, maintain block-wise database of private medical practitioners whose credentials may be certified by Indian Medical Association (IMA).

   ❖ Revive the earlier system of licensed medical practitioners who, after appropriate certification from IMA, may

participate in the provision of clinical services

❖ Involve nonmedical fraternity in counseling and advocacy

❖ Modify the under/postgraduate medical, nursing and paramedical professional course syllabic and curricula in consultation with the relevant apex body (AMA, INC, etc), in order to reflect the concepts and implementation strategies of the reproductive and child health program and the national population policy

❖ Encourage the efficient functioning of the first referral units, i.e. 30-bed hospitals at block levels which provide emergency obstetric and child health care, to bring about reductions in maternal mortality rate (MMR) and infant mortality rate (IMR).

7. **Collaboration with and commitment from the nongovernment sector to augment advocacy, counseling and clinical services**

   ❖ Collaboration between the voluntary sector and the NGOs will facilitate dissemination of efficient service delivery to village levels

   ❖ Encourage voluntary sector to motivate village-level self-help groups to participate in community activities

   ❖ Specific collaboration in social marketing of contraceptives to reach village levels.

8. **Mainstreaming of Indian systems of medicine and homeopathy**

   ❖ Utilize the ISMH institutions, dispensaries and hospitals for health and population related programs

   ❖ Utilize the ISM "barefoot doctors" after appropriate training and orientation for providing advocacy and counseling for disseminating supplies and equipment, such as depot holders at village levels.

9. **Promotion of research on contraceptive technology and RCH**
   Promote and finance studies and research projects related to maternal and child

health services and contraceptive technology.

10. **Providing for older population**
11. **Promoting information, education and communication**
    - ❖ Optimal use of folk media to successfully mobilize local population.
    - ❖ Involve departments of rural development, social welfare, transport, co-operatives and education with special reference to schools to improve clarity and focus of the IEC effort and to extend coverage and outreach. Health and population education must be included from the school level
    - ❖ Utilize radio and television as the most powerful media for disseminating relevant socio-demographic messages
    - ❖ Involve civil society for disseminating information, counseling and spreading education about small family norm, need for fewer but healthy babies, higher female literacy and later marriages for women. Civil society could also be of assistance in monitoring the availability of contraceptives, vaccines and drugs in rural areas and in urban slums.

NATIONAL FAMILY WELFARE PROGRAM

India launched the National Family Welfare Program in 1951, with the objective of reducing the birth rate to the extent necessary to stabilize the population at a level consistent with the requirement of the national economy. The family welfare program in India is recognized as a priority area and is being implemented as a 100 percent centrally sponsored program.

Evaluation of the Family Welfare Program

The approach under the program during the first and second five year plan was mainly 'clinical' under which facilities for provision of services were created. However, on the basis of data brought out by the 1961 census, clinical approach adopted in the first-two plans was replaced by 'Extension and Education Approach' which envisaged expansion of service facilities along with spread of message on small family norm.

In the 4th plan (1961–1970) high priority was accorded to the program and it was proposed to reduce birth rate from 35 per 1000 to 32 per 1000 by the end of the plan. 16.5 million couples, constituting about 16.5 percent of the couples in the reproductive age group were protected against conception by the end of 4th plan.

The objective of the 5th plan (1974–1979) was to bring down the birth rate to 30 per 1000 by the end of 1978-1979 by increasing integration of family planning services with those of Maternal and Child Health (MCH) and Nutrition so that, the program become more, readily acceptable.

There was phenomenal increase recorded in the performance of sterilization in 1975-1977 periods. In view of the rigidity of enforcement of targets by field functionaries and an element of coercion in the implementation of the program in some areas the program received a set back during 1977-1978.

This led to a change in approach and the government made it clear that there was no place for force or coercion or pressure of any sort and the program had to be implemented as an integral part of Family Welfare relying solely on mass education and motivation. The name of the program was changed to family welfare from family planning.

In the 6th plan (1980-1985), certain demographic goals of reaching net reproduction rate of unity were envisaged. These were to achieve the following by the year 2000:
- ❖ Reduction of average family size from 4.4 children in 1995 to 2.3 children
- ❖ Reduction of birth rate to 21 from the level of 33 in 1978 and death rate to 9 from 14, and infant mortality to 67 from 127
- ❖ Increasing the couple protection level from 22 to 60 percent.

The Family welfare program during the 7th five year plan (1985-1990) was continued on a purely voluntary basis with emphasis on promoting spacing methods, securing maximum community participation and promoting maternal and child health care. In order to provide facilities/services nearer to the door steps of population, the following initiatives were taken.

❖ To have one subcenter for every 5000 population in plain areas and for 3000 population in hilly and tribal areas. At the end of 7th plan, i.e. 1990, 1.3 lakhs subcenters were established in the country

❖ To extend the postpartum program progressively to subdistrict level hospitals. At the end of 7th plan 1012 subdistrict level hospitals and 870 health posts were established

❖ To extend the universal immunization program (UIP) to cover all the districts in the country by 1990

❖ To improve primary health care in urban slums in the cities of Mumbai and Chennai with assistance from World Bank

❖ To implement area development projects in selected districts in 15 major states.

The achievements of the family welfare program at the end of 7th plan were:

❖ Reduction in crude birth rate from 41.7 (1951-1961) to 30.2 (1990)

❖ Reduction in total fertility rate from 5.97 (1950-1955) to 3.8 (1990)

❖ Reduction in infant mortality rate from 146 (1970-1971) to 80 (1990)

❖ Increase in couple protection rate 10.4 percent (1970-1971) to 43.3 percent (1990)

❖ Setting up of a large network of service delivery infrastructure

❖ Over 118 million births were averted by the end of March 1990.

In the 8th five year plan (1992-1997), several new initiatives were introduced to introduce new dynamism to the Family Welfare Program. On going schemes were revamped and new initiatives were introduced as under:

❖ World Bank assisted Area Projects which seek to upgrade infrastructure and development of trained manpower. Indian Population Project (IPP) 8th and 9th were initiated during the 8th plan. The IPP 8th project aims at improving health and family welfare services in urban slums of Delhi, Kolkata, Hyderabad and Bengaluru. IPP 9th will operate in the states of Rajasthan, Assam and Karnataka.

❖ An USAID assisted project named "Innovations in Family Planning Services" was taken up in Uttar Pradesh with the specific objective of reducing total fertility rate (TFR) from 5.4 to 4 and increasing couple protection rate (CPR) from 35 to 50 percent over 10 years project period.

❖ Realizing that Government efforts alone in propagating and motivating the people for adoption of small family norm would not be sufficient, greater stress was laid on involvement of NGOs to supplement and complement the Government efforts.

The Universal Immunization Program (UIP) was launched in 1985 to provide universal coverage of infants and pregnant women with immunization against identified vaccine preventable diseases. From the year 1992 – 1993, the UIP has been strengthened and expanded into the Child Survival and Safe Motherhood (CSSM) project. It involves sustaining the high immunization coverage level under UIP, and augmenting activities under Oral Rehydration Therapy (ORT), prophylaxis for control of blindness in children and control of acute respiratory infections. Under the safe motherhood component, training of traditional birth attendants (TBA), provision of aseptic delivery kits and strengthening of first referral units to deal with high-risk and obstetric emergencies were taken up.

The targets fixed for the 8th plan of national level birth rate of 26 was achieved by all states except the states of Assam, Bihar, Haryana, Madhya Pradesh, Orissa, Rajasthan and Uttar Pradesh.

In the 9th five year plan (1997-2002), reduction in the population growth has been recognized as one of the priority objectives. The objectives were:

❖ To meet all the felt needs for contraception.

❖ To reduce the infant and maternal morbidity and mortality so that, there is a reduction in the desired level of fertility.

The strategies during the plan would be:

❖ Assess the needs for reproductive and child health at PHC level and undertake area-specific micro planning.

❖ To provide need-based demand-driven, high quality, integrated reproductive and child health care.

The expected levels of achievement by the terminal year of 2002 were:

– Crude birth rate (CBR) 23/1000
– Infant mortality rate (IMR) 50/1000
– Total fertility rate (TFR) 2.6
– Couple protection rate (CPR) 60 percent
– Neonatal mortality rate (NNMR) 35/1000
– Maternal mortality rate (MMR) 3 /1000.

Implementation of the FWP

The following were the main components of Family Welfare Program:

❖ Maternal health
❖ Child health
❖ Population control/stabilization.

The following were the schemes and programs for implementation of national family welfare:

❖ Reproductive and child health program (RCH)
❖ Janani Suraksha Yojana
❖ Vandemataram Scheme
❖ Safe Abortion Services
❖ National Rural Health Mission (NRHM)
❖ Integrated Child Development Services (ICDS).

REPRODUCTIVE AND CHILD HEALTH PROGRAM (RCH)

Population growth and health of women and children had been a major problem in India despite implementation of several programs since 1951. Maternal and Child Health (MCH) and Child Survival and Safe motherhood (CSSM) programs were implemented through organized health care systems.

In 1994, during the International conference on Population Development (ICPD), a new approach to tackle the problem was recommended. The government of India adopted the Reproductive Health Approach and launched the RCH program in October 1997.

The objective of the RCH program was to provide quality, integrated and sustainable primary health care services to women in the reproductive age group and children with special focus on family planning and immunization.

Essential Components of RCH Program

❖ Prevention and management of unwanted pregnancy
❖ Services for mothers during pregnancy, childbirth and postpartum period
❖ Child survival services for newborns and infants
❖ Management of reproductive tract infections (RTI) and sexually transmitted diseases
❖ Establishment of an effective referral system
❖ Reproductive services for adolescent health
❖ Health services including counseling on sexuality and family life.

Services Included in the Program for Mothers and Children

1. **Essential care for all mothers and children**
   ❖ Registration by 12th to 16th week of pregnancy
   ❖ Antenatal check-up at least three times during pregnancy
   ❖ Tetanus toxoid to all women as early as possible during pregnancy with two doses at one month interval
   ❖ Iron and folic acid tablets daily for 100 days. Women with clinical signs of anemia to receive 2 tablets daily for 100 days
   ❖ De-worming with Mebendazole during 2nd or 3rd trimester in areas where hookworm infestation is common

- ❖ Safe and clean delivery services
- ❖ Preparation of women for exclusive breast feeding and timely weaning
- ❖ Postpartum care, including advises and services for limiting and spacing births.

2. **Early detection of complications**
   - ❖ Clinical examination to detect anemia
   - ❖ Referral and transportation to the nearest hospital of women with hemorrhage or complications
   - ❖ Referral of all women identified as having pregnancy induced hypertension (BP > 140/90 mm Hg and weight gain > 3 kg/month)
   - ❖ Referral of all women who develop signs of infection following delivery or abortion
   - ❖ Transfer of women in labor for more than 12 hours to the nearest hospital that has facilities for cesarean delivery.

3. **Emergency care to those who need it**
   - ❖ Early identification of obstetric emergencies
   - ❖ Initial management of emergencies and transfer to referral hospital without delay using the fastest available mode of transport.

4. **Care to women in the reproductive age group**
   - ❖ Counseling on:
     - Optimal timing and spacing of birth
     - Small family norm
     - Use and choice of contraceptives
     - Prevention of sexually transmitted diseases and reproductive tract infections
     - Importance of girl child.
   - ❖ Information on availability of:
     - Medical termination of pregnancy (MTP) services
     - IUCD and sterilization services.
   - ❖ Family planning services:
     - Condom distribution
     - Oral contraceptive dispensing
     - IUCD services.
   - ❖ Recognition and referral of clients with sexually transmitted diseases and reproductive tract infections.

5. **Provision of clean and safe delivery practices at the community level**
   - ❖ Creation of awareness about the need for clean and safe deliveries
   - ❖ Deliveries by trained personnel
   - ❖ Provision of disposable delivery kits for deliveries
   - ❖ Promotion of institutional deliveries
   - ❖ Early identification and referral of high-risk cases.

6. **Newborn care**
   - ❖ Weighing all newborns at birth. Normal weight 2500 to 2800 gm. Referral of newborns weighing > 2000 gm
   - ❖ Resuscitation of asphyxiated newborns using mucus sucker or breathing as required
   - ❖ Prevention of hypothermia
   - ❖ Breastfeeding within one hour of birth
   - ❖ Referral of newborns who show signs of illness
   - ❖ Education of mother on newborn care and feeding.

7. **Immunization**
   Infants
   - ❖ BCG one dose at birth
   - ❖ DPT: three doses, beginning at 6th week at monthly interval
   - ❖ Polio: '0' dose at birth for all institutional deliveries and 3 doses at one month interval
   - ❖ Measles: one dose at completion of 9 months
   - ❖ Vitamin A: First dose of 100,000 IU along with measles vaccination.

   Children 1 to 3 years
   - ❖ DPT
   - ❖ OPV booster dose at 16th to 18th month
   - ❖ Vitamin A
     - 2nd dose 200,000 IU at 16th to 18th month
     - 3rd to 5th doses 200,000 IU each at 6 monthly intervals

   Children 3 to 5 years
   - ❖ Iron and folic acid (smaller dose) for children with signs of anemia
   - ❖ Treatment for worm infestation with mebendazole.

8. **Prevention of deaths due to diarrheal diseases**
   ❖ Correct management
   ❖ Teaching mothers to increase body fluid with ORS (Oral rehydration solution), and normal feeding
9. **Prevention of deaths due to pneumonia**
   ❖ Correct management of all cases of acute respiratory infections
   ❖ Referral of children with severe pneumonia or severe illness.

RCH phase II began in April 2005. The focus of the program was to reduce maternal and child morbidity and mortality with emphasis on rural health care. The major strategies of the second phase of RCH are:

1. Essential obstetric care
   a. Institutional delivery
   b. Skilled attendance at delivery
   c. Policy decisions
2. Emergency obstetric care
   a. Operationalizing first referral units
   b. Operationalizing PHCs and CHCs for round the clock delivery services.
3. Strengthening the referral system.

1. **Essential obstetric care**
   a. *Institutional delivery:* In order to promote institutional deliveries, it is envisaged that 50 percent of the PHCs and all the CHCs would be made operational as 24-hour delivery centers in a phased manner by 2010. Basic emergency obstetric care essential newborn care and basic newborn resuscitation services will be provided in these centers round the clock.
   b. *Skilled attendance at delivery:* Guidelines for conducting normal delivery and management of obstetric complications at PHC and CHC for medical officers and for skilled attendance at birth for ANM and LHVs have been formulated and disseminated to the states.
   c. *Policy decisions regarding use of drugs and interventions:* ANMs, LHVs and SNs have now been permitted to use certain drugs in specific emergency situations to reduce maternal mortality. They have also been permitted to carry out certain emergency interventions when the life of the mother is at stake.

2. **Emergency obstetric care**
   The first referral units (FRU) will be made operational/functional with following services on a 24-hour basis.
   ❖ 24-hour delivery services including normal and assisted deliveries.
   ❖ Emergency obstetric care including surgical interventions like cesarean sections:
      – Newborn care
      – Emergency care of sick newborns
      – Full range of family planning services including laparoscopic services
      – Safe abortion services
      – Treatment for sexually transmitted infections and respiratory tract infections
      – Blood storage facility
      – Essential laboratory services and
      – Referral (transport) services.

   In order to perform full range of FRU functions a health facility must have:
   a. Minimum bed strength of 20 to 30
   b. Fully functional operation theater
   c. Fully functional labor room with well equipped care area
   d. A functional laboratory and blood storage facility
   e. 24-hour water and electricity supply
   f. Arrangements for waste disposal
   g. Ambulance facility.

3. **Strengthening referral system**
   In order to improve referral linkage practiced in RCH Phase I, new initiatives were added.
   ❖ Training of MBBS doctors in life-saving anesthetic skills for emergency obstetric care
   ❖ Setting up of blood storage centers at FRUs according to Government of India guidelines
   ❖ Janani Suraksha Yojana: The national maternity benefit scheme has been modified into a new scheme called Janani Suraksha Yojana.

JANANI SURAKSHA YOJANA

This program was launched on 12th April 2005. The objectives of the scheme are: reducing maternal mortality and infant mortality through encouraging delivery at health institutions and focusing at institutional care among women below poverty line families.

Salient Features of the JSY

❖ It is a 100 percent centrally sponsored scheme
❖ Benefit of cash assistance with institutional care during antenatal, delivery and post-partum care to all women both rural and urban belonging to below poverty line households and aged 19 years or above, up to first two live births. In ten low performing states, the cash benefit will be extended up to the third child, if the mother chooses to undergo sterilization in the health facility where she delivered. The accredited social health activist (ASHA) will be responsible for making institutional care available. She would also be responsible for escorting the pregnant woman to the health center.

The cash assistance will be ₹ 1,400 to all mothers in rural areas of low performing states and ₹ 1,200 to mothers in urban areas. All women including those from SC and ST families delivering in government institutions or accredited private institutions are eligible for cash assistance. Women from rural areas of high performing states get ₹ 700 while those from urban areas get ₹ 600.

The Yojana gives cash assistance of ₹ 250 for transportation of women to the nearest health center for delivery. The women get a subsidy of ₹ 1,500 for cesarean deliveries and management of obstetric complications. According to the government report of 2008, in the years 2006–2008 about 28.11 lakhs pregnant women received benefits from this scheme, out which 18.72 lakhs had institutional deliveries.

VANDEMATARAM SCHEME

This is a voluntary scheme wherein any obstetric or gynec specialist, maternity home or nursing home lady doctor or MBBS doctor can volunteer herself/himself for providing safe motherhood services. The enrolled doctor will display "Vandemataram logo" at the clinic. Iron and folic acid tablets, oral pills, TT injections, etc. will be provided by the respective District Medical Officers (DMO) to the "Vandemataram doctors or clinics" for distribution to beneficiaries. The cases needing special care and treatment can be referred to the government hospitals that have been adviced to take due care of such patients coming with Vandemataram cards.

SAFE ABORTION SERVICES

In India abortion is a major cause of maternal morbidity and mortality and accounts for nearly 8.9 percent of maternal deaths. Majority of abortions take place outside authorized health services and/or by unauthorized and unskilled persons. Under RCH Phase II, following facilities are provided:

❖ *Medical method of abortion:* Termination of early pregnancy with drugs – Mifepristone (RU486) followed by misoprostol; Currently, the use of these two drugs are recommended up to 7 weeks (49 days) of amenorrhea in a facility with provision for safe abortion services and blood transfusion. Termination of pregnancy using these two drugs is offered to women under the preview of the MTP Act 1971.
❖ *Manual Vacuum Aspiration (MVA):* Manual vacuum aspiration is a safe and simple technique for termination of early pregnancy, and is feasible to be used in primary health centers or comparable facilities, thereby increasing the access to safe abortion services.

All the below listed interventions included in RCH phase I will continue in the phase II implementation period.

– Appointing additional public health nurses, ANMs, anesthetists, and safe motherhood consultants
– Providing 24-hours delivery services at PHCs and CHCs

- Providing referral transport, and integrated financial package.
- Conducting RCH camps, and training of Dais.
- Implementing interventions for newborn care and child health (Immunization, control of ARI and diarrhea, vitamin A and iron supplementation, etc).

NATIONAL RURAL HEALTH MISSION (NRHM)

The government of India launched National Rural Health Mission (NRHM) on 5th April 2005 for a period of 7 years (2005–2012) in order to improve the quality of life of its citizens. The mission seeks to improve the health care delivery system. It is operational in the whole country with special focus on North East states.

The main aim of NRHM is to provide accessible, accountable, effective and reliable primary health care and to bridge the gap in rural health care through creation of a cader of Accredited Social Health Activists (ASHA), and strengthening the services of sub-centers, primary health centers and community health centers.

The Goals to be Achieved by NRHM

A. At national level

- Reduction of infant mortality rate to 30/1000 live births
- Reduction of maternal mortality rate to 100/100,000
- Reduction of total fertility
- Reduction of mortality rates of Malaria, Filaria, Dengue, Kala-azar and Japanese encephalitis
- Reduction of prevalence rates of leprosy and tuberculosis
- Upgrading community health centers to Indian Public Health standards
- Increasing first referral units from less than 20 to 75 percent.
- Engaging 250,000 female Accredited Social Health Activists.

B. At community level

- Availing trained community level workers at village level with a drug kit for general ailments
- Provision of immunization, antenatal and postnatal check ups, and services related to health of mother and child including nutrition at anganwadi level
- Availing of generic drugs for common ailments at sub-center level
- Providing good hospital care through assured availability of doctors, drugs and quality services at PHC and CHC level
- Improved access to universal immunization
- Improved facilities for institutional deliveries
- Availability of assured health care at reduced financial risk
- Improved outreach services through mobile medical units at district level
- Provision of household toilets.

Plan of Implementation of NRHM

Implementation of the NRHM program will be through ASHAs and ANMs.

Selection of ASHA

ASHA must be a resident of the village—a woman (married/widowed/divorced) preferably in the age group of 25–45 with formal education up to eight class, having communication skills and leadership qualities. The general norm will be one ASHA for 1,000 populations. In tribal, hilly and desert areas, the norm could be relaxed to one ASHA per habitation. The selected ASHAs will be trained to carry out specific responsibilities.

Roles and Responsibilities of ASHA

The ASHA will function as a health activist in the community and carry out the following responsibilities:

- Take steps to create awareness and provide information on health determinants such as nutrition, basic sanitation and hygienic practices, healthy living and the need for utilization of existing health and family welfare services
- Counsel women on birth preparedness, safe delivery, breastfeeding, complementary

feeding, immunization, contraception and prevention of common infections including reproductive tract infections and sexually transmitted infections

- Mobilize community in accessing health related services available at the anganwadi, subcenter, and primary health center such as immunization, antenatal check-up, postnatal check-up, supplementary nutrition, sanitation and other services being provided by the government
- Identify women in families below poverty line (BPL) as beneficiaries of the scheme (NRHM) and assist them to obtain BPL registration
- Ensure that the Janani Suraksha Yojona (JSY) card is filled up at least 16–20 weeks prior to delivery
- Work with the village health and sanitation committee of the Gram Panchayat to develop comprehensive village health plan
- Arrange escort/accompany pregnant women and children requiring treatment/ admission to the nearest pre-identified health facility (sub-center or PHC)
- Provide primary medical care for minor ailments such as fever, diarrhea, and first aid for minor injuries
- Be a provider of 'directly observed treatment short-course' (DOTS) under national tuberculosis control program
- Will act as a direct depot holder for essential provisions like oral rehydration solution (ORS), iron and folic acid tablets, chloroquin, disposable delivery kits, oral pills and condoms and keep a medicine kit with AYUSH and allopathic formulations recommended by the technical/expert advisory group of the government
- Ensure registration of births and deaths in her village, any unusual health problems or disease outbreaks in the community
- Promote construction of household toilets under total sanitation campaign.

Role and Integration with ANM

The auxiliary nurse midwife will guide ASHA in performing her functions through activities such as:

- Holding weekly/fortnightly meetings to discuss activities
- Acting as resource person for training of ASHA
- Guiding ASHA regarding arrangement for outreach programs
- Participating and guiding ASHA in organizing health days in anganwadi center.
- Utilizing ASHA to motivate pregnant women to go to the subcenter for check ups, take full course of iron and folic acid tablets and tetanus toxoid injections.

The ANMs will inform ASHA on date, time and place for initial and periodic training schedule and also ensure that ASHA gets the compensation for performance and TA /DA for attending training.

INTEGRATED CHILD DEVELOPMENT SERVICES (ICDS)

This program adopts a multi-sectoral approach to child well-being incorporating health education and nutrition interventions and is implemented through a network or anganwadi centers at the community level. Malnutrition is fought through interventions targeted at unmarried adolescent girls, pregnant women, mothers and children up to 6 years.

The key services provided through ICDS are:

- Supplementary feeding
- Immunization
- Health and nutrition education
- Micronutrient supplementation
- Preschool education for 3 to 6 year olds
- Nutrition, health awareness and skills development for adolescent girls
- Income generation schemes for women.

Supplementary nutrition service includes growth monitoring, prophylaxis against vitamin A deficiency and control of nutritional anemia. All families in the community are surveyed to identify children below the age of six, pregnant and nursing mothers. They are given supplementary nutritional support for 300 days in a year. The program aims to bridge the caloric gap between the national recommended and average intake of children and women in low income and disadvantaged groups.

Children below the age of three are weighed once a month and children below 3 to 6 are weighed quarterly. Growth rate and nutritional status are assessed and malnourished children are given supplementary feeding and referred to medical centers.

Immunization of pregnant women against tetanus is undertaken towards reducing maternal and neonatal mortality. Vaccination of infants and children for six vaccine preventable diseases—poliomyelitis, diphtheria, pertussis, tetanus, tuberculosis and measles are also included.

Health check-ups are offered to children up to 6 years, and expectant and nursing mothers. The services are provided by anganwadi workers and primary health center (PHC) staff and include weight checking, immunization, management of malnutrition, treatment of diarrhea, de-worming and distribution of simple medicines. Through the 1.4 million anganwadi centers, the education component of the ICDS program is implemented. The early learning provides foundation for cumulative, life-long learning and development. This also contributes to universalization of primary education. Providing to children the necessary preparation for primary schooling, nutrition, and health education are key elements of the work of anganwadi workers. Capacity building of women, especially in the age group of 15 to 45 years is a long-term goal to be achieved.

The ICDS Team

The ICDS team comprises the anganwadi workers, anganwadi helper, supervisors, child development project officers (CDPOs) and district program officers (DPOs). Anganwadi workers are ladies selected from the local communities and as such community-based front line workers of the ICDS program. The health teams include medical officers, auxiliary nurse midwives (ANMs) and accredited social health activists (ASHAs) as functionaries of ICDS to provide different services.

60 Obstetric and Gynecological Instruments

Sponge Holding Forceps (Fig. 60.1)

Specifications and Uses

❖ A heavy metal instrument 23 to 75 cm in length
❖ Shafts are thin and blades are fenestrated
❖ Has a catch-lock, which gives firmness while holding any material
❖ Has ring shaped tips, which may be serrated or smooth
❖ Used for cleaning the operative field
❖ Used for swabbing or packing body cavities like vagina
❖ Can be used to catch hold of soft organs like ovary and cervix in pregnancy
❖ Can be substituted in the place of an ovum forceps

Fig. 60.1: Sponge holding forceps

❖ Used for deep moping to clear the area during surgery.

Kocher's Hemostatic Forceps (Figs 60.2A and B)

Specifications and Uses

❖ A strong, straight metal instrument
❖ Has a catch-lock to bring the blades together for locking
❖ Inner surface of both blades are transversely serrated

Figs 60.2A and B: (A) Kocher's forceps; (B) Toothed distal end

- It may be straight or curved
- Single toothed at distal end
- Used to catch the edges of the incision while suturing skin
- Used for artificial rupture membranes
- Used to clamp the umbilical cord.

Hemostats (Artery Forceps) (Figs 60.3A and B)

Specifications and Uses

- Artery forceps may be small or mosquito, straight or curved, strong metal instrument
- Medium or large in size
- Blades are tapering to the distal end but blunt
- Has a catch-lock to bring the blades together and to lock it
- Inner surface of the blades are transversely serrated and when locked, the blades are well in apposition
- Blades are roughly half the size of the handle
- Used to stop bleeding by catching the blood vessel
- Used as a clamp for pedicles of internal organs like kidney, spleen, ligaments of uterus, etc.
- Used to enlarge the opening of an abscess in the absence of a sinus forceps
- Can be used to substitute a needle holder
- Used to hold the incised edges of skin and fascia
- Used to hold the free ends of sutures at the beginning of suturing and to hold the cut ends of tension sutures before tying
- Used to hold the tape of abdominal pads or sponges during surgeries to prevent them missing in the cavity

- Mosquito forceps are used to hold the small bleeding points
- Used for blunt dissection by holding swabs.

Ovum Forceps (Figs 60.4A and B)

Specifications and Uses

- A moderately heavy metal instrument having cupped blades with linear fenestrations
- The size and type of blades can hold a reasonable amount of tissues in between with good grip
- The length is about 30 cm
- Used for removing products of conception from the uterus in incomplete abortion

Figs 60.4A and B: Ovum forceps

Figs 60.3A and B: (A) Straight artery forceps; (B) Curved artery forceps

❖ Used to remove any foreign body from the uterine cavity, e.g. intrauterine device when threads are broken

❖ Used to remove any retained placental bits or membrane pieces from the uterus after delivery.

Vulsellum Forceps (Fig. 60.5)

Specifications and Uses

❖ An average sized metal instrument resembling forceps at the distal end

❖ The proximal end has a lock for fixing and distal end has multiple sharp teeth for firm grip

❖ The curvature of blades helps to retract the anterior vaginal wall when the instrument is pulled up after holding the cervical lip for better visualization

❖ Used for holding the anterior or posterior lip of cervix in operations like dilatation and curettage (D & C) and cauterization of cervix

❖ Used to test the mobility of cervix and laxity of ligaments in prolapse of uterus

❖ Used to bring down the fundus of uterus in vaginal hysterectomy

❖ Used to hold the cervical lip for procedures like tubal insufflation or introduction of laminaria tent.

Fig. 60.5: Vulsellum forceps

Green Armytage's Forceps (Figs 60.6A and B)

Specifications and uses

❖ A metal instrument resembling any other forceps except for triangular blades with serrated edges

Figs 60.6A and B: Green Armytage's forceps

❖ Has small space between the blades, even when the forceps is locked and fully closed

❖ Used in lower segment cesarean section (LSCS) to hold the retracted edges of the uterine wall for easy stitching

❖ While holding the edges it acts as a hemostat to decrease bleeding from the incision.

Uterine Packing Forceps/Uterine Dressing Forceps (Fig. 60.7)

Specifications and Uses

❖ A curved forceps about 35 cm in length, the curvature corresponding to axis of birth canal for easy packing

❖ Has blades, handles and finger bows

❖ The blades are provided with slight groves on inner surfaces

❖ Used for vaginal packing to control bleeding from lacerations in birth canal due to trauma

❖ Used to swab uterine cavity following dilatation and evacuation with small gauze pieces

❖ Used to pack the uterine cavity following D and C or delivery to control bleeding

❖ Used for application of drug into the uterine cavity.

Fig. 60.7: Uterine packing forceps

Fig. 60.9: Tenaculum forceps

Fig. 60.8: Allis tissue forceps

Allis Tissue Forceps (Fig. 60.8)

Specifications and Uses

❖ An instrument with straight blades and catch-lock

❖ Have sharp teeth at the tip, with interlock on closing

❖ The tips are slightly curved or angulated for better grip of tissues

❖ It is used to:
  – Catch hold of the anterior lip of the cervix during D & C operation
  – Hold the apex of the episiotomy wound during repair
  – Catch hold of the torn ends of the *sphincter ani prior* to suturing in repair of complete perineal tear
  – Catch hold of the margins and angles of the uterine flaps in LSCS after delivery of the baby
  – Hold thinner structures like skin, deep fascia and layers of rectus sheath.

Tenaculum Forceps (Fig. 60.9)

Specifications and Uses

❖ An instrument resembling vulsellum forceps except there is a single tooth at the distal end

❖ Used to hold the tissues at one point only so as to minimize bleeding

❖ Used to hold the anterior lip of cervix transversely, while doing Rubin's test in order to fit the cannula airtight in the cervix.

Laminaria Tent Introducing Forceps (Fig. 60.10)

Specifications and Uses

❖ A metal instrument with a handle and lock

❖ Almost similar to uterine dressing forceps

❖ Has a grove on either blade to catch the Laminaria Tent

❖ Used to hold and introduce the Laminaria Tent conveniently into the cervix.

Fig. 60.10: Laminaria tent introducing forceps

Laminaria Tent (Fig. 60.11)

Specifications and Uses

❖ It is dehydrated, compressed, Chinese seaweed

❖ It is sterilized by keeping it immersed in absolute alcohol

Fig. 60.11: Laminaria tent

❖ Tents are about 7 to 10 cm in length, with an eye at one end, and a thread hanging through the eye of each tent
❖ The thread attached to the tent facilitates easy removal
❖ Laminaria Tents (more than one) are introduced into the cervical canal and kept for 12 to 24 hours
❖ The tent being hygroscopic swells up by absorbing fluid from cervix causing slow dilatation of cervical canal
❖ Used for dilating cervical canal in cases of spasmodic dysmenorrhea, and for expulsion of products of conception in MTP, incomplete abortion and hydatidiform mole.

Dissecting Forceps (Figs 60.12A and B)

Specifications and Uses

❖ It has two equal, flat shafts with a sharp curve at the middle and joined at the proximal end
❖ Toothed dissecting forceps have tooth in the inner surface of the distal end
❖ On pressing the shafts, the pointed tips are well apposed so that they do not slip against each other
❖ The outer surface of shafts is made rough and irregular to get a firm grip while holding in the hand
❖ Plain dissecting forceps are used to hold delicate structures like peritoneum, vessels, bowel wall, etc. for suturing and to lift swabs and gauze pieces for dressing
❖ Toothed dissecting forceps are used to hold tough structures like skin or fascia while suturing

Figs 60.12A and B: (A) Non-toothed dissecting forceps; (B) Toothed dissecting Forceps

❖ It is used to lift the knots of sutures while removing them after the wounds are healed. It is used to dissect soft, friable tissues.

Doyen's Towel Clip (Fig. 60.13)

Fig. 60.13: Doyen's towel clip

Specifications and Uses

❖ It is a light and strong metal instrument
❖ It has a catch lock to fix the grip of drapes
❖ The tips are sharply pointed for better grasping
❖ Used to fix drapes in order to expose only the required area
❖ Used to fix tubing such as suction tubes to drapes preventing displacement

❖ It can be used as tongue holding forceps in emergency situations but it will perforate the tongue.

Doyen's Retractor (Fig. 60.14)

Specifications and Uses

❖ It is a metal instrument with flat solid blade on one end and a long handle
❖ Used to retract pelvic organs during cesarean section
❖ It is temporarily taken off while delivering the baby and then reintroduced till toileting of peritoneal cavity is done.

Fig. 60.14: Doyen's retractor

Anterior Vaginal Wall Retractor (Fig. 60.15)

Specifications and Uses

❖ A metal instrument with two oval shaped and fenestrated ends
❖ The fenestrated end has transverse serrations
❖ The oval shaped ends are connected at an angle of 45°C to both ends of the shaft
❖ It is used with Sim's speculum to retract the anterior vaginal wall for exposing the cervix and anterior fornix.

Fig. 60.15: Anterior vaginal wall retractor

Kelly's Deep Retractor (Fig. 60.16)

Specifications and Uses

❖ A large metal retractor with a broad and slightly curved blade
❖ Handle is long and end is curved like a hook, which provides better grip
❖ This type of retractor is available in various sizes
❖ It is used for retracting intra-abdominal viscera like liver and spleen during surgeries like cholecystectomy
❖ Smaller size retractor is used to retract the bladder walls in intravesical operations
❖ It is used to retract pelvic structures during surgery of appendix, cecum, etc. to prevent injury to pelvic organs.

Fig. 60.16: Kelly's deep retractor

Sim's Double Bladed Vaginal Speculum (Fig. 60.17)

Specifications and Uses

❖ A moderately heavy metal instrument
❖ It has two thick blades of unequal breadths to facilitate introduction according to the size of vagina

Fig. 60.17: Sim's double bladed vaginal speculum

* It is used to:
  - Toilet the vagina following delivery
  - Visualize any injured site on the cervix or vagina
  - Inspect the cervix to exclude any local lesion causing bleeding in suspected cases of abortion, APH or PPH.
* Used in operations of the cervix and vagina in lithotomy position
* Used in D & C and D & E surgery
* Used for taking biopsy from genital tract and for cauterization of erosions of cervix.

Cusco's Bivalved Speculum (Fig. 60.18)

Specifications and Uses

* A self-retaining speculum with a special screw arrangement
* It has two blades, which can be opened laterally and adjusted at various angles by adjusting the screw after introducing in the vagina
* It is introduced into the vagina with its blades closed in vertical position and then made horizontal, opened and locked in position. It can be closed and rotated further and opened again to see other sides of vagina after locking in required position
* Can be used without any assistance
* Used to visualize or inspect vagina and cervix
* Can be used without bringing the patient to the edge of bed
* Used in insertion of intrauterine contraceptive device

Fig. 60.18: Cusco's bivalved speculum

* Used to reach into the cervix to apply medications to take swabs for culture and sensitivity to get biopsy specimens and to do electrocautery in the cervix.

Auvard's Weighted Vaginal Speculum (Fig. 60.19)

Specifications and Uses

* It is weighted vaginal speculum for retaining
* The weight is due to the metal weight attached to the handle
* There is a channel in the handle for collection of discharges and curette material
* It is used to retract the posterior vaginal wall in operations of the cervix and vagina in lithotomy position such as dilatation and curettage, dilatation and evacuation or dilatation and insufflation.

Fig. 60.19: Auvard's weighted vaginal speculum

Sim's Double Ended Uterine Curette (Fig. 60.20)

Specifications and Uses

* A flat metal instrument with small spoon-like arrangement for scarping
* Both ends are spoon-shaped with fenestrations in the middle
* One end is blunt and the other end is sharp for curetting
* Used to take out the endometrium by curetting the uterine cavity for diagnostic or therapeutic purpose
* Used to empty the uterus by curetting the products of conception in incomplete or missed abortion.

Fig. 60.20: Uterine curette

Das's Cervical Dilators (Fig. 60.21)

Specifications and Uses

❖ Heavy metal instruments of gradually increasing sizes
❖ Has smooth, round body and tip having two different sizes in a single dilator
❖ The marking on the dilators indicates the circumference in millimeters
❖ Available in a set of 24 sizes from 2 mm upwards
❖ Used for dilating the cervix for curetting uterine contents in evacuation of the products of conception in MTP or incomplete abortion
❖ Used for dilating cervix.

Fig. 60.21: Das's cervical dilators

Flushing Curette (Figs 60.22A and B)

Specifications and Uses

❖ A curette with small spoon-like arrangement at one end for scraping
❖ The stem of the curette is hollow for the passage of any fluid to the interior of the spoon-like end
❖ To the other end (proximal), rubber tubing can be attached from a reservoir to pass fluids through the hollow area to the curetting end, which is blunt
❖ Used to wash out the uterine cavity, usually with warm antiseptic solution.

Figs 60.22A and B: Flushing curette

Drew-Smythe Catheter (Membrane Perforator) (Fig. 60.23)

Specifications and Uses

❖ It is a S-shaped, double curved metal catheter with a blunt stilet
❖ It has two openings–one inlet and one outlet, and double tube–one inner tube and one outer tube

Fig. 60.23: Drew-smythe catheter

❖ It is used for high rupture of membranes
❖ It allows controlled escape of liquor amni through it
❖ It can be passed between the membranes and uterus some length before puncturing
❖ The high rupture of membranes accomplished preserves the dilating effect of bag of waters and reduces the chances of infection and prolapse of the cord.

Uterine Sound (Fig. 60.24)

Specifications and Uses

❖ A slender, graduated, malleable metallic instrument
❖ It has an olive pointed tip and a broad handle
❖ The body is graduated and it can be used as a first dilator to dilate the cervix
❖ It is used to note the position of uterus and to measure the length of uterine cavity prior to dilatation and evacuation procedure

Fig. 60.24: Uterine sound

❖ It can be used to sound the uterine cavity to locate the IUCD with missing threads.

Scissors (Figs 60.25A to C)

Specification and Uses

❖ Scissors are used for blunt or sharp dissection
❖ Straight or curved Mayo scissors, which are very smooth at the ends, are sued to cut the tissues and internal organs so that adjacent tissues are protected while using
❖ Episiotomy scissors are used for cutting the perineum to enlarge the vaginal opening to deliver the fetal head
❖ Umbilical cord cutting scissors with broad rounded end are used for cutting umbilical cord.

Figs 60.25A to C: (A) Straight Mayo scissors; (B) Episiotomy scissors; (C) Umbilical cord cutting scissors

Bulb Syringe (Fig. 60.26)

Specifications and Uses

- A rubber bulb with elongated tip
- Used to remove secretions from mouth and nostrils of neonates following delivery of head.

Fig. 60.26: Bulb syringe

Mucus Sucker (Fig. 60.27)

Specifications and Uses

- A plastic device with graduated barrel and tubes
- Used to suck secretions from oropharynx and hypopharynx of neonates following birth, prior to the attempt of respiration.

Fig. 60.27: Mucus sucker

Cord Clamp (Fig. 60.28)

Specifications and uses

- A plastic device fused to clamp the umbilical cord
- It is kept in place until the cord dries and falls off. The clamp falls off with the detached cord stump.

Fig. 60.28: Disposable cord clamp

Wrigley's Outlet Forceps (Fig. 60.29)

Specifications and Uses

- A metal instrument in two pieces (halves) articulated by lock
- Each piece has a handle, lock, shaft and a fenestrated expanded blade
- The fenestrated portion of the blade allows good grip of the fetal head
- It is used to deliver the fetal head presenting at the pelvic outlet
- Delivery of the head is accomplished by extending it.

Fig. 60.29: Wrigley's forceps

Das's Long Curved Obstetric Forceps (Fig. 60.30)

Specifications and Uses

- A heavy metal instrument about 37 cm (15 inches) long. Its parts are blade, shank, lock and handle
- The blades are named left or right in relation to maternal pelvis in which they lie when applied
- Each blade has a cephalic curve to grasp the fetal head without compression and a

Fig. 60.30: Long curved forceps

pelvic curve to fit the curve on the axis of pelvic canal (curve of Carus)

❖ In order to lock the two halves after application, the left blade needs to be inserted first

❖ It is used in low forceps operation.

Axis Traction Forceps (Figs 60.31A and B)

Specifications and Uses

❖ It includes two axis traction rods (right and left) and a traction handle

❖ The rods are assembled in the blades of long curved obstetric forceps prior to

Figs 60.31A and B: (A) Axis traction devices; (B) Long curved forceps with axis traction device

introduction and lastly the handle is attached to the rods

❖ The devices are required (used) where much force is necessary for traction as in mid-forceps operation

❖ It provides traction in the correct axis of the pelvic curve and as such less force is necessary to deliver the head.

Keilland's Forceps (Fig. 60.32)

Specifications and Uses

❖ It is a long, almost straight (very slight pelvic curve) obstetric forceps with a sliding lock

❖ Usually used as rotation forceps in deep transverse arrest of occipito-posterior position of the head

❖ Facilitates grasping and correction of an asynclitic head because of its sliding lock.

Fig. 60.32: Keilland's forceps

Ventouse Cup with Traction Device/ Vacuum Extractor (Figs 60.33A and B)

Specifications and Uses

❖ An instrumental device designed to assist delivery by creating a vacuum between it and the fetal scalp

❖ The bell-shaped cups are of 4 sizes (30, 40, 50 and 60 mm)

❖ The cups have metallic plates at their apex. Each cup has a traction tube (rubber tube through which the traction chain passes) and a traction bar

❖ The traction devise is used with a vacuum pump

❖ It is used in the operation of vacuum extraction of the fetal head

Figs 60.33A and B: (A) Metal suction cups with metal chain, vacuum bottle and vacuum pump and tube; (B) Silastic vacuum cup

* The cup is to be fitted to the scalp of the fore coming head by producing a "chignon" with the help of vacuum
* A manometer connects the traction bar and suction bottle
* It can be used with lesser force (10 kg) than required for forceps application to accomplish delivery of the head
* Silastic vacuum cups are softer, less traumatic and safer to use
* Vacuum extractor is used as an alternative to forceps
* It can be used on a fetal head at a higher station and not well rotated.

Simpson's Perforator (Fig. 60.34)

Specifications and Uses

* A heavy metal instrument with spear-shaped sharp blades and handles with ridges
* With the blades closed, it is introduced into the vagina and fetal skill is perforated using rotary movements
* It is used to churn the brain matter before withdrawal to facilitate evacuation of brain matter.

Cranioclast (Fig. 60.35)

Specifications and Uses

* A heavy metal instrument with two blades. One blade is solid and the other fenestrated
* Used to compress the head following perforation
* The solid blade is introduced inside the cranium and the fenestrated blade outside for compression and extraction by traction.

Fig. 60.35: Cranioclast

Embriotomy Scissors (Fig. 60.36)

Specifications and Uses

* A heavy scissors used in destructive operation
* It is used to cut the thoracic cage or the abdominal wall during evisceration or to cut

Fig. 60.34: Simpson's perforator

Fig. 60.36: Embriotomy scissors

the remnant of the soft tissue of neck behind, during decapitation or in cleidotomy or spondylotomy operation
❖ With this instrument, only the tissues of the baby are cut.

Breech Hook and Crochet (Fig. 60.37)

Specifications and Uses

❖ A metal instrument, which has curves at both ends. One end is acutely curved (the crochet) and the other gradually bent (breech hook)
❖ The hook is used to give traction to groin of a dead baby when breech is impacted at the outlet
❖ The crochet is used to deliver the decapitated head by hooking the mandible through mouth or through a hole in the skull
❖ The middle portion is ridged to act as a handle and both ends may be used.

Fig. 60.37: Breech hook and crochet

Jardine's Decapitation Hook (Fig. 60.38)

Specifications and Uses

❖ This instrument has a handle and a head
❖ It is used in decapitation operation in neglected transverse lie or in impacted shoulder presentation where the fetal neck is accessible per vagina
❖ The hook with knife is used to severe both the vertebral column and soft tissue. In locked twins where disengagement is impossible, it is used to perform decapitation to save the second twin
❖ It is used in rare cases of double-headed fetus to facilitate extraction.

Fig. 60.38: Decapitation hook

Combined Cranioclast and Cephalotribe (Fig. 60.39)

Specifications and Uses

❖ The instrument consists of three parts, which can be adjusted and locked by a screw
❖ The central piece is placed within the skull through the opening made by a perforator
❖ The other two blades are almost straight without any pelvic curve
❖ They are placed externally over the skull and brought together by a butterfly screw prior to extraction of a dead fetus.

Fig. 60.39: Cranioclast and cephalotribe

External Pelvimeter (Fig. 60.40)

Fig. 60.40: Pelvimeter

Specifications and Uses

❖ A metal instrument with a joint at one end and a graduated bar
❖ Used to determine the external pelvic measurements
❖ Used to measure fundal height from symphysis pubis.

Pinard's Stethoscope/Fetoscope (Fig. 60.41)

Specifications and Uses

❖ A light, aluminium instrument
❖ It has an open abdominal end and an aural end
❖ When used to listen to fetal heart tones, it should be held firmly at right angle to the point on abdominal wall
❖ While listening to the fetal heart tones, the fetoscope should not be touched by hand.

Fig. 60.41: Fetoscope

Needle Holder (Fig. 60.42)

Specifications and Uses

❖ The instrument has long handles and small blades and resembles an artery forceps
❖ The blades have cross serrations
❖ It has a groove for catching the needle on its inner surface
❖ It may be straight or curved
❖ Used to hold the needle for suturing
❖ Straight type is used for holding needles while suturing a surface; curved type is used to work at depth or inside the cavity.

Fig. 60.42: Needle holder

Female Metal Catheter (Fig. 60.43)

Specifications and Uses

❖ A hollow, metallic tube, which may be straight or curved, tapering at the tip with an opening in the side and a ring at the base
❖ Used to evacuate the bladder in labor when rubber or flexible catheter cannot be inserted into the bladder
❖ Used to differentiate between a vesico-vaginal fistula and an urethro-vaginal fistula
❖ Used to ascertain the lower limit of the bladder before operations for genital prolapse
❖ Used only when other softer catheters cannot be used or when urethra is obstructed. Gentle manipulation is needed as it can cause injury.

Fig. 60.43: Female metal catheter

Ring Pessary (Fig. 60.44)

Specifications and Uses

❖ A round, flexible, rubber instrument.
❖ Used to support the uterus in following conditions:

Fig. 60.44: Ring pessary

Fig. 60.45: Hodge–smith pessary

- Prolapse in older age group
- Prolapse associated with pregnancy
- Puerperal prolapse or retroversion
- Prolapse when patient is a surgical risk or refuses to undergo surgery
❖ Used as a temporary measure to support uterus
❖ The watch-spring, inside the rubber ring of the instrument stretches the vaginal walls, which can thus act as a better support.

Hodge–Smith Pessary (Fig. 60.45)

Specifications and Uses

❖ A rubber or plastic device shaped as ring with one end broader
❖ Used to support uterus in the following conditions:
  - Symptom-producing, mobile, uncompli-cated retroverted uterus
  - Retroverted uterus in puerperal period
  - Retroverted gravid uterus up to 24th week of gestation.

Babcock's Tissue Forceps (Fig. 60.46)

Specifications and Uses

❖ A light and delicate instrument
❖ It is a non-traumatizing type of tissue forceps
❖ The blades are curved and fenestrated
❖ Tips of the blades are in the form of transverse bars with transverse serrations on its inner aspects
❖ It is used to hold soft and delicate tissues such as fallopian tubes, ureters, appendix and gut wall as in gastrostomy and colostomy

Fig. 60.46: Babcock's tissue forceps

❖ It can be used as a hemostat when the bleeder is difficult to pinpoint. The whole chunk of tissue is held with Babcock's forceps to cause temporary hemostasis.

BIBLIOGRAPHY

1. Bhowmik A, Chatterjee. Medical Instruments, 3rd edn. New Delhi: BI Publications (Pvt) Ltd, 2005.
2. Dutta DC. Textbook of Obstetrics, Calcutta; New Central Book Agency (P) Ltd, 2006.
3. Pilliteri Adele. Maternal and Child health nursing, 5th edn. Philadelphia: Lippincot Williams & Wilkins, 2007.
4. Thresiamma CP. Operating Room Technique and Anesthesia for GNM Course, 2nd edn. New Delhi: Jaypee Brothers Medical Publishers (Pvt) Ltd 2003.
5. Yadav Arun, Arora VS. Synopsis of Medical Instruments and Procedures, New Delhi: BI Publications (Pvt) Ltd, 2003.

Gynecological Nursing

61

Menstrual Cycle Disorders and Abnormal Bleeding

Learning Objectives

Upon completion of this chapter, the learner will be able to:
- Discuss the subjective and objective data, laboratory test results and investigations for menstrual cycle disorders
- Discuss the therapeutic interventions for menstrual cycle disorders
- Discuss the nursing process appropriate for patients with menstrual disorders.

Abnormal conditions of the menstrual cycle are deviations from what is normal for an individual woman. The condition may occur in the frequency or length of the cycle, volume or length of menstrual follow or the total number of years of menstruation. Menstrual cycle conditions may be classified as amenorrhea, Mittelschmerz's, syndrome, dysmenorrhea, dysfunctional uterine bleeding and premenstrual syndrome.

AMENORRHEA

Amenorrhea is the absence or lack of menses during the reproductive years. Normal causes of amenorrhea include pregnancy, lactation and menopause. Other causes can be pathologic and may include stress, excessive exercise, eating disorders, weight loss, a low body mass index (BMI) or other potentially life-threatening disorders.

Classification

1. **Primary amenorrhea:** Primary amenorrhea is the absence of menarche until age 16 or the absence of the development of secondary sex characteristics and menarche till age 14.

Causes

Causes of primary amenorrhea include:
- Hypothalamic, pituitary or enzymatic problems
- Chromosomal abnormalities
- Genitourinary abnormalities
- Drugs.

Symptoms

- Failure to experience menarche when there has been development of secondary sex characteristics
- No menarche and absence of development of secondary sex characteristics as in Turner's syndrome.

Management

Therapeutic interventions depend on the cause of amenorrhea.
- Estrogen replacement therapy (ERT) to stimulate development of secondary sex characteristics and to prevent osteoporosis.

2. **Secondary amenorrhea:** Secondary amenorrhea is the absence of menses for at least six months or for three cycles after menarche.

Causes

- Physiologic response to pregnancy, lactation or anovulation
- Hypothyroidism or hyperthyroidism

- Adrenal disease
- Chronic renal disease
- Polycystic ovary syndrome
- Chronic hepatic disease
- Anorexia nervosa
- Malnutrition
- Vigorous athletic training.

Investigations

- Thyroid function tests
- Blood glucose level
- Laparoscopy to check ovarian pathology
- Ultrasound to check polycystic ovary syndrome.

Management

- Cyclic progesterone therapy if the cause is anovulation
- Oral contraceptives for women who desire contraception
- Bromocriptine if there is hyperprolactinemia
- Gonadotropin releasing hormone (GnRH) when the cause is hypothalamic failure
- Thyroid hormone replacement for hypothyroidism
- Calcium and estrogen to prevent development of osteoporosis.

DYSMENORRHEA

Dysmenorrhea is painful menses or cramping during menstruation. Typically dysmenorrhea begins upto 48 hours before onset of menses and resolves with in 2 to 4 days of onset or by the end of menstrual period. Dysmenorrhea can be classified as primary (spasmodic) or secondary (congestive).

Primary Dysmenorrhea

Primary dysmenorrhea is one where there is no pelvic pathology. Usually occurs within 1 to 3 years of menarche.

Causes

Painful uterine contractions stimulated by prostaglandin produced by the endometrium during menses.

Symptoms

- Sharp, intermittent suprapubic pain radiating to the back or thighs
- Headache and backache
- Fatigue, dizziness and syncope
- GI symptoms: nausea, vomiting and bloating.

Treatment

Women often experience reduction in dysmenorrhea after pregnancy. Therapeutic interventions include:

- NSAIDs started one to three days before the onset of menstruation (to decrease prostaglandin production)
- Oral contraceptives to decrease endometrial proliferation and production of prostaglandin.

Secondary Dysmenorrhea

Secondary, dysmenorrhea is painful menstruation resulting from a pathologic process. The pain may be related to increasing tension in the pelvic tissues due to pelvic congestion or increased vascularity in the pelvic organs. Patients are usually in thirties and parous.

Causes

- Chronic pelvic infection
- Pelvic endometriosis
- Pelvic adhesions
- Uterine fibroids
- Endometrial polyp
- IUCD in utero.

Symptoms

- Dull pain situated in the back and front
- Pain starts 3 to 5 days prior to onset of menstruation and relieves with the start of bleeding
- Symptoms of associated pathology and no systemic discomfort.

Treatment

Treatment involves correction of the cause. The type of treatment depends on the severity, age and parity of the patient.

MITTELSCHMERZ'S SYNDROME (OVULAR PAIN)

Mittelschmerz's syndrome is a mid menstrual pain that occurs around the time of ovulation in menstruating women. The pain is usually situated in the hypogastrium or one iliac fossa.

Characteristics

❖ The pain is usually located on one side and does not change according to which ovary is ovulating.
❖ The pain usually lasts for about 12 hours.
❖ It may be associated with slight vaginal bleeding or excessive mucoid vaginal discharge.

Probable Causes

❖ Increased tension of the Graafian follicle prior to rupture
❖ Peritoneal irritation by the follicular fluid following ovulation
❖ Contraction of the fallopian tubes and uterus.

Treatment

❖ Analgesics and reassurance
❖ Contraceptive pills to make the cycle anovular in obstinate cases.

DYSFUNCTIONAL UTERINE BLEEDING (DUB)

Dysfunctional uterine bleeding is abnormal uterine bleeding without any clinically detectable cause. DUB occurs more often in adolescents and perimenopausal women.

Causes

❖ Hormonal abnormalities such as anovulation
❖ Pelvic inflammatory disease
❖ Endometriosis
❖ Neoplasms.

Pathophysiology

Abnormal bleeding is probably due to local causes in the endometrium. There is disturbance of the endometrial blood vessels and capillaries and coagulation of blood in and around these vessels. These are probably related to alteration in the ratio of endometrial prostaglandins which are delicately balanced in homeostasis of menstruation.

Clinical Manifestations

❖ Polymenorrhea (Frequent menses)
  This occurs following childbirth and abortion, during adolescence and premenopausal period
❖ Oligomenorrhea (light or infrequent menses)
  This occurs in adolescence and preceding menopause
❖ Menorrhagia (Excessive and prolonged menses).

Investigations

❖ History of the nature of menstrual abnormity
❖ Internal examination including speculum examination
❖ Blood tests: Hemoglobin, CBC, platelets, prothrombin time, bleeding time, partial thromboplastin and thyroid function tests.
❖ Ultrasound and color Doppler: Transvaginal sonography and saline infusion sonography to detect abnormalities like fibroids and adenomyosis
❖ Endometrial biopsy through hysteroscopy to rule out endometrial cancer
❖ Laparoscopy to exclude pelvic pathology.

Management

❖ General: Correction of anemia by diet, hematinics and blood transfusion if required
❖ Oral contraceptives for menstrual cycle regulation
❖ Cyclic progesterone for anovulatory bleeding
❖ Nonsteroidal anti-inflammatory drugs (NSAIDs) to reduce the amount of menstrual bleeding
❖ GnRH agonists: If the woman is infertile and wants pregnancy. In low dosess, it reduces blood loss and produces hypo-estrogenic features

- Endometrial ablation (separation) to decrease or eliminate tissue sloughing
- Anti-progesterone: Mifepristone (Ru486) to inhibit ovulation, induce amenorrhea and reduce myoma size
- Hysterectomy when abnormal uterine bleeding cannot be corrected by conservative treatment and the blood loss impairs the health of the patient.

PREMENSTRUAL SYNDROME (PMS)

Premenstrual syndrome is a cyclic cluster of behavioral, emotional and physical symptoms that occurs just prior to menstruation that is in the luteal phase of the menstrual cycle. There is a cyclic appearance of large number of symptoms during the last 7 to 10 days of the menstrual cycle. The symptoms must be sufficiently severe and fulfill the following criteria before the diagnosis can be made

- Not related to any organic lesion
- Occurs regularly during the luteal phase of each ovulatory menstrual cycle
- Symptom- free period during the rest of the cycle.

Pathophysiology

The probable causes of the conditions are:

- Alteration in the level of estrogen and progesterone starting from the mid-luteal phase
- Neuroendocrine factors such as decreased synthesis of serotonin and withdrawal of endorphins (neurotransmitters) during the luteal phase.
- Psychological and psychosocial factors producing behavioral changes.

Clinical Features

Related to water retention:

- Abdominal bloating
- Breast tenderness
- Swelling of extremities
- Weight gain.

Neuroendocrine and Psychological Related

- Irritability, tearfulness
- Depression, anxiety

- Tension, mood swings
- Rejection sensitivity
- Insomnia/hypersomnia
- Decreased concentration
- Forgetfulness, confusion
- Restlessness
- Headache
- Increased appetite
- Change in libido.

Autonomic Symptoms

- Nausea, anorexia
- Diarrhea
- Palpitation
- Perspiration.

Behavioral Symptoms

- Fatigue, decreased motivation
- Tiredness, social isolation
- Clumsiness, paresthesia (numbness or tingling).

Treatment

Treatment is aimed at alleviation of symptoms since PMS is not a disease. No single treatment may be effective. Drugs like tranquilizers, diuretics and antidepressants are used based on individual needs. Women are taught the following measures to reduce the intensity of symptoms:

- Modify diet
- Increase exercise
- Alleviate stress
- Change activities of daily living
- Reduce fatigue
- Enhance ability to sleep.

Nursing Process for Client with Menstrual Cycle Disorders

Nursing assessment for menstrual conditions involves careful medical and gynecologic history, assessment of symptoms, and assessment for specific suspected condition. The physical assessment focuses on collection of data regarding the suspected menstrual cycle abnormality including collection of data from laboratory tests and special investigations.

Applicable nursing diagnoses may include:
- ❖ Pain related to the specific menstrual condition
- ❖ Fear related to the medical diagnosis
- ❖ Anxiety related to unknown outcomes
- ❖ Deficient knowledge related to limited experience regarding specific menstrual cycle disorder.

Planning includes specific actions the woman should complete to achieve the highest level of wellness. Plans prepared in collaboration with the client may include the following:
The client will:
- ❖ Consume correct proportions of recommended food as evidenced by a 24-hour diet recall
- ❖ Exercise by walking 30 minutes each day
- ❖ Take prescribed medications according to instructions
- ❖ Return to the health care facility as scheduled for follow-up visits
- ❖ Contact the physician if symptoms do not improve
- ❖ Understand the health promotion counseling.

MENORRHAGIA

Definition

Menorrhagia is an abnormally heavy and prolonged menstrual period at regular intervals. Normal menstrual cycle is 25 to 35 days in duration with bleeding lasting an average of 5 days and a total blood flow between 25 and 80 ml. A blood loss greater than 80 ml or lasting longer than 7 days constitutes menorrhagia (also called *Hypermenorrhea*).

Causes

Usually no causative abnormality can be identified and treatment is directed to the symptom rather than a specific mechanism. An overview of causes includes:

Uterine

- ❖ Endometrial polyp
- ❖ Submucosal fibroid
- ❖ Endometrial hyperplasia
- ❖ Endometrial adenomyosis.

Ovarian

- ❖ Ovulatory DUB
- ❖ Anovulatory DUB
- ❖ Polycystic ovary syndrome
- ❖ Granulosa cell tumor of ovary.

Others

- ❖ Hematological causes
- ❖ Von Willebrand's disease
- ❖ Hypothyroidism, hyperthyroidism
- ❖ Leukemia.

Diagnosis

- ❖ Pelvic and rectal examination
- ❖ Pap smear
- ❖ Pelvic ultrasound scan is the first line diagnostic study for identifying structural abnormalities
- ❖ Endometrial biopsy to exclude atypical hyperplasia or endometrial cancer
- ❖ Hysteroscopy.

Treatment

Where underlying cause can be identified, treatment may be directed at this. Clearly heavy periods at menarche and menopause may settle spontaneously.

Medications

- ❖ Iron supplements to counter anemia.
- ❖ Nonsteroidal anti-inflammatory drugs (NSAIDs) to reduce blood loss
- ❖ Hormonal treatment for DUB
  - – Oral contraceptives, usually combined estrogen—progesterone pills for few months.
  - – Progesterone only pills or injection Depo-provera.
  - – Progesterone releasing intrauterine system (IUS).
- ❖ Other options
  - – Antifibrinolytics: Gonadotropin-releasing hormone (GnRH) agonists.

Surgery

Surgical treatment is rarely resorted to:
- ❖ Endometrial ablation
- ❖ Dilatation and curettage

- ❖ Hysteroscopic myomectomy to remove fibroids.

POLYMENORRHEA (EPIMENORRHEA)

Polymenorrhea or epimenorrhea is defined as cyclic bleeding, where the cycle is reduced to an arbitrary limit of less than 21 days and remain constant at that rate. If the frequent cycle is associated with excessive and or prolonged bleeding, it is called epimenorrhea.

Causes

- ❖ Dysfunctional uterine bleeding
  Common in adolescence, preceding menopause and following delivery and abortion. Hyperstimulation of ovaries by the pituitary hormone may be the causative factor
- ❖ Ovarian hyperemia.
  Seen in pelvic inflammatory disease (PID) or ovarian endometriosis.

Treatment

Hormone therapy.

METRORRHAGIA

Metrorrhagia is defined as irregular, acyclic bleeding from the uterus. It is mostly related to surface lesions in the uterus. When the bleeding is so irregular and excessive that the menses (periods) cannot be identified, it is called as *menometrorrhagia*.

Causes

Acyclic Bleeding

- ❖ DUB (during adolescence, following childbirth or abortion and preceding menopause)
- ❖ Submucous fibroid
- ❖ Uterine polyp
- ❖ Endometrial or cervical cancer.

Contact Bleeding

- ❖ Carcinoma cervix
- ❖ Mucous polyp of cervix

- ❖ Infections: chlamydial or tubercular cervicitis
- ❖ Cervical endometriosis.

Intermenstrual Bleeding

- ❖ Urethral caruncle
- ❖ IUCD *in utero*
- ❖ Breakthrough bleeding in pill users
- ❖ Ovular bleeding.

Treatment

Treatment is directed to the underlying pathology.

OLIGOMENORRHEA

Oligomenorrhea is defined as bleeding occurring more than 35 days apart and which remains constant at that frequency.

Causes

- ❖ Age related: During adolescence and preceding menopause
- ❖ Obesity
- ❖ Vigorous exercise
- ❖ Endocrine disorders: PCOS, Hypoprolactinemia, hyperthyroidism
- ❖ Androgen producing tumors – ovarian, adrenal
- ❖ Tubercular endometritis.

Treatment

Treatment according to the cause identified.

HYPOMENORRHEA

Hypomenorrhea is defined as menstrual bleeding that is unduly scanty and lasts for less than 2 days.

Causes

- ❖ Uterine synechiae
- ❖ Endometrial tuberculosis
- ❖ Use of oral contraceptives
- ❖ Thyroid dysfunction
- ❖ Malnutrition
- ❖ Premenopausal period.

Treatment

Treatment is directed to the specific cause.

62

Displacement of Uterus

The uterus is not in a fixed position in pelvis. Minor variations in position occur with changes in posture with straining and with full bladder or rectum. When the uterus rests habitually in a position beyond the limit of normal variation, it is called displacement. The commonly occurring displaced positions are retroversion, prolapse and inversion of uterus.

RETROVERSION OF UTERUS (FIGS 62.1A TO C)

Retroversion is the turning backward of the uterus with the long axis of the corpus and cervix in line and the whole organ turns backwards in relation to the long axis of the birth canal. Retroflexion is a bending backwards of the corpus on the cervix at the level of the internal os. The two conditions are usually present together and are referred to as retroversion-flexion or retrodisplacement.

Degrees of Displacement

- ❖ *First degree*: The fundus is vertical and pointing towards the sacral promontory
- ❖ *Second degree*: The fundus lies in the sacral hollow but not below the internal os
- ❖ *Third degree*: The fundus lies below the level of internal os.

Causes

- ❖ *Developmental defects:* The infantile position of the uterus is retained. There is lack of uterine muscle tone and the condition is associated with short vagina with shallow anterior vaginal fornix
- ❖ *Puerperal:* Due to stretched ligaments caused by childbirth
- ❖ Prolapse caused by traction following cystocele
- ❖ Fibroid tumor in the anterior or posterior wall of the uterus produces heaviness making it fall behind
- ❖ *Pelvic adhesions:* Adhesions either inflammatory, operative or due to endometriosis pull the uterus posteriorly.

Incidence

The condition is seen in about 15 to 20 percent of normal women.

Signs and Symptoms/Clinical Presentation

- ❖ Chronic premenstrual pelvic pain due to varicosities in broad ligament produced by the kinks.
- ❖ Dyspareunia due to direct thrust by the penis against the retroflexed uterus or

Figs 62.1A to C: Retroversion and retroflexion of the uterus: (A) The most common position; (B) Retroversion of uterus; (C) Retroversion and retroflexion of uterus

prolapsed ovaries lying in the pouch of Douglas

❖ Infertility as the external os is away from the seminal pool at the posterior fornix during coitus or it may be occluded by the anterior vaginal wall

❖ On bimanual examination, body of the uterus is felt in the posterior fornix and cervix directed upwards

❖ On speculum examination, the cervix is viewed easily and the external os points forwards.

Prevention

The following are guidelines to be followed during the weeks after childbirth or abortion to prevent retroversion.

❖ Empty the bladder regularly

❖ Increase the tone of the pelvic muscles by regular exercise

❖ Encourage lying in prone position for 30 to 60 minutes twice daily in 2nd to 4th week postpartum.

Corrective Treatment

❖ Hodge-Smith pessary for stretching the uterosacral ligaments so as to pull the cervix backwards

❖ Surgical correction
Ventrosuspension of the uterus by plicating the round ligaments of both sides extra-peritoneally to the under surface of the anterior rectal sheath. This will pull the uterus forwards and maintains it permanently.

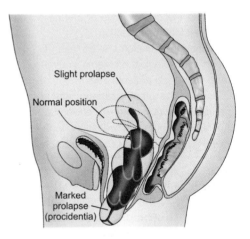

Fig. 62.2: Degrees of uterine prolapse

UTERINE PROLAPSE (FIG. 62.2)

Definition

Prolapse of uterus refers to a collapse, descend or change in the position of the uterus in relation to surrounding structures in the pelvis.

Description

Uterine prolapse occurs when pelvic floor muscles and ligaments stretch and weaken providing inadequate support for the uterus. The uterus then descends into the vaginal canal. Uterine prolapse usually happens in women who have had one or more vaginal births. Congenital or nulliparous prolapse is a rare type of prolapse seen in young women.

Associated Conditions (Figs 62.3 and 62.4)

Other conditions associated with prolapsed uterus occur due to weakness of muscles that hold the uterus in place.

❖ *Cystocele (Figs 62.3A and B):* It is a herniation or bulging of the upper two-thirds of the anterior vaginal wall, where a part of the bladder budges in to the vagina. This leads to urinary frequency, urgency, retention and incontinence.

❖ *Urethrocele:* There is herniation of the anterior vaginal wall. This may appear independently or along with cystocele and is called urethrocystocele.

❖ *Enterocele:* There is herniation of the upper posterior vaginal wall, where a portion of small bowel bulges in to the vagina. Standing leads to a pulling sensation and backache and this is relieved on lying down.

❖ *Rectocele (Fig. 62.4):* There is herniation of the middle third of the posterior vaginal wall where the rectum bulges into the vagina. This makes bowel movements difficult to the point that the woman may need to push on the inside of vagina to empty the bowel.

❖ *Relaxed perineum:* There is gaping of the introitus produced by torn perineal body with bulge of the lower part of the posterior vaginal wall.

Fig. 62.4: Rectocele (*For color version see Plate 7*)

Degrees of Prolapse (Figs 62.2 and 62.5)

Prolapse of the uterus may be one of three types, depending on severity.

❖ *First degree:* The uterus sags downward from the normal anatomic position into the upper vagina. The external os remains inside the vagina.

❖ *Second degree:* The cervix is at or outside the vaginal introitus, but the uterine body remains inside the vagina.

Figs 62.3A and B: (A) Cystocele and uterovaginal prolapse; (B) Cystocele and enterocele (*For color version see Plate 7*)

A   **B**

Figs 62.5A and B: Complete uterine prolapse (*For color version see Plate 8*)

❖ *Third degree:* This type is also referred to as complete prolapse or procidentia. The entire uterus descends to lie outside the introitus.

Causes

The uterus is held in position in the pelvis by muscles, special ligaments and other tissue. The uterus prolapses into the vaginal canal when these muscles and connective tissue weakens.

❖ Stretching of the pelvic support system: Long and difficult childbirth or multiple childbirth causes the muscles and ligaments that normally hold the uterus in place to become stretched and slack.

❖ Pelvic relaxation that happens during pregnancy: There is softening of the pelvic tissues and laxity of the supports during pregnancy as the weight of the gravid uterus continuously bears down upon the pelvic diaphragm.

❖ Chronic increase in intra-abdominal pressure such as may be associated with obesity, abdominal or pelvic tumors, ascites or repetitive downward thrust of intra-abdominal pressure due to constipation or chronic cough.

❖ Normal aging and lack of estrogen hormone after menopause.

Symptoms

❖ A feeling of something coming down per vagina, especially while moving about. There may be variable discomfort on walking when the mass comes out of the introitus

❖ Backache or dragging pain in the pelvis; which may be relieved on lying down

❖ Dyspareunia

❖ Urinary symptoms (in presence of cystocele)
  – Difficulty in passing urine. Patient may have to elevate the anterior vaginal wall for emptying the bladder
  – Incomplete emptying of the bladder, causing frequent desire to pass urine
  – Urgency and frequency of micturition which may also be due to cystitis
  – Stress incontinence usually due to associated urethrocele
  – Retention of urine may rarely occur.

❖ Bowel symptoms (in presence of rectocele)
  – Difficulty in passing stool. Patient may have to push back the posterior vaginal wall to complete the evacuation of feces Fecal incontinence may be associated.
  – Excessive white or blood stained discharge per vagina due to associated vaginitis or ulceration.

Examination and Diagnosis

* *Inspection and palpation:* Vaginal, rectal and rectovaginal examination
* Pelvic examination in dorsal and standing positions. Patient may be asked to perform Valsalva maneuver during examination.
* Examination in squatting position if reconfirmation is required.
* Examination under anesthesia if difficult to arrive at a conclusion.

Management of Uterine Prolapse

Preventive

* Adequate antenatal and intranatal care: To avoid injury to the supporting structures during vaginal delivery, either spontaneous or instrumental.
* Adequate postnatal care: To encourage early ambulation and pelvic floor exercises (Kegel's exercises) during puerperium.
* General measures: To avoid strenuous activities, chronic cough, constipation and heavy weight lifting.
* Limiting and spacing pregnancies help avoid pelvic relaxation.

Conservative

* Estrogen replacement therapy may improve minor degree prolapse in post-menopausal women.
* In mild cases, exercises to strengthen pelvic floor muscles may help.
* Obese patients may be instructed to reduce weight in order to reduce pressure on pelvic organs.
* To avoid wearing constrictive clothing such as girdles.

Non-surgical management: A pessary may be placed inside the vagina to support the pelvic organs for patients who do not desire surgery.

This serves to relieve the symptoms but does not cure the condition. Pessary may also be used for patients waiting for surgery or unfit for surgery.

Surgical management: Surgical management depends on the anatomical alteration of structures and the degree of prolapse.

Patients age and reproductive and sexual functions are also considered.
  – Anterior colporrhaphy for correction of cystocele and urethrocele.
  – Perineorrhaphy/colpoperineorrhaphy to repair the prolapse of posterior vaginal wall which may include repair of *relaxed perineum, rectocele* and *enterocele.*
* *Fothergill's or Manchester operation:* This is designed to correct uterine descend associated with cystocele and rectocele where preservation of uterus is desired. The operation combines repair of anterior and posterior vaginal walls with amputation of cervix and plication of Mackenrodt's ligaments in front of the cervix.
* Vaginal hysterectomy with pelvic floor repair.
* Cervicopexy or Purandare's operation for congenital or nulliparous prolapse without cystocele.

Possible Complications Following Surgical Management

Immediate

Hemorrhage within 24 hours following surgery (primary) or between 5th to 10th days (secondary)
* Retention of urine
* Infection leading to cystitis
* Wound sepsis
* Vault cellulitis.

Late

* Dyspareunia
* Recurrence of prolapse
* VVF following bladder injury
* RVF following rectal injury
* Cervical stenosis-hemometra
* Infertility
* Cervical incompetency.

CHRONIC INVERSION OF UTERUS

Definition

This type of inversion is a condition where the uterus becomes turned inside out, the fundus prolapsing through the cervix.

Causes

❖ Incomplete obstetric inversion unnoticed or left uncared following failure to reduce it for a variable period of 4 weeks or more
❖ Submucous myomatous polyp arising from the fundus causing traction effect
❖ Sacromatous changes of fundal fibroma causing infiltration of malignancy into the myometrium leading to softening of the wall
❖ Senile inversion following high amputation of the cervix.

Types of Inversion

❖ *Incomplete inversion:* The fundus protrudes through the cervix and lying inside the vagina.
❖ *Complete inversion:* Whole of the uterus including the cervix are inverted. The vagina may also be involved.

Symptoms and Signs

❖ Sensation of something coming down per vagina
❖ Irregular vaginal bleeding
❖ Offensive vaginal discharge
❖ On inspection, the protruding mass appears globular with no opening in the leading part. A tumor may be present at the bottom
❖ On vaginal examination, the cervical rim is either felt high up or not felt. A cup-shaped depression felt at the fundus or the uterus is not felt in position

❖ On rectoabdominal examination, displacement of uterus or fundal depression is felt
❖ Uterine sound test demonstrates shortness or absence of uterine cavity
❖ Examination under anesthesia (EUA) may be needed to confirm the diagnosis. When the inversion is secondary to a fibroid polyp or sarcoma and the inversion is incomplete, filling the vagina, diagnosis is more difficult.

Treatment

Rectification of inversion by surgery or removal of the uterus is determined by such factors as age, parity and associated complications.

Improvement of general condition by treating anemia and local sepsis is done if required prior to surgery.

❖ Haultain's operation: Rectification per abdomen
❖ Spinelli's operation: Rectification per vagina
❖ Hysterectomy following rectification.

Nursing Implications

Nursing diagnoses are individualized to each client and her specific condition. Applicable diagnoses may include:

❖ Pain related to specific gynecologic condition.
❖ Fear related to diagnostic and therapeutic procedures.
❖ Anxiety related to treatment outcome.
❖ Deficient knowledge regarding the pelvic condition, treatment and prognosis.

63

Infectious Conditions of Pelvic Organs

Infection and inflammation affect upper genital tract organs together and individual organs of both upper and lower genital tracts. Depending on the causative organisms, pathological changes in the organs and nature and severity of the condition, medical and/or surgical management are required.

PELVIC INFLAMMATORY DISEASE (PID)

Pelvic inflammatory disease is a spectrum of infection and inflammation of the upper genital tract organs typically involving the endometrium, fallopian tubes, ovaries, pelvic peritoneum and surrounding structures.

Risk Factors

- Menstruating teenagers—ascending infections especially *E. coli*, group B *Streptococcus* and *Staphylococcus*
- Previous history of acute PID
- Use of intrauterine contraceptive devices (IUCD)
- Multiple sex partners.

Types of Infections

- Uterus
  - Acute endometritis
  - Chronic endometritis
  - Atrophic (senile) endometritis
  - Pyometra (collection of pus in the uterine cavity)
- Fallopian tubes
  - Acute salpingitis
  - Chronic salpingitis
- Ovaries
  - Oophoritis.

Causative Organisms

Acute PID is usually a polymicrobial infection caused by organisms ascending from the lower genital tract. The primary organisms are usually sexually transmitted and the secondary organisms are those normally found in the vagina.

- Sexually transmitted organisms:
  - *Gonococcus*
  - *Chlamydia trachomatis*
  - *Mycoplasma hominis.*
- Pyogenic infection
  - *Streptococcus*
  - *Staphylococcus*
  - *E. coli*
  - *Actinomycosis*
  - *Bacteroides species—fragilis and bivius, Peptostreptococcus and Peptococcus.*

Pathology

The pathological process is initiated in the endosalpinx with gross destruction of the epithelial cells, cilia and microvilli. In severe infection, it involves all the layers of the tube and produces acute inflammatory reaction; becomes edematous and hyperemic. The abdominal ostium is closed due to inflammatory adhesions. Depending upon the virulence, the exudate may be watery producing hydrosalpinx or purulent producing pyosalpinx.

On occasions, the exudate pours through the abdominal osteum to produce pelvic peritonitis and pelvic abscess or may affect the ovary producing ovarian abscess.

Clinical Features

Symptoms usually appear at and immediately following menses in acute infections:

- Bilateral lower abdominal and pelvic pain
- Fever—temperature > 38.3°C
- Tiredness and headache
- Irregular and excessive vaginal bleeding due to endometritis
- Increased vaginal discharge usually mucopurulent
- Nausea and vomiting
- Dyspareunia and dysuria
- Dysmenorrhea
- Postcoital spotting
- Cervical motion tenderness
- Hypoactive bowel sounds
- Adnexal fullness and tenderness
- Cervical friability
- Congested vulva, urethral meatus and openings of Bartholin's ducts
- Elevated ESR and C-reactive protein
- Ultrasound evidence of fluid or pus collection.

Investigations

- Identification of organisms from the materials collected from the affected organ.
- Blood tests for WBC (leukocitosis and elevated ESR)
- Sonography; dilated fluid filled tubes, adnexal mass or fluid in the pouch of Douglas is suggestive of PID
- Laparoscopic examination in severe cases
- Culdocenesis and examination of the fluid.

Treatment

Patients with severe infection are hospitalized for management.

- Best rest
- Restricted oral feeding
- Intravenous fluid to correct dehydration and acidosis
- Antibiotics intravenously; cefoxitin or gentamicin and metronidazole
- Draining of collected fluid or pus via laparotomy
- Nasogastric suction in the presence of ileus or abdominal distention.

Indications for Surgical Interventions

Need for surgical intervention is rare and indicated in:

- Generalized peritonitis
- Pelvic abscess
- Tubo-ovarian abscess which does not respond to antimicrobial therapy for 48 to 72 hours.

Complications

With chronic PID which is diagnosed and treated late, there is increased risk of developing complications such as:

- Infertility
- Ectopic pregnancy
- Chronic pelvic pain.

Measures to Prevent Reinfection

Patients should be educated on following measures to prevent repeat infection.

- Avoid multiple sexual partners
- Use condom for sexual intercourse
- Get the sexual partner investigated and treated
- Have follow-up smears and culture tests until it becomes negative for infecting organisms. The tests are usually repeated following menstrual period until it becomes negative for three consecutive reports.

ENDOMETRITIS

Endometritis is an inflammation of the lining of the uterus—the endometrium.

Causes

Endometritis can stem from several underlying causes the most prevalent of which are bacterial infections.

- Remnant tissues such as the placenta retained after a delivery or abortion is the most common cause of postpartum infection. Such infection may spread to the entire uterus, ovaries and pelvis
- Amniotic fluid can become infected from stool excreted by the fetus or from other sources of pathogenic bacteria during pregnancy
- Sexually transmitted diseases (STDs) such as gonorrhea and *Chlamydia* are often the causes
- Pelvic inflammatory disease (PID) may also lead to endometritis
- Tuberculosis
- Normal vaginal bacteria can be a reason for endometritis.

Risk Factors

The risk of developing endometritis increases by number of factors:

- A cesarean section significantly heightens the chances of postpartum infection
- Extended labor or premature rupture of fetal membranes
- Anemia may be a pre-existing condition or it may result from heavy bleeding during labor.
- Steroid medications: Sometimes used to assist fetal lung development and functioning when premature birth is expected, are another risk factor.
- The presence of an intrauterine device (IUD) can induce or exacerbate inflammation
- Use of special instruments and procedures such as hysteroscopy and D&C can induce inflammation.

Signs and Symptoms

Postpartum endometritis develop in 49 to 72 hours.

- Abdominal distention or swelling
- Abnormal vaginal bleeding
- Abnormal vaginal discharge often with a foul odor
- Lower abdominal or pelvic pain
- Fever with chills (Temp 100 – 104° F)
- Discomfort with bowel movement (constipation may occur)
- Malaise and general discomfort.

Tests and Investigations

- Abdominal palpation to discover tenderness or soreness
- Pelvic examination
- Blood tests; WBC, CBC, ESR
- Cultures from cervix for organisms
- Pap smear to detect the presence of abnormal cells
- Laparoscopy/hysteroscopy and endometrial biopsy
- CT scan to assess the uterus and other internal organs.

Treatment

Patients with serious symptoms and postpartum infection need to be hospitalized and treated. Treatment measures include:

- Administration of intravenous antibiotics for two to seven days
- Administration of oral or intravenous fluids to prevent dehydration
- Aspiration to drain pus from uterus
- Evacuation of remnant tissue from the uterus (placenta, membranes)
- Adequate rest
- A postpartum hysterectomy to remove a hopelessly damaged or infected uterus
- Analgesics for pain and fever and isolation to avoid cross-infection are often instituted. Mild cases may be treated on an outpatient basis.

Prognosis

Most cases of endometritis clear up with antibiotics. Untreated endometritis can lead to more serious infection and complications with pelvic organs, reproduction and general health.

Possible Complications

❖ Infertility
❖ Pelvic peritonitis
❖ Pelvic or uterine abscess formation
❖ Septicemia
❖ Septic shock

Prevention

Endometritis caused by sexually transmitted infections, can be prevented by:
❖ Early diagnosis and complete treatment of sexually transmitted diseases
❖ Educating women on safe sex practices.

The risk of endometritis will be reduced by following sterile techniques by health care workers while delivering a baby or performing an abortion, IUD placement or other gynecological procedures.

CERVICITIS

Cervicitis refers to infection of the endocervix including the glands and stroma. The infection may be acute or chronic and usually occurs following childbirth, abortion or any operation on the cervix. The infection may be acute or chronic.

Causative Organisms

Organisms causing cervicitis include *Streptococcus, Staphylococcus, E. coli, Gonococcus* and *Chlamydia trachomatis*. The organisms gain entry in to the glands of the endocervix and produce acute inflammatory changes. The infection may be localized or spread upwards to involve the fallopian tubes and parametrium.

Clinical Features

❖ Spotting after sexual intercourse
❖ Yellowish-white discharge
❖ Red, edematous, friable cervix
❖ Cervical motion tenderness
❖ Vaginal examination is painful.

Treatment

❖ Antibiotic therapy based on identified drug sensitivity (High vaginal and endocervical swabs are taken for bacteriological identification and drug sensitivity)
❖ In chronic cervicitis, the diseased tissue may be destroyed by electro or diathermy cauterization or laser or cryosurgery
❖ Any associated cervical tear if present may be reconstructed
❖ Cervical scrape cytology must be done to exclude malignancy.

VULVAL AND VAGINAL INFECTIONS

Vulval and vaginal infections occur when the defense is lost following constant irritation by vaginal discharge or urine (incontinence) or following menopause when there will be atrophic changes.

Common Infectious Conditions

❖ Bartholinitis, Bartholin abscess and Bartholin cysts
❖ Vaginitis: Bacterial, viral, Monilial and atrophic (postmenopausal)
❖ Vulvovaginitis.

Causative Organisms and Clinical Manifestations

❖ Bacterial infections are caused by sexually transmitted organisms such as gonorrhea, *Chlamydia trachomatis* and syphilis:
  – Increased vaginal discharge
  – Musty or fleshy odor of discharge following sexual intercourse
  – Homogeneous, gray-white discharge Bacterial infections are treated with local antiseptics and systemic antibiotics.
❖ Monilial infections—caused by *Candida albicans*. Manifestations are:
  – Itching and burning
  – Thick curd-like discharge
  – Dyspareunia
  – Vulvar and/or vaginal erythema
  – Edematous cervix.

Monilial infection is treated with local fungicidal preparations such as nistatin, clotrimazole, miconazole or econazole or fluconazole oral therapy.

- Vulval infection: It is usually by *Varicella-zoster* virus. It produces painful eruptions of groups of vesicles distributed over the skin. Vesicles may rupture or become dry with scab formation.

  It is treated with analgesics to relieve pain, antibiotics to prevent secondary infection and acyclovir as antiviral drug.

- *Atrophic vulvovaginitis:* This type of infection is seen in postmenopausal women. There is atrophy of the vulvovaginal structures due to deficiency of estrogen. Vaginal mucosa is thin and more susceptible to trauma and infection.

Clinical Features

- Dryness and soreness
- Itching and burning
- Vulvar and vaginal atrophy
- Pale, thin, friable vaginal mucosa
- Sparse pubic hair
- Dyspareunia
- Yellowish or blood stained discharge.

Treatment

- Intravaginal applications of estrogen cream
- Systemic estrogen if there is no contra-indication
- Treatment of local infection if present.

Nursing Process for Clients with Pelvic Infections

Nursing assessment for genital infections include assessment for risk, symptoms, medical history, gynecologic history and lifestyle behaviors. Physical assessment focuses on data from assessment and investigation findings to aid diagnosis of specific infection. Nursing diagnoses are formulated after diagnosis of infection. Applicable nursing diagnoses may include the following:

- Pain related to infection
- Fear related to the diagnosis
- Deficient knowledge related to the experience regarding the diagnosis.

Nursing care plans include specific actions the client completes to achieve the highest level of wellness possible. Sample goals may include the following:

The Client

- Takes the prescribed medications correctly
- Returns to health care facility/physician as scheduled for follow-up assessment of infectious status
- Notifies physician of any failure of symptoms to improve as expected or adverse effects of prescribed medications
- Adopts recommended changes in lifestyle behaviors to prevent recurrent infection
- Learns measures for health promotion.

Nursing interventions include teaching and counseling for prevention and explaining prescribed medications.

64

Benign Pelvic Conditions

Learning Objectives

Upon completion of this chapter, the learner will be able to:
* List the benign pelvic conditions that are structural and functional
* Explain the common tumors of uterus and ovary
* Describe polyps and cystic conditions of pelvic organs
* Describe polycystic ovary disease and management of patients
* Explain the nursing management of clients with benign pelvic conditions.

Benign pelvic conditions can be categorized as structural and functional growths. Common structural conditions include fibroid tumors, ovarian tumors, cysts and polyps. Common functional condition is polycystic ovary syndrome (PCOS).

FIBROID TUMORS

Fibroid tumors are benign tumors arising in the myometrium which can protrude into the uterine cavity, bulge through the outer layer or grow within the myometrium.

Growth of Fibroids

* Fibroids develop due to proliferation of smooth muscle cells. The tumors usually grow very slowly, about 1 to 2 cm per year.
* Fibroids are estrogen dependent and thus grow rapidly during pregnancy. They do not occur before menarche and growth cessation occurs after menopause.

Incidence

The tumors are found most often during the 4th and 5th decades of life. The incidence of symptomatic fibroid is about 3 percent in Indian women. The incidence is higher in women in USA and UK. Fibroids occur more often in nulliparous women or in those having secondary infertility. Higher incidence is seen in obese women and oral pill users.

Types of Fibroids (Fig. 64.1)

1. Interstitial or intramural fibroids 75 percent. These are fibroids that grow with in the myometrium.
2. Subserous or subperitoneal fibroids 15 percent. These are intramural fibroids that are pushed outwards towards the peritoneal cavity. They are partially or completely

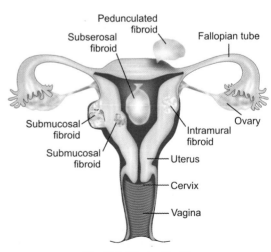

Fig. 64.1: Uterine fibroids

covered by peritoneum. If the fibroid has a pedicle, it is called pendunculated subserous fibroid.

3. Submucous fibroids 15 percent. When the tumor protrudes into the uterine cavity and lies underneath the endometrium, it is called submucous fibroid. This can make the uterine cavity irregular and distorted. Pedunculated submucous fibroid may come out through the cervix.

Clinical Features

❖ Majority of fibroids (75%) remain asymptomatic and are detected during routine examination or at laparotomy or laparoscopy
❖ The uterus reaches a 4 to 5 months gestation size without symptoms in most cases
❖ In symptomatic type, menorrhagia is the classic symptom
❖ Metrorrhagia or irregular bleeding is seen in some women
❖ Dysmenorrhea is a symptom when it is associated with pelvic congestion or endometriosis
❖ Infertility is seen in about 30 percent of women
❖ Recurrent pregnancy loss (Miscarriage or preterm labor)
❖ Lower abdominal or pelvic pain.

Diagnosis

❖ Majority of uterine fibroids can be diagnosed from history and pelvic examination
❖ Ultrasound and color Doppler are used to locate the fibroids accurately. Laparoscopy is useful if the uterine size is less than 12 weeks and associated with pelvic pain and infertility
❖ Uterine curettage is done in the presence of irregular bleeding to detect any co-existing pathology and to study the endometrial pattern.

Management

Therapeutic intervention depends on the woman's desire for future pregnancy and the tumor size.

❖ *Medical management*: Hormone therapy may be used as a short term intervention to decrease the size of fibroid and to minimize blood loss. Drugs used are antifibrinolytics, antiprogesterones, Danazol, GnRH analogous and prostaglandin synthetic inhibitors. Use of hormones for more than 6 months can increase the risk of osteoporosis.
❖ *Surgical management*:
  – Myomectomy to remove submucous fibroid for women who desire future childbearing
  – Hysterectomy for women who do not desire future pregnancies and with tumors which are large.

BENIGN OVARIAN TUMORS

Benign ovarian neoplasms commonly seen are Mucinous cyst adenoma, serous cyst adenoma, Brenner tumor and dermoid cyst.

❖ *Mucinous cyst adenoma:* It arises from the totipotent (cells that have ability to differentiate into any type of cells) surface epithelium of the ovary as a mucinous metaplasia of the epithelial cells. The tumors are bilateral in about 10 percent of cases. It may attain a huge size if left uncared for. It is the largest benign ovarian tumor. The content inside is thick, viscid mucin (a glycoprotein which is colorless unless complicated by hemorrhage). The chance of malignancy is about 10 percent.
❖ *Serous cyst adenoma:* Serous cyst arises from the totipotent surface epithelium of the ovary. This type of adenoma is quite common and accounts for 40 percent of ovarian tumors. It is bilateral in about 40 percent. The cyst appears smooth, shiny and grayish-white. The content fluid is clear and rich in serum proteins—albumin and globulin.
❖ *Brenner tumor:* Brenner tumor accounts for 1 to 2 percent of all ovarian tumors. About 8 to 10 percent is bilateral and is seen in women over the age of 40. Majority are solid, similar to that of fibroma and measure less than 2 cm in diameter. The cells look like

coffee bean as the nuclei have longitudinal groves. Estrogen is secreted by the tumor and the women may present with abnormal vaginal bleeding.

* *Dermoid cyst:* Dermoid cyst arises from the germ cells arrested after first meiotic division. Its incidence is about 15 to 20 percent amongst ovarian tumors. The tumor is bilateral in about 15 to 20 percent. The cyst usually is of moderate size with tense, smooth capsule. The content is predominantly sebatious material with hair.

Clinical Features of Benign Tumors and Cysts of Ovary

* Generally manifests in the late childbearing period. Dermoid cyst is more common in pregnancy
* Often seen related with nulliparity
* Tumors are asymptomatic and usually detected during routine abdominal or pelvic examination, laparoscopy or laparotomy
* When the tumor becomes symptomatic, they present with:
  - Heaviness in the lower abdomen
  - Gradual growth of size of abdomen
  - Dull, aching pain in abdomen.
* Gastrointestinal symptoms like nausea and indigestion in neglected cases when the tumor becomes big enough to fill the whole abdomen
* With large mucinous cyst adenoma, patient may be cachetic due to protein loss
* Pitting edema of legs when a huge tumors press on great veins.
* On abdominal examination, the tumor is nontender, which can be moved from side to side.
* On pelvic examination, the tumor mass is felt separated from the uterus and not movable when the cervix is moved. Lower pole of the cyst can be felt through the fornix.

Special Investigations

* Sonography: Transvaginal sonography with color Doppler to note the tumor volume and vascularity.

* Straight X-ray of the abdomen for evidence of teeth or bone tissue in dermoid cyst
* CT scan to identify presence of fat, calcification and teeth
* Laparoscopy if there is pain and suspicion of ectopic pregnancy
* Cytology when the patient presents with ascites or pleural effusion.

Complications of Benign Ovarian Tumors

* Torsion of the pedicle
* Intracystic hemorrhage
* Infection
* Rupture
* Pseudomyxoma peritonei (Peritoneal mass composed of mucus resembling myxoma)
* Malignancy.

Management

* Ovarian cystectomy, leaving behind the healthy ovarian tissue in young patients
* Salpingo-oophorectomy for a big tumor that has destroyed most of the ovarian tissues or for a gangrenous cyst
* Total hysterectomy with bilateral salpingo-oophorectomy for parous women above 40 years.

POLYPS

A polyp is a tumor attached by a pedicle. Two types of polyps are commonly seen; mucoid polyp and fibroid polyp.

Mucoid Polyp

This type of polyp arises from the body of uterus or from the cervix. The pedicle may at times be long enough to make the polyp protrude from the cervix or reach up to the vaginal introitus.

Clinical Features

* There may not be any symptom. Polyps are usually discovered during speculum examination, hysteroscopy or hystero-salpingography.
* Irregular uterine bleeding—either pre-or postmenopausal.

❖ Contact bleeding if the polyp is at or outside the cervix

❖ Excessive vaginal discharge which may be offensive

❖ On speculum examination, the polyp looks reddish in color, attached usually by a slender pedicle. The size may be about 1 to 2 cm.

Fibroid Polyp

The fibroid polyp may arise from the body of the uterus or from the cervix. It is an extrusion of a submucous fibroid from the uterine cavity. The polyp is usually single and of varying sizes. There may be infection, necrosis and hemorrhage at the tip.

Clinical Features

Patients are usually in reproductive period.

❖ Intermenstrual bleeding

❖ Colicky pain in lower abdomen

❖ Excessive vaginal discharge which may be offensive

❖ Sensation of something coming down when the polyp becomes big distending the vulva

❖ Uterus may feel bulky

❖ Pale or hemorrhagic polyp can be visualized on speculum examination.

Management

❖ Small polyps such as mucus polyps are removed by twisting, after catching it with an Allis forceps or tissue forceps

❖ Polyps with thick pedicles are removed by placing a transfixation suture in the pedicle and then cutting it distal to the ligature

❖ Big fibroid polyp lying in the vagina is removed by morcellation (piecemeal).

POLYCYSTIC OVARY SYNDROME (PCOS)

Polycystic ovary syndrome is a complex endocrine disorder associated with long-term anovulation and an excess of androgen circulation in the blood. The syndrome is characterized by in formation of cysts in the ovaries. PCOS is the feading cause of amenorrhea in young reproductive age group women (20 to 30%).

Clinical Features

❖ Increasing obesity, especially central obesity

❖ Menstrual abnormalities in the form of oligomenorrhea, amenorrhea or dysfunctional uterine bleeding

❖ Infertility

❖ Hirsutism and acne

❖ Ancanthosis nigricans (thickened, pigmented skin) over nape of neck, inner thighs and axilla.

Causes

The disorder is characterized by excessive androgen production by the ovaries which interfere with reproductive, endocrine and metabolic functions.

The syndrome begins with an imbalance of luteinizing hormone (LH) and follicle stimulating hormone (FSH). LH is seen elevated and FSH low to normal.

The result of hormonal imbalance is continued follicular development, elevated estrogen levels, anovulation and multiple cysts. Diagnosis is based on the presence of any two of the following three criteria:

❖ Oligo and/or anovulation

❖ Hyperandrogenism

❖ Polycystic ovaries.

Investigations

❖ Sonography: Transvaginal sonography will show enlarged ovaries with peripherally arranged cysts

❖ Serum values:
  – LH level is elevated, and LH: FSH ratio is elevated (>3:1)
  – Raised level of estradiol and estrone
  – Reduced level of sex hormone binding globulin (SHBG)
  – Raised serum testosterone (> 150 ng/dl)
  – Raised fasting insulin levels > 25 µIU/ml
  – Raised level of prolactin.

❖ Laparoscopy: Bilateral polycystic ovaries.

Possible Late Sequelae

❖ Risk of developing diabetes mellitus due to insulin resistance (15%)

❖ Risk of developing endometrial carcinoma due to persistently elevated level of estrogens
❖ Risk of hypertension and cardiovascular disease due to abnormal lipid profile (dyslipidemia)
❖ Postmenopausal breast cancer.

Management

Management of PCOS needs to be individualized. It depends on her presenting symptoms like menstrual disorder, infertility, obesity, hirsutism or combined symptoms.

Medical Management

❖ Correction of biochemical abnormalities with combination oral pills, GnRH agonists and medroxyprogesterone (provera)
❖ For patients wanting pregnancy
Ovulation induction by giving clomiphene citrate with or without dexamethasone or bromocripine
❖ For patients with hyperinsulinemia, metformin is given with clomiphene.

Surgical Management

Surgical treatment is indicated for those resistant to medical therapy. Endoscopic cauterization or CO_2 laser vaporization of multiple cysts is usually done.

Nursing Process

Nursing assessment for pelvic conditions involves assessing risk factors, presenting symptoms and medical and gynecological history. Data from physical assessment, laboratory tests and diagnostic procedures are considered. Nursing diagnoses are formulated based on assessment data and findings. Applicable nursing diagnoses may include:

❖ Pain related to pelvic condition
❖ Fear related to procedures and treatment
❖ Anxiety related to effects of condition or treatment
❖ Anxiety related to future childbearing
❖ Deficient knowledge regarding specific pelvic condition.

Nursing care plans include specific actions the client will complete to achieve the highest level of wellness. Goals for the client may be that she will:

❖ Develop strategies for coping with pain
❖ Reduce stress and promote wellness by following exercise regimens
❖ Consume recommended food to control obesity and maintain optimum body weight
❖ Return to physician for follow-up care
❖ Notify physician of response to therapy and improvement or lack of it
❖ Be informed about the choices of medical management and expected outcomes of therapy.

Nursing interventions include education about the condition, specific procedures, expected outcomes of therapy and providing emotional support.

65 Gynecological Examinations and Diagnostic Procedures

Upon completion of the chapter, the learner will be able to:

❖ Gather patient information and relevant history from gynecological patients for identifying health problems

❖ Describe the gynecological examinations that are performed for clients with various problems

❖ Discuss the tests and procedures in gynecology for diagnostic and therapeutic purposes.

Examination of a gynecological patient includes history taking as well as general, abdominal and internal examinations. A detailed and composite history using different formats can be obtained.

HISTORY

❖ **Demographic Data**
  Name ....
  Age ....
  Marital Status ....
  Education..
  Occupation..
  Income ....
  Religion ....
  Address ....

❖ **Menstrual History**
  Age of menarche..
  Regularity of cycle......................................
  Duration of period ....
  Length of cycle ....
  Amount of bleeding ....
  Menstrual discomfort...................................
  Amenorrhea..
  Last menstrual period ....

❖ **Past medical history:** Information regarding relevant medical disorders such as systemic illness, metabolic or endocrine disorder and infection.

❖ **Past surgical history:** General, obstetrical or gynecological surgeries, postoperative recovery and any special information related to investigations are included.

❖ **Personal history:** Data related to occupation, marital status, sexual life, contraceptive practices, any infertility problems and if not married status of genitourinary functions are included. History of medications taken in the past and currently and any allergies are also entered.

❖ **Obstetrical History**

S/no.	Date of delivery	Duration of pregnancy	Abnormalities in pregnancy	Delivery (vaginal/ cesarean)	Puerperium, baby (alive/stillborn)

* **Family history:** Information on diseases in family that can have some value such as malignancies of genital organs, colon, tubercular infections, etc. is taken.

Examination

Examination of a gynecologic patient includes general and systemic examination, and gynecological examination.

* *General and systemic examination:* Aspects included in this examination are:
  - General body built (obese/thin)
  - Development of social characteristics
  - Appearance—inspection (head to foot)
  - Systems examination—gastrointestinal, cardiovascular, respiratory
  - Vital signs.
* *Gynecological examination:* Breast examination is done especially for women above 30 years with special attention to the presence of any lump or pathology.
* *Abdominal examination:* Using different methods such as *inspection, palpation, percussion and auscultation,* abdominal and pelvic organs and their functions are assessed. Some of the important observations include presence of old scar, striae, prominent veins, hernia and abnormal distention of abdomen. **Palpation** can reveal muscle tension, rigidity or guarding. Any tumor or growth if felt may be further tested for consistency, mobility and location. **Percussion** may be useful to study the details of any tumor or fluid collection palpated. **Auscultation** method is used to identify intestinal sounds, uterine soufflé over a vascular fibroid or pregnant uterus and FHR over a pregnant uterus.
* *Pelvic examination:* Internal examination for gynecological patients includes:
  - Inspection of the external genitalia
  - Vaginal examination
  - Rectal examination
  - Retrovaginal examination.
* *Inspection of vulva:* This is done to note any anatomical abnormality, visible pathological changes, discharges, genital prolapse, stress incontinence and hemorrhoids.

Vaginal examination is done for inspection of vagina and cervix. A speculum examination followed by a bimanual examination is done by the physician to evaluate the structures. Cervical scrape cytology and endocervical sampling for cytological testing are done in all or selected gynecological patients. Digital examination of the vagina using a gloved index finger lubricated with sterile lubricant is done to palpate any swelling in the labia or adjacent structures. In virgins with intact hymen, this examination is done only under anesthesia.

The vaginal cervix is examined for following features:

Direction	–	Anteverted or retroverted
Station	–	External os at the level of ischial spines or not
Texture	–	firm like tip of nose or soft
Shape	–	conical or cylindrical
External os	–	Round or dilated
Movement	–	Painful or not

Tendency to Bleed on Touch—Present or not

Integrity and tone of the perineal body are checked by flexing the internal finger posteriorly and palpating it with the thumb placed externally. A bimanual examination will be done to palpate the uterus, uterine appendages and pouch of Douglas.

* *Rectal examination:* Rectal examination is done in isolation or as an adjunct to vaginal examination. It is indicated in:
  - Children or adult virgins
  - Painful vaginal examination
  - Carcinoma cervix
  - Vaginal atresia
  - Rectocele or Enterocele.

Rectovaginal or bimanual examinations may also be performed when indicated, e.g. adnexal mass.

* *Blood investigations:* Commonly included blood tests are:
  - Hemoglobin estimation
  - White blood cells counts
  - Erythrocyte sedimentation rate
  - VDRL

- Platelet count
- Bleeding and coagulation time.
- ❖ *Urine examination*
  - Routine examination
  - Culture and drug sensitivity.
- ❖ *Vaginal or cervical discharge and scraping*
  - Microscopic examination
  - Culture examination.
- ❖ *Cervical smear for cytological and hormonal study.*
  - Cervical mucous for bacteriological study, hormonal status and infertility investigation.

Diagnostic Procedures

Colposcopy

Colposcopy is examination of the cervix and vagina using an instrument called colposcope and colpomicroscope.

Patient Selection
- ❖ Women with abnormal smear report
- ❖ Women with history of contact bleeding despite negative smear.

Procedure
- ❖ Patient is placed in lithotomy position after ensuring that her urinary bladder is empty
- ❖ Cusco's speculum is placed to visualize the cervix
- ❖ Colposcope is inserted and cervix and vagina examined using low power magnification
- ❖ During examination, cervix is wiped with normal saline and 3 percent acetic acid for better assessment. Findings include – normalcy of epithelium, and changes due to condyloma or papilloma.

X-ray Examination

Plain X-ray of pelvis is used to locate an IUCD or shadows of teeth or bone in a cystic teratoma. Special X-rays used for gynecologic patients are:
- ❖ Hysterosalpingography to note tubal potency.
- ❖ Lymphangiography to locate the lymph glands involved in pelvic malignancy.

Ultrasound Examinations

Ultrasonographic examinations are common diagnostic modalities in gynecology.

- ❖ Transabdominal sonography (TAS) is used in conditions where patient has large masses like fibroid or ovarian tumor.
- ❖ Transvaginal sonography (TVS): This is done with a probe which is placed close to the target organ. Detailed evaluation of pelvic organs (within 10 cm of the field) is possible with TVS. This method is not suitable for use in women with narrow vagina as in virgins, postmenopausal women or postradiation vaginal stenosis.
- ❖ Transvaginal color Doppler sonography: This examination provides additional information of blood flow to, from or within an organ (uterus or adnexal). This flow can be measured by analysis of the waveform using the pulsatility index
- ❖ Use of ultrasound examinations:
  - Infertility work up: Monitoring of follicular maturation and ovulation for induction of ovulation, artificial insemination and ovum retrieval in IVF and GIFT programs.
  - Detection of ectopic pregnancy as a 'tubal ring' separate from ovary in a patient with empty uterine cavity.
  - Detection of pelvic mass such as uterine fibroid, ovarian mass, endometriomas, tubo-ovarian mass etc. with regard to its location and consistency (TV – CDS) can assess the vascularity of the mass that raises suspicion of malignant tumor.
  - Detection of submucous fibroids and polyps using sonohysterographic studies which involve instillation of saline in the uterine cavity and aspiration of material from cysts and masses.

Computed Tomography (CT Scan)

CT scan provides high resolution, two dimensional images. CT scan differentiates tissue densities and these gray-scale pictures can be read on X-ray film or a television monitor. Pelvic organs can be differentiated from gastrointestinal and urinary systems using contrast media given orally, IV or rectally.

CT scan is most useful in the diagnosis of lymph node metastasis, depth of myometrial invasion in endometrial cancer, ovarian mass and myomas. CT scan also facilitates the percutaneous needle biopsy of suspicious lymph nodes. CT scan is also useful in assessing tumor extent and detecting metastases. It is useful in staging of ovarian cancer and deposits of cancer cells in other organs such as the liver.

Magnetic Resonance Imaging (MRI)

MRI creates cross-sectional images of body using a combination of radio waves (non-ionizing radiation) and magnetic fields.

In gynecology, MRI is found superior to CT scan in the delineation of pelvic organs in multiple planes.

Uses of MRI

- It is used to measure the depth of myometrial penetration of endometrial cancer preoperatively
- It can detect accurately the parametrial invasion of cervical cancer and distinguish post-treatment fibrosis and recurrence
- Tumor volume can be measured with 3D imaging system. MRI is thus useful in determining the invasion of bladder, rectum, parametrium and uterine body
- Leiomyomas are better diagnosed with MRI
- MRI is useful in the diagnosis of endometriosis as it can measure the depth of penetration which is responsible for pelvic pain
- MRI is useful and even superior in the evaluation of metastatic lymph nodes or recurrent pelvic tumor

Positron Emission Tomography (PET)

PET is based on the tissue uptake of 18-fluro-2 deoxyglucose. FDG-PET can measure the difference between the normal tissue and cancerous tissue. The glucose analog is given IV The scan is then done and images are interpreted

The scan is more sensitive for detection of metastatic diseases and recurrence of ovarian malignancy. It is also useful to assess the response following tumor therapy.

Surgical Methods

- *Endometrial sampling:* Endometrial sampling is one of the diagnostic tests done in the clinical work up of women with infertility or abnormal uterine bleeding or for periodic screening during hormone replacement therapy. A uterine sampler which has a thin plastic cannula and plunger is used to obtain a sample of endometrium. Endometrial sample obtained by suction from the fundus and upper part of the body is used for the test.
- *Endometrial biopsy:* This is the method of obtaining endometrium by curettage after dilatation of the cervix. It is usually performed under general anesthesia.
- *Cervical biopsy:* Cervical biopsy is done to confirm the clinical diagnosis of cervical pathology. Biopsy can be taken in the outpatient unit, if the pathology is detectable, but for wider tissue excision as in cone biopsy, it is done as an inpatient procedure.
- *Culdocentesis:* Culdocentesis is the transvaginal aspiration of peritoneal fluid from the cu-de-sac or pouch of Douglas. The procedure is done in suspected ectopic pregnancy or other conditions producing hemoperitoneum and pelvic abscess.
- *Laparoscopy:* Laparoscopy is a technique of visualization of peritoneal cavity by means of a fiber optic endoscope introduced through the abdominal wall. Prior to introducing the endoscope pneumoperitoneum is achieved by introduction of carbon dioxide or air. Either local or general anesthesia may be used for performing the procedure.
- *Hysteroscopy:* Hysteroscopy is an operative procedure for visualizing the endometrial cavity with the aid of fiber optic telescope. Uterine distension is achieved by carbon dioxide, normal saline or glycine. The instrument is passed transcervically after paracervical block or general anaesthesia. Hysteroscopy is done for the following indications:
  - Unresponsive irregular uterine bleeding
  - Recurrent abortion

- Missing threads of IUCD
- Intrauterine adhesions (uterine syne–chiae)
- To visualize transformation zone with colpomicrohysteroscopy when colposcopic finding is unsatisfactory.

❖ *Salpingoscopy:* In Salpingoscopy, a firm telescope is inserted through the abdominal osteum of the fallopian tube so that the tubal mucosa can be visualized by distending the lumen with saline infusion. The telescope is introduced through laparoscope. This is used to study the anatomy and physiology of the tubal epithelium for selecting patients for IVF.

❖ *Cystoscopy:* The use of cystoscopy in gynecology is to evaluate cervical cancer prior to staging and to investigate the urinary symptoms including hematuria, incontinence and fistulae.

❖ *Culdoscopy:* Culdoscopy is the procedure of visualizing the pelvic structures through an incision in the pouch of Douglas. Use of culdoscope is limited as compared to laparoscope.

❖ *Proctoscopy:* Proctoscopy is done following a digital examination of the rectum in cases of rectal involvement of genital malignancy.

❖ *Examination under anesthesia (EUA):* EUA is indicated where bimanual examination cannot be conducted properly either because of extreme tenderness or inadequate relaxation of abdominopelvic muscles or noncooperative patient. It is also done in cases of uterine malignancy for clinical staging and also to examine virgins and children with gynecological problems.

❖ *Laser (Light amplification by stimulated emission of radiation):* Laser is used in gynecology for the purpose of tissue cutting, coagulation or vaporization. It is used widely in genital tract surgeries and with endoscopic surgeries.

66 Congenital Malformations of Female Genital Organs

Learning Objectives

Upon completion of the chapter, the learner will be able to:
- List the common congenital malformations of female genital organs
- Describe the manifestations of malformations of different organs
- Describe the management of different congenital problems
- Describe the nursing managements of clients and families facing problems related to congenital malformations of genital organs.

Congenital malformations are anomalies which may be either hereditary or occurring during gestation and evident at the time of birth. Development of the female genital tract is a complex process dependent upon a series of events involving cellular differentiation, migration, fusion and canalization. Failure of any one of these processes results in a congenital anomaly.

The development of female genital tract begins at three weeks of gestation and continues into the second trimester of pregnancy.

While major abnormalities escape attention, the moderate and severe ones produce gynecologic and obstetric problems. Female genital abnormalities often do not present until or well after puberty. Although genital abnormalities may be isolated, careful assessment for possible underlying disorders particularly chromosomal or metabolic is essential.

UTERINE ABNORMALITIES

The most common types of uterine abnormalities are caused by incomplete fusion of the *Müllerian ducts*.

Complete failure is less and results in double vagina, double cervix and double uterus. Variants may occur depending on the degree of malformation of the Müllerian ducts. More extensive fusion of the Müllerian ducts results in a single vagina, single cervix and double or single-horned uteruses which are partially fused.

Prevalence

The prevalence of uterine malformation is estimated to be 6.7 percent in the general population, slightly higher (7.3%) in the infertility population and significantly higher in a population of women with a history of recurrent miscarriages (16%).

Types

There are six different uterine malformations:
1. *Arcuate uterus*: The arcuate uterus has a depression at the fundus. A woman with an arcuate uterus carries a baby to full-term pregnancy. However, this condition is associated with a higher risk for miscarriage and premature births.
2. *Bicornuate uterus (uterus with two horns) (Fig. 66.1B)*: Bicornuate uterus is heart shaped with a marked indentation and is separated into two cavities. The part of the Müllerian duct that forms the upper part of the uterus fails to fuse. Thus, the caudal part of the uterus is normal, the cranial part is bifurcated.

   The primary risk with having a bicornuate uterus is preterm labor and cervical incompetency during the second

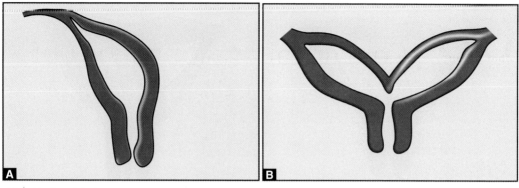

Figs 66.1A and B: Uterus with horns: (A) Unicornuate uterus; (B) Bicornuate uterus *(For color version see Plate 8)*

trimester of pregnancy. In some cases, a woman with this type of uterus can carry the baby to full term with no complications.

3. *Didelphic uterus (double uterus):* The double uterus has a duplication of the uterus and a duplication of the cervix. In this malformation, there are two uterine cavities and two cervixes accompanying each cavity. Women with this type of uterus often suffer dysmenorrhea and dyspareunia. Premature births and malpresentations are common.

Twin pregnancies are commonly associated with didelphic uterus. There is a good chance that the births can occur at separate times (days or weeks apart).

4. *Unicornuate uterus (one-sided uterus) (Fig. 66.1A):* Only one side of the Müllerian duct forms. There is a single uterine cavity with a cervix and one fallopian tube coming out of the uterus. Only one side of the uterus forms and the other side may have a rudimentary horn. The uterus has a typical "penis shape" on imaging systems.

5. *Septate uterus (uterine partition) (Figs 66.2A and B):* A septum separates the uterine cavity into two separate cavities. The septum will arise at the top of the uterine cavity and then extend down to the cervix and vagina. This develops when the two Müllerian ducts have fused, but the partition between them persisted splitting the system into two parts.

When the defect is partial, the septum affects only the cranial (top) part of the uterus. Uterine septum is the most common form of malformation and a cause for abortion. There is a chance of preterm labor if pregnancy progresses.

6. *Absent uterus (uterine agenesis):* This is the most severe form of uterine malformation. There is failure of uterus, cervix and vagina to develop. A girl with this malformation will experience puberty with the absence of menstruation. The woman will have only a small dimple in the place where the vagina should be at. The external view of the genitals will be normal; with closer examination, a shallow vagina will be noticed. There is, greater chance for abnormalities of kidneys and/or bones to be present with this malformation. The woman with this malformation can have sexual intercourse after having a surgical procedure to extend the length of vagina.

Diagnosis

❖ Ultrasound examination
❖ Hysterosalpingography which allows evaluation of the uterine cavity and tubal patency
❖ MRI scan is considered the best imaging technique for uterine abnormalities
❖ Hysteroscopy.

Complications

❖ Dysmenorrhea
❖ Hematometra
❖ Complications during pregnancy and labor: late miscarriage, premature labor, uterine rupture, malpresentations, obstructed labor, retained, placenta, postpartum hemorrhage.

Figs 66.2A and B: Septate uterus: (A) Partial septum; (B) Complete septum *(For color version see Plate 8)*

❖ Fertility is unaffected except for uterine agenesis.

Management

❖ Surgical intervention depending on the type of abnormality on enabling a viable pregnancy
❖ A septate vagina and rudimentary horn of a bicornuate uterus are usually removed
❖ A uterine reconstruction may be done for a bicornuate or septate uterus (Metroplasty) which is considered to be the cause of recurrent miscarriages.

VAGINAL MALFORMATIONS

The significant abnormalities of the vagina are:
1. Vaginal agenesis
2. Vaginal atresia
3. Vaginal septum
4. Hymen abnormalities
5. Narrow introitus
6. Associated abnormalities.

Vaginal Agenesis/Hypoplasia

Vaginal agenesis occurs in approximately 1 in 5000 to 7000 female births. It results from a problem during the early development of the reproductive system of a fetus. The condition is also known as Rokinansky syndrome. It is often associated with hypoplasia which is less development than usual. There is absence of vagina, fallopian tubes, cervix and uterus.

Some women have incompletely developed uterine remnants or horns. The ovaries and external genitalia are normal and the chromosome make up is normal. The syndrome (complete agenesis) is known as Rokinansky-Mayer-Kuster-Hauser syndrome (RMKH).

Diagnosis

Diagnosis of vaginal agenesis or hypoplasia is commonly made between the ages of 15 to 18 years when women present themselves with concerns that they have not started menstruating.

As they have normal functioning ovaries they would have gone through puberty and have normal breasts and pubic hair. Careful physical examination, hormonal and genetic tests, imaging studies such as ultrasound, MRI and IVP are done to confirm the diagnosis.

Treatment

❖ Reconstructive operation (vaginoplasty) is done if the patient wishes to marry.
❖ Pressure dilatation: Expanding and enlarging the tissue already present at the vaginal entrance by applying pressure over an extended period of time.

Vaginal Atresia

The lower portion of the vagina consists of fibrous tissue. Some methods of correction as for vaginal hypoplasia can be done.

Vaginal Septum

Transverse vaginal septa can be present as single or multiple in the upper or lower segments and may be complete or patent. Septum located in the lower vagina is often complete and can be the cause of hematometra or other fluid collections. Septum located in the upper vagina is often perforated. Longitudinal septum of vagina may be present when the distal parts of the Müllerian ducts fail to fuse. It may be associated with double uterus and double cervix. This may cause dyspareunia or may obstruct delivery. Management depends on the type of septum. Incision or excision of the septum is done for relief of symptoms.

Hymen Abnormalities

Imperforate hymen is the common abnormality. It is due to failure of disintegration of the central cells of the Müllerian eminence that projects into the urogenital sinus. This may first present with obstruction of menstrual flow after puberty. The menstrual blood collects behind the hymen (cryptomenorrhea). The accumulated blood first distends the vagina (hematocolpos). The uterine cavity gets filled after that (Hematometra). In late and neglected cases, the tubes may also get distended after the fimbrial ends become closed by adhesions (hematosalpinx).

Clinical Features

Girls aged about 14 to 16 present with:
* Periodic lower abdominal pain
* Primary amenorrhea
* Urinary frequency, dysuria or retention
* Suprapubic swelling
* On vaginal examination, the bulging bluish membranes which may be the transverse vaginal septum close to the inner aspect of hymen.

Ultrasonography can be used to make the diagnosis of the condition. Treatment is draining the collected blood through a cruciate incision in the hymen. Antibiotic therapy and treatment of any residual pathology are generally required.

Narrow Introitus

The existence of this is revealed after marriage when the woman complains of dyspareunia or during investigation for infertility. Treatment is manual stretching under general anesthesia or surgical enlargement (Perineoplasty).

Associated Abnormalities

Abnormalities associated with congenital malformations of vagina are vesicovaginal fistula, rectovaginal fistula and persistent urogenital sinus.

Vesicovaginal fistula is formed when the Müllerian eminence ruptures into the vesicoureteral part of the cloaca instead of the pelvic part of the urogenital sinus.

Rectovaginal fistula forms when the Müllerian eminence opens in the dorsal segment of the endodermal cloaca. Persistent urogenital sinus presents with various irregularities of urethral and vaginal orifices.

ABNORMALITIES OF EXTERNAL GENITALIA

Labia Minora Abnormalities

This can have *Labial fusion* or *hypertrophy* in otherwise normal females. Hypertrophy can be unilateral or bilateral and may occasionally require surgical correction.

Labia Majora Abnormalities

This can be hypoplastic or hypertrophic. Abnormal fusion is usually associated with *ambiguous genitalia* of female and *pseudo-hermaphroiditism* due to congenital adrenal hyperplasia.

Clitoral Abnormalities

These are generally rare and are double clitoris or bifid clitoris. Hypertrophy can be associated with a number of *intersex disorders*.

ANOMALIES OF THE OVARIES

Ovarian Agenesis/Dysgenesis

* This includes *Turner's syndrome* and a wide range of chromosomal anomalies
* This results in the production of *streak ovaries* and is associated with a number of other somatic abnormalities

- Neonates with streak ovaries often have oedema of the hands and feet. Many present in adolescence with short stature
- Girls with Turner's syndrome have genital infantilism, webbing of the neck cubitus valgus and retarded growth
- Girls with streak (indistinct) ovaries have shield chest, obesity, high palate, micrognathia, epicanthal folds, low set ears, hypoplasia of nails, osteoporosis, pigmented moles, hypertension, lymph edema, coarctation of aorta, deafness and mental retardation
- There are also patients of normal height without those abnormalities but with gonadal streaks in which there are two cell types—one with two normal sex chromosomes and another with only a single X chromosome
- Follicle stimulating hormone (FSH) and leuteinizing hormone (LH) are raised, estrogens are low and nongonadal endocrine functions are normal
- Treatment is with estrogen for development of secondary sex characteristics, growth hormone to increase height and surgical removal of gonadal streaks to prevent malignant degeneration.

True Hermaphroditism

This is characterized by the presence of both ovarian and testicular tissue in a single patient. The testes will develop in the presence of a single Y chromosome even with more than a single X chromosome. No single clinical feature can distinguish the condition from other forms of intersexuality. Diagnosis is possible after hormone assay and ultrasonography.

Often patients are reared as males because of appearance of external genitalia. However, with early diagnosis and treatment with hormones most can be reared as females.

Many menstruate and some who had testicular tissue removed have become pregnant. Treatment is to remove contradictory organs and reconstruct external genitalia corresponding to the sex of rearing.

Female Hermaphroditism due to Congenital Adrenal Hyperplasia

Usually this is due to a genetic defect in the synthesis of the enzyme required for the synthesis of cortisol. Adrenal glands secrete abnormally large amounts of virilizing steroids, even in the fetus. The baby is born with scrotolabial folds fused and a greatly enlarged clitoris that can easily be mistaken for a penis. No testes are palpable. Normally only a single urinary meatus at the base of the phallus is seen with the vagina entering a urogenital sinus.

Babies exhibit rapid growth in infancy but this stops early creating short structure. Pubic hair can appear as early as two years but generally later than this followed by the appearance of pubic and facial hair and acne. Puberty does not occur and there is no breast development. Diagnosis is by pelvic ultrasound in the newborn in the presence of ambiguous external genitalia, assay of urinary *17–ketosteroid* and serum *17–hydroxyprogesterone*. Treatment is with hydrocortisone and surgical correction of external genitalia.

Accessory Ovary and Supernumerary Ovaries

Accessory ovary occurs due to division of the original ovary into two. This is seen very rarely. Supernumerary ovaries may be found in the broad ligament or elsewhere. This can explain a rare event where menstruation continues even after removal of two ovaries.

67

Genital Fistulae

GENITOURINARY FISTULA

Definition

Genitourinary fistula is an abnormal communication between the urinary and genital tract either acquired or congenital with involuntary escape of urine into the vagina.

Types (Fig. 67.1)

The communication may occur between the bladder, urethra or ureter and genital tract.

Bladder

❖ Vesicovaginal (commonest)
❖ Vesicourethrovaginal
❖ Vesicouterine
❖ Vesicocervical.

Ureter

❖ Ureterovaginal
❖ Ureterouterine
❖ Ureterocervical.

Vesicovaginal Fistula

There is communication between the bladder and the vagina and urine escapes into the vagina causing true incontinence. This is the commonest type of genitourinary fistula.

Causes

1. *Obstetrical*: The commonest cause is obstetrical and constitutes 80 to 90 percent of cases in developing countries as against 5 to 15 percent in developed countries. The fistula may occur due to ischemia or following trauma
   a. *Ischemic*: The fistula results from prolonged compression effect on the bladder base between the fetal head and symphysis pubis in obstructed labor. The compression causes ischemic necrosis, infection, sloughing and fistula in 3 to 5 days following delivery.
   b. *Traumatic*: This may be caused by:
      ❖ Instrumental vaginal delivery such as destructive operations or forceps, especially with Kielland's forceps
      ❖ Abdominal operations such as hysterectomy for rupture uterus or cesarean hysterectomy. Traumatic fistula usually follows soon after delivery.
2. *Gynecological*: Fistulae due to gynecological causes are rare in the developing countries and is the commonest in the developing countries.

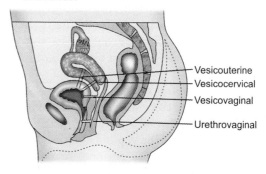

Fig. 67.1: Types of genitourinary fistula

- Vesicouterine
- Vesicocervical
- Vesicovaginal
- Urethrovaginal

* *Operative injury*: During operations like anterior colporrhaphy, abdominal hysterectomy or removal of Gartner's cyst
* *Traumatic*: Injury to anterior vaginal wall and the bladder wall following fall on a pointed object, use of a stick for criminal abortion, following fracture to pelvic bone or due to retained pessary
* *Malignancy*: Advanced carcinoma of the cervix, vagina and bladder may produce fistula by direct spread
* *Radiation*: Ischemic necrosis may occur when carcinoma cervix is treated by radiation in 1 to 2 years
* *Infective*: Chronic granulomatous lesions such as vaginal tuberculosis, lymphogranuloma venerium and actinomycosis may produce fistula.

Sites of VVF

* *Juxtacervical (close to the cervix)*: The communication is between the supratrigonal region of the bladder and the vagina.
* *Midvaginal*: The communication is between the base (trigone) of the bladder and vagina.
* *Juxtaurethral*: The communication is between the neck of the bladder and vagina (may involve the upper urethra as well).

Clinical Features

* Patient profile
  The patients are usually young primiparous with history of difficult labor or instrumental delivery in recent past. In others it is related with relevant events.
* Continuous escape of urine per vagina is the classic symptom. The patient has no urge to pass urine. If the fistula is small, the escape of urine occurs in certain positions and the patient can also pass urine normally.
* Pruritus vulva
* Escape of watery discharge per vagina of ammoniacal smell
* Excoriation of the vaginal skin
* Varying degrees of perineal tear may be present

Fig. 67.2: Three swab test using methylene blue

* On speculum examination; the bladder mucosa may be seen prolapsed through a big fistula. Puckered area of vaginal mucosa is evidenced in tiny fistula.

Diagnosis of Fistula (Fig. 67.2)

* Examination under anesthesia (EUA)
* Examination in Sim's or knee-chest position: Bubbles of air are seen through the tiny fistula when the woman coughs
* Dye test: A speculum is introduced and the anterior vaginal wall is swabbed dry When the Methylene blue solution is introduced into the bladder by a catheter, the dye will be seen coming out through the opening
* Catheter test: A metal catheter passed through the external urethral meatus, when passes out through the fistula, VVF is confirmed
* Three swab test (Table 67.1)
  Three cotton swabs are placed in the vagina: one at the vault, one at the middle and one just above the introitus. Methylene blue is instilled into the bladder through a rubber catheter and the patient is asked to walk about for 5 minutes. She is then asked to lie down and the swabs are removed for inspection.

Investigations

* Intravenous urography: For the diagnosis of ureterovaginal fistula
* Retrograde pyelography: For the diagnosis of exact site of ureterovaginal fistula
* Cystography: In complex fistula or vesicouterine fistula where lateral view of uterine cavity may be seen (done rarely)

Table 67.1	Three swab test	

Observation	Inference
Upper most swab socked with urine, but unstained with dye. The lower two swabs remain dry	Ureterovaginal fistula
Upper and lower swabs remain dry, but the middle swab stained with dye	Vesicovaginal fistula
The upper two swabs remain dry but the lower swab stained with dye	Urethrovaginal fistula

❖ Endoscopy studies to identify the exact location of the fistula and its relationship to ureteric orifices and bladder neck (done rarely).

Treatment of VVF

❖ Preventive
Obstetric fistula is prevented with safe motherhood initiative. Gynecologic fistula can be prevented with better anticipation and improved surgical skill.
The measures to be taken are:
– Adequate antenatal screening to identify "at risk" mothers likely to develop obstructed labor
– Anticipation, early detection and ideal approach in the method of delivery in relieving the obstruction
– Continuous bladder drainage for 5 to 7 days following delivery either vaginally or abdominally in a case of long-standing obstructed labor
– Care to avoid injury to the bladder during pelvic surgery-obstetrical or gynecological.
❖ Immediate management
Once the diagnosis is made, catheterization and continuous bladder drainage for 6 to 8 weeks is maintained. This may cause spontaneous closure of the fistula tract that is small, with minimal tissue damage.
❖ Operative management
Local repair of the fistula is the surgery of choice.
– Preoperative assessment includes identifying the site, size, number and status of the margins of the fistula, and urethral involvement

– Improvement of general condition is essential as most patients may be of poor socioeconomic status
– Local infection in the vulval region if present should be treated with local application of bland ointments or glycerine
– Urinary infection if any should be treated
– Psychological preparation of the patient and family with adequate explanation of the expected management and recovery.
The ideal time for surgery is after 3 months following delivery in case of old VVF. Surgical fistula recognized within 24 hours may be repaired immediately provided it is small.
Repair is done by flap splitting method or by using tissue graft depending on the site and size of the fistula.

Postoperative Care

Special care following VVF repair include:
❖ Urinary antiseptic either at random or appropriate to the sensitivity report
❖ Continuous bladder drainage for about 10 to 14 days
❖ Advice to pass urine 2 hourly following removal of catheter. The interval to be increased gradually.

Instructions during Discharge from Hospital are:
❖ To pass urine more frequently
❖ To avoid intercourse for at least 3 months
❖ To differ pregnancy for at least one year
❖ If conception occurs to report to the physician and must have mandatory antenatal check-up and hospital delivery.

URETHROVAGINAL FISTULA

Causes

The causes are the same as those of VVF. Part or whole of the urethra is involved along with the bladder.

Small isolated urethrovaginal fistula is caused by:
❖ Injury inflicted during anterior colporrhaphy, urethroplasty or sling operation for stress incontinence
❖ Residual fistula left behind following repair of vesicourethrovaginal fistula.

Diagnosis

❖ The patient has urge to pas urine but urine dribbles out into the vagina during the act of micturition.
❖ A sound or a metal catheter passed through the external urethral meatus comes out through the communicating urethrovaginal opening.
❖ 'Three swab test' may be employed to confirm the diagnosis.

Treatment

❖ Surgical repair in two layers followed by continuous bladder drainage as outlined for VVF is done
❖ Prior suprapubic or vaginal cystostomy ensures better success
❖ In cases of complete destruction of the urethra, reconstruction of urethra is performed
❖ Stress incontinence may occur in 10 to 15 percent of cases following repair.

URETEROVAGINAL FISTULA

Causes

❖ *Congenital*: The aberrant ureter may open into the vault of vagina, uterus or into urethra
❖ *Acquired*: This is the commonest type and usually follows trauma during pelvic surgery. It is commonly associated with difficult surgery like abdominal hysterotomy in cervical fibroid, broad ligament fibroid, endometriosis, ovarian malignancy or radical hysterectomy.

Diagnosis

❖ Signs and symptoms are subtle and often overlooked Patient may develop fever, flank pain, hematuria, and abdominal distension, urine leakage through vagina, peritonitis and retroperitoneal urinoma.

Investigations

a. Three swab test.
b. Intravenous indigo carmine test: Indigo carmine is injected intravenously. If urine in the vagina becomes blue in 4 to 5 minutes, the diagnosis of ureterovaginal fistula is established.
c. Cystoscopy—to determine the side of ureterovaginal fistula.
d. Excretory urogralphy (IVU) confirms the side, site and tract of ureterovaginal fistula.
e. Renal ultrasound.
f. Computed tomography (CT).

Management

When injury is recognized during operation:
❖ Ureteral sheath denudation: No intervention and rarely ureteral stenting, if a long segment is involved
❖ Ureteral kinking (due to closely placed sutures): Immediate removal of suture
❖ Ureteral ligation: Immediate delegation—assessment of viability by blood flow and ureteral peristalsis. Stenting may be needed if any doubt
❖ Extraperitoneal drainage
❖ Ureteric implantation into the bladder if the length of ureter is sufficient
❖ Bladder flap procedure when the ureter is short or injury is at the level of pelvic brim.

Complications Following Repair of Ureteric Injury

❖ Stricture
❖ Infection
❖ Ureteric obstruction
❖ Reflux of urine
❖ Stent or flap complications.

RECTOVAGINAL FISTULA (RVF)

Causes

Abnormal communication between the rectum and vagina with involuntary escape of flatus and/or feces into the vagina is called rectovaginal fistula.

Acquired RVF

Obstetrical

a. Incomplete healing or unrepaired recent complete perineal tear (CPT).
b. Obstructed labour causing pressure necrosis → infection → sloughing → fistula.
c. Instrumental injury inflicted during destructive operation.

Gynecological

a. Following incomplete healing of repair of old CPT (commonest).
b. Trauma inflicted inadvertently and remains unrecognized in pelvic operations like perineorrhaphy, repair of enterocele, vaginal tubectomy, posterior colpotomy, reconstruction of vagina, etc.
c. Fall on sharp pointed object.
d. Malignancy of the vagina, cervix or bowel.
e. Radiation.
f. Lymphogranuloma venerium or tuberculosis of vagina.
g. Diverticulitis of the sigmoid colon, when the abscess bursts into the vagina.
h. Crohn's disease involving the anal canal or lower rectum.

Congenital

The anal canal may open into the vestibule or into the vagina.

Diagnosis

❖ Involuntary escape of flatus and/or feces into the vagina
❖ Rectovaginal examination reveals the size and site of fistula
❖ Dye test: Methylene blue introduced into the rectum is seen escaping through the fistula into the vagina
❖ Probe test: Passing a probe through the vagina into the rectum
❖ Examination under anesthesia.

Investigations

❖ Barium enema.
❖ Barium meal and follow through to confirm the site of intestinal fistula
❖ Sigmoidoscopy and proctoscopy in case of inflammatory bowel disease for taking biopsy of fistula edge.

Treatment

Preventive

❖ Good antenatal care
❖ Identification of complete perineal tear and effective repair
❖ Care to prevent injury during gynecologic surgeries.

Definitive

❖ Extension to CPT and repair if the defect is situated low down
❖ Repair by flap method for injury situated in the middle third
❖ For defect situated high up, preliminary colostomy → local repair after 3 weeks and → closure of colostomy after 3 weeks.

68

Perioperative Care of Gynecological Patient

Learning Objectives

Upon completion of this chapter, the learner will be able to:

❖ Describe the phases of perioperative period
❖ Discuss various types of surgery according to degree of urgency, risk and purpose
❖ Identify essential aspects of perioperative assessment of gynecological patient
❖ Identify nursing responsibilities in planning perioperative nursing care
❖ Describe essential preoperative preparation including teaching
❖ Identify essential nursing assessments and interventions for the postoperative patient.

Surgery is a unique experience of planned physical alteration encompassing three phases: *Preoperative, intraoperative* and *postoperative are* three phases and together referred to as the *perioperative* period.

The preoperative phase begins when the decision to have surgery is made and ends when the patient is transferred to the operating table. Nursing activities associated with this phase include assessing the patient, identifying potential or actual health problems, planning specific care based on the individual's needs and providing preoperative teaching for the patient and family.

The intraoperative phase begins when the patient is transferred to the operating table and ends when the patient is transferred to the recovery or postanesthetic room. Nursing activities related to this phase include a variety of special procedures to maintain the health status of the patient.

The postoperative phase begins with the admission of the patient in the postoperative unit or ward and ends when the healing is complete. Nursing activities during this period include assessing the patient's response (physiologic and psychologic) to surgery, performing interventions to facilitate healing and preventing complications, teaching and providing support and planning for home care.

Some gynecological operations are per-formed in an outpatient setting. In such situations, the three phases of perioperative period are shortened and the postoperative period continues at home. With such patients, the nurses' role in assessing, teaching and following up is vital to successful outcome for the patient.

TYPES OF SURGERY

Surgical procedures are commonly grouped according to purpose, degree of urgency and degree of risk.

1. Purposes of surgical procedure
   ❖ *Diagnostic*: Confirms or establishes diagnosis; for example, biopsy of a mass or growth
   ❖ *Palliative*: Relieves or reduces pain or symptoms of a disease but does not cure; for example, draining a hematoma
   ❖ *Ablative*: Removes a diseased body part; for example, removal of breast (mastectomy)
   ❖ *Constructive*: Restores function or appearance that has been lost or reduced. For example, perineoplasty.

2. Degrees of urgency: Surgery is classified by its urgency and necessity to preserve the patient's life, body part or function.

   ❖ Emergency surgery is performed immediately, e.g. rupture of an ectopic pregnancy

   ❖ Elective surgery is performed when surgical intervention is the preferred treatment for a condition that is not immediately life-threatening. An example is hysterectomy for fibroids in the uterus.

3. Degree of risk: Surgery is classified as major or minor according to the degree of risk to the patient. The degree of risk involved in a surgical procedure is affected by the patient's age, general health, nutritional status, use of medications for conditions unrelated to the indication for surgery and the mental status (disorders that affect cognitive function). Some surgeries are thus referred to as high-risk surgeries.

MANAGEMENT IN PREOPERATIVE PHASE

The overall goal of nursing care during the preoperative phase is to prepare the patient mentally and physically for surgery. Pre-operative evaluation of a patient includes a detailed *history* (general, medical and surgical), a complete *physical examination* and *laboratory investigations*.

1. History:

   ❖ Age: Very young and older patients are greater surgical risks than children and adults

   ❖ General health: Surgery is least risky when the client's general health is good. Any infection or pathophysiology increases the risk

   ❖ Nutritional status: Adequate nutrition is required for normal tissue repair. Surgery increases the body's need for nutrients for the needed tissue healing and prevention of infection during the postoperative period. Obesity contributes to postoperative complications such as pneumonia and wound infection. A malnourished client also is at risk for delayed wound haling. If the surgery cannot be delayed, parenteral or enteral nutrition may be initiated

   ❖ Medications: Regular use of certain medications can increase surgical risk. Examples are anticoagulants, tranquillizers, corticosteroids and diuretics. Information related to the use of such medications can help the surgeon plan relevant management

   ❖ Allergies: Allergies to drugs, food, latex, antiseptics, etc. can alert the hospital staff in using medications and procedures

   ❖ Previous surgeries: Previous surgical experiences may influence the client's physical and psychological responses to surgery

   ❖ Mental status: Clients mental status and ability to understand and respond appropriately can affect the entire perioperative experience

   ❖ Smoking: Smokers may have more difficulty clearing respiratory secretions after surgery; increasing the risk of postoperative pneumonia and atlectasis

   ❖ Alcohol and other mind altering substances: Use of these can affect the central nervous system, liver and other body systems

   ❖ Family and social resources: Availability of family, care givers and social support are important for recovery

   ❖ Coping: Patients with healthy self-concept and coping mechanisms deal better with stressors of surgery.

2. Physical examination and investigations: Assessment of physiological status is done by review of body systems such as respiratory system, circulatory system, gastrointestinal system, neurological system, etc.

Routine Investigations

Routine investigations are:

❖ Blood—hemoglobin and hematocrit:
   – Total and differential leukocyte count and platelet count
   – Blood group and cross, matching
     For older patients:
   – Liver function, renal function, serum electrolytes, and blood glucose

❖ Urine: Routine and microscopic analysis which includes tests for protein, glucose, casts and pus cells

❖ Chest X-ray and electrocardiogram for patients over 40 years. If there is history of any systemic disease, relevant investigations such echocardiography, blood coagulation profile, etc. will be required

❖ Special investigations which are appropriate for certain lesions such as VVF or malignancy may be included

❖ Screening for HIV antibodies and Hepatitis B virus may be included for patients in high-risk group.

3. Preoperative consent: Prior to any surgical procedure, the patient must sign a consent form which is generally, supplied by the hospital or health care facility.

   Although the surgeon maintains legal responsibility for ensuring that the client gives informed consent, the nurse may witness the client's signature on the consent form. A preoperative informed consent form should include the following information:

   ❖ Nature and intention of the surgery
   ❖ Name and qualification of the surgeon
   ❖ Risks including tissue damage, disfigurement or even death
   ❖ Chances of success
   ❖ Possible alternative measures
   ❖ The right of the client to refuse consent or later withdraw consent.

4. Preoperative teaching: Preoperative teaching should include information about the specific gynecologic condition of the patient, for which she needs surgery, role of the client through out the perioperative period, expected discomforts and training for the postoperative period and psychological support. Teaching for postoperative period should include moving, leg exercises and coughing and deep breathing exercises to prevent postoperative complications.

5. Physical preparation: Physical preparation for the surgical patient will include special attention to meet her needs of nutrition and fluids, elimination, hygiene, rest, medications and surgical skin preparation.

❖ Light diet in the previous evening and nothing in the morning of operation. Nothing by mouth for at least 8 hours to keep the stomach empty at the time of anesthesia

❖ A cleansing enema in the evening before surgery. If bowel involvement is suspected, additional bowel preparation with osmotic oral purgative may be prescribed

❖ Skin preparation (local preparation) by shaving of the operative area or clipping of hair is done to reduce the chance of wound infection. Cleansing with soap and water, and povidone iodine will be done in the ward and in the operating room.

6. Preoperative checklist: A preoperative checklist is completed before the patient goes to operating room. This is a guide to the adequacy of patient preparation and documentation.

7. Presurgery medications include:
   ❖ Tranquillizer or sedative medication in the night before surgery
   ❖ Tranquillizer and pre-anesthetic medication 2 hours before surgery
   ❖ Prophylactic antibiotics.

INTRAOPERATIVE PHASE

The overall goal of nursing care during the intraoperative phase is maintaining the patient's safety. Anesthesia may be general or regional. Regional anesthesia includes topical, local, nerve block, spinal anesthesia (subarachnoid block) and epidural anesthesia.

❖ A surgical skin preparation should be carried out as close to the time of surgery as possible. Intravenous line will be established if not already done

❖ Positioning of patient: Dorsal or lithotomy position is chosen according to type of operation

❖ Draping is done using sterile linen and towel clips as required for the specific surgery

❖ The surgeon then makes an appropriate incision and performs the intended procedure (surgery) and closure of the incision.

❖ In the case of minor or day care surgery, patients are admitted, operated and discharged on the same day.

Common 'day care' gynecological operations are:
❖ Dilatation and curettage (D&C)
❖ Dilatation and evacuation (D&E)
❖ Biopsy procedures
❖ Examination under anesthesia (EUA)
❖ Endoscopic procedures.

Immediate postanesthetic care focuses on assessment and monitoring parameters to prevent complications from anesthesia or surgery.

POSTOPERATIVE PHASE

The overall goals of nursing care during the postoperative period are to promote comfort and healing, restore the highest possible wellness and prevent associated risks such as infection or respiratory and cardiovascular complications.

Initial and ongoing assessment of the postoperative patient includes:
❖ Level of consciousness
❖ Vital signs
❖ Oxygen saturation
❖ Skin color and temperature
❖ Comfort
❖ Fluid balance
❖ Dressings and drains.

Ongoing postoperative nursing interventions include:
❖ Managing pain
❖ Appropriate positioning
❖ Encouraging deep breathing and coughing exercises
❖ Promoting leg exercises and ambulation
❖ Maintaining adequate hydration and nutrition status
❖ Promoting urinary elimination
❖ Providing wound care.

Surgical aseptic technique (sterile technique) is used when changing dressing on surgical wounds to promote healing and to reduce risk of infection.

Sutures or clips used to approximate skin and underlying tissue after surgery are generally, removed 7 to 10 days after surgery. Instructions for home care and follow-up are reviewed with the patient and family prior to discharge from the hospital.

69

Infertility and its Management

Learning Objectives

Upon completion of this chapter, the learner will be able to:

❖ Explain the factors related to male and female infertility
❖ Enumerate the investigations for infertile couples
❖ Discuss the regimens to treat infertility of male and female partners.
❖ Explain the procedures of assisted reproductive technology.

DEFINITIONS

Infertility is defined as a failure to conceive within one or more years of regular un-protected intercourse.

Subfertility refers to a state in which a couple has tried unsuccessfully to have a child for a year or more. The term subfertile means less fertile than a regular couple.

Primary infertility denotes couples who have never been able to conceive.

Secondary infertility indicates difficulty conceiving after already having conceived (and either carried the pregnancy to term or had a miscarriage).

Incidence

Generally, worldwide it is estimated that one in seven couples have problems conceiving. Eighty percent of couples achieve conception, if they so desire within one year of having regular intercourse with adequate frequency (4 – 5 times a week). Another 10 percent will achieve the objective by the end of second year. About 10 percent remain infertile by the end of 3rd year.

Factors Required for Fertility (Male and Female)

❖ Healthy spermatozoa should be deposited high in the vagina at or near the cervix
❖ Capacitation and acrosome reaction: Spermatozoa should undergo changes and acquire motility in cervical canal
❖ Motility: Spermatozoa should ascend through the cervix into the uterine cavity and fallopian tube
❖ Ovulation: Ovum should reach the fimbriated end of the tube
❖ Patent fallopian tube: Fertilization should occur at the ampulla of the tube.
❖ Transportation of fertilized ovum to uterine cavity; in 3 and 4 days the fertilized ovum should reach the uterine cavity for nidation.

Cause of Infertility

Conception depends on the fertility potential of both male and female partner. For infertility, male factor contribution is about 30 to 40 percent, female factor 40 to 55 percent and combined factor about 10 to 15 percent. In about 10 percent of the couple, the cause is unexplained. About 4 out of 10 in the unexplained group conceive within 3 years without any specific treatment.

Male Factors that Cause Infertility

1. Defective spermatogenesis: Spermato-genesis and sperm maturation need a high androgenic environment. Spermatogenesis is predominantly controlled by the genes on the 'y' chromosome. The process of sperma-togenesis takes approximately 74 days for

completion. Additional 12 to 20 days are needed for spermatozoa to travel the epididymis. The causes of defective spermatogenesis are:

- ❖ Congenital: Undescended testes is a congenital condition in which spermatogenesis is depressed. Vas deferens is absent bilaterally in 1 and 2 percent of such men
- ❖ Hypospadias causes failure to deposit sperm high in the vagina. In Kartager syndrome (autosomal disease), there is loss of ciliary function and sperm motility.
- ❖ Thermal factor: The scrotal temperature has to be 1 and 2°F less than the body temperature. It is raised in conditions such as varicocele, big hydrocele or filariasis. Other causes are using tight undergarment or working in hot atmosphere
- ❖ Infection: Mumps orchitis after puberty may permanently damage spermatogenesis. In chronic systemic illnesses like bronchiectasis, the quality of sperm is adversely affected. Infection of the seminal vesicle or prostate depresses sperm count
- ❖ Gonadotrophin suppression: This happens in chronic debilitating diseases, malnutrition, heavy smoking and with high alcoholic consumption
- ❖ Endocrine factors: FSH level is seen raised in idiopathic testicular failure. Hypoprolactinemia is associated with impotence
- ❖ Loss of sperm motility (asthenozoospermia and abnormal sperm morphology are seen in some males)
- ❖ Genetic: Common chromosomal abnormality, in azoospermic male is Kleinfelter's syndrome (47 XXY)
- ❖ Iatrogenic: Radiation, cytotoxic drugs, nitrofurantoin, cimetidine, β-blockers, antihypertensives, anticonvulsants and antidepressant drugs are likely to hinder spermatogenesis
- ❖ Immunological factor: Antibodies against spermatozoa surface antigens may cause infertility. This causes clumping of spermatozoa after ejaculation.

Table 69.1 Normal semen values as given by WHO (2002)

Volume	: 20 ml or more
pH	: 7.2 to 7.8
Sperm concentration	: 20 million per ml or more
Motility	: 50% or more with progressive forward motility
Morphology	: 15% or more in normal form
Viability	: 75% or more living
Leukocytes	: Less than one million per ml
Sperm agglutination	: < 2

2. Obstruction of the efferent ducts: The efferent ducts may be obstructed by gonococcal or tubercular infections. Surgical trauma during vasectomy or herniorraphy may lead to obstruction.

3. Failure to deposit sperm high in the vagina (coital problems)
   - ❖ Erectile dysfunction
   - ❖ Ejaculatory defects such as premature, retrograde or absence of ejaculation.
   - ❖ Hypospadias.

4. Errors in seminal fluid
   - ❖ Unusually high or low volume of ejaculate (Normal volume is 2 ml or more).
   - ❖ Low fructose content.
   - ❖ High prostaglandin content.
   - ❖ Undue viscosity.

Normal semen values as determined by WHO are given in Table 69.1.

Causes of Female Infertility

Ovarian Factors

- ❖ Anovulation or Oligo-ovulation: Ovarian activity depends on gonadotrophins which are related to the release of GnRH from hypothalamus (hypothalamopituitary—ovarian axis).

  Disturbance of these may result in anovulation, oligomenorrhea or even amenorrhea. In these conditions there is inadequate growth and function of the corpus luteum.

- ❖ Tubal and peritoneal factors: Tubal and peritoneal factors are responsible for about 30 to 40 percent of cases of female infertility. These include:
  - – Peritubal adhesions
  - – Endosalpingeal damage

- Previous tubal surgery or sterilization
- Salpingitis
- Tubal or peritoneal endometriosis
- Polyps within the lumen
- Tubal spasm.

Uterine Factors

These include factors that interfere with reception and nidation of fertilized ovum (unfavorable endometrium).

Common Conditions are:

- Uterine hyperplasia
- Inadequate secretary endometrium
- Fibroids
- Endometritis
- Uterine synechiae
- Congenital malformations.

Cervical Factors

Ineffective sperm penetration due to following factors:

- Chronic cervicitis
- Presence of antisperm antibodies
- Congenital elongation of cervix
- Second degree uterine prolapse
- Acute retroversion of uterus
- Occlusion of cervical canal with polyp
- Pinhole os
- Scanty vaginal mucus
- Abnormal constituents in the mucus (excessive, viscous or purulent).

Vaginal Factors (Implicated)

- Atresia (partial or complete)
- Septum
- Narrow introitus.

Combined Factors

These include presence of factors both in female and male factors causing infertility:

- Age of wife beyond 35 years and advancing age in men
- Infrequent intercourse (less than 4 – 5 per week) during fertile period (around ovulation)
- Apareunia (failure of emission of semen/ejaculation) and dyspareunia

- Anxiety and apprehension
- Use of lubricants during intercourse which may be spermicidal
- Immunological factors (Antisperm antibodies).

Investigations of Female

History

- History: Age, duration of marriage, history of previous marriage with proven infertility if any
- Medical history: Of tuberculosis, STD, pelvic inflammatory disease, diabetes
- Surgical history: Abdominal or pelvic surgery that can cause peritubal adhesions
- Menstrual history: Hypomenorrhea or oligomenorrhea that are associated with hypothalamopituitary ovarian axis which may be either primary or secondary to adrenal or thyroid dysfunction
- Previous obstetric history: In the case of secondary infertility, history of previous pregnancies, interval, premature rupture of membranes or puerperal sepsis are taken
- Contraceptive practice: Use of IUCD that have chance to produce PID
- Sexual problems: Dyspareunia and loss of libido.

Examinations

- General examination: Obesity or marked reduction in weight, abnormal distribution of hair and underdevelopment of secondary sex characteristics
- Systemic examination: Hypertension, organic heart disease, chronic renal lesion or endocrinopathies
- Gynecologic examination: To look for adequacy of hymenal opening, evidence of vaginal infection, undue elongation of cervix, uterine size, position and mobility. Presence of adnexal mass and nodules in the pouch of Douglass
- Speculum examination: For presence of cervical discharge, which if present needs to be tested for infection.

Diagnostic Evaluation

In the presence of major fault in male partner such as azoospermia or intersex, there is very little scope in investigating the female partner. However, considering the scope of Assisted Reproductive Technology (ART), investigations may be done, if the couple so desire. Similarly, if a major defect is identified in female partner such as Müllerian agenesis or intersex, further investigations may be suspended. Any correctable abnormality found should be rectified prior to investigations, e.g. narrow vaginal introitus, hypothyroidism or diabetes mellitus. Noninvasive and minimal invasive methods are to be carried out prior to major invasive ones.

❖ Menstrual history: Look for evidences of ovulation such as:
  – Regular, normal menstrual loss between the ages of 20 to 35
  – Midmenstrual bleeding (spotting) or pain or excessive mucoid vaginal discharge suggestive of Mittel-schmerz's syndrome
  – Features of primary dysmenorrhea or PMS.
❖ Basal body temperature (BBT).

Patient is instructed to take and record body temperature daily on waking in the morning, before rising out of bed. The body temperature maintaining throughout the first half of the cycle, drops about 0.5°F about middle of cycles then is raised to 0.5° to 1°F (0.2-0.3°C) following ovulation. The rise is sustained throughout the second half of the cycle and falls about 2 days prior to the next period.

The drop in temperature of 0.5°F before the rise coincides with either LH surge or ovulation. Maintenance of BBT chart helps in determining ovulation and timing of postcoital test, endometrial biopsy, cervical mucus or vaginal cytology test for ovulation. It also helps the couple to determine the most fertile period, if the cycle is regular.

❖ Cervical mucus study: Alteration of the physiochemical properties of the cervical mucus occurs due to the effect of estrogen and progesterone. Disappearance of fern pattern of the mucus beyond 22nd day of cycle, progesterone causes dissolution of sodium crystals. Following ovulation there is loss of stretchability or elasticity which was present in the midcycle. This loss of elasticity is an evidence of ovulation. Fern test during the cycle aids in determining ovulation.

❖ Hormone estimation:
  – Serum progesterone: Estimation on day 8 and 21 of cycle. An increase in value from 1 mg/ml to greater than 6 mg/ml suggests ovulation
  – Serum LH: Daily estimation of serum LH at midcycle can detect LH surge. Ovulation occurs about 34 to 36 hours after beginning of LH surge and coincides about 10 to 12 hours after the LH peak
  – Serum estradiol: This hormone attains peak rise approximately 24 to 36 hours prior to ovulation (these tests are used for *in vitro* fertilization)
  – Urinary LH: Ovulation usually occurs within 14 to 26 hours of detection of urine LH surge and almost always within 48 hours (the test should be done on a daily basis, starting 2-3 days before the day of expected surge).

❖ Endometrial biopsy: Biopsy is done on 21st to 23rd day of the cycle (If the cycle is irregular, it is done within 24 hours of the period). Evidence of secretary activity of the endometrial glands in the second half of the cycle gives the diagnosis of ovulation. The secretary changes are due to the action of progesterone on the estrogen primed endometrium

❖ Sonography: Serial sonography during midcycle can precisely measure the Graafian follicle just prior to ovulation (18 to 20 mm). The features of recent ovulation are collapsed follicle and fluid in the pouch of Douglas

❖ Laparoscopy: Laparoscopic visualization of recent corpus luteum or detection of the ovum from the aspirated peritoneal fluid from the pouch of Douglas is the direct evidence of ovulation

❖ Insufflation test (Rubin's test): It is done to see the patency of fallopian tubes. It is done by pushing air or carbon dioxide under-pressure through the cervical canal. If the tubes are patent air reaches the peritoneal cavity.

It is done in the postmenstrual period, at least 2 days after stoppage of menstrual bleeding. Positive findings include:

- Fall in the pressure when raised beyond 120 mm Hg
- Hissing sound heard on auscultation on either iliac fossa
- Shoulder pain experienced by the patient due to irritation of diaphragm by air.

The procedure should not be done in the presence of pelvic infection. In about 1/3rd of cases the test gives false—negative findings and hence not very reliable. This test is not commonly alone these days.

❖ Hysterosalpingography (HSG): In this test, instead of air or carbon dioxide, dye is introduced transcervically. The test is done in the postmenstrual phase, two days after the stoppage of menstruation. It is avoided if the woman has pelvic infection.

HSG has definite advantages over-insufflation test. It can precisely detect the site of block in the tube. It can reveal any abnormality in the uterus such as fibroid or synechiae. Disadvantage of HSG is radiation risk

❖ Laparoscopic chromotubation: This is an invasive investigation and hence performed only after male factors and ovulation functions have been found normal or corrected. It involves checking for tubal patency laparoscopically by injecting methylene blue through the cervix into the fallopian tubes to confirm spillage of the dye into the pelvic cavity. It also helps in the detection of PID, endometriosis and pelvic adhesions along with tubal patency. Chromotubation is a diagnostic and therapeutic procedure as it can allow for release of peritubal adhesions and fimbrial block. Appropriate surgery for infertility can be planned based on the findings

❖ Sonosalpingography: This test involves a slow injection of physiological saline into the uterine cavity using a pediatric Foley's

catheter. The catheter balloon is inflated at the level of the cervix to prevent fluid leak. Ultrasonography of the uterus and fallopian tubes is then done. Ultrasound can follow the fluid through the tube up to the peritoneal cavity and in the pouch of Douglas.

Management of Infertility

Management of infertility or subfertility would depend upon the cause identified, duration and age of the couple, especially the female.

General Instructions

When minor defects are detected in both the husband and wife, each of which alone could not cause infertility, but in combination they decrease the fertility potential, the faults should be treated simultaneously.

❖ Body weight: Overweight or underweight of any partner should be adequately dealt with to obtain an optimal body weight
❖ Smoking and alcohol: Excess smoking or alcohol consumption to be avoided
❖ Ideal coital frequency: Intercourse on multiple days during the fertile window period which includes the 5 preceding and the day of anticipated ovulation should be reviewed with the couple
❖ Use of at home "fertility monitor" and checking of vaginal mucus discharge to determine the optimal timing of intercourse may be most helpful
❖ Use of LH surge kit: Use of the kit can detect LH surge in urine by getting a deep blue color of dipstick. The test performed between 12th to 16th day of regular cycle and timed intercourse over 24 to 36 hours after the color change reasonably succeeds to conception
❖ Avoidance of lubricants and douches to be stressed
❖ The use of fertility impairing medica-tions should be avoided by both partners if possible, e.g. hormones
❖ Psychological support should be offered as the couple may face significant stress and sadness as the investigations and consultations progress.

Management of Male Infertility

The treatment of male partner is indicated in *extreme oligospermia, azoospermia, low volume ejaculate* and *impotency.*

Measures to improve spermatogenesis are advised:

General Care

❖ Improvement of general health:
  – Reduction of weight in obese
  – Avoidance of alcohol and heavy smoking
  – Avoidance of tight and warm under-garments
  – Avoidance of occupation that may elevate testicular temperature.
❖ Avoiding medications that interfere with spermatogenesis such as:
  – Cytotoxic drugs, nitrofurantoin, cimetidine, anticonvulsants, antide-pressants and β-blockers.
❖ Medications to treat specific causes:
  – hCG and hMG for hypogonadism
  – Dopamine agonist (cabergoline) for hyperprolactinemia and altered test-osterone level and to improve libido, potency and fertility
  – GnRH therapy for hypogonadism
  – Clomiphene citrate to increase serum levels of FSH, LH and testosterone
  – Antibiotics for genital tract infections.
❖ Special treatments for causes identified such as:
  – Intrauterine insemination (IUI)
  – *In vitro* fertilization or (IVF)
  – Intracytoplasmic sperm injection (ICSI)
  – Artificial insemination with donor sperm (AID).
❖ Surgical treatment:
  – In men whose testicular biopsy shows normal spermatogenesis and obstruction is suspected, vasoepididymostomy or vasovasostomy may help
  – Correction of hydrocele.

Management of Female Infertility

Treatment for females is also according to the disorders identified.

❖ Ovulatory dysfunction:
  – Induction of ovulation using drugs such as clomiphene citrate, letrozole, FSH, hCG and GnRH
  – Correction of biochemical abnormality: Metformin for hyperinsulinemia, dexamethasone for androgen excess, bromocriptine for prolactin excess
  – Substitution therapy: Thyroxin for hypothyroidism, antidiabetic drugs for diabetes mellitus.
❖ Surgery:
  – Laparoscopic ovarian drilling (LOD) or laser vaporization for polycystic ovarian syndrome (PCOS)
  – Surgical removal of virilizing or func-tioning ovarian or adrenal tumor
  – Tubotubal anastomosis for adhesion in tube
  – Cannulation and balloon tuboplasty for block in tube
  – Fimbrioplasty for fimbrial adhesion
  – Adhesiolysis for separation or division of adhesion
  – Salpingostomy to create an opening in tube in a completely occluded tube.

Management of Unexplained Infertility

Unexplained or persistent infertility refers to those couples who have undergone complete basic infertility work up and in whom no abnormality has been detected and still remains infertile. The reported evidence is about 10 to 20 percent. About 60 to 80 percent of those couples become pregnant within 3 years without any treatment.

The recommended treatment for unexpl-ained infertility is induction of ovulation, intrauterine insemination (IUI), and super ovulation combined with IUI.

ASSISTED REPRODUCTIVE TECHNOLOGY (ART)

Assisted reproductive technology encompasses all methods used to achieve pregnancy by artificial or partially artificial means. It involves manipulation of gametes and embryos outside the body for the treatment of infertility.

In ART, the process of intercourse is bypassed either by intrauterine insemination (IUI) or fertilization of the oocytes in the laboratory environment as in *in vitro* fertilization (IVF).

Different Techniques of ART

- ❖ Intrauterine insemination (IUI)
- ❖ *In vitro* fertilization and embryo transfer (IVF - ET)
- ❖ Gamete intrafallopian transfer (GIFT)
- ❖ Zygote intrafallopian transfer (ZIFT)
- ❖ Intracytoplasmic sperm injection (ICSI).

Intrauterine Insemination (IUI)

Intrauterine insemination involves placing increased concentration of motile sperms close to the fallopian tubes bypassing the endocervical canal which is abnormal. IUI may be *artificial insemination husband, artificial insemination donor or insemination with donor egg.*

Indications

- ❖ Hostile cervical mucus
- ❖ Cervical stenosis
- ❖ Oligospermia or athenospermia
- ❖ Immune factor (male or female)
- ❖ Male factor impotency or anatomical defect, but normal ejaculate can be obtained, e.g. hypospadias (AIH)
- ❖ Unexplained infertility.

Technique

About 3 ml of washed and concentrated sperms are injected through a flexible polyethylene catheter within the uterine cavity around the time of ovulation. The processed sperms for insemination should at least be one million. Fertilizing capacity of spermatozoa is 24 to 48 hours. The procedure may be repeated 2 to 3 times over a period of 2 and 3 days. Generally, 4 to 6 cycles of insemination with or without super ovulation are advised.

When large volumes of washed and processed sperms are placed within the uterine cavity, around the time of ovulation, it causes perfusion of the fallopian tubes with spermatozoa. Hence this method is known as *fallopian tube sperm perfusion.*

In conjunction with ovulation induction, pregnancy rate is 25 to 30 percent per cycle.

Artificial Insemination Donor (AID)

When the semen of a donor is used for insemination, it is called *artificial insemination donor.*

Indications

- ❖ Untreatable azoospermia or athenospermia of husband
- ❖ Genetic disease affecting spermato-genesis in husband
- ❖ Rh – sensitization of the woman.

Technique

The donor should be healthy and serologically and bacteriologically free from venereal disease, HIV and hepatitis. The recipient and donor must be matched for blood group and Rh typing. Either fresh or frozen semen is used.

About 3 to 6 cycles may be used for success. Insemination when combined with super ovulation enhances success rate. Two inseminations 18 and 42 hours after hCG administration (for ovulation) give higher result when compared to single insemination after 36 hours.

Artificial Insemination Husband (AIH)

An artificial insemination with husband's semen is done for 4 cycles. The results are better, if combined with ovulation induction for multiple ovulations.

Indications

- ❖ Oligospermia
- ❖ Impotency
- ❖ Premature ejaculation or retrograde ejaculation
- ❖ Hypospadias
- ❖ Antisperm antibodies in cervical mucus
- ❖ Unexplained infertility
- ❖ X-Y fractionizaton of sperms for sex selection in genetic and chromosomal abnormalities.

Technique

Semen collection, washing, centrifugation and swim up methods are done. Washed and concentrated sperm is then placed in uterine cavity as in AID technique.

In virto Fertilization and Embryo Transfer (IVF-ET)

Fertilization of an ovum outside the body is a technique used when a woman has blocked fallopian tubes or some other impediment to the union of sperm and ovum in the reproductive tract. The woman is given hormone therapy causing a number of ova to mature at the same time (super ovulation). Several of them are then removed from the ovary through a laparoscope.

The ova are mixed with spermatozoa from her spouse and incubated in a culture medium until a blastocyst is formed. The blastocyst is then implanted in the mother's uterus and the pregnancy allowed to continue normally.

❖ Indications:
  − Tubal disease or block
  − Endometriosis
  − Cervical hostility
  − Unexplained infertility
  − Ovarian failure (donor oocyte IVF).

Donor oocyte IVF is done for women with no eggs due to surgery, chemotherapy, genetic causes or poor egg quality.

❖ Patient selection:
  − Age of women (egg donor) less than 35 years
  − Presence of at least one functioning ovary
  − Normal seminogram for husband.
  − Couple negative for HIV and hepatitis.

❖ Technique/procedure steps:
  − Induction of superovulation using drugs clomiphene citrate and gonadotropin releasing hormone (GnRH)
  − Monitoring of follicular growth: This is done by cervical mucus study, Sonographic measurement of the follicle and serum estriol estimation
  − Ovum retrieval: This is done either laparoscopically or vaginally. If vaginal route is used, a small needle is inserted

through the back of the vagina and guided via ultrasound into the ovarian follicle to collect the fluid that contains the ova about 36 hours after hCG administration but before ovulation occurs

− Fertilization (*in vitro*): The sperm for insemination *in vitro* is prepared by the wash and swim technique. Approximately 50,000 to 100,000 sperms are placed into the culture media containing the oocyte within 4 to 6 hours of retrieval. The semen is collected just prior to ovum retrieval. Sperm density and motility are most important criteria for successful IVF

− Embryo transfer: The fertilized ova at the 4 to 8 cell stage are placed into the uterine cavity close to the fundus about 48 to 72 hours later though a fine flexible tube transcervically. Not more than three embryos are transferred per cycle to minimize multiple pregnancies.

Gamete Intrafallopian Transfer (GIFT)

In this procedure, both the sperm and the unfertilized oozyte are transferred into the fallopian tubes using laparoscopy following transvaginal ovum retrieval. Fertilization is then achieved *in vivo*.

The prerequisite for GIFT procedure is to have normal fallopian tubes. The result is poor in male factor abnormality. Superovulation is done as in IVF. Two hours prior to ovum retrieval, semen specimen is obtained. The semen is washed by "swim up" technique and the most fertile fraction of the sperm is obtained and used for transfer.

Zygote Intrafallopian Transfer (ZIFT)

In zygote Intrafallopian transfer, egg cells are removed from the woman's ovaries and fertilized in the laboratory. The resulting zygote is then placed in the fallopian tube following one day *in vitro* fertilization through laparoscope or through a uterine opening under ultrasonic guidance.

The technique is a suitable alternative of GIFT. GIFT procedures are avoided when tubal factors of infertility are present.

Intracytoplasmic Sperm Injection (ICSI)

This method is beneficial in the case of male factor infertility where the sperm counts are very low or failed fertilization with previous IVF attempts. The ICSI procedure involves a single sperm carefully injected into the center of an egg using a microneedle. Sperm is retrieved from the ejaculate or by testicular sperm extraction (TESE) or by microsurgical epididymal sperm aspiration (MESA). Indications are azoospermia, severe oligospermia, sperm antibodies and obstruction of afferent duct system and failure of IVF.

Prognosis of Artificial Reproductive Methods

The pregnancy rate within two years after the start of investigations ranges from 30 to 40 percent. The rate is higher, if AID cases are included. However, if pregnancy occurs, there is two-fold increased chance of abortion, five times ectopic pregnancy and the perinatal mortality doubles.

Role of Nurses in Management of Infertility

Nurses meet couples seeking help for treatment of infertility in special centers or clinics where such services are available. Those working in infertility centers usually are the first contact persons who co-ordinates various activities for the couple's treatment. Their role with such couples includes assessing, educating and counseling in addition to therapeutic assistance as they undergo tests and procedures.

When a couple presents with concerns about infertility, it is important for the nurse to understand that men and women are very concerned and possibly emotionally fragile.

Entering a medical facility for evaluation is in itself for some an admission of failure.

Before even beginning the medical aspects of care it is important to understand and assist the couple to understand their motivation for pregnancy and to offer support. The couple should understand and accept that the evaluation and treatment for infertility will be stressful and will involve both partners throughout the process. It is important to meet the couple together.

An important step in evaluation for infertility is taking a detailed medical and family history from each partner. Treatment may be individualized for each partner. Nursing interventions include assisting in reducing stress in the relationship, encouraging cooperation, protecting privacy and fostering understanding. Because infertility evaluations and treatments are expensive, time consuming, invasive, stressful and not always successful, couples need great support in working together to deal with the process. During the period of therapy, couples need to avoid smoking, continue good diet, exercise, maintain health and take folic acid supplements if prescribed.

BIBLIOGRAPHY

1. Baram DA. Sexuality and Sexual Function, Novak's Gynecology 13th edn. Baltimore: Williams & Wilkens.
2. Dutta DC. Textbook of Gynecology, 5th edn. New Kolkata: Central Book Agency, 2008.
3. James CA. The Nursing role in assisted reproductive technologies, NAACOGS, Clinical issues in perinatal women's health nursing 1992;3(2) 328-44.
4. Jorka J, Schutte S, Foxhall MJ. Loneliness and social support in infertile couples, Journal of Obstetric, Gynecologic and Neonatal Nursing 1966;25(1)55-60.
5. Kolplan CR. Work-up of infertility diagnosis and treatment of anovulation, The Female Patient 1966;21(3):35-42.
6. Littleton LY, Engebreton. Maternity Nursing Care, Thomson Delmar Learning 2005.

70

Genital Malignancies

Cancer is a disease in which cells of the body grow out of control. The new growth is termed neoplasm and that with locally invasive, destructive and metastatic properties is termed a malignancy. A malignant growth or cancer is always named for the part of the body where it starts even if it spreads to other parts later. Genital cancers develop in the ovaries, uterus, cervix, vulva, vagina and fallopian tubes.

OVARIAN CANCER

Ovarian cancer is a term that includes a variety of malignant growths that originate in the ovary. There are about 20 microscopically distinct types. They can be classified into three large groups; *epithelial cancers, germ-cell tumors and specialized stromal cell cancers*. There are three such groups because the ovary contains collections of cells with three distinct origins and functions.

Incidence

Ovarian malignancy constitutes about 15 to 20 percent of genital malignancy. It is more prevalent in the USA and Scandinavian countries, but much less in Oriental or Latin American and Asian countries including Japan and India.

Epidemiology

Nulligravidas carry a higher risk for ovarian malignancy. Repeated ovulatory trauma to the ovarian epithelial lining is seen as a promoting factor for carcinogenesis. There is a significant reduction in the risk with increasing parity. Combined oral contraceptive pills reduce the risk significantly as also repeated pregnancies.

The use of coffee, tobacco, alcohol and dietary fat has also been associated with reduction in the risk.

Origin of Ovarian Cancers

During embryonic development, when the fetus is about 8 weeks postconception, the organ systems begin to form. There is on each side of the abdominal cavity, an area that is destined to become ovary. Into this area, special cells migrate from the yolk sac, which are destined to become ova. These cells are called *germ cells*. Also in these two areas are cells specialized for manufacture of steroid hormones. Covering all these is the mesothelium which becomes the peritoneum—the lining of abdominal cavity that contains all of the intestines, liver and in women, the uterus and ovaries. From puberty and through adult life the ovary will function as a producer of ova and steroid hormones—estrogen and progesterone.

During each menstrual cycle, a germ cell will mature into an ova or egg contained in a follicle or cyst. While maturing the ova, the ovary produces estrogen. The follicle cyst is covered with the epithelium that once was the mesothelium. At ovulation the follicle breaks and releases the ova. The remnant of the follicle cyst called corpus luteum produces progesterone.

The epithelial covering gives rise to *epithelial ovarian cancers*, the germ cells to the *germ cell tumors* and the steroid producing cells to the *specialized stromal cells cancers*.

About 80 percent of ovarian cancers are epithelial, 10 to 20 percent are of germ cell origin and very little are of stromal cell origin, 3 to 5 percent.

Genetics and Ovarian Malignancy

Hereditary ovarian cancer occurs in two forms:
1. Hereditary breast ovarian cancer syndrome (BOC): When gene mutation occurs to chromosome 17q, it is called BRCA - 1. When gene mutation happens in chromosome 13q, it is BRCA - 2. These produce serous carcinoma in early age.
2. Hereditary nonpolyposis colorectal cancer (HNPCC) or Lynch syndrome: This is an autosomal dominant transmission. Women with HNPCC have life time risk of bout 50 percent for endometrial cancer and 12 percent for ovarian cancer. However, majority of epithelial ovarian cancers are not familial or hereditary. They are less than 10 percent of all ovarian cancers.

Classification of Ovarian Cancers

* Epithelial ovarian cancers
  - Serous
  - Endometrioid
  - Clear cell
  - Papillary serous
  - Brenner cell
  - Undifferentiated adenocarcinoma and sarcoma.
* Stromal cell cancers
  - Immature teratoma
  - Mature teratoma

- Carcinoid tumor
- Dysgerminoma
- Embryonal cell carcinoma
- Endodermal sinus tumor
- Primary choriocarcinoma
- Gonadoblastoma
* Specialized stromal cell cancers
  - Granulosa cell tumor
  - Theca cell tumor
  - Sertoli - Leydig cell tumor
  - Hilar cell tumor

In addition, there are others that are very rare. These rare tumors are not discussed in this chapter. The ovary is also a site for metastasis from other cancers, especially the intestinal cancer and breast cancer. Cancers metastatic to the ovaries are called as *Krukenberg tumors*.

Features of Specific Types of Tumors
Epithelial Cancers

* Malignant epithelial tumors are both cystic and solid types, with the cystic type more common.
* These are bilateral in about 50 percent.
* These may arise *de novo* as malignant or more commonly result from malignant changes of benign cystic tumors.
* In 20 percent, it is seen associated with endometrial carcinoma and in 10 percent with ovarian endometriosis. In less than 5 percent, it may arise from an endometrial cyst.

Germ Cell Tumors

* These tumors commonly occur in young women. 50 percent are women younger than 21 years of age
* These are very aggressive and virulent cancers
* The teratomas have the potential to form complete adult type tissues
* The mature teratoma is called "dermoid" and can contain hair, teeth, bone and brain tissue. Often they are full of skin
* They are generally not malignant but very rarely can have a secondary malignancy such as melanoma or squamous cell cancer of skin.

❖ Some contain thyroid tissue and can cause hyperthyroidism
❖ If the tissues remain immature or fetal in appearance, then they are malignant.

Specialized Stromal Cell Tumors

❖ Granulosa and theca cell tumors are often mixed and can produce estrogen
❖ If it occurs in a young girl, it can produce premature sexual development which will also stop the bones from growing, causing short stature
❖ Sertoli-Leydig cell tumors produce male hormones and will cause defeminization, then masculinization with male pattern baldness, deep voice, excessive hair growth and enlargement of clitoris
❖ The specialized stromal cell cancers are not aggressive cancers and usually involve only one ovary.

Risk Factors for Ovarian Cancer

Majority of ovarian cancers are epithelial cell type cancers.

❖ Epithelial ovarian cancers tend to be a cancer of affluent societies where expected life spans are long. Most ovarian cancers occur in women over age 50
❖ An increased risk factor other than age is nulliparity or delayed child bearing
❖ Use of fertility drugs that induce ovulation
❖ Familial cancers: breast, endometrial, ovarian, colorectal
❖ History of removal of benign ovarian tumor or breast carcinoma
❖ Postmenopausal palpable ovary (volume > 8 cm^2
❖ Women workers in asbestos related industries
❖ A decreased risk is seen with multiparity and with prolonged use of birth control pill. The mechanism for this protective effect may be that the number of ovulations is reduced. Each ovulation requires the breakage of the ovarian follicle and the repair of the ovarian surface. A repair process means increased cell divisions or mitosis. Each mitotic division is a time of risk for mutation to occur.

Clinical Features

Ovarian cancer is very difficult to detect in its early stages because at first there are often no obvious symptoms. A cyst can break and bleed and can cause enough symptoms to cause the woman to seek help. Otherwise the cancer is usually far advanced before it is diagnosed. When symptoms do appear, they may include:

❖ An ongoing feeling of abdominal discomfort or pain which the patient may express as gas, indigestion, bloating, swelling or cramps
❖ Nausea, diarrhea, constipation
❖ Loss of appetite
❖ Feeling full even after a light meal
❖ Sudden loss of weight
❖ Urinary frequency or incontinence
❖ Abnormal vaginal bleeding
❖ Pelvic pain, back pain
❖ Fatigue and pallor
❖ Edema leg or vulva
❖ Respiratory distress due to ascitis or pleural effusion.

Special Investigations

Investigations are aimed at identifying the extent of lesion to detect the primary site and to confirm malignancy prior to surgery.

❖ Cytology examination of fluid collected from abdominal paracentesis or cul-de-sac aspiration
❖ Blood test for CA 125 tumor maker. Level >35 u/ml with a pelvic mass may be suggestive of epithelial ovarian cancer
❖ Chest X-ray to exclude pleural effusion and chest metastasis
❖ Barium enema to detect any lower bowel malignancy
❖ Sonography to detect involvement of the omentum or contralateral ovary
❖ Computed tomography for retroperitoneal lymph node assessment and to detect metastasis in liver or omentum
❖ Magnetic resonance imaging (MRI) to detect involvement of lymph nodes relapse following initial treatment
❖ Positron emission tomography (PET) is a more sensitive test than MRI or CT scan to

differentiate normal tissues from cancer tissues

❖ Intravenous pyelography

❖ Diagnostic uterine curettage (D&C)

In all but the earliest cancers, there is often some cancer remaining after surgery. This is because it spreads throughout the abdomen in little nodules, some are only barely visible and others are too small to see.

The surgical goal is not to leave any nodule larger than 1 cm. If the residual is smaller, debulking or cryoreduction may be done. If small nodules are detected on the intestine, then removal of a piece of intestine and even a colostomy may be necessary to achieve the goal.

In addition to stage (size and extent of spread) the grade (microscopic appearance) is also important. Grade "O" refers to an epithelial carcinoma of low malignant potential which is borderline cancer.

Grade I adenocarcinoma is easily identified as being from a glandular origin. Grade III cancers are difficult to identify as glandular and are poorly differentiated and expected to behave the worst. Grade II cancers are intermediate in appearance.

Preventive Management

Primary Prevention

❖ Genetic screening for BRCA for women who are at high-risk for breast and ovarian cancer.

❖ Annual mammographic screening for women with strong family history of breast cancer

❖ Periodic screening for other malignancies. For example, colonoscopy and endometrial biopsy for women with Lynch II syndrome (HNPCC)

❖ Combined contraceptive pills for women belonging to HNPCC families

❖ Prophylactic oophorectomy with hysterectomy in high-risk women such as:
  – Nulliparous women >45 years
  – Women with history of ovarian, endometrial or colonic cancer in the first degree relative (mother, sister)

– Grossly abnormal ovary in premenopausal women (ovarian volume > 20 cm^2)
– Women who had one ovary removed for neoplasm
– Previous history of breast carcinoma
– Any woman with radiation induced menopause.

❖ Careful follow-up of any ovarian enlargement ≥ 8 cm during child bearing period

❖ In postmenopausal women any ovarian enlargement should be assessed by CA 125 and transvaginal sonography.

❖ Follow-up of women who had ovarian cyst with ultrasound and serum CA 125 at an interval of 4 months

❖ Laparotomy for any enlargement of ovary beyond 8 cm and symptomatic ovarian tumor, while the woman is under observation.

Secondary Prevention

Screening as secondary preventive measure aims at detecting early ovarian malignancy in asymptomatic women.

❖ Tumor marker: Test for Specific antigen CA 125. Values more than 35 u/ml are suggestive of epithelial ovarian cancer.

❖ Transvaginal ultrasonography and study of vascular parameters.

Treatment

❖ **Surgery** is the key treatment for ovarian malignancy. Chemotherapy, radiotherapy and combination therapy are used according to the stage and degree of the malignancy (Table 70.1).

1. *Borderline ovarian cancer*: This category of epithelial ovarian cancers are of low malignant potential and slow growing. Recurrence after surgery may not develop for 15 to 20 years or may not recur at all. Most are Stage I but can be Stage III when diagnosed. These are usually treated only by surgery.

2. *Epithelial ovarian cancer*: For this type of cancer, the initial treatment is surgery, which is removal of uterus, tubes and ovaries as well as any large nodules of cancer.

Table 70.1	Surgical stages of ovarian cancer (FIGO)
Stage I	Limited to the ovaries
Stage I A	One ovary involved
Stage I B	Both ovaries involved
Stage I C	One or both ovaries involved but with cancer on the surface of an ovary, rupture of an ovarian cyst, malignant ascitis or positive abdominal washings
Stage II	Spread to adjacent pelvic structures
Stage II A	Spread to uterus or fallopian tubes
Stage II B	Spread to pelvic peritoneum
Stage II C	Confined to the pelvis but with malignant ascitis or positive abdominal washings
Stage III	Spread to the upper abdomen
Stage III A	Microscopic spread to the upper abdomen
Stage III B	Cancer nodules less than 2 cm
Stage III C	Nodules more than 2 cm or positive pelvic or aortic lymph nodes
Stage IV	Distant spread beyond the abdomen, liver, lung, etc.

Removal of only one ovary is done in the following situations:

– The patient has strong desire for further childbearing
– The cancer is Stage IA grade '0' or Stage II epithelial cancer
– The cancer is Stage I germ cell or a specialized stromal cell type.

When unilateral oophorectomy is done, the woman is advised to have the remaining ovary removed when childbearing is completed. All ovarian cancer patients will receive a maximal surgical effort so that the residual is small and there is a better chance for complete response to chemotherapy. In advanced stage, a segment of intestine may be removed with a colostomy.

❖ **Chemotherapy** is accomplished by giving chemotherapeutic drugs soon after surgery. The drugs are repeated every 3 to 4 weeks and usually six courses are given. Single agent drugs commonly used are Melphelan, Cisplatin, Carboplatin and Paclitaxel. For combination therapy the drugs used are Cyclophosphamide, Adriamycin and Cisplatin.

❖ **Radiation:** Radioactive isotope of phosphorus called p-32 is instilled in the abdominal cavity. This is used when micro-scopic amount of cancer only is present. With a one-time instillation, the entire abdominal contents receive a dose of several thousand RADs to a depth of several millimeters.

❖ **Immunotherapy:** Use of cytokines, interferon or interleukin – 2 has shown improvement in response rate.

Prognosis

❖ Stage I A and I B grade I cancers require no further treatment after surgery. The five year survival rate is 95 percent.

❖ All stage I C and all Stage III cancers receive treatment either with chemotherapy or p-32. The prognosis is usually good with cure rate of 65 to 80 percent.

❖ All Stage II and Stage III cancers with minimal or microscopic residual receive chemotherapy. The five year survival is 30 to 35 percent.

❖ For those with Stage III and IV cancers with bulky residual, the short term response is good, but the long term outlook is poor.

UTERINE CANCER

Uterine cancer also called as endometrial cancer and uterine adenocarcinoma involves a malignant growth that originates in the lining of the uterus—the endometrium. Endometrial cancer is the most common cancer of the female reproductive system. Cancer of the uterus mainly affects postmenopausal women between the ages of 50 and 60 and is uncommon below 40 years.

Incidence

The incidence is higher amongst the white population of United States of America and lowest in India and Japan. The high incidence within a few decades of menopause is associated with excessive exposure to estrogen.

Etiology

The following are found to be related to carcinoma body of the uterus:

❖ Estrogen: Persistent stimulation of endometrium with unopposed estrogen is the single most important factor for the development of endometrial cancer.

- Age: About 75 percent postmenopausal cancers are diagnosed at median age of 60. About 10 percent of women with postmenopausal bleeding have endometrial cancer.
- Parity: It is more common in unmarried and nulliparous women (about 30%)
- Late menopause: The chance of carcinoma increases if menopause fails to occur beyond 52 years
- Corpus cancer syndrome: Encompasses obesity, hypertension and diabetes
- Obesity: Leads to high level of free estradiol as the sex hormone binding globulin level is low
- Unopposed estrogen stimulation that occurs in conditions such as functioning ovarian tumor, polycystic ovarian disease (PCOD), and estrogen replacement therapy in postmenopausal women is associated with endometrial cancer
- Tamoxifen used for treatment of breast cancer is noted as contributing to endometrial cancer due to its weak estrogenic effect
- Family history or personal history of colon, ovarian or breast cancer increases the risk of endometrial cancer
- Fibroid is associated in 30 percent of cases.

Classification

Carcinoma

Most endometrial cancers are **carcinomas** usually **adenocarcinomas** meaning that they originate from the single layer of epithelial cells that line the endometrium and form the endometrial glands. The microscopic type of endometrial carcinoma include the:
- Endometrioid type
- Papillary serous carcinoma
- Clear cell endometrial carcinoma.

Sarcoma

Endometrial stromal sarcomas are cancers that originate in the nonglandular connective tissue of the endometrium.

Carcinosarcoma

This is a rare uterine cancer that contains cancerous cells of both glandular and sarcomatous appearance. In this case, the cell of origin is unknown.

Signs and Symptoms

- Vaginal bleeding and/or spotting in postmenopausal women
- Abnormal uterine bleeding and abnormal menstrual periods
- Bleeding between normal periods in premenopausal women. Extremely long, heavy or frequent episodes of bleeding may indicate premalignant changes
- Anemia caused by chronic loss of blood
- Lower abdominal pain or cramping
- Thin white or clear vaginal discharge in postmenopausal women
- Abdominal mass
- Pain during sexual intercourse.

Risk Factors

- High level of estrogen
- Endometrial hyperplasia
- Obesity, diabetes, hypertension
- Polycystic ovary syndrome
- Nulliparity and infertility
- Early menarche
- Late menopause
- Endometrial polyps or other benign growths of uterine lining
- History of irregular and excessive premenopausal bleeding
- Use of Tamoxifen for breast cancer treatment
- High intake of animal fat
- Pelvic radiation therapy
- Ovarian cancer
- Anovulatory cycles.

Diagnosis

- History and clinical examination
- Pap smear may be either normal or show abnormal cellular changes
- Endometrial biopsy using a Sharman Curette or aspiration using a soft, flexible plastic suction cannula
- Transvaginal ultrasound and color Doppler to evaluate the endometrial thickness in women with postmenopausal bleeding
- Hysteroscopy and direct visualization of the uterine cavity to take biopsy

- Fractional curettage to detect the extent of growth.

Preoperative Evaluation

- Complete medical history, physical examination and pelvic examination
- Blood examination—hemoglobin, complete blood count, blood glucose, urea, creatinine and electrolytes
- Urine examination—routine examination for protein, sugar and pus cells
- Chest X-ray and ECG
- Pelvic ultrasonography
- Liver and renal function tests
- Serum tumor marker – C 125.

Treatment

Choice of treatment is based on the surgical staging (Table 70.2).

The primary treatment is surgery.

- Surgical treatment consists of:
  - Cytologic sampling of the peritoneal fluid
  - Abdominal exploration
  - Palpation and biopsy of suspicious lymph nodes
  - Abdominal hysterectomy
  - Bilateral Salpingo-oophorectomy and Lymphadenectomy (pelvic and para-aortic Lymph nodes) if the tumor has high-risk features or extension to the cervix or adnexa.
- Surgery in combination with radiotherapy for women with Stage I disease that are at risk for recurrence and for those with Stage II cancer

Table 70.2	Staging of endometrial carcinoma FIGO 2010
Stage I A	Tumor confined to the endometrium
Stage I B	Invasion of less than half the endometrium
Stage I C	Invasion of more than half the endometrium
Stage II A	Endocervical glandular involvement only.
Stage II B	Cervical stromal invasion
Stage III A	Tumor invades serosa or adnexa
Stage III B	Vaginal and /or parametrial involvement
Stage III C$_1$	Pelvic node involvement
Stage III C$_2$	Para-aortic lymph node involvement with or without pelvic node involvement
Stage IV A	Tumor invasion to bladder and/or bowel mucosa.
Stage IV B	Distant metastasis including abdominal metastasis and/or inguinal lymph nodes.

- Chemotherapy for those with Stage III and IV disease
- Hormonal therapy with progestins and antiestrogens for treatment of endometrial and stromal sarcomas.

Complications of Treatment

- Uterine perforation may occur during a D&C or an endometrial biopsy.
- Asherman's syndrome: Intrauterine adhesions may occur from D&C, resulting in infertility and an increased risk of future obstetric complications.

Prognosis

- Prognosis is poor for tumors that are poorly differentiated with greater degree of myometrial penetration, lymphovascular space invasion and advanced stages
- Anuploid tumors are prognostically worse.

GESTATIONAL TROPHOBLASTIC DISEASE (GTD)

Gestational trophoblastic disease/neoplasia is a generic name for a group of pregnancy related disorders that arise from trophoblasts (primitive cells which are placental stem cells). When there is persistence of GTD beyond pregnancy, the condition is referred to as *gestational trophoblastic neoplasia* (GTN).

Types

GTD is the common name for five closely related tumors, most of which are malignant. Benign – Hydatidiform mole.

Malignant

a. Invasive mole
b. Choriocarcinoma
c. Placental site trophoblastic tumor
d. Persistent trophoblastic disease

The tumors arise from trophoblastic cells. Trophoblast is the membrane that forms the wall of the blastocyst in the early development of the fetus. In a normal pregnancy, tropho-blastic cells aid the implantation of the fertilized egg into the uterine wall. But in GTD, they develop into tumor cells.

Invasive Mole (Choriocarcinoma Destruens)

Invasive mole consists of 15 percent of all gestational trophoblastic neoplasms.

Features of invasive mole are:

❖ Abnormal penetration through the muscle layers of the uterus
❖ Perforation of the uterine wall at multiple areas showing purple fungating growth
❖ Intraperitoneal hemorrhage
❖ Metastasis to vagina or distant sites as in choriocarcinoma.

Diagnosis

❖ On laparotomy
 – Perforation of the uterus through which purple fungating growth is visible
 – Hemoperitoneum
 – On histological examination, hyperplasic, trophoblastic cells which still retain villus structure are seen
 – Persistent high level of urinary and serum hCG.

Choriocarcinoma

Choriocarcinoma is a highly malignant and aggressive cancer arising from the chorionic epithelium. The abnormal cells start in the tissue that would normally become placenta. About 3 to 5 percent of all patients with molar pregnancy develop choriocarcinoma. Choriocarcinoma of the placenta is preceded by – Hydatidiform mole in 50 percent of cases, spontaneous abortion in 20 percent of cases, Ectopic pregnancy in 20 percent of cases and Normal term pregnancy in 20 to 30 percent cases.

Pathology

Characteristic feature is the identification of intimately related syncytiotrophoblasts and cytotrophoblasts without formation of definite placenta type villi.

Placental Site Trophoblastic Tumor

The tumor arises from the trophoblasts of the placental bed. Incidence is about 1 percent of all patients with GTN. 15 to 20 percent of these patients develop metastasis. Intermediate trophoblast cells are predominant. α-hCG secretion is low but human placental lactogen (HPL) is secreted and this is monitored during follow-up. Hysterectomy is the preferred treatment. This neoplasm is not responsive to chemotherapy.

Persistent Trophoblastic Disease (PTD)

The term persistent trophoblastic disease (PTD) is used when after treatment of a molar pregnancy, some molar tissue is left behind which again starts growing into a tumor. Patient presents with irregular vaginal bleeding, subinvolution of uterus, persistence of theca lutein cysts and elevation of hCG (after molar evacuation serum β-hCG becomes normal in about 7 to 9 weeks). Majority of these patients need treatment with chemotherapy (90%). About 10 percent of patients can be treated successfully with a second curettage.

Spread of GTN

Apart from the local spread, vascular erosion takes place early and hence metastases occur rapidly. The common sites of metastases are lungs, anterior vaginal wall, brain, and liver.

Clinical Features of GTN

Clinical features depend on the location of the primary growth and on its secondary deposits.

❖ History of molar pregnancy in the recent past. It is rarely related to a term pregnancy, abortion or ectopic pregnancy. GTN after a molar pregnancy is always a choriocarcinoma
❖ Persistent ill health
❖ Hyperemesis
❖ Irregular vaginal bleeding, at times brisk
❖ Uneven swelling of the uterus
❖ Cough breathlessness and hemoptysis with lung involvement
❖ Head ache, convulsion and paralysis with cerebral involvement
❖ Epigastric pain and jaundice with liver involvement
❖ Pallor of varying degree
❖ On bimanual examination—subinvolution of uterus is seen. There may be a purplish-red

Table 70.3	FIGO anatomical staging of gestational trophoblastic tumor (GTT)
Stage I	The lesion is confined to the uterus.
Stage II	The lesion spreads outside the uterus, but is confined to the genital organs.
Stage III	The lesion metastasizes to the lungs.
Stage IV	The lesion metastasizes to sites such as brain, liver or gastrointestinal tract.

nodule in the lower-third of the anterior vaginal wall. Unilateral or bilateral enlarged ovaries palpable through lateral fornices.

❖ On chest X-ray, multiple infiltrates of various shapes in both lungs giving a "snow storm" appearance and pleural effusion may be present.

❖ Raised level of serum hCG and urine hCG.

❖ Pelvic sonography helps to localize the lesion.

The anatomical staging is described in Table 70.3.

Management of GTN

Preventive

❖ Prophylactic chemotherapy following evacuation of molar pregnancy to "at risk" women who are:
  – Age over 35 years
  – Initial serum hCG ≥100,000 u/ml
  – hCG level fails to become normal in 7 to 9 weeks or there is an elevation
  – Previous history of molar pregnancy
  – Unable for follow-up.

❖ Meticulous follow-up following evacuation of hydatidiform mole for at least 6 months, to detect early evidence of GTN

❖ Selective hysterectomy in hydatidiform mole—women over 35 years

❖ Diagnostic uterine curettage in unexplained abnormal bleeding 8 weeks following term delivery or abortion.

Curative

❖ Chemotherapy
  – Single drug regimen in low-risk cases (Stage I) using Methotrexate or Folinic acid.
  – Combination therapy for stages II, III and IV based on individualized assessment. Drugs include Methotrexate, Folinic acid, Actinomycin D, Cyclophosphamide and Vincritine.

❖ Surgery
  – Hysterectomy for lesions confined to the uterus in women above 35 years, with intractable hemorrhage or in whom accidental perforation occurred during uterine curettage
  – Lung resection in pulmonary metastasis, in drug resistant cases
  – Craniotomy for control of bleeding.

❖ Radiation
  – Whole brain radiation for patient's with brain metastasis
  – Whole liver radiation along with chemotherapy in hepatic metastasis.

Prognosis: Most women whose cancer has not spread can be cured and will maintain reproductive function. Complete cure is harder if:
  – The disease has spread to liver or brain.
  – hCG level is > 40,000 m U/L when treatment begins
  – Cancer recurred after chemotherapy
  – Carcinoma occurred after a pregnancy that resulted in the birth of a baby (GTD coexisting with a normal fetus).

Prevention of Recurrence and Follow-up

For prevention of recurrence, additional chemotherapy following normalization of hCG level is recommended as follows:

Non metastatic disease—one cycle

Metastatic disease: Two to three cycles based on the assessment of prognosis.

Follow-up is mandatory for all patients at least for 2 years. Serum hCG levels are to be monitored weekly for three months, monthly for six months and six monthly for life. Future conception is recommended after one year of completion of treatment with instruction for regular check ups.

CANCER OF CERVIX

Cancer cervix is the most common cancer in women of the developing countries where screening facilities are inadequate. It is a preventable disease as the different screening, diagnostic and therapeutic procedures are effective. Incidence of cervical cancer is steadily decreasing in the developed world.

The incidence in India according to the 2004 ICMR report was between 14 to 24 percent of all female cancers. Major factors affecting the prevalence of carcinoma cervix in a population are economic factor, sexual behavior and degree of effective screening.

Epidemiology

Worldwide, cervical cancer is twelfth most common and fifth most deadly cancer in women. It affects about 16 per 100,000 women per year and kills about 9 per 100,000 each year. Approximately 80 percent of cervical cancers occur in developing countries.

Causes

Human papilloma virus infection (HPV) is a necessary factor in the development of all cases of cervical cancer.

Other co-factors and risk factors provided by the American Cancer Society include:

- HIV infection, Chlamydia infection, hormonal contraception, exposure to the hormonal drug diethyl stillbestrol and family history of cervical cancer
- Early age at first intercourse and first pregnancy are also considered risk factors.

Signs and Symptoms

Patients are usually multiparous, in premenopausal age group. The early stages of cervical cancer may be completely asymptomatic. They have previous history of postcoital or intermenstrual bleeding which they ignored.

- Vaginal bleeding: Irregular or continued and contact bleeding
- Offensive vaginal discharge
- Pelvic pain of varying degree due to involvement of uterosacral ligament or sacral plexus
- Leg edema due to progressive obstruction of lymphatics and/or ileofemoral veins by the tumor
- Back pain and leg pain

- Bladder symptoms such as frequency of micturition, dysuria, hematuria or true incontinence due to fistula formation
- Rectal involvement symptoms such as diarrhea, rectal pain, bleeding per rectum or even rectovaginal fistula
- Frequent attacks of pyelonephritis due to ureteric obstruction
- In late stages, patient may be cachetic and anemic with edema of legs
- Uremia in advanced stage.

Diagnosis

- Pap smear is an effective screening test
- Speculum examination reveals the nature of the growth: Ulcerative or fungating or bleeds on touch
- Bimanual examination reveals the induration and extent of growth to the vagina and to the sides
- Rectal examination to note the involvement of parametrium and extent to the lateral pelvic wall
- Biopsy for confirmation of diagnosis. Wedge biopsy is done for small lesion which includes a portion of the healthy tissue as well. If the lesion is big and infected, a bit of tissue from the noninfected area is taken
- Ancillary aids for staging are cystoscopy, chest X-ray, intravenous pyelography and proctoscopy
- MRI and PET scanning are used to detect parametrial extension and to define the tumor volume.

Diagnosis of Precancerous Lesions

Cervical intraepithelial neoplasia (CIN), the potential precursor to cervical cancer is often diagnosed on examination of biopsies. For premalignant dysplastic changes, the CIN grading is used. It classifies mild dysplasia as CIN_1, moderate dysplasia as CIN_2 and severe dysplasia as CIN_3 in a pathology report. Histologic subtypes of invasive carcinoma of cervix are the following:

- Squamous cell carcinoma
- Adenocarcinoma
- Adenosquamous carcinoma
- Small cell carcinoma
- Neuroendocrine carcinoma

Staging

Cervical cancer is staged by the International Federation of Gynecology and Obstetrics (FIGO) based on clinical examination (Table 70.4). Diagnostic tests used in determining the stages are colposcopy, proctoscopy, endometrial curettage, hysteroscopy, cystoscopy, intravenous urography, X-ray of lungs and skeleton and cervical conization.

Complications

The following complications may occur sooner or later as the lesion progresses.
❖ Hemorrhage
❖ Frequent attacks of ureteric pain due to pyometra especially with endocervical variety
❖ Vesicovaginal fistula
❖ Rectovaginal fistula—this is a comparatively rare complication.
❖ Cystitis pyelonephritis and bladder dysfunction.

Management

Primary Prevention

❖ Identifying high-risk women
  – History of early sexual intercourse
  – History of age of first pregnancy
  – History of too many or too frequent birth
  – Low socioeconomic status
  – Poor maintenance of local hygiene
  – Sexually transmitted oncogenes (HPV and HSV type II).
❖ Identifying high risk men (spouses)
  – Multiple sex partners
  – Previous wife died of cancer.
❖ Employing positive measures.
  – Use of condom during early intercourse
  – Raise the age of marriage and first childbirth
  – Limitation of family size
  – Maintenance of local hygiene
  – Effective treatment of STD.

Secondary Prevention

❖ Screening: The widespread introduction of screening for cervical cancer using. Papanicolau test (papsmear) has been found to reduce the incidence and mortality of cervical cancer in developed countries. It is recommended to start testing 3 or more years after first sex.

Treatment

The types of treatment employed for the invasive cancer are:
– Primary surgery
– Primary radiotherapy
– Chemotherapy and
– Combination therapy.
❖ Stage IA (Microinvasive cancer) is usually treated by hysterectomy (removal of the whole uterus including part of the vagina)
❖ Stage IA$_2$: In addition to hysterectomy, the lymph nodes are also removed. For patients who desire to remain fertile, a local surgical procedure called *"loop electrical excision procedure"* (LEEP) or cone biopsy is done. Another surgical option for patients who want to preserve fertility is *trachelectomy*
❖ For Stages IB$_1$ and IIA less than 4 cm can be treated with *radical hysterectomy* with removal of lymph nodes and radiation therapy. Radiation therapy with or without chemotherapy is given for patients who show high-risk features on pathologic

Table 70.4	Staging of cervical cancer FIGO
Stage 0	Full thickness involvement of the epithelium without invasion into the stroma (cancer *in situ*)
Stage I	Limited to the cervix
Stage IA	Diagnosed only by microscopy; no visible lesions
Stage IA$_1$	Stromal invasion less than 3 mm in depth and 7 mm or less in horizontal spread
Stage IB	Visible lesion or a microscopic lesion with more than 5 mm of depth or horizontal spread of more than 7 mm
Stage IB$_1$	Visible lesion 4 cm or less in greater dimension
Stage IB$_2$	Visible lesion more than 4 cm
Stage II	Invades beyond cervix
Stage IIA	Without parametrial invasion but involve upper 2/3 of vagina
Stage IIB	With parametrial invasion
Stage III	Extends to pelvic wall or lower third of vagina
Stage IIIA	Involves lower third of vagina
Stage IIIB	Extends to pelvic wall and/or causes hydronephrosis or nonfunctioning kidney
Stage IV	Extends outside the vagina
Stage IVA	Invades mucosa of bladder or rectum
Stage IVB	Distant metastasis

examination. Tumors more than 4 cm can be treated with radiation therapy and cisplatin based chemotherapy followed by hysterectomy.

Prognosis

Prognosis depends on the stage of cancer. With treatment, the 5 year relative survival rate for the earliest stage of invasive cancer is 92 percent and overall (all stages combined) 5 year survival rate is 72 percent.

According to the International Federation of Gynecology and obstetrics (FIGO), survival improves when radiotherapy is combined with Cisplatin based chemotherapy.

As the cancer metastasizes to other parts of the body, prognosis drops drastically because treatment of local lesions is generally more effective than the whole body treatment such as chemotherapy.

CANCER OF THE VULVA

Vulval cancer is an abnormal growth of malignant cells (neoplasm, tumor) in the vulva. The vulva is defined as the female external genitalia and includes the labia majora, labia minora, clitoris and vestibule.

Incidence

The lesion is rare, about 1.7/100,000. About 70 percent of vulval cancers involve the labia majora, 15 to 20 percent involves the clitoris and another 15 to 20 percent involves the perineum. In about 5 percent of cases, the cancer is present at more than one site.

Etiology

The etiology remains unclear but the following factors are seen related.

- Usually seen in postmenopausal women with median age of 60
- More common among whites
- Increased association with obesity, diabetes, hypertension and nulliparity
- Associated with local lesions such as chronic vulval dystrophy of atypical type
- Human papilloma virus
- Condyloma accuminata, herpes simplex, syphilis and lymphogranuloma venereum

- Chronic pruritus and poor hygiene
- Malignancies in other sites of genital tract.

Types of Vulval Cancer

- Squamous cell carcinoma: The vast majority (90%) of vulval cancers are squamous cell carcinomas which originate from the epidermis of the vulval tissue. Carcinoma *in situ* is a precursor stage of squamous cell cancer prior to invading through the basement membrane. Most lesions originate in the labia majora. Other areas affected are the clitoris, fourchette and the local glands. Squamous cell lesions tend to grow with local extension and spread via local lymph system. The tumor may also invade adjacent organs such as the vagina, urethra and rectum and spread via their lymphatics.
- Melanoma: About 5 percent of vulval malignancy is caused by melanoma of the vulva. Such melanomas behave like melanomas in other locations and may affect a much younger population. Melanomas have a risk of metastasis unlike squamous cell carcinomas.
- Basal cell carcinoma: Basal cell carcinoma constitute about 1 to 2 percent of vulval cancer. It is a slowly growing lesion and affects the elderly. It behaves similar to basal cell carcinoma in other locations that is it spreads to grow locally with low potential of deep invasion or metastasis.
- Other lesions: Vulvar lesion can be caused by other lesions such as adenocarcinoma or sarcoma.

Clinical Features

- The lesion is present in the form of a lump or ulceration, often associated with itching, irritation and some times local bleeding and discharge
- Dysuria, dyspareunia and pain in the vulvar region
- Melanomas have a typical dark discoloration
- Adenocarcinomas may arise from the Bartholin gland and appear as a painful lump

- Inguinal lymph glands of one or both sides may be enlarged and palpable if there is associated infection.
- Vulval ulceration which bleeds on touching.
- Edematous, indurated tissue surrounding the lesion.

Diagnosis

- Examination of the vulva
- Biopsy from the margin
- Supplemental evaluation including chest X-ray, IVP, cystoscopy and proctoscopy.

Staging

The clinical staging as outlined by FIGO is tabulated below (Table 70.5).

Table 70.5	Staging of vulval carcinoma, FIGO 1995
Stage 0	Carcinoma-*in situ*, Intraepithelial carcinoma (VIN-3)
Stage I	Tumor confined to the vulva and/or perineum – 2 cm or less in greatest dimension, nodes are not palpable
Stage I A	Stromal invasion no greater than 1 mm
Stage I B	Stromal invasion greater than 1 mm
Stage II	Tumor confined to the vulva and/or perineum – more than 2 mm in greatest dimension. Nodes are not palpable
Stage III	Tumor of any size with: (1) Adjacent spread to the lower urethra and/or vagina or the anus (2) Unilateral regional node metastasis.
Stage IV	A. Tumor invades any of the following: Upper urethra, bladder mucosa, rectal mucosa, pelvic bone and/or bilateral regional node metastasis B. Any distant metastasis including pelvic lymph nodes.

Treatment

- Adequate treatment for persistent pruritus vulva in postmenopausal women
- Simple vulvectomy for advanced cancers, where the disease has spread to adjacent organs such as urethra, vagina and rectum
- Radiation therapy and chemotherapy are usually not a primary choice of therapy but may be used in selected cases of advanced cancer
- Chemotherapy followed by surgery, radiotherapy or both.

Prognosis

With negative groin nodes, the 5 year survival rate is about 75 percent of course it depends on factors such as stage, and type of lesion, age and general health. Five year survival rate is about 20 percent when pelvic lymph nodes are involved.

BARTHOLIN GLAND CANCER

A distinct mass or lump on either side of the opening to the vagina can be the sign of Bartholin gland carcinoma. A lump in this area may some times be a Bartholin gland cyst which is more common. Treatment is surgery like that of squamous cell carcinoma of the vulva.

VAGINAL CANCER

There are two main types of primary vaginal cancers and they are named after the cells from which they develop:
- Squamous cell carcinoma: This is the most common type of vaginal cancer and found in the upper part of the vagina. It affects women between the ages of 50 and 70. Exact etiology is unknown. Following factors are often related.
  - Human papilloma virus
  - Progression from vaginal intraepithelial neoplasia (VIN)
  - Previous irradiation therapy to the vagina or immunosuppression
  - Prolonged use of pessary.
- Clear cell carcinoma: This type of carcinoma is found in adolescent girls who have had history of intrauterine exposure to diethyl stillbestrol in first trimester.

The risk of developing clear cell adenocarcinoma of the vagina following DES exposure is 1 in 1000 or less. These patients are more likely to develop adenomyosis and rarely adenocarcinoma. The lesion usually involves the upper third of the anterior vaginal wall.

Treatment is radical hysterectomy and vaginectomy with pelvic lymphadenectomy. Radio therapy is reserved for advanced cases.

Signs and Symptoms of Primary Vaginal Cancer

The mean age of the patient is 55 years. The cancer may be asymptomatic, being accidentally discovered during routine screening procedure. The most common symptoms are:

* Blood stained vaginal discharge
* Postcoital vaginal bleeding and pain
* Urinary frequency, nocturia and hematuria
* Foul smelling vaginal discharge
* Rectal pain.

On vaginal examination:

* Ulcerative, nodular or exophytic growth.

Diagnosis

* Smear test for cytology
* Colposcopic examination and biopsy
* Biopsy from clinically suspected lesion
* CT scan
* MRI scan.

Staging

The clinical staging as outlined by FIGO is tabulated below (Table 70.6)

Table 70.6	Staging of vaginal carcinoma, FIGO 1995
Stage 0	Carcinoma *in situ*
Stage I	Carcinoma is limited to the vaginal wall
Stage II	Carcinoma has involved subvaginal tissue, but has not extended to the pelvic wall
Stage IV	Carcinoma has extended beyond the true pelvis or has involved the mucosa of bladder or rectum
Stage IVA	Adjacent organs are involved—bladder, rectum
Stage IVB	Distant organs are involved.

Treatment

The treatment for vaginal cancer depends on a number of factors including age, general health, stage (size and extent of spread) grade (microscopic appearance) and the type of cancer. Radiotherapy, surgery and chemotherapy are used separately or in combination.

Surgery

* For growth limited to upper-third: Radical hysterectomy, partial vaginectomy, bilateral vaginal lymphadenectomy

* For growth limited to the lower-third: Radical vulvectomy with removal of bilateral inguinofemoral lymph nodes along with partial vaginectomy
* For growth limited to middle-third: Radiation by external beam therapy with intracavity or interstitial radiation: Care to be taken to prevent bladder or rectal injury.
* In cases of failure with radiation therapy, pelvic exteneration operation (very extensive surgery) can be done.

Radiotherapy

For many patients with cancer vagina, radiotherapy is the most suitable treatment. In younger women, radiotherapy may be combined with chemotherapy which is known as chemoradiation.

Teletherapy, a method of external radiation is administered on the pelvis encompassing the vagina. Additional radiation is delivered locally in the form of interstitial therapy or brachytherapy with iridium.

External radiation reduces the tumor volume and sterilizes the regional lymph nodes. Complications of radiotherapy include vaginal stenosis, and bladder and rectal fistulae.

Prognosis

The overall 5 year survival rate ranges from 80 percent for stage I disease to 10 percent for stage IV disease.

CANCER OF FALLOPIAN TUBE

Primary fallopian tube cancer is the rarest of all gynecologic cancers representing less than 1 percent. It is an abnormal growth of malignant cells in one or both of a woman's fallopian tubes.

Fallopian tube cancers are found in women between 60 and 64 years of age but can also manifest in women in their mid 80's.

Pathology

The site is usually the ampullary part and the mucosa. Fimbrial end usually gets blocked resulting in hydrosalpinx. It is unilateral in 80 percent and mostly adenocarcinoma. In most cases, cancer that affects the fallopian tubes originates from some other part of the uterus like the cervix or endometrium. The cancer cells metastasize and then spread to the tubes.

Clinical Manifestations

* Patients are usually postmenopausal and nulliparous.
* History of infertility and pelvic infection.
* Vaginal bleeding after menopause.
* Colicky pain in lower abdomen
* Intermittent vaginal discharge that is white, clear, watery or pink in color
* On bimanual examination, unilateral mass which may be tender.

Diagnosis

* Many cases of fallopian tube cancer are accidentally discovered on laparotomy and histologic examination of the excised tube
* Clinical features as mentioned above
* CA 125 test which measures the level of blood protein that is linked to certain gynecological cancers
* A CT scan and ultrasound examination of the pelvic region and uterus
* Laparoscopy in case of persistent post-menopausal bleeding with a negative cervical and endometrial pathology
* Ultrasound can help in the peoperative diagnosis.

Treatment

* Total hysterectomy with bilateral salpingo-oophorectomy along with omentectomy
* External pelvic radiation following surgery
* Chemotherapy after surgery to destroy residual tumor cells.

Prognosis

The prognosis is mostly unfavorable due to late diagnosis. The five year survival ranges between 25 to 40 percent.

SECONDARY FALLOPIAN TUBE CANCER

Secondary fallopian tube cancers are more common (90%) than the primary. The common primary sites are ovary, uterus, breast and gastrointestinal tract. The mode of spread from the ovary or uterus is probably by lymphatics rather than direct spread. Diagnosis and treatment are same as for primary fallopian tube cancer.

Nursing Management of Patients with Genital Malignancies

Nursing management includes those related to the patient's treatment plan which may include surgery, chemotherapy, radiation, palliation or combination of these. Emotional support, comfort measures, and information plus attentiveness and caring are important components of nursing care for the patient and her family.

Nursing interventions after pelvic surgery to remove the tumor are similar to those after other abdominal surgeries. Patients with pelvic organ cancer may develop ascites and pleural effusion. Nursing care may include administering IV fluids prescribed to alleviate fluid and electrolyte imbalance, administering parenteral nutrition to provide adequate nutrition, providing postoperative care after intestinal bypass to avoid any obstruction, controlling pain and managing drainage tubes. Comfort measures may include providing small frequent meals, decreasing fluid intake, administering diuretic agents and providing rest.

Nursing Diagnoses

The possible, major nursing diagnoses include the following:

* Anxiety related to the diagnosis of cancer and surgery
* Acute pain related to the surgical incision and subsequent wound care
* Impaired skin integrity related to the wound and drainage
* Sexual dysfunction related to change in body image
* Self-care deficit related to lack of understanding of health status and care needs
* Deficient knowledge of the perioperative aspects and postoperative self-care.

71

Special Gynecological Conditions

Learning Objectives

Upon completion of this chapter, the learner will be able to:
* Discuss the pathological changes manifestations and management of adenomyosis, endometriosis and dyspareunia
* Describe the physiological changes, symptoms and management of females in puberty and menopause.

ADENOMYOSIS

Adenomyosis is a condition where there is ingrowth of the endometrium directly into the myometrium. It is an ectopic occurrence of adenomatous tissue in the uterine muscle.

Pathology

The growth and tissue reaction in the endometrium depend on the response of ectopic endometrial tissue to the ovarian hormones. The response to hormones is minimal if the basal layer only is involved and marked if the functional layer is involved. There is hyperplasia of the myometrium producing diffuse enlargement of the uterus sometimes symmetrically but at times more on the posterior wall. The growth may be localized or diffuse. When localized, it may grow to the size of a large orange or 12 to 14 weeks pregnant uterus. Unlike fibroid, there is no capsule surrounding the growth.

Clinical Features

In about one-third, the condition remains asymptomatic. Patients are usually parous with age over 40.

* Menorrhagia (70%): Excessive bleeding occurs due to bigger uterine cavity associated with endometrial hyperplasia and inadequate uterine contraction
* Dysmenorrhea (30%) colicky pain during menses probably due to disturbed myometrial contraction
* Frequency of micturition
* Dyspareunia
* On abdominal examination, mass may be felt in the midline arising out of the pelvis
* On pelvic examination, uniform uterine enlargement
* Ultrasound and Color Doppler examination may reveal: heterogenous echogenecity, hypoechoic myometrium with multiple small cysts and increased vascularity within the myometrium
* Magnetic resonance imaging will reveal thickened junctional zone in the myometrium.

Treatment

* Levonorgestrel—releasing IUS to improve the menorrhagia and dysmenorrhea.
* Conservative surgery for partial resection of adenomyomata.
* Hysterectomy for parous and aged women.

ENDOMETRIOSIS

Endometriosis is a chronic disorder resulting from the implantation of endometrial tissue (glands and stroma) outside the uterus.

Common Sites (Fig. 71.1)

* Pelvic sites of endometrial tissue include the cervix, pouch of Douglas, ovaries,

Fig. 71.1: Common sites of endometriosis

fallopian tubes, pelvic peritoneum, broad ligaments and sigmoid colon

❖ Distant sites of endometrial tissue implantation occur less commonly and can include the abdominal wall, kidneys, spleen, gall bladder, diaphragm, lungs, stomach or breasts.

Prevalence

The disorder affects nearly one in 10 women of childbearing age. The incidence is high in infertile women, about 30 to 40 percent. Delayed marriage, postponement of first conception and adoption of small family norm are contributing factors for increased prevalence.

Pathology

❖ The endometrium in the ectopic sites has the potentiality to undergo changes under the action of ovarian hormones

❖ Cyclic growth and shedding continue till menopause (Each of the sites will bleed during the menstrual cycle). The periodically shed blood may remain encysted or the cyst may become tense and rupture

❖ There is dense tissue reaction surrounding the lesion (where bleeding occurred) with fibrosis. If the fibrosis occurs on the pelvic peritoneum, it produces adhesions

❖ If the blood gets encysted, the cyst enlarges with cyclic bleeding and the content inside becomes chocolate colored. Those are called endometrial cysts or endometriomas. Because of the color the term 'chocolate cysts' may also be used

❖ Depending on the location, size and reaction, the lesions appear differently as:
  – Small, black dots like 'powder burns' on uterosacral ligaments and pouch of Douglas
  – Red flame shaped, red polypoid or yellow brown patches on the peritoneum and surrounding tissues
  – Bluish lesions for endometriomas (chocolate cysts) in ovaries.

Clinical Features

❖ Patients are mostly nulliparous or have had one child

❖ Age is between 30 to 45

❖ Infertility or voluntary postponement of conception till late age

❖ Abnormal menstruation: Short menstrual cycles (less than 28 days), increased duration of bleeding (7 days or more), excessive bleeding (for at least 5 days) and significant cramping

❖ Pain, inflammation or pelvic heaviness depending on the location of endometrial tissue implantation, duration of the disorder and the phase of menstrual cycle

❖ Bladder-frequency, dysuria or hematuria

❖ Sigmoid colon and rectum—painful defecation (dyschezia), diarrhea, rectal bleeding, dyspareunia

❖ Chronic fatigue and premenstrual syndrome.

Diagnosis

❖ Classic symptoms of progressively increasing dysmenorrhea, dyspareunia and infertility

❖ Pelvic examination findings of nodules in the pouch of Douglas, uterosacral ligaments, fixed retroverted uterus and unilateral or bilateral adnexal mass

❖ Ultrasonography: Transvaginal and endorectal ultrasound are found better for diagnosing rectosigmoid endometriosis

❖ Laparoscopy and biopsy.

Complications

The following complications may occur:
- Infertility
- Rupture of chocolate cysts
- Infection of chocolate cyst
- Obstructive features
  - Ureteral infection → hydroureter → hydronephrosis → renal infection
  - Intestinal obstruction.

Treatment

Therapeutic interventions are focused on stopping the progressive destruction of pelvic organs caused by endometrial implants and preserving fertility options for the woman.

Medical

- Encourage married women with family history of endometriosis not to delay first conception and to complete the family
- NSAIDS to control pain by reducing prostaglandin production by the endometrial implants during menses
- Gonadotropin releasing hormone (GnRH) to prevent release of luteinizing hormone (LH), thus causing temporary cessation of menstruation
- Combined estrogen and progesterone: Low dose oral contraceptives help to reduce the growth and pain of endometriosis.

Surgical

Endometriosis with severe symptoms unresponsive to hormone therapy is treated surgically.
- Endometrial ablation or removal of endometrial implants with laser or electrocautery for those who need to preserve childbearing capacity
- Hysterectomy with bilateral salpingo-oophorectomy along with resection of endometrial tissues as complete as possible for women who have completed the family.

DYSPAREUNIA

Dyspareunia is a sexual dysfunction characterized by difficult and painful sexual intercourse.

Male Causes

- Impotence
- Premature ejaculation
- Congenital anatomic defect of the penis
- Improper technique of coital act.

Female Causes

a. Superficial or entrance dyspareunia
   - Narrow introitus
   - Tough hymen
   - Bartholin gland cysts
   - Tender perineal scar
   - Vulval infection
   - Urethral infection
   - Vestibulitis.
b. Vaginal causes: This produces burning pain along the barrel of vagina either during intercourse or following intercourse. The conditions are:
   - Vaginitis
   - Vaginal septum
   - Tender scar following delivery or gynecological operation
   - Secondary vaginal atresia
   - Vaginal atrophy due to menopause
   - Growth or tumor.
c. Deep causes: With deep causes the patient experiences pain while the penis penetrates deep into the vagina. Deep pain usually results from pathology of paravaginal tissues or pelvic organs. Such lesions are:
   - Endometriosis on rectovaginal septum
   - Chronic cervicitis
   - Chronic PID
   - Retroverted and fixed uterus
   - Ovary prolapsed in the pouch of Douglas.

Treatment

Treatment is given according to the cause and the measures are:
- Sex education of both partners
- Treatment of the infective lesion
- Excision of scar tissue on the perineum and vagina
- Surgical correction of retroversion of uterus or prolapsed ovary.

PUBERTY

Puberty is the period of life during which secondary sex characteristics develop and the capability of sexual reproduction are attained. It is the period which links childhood to adulthood.

Physical Changes in Girls

Certain important physical changes are evident during puberty. These are breast development, pubic and axillary hair growth, growth in height and starting of menstruation. Most of the changes occur gradually and only menarche can be dated. The changes follow a common order beginning with a growth spurt and the last one is menstruation.

The factors that control the onset of puberty are genetic, nutrition, body weight, psychological state, social and cultural back ground and exposure to light.

Pubertal Changes in Boys

In male, pubertal sexual maturation is based on genital size and pubic hair development. The changes are:
- Testicular enlargement
- Increase in length and diameter of penis
- Growth of curly hair around the base of penis and over the genital area
- Symmetric or asymmetric gynecomastia
- Appearance of mature spermatozoa in microscopic urinalysis.

Stages of Pubertal Development in Girls (Tanner Stages)

Stage: 1 Prepubertal Stage

No palpable breast tissue, areola generally less than 2 cm in diameter. Nipples may be inverted, flat or raised. No pubic hair.

Stage: 2

Breast budding occurs with a visible and palpable mound of breast tissue. The areolae begin to enlarge and nipples develop to varying degree. Sparse long hair on either side of labia majora

Stage: 3

Further growth of entire breast tissue: Darker, coarser and curly hair over the mons pubis

Stage: 4

Secondary mound of areola and papillae projecting over the breast tissue, Adult type hair covering the mons pubis

Stage: 5

Areola recessed to general contour of breast. Adult hair with an inverse triangle distribution.

Endocrinology in Puberty

- Hypothalamopituitary gonadal axis: As puberty approaches, the hypothalamic centers involved in the release of gonadotropin releasing hormone (GnRH) becomes more and more sensitive to the feedback of ovarian steroids. There is augmented GnRH pulse release. This results in gradually increasing gonadotropin secretion → increasing ovarian stimulation → increasing estrogen levels → tonic and pulsatile release of gonadotropins. This increasing level of estrogen is responsible for the growth and initiation of thelarche (breast budding) and finally menarche
- Thyroid gland plays an active role in the hypothalamopituitary gonadal axis
- Adrenal glands increase their activity of sex steroid synthesis (androstenedione). Increased sebum formation, pubic and axillary hair and change in voice are primarily due to adrenal androgen production
- Gonadal estrogen is responsible for the development of uterus, vagina, vulva and also the breasts in girls
- Testosterone secretion from testes increases in boys
- Growth hormone secretion increases along with gonadotropin at the onset of puberty.

Menarche

Menarche is the onset of first menstruation in life. It may occur any time between 10 and 16 years, the peak time being 13 years. The endometrium which proliferates due to stimulation of ovarian estrogen sheds when the level (of estrogen) drops and visible bleeding occurs.

The first period is usually anovular and ovulation may be irregular for a variable period following menarche. The menses may be irregular and short to start with and it may take about two years for regular ovulation to occur.

Growth

Growth in height in an adolescent girl occurs mainly due to hormones. The important hormones are growth hormone, estrogen and insulin-like growth factor.

Genital Organ Changes

Ovaries: Shape changes from elongated to ovoid and becomes bulky due to follicular enlargement and proliferation of stromal cells.

Uterus: Enlargement of the body of uterus occurs. Uterine body to cervix ratio becomes 1:1 when menarche occurs and thereafter rapid enlargement of the body occurs so that the ratio becomes 2:1.

Vagina: The epithelium becomes thick with many layers. The cells become rich with glycogen. Doderlein's bacilli appear which convert glycogen into lactic acid. The vaginal pH becomes acidic ranging between 4 and 5.

Vulva: Vulva becomes more reactive to steroid hormone.

Mons pubis and labia minora: Increase in size.

Breast changes: Marked proliferation of duct systems and deposition of fat occurs under the influence of estrogen. Breasts become prominent and round. Under the influence of progesterone the development of acini increases.

The commonly seen disorders of puberty are precocious puberty and delayed puberty.

In precocious puberty, girls exhibit secondary sex characteristics before the age of 8 or menstruate before the age of 10.

In delayed puberty, development of breast tissue and/or pubic hair does not occur by 13 to 14 years or menarche does not happen as late as 16 years.

These conditions need to be investigated to find the cause which may often be hormonal and treated accordingly.

MENOPAUSE

Menopause is defined as permanent physiologic cessation of menstruation at the end of reproductive life due to loss of ovarian follicular activity. It is the point of time when last and final menstruation occurs.

Climacteric is the phase of aging process during which a woman passes from the reproductive to the nonreproductive stage. This phase covers 5 to 10 years on either side of menopause.

Premenopause is the part of the climacteric before menopause, when the menstrual cycle is likely to be irregular. Postmenopause is the phase that comes after the menopause.

Age of Menopause

Age of menopause is genetically predetermined. The age of menopause ranges between 45 to 55 years, average being 50 years. Cigarette smoking and severe malnutrition may cause early menopause.

Endocrinology of Climacteric and Menopause

❖ Few years prior to menopause, depletion of ovarian follicles occurs and the existing follicles become resistant to gonadotropins. This results in impaired folliculogenesis and diminished estradiol production. The serum estradiol level falls from 50 to 300 pg/ml before menopause to 10 to 20 pg/ml after menopause. This decreases the negative feedback effect on hypothalamopituitary axis resulting in increase in FSH

❖ The diminished folliculogenesis result in anovulation, oligo-ovulation and corpus luteum insufficiency. The sustained level of estrogens may cause endometrial hyperplasia and menstrual abnormalities

- Shortening of the follicular phase leads shorter menstrual cycles
- There is fall in the levels of prolactin and inhibitin
- Ultimately, there are no more follicles responsive to gonadotropins. Estradiol production drops and endometrial growth stops resulting in absence of menstruation.

Organ Changes

- Genitourinary system
  - *Ovaries* shrink in size, become wrinkled and white. Thinning of cortex and abundance of stroma cells occur
  - *Fallopian tubes* show features of atrophy. The muscle coat becomes thinner, the cilia disappear and the plicae become less prominent
  - *The uterus* becomes smaller, endometrium becomes thin and atrophic. The cervical secretion becomes scanty
  - *The vagina* becomes narrower due to gradual loss of elasticity. The rugae progressively flatten. There is no glycogen and Doderlein's bacillus. The vaginal pH becomes alkaline
  - *The vulva* shows features of atrophy. The labium becomes flattened and the pubic hair becomes scantier resulting in a narrow introitus
  - *Breast* fat gets reabsorbed and the glands atrophy. The nipples decrease in size, the breasts become flat and pendulous
  - *Bladder and urethra:* The epithelium becomes thin and is more prone to damage and infection
  - *Loss of muscle tone* leads to pelvic relaxation, uterine descend and anatomic changes in the urethra and neck of bladder.
- Skeletal system: Following menopause, there is loss of bone mass by about 3 to 5 percent per year due to deficiency of estrogen leading to osteoporosis.
- Cardiovascular system: Deficiency of estrogen increases the risk of cardiovascular disease because of its function of

decreasing HDL cholesterol and antioxidant property.

Menstruation Pattern Prior to Menopause

Any of the following patterns may be observed prior to menopause.
- Abrupt cessation of menstruation
- Gradual decrease in both amount and duration
- Irregular with or without excessive bleeding.

Menopausal Symptoms

Majority of women do not experience any symptom apart from cessation of menstruation. Some women experience symptoms and health concerns.
- Vasomotor symptoms: The characteristic symptom of menopause is "hot flush". It is characterized by sudden feeling of heat followed by profuse sweating with cutaneous vasodilatation.
- Genital and urinary symptoms: Atrophy of the epithelium of vagina, urinary bladder and urethra causes dyspareunia, vaginal infections, dryness, pruritus and leukorrhea. Urinary symptoms include urgency, dysuria, stress incontinence and frequent urinary tract infections.
- Psychological symptoms: Estrogen deficiency is associated with decreased sexual desire. There may be psychological changes such as increased anxiety, headache, insomnia, irritability, dysphasia and depression. Dementia, mood swings and inability to concentrate are also seen.
- Osteoporosis: Osteoporosis occurs in postmenopausal women due to estrogen loss, deficiency of calcium and vitamin D or hereditary. Osteoporosis may lead to back pain, loss of height and kyphosis and fracture of bones. Fracture may involve vertebral body, femoral neck or distal forearm.
- Cardiovascular and cerebrovascular effects: Risks of ischemia, heart disease, coronary artery disease and stroke are increased due to atherosclerotic changes, vasoconstriction and thrombus formation.

Diagnosis of Menopause

❖ Cessation of menstruation for twelve consecutive months during climacteric
❖ Occurrence of hot flushes and night sweats
❖ Features of low estrogen on vaginal cytology
❖ Serum estradiol < 20 pg/ml
❖ Serum FSH and LH > 40 mlU/ml at one week interval for 3 times.

Management

❖ Counseling: Adequate explanation to every woman with symptoms may help understand and accept the changes. Those who have artificial and early menopause due to bilateral oophorectomy or radiation may require more reassurance.
❖ Nonhormonal treatment
 – Nutritious diet—balanced with protein and calcium
 – Supplementary calcium—total daily requirement of calcium is 1.5 gm
 – Exercise—walking, jogging and weight bearing exercises.
❖ To follow healthy lifestyle, health promotion and regular health screening.
 – Supplementation with vitamin D 400 – 800 IU/day
 – Cessation of smoking and alcohol
 – Hormone replacement therapy (HRT) – Replacement of estrogen and progestin are prescribed for women with premature ovarian failure, gonadal dysgenesis and surgical or radiation menopause.

Abnormal Menopause

❖ Premature menopause occurs at or below the age of 40. Treatment by substitution therapy is usually followed
❖ Delayed menopause—menopause does not occur beyond 55 years of age. Detailed investigations for any pelvic pathology and appropriate treatment are indicated
❖ Artificial menopause—permanent cessation of ovarian function as a result of surgical removal of ovaries or by radiation.

Nursing Implications for Menopausal Conditions

Nursing diagnoses are individualized to each woman and her specific menopausal condition. Applicable diagnoses may include:
❖ Pain (mild or moderate) related to specific menopausal condition
❖ Grief related to mid to late life losses
❖ Deficient knowledge related to limited experience regarding specific menopausal condition
❖ Ineffective coping related to lack of acceptance of prognosis (for specific menopausal condition).

Nursing Interventions for Women with Menopausal Conditions Include

❖ Education regarding reduction of risk factors
❖ Emphasizing prevention strategies
❖ Explaining therapeutic interventions to ensure successful compliance
❖ Education to focus on health promoting nutrition, maintenance of appropriate weight for height (BMI) and exercise.

BIBLIOGRAPHY

1. Bowmik AC. Medical instruments 3rd edn, New Delhi, BI publications (Pvt) Ltd 2005.
2. Dutta DC. Textbook of Gynecology, 5 edn, Kolkata; New Central Book Agency 2009.
3. Dutta DC. Textbook of Obstetrics, 5th edn, Kolkata; New Central Book Agency 2001.
4. Rao K. Textbook of Midwifery and Obstetrics for Nurses, Noida; Reed Elsevier India Private Limited 2011.
5. Kozier B, Erab G, et al. Fundamentals of Nursing, 3rd Edn, New Delhi; Dorling Kindersley (India) Pvt Ltd 2007.
6. Kumari N, Sharma S and Gupta P. A Textbook of Midwifery and Gynecological Nursing, Jalandhar City; S Vikas and Company, India 2010.
7. Littleton LY, Engebretsn JC. Maternity Nursing Care, Canada; Thmsn Delmar Learning, 2005.
8. Skidmore-Roth L Mosby's 2009 Nursing Drug Reference, NOida; Reed Elsevier India Private Limited 2009.
9. Smeltzer SC, Bare BG, et al. Textbook of Medical Surgical Nursing 11th Edn, New Delhi; Wolters Kluwer (India) Pvt Ltd 2008.
10. Pilliteri A. Maternal and Childhealth Nursing, 5th edn. Philadelphia; Lippincot Williams & Wilkins 2007.
11. Yadav A, Arora VS. Synopsis of Medical Instruments and Procedures, New Delhi; BI Publications (Pvt) Ltd 2003.

Appendix

Nursing Care Plans for Maternal-Neonatal Clients

I. NURSING DIAGNOSES FOR PRENATAL CLIENTS

Deficient Knowledge Related to Self-care Activities during Pregnancy

Definition

Inadequate understanding of information needed to practice health-related behaviors during pregnancy.

Assessment

- Age of patient
- Psychosocial aspects such as health beliefs, knowledge regarding pregnancy and learning ability
- Previous obstetric history, support system and coping pattern
- Mental status and orientation and memory.

Defining Characteristics

- Inability to follow through with instructions
- Inappropriate or exaggerated behaviors such as hostility, apathy and agitation
- Inadequate knowledge of care to be taken during pregnancy
- Verbalization of problems.

Expected Outcomes

- Patient will communicate need for more information
- Patient will demonstrate understanding of information taught
- Patient will demonstrate ability to perform new bahaviors learned
- Patient will continue to practice appropriate health-related behaviors after pregnancy.

Nursing Interventions

- Establish a trusting relationship and respect so that patient will be relaxed and be receptive to learning
- Communicate and negotiate realistic learning goals with the patient
- Assess patient's knowledge of pregnancy to establish a basis for nursing care plans
- Provide information/teaching tailoring the content to suit the patient's level of understanding
- Provide instructions to seek appropriate resource persons for obtaining comprehensive care during pregnancy
- Review exercise routines designed for pregnant women to enhance well being and improve muscle tone in preparation for child birth
- Review dietary intake during pregnancy based on physician's recommendations. Explain to patient that she needs an extra 300 calories per day, for a total of 2100 to 2400 calories per day.
- Instruct patient to avoid wearing constrictive clothing, using high-heeled shoes and taking nonprescription drugs. Constrictive clothing can decrease venous circulation and high-heeled shoes can increase the likelihood of back strain
- Discuss dangers of exposure to toxic chemicals or gases to avoid possible teratogenic effects on fetus
- Instruct the woman to contact physician or go to hospital if she experiences any danger signs or symptoms like:
  – Severe vomiting
  – Frequent and severe headache

- Epigastric pain
- Vision disturbances
- Swelling of fingers and face
- Altered or absent fetal movements after quickening
- Signs of vaginal tract or urinary infection
- Unusual or severe abdominal pain
- Fluid discharge from vagina
- Vaginal bleeding.

Evaluations for Expected Outcomes

❖ Patient expresses need for more information about self-care
❖ Patient establishes realistic goals
❖ Patient demonstrates understanding of matters taught
  - Follows appropriate exercises
  - Limits or stops smoking and/or consumption of alcohol if indicated
  - Obtains sufficient rest
  - Avoids areas that may contain toxic chemicals or gases
  - Stops wearing constrictive clothing and high-heeled shoes
  - Reports danger signals to physician promptly
  - Takes prenatal vitamins as prescribed.
❖ Patient demonstrates ability to perform health related behaviors learned
❖ Patient continues to practice health related behaviors after pregnancy.

Documentation

❖ Patient's knowledge of self-care activities
❖ Expressions indicating motivation to learn
❖ Teaching carried out and methods of teaching used
❖ Dietary intake reported or observed.
❖ Demonstration or return demonstration of skills
❖ Response to teaching observed.

Nausea and Vomiting Related to Physiological Changes of Pregnancy

Definition

A minor disorder of pregnancy is experienced by pregnant women between 4th and 16th week of gestation.

Assessment

❖ Characteristics and patterns of occurrence of nausea and vomiting
❖ Types of food and smell to which patient has intolerance
❖ Physical health status
❖ Patient's understanding of the physiological changes of pregnancy
❖ Support system available.

Defining Characteristics

❖ Change in appetite and pattern of eating
❖ Vomiting in the morning and/or later in the day
❖ Increased salivation
❖ Inability to retain food and fluids
❖ Fatigue and signs of dehydration.

Expected Outcomes

❖ Patient will identify the factors that aggravate vomiting
❖ Patient will appreciate the physiological changes of pregnancy that cause vomiting
❖ Patient will modify her eating habits
❖ Patient will adopt appropriate measures to obtain relief
❖ Patient will experience cessation of vomiting and improvement of general health.

Nursing Interventions

❖ Assess and document the extent of nausea and vomiting to have a database
❖ Reassure patient that nausea will usually subside by the 4th month of pregnancy in order to reduce her anxiety
❖ Instruct patient to eat dry, unsalted crackers before rising in the morning to prevent nausea from an empty stomach
❖ Instruct patient to avoid greasy or spicy food, which irritate the stomach. Fats with meals depress gastric motility and secretion of digestive enzymes and slow intestinal peristalsis causing gastroesophageal reflux
❖ Advise patient to avoid cooking odors that precipitate nausea
❖ Advise mothers to eat six small meals instead of three large ones to avoid overloading the stomach

❖ Advise mothers to eat foods high in carbohydrates as they are easier to digest.

❖ Instruct her to take iron pills and vitamins after meals to avoid irritating the stomach.

❖ Advise to take frequent walks outside, as fresh air reduces nausea and helps reinforce a positive outlook

❖ Instruct to separate food and fluid intake by 1/2 hour. Drinking excessive fluids with food distends stomach, predisposing to nausea

❖ Advise client to avoid very cold food and fluids at meal times as they may cause nausea and abdominal cramping

❖ Instruct her to consult physician before taking over-the-counter medications for nausea and vomiting to avoid harmful effects on fetus.

Evaluations for Expected Outcomes

❖ Patient identifies factors and food habits that aggravate nausea and vomiting

❖ Patient modifies her eating habits

❖ Patient adopts measures to obtain relief from nausea

❖ Patient experiences reduction in nausea and cessation of vomiting

❖ Patient experiences improvement of general health.

Documentation

❖ Patient's description of nausea, vomiting and aggravating factors

❖ Patient's general health observed

❖ Instructions given to patient and her response to teaching

❖ Change in eating and drinking habits observed and reported by patient

❖ Expected outcomes evaluated.

Acute Pain—Backache Related to Physiological Changes of Pregnancy

Definition

Discomfort experienced by some pregnant women during pregnancy in the lower back region.

Assessment

❖ Patient's posture, lifting techniques and footwear

❖ Life style and exercise pattern

❖ Type and duration of pain

❖ Relief measures.

Defining Characteristics

❖ Strain of muscles in the lower back

❖ Difficulty in changing position and lifting objects

❖ Anxiety due to disruption of normal activities

❖ Anxiety due to inability to continue exercises.

Expected Outcomes

❖ Patient will identify characteristics of pain

❖ Patient will verbalize factors that intensify pain and modify behaviors, accordingly

❖ Patient will carry out appropriate interventions for pain relief.

Nursing Interventions

❖ Instruct patient to maintain good posture, hold her shoulders back and to wear low heeled shoes to decrease spinal curvature which may reduce backache

❖ Instruct the patient in proper body mechanics to help her avoid stress to her lower back

❖ Advise patient to rest in recumbent position or with her legs bent and elevated on a bed or chair to relieve strain in the lower back

❖ Instruct the patient to perform moderate daily exercises to tone and maintain muscle strength in the lower back

❖ Explain the benefits of massaging and applying warm, moist heat to the lower back to relax and soothen tight muscles.

Evaluation for Expected Outcomes

❖ Patient identifies characteristics of back pain

❖ Patient lists factors that intensify pain and modifies behavior accordingly

❖ Patient carries out appropriate interventions for pain relief.

Documentation

❖ Patient's description of pain and expression of feelings about pain
❖ Observations about patient's responses to pain
❖ Comfort measures and medications provided to reduce pain
❖ Effectiveness of interventions for pain relief.
❖ Patient teaching carried out about pain relief measures
❖ Expected outcomes observed and reported by patient.

Urinary Frequency and Dysuria Related to Physiological Changes of Pregnancy

Definition

Frequency, urgency and pain on urination experienced by some women during pregnancy.

Assessment

❖ Nature and duration of urinary frequency
❖ Daily fluid intake
❖ Symptoms of UTI such as pain on micturition, and fever
❖ Patient's understanding of the physiological changes in pregnancy.

Defining Characteristics

❖ Frequency and urgency of urination
❖ Dysuria if associated infection present
❖ Sleep disturbance due to urinary frequency
❖ Occurrence of complaints in the early and late months of pregnancy.

Expected Outcomes

❖ Patient will experience relief from frequency of urination and dysuria
❖ Patient will increase her fluid intake during day time
❖ Patient will practice measures to prevent bladder distention and urinary stasis
❖ Patient will learn to report signs of developing urinary tract infections.

Nursing Interventions

❖ Reassure patient that urinary frequency is normal in the early and late months of pregnancy because the enlarging uterus places pressure on the bladder
❖ Instruct patient to avoid drinking large amounts of fluids within 2-3 hours of bedtime to prevent nocturnal urination and sleep loss
❖ Instruct client to ingest the required amount of fluid early in the day to reduce the need for evening liquids
❖ Instruct client to void whenever the urge occurs, to prevent bladder distention and urinary stasis which may predispose to urinary tract infection
❖ Teach patient signs and symptoms of UTI
❖ Teach patient to report signs and symptoms of UTI promptly.
   Early detection of UTI allows early treatment and helps prevent complications such as pyelonephritis.

Evaluations for Expected Outcomes

❖ Patient develops knowledge of the causes of urinary frequency
❖ Patient adapts and adjusts to the change in urinary elimination
❖ Patient modifies her fluid intake pattern
❖ Patient learns to identify and report signs of UTI if she develops it
❖ Patient experiences more rest during night and relaxation during day time.

Documentation

❖ Patient's description of urinary frequency and dysuria
❖ Measures of relief explained and response of patient
❖ Relief measures observed and reported
❖ Health instructions given.

Acute Pain—Leg Cramps Related to Physiological Changes of Pregnancy

Definition

A minor disorder of pregnancy experienced as sudden severe pain in leg muscles.

Assessment

❖ Dietary pattern
❖ Pain status such as location, time and duration

- Activity and rest pattern
- Relief measures
- Body mechanics and exercise practices.

Defining Characteristics

- Contraction of muscle and severe pain
- Inability to change position
- Anxiety due to the acute pain
- Fear of recurrence of pain
- Lack of knowledge of measures for relief of cramps.

Expected Outcomes

- Patient will identify factors that cause leg cramps
- Patient will discuss the measures to deal with episodes of leg cramps
- Patient will increase her intake of calcium containing foods and decrease the consumption of phosphorous
- Patient will practice exercises to increase general circulation
- Patient will stop getting cramps.

Nursing Interventions

- Reassure patient that leg cramps are normal during pregnancy to help reduce her anxiety
- Assess dietary pattern for inadequate dairy protein and excessive soft drink intake as alteration of calcium-phosphorus ratio can lead to leg cramps
- Instruct patient to increase the intake of milk and other sources of calcium rich food items
- Instruct patient to elevate her legs periodically and to avoid lying with toes pointed. Lying prone with toes pointed predisposes to blood vessel occlusion and subsequent cramping
- Instruct patient to exercise and use good body mechanics to prevent leg cramping by increasing general circulation
- Advice patient to take warm bath at bedtime to relax muscle fibers and increase blood flow to muscles
- Teach patient what she needs to do when cramping occurs; straighten the affected leg and dorsiflex the foot. These measures pull the contracted muscles taut, thus relieving a cramp caused by contraction
- Caution the mother not to rub the affected calf to avoid the risk of dislodging any undetected thrombus.

Evaluations for Expected Outcomes

- Patient expresses understanding of factors that cause leg cramps
- Patient verbalizes the measures she will practice to reduce the occurrence of leg cramps
- Patient discusses the measures to practice when cramping occurs
- Patient reports changes in dietary pattern and exercises
- Patient reports relief from occurrence of leg cramps.

Documentation

- Patient's knowledge of causes and measures to deal with leg cramps
- Instructions given and patient's response
- Patient's report of lifestyle changes to avoid leg cramps
- Changes reported by patient regarding reduction of the problem of leg cramps.

Acute Pain—Heartburn Related to Physiological Changes of Pregnancy

Definition

Uncomfortable sensation in the abdomen experienced in relation to food intake during pregnancy.

Assessment

- Dietary patterns
- Intake of greasy and spicy foods
- Pattern of fluid intake
- Occurrence of heartburn in relation to food intake.

Defining Characteristics

- Onset of heartburn after eating heavy meals
- Onset after greasy and spicy food
- Discomfort in supine position
- Discomfort after consuming cold foods.

Expected Outcomes

❖ Patient will change eating pattern to small, frequent meals
❖ Patient will avoid high fat content in food
❖ Patient will avoid unhealthy posture after meals
❖ Patient will avoid drinking very cold fluids and fluids with meals.

Nursing Interventions

❖ Assess patient's nutritional habits for selection of appropriate interventions
❖ Reassure patient that normal changes in pregnancy can cause heartburn to reduce her anxiety
❖ Instruct patient to eliminate greasy and spicy foods and to avoid fats. Such foods decrease stomach motility and increase gastric acidity
❖ Instruct patient to reduce fluid intake with meals as it tends to inhibit gastric juices
❖ Instruct her to avoid very cold foods as they may cause gastric reflux
❖ Instruct her to drink low fat or skimmed milk rather than whole milk
❖ Instruct mother to avoid assuming supine position after eating to provide more room in stomach for function
❖ Instruct patient to take small, frequent meals to avoid overloading the stomach
❖ Instruct to avoid bending over whilst doing house keeping activity
❖ Instruct her to remain upright for 3 to 4 hours after each meal to decrease the possibility of reflux
❖ Instruct her to take antacids if prescribed by physician for relief of discomfort.

Evaluations for Expected Outcomes

❖ Patient expresses understanding of the physiological changes in pregnancy that cause heartburn
❖ Patient expresses measures she will adapt for reducing heartburn
❖ Patient reports decreased discomfort from heartburn
❖ Patient demonstrates signs of reduced anxiety.

Documentation

❖ Patient's description of discomfort due to heartburn
❖ Patient's description of relief measures she uses
❖ Change in eating and drinking habits reported and observed
❖ Expected outcomes evaluated.

II. NURSING DIAGNOSES FOR LABOR AND DELIVERY CLIENTS

Acute Pain—Related to Physiological Response to Labor

Definition

An unpleasant sensory and emotional experience arising from actual or potential tissue damage; pain may be sudden or slow in onset, vary in intensity from mild to severe and constant or recurring.

Assessment

❖ Characteristics of pain including location, intensity and source of relief
❖ Physiological variables including age, and pain tolerance.
❖ Psychological variables including personality, previous experience with pain and anxiety
❖ Sociocultural variables such as cognitive style, culture, attitudes and values
❖ Knowledge and expectations of labor and delivery.

Defining Characteristics

❖ Alteration is muscle tone-listless to rigid.
❖ Autonomic response such as diaphoresis, change in blood pressure and respiratory rate, dilated pupils
❖ Change in appetite
❖ Communication of pain
❖ Behavior such as pacing and seeking out other people
❖ Expressions of pain such as moaning and crying
❖ Grimacing and other facial expressions
❖ Guarding or protective behavior

- Narrowed focus such as altered perception, impaired thought process and withdrawal from people
- Self focusing
- Sleep disturbance.

Expected Outcomes

- Patient will identify characteristics of pain
- Patient will describe factors that intensify pain
- Patient will modify behavior to decrease pain
- Patient will express decrease in intensity of pain
- Patient will express satisfaction of her performance during labor and delivery.

Nursing Interventions

- Orient patient to labor and delivery rooms on admission
- Explain admission protocol and labor process
- Show patient her room, bed and facilities such as call bell, toilet, television etc, to allay her fear and anxiety
- Assess patient's knowledge of labor process to plan nursing interventions
- Explain availability of analgesics and/or anesthesia (epidural) to patient and family for reducing anxiety
- Encourage support person or family member to remain with patient if hospital policy permits
- Instruct patient and support person in techniques to decrease the discomfort of labor
  - Discuss techniques of conscious relaxation.
  - Instruct to concentrate on an internal or external focal point.
  - Instruct in deep chest breathing during contractions.
  - Instruct in shallow chest breathing and slow panting like breathing which will avoid hyperventilations.
  - Instruct patient in effleurage.
- In early labor, provide patient with diversional activities such as watching television if possible to reduce anxiety

- As labor progresses to active phase, modify environment to reduce distractions and promote concentration, e.g. close curtains and door, turn off television
- Apply sacral pressure if needed to decrease back pain
- Assist to change position and provide additional pillow to reduce stiffness and promoter comfort
- Assess bladder for distention and encourage to void every two hours to reduce discomfort during contractions and facilitate fetal descend
- Provide frequent mouth care. Provide ice chips or wet gauze for dry lips caused by breathing techniques and nil-by-mouth
- Apply cool, damp wash cloth to forehead to relieve diaphoresis
- Provide clean gown and bed linen as needed. Diaphoresis and vaginal discharge can dampen bed lines and gown
- Encourage patient to rest and relax between contractions to decrease discomfort
- Discuss with patient and support person that pain medications are available if alternate pain control methods provide inadequate relief
- When required, administer prescribed analgesics to cope with labor process.

Evaluations

- Patient identifies characteristics of pain and describes factors that intensify it
- Patient modifies behaviors to decrease pain and discomfort such as using breathing techniques, asking for analgesia and assuming comfortable position
- Patient reports decrease in discomfort
- Patient expresses satisfaction with her performance during childbirth.

Documentation

- Patient's childbirth preparation
- Patient's description of pain and discomfort
- Observation of patient's response to labor
- Nursing interventions carried out to decrease discomfort
- Patient's response to nursing interventions.

Deficient Knowledge Related to Information About Birth Process

Definition

Inadequate understanding of or inability to perform skills needed to cope effectively with the process of labor.

Assessment

* Age of patient
* Psychosocial status such as expectations of the birth process and interest in learning
* Current knowledge about pregnancy, birth and recovery
* Ability to learn and attention span
* Support system including presence of support person interested in helping the patient.

Defining Characteristics

* Inability to follow through with instructions
* Inappropriate or exaggerated behaviors such as hysteria, hostility, agitation and apathy
* Verbalization of problems.

Expected Outcomes

* Patient will recognize that increased knowledge and skill will help her cope better with birth process
* Patient will demonstrate understanding of what is taught
* Patient will demonstrate ability to perform skills needed for coping with labor
* Patient will express realistic expectations about birth process
* Patient will express satisfaction with her increased knowledge.

Nursing Interventions

* Find a quite, private place to teach the patient
* Establish a trusting relationship with the patient and develop mutual goals for learning
* Select appropriate teaching methods and materials such as discussions and demonstrations using audiovisual aids

* Teach information and skills needed for understanding and coping during birth to increase the patient's sense of competence.

Evaluations for Expected Outcomes

* Patient expresses desire to put knowledge into practice during labor
* Patient describes birth process in her own words
* Patient responds to labor without undue anxiety and uses breathing, relaxation and position changes
* Patient voices satisfaction with newly acquired knowledge and skills.

Documentation

* Patient understands about birth process
* Patient's expression of need for better understanding
* Learning goals established with the patient
* Information and skills taught to patient
* Teaching methods used
* Patient's response to teaching
* Patient's mastery of knowledge and skills demonstrated
* Evaluation of expected outcomes observed.

Ineffective Coping Individual Related to Labor and Delivery

Definition

Inability to use adaptive behaviors in response to labor and delivery.

Assessment

* Age, health beliefs, feelings about pregnancy, decision making ability motivation to learn and obstacles to learning
* Pain threshold, perception of pain and response to analgesia
* Stage and length of labor, complications, ability to concentrate and use techniques, presence and effectiveness of support person
* Mode of delivery
* Previous experience with pregnancy, labor and delivery and knowledge of birth process
* Pre-existing pregnancy induced or medical conditions.

Defining Characteristics

- ❖ Expressed inability to cope
- ❖ Fatigue
- ❖ Inability to meet basic needs and role expectations
- ❖ Poor concentration and problem solving abilities
- ❖ Destructive behavior towards self or others.

Expected Outcomes

- ❖ Patient will express need to develop better coping behaviors
- ❖ Patient will set realistic learning goals
- ❖ Patient will use learned coping skills
- ❖ Patient will communicate feelings about pregnancy, labor and delivery
- ❖ Patient will maintain appropriate sense of control throughout the course of labor and delivery
- ❖ Patient will demonstrate ability to cope with unexpected changes.

Nursing Interventions

- ❖ Establish a relationship of mutual trust and respect to enhance patient's learning
- ❖ Develop learning goals with the patient to foster a sense of control
- ❖ Select appropriate teaching strategies to encourage compliance
- ❖ Teach skills that the patient can use during labor and delivery and have her give a return demonstration of each skill
- ❖ During the latent phase of labor (dilatation 1-4 cm)
  - − Encourage patient to participate in her own care
  - − Review breathing techniques she can use during labor
  - − Involve support person in care and comfort measures
  - − Provide continuous or frequent monitoring to identify any deviation from normal.
- ❖ During the active phase of labor (dilatation 4-8 cm)
  - − Encourage patient to assume comfortable position to promote relaxation between contractions

- − Assist patient with breathing techniques to reduce anxiety and prevent hyperventilation
- − Encourage the support person to participate in patient care such as changing soiled linen, providing sacral pressure, back rub and offering ice chips to moisten lips
  Administer analgesia as ordered to reduce pain
- − Reassure patient about fetal status.
- ❖ During the transitional phase of labor (dilatation 8-10 cm)
  - − Assist patient with breathing during contractions
  - − Encourage rest between contractions
  - − Explain all procedures and treatments and answer patient's questions to allay fears.
- ❖ During delivery of the placenta
  - − Encourage patient to maintain her position to facilitate delivery of placenta
  - − Show the neonate to the patient and reassure about the neonate's condition to provide emotional support
  - − Allow the patient to hold the neonate if permitted
  - − Allow her to breast feed neonate if she desires to promote bonding
- ❖ In a delivery, allow the patient to express her feelings and explain to her the care being provided to enable her cope with the task of motherhood.

Evaluation for Expected Outcomes

- ❖ Patient participates in establishing learning goals
- ❖ Patient successfully uses breathing and relaxation techniques during labor and delivery
- ❖ Patient maintains appreciable sense of control during labor and delivery
- ❖ Nurses and support persons provide effective comfort to patient during labor and delivery
- ❖ Patient demonstrates ability to cope with unexpected changes.

Documentation

- ❖ Patient's knowledge of labor and delivery
- ❖ Patient's expressions of motivation to learn.

❖ Methods used to teach patient
❖ Information taught and skills demonstrated
❖ Patient's level of satisfaction with delivery
❖ Evaluation for expected outcomes.

Anxiety Related to Hospitalization and Birth Process

Definition

Feeling of threat or danger to self related to pregnancy or delivery.

Assessment

❖ Expressed worries fears and concerns
❖ Expectations of labor experience
❖ Reactions to uterine activity, fetal movement, and interactions with nurse and significant others
❖ Ability to concentrate, learn and remember.
❖ Physiologic status
❖ Usual coping methods
❖ Mood and personality
❖ Progress of labor.

Defining Characteristics

❖ Excessive attention to uterine activity and fetal movements
❖ Excessive reaction to uterine contractions
❖ Expressed concern about childbirth
❖ Expressed fear of unspecified negative outcomes
❖ Expressed feelings of helplessness
❖ Fear and apprehension
❖ Inability to concentrate and remember
❖ Increased muscle tension in body
❖ Increased perspiration
❖ Rapid pulse rate
❖ Restlessness, shakiness and trembling.

Expected Outcomes

❖ Patient will express feelings of anxiety
❖ Patient will identify causes of anxiety
❖ Patient will make use of available emotional support
❖ Patient will show fewer signs of anxiety
❖ Patient will identify positive aspects of her efforts to cope during childbirth
❖ Patient will acquire increased knowledge about childbirth

❖ Patient will be better prepared to cope with future births.

Nursing Interventions

❖ Assess the patient's knowledge and expectations of labor to identify the precise source of anxiety
❖ Discuss normal labor progression with patient and explain what to expect during labor to help her to understand her own experience
❖ Involve the patient in making decisions about care to reduce the sense of powerlessness
❖ Share information about progress of labor and neonate's condition with patient to provide reassurance and to increase her sense of participation
❖ Interpret to patient, sights and sounds in labor room such as fetal heart sounds, fetal monitor strip and activities to reduce anxiety and increase confidence
❖ Attend to the patient's comfort needs to increase her trust
❖ Encourage patient to use coping skills such as breathing relaxation and positioning to increase her sense of power and control
❖ Provide adequate explanation regarding all procedures performed on her in the labor room
❖ Spend as much time as possible with the patient to provide comfort and assistance, thereby promoting the patient's sense of security
❖ Allow family member to participate in care to promote comfort and help patient cope with labor.

Evaluation for Expected Outcomes

❖ Patient expresses feelings of anxiety about pregnancy and childbirth
❖ Patient identifies causes of anxiety
❖ Patient communicates with nurse and family members to gain reassurance and emotional support
❖ Patient's physiologic and behavioral signs return to normal
❖ Patient express satisfaction with her behavior while giving birth.

Documentation

- ❖ Patient's expression of anxiety
- ❖ Patient's statement of reason for anxiety
- ❖ Observations of physical and behavioral signs of anxiety
- ❖ Interventions to assist patient with coping
- ❖ Patient's response to interventions
- ❖ Evaluations of expected outcomes observed.

Risk for Infection Related to Labor and Delivery

Definition

Presence of internal or external hazards that threaten maternal and neonatal well being.

Assessment

- ❖ Maternal vital signs
- ❖ Fetal heart rate
- ❖ Health history including previous infection
- ❖ Detail regarding rupture of membranes such as time of rupture and characteristics of amniotic fluid (amount, color an odor)
- ❖ Laboratory findings such as WBC, platelet count, clotting factors, hemoglobin, hematocrit and culture of blood and urine
- ❖ Signs and symptoms of chorioamnionitis such as maternal pulse rate over 160 beats per minute, foul smelling amniotic fluid, increasing uterine tenderness and fetal tachycardia.

Associated Medical Conditions

- ❖ Early rupture of membranes
- ❖ Peritonitis
- ❖ Pyelonephritis
- ❖ Urinary tract infection.

Expected Outcomes

- ❖ Patient will maintain good hygiene
- ❖ Patient will remain free from infection
- ❖ Patient's temperature will remain within normal range.

Nursing Interventions

- ❖ Monitor and record the patient's temperature every 4 hours before rupture of membranes and every 2 hours after they rupture to detect early signs of infections

- ❖ Monitor fetal heart rate continuously if a monitor is used and every 30 minutes otherwise. Report rates over 160 beats per minute and variability under 3 to 5 beats per minute as these are signs of maternal fever
- ❖ Wash hands thoroughly before and after providing care to mother to prevent spread of infection
- ❖ Wear gloves when contact with patient's blood and body fluids is expected for prevention of spread of infection
- ❖ Use strict sterile technique for procedures such as applying scalp electrode, inserting urinary catheter and inserting IV lines to reduce the likelihood of nosocomial infection
- ❖ Minimize vaginal examinations after rupture of membranes and always use sterile gloves to reduce the risk of chorioamnionitis
- ❖ Clean perineal area and maintain good hygiene, clean from front to back to reduce the risk of infection
- ❖ Monitor intake and output to assess for dehydration.

Evaluation for Expected Outcome

- ❖ Patient maintains good hygiene
- ❖ Patient remains free from infection as evidenced by clear, odorless, sediment-free urine, WBC count within normal limits and cultures free from pathogens
- ❖ Patient's temperature stays between 97° and 99°F (36.1-37.2°C).

Documentation

- ❖ Maternal vital signs
- ❖ Fetal heart rate and variability
- ❖ Date, time and sites of catheter insertions
- ❖ Nursing interventions performed to reduce risk of infection
- ❖ Evaluations of expected outcomes.

Risk for Injury Related to Induction of Labor

Definition

Increased risk to maternal or fetal wellbeing resulting from oxytocin stimulation.

Assessment

- History of previous pregnancies
- Prenatal history of present pregnancy (including laboratory findings, pelvic measurements, allergies, weight gain, last menses and estimated date of confinement)
- Physical examination including vital signs, Leopold's maneuvers, uterine contractions, vaginal examination and fetal heart rate
- Diagnostic studies as ultrasound test (to determine gestational age and fetal size, and non-stress or contraction stress test to assess fetal-placental function)
- Laboratory studies including complete blood count, blood type and Rh factor, platelets and urine test for protein and glucose levels.
- Contraindications such as Cephalopelvic disproportion, fetal distress, grand multiparity, over distention of uterus from multiple gestation or polyhydramnios, vaginal bleeding and unfavorable fetal presentation or position.

Risk Factor

- Dysfunctional labor
- Hypotonic contractions
- Post maturity
- Previous precipitous delivery
- Prolonged rupture of membranes.

Expected Outcomes

- Patient will have effective uterine contractions, i.e. every 2 to 3 minutes for 30 to 40 seconds or with intensity of 40 to 60 mm Hg by electronic monitor
- Continuous fetal monitoring will show fetal heart rate variability of 6 to 10 beats per minute with reassuring pattern
- Patient will achieve good labor pattern and neonate will be delivered without complications
- Patient and fetus will maintain optimal well being.

Nursing Interventions

- Explain oxytocin protocol to the patient and her support person. (Explain that oxytocin induced contractions may peak more quickly and last longer than spontaneous contractions to reduce apprehension and encourage patient participation)
- Encourage patient to void before applying fetal monitor and administering oxytocin. (Palpate bladder for distention every two hours to avoid discomfort during induction period)
- Monitor intake and output and measure urine specific gravity to detect urine retention which may delay descend
- Place patient in comfortable position as possible and in left lateral (as it relieves pressure of gravid uterus on the inferior vena cava and promotes blood flow to the placenta)
- Apply the fetal monitor and obtain a 15 to 20 minute baseline strip
- Start a primary IV line with an 18G or 20G catheter
- Prepare oxytocin as ordered. Add the drug to a 5 percent dextrose or normal saline solution (10 units to 1000 ml solution initially). Label the bottle with the patient's name, amount of oxytocin, date and time prepared and the nurse's name
- Piggyback the oxytocin solution to the primary IV line. Use an IV infusion pump to control the flow rate. The infusion pump guarantees exact dose administration for accurate assessment of uterine response
- Begin infusion at the rate of 0.5 to 1 mg/minute and remain with the patient during the first 20 minutes to evaluate the patient's response to uterine stimulation
- Increase the oxytocin infusion as ordered, by increments of 1 to 2 mU/minute as ordered, every 30 to 60 minutes until the desired contraction pattern is achieved and cervix is dilated 5 to 6 cm. Monitor blood pressure before and after each increase
- Monitor the contraction pattern and fetal rate every 15 minutes. Document the fetal heart rate, variability and any fetal strip changes
- If the patient responds poorly to oxytocin infusion, check the IV mixture and IV lines for patency. Increase the flow rate according to agency policy and physician's order

❖ Observe for hypertonicity; contractions lasting longer than 90 seconds and occurring less than 2 minutes a part and a reaching (on minor strip) greater than 75 mm Hg. If detected discontinue infusion immediately check maternal vital signs and notify physician. Increase the flow rate of primary IV solution and position the patient on her left side. These measures help arrest hypertonicity

❖ Monitor continuously for loss of variability, late decelerations or persistent bradycardia to detect fetal distress resulting from impaired uteroplacental perfusion caused by increased tonicity of contractions

❖ If signs of fetal distress are noted, take the following steps:
  – Discontinue oxytocin infusion Administer oxygen using a rebreathing mask at 8 to 12 per minute to increase the oxygen supply to fetus
  – Increase the flow rate of primary IV line to increase fluids
  – Reposition patient on her left or opposite side to increase placental blood flow.

❖ Assess the patient's intake and output and monitor the amount of oxytocin administered. Total fluid intake should not exceed 125 ml/hour. (The antidiuretic effect of oxytocin and large volume of electrolyte free solution can lead to water intoxication).

Evaluation of Expected Outcome

❖ Patient has contractions every 2 to 3 minutes that last for 30 to 60 seconds and are of moderate intensity with adequate resting tonus

❖ Continuous fetal monitoring shows reassuring fetal heart pattern with variability of 6 to 10 beats

❖ Patient achieves good labor pattern and delivers neonate without complications

❖ Patient maintains fluid balance

❖ Patient and fetus maintain optimal well begin during labor and delivery.

Documentation

❖ Vital signs on admission and every 15 to 30 minutes according to facility policy

❖ Baseline assessment of uterine activity (frequency, intensity, interval, duration and tonus) before oxytocin stimulation and every 30 minutes thereafter via continuous electronic fetal monitoring

❖ Assessment of fetal heart rate including baseline rate, long-term variability, short-term variability, accelerations and periodic changes using internal or external monitoring

❖ Patient's physical and emotional response to induction or augmentation or labor.

Deficient Knowledge Related to Premature Labor

Definition

Inadequate understanding of, or inability to perform, skills needed to cope with premature labor.

Assessment

❖ Age of patient
❖ Health beliefs
❖ Knowledge regarding pregnancy and birth process
❖ Previous experience with premature labor
❖ Financial resources
❖ Learning ability
❖ Support system

Defining Characteristics

❖ Inappropriate or exaggerated behaviors, e.g. hysteria, hostility, agitation
❖ Inability to follow instructions
❖ Inadequate knowledge of the condition
❖ Verbalization of the problems.

Expected Outcomes

❖ Patient will express desire to learn about premature labor
❖ Patient will express understanding of causes, signs and symptoms and management of premature labor
❖ Patient will identify and report danger signals without delay
❖ Patient will use available support systems

❖ Patient will cope successfully with premature labor
❖ Pregnancy will result in positive outcome.

Nursing Interventions

❖ Provide measures to reduce anxiety such as:
  – Introducing staff members to patient and family
  – Providing orientation to surroundings and routine
❖ Establish mutual trust and respect which will calm the patient
❖ Assist patient to develop realistic goals
❖ Assess patient's understanding of pregnancy and premature labor using appropriate teaching strategies
❖ Remain with patient for uninterrupted period of time and project a warm and caring attitude
❖ Include patient in decision making when possible to give her a sense of participation and control
❖ Provide information related to health status and condition of fetus to relieve her anxiety
❖ Teach patient the danger signs and symptoms to be reported immediately such as:
  – Contractions occurring every 10 minutes or less for one hour
  – Fluid leaking from vagina
  – Reduced or lack of or fetal movements
❖ Prompt reporting helps avoid premature labor
❖ Review discharge instructions if patient are discharged for home before delivery
❖ Emphasize taking prescribed medications limiting activities and reporting danger signs.

Evaluation for Expected Outcomes

❖ Patient express desire to learn about premature labor
❖ Patient demonstrates ability to identify causes and signs and symptoms of premature labor
❖ Patient expresses understanding of methods of management of premature labor

❖ Patient reports promptly danger signals and receive appropriate interventions
❖ Patient uses available support systems
❖ Patient successfully copes with premature labor as demonstrated by verbal and nonverbal behaviors
❖ Pregnancy results in positive outcome.

Documentation

❖ Patient's understanding of premature labor expressed in her own words
❖ Methods used to teach patient and family support person
❖ Response to teaching demonstrated by patient and family
❖ Maternal and fetal physical status
❖ Evaluations of expected outcomes.

Deficient Fluid Volume Related to Altered Intake during Labor

Definition

Inadequate hydration resulting from reduced intake or excessive loss of body fluids.

Assessment

❖ Vital signs such as temperature, pulse rate, respiration and blood pressure
❖ Fluid and electrolyte status including weight, intake and output, urine specific gravity, skin turgor, mucus membranes, electrolytes and blood urea levels.

Defining Characteristics

❖ Change in mental status
❖ Decreased pulse volume and pressure
❖ Decreased urine output
❖ Decreased venous filling
❖ Dry skin and mucous membranes
❖ Increased body temperature
❖ Increased hematocrit
❖ Increased pulse rate
❖ Increased urine concentration
❖ Low blood pressure
❖ Poor skin turgor
❖ Sudden loss of weight
❖ Increased weakness.

Associated Medical Conditions

❖ Diabetes mellitus
❖ Hemorrhage
❖ Pregnancy induced hypertension (PIH)
❖ Premature rupture of membranes
❖ Shock.

Expected Outcomes

❖ Patient will maintain fluid balance
❖ Patient will demonstrate optimal hydration
❖ Patient will show no sign of dehydration.

Nursing Interventions

❖ Monitor vital signs at frequency intervals according to the policy of the institution
❖ Assess skin turgor and examine oral mucous membrane for dryness periodically
❖ Monitor intake and output according to protocol
❖ Administer and monitor parental fluids (usually 125-175 ml/hour). Output should approximate intake in order to help ensure adequate hydration
❖ Monitor electrolyte values and report abnormal values
❖ Provide patient with ice chips and cold compress to increase comfort and decrease mouth dryness
❖ Measure the amount and character of vomitus and assess the need for an antiemetic (when labor begins GI motility and absorption decreases as blood is rerouted to meet the energy needs of contracting uterus causing food to remain in the stomach for up to 12 hours. This predisposes to nausea and vomiting especially during the transition phase of labor)
❖ Administer antiemetics as ordered
❖ Keep patient cool and comfortable by changing soiled linen and applying cold compress to face and body to reduce discomfort caused by diaphoresis
❖ Position patient on her left side to aid kidney perfusion and increase cardiac and urine output.

Evaluation

❖ Patient maintains fluid balance with intake approximately equaling output
❖ Patient maintains optimal hydration

❖ Patient has no signs of dehydration
  – Mucous membranes remain pink and moist
  – Skin turgor remains optimal
  – Vital signs stay within normal limits
  – Urine output is at least 30 ml/hour or 100 ml in 4 hours.

Documentation

❖ Vital signs
❖ Observation of fluid volume status
❖ Intake and output
❖ Nursing intervention and patient's response
❖ Evaluation of expected outcomes.

III. NURSING DIAGNOSES FOR POSTPARTUM CLIENTS

Deficient Knowledge Related to Postpartum Care

Definition

Inadequate understanding of postpartum self care activities or inability to perform skills needed to practice health related behaviors.

Assessment

❖ Age and learning ability
❖ Decision making ability
❖ Interest in learning
❖ Knowledge and skill regarding postpartum self care
❖ Obstacles to learning
❖ Support systems and usual coping pattern
❖ Physical abilities to perform self care activities.

Defining Characteristics

❖ Inability to follow through with instructions
❖ Inappropriate or exaggerated behaviors such as hostility, agitation or apathy
❖ Poor knowledge level
❖ Verbalization of problem.

Expected Outcomes

❖ Patient will express desire to learn how to care for herself after delivery

- Patient will verbalize or demonstrate understanding of what she has learned about self care
- Patient will incorporate newly learned skills into daily routine
- Patient will make changes in postpartum routine
- Patient will seek help from health care professional if required.

Nursing Interventions

- Establish mutual trust and respect to enhance patient's learning
- Assess patient's level of understanding of postpartum self care activities to establish a baseline for learning
- Assist patient in making decisions regarding target dates for mastering postpartum self care skills
- Select teaching strategies best suited for patient's individual learning style to enhance learning
- Teach skills which the patient can incorporate into her daily life such as perineal care, sitz bath, application and removal of perineal pads and breast care
- Teach patient about the process of involution that help her to understand postpartum changes
- Teach the patient about importance of adequate nutrition and hydration to ensure proper urinary and bowel elimination
- Discuss the importance of adequate rest to promote emotional and physical stability
- Help the patient to incorporate learned skills into her daily routine during hospitalization
- Encourage patient to continue hygienic practices even after discharge from hospital.

Evaluation for Expected Outcomes

- Patient expresses motivation to learn
- Patient establishes realistic learning goals
- Patient demonstrates understanding of what she has learned
- Patient incorporates what she has learned into her daily routine such as breast care, perineal care and obtaining adequate rest and sleep

- Patient states intention of making changes in daily routine
- Patient expresses intention to seek help from health professional if required.

Documentation

- Patient's understanding and skill in postpartum self care
- Patient's expressions which indicate her motivation to learn
- Methods used to teach patient
- Information taught to patient
- Skills demonstrated to patient
- Patient's response to teaching
- Evaluation of expected outcomes.

Pain Related to Postpartum Physiological Changes

Definition

An unpleasant sensory and emotional experience that arises from actual or potential tissue damage.

Assessment

- Patient's description of pain
- Patient's age, parity and pain tolerance
- Previous experience with pain in post-delivery period
- Presence of physical factors such as breast engorgement, cracked nipples and hemorrhoids.

Defining Characteristics

- Alteration in vital signs, diaphoresis, etc.
- Communication of pain in verbal and non-verbal forms.
- Behavior changes such as pacing and repetitive actions
- Expressions of pain such as crying, groaning and grimacing
- Sleep disturbance.

Expected Outcomes

- Patient will identify characteristics of pain and describe the factors that intensify it
- Patient will carry out appropriate interventions for pain relief

❖ Patient will express relief from pain and comfort.

Nursing Interventions

❖ Assess patient's pain symptoms

❖ Discuss the reasons for pain and its expected duration to reduce the patient's anxiety

❖ Inspect the presence of hemorrhoids and provide instructions for hemorrhoid care if indicated

❖ Assess for uterine tenderness and presence and frequency for afterbirth pains every 4 hours for first 24 hours and every shift thereafter as indicated. Oxytocin administration, multiparity and breastfeeding are factors that may intensify uterine contractions

❖ Instruct breastfeeding mother to wear supportive bra to increase comfort

❖ If breastfeeding mother is engorged instruct her to use warm compress or take warm shower to simulate the flow of milk and help relieve stasis and discomfort

❖ If nipples become sore, instruct mother to air dry the nipples for 20 to 30 minutes after feeding to roughen the nipples

❖ Apply breast cream as ordered to soften nipples and relieve pain

❖ Instruct non-breastfeeding mother to wear tight, supportive bra or breast binder and apply ice packs as needed to prevent or reduce lactation.

Evaluations for Expected Outcomes

❖ Patient describes pain and factors that intensify it

❖ Patient carries out appropriate interventions for pain relief as instructed

❖ Patient expresses relief of pain and discomfort

❖ Patient's breasts remain soft and lactation continues to be adequate

❖ Patient expresses understanding of instructions and follows through.

Documentation

❖ Patient's description of pain and discomfort

❖ Observations of pain manifestations

❖ Comfort measures and medications provided for pain relief

❖ Effectiveness of interventions carried out

❖ Instructions provided to patient about pain and pain relief measures

❖ Evaluations of expected outcome.

Deficient Fluid Volume Related to Postpartum Hemorrhage

Definition

Excessive fluid and electrolyte loss resulting from excessive postpartum bleeding.

Assessment

❖ History of problems that can cause fluid loss such as hemorrhage, vomiting and diarrhea

❖ Vaginal signs such as visible bleeding and lacerations

❖ Fluid and electrolyte status including weight, intake and output, urine specific gravity, skin turgor, mucous membranes and serum electrolytes and blood urea nitrogen levels

❖ Laboratory values such as hemoglobin (Hb) level and hematocrit (Hct) value

❖ Risk factors such as grand multiparty, overdistended uterus, prolonged labor, previous history of postpartum hemorrhage, traumatic delivery, uterine fibroids, and bleeding disorders.

Defining Characteristics

❖ Decreased pulse volume and pressure

❖ Decreased urine output and increased concentration

❖ Dry skin and mucous membranes

❖ Increased hematocrit

❖ Increased pulse rate

❖ Low blood pressure

❖ Poor skin turgor

❖ Thirst

❖ Weakness

❖ Change in mental status.

Expected Outcomes

❖ Patient's vital signs will remain stable

❖ Patient's hematology values will be within normal range

- Patient's uterus will remain firm and contracted
- Signs of shock will be identified quickly and treatment initiated immediately by medical personnel
- Patient's blood volume will return to normal
- Patient's urinary output will return to normal.

Nursing Interventions

- Following delivery, monitor the color, amount and consistency of lochia every 15 minutes for one hour, every 4 hours for 24 hours and then every shift until discharge
- Count or weigh sanitary pads if lochia is excessive
- Monitor and record vital signs every 15 minutes for one hour, every hour for 4 hours and every 4 hours for 24 hours to detect signs of hemorrhage and shock
- Immediately after delivery, palpate the fundus every 15 minutes for one hour, every hour for 4 hours, every 4 hours for 24 hours and then every shift until discharge to note its location and muscle tone. Lack of uterine muscle tone or strength (atony) is the most common cause of postpartum hemorrhage
- Gently massage a boggy fundus, to make it become firm (overstimulation can cause relaxation)
- Teach patient to assess and gently massage the fundus and notify if bogginess persists
- Explain to patient the process of involution and the need to palpate the fundus to decrease her anxiety and increase cooperation
- Evaluate postpartum hematology studies and report abnormal values to plan required interventions
- Administer fluids, blood or blood products or plasma expanders as ordered to replace lost blood volume
- Monitor patient's intake and output every shift
- Note bladder distention and catheterize as ordered as distended bladder interferes with involution of uterus

- Administer oxytocic agents such as ergometrine as ordered as distended bladder interferes with involution of uterus
- Assess patient regularly for signs and symptoms of shock such as rapid thready pulse, increased respiratory rate, decreased blood pressure and urine output and cold, clammy, pale, skin.

Evaluations for Expected Outcomes

- Patient's vital signs remain stable
- Results of hematology studies are within normal range
- Patient's uterus remains firm
- Patient does not develop distended bladder
- Patient's blood loss after delivery is less than 500 ml
- Patient's blood volume is replenished
- Quick identification and prompt treatment are provided if patient develops shock.

Documentation

- Estimation of blood loss
- Location and tone of fundus
- Laboratory results
- Replacement of lost fluid
- Nursing interventions to control active blood loss
- Vital signs, intake and output
- Patient's response to nursing interventions.

Risk for Infection Related to Altered Primary Defenses during Postpartum Period

Definition

Presence of internal or external hazards which threaten maternal well being during postpartum period.

Assessment

- Laboratory values including WBC and platelet count, hemoglobin level, hematocrit, blood and body fluid culture.
- History of labor and delivery such as episiotomy and premature rupture of membranes.
- Presence of medical conditions such as diabetes mellitus that increase the likelihood of infection.

❖ Signs and symptoms of infection such as pallor, fatigue, malaise, anorexia, fever with hills, foul-smelling lochia, calf tenderness, dysuria, abdominal tenderness and tender, reddened breasts.

Risk Factors

❖ Chronic illness
❖ Exposure to pathogens during and prior to labor
❖ Inadequate primary defenses such as broken skin
❖ Invasive procedure
❖ Lack of knowledge about causes of infection
❖ Malnutrition
❖ Premature rupture of membranes
❖ Tissue destruction and trauma.

Expected Outcomes

❖ Patient's vital signs will remain within normal range
❖ Results of laboratory studies will not indicate infection
❖ Patient's urine and body secretions such as lochia will not show evidence of infection
❖ Patient's episiotomy or abdominal incision site will remain free from infection
❖ Patient's IV site will not become inflamed.
❖ Patient will maintain good personal hygiene
❖ Patient will state risk factors that can lead to infection
❖ Patient will remain free from signs and symptoms of infection.

Nursing Interventions

❖ Minimize the patient's risk of infection by:
 – Washing hands before and after providing care.
 – Wearing gloves to maintain asepsis when giving direct care and when in contact with blood and body fluids.
❖ After delivery monitor vital signs
 – Every 15 minutes for one hour then every 4 hours for 24 hours and then every shift until discharge and report any abnormal change.
❖ Elevated vital signs indicate infection.

❖ A temperature greater than 100.4° F (38° C) on two consecutive readings after the first 24 hours post-delivery may indicate endometriosis, mastitis or other infection
❖ Monitor WBC count as ordered and report abnormal values as it indicates increased production of leukocytes in response to bacterial pathogens
❖ Culture urine, wound drainage, lochia or blood as ordered to identify pathogens for antibiotic therapy
❖ Instruct patient in proper personal hygiene such as perineal wash, sitz bath, hand washing and breast care to reduce risk of infection
❖ Teach patient how to apply perineal pads front to back and how to remove them back to front and to clean perineum from front to back after elimination. These measures reduce bacterial concentrations and help prevent genitourinary tract infection
❖ Follow universal precautions to prevent nosocomial infections
❖ Use strict sterile technique while performing invasive procedures such as IV line insertion or urinary catheterization to minimize the risk of infection
❖ Assess IV site every shift for redness or warmth and change IV tubing and site every 72 hours or according to hospital policy
❖ Instruct postoperative patient to deep breathe and cough to help remove secretions and prevent respiratory complications
❖ Assess the patient for generalized signs of infection such as pallor, fatigue, malaise and anorexia and chills every shift and instruct her to report danger signs immediately

Evaluation for Expected Outcomes

❖ Patient's vital signs remain within normal limits
❖ Patient's WBC count and differential remain within normal range
❖ Patient's respiratory secretions are clear and odorless, urine is clear, yellow and odorless, and sediment free
❖ Patient's IV site does not become inflamed

- Patient's lochia discharge remains normal in color, consistency and odor
- Patient performs personal hygiene correctly at regular intervals
- Patient discusses risk factors that can cause infection
- Patient remains free from infection.

Documentation

- Vital signs
- Appearance of episiotomy or abdominal incision site
- Date, time and sites of culture if done
- Appearance of IV site
- Patient teaching about infection control
- Interventions performed to reduce risk of infection
- Patient's response to nursing interventions
- Evaluations for expected outcome.

Pain Related to Episiotomy or Cesarean Incision

Definition

An unpleasant sensory and emotional experiences arising from tissue damage which vary in intensity from mild to severe and be constant or recurring.

Assessment

- Patient's description of pain including quality and intensity
- Patient's age and pain tolerance
- Patient's anxiety level and any symptoms of secondary gain.

Defining Characteristics

- Alteration in vital signs, diaphoresis or dilated pupils
- Change in appetite and eating
- Communication of pain in verbal and non-verbal forms
- Expressions of pain such as crying, moaning and grimacing
- Guarding or protective activities
- Sleep disturbance.

Expected Outcomes

- Patient will describe nature of pain and intensity
- Patient will understand and carry out appropriate interventions for pain relief
- Patient will express comfort and relief from pain.

Nursing Interventions

- Examine the episiotomy site for redness, edema, ecchymosis, drainage and approximation to detect trauma to perineal tissues or developing complications
- Discuss reasons for pain and discomfort and measures to be carried out for relief
- Apply ice pack to the episiotomy site for the first 24 hours to increase vasoconstriction and reduce edema and discomfort
- Provide warm sitz bath (temperature 100°-105°F/37.8-40.6°C) from 2nd postpartum day. Instruct patient to take sitz baths three times a day with each lasting for 20 minutes. Sitz bath increases circulation, reduces edema and promotes healing.
- Provide infrared light to perineum if ordered to reduce discomfort
- Apply any prescribed sprays, creams or ointments for reduction of swelling and discomfort
- Instruct patient to tighten buttocks before sitting and to sit on flat firm surface. This reduces stress and direct pressure on the perineum
- Administer prescribed pain medications to provide pain relief
- For post cesarean patients, provide an additional pillow and teach to splint the incision site when moving or coughing to provide support for abdominal muscles.

Evaluations for Expected Outcomes

- Patient reports characteristics and intensity of pain
- Patient carries out appropriate interventions for pain relief as instructed.
- Patient expresses relief of pain and discomfort

❖ Episiotomy or cesarean incision heals normally

❖ Patient expresses understanding of instructions given and implements care activities.

Documentation

❖ Patient's description of pain and pain relief experienced

❖ Nurse's observation of patient's response to interventions for pain relief

❖ Comfort measures and medications provided for pain relief

❖ Instructions provided to patient for self care activities.

Impaired Skin Integrity Related to Episiotomy or Abdominal Incision

Definition

Interruption in skin integrity resulting from surgical incision in the perineum or abdomen made for delivering the fetus.

Assessment

❖ Vital signs

❖ Integumentary status such as color, hygiene, drainage and texture

❖ Extent of interruption of skin integrity because of delivery

❖ Health history including past skin problems, trauma and surgery

❖ Dietary intake, appetite, hydration and weight

❖ Laboratory data such as hemoglobin, hematocrit and WBC levels

❖ Patient's understanding of her condition and readiness to learn

❖ Presence of any medical condition that may interfere with healing.

Defining Characteristics

❖ Destruction of skin layers surrounding episiotomy or abdominal incision

❖ Disruption of skin surfaces

❖ Signs of infection (invasion by pathogens) such as elevation of temperature local inflammation, discharge, etc.

Expected Outcomes

❖ Patient will demonstrate understanding of self care activities

❖ Patient will perform skin care routine

❖ Patient will identify possible danger signs and report immediately

❖ Patient will regain skin integrity

❖ Patient's episiotomy or abdominal incision will heal without infection.

Nursing Interventions

❖ Inspect the incision every shift for redness, edema, ecchymosis, discharge and approximation (REEDA) to detect signs of possible infection

❖ Instruct and assist the patient with hygienic practices such as hand washing and toileting practices to prevent wound contamination

❖ Carry out prescribed treatment such as cleaning and applying medications and dressing changes to decrease bacterial contamination

❖ Instruct and assist the patient in performing perineal wash/perineal care and sitz baths 3 to 4 times a day to maintain cleanliness and promote healing

❖ Teach patient how to apply and remove perineal pad. Clean pad to be applied front to back and soiled pad to be removed from back to front to reduce the risk of contaminating the vaginal area

❖ Maintain infection control standards to reduce the risk of nosocomial infections

❖ Instruct patient to report possible danger signs and symptoms such as temperature above 100.4°F (38°C), incision drainage, increased discomfort at the episiotomy or incision site and reddened, warm skin surrounding the incision site.

Evaluations for Expected Outcomes

❖ Patient demonstrates correct self care practices

❖ Patient performs skin care or episiotomy care routine

❖ Patient identifies and reports to physician possible danger signs

❖ Patient regains skin integrity

❖ Patient's episiotomy or abdominal incision shows no sign of infection.

Documentation

- Patient's expressed concerns about change in skin integrity
- Patient's ability to perform self care practices
- Observations of episiotomy or abdominal incision site
- Response to treatment and nursing care
- Instructions regarding treatment and self care
- Prescribed treatment carried out
- Nursing interventions and supportive care carried out and patient's response
- Self care practices performed by patient
- Expected outcomes evaluated.

IV. NURSING DIAGNOSES FOR NEONATAL CLIENTS

Risk for Aspiration Related to Immature Cough or Gag Reflex

Definition

Entry of oropharyngeal and GI secretions or exogenous fluids into neonate's tracheobronchial passages.

Assessment

- Gestational age of neonate
- Weight of neonate in relation to gestational age
- Maternal sedation during labor (before delivery)
- Neonate's health status including pre-existing conditions, intrauterine environment, cardiovascular status, respiratory status, GI status and anomalies
- Laboratory values of the neonate such as fluid, electrolyte and blood gas levels
- Vital signs of the neonate
- Nutritional status of the neonate.

Risk Factors

- Decreased GI mobility and delayed gastric emptying
- Depressed cough and gag reflexes
- Impaired swallowing
- Incompetent lower esophageal sphincter
- Increased gastric residual contents
- Conditions contraindicating elevation of upper body

- Surgery or trauma to face, mouth or neck
- Tracheostomy or endotracheal tube
- GI tubes.

Expected Outcomes

- Neonate will maintain clear airway (through suctioning as needed)
- Neonate will not exhibit gastric distention
- Neonate will demonstrate minimal quantity of nasopharyngeal and oropharyngeal secretion
- Neonate will tolerate initial feeding
- Neonate will demonstrate appropriate suck and swallow reflex
- Neonate will not exhibit signs and symptoms of aspiration
- Neonate will have no abnormal breath sounds.

Nursing Interventions

- Assess the neonate's respiratory status until stable after birth, to evaluate the respiratory system during transition to extrauterine life
- Monitor vital signs according to agency protocol to determine the neonate's adjustment to extrauterine existence
- Suction as needed to keep the upper and lower airway clear. In the labour room, suction the oropharynx and nasopharynx with a bulb syringe, DeLee catheter or suction catheter attached to wall suction
- Assist physician with laryngoscopy to suction below vocal cord, if the neonate aspirates meconium
- Perform a head-to-toe physical assessment to detect abnormalities in other systems that may affect respiratory effort
- Withhold oral feedings and provide IV fluids if signs of respiratory distress occur
- Observe for sucking and swallowing reflex, gag and cough reflex and color changes when offering the initial feeding
- Keep the head of bed elevated during and after gavage feeding if not contraindicated
- Monitor residual gastric contents and follow parameters for withholding feedings
- Measure abdominal girth every shift to check for distention and stop feeding imme-

diately if aspiration is suspected. Perform suctioning as needed

- Explain to parents the reasons for these interventions
- Instruct mother in feeding techniques that will help prevent a distended abdomen leading to aspiration
  - Instruct mother to avoid overfeeding and to burp the neonate at frequent intervals (after intake of ½-1 oz)
  - Instruct mother to position the neonate on his right side with the head of the bed elevated for 30 to 60 minutes after feeding.

Evaluations for Expected Outcomes

- Neonate receives suctioning as needed and maintains patent airway
- Neonate does not have gastric distention
- Neonate tolerates initial feeding
- Neonate does not manifest color changes during feeding
- Neonate has appropriate sucking and swallowing reflex
- Neonate has no adventitious (abnormal) breath sounds
- Neonate shows no signs and symptoms of aspiration.

Documentation

- Neonate's tolerance of initial feeding and gavage feedings
- Residual gastric contents after gavage feeding
- Episodes of vomiting, aspiration or both
- Breath sounds
- Observations of physical findings including heart rate and respirations
- Interventions performed to prevent aspiration
- Expected outcomes evaluated.

Ineffective Breastfeeding Related to Difficulty with Breastfeeding Process

Definition

State in which mother or neonate experiences dissatisfaction or difficulty with breastfeeding process.

Assessment

- Maternal status such as age, parity, previous bonding history and breastfeeding preparation in prenatal period
- Adequacy of milk supply, nipple shape and perceptions about breastfeeding
- Neonate's growth rate and age-weight relationship.

Defining Characteristics

- Inadequate milk supply
- Arching and crying when at breast
- Evidence of inadequate milk intake
- Fussiness and crying within an hour of breastfeeding
- Inability to latch on to nipple correctly
- Lack of sustained sucking at breast
- Insufficient emptying of breasts
- Lack of response to other comfort measures
- Sore nipples for mother after first week of breastfeeding.

Expected Outcomes

- Mother will express satisfaction with breastfeeding techniques and practice
- Mother will show decreased anxiety and apprehension
- Neonate will feed well on both breasts and appear satisfied for at least two hours after feeding
- Neonate will grow and thrive.

Nursing Interventions

- Educate mother in breast care and breastfeeding techniques
- Be available and encourage mother during initial breastfeeding episodes
- Teach techniques for encouraging the letdown reflex such as warm shower before feeding, breast massage and holding the neonate close to the breasts
- Provide quiet, private, comfortable, environment for mother and baby to promote successful breastfeeding
- Encourage mother to clarify questions regarding successful breastfeeding.

Evaluations for Expected Outcomes

- Mother expresses satisfaction with breastfeeding practices

- Mother will exhibit decreased anxiety and apprehension
- Neonate feeds successfully on both breasts and appears satisfied for at least two hours after feeding
- Neonate grows and thrives.

Documentation

- Mother's expressions of satisfaction and comfort with breastfeeding ability
- Observations of bonding and breastfeeding processes
- Teaching and instructions given
- Neonates weight and growth
- Expected outcomes evaluated.

Interrupted Breastfeeding Related to Contraindicating Conditions

Definition

Break in the continuity of breast feeding resulting from inability or inadvisability to feed the baby from breasts.

Assessment

- Maternal status such as nipple anomaly, psychological stress, presence of infection and use of medication
- Neonatal status such as age-weight relationship, respiratory status, suck reflex, prematurity, hyperbilirubinemia and anomalies that interfere with proper sucking (e.g. cleft lip or palate).

Expected Outcomes

- Mother will express her understanding of factors that necessitate interruption of breastfeeding
- Mother will express understanding that she may resume breastfeeding
- Mother will express and store breast milk appropriately
- Mother will resume breastfeeding when interfering factors cease
- Mother will have adequate milk supply when breastfeeding resumes
- Mother will experience relief from discomfort associated with engorgement
- Neonate's nutritional needs will be met.

Nursing Interventions

- Assess the mother's understanding of the reasons for interrupting breastfeeding
- Teach mother about alternate methods to meet the nutritional needs of the baby
- Assess mother's desire to resume breastfeeding
- Instruct mother in techniques of expressing and storing breast milk to ensure adequate milk supply
- Teach the use of breast pump to empty the breasts
- Educate mother to save her breast-milk in a sterile container and store it in the refrigerator for future feedings
- Instruct her in ways to relieve breast engorgement
- Instruct mother in use of devices such as nipple shield in case of flat or inverted nipple
- If the mother does not wish to resume breastfeeding instruct her to wear supportive bra/binder, apply ice and take mild analgesic to alleviate discomfort related to engorgement.

Evaluations for Expected Outcomes

- Mother describes factors that necessitate interruption in breastfeeding
- Mother explains her decision about whether to resume breastfeeding
- Mother demonstrates proper milk expression and storage techniques
- Mother resumes breastfeeding when interrupting factors are eliminated
- Mother has adequate milk supply when breastfeeding resumes
- Mother obtains relied from discomfort associated with engorgement
- Infant's nutritional needs are met as evidenced by appropriate weight gain (e.g. one oz. per day for first six months of life).

Documentation

- Factors that necessitate interruption of breastfeeding
- Mother's feeling expressed about need to interrupt breastfeeding
- Mother's decision whether to continue breastfeeding when possible

- Mother's efforts to ensure adequate milk supply
- Mother's response to nursing interventions
- Neonate's weight and growth
- Expected outcomes evaluated.

Ineffective Breathing Pattern Related to Adjustment to Extrauterine Existence

Definition

State in which a neonate's initial breathing pattern does not provide adequate lung expansion for successful transition to extra-uterine life.

Assessment

- Gestational age
- Weight in relation to gestational age
- Maternal sedation before delivery
- Pre-existing conditions such as anomalies, adverse intrauterine environment and prematurity
- Assessment of cardiovascular, respiratory and GI status and fluid and electrolyte balance
- History of meconium aspiration or neonatal asphyxia.

Defining Characteristics

- Use of accessory muscles for breathing
- Altered chest excursion (increased chest movement)
- Altered respiratory rate or depth or both
- Dyspnea
- Nasal flaring
- Retractions of chest wall
- Shortness of breath.

Expected Outcomes

- Neonate will establish normal respiratory rate (40-60 breaths/minute) within one hour of birth
- Neonate will have no signs of respiratory distress one hour after birth
- Neonate will not require assisted ventilation or supplemental oxygen
- Neonate will have Apgar score of 8 to 10 at 1 and 5 minutes of age

- Neonate will make successful transition to extrauterine life with adequate respiratory function.

Nursing Interventions

- Carry out the following immediately after delivery:
  - Dry the baby and place him under a radiant warmer
  - Suction the oropharynx and nasopharynx as needed with a bulb syringe, DeLee catheter or suction catheter connected to wall suction
  - Obtain 1 minute and 5 minute Apgar scores
  - Provide oxygen if indicated
  - Remove wet blankets and replace them with dry ones
  - Observe for signs of respiratory distress such as nasal flaring, tachypnea, retractions, grunting and use of accessory muscles for breathing
  - Provide or assist with resuscitative measures, as indicated including bag and mask ventilation, administration of narcan (naloxone), intubations and suctioning below the vocal cords.
- Transfer the neonate to nursery when condition is stable or if the neonate needs more extensive resuscitative measures
- On admission to the nursery carry out the following:
  - Obtain vital signs
  - Observe central and peripheral color
  - Note signs of respiratory distress
  - Perform a physical assessment noting anomalies or abnormal findings
  - Maintain a neutral thermal environment
  - Obtain a brief history of labor and delivery and condition of the neonate before arrival in nursery to identify the risk factors
  - Obtain laboratory studies as ordered
  - Provide resuscitative measures if needed
  - Monitor vital signs until stable and then routinely
- Continually assess the need to repeat suctioning to maintain a patent airway.

Evaluations for Expected Outcome

❖ Neonate establishes respiratory rate of 40 to 60 breaths/minute within one hour of birth

❖ Neonate has no signs of respiratory distress 1 hour after birth. Neonate does not require assisted ventilation or supplemental oxygen

❖ Neonate has Apgar score of 8 to 10 at 1 and 5 minutes of age

❖ Neonate makes successful transition to extrauterine life.

Documentation

❖ Vital signs

❖ Physical findings

❖ Interventions performed to enhance neonate's ability to breathe effectively

❖ Neonate's response to nursing interventions

❖ Expected outcomes evaluated.

Ineffective Breastfeeding Related to Limited Maternal Experience

---

Definition

State in which mother or neonate experiences dissatisfaction or difficulty with breastfeeding process.

Assessment

❖ Age and maturity of mother

❖ Previous bonding history-parity

❖ Level of prenatal breastfeeding preparation.

❖ Previous breastfeeding experience

❖ Actual or perceived inadequate milk supply

❖ Nipple shape such as inverted nipple

❖ Stressors such as family and career

❖ Views on breastfeeding

❖ Support from spouse and family members

❖ Satisfaction and contentment of neonate.

Defining Characteristics

Mother

❖ Actual or perceived inadequate supply of milk

❖ Insufficient emptying of each breast

❖ Lack of observable signs of oxytocin release

❖ Sore nipples after first week of breast-feeding.

Baby

❖ Arching and crying when at breast

❖ Evidence of inadequate intake of milk

❖ Fussing and crying within one hour after feeding

❖ Inability to latch on to nipple correctly

❖ Lack of response to comfort measures and efforts at pacifying

❖ Lack of sustained sucking at breast

❖ Resistance to latch on to breast

❖ Unsatisfactory breastfeeding process.

Expected Outcomes

❖ Mother will express understanding of breastfeeding techniques and practice

❖ Mother will display decreased anxiety and apprehension

❖ Mother and baby will experience successful breastfeeding

❖ Neonate's initial weight loss will be within accepted norms

❖ Neonate's nutritional needs will be met adequately.

Nursing Interventions

❖ Assess mother's knowledge of breastfeeding

❖ Educate mother in breast care and breast-feeding techniques

❖ Provide written materials and audiovisual aids which illustrate proper feeding techniques

❖ Teach techniques for encouraging the let-down reflex such as; warm shower, breast massage, relaxation, holding neonate close to the breasts and initiating sucking

❖ Stay with mother during feeding and encourage asking questions to increase understanding

❖ Evaluate nipple position in neonate's mouth and sucking motion

❖ Ensure that the neonate is awake and alert when feeding, unwrap as needed

❖ Evaluate neonate for anomalies that may interfere with breastfeeding ability such as cleft lip or palate

❖ When ready to start feeding, let a drop or two of breast milk fall on baby's lips. The neonate may open his mouth on tasting the milk

- Instruct the mother in breast care techniques such as wearing supportive bra, washing and air drying nipples to prevent cracking, soreness and bleeding which interfere with feeding
- Teach mother on ways to prevent breast engorgement
- Teach mother the factors that enhance mild production as well as those that can alter production and quality of milk
- Provide positive reinforcement for the mother's efforts in order to decrease her anxiety and increase her confidence and self esteem.

Evaluations for Expected Outcomes

- Mother properly positions baby during breastfeeding
- Uses appropriate techniques to encourage attachment to nipple
- Mother expresses decreased anxiety and increased enthusiasm for breastfeeding
- Neonate feeds successfully on both breasts and appears satisfied for at least two hours after feeding
- Neonate's nutritional needs are met
- Neonate's initial weight loss remains within accepted norms.

Documentation

- Mother's level of knowledge related to breastfeeding
- Mother's expression of dissatisfaction with breastfeeding ability
- Mother's breastcare practices
- Maternal conditions that interfere with breastfeeding such as inverted nipples
- Mother's and neonate's behavior during and after breastfeeding such as positioning on breasts and baby's level of satisfaction
- Frequency and duration of breastfeeding
- Teaching and instructions given and mother's response to teaching
- Neonate's weight and growth
- Mother's and neonate's response to nursing interventions.

Risk for Infection Related to Neonate's Immature Immune System

Definition

Presence of internal or external hazards that threaten neonate's health.

Assessment

- Gestational age of neonate
- Temperature, heart rate and respirations
- Labor and delivery record including maternal fever, premature rupture of membranes and foul smelling amniotic fluid
- Recent or current maternal infections
- Signs of infection of umbilical cord and skin at base of cord such as redness, odor and discharge
- Signs and symptoms of developing infections such as lethargy, jaundice, skin lesions, thrush, unstable body temperature, hypoglycemia, diarrhea, vomiting, poor feeding patterns, cyanosis and mottling of skin
- Signs of respiratory distress such as grunting, retractions, nasal flaring and cyanosis
- Evidence of chronic intrauterine infections such as growth retardation and hepatosplenomegaly.

Risk Factors

- Early rupture of amniotic membranes
- Environmental exposure to pathogens during birth process
- Inadequate primary responses such as broken skin
- Invasive procedures
- Poor feeding pattern
- Tissue destruction
- Trauma
- Medication use.

Expected Outcomes

- Neonate's vital signs will remain within normal range
- Neonate will be alert and active
- Neonate will remain free from signs and symptoms of infection
- Neonate's umbilical cord will remain free of infection and heal properly

❖ Mother and family members will practice good handwashing technique before handling neonate.

Nursing Interventions

❖ Review the maternal chart and delivery record to detect risk factors that predispose the neonate to infection

❖ Assess the neonate's gestational age. [As passive immunity via the placenta increases significantly in last trimester, premature neonates are more susceptible to infection]

❖ Follow sterile techniques: Remove rings, wrist watch and bracelet before handling the neonate

❖ Scrub hands and arms with antimicrobial preparation before entering nursery and after contact with contaminated material

❖ Wash hands after handling the neonate and instruct parents in handwashing techniques

❖ Perform umbilical cord care with each diaper change or as facility policy dictates in order to promote healing

❖ Assess respirations, heart rate and temperature every 15 minutes for first hour, then every hour for four hours, then every four hours for 24 hours, then every shift or as indicated. [Unstable vital signs, persistent elevations in temperature or hypothermia may indicate neonatal infection]

❖ Observe neonate for signs and symptoms of infection and notify physician if signs and symptoms of infection appear

❖ Observe standard precautions: Wear gloves for neonate's first bath and when in contact with blood and body secretions.[These actions prevent cross-contamination and transmission of pathogens]

❖ Encourage mother to begin breastfeeding early. Colostrum and breast milk provide passive immunity and helps reduce infection.

Evaluations for Expected Outcomes

❖ Neonate's vital signs remain within normal range

❖ Neonate remains alert and active

❖ Neonate is free from signs and symptoms of infection

❖ Umbilical cord is clean, dry and healing

❖ Mother and family members demonstrate proper hand-washing technique before handling neonate.

Documentation

❖ Vital signs
❖ Appearance of umbilical cord
❖ Feeding pattern and weight gain
❖ Condition of oral mucosa
❖ Skin colour and rashes
❖ Elimination pattern
❖ Activity pattern
❖ Interventions performed to reduce risk of infection
❖ Neonates response to nursing interventions
❖ Evaluations of outcomes observed.

Imbalanced Nutrition Less than Body Requirement Related to Ineffective Suck Reflex

---

Definition

Inability to ingest sufficient fluids and nutrients resulting from ineffective sucking reflex.

Assessment

❖ Gestational age
❖ Perinatal history
❖ Apgar score
❖ Suck and swallow reflex
❖ GI assessment including vomiting, regurgitation and stool characteristics
❖ Examination of abdomen including inspecting auscultation of bowel sounds, percussion and palpation for abnormalities
❖ Nutritional status including intake and output, weight changes, skin turgor and urine characteristics, signs of dehydration and feeding pattern
❖ Laboratory studies such as urine glucose levels, urine bilirubin levels and urine specific gravity
❖ Adequacy of breastfeeding techniques (practices) of mother such as condition of nipple and positioning of neonate.

Defining Characteristics

❖ Lack of interest in feeding
❖ Weight loss more than expected normal for the neonatal period

❖ Diarrhea
❖ Inadequate intake
❖ Pale conjunctiva and mucous membranes
❖ Signs of abdominal pain or cramping.

Expected Outcomes

❖ Mother will demonstrate effective feeding technique
❖ Neonate will not lose more than 10 percent of birth weight
❖ Neonate will retain entire feeding without vomiting or regurgitating
❖ Neonate will establish effective sucking and swallowing reflexes allowing for adequate nutritional intake
❖ Neonate will maintain good skin turgor, moist mucous membranes, adequate urine output and flat soft fontanelles.

Nursing Interventions

❖ Check neonate's weight at the same time each day
❖ Record feedings accurately. If breastfeeding, number of minutes at each feeding and if bottlefeeding, amount ingested at each feeding
❖ Teach mother how to position the neonate during and after feeding and how to burp the neonate
❖ Regularly assess the neonate's sucking pattern and provide teaching as needed
❖ Instruct mother to make sure that the neonate is awake before feeding. Unwrap the blanket and tap the soles of the feet
❖ Record the number of stools and amount of urine voided in each shift
❖ Monitor the neonate for signs of dehydration such as poor skin turgor, dry mucus membranes, decreased or concentrated urine and sunken fontanelles and eyeballs
❖ Assess the need for gavage feeding.

Evaluations for Expected Outcomes

❖ Mother demonstrates competence when feeding neonate
❖ Neonate retains entire feeding
❖ Neonate establishes effective sucking and swallowing reflexes
❖ Neonate maintains good skin turgor, moist mucous membranes, adequate urine output and soft fontanelles

❖ Neonate regains the birth weight by 10 days after birth.

Documentation

❖ Frequency, bold amount and type of feeds taken
❖ Incidence of regurgitation and vomiting
❖ Frequency of bowel elimination and urination
❖ Effectiveness of suck reflex
❖ Neonate's daily weight
❖ Care given and bonding pattern by mother/parents
❖ Signs of dehydration
❖ Nursing interventions carried out and neonate's response
❖ Expected outcomes evaluated.

Hypothermia Related to Cold Stress or Sepsis

Definition

State in which neonate's body temperature is below normal range.

Assessment

❖ Gestational age
❖ Intrapartal history
❖ Presence of maternal risk factors such as fever, diabetes mellitus dystocia and perinatal asphyxia
❖ Vital signs including core temperature, heart rate respiration and blood pressure
❖ Lab values such as arterial blood gas values, serum glucose and electrolytes
❖ Skin colour: Central and peripheral
❖ Birth weight.

Defining Characteristics

❖ Body temperature below normal level
❖ Cool, pale skin
❖ Cyanotic nail beds
❖ Increased heart rate and blood pressure
❖ Piloerection
❖ Shivering
❖ Slow capillary refill.

Expected Outcomes

❖ Neonate will exhibit normal body temperature

- ❖ Neonate will have warm, dry skin and normal capillary refill
- ❖ Neonate will not develop complications of hypothermia
- ❖ Neonate will not shiver
- ❖ Neonate will maintain normal body temperature
- ❖ Mother will verbalize knowledge of how hypothermia develops and will state measures to prevent recurrence of hypothermia.

Nursing Interventions

- ❖ Monitor body temperature every hour by axillary route. If using a radiant warmer, monitor the device's temperature reading hourly and compare it with the neonates body temperature
- ❖ Monitor and record vital signs every 1 to 4 hours. Perform continuous electronic cardiorespiratory monitoring as appropriate
- ❖ *For mild hypothermia*, dress the baby with a shirt, diaper, stockinette cap or knitted hat and wrap in double blankets
- ❖ Avoid overheating and wet diaper
- ❖ Perform all procedures under a radiant warmer if possible
- ❖ Postpone bathing
- ❖ For severe hypothermia, place the neonate in an isolette or overhead radiant warmer bed and provide supportive measures
  - – Keep the neonate undressed
  - – Set the isolette temperature at 36 to 36.6 °C (96.8-97.8°F)
  - – Attach a skin probe to the right upper quadrant of the neonate's abdomen

- – Monitor carefully for evaporative and insensible fluid loss
- ❖ Carry out prescribed treatment regimen such as administering IV fluids and small frequent feeding
- ❖ Discuss precipitating factors with mother and family members to prevent recurrence
- ❖ Instruct family members in preventive measures such as dressing the neonate appropriately and providing adequate nutrition for neonate's growth needs.

Evaluations for Expected Outcomes

- ❖ Neonate's temperature returns to normal
- ❖ Neonate exhibits warm, dry skin and normal capillary refill time
- ❖ Neonate does not develop complications of hypothermia
- ❖ Neonate does not demonstrate signs of hyperthermia related to radiant heat source
- ❖ Neonate is successfully weaned from isolette or radiant warmer
- ❖ Parents verbalize understanding of causes of hypothermia and preventive measures
- ❖ Mother demonstrates proper temperature measurement technique.

Documentation

- ❖ Neonate's physical findings such as cardiovascular status and temperature
- ❖ Nursing interventions carried out
- ❖ Neonate's response to interventions
- ❖ Mother's and family members' willingness and ability to provide adequate care at home
- ❖ Expected outcomes evaluated.

Glossary

ABO Incompatibility: A condition that may lead to neonatal hemolytic disease. The mother who has type 'O' red cells has antibodies to type 'A' and type 'B' red cells. These antibodies are transferred to the fetus and cause destruction of fetal red blood cells. The hemolytic disease resulting from ABO incompatibility is usually less severe than the disease caused by Rh incompatibility. Unlike Rh incompatibility, ABO incompatibility cannot be prevented by giving the mother Rh immune globulin.

Abortion: The termination of pregnancy by expulsion of the products of conception prior to viability (the ability to survive, if born), which is less than 28th week of gestation. The international acceptance is either 20th week or fetus weighing 500 gm.

Abruptio Placentae: Premature separation or detachment from the wall of the uterus of a normally situated placenta; can be partial or complete separation.

Acceleration: Refers to a periodic rise in fetal heart rate from the baseline in response to stress of lowered oxygen availability or fetal movement.

Acidosis: A decrease in the pH of the blood. The range of pH in a neonate is between 7.30 and 7.40. A blood pH of 7.20 or lower is considered severe acidosis. If a baby is gasping, the pH is probably 7.0 or less.

Acrocyanosis: The slightly bluish, grayish discoloration of a newborn's hands and feet within the first 24 hours of birth.

AGA: Abbreviation for 'Appropriate for Gestational Age', when a newborn's birth weight is within the 10th to 90th percentile expected for that length gestation.

Albumin: The major protein in blood. In 5 percent concentration, it is used as an emergency blood volume expander in the treatment of shock.

Alkalosis: An increase in the pH of blood. Alkalosis may result from a high (above 7.40) serum bicarbonate or, more commonly, if the carbon dioxide concentration in the baby's blood is lowered by hyperventilation (assisting the baby's breathing at an excessively fast rate).

Alpha-Fetoprotein: A glycoprotein and a major component of fetal blood; small amounts are found in the amniotic fluid of normal fetuses. Elevated levels may indicate neural tube malformations.

Amniocentesis: A procedure for removing amniotic fluid from the amniotic sac by inserting a needle through the abdominal wall usually to assess fetal health or maturity.

Amniotomy: The artificial rupture of amniotic membranes when an amnihook or other rupturing device is introduced into the vagina and a small tear is made in the membranes.

Anencephaly: A congenital anomaly in which there is partial or complete absence of the skull and brain.

Anomaly: An abnormal occurrence or malformation. For example, a cleft lip is an anomaly.

Anoxia: Absence or deficiency of oxygen, as reduction of oxygen in body tissues below physiologic levels.

Antenatal Period: The time of pregnancy from the first day of last menstrual period (LMP) to the start of true labor.

Anterior Fontanelle: Diamond shaped fontanelle located at the juncture of the coronal, frontal and sagittal sutures.

Antibody Titers: A test used to indicate the relative concentration of a particular antibody present in a person's blood. For example, a high rubella titer indicates a person has been exposed to rubella (German measles) and has formed a significant amount of antibody against the rubella virus and therefore, will most likely be able to ward off another attack of the virus without becoming ill.

Apgar: A five part scoring system to assess newborns at one minute and five minutes after birth regarding heart rate, respiratory effort, muscle tone, reflex irritability, and color.

Appropriate for Gestational Age: When a newborn's birth weight is within the 10th to 90th percentile expected for that length gestation (see AGA).

Asphyxia: A decrease in the amount of oxygen and an increased amount of carbon dioxide in the body because of some interference with respiration.

Attachment: The establishment of a reciprocal relationship between the parents and the newborn after a period of bonding; development of a deeper intimacy, which grows over time.

Attitude: The relationship of the fetal head and limbs to its trunk.

Autosomes: The chromosomes in the body other than the sex (X and Y) chromosomes.

Azoospermic: A condition in which sperm is absent in the semen.

Baby-Blues: A common transient mild depression or emotional disturbance affecting the mother after delivery due to hormonal changes, sleep deprivation and emotional let-down.

Ballottement: When palpated, the fetus floats way then returns to touch the examiners fingers.

Bicornuate uterus: A double uterus.

Bilirubin: The orange or yellow-colored pigment in bile produced by the breakdown of hemoglobin and excreted by the liver cells.

Biophysical Profile (BPP): A combination of measures used to evaluate fetal well-being; each of the five components (non-stress test, ultrasound evaluation of amniotic fluid volume, fetal body movements, muscle tone and respirations) are scored; these scores are added together for the final BPP score.

Bishop's Score: A pre-labor scoring system with five components (cervical dilatation, effacement, consistency, position and fetal station) to help determine if induction of labor will be effective.

Bloody Show: Rupture of the small cervical capillaries when the cervix begins to dilate and efface; when the mucus plug is lost the resultant cervical drainage is pink-tinged.

Bonding: The initial attraction and period of exploration between the parents and newborn; becoming acquainted.

Bradycardia (Slow Heart Rate): (1) *Fetal*: A sustained heart rate less than 100 beats per minute (bpm), (A heart rate less than 120 bpm may also be abnormal depending upon the clinical situation). (2) *Neonatal*: A sustained heart rate less than 100 beats per minute.

Braxton Hicks: The intermittent, irregular painless uterine contractions which occur during pregnancy; they do not dilate and efface the cervix (see true labor).

Breech Presentation: The feet-first or buttocks-first presentation of the fetus; the position is termed breech whether one foot, both feet or the buttocks are born first; frank breech is the buttocks-first presentation.

Brown Fat: Fat tissue, which has a rich blood and nerve supply. Babies have proportionately more brown fat than do adults and metabolize or "burn" it as their main source of heat production, while adults produce heat by shivering. Extra oxygen and calories are used when brown fat is metabolized.

Bubble: An acronym standing for the five most important assessment areas of a postpartum woman; breasts, uterus, bowels, bladder, lochia, episiotomy and extremities.

Cesarean Delivery: Surgical delivery of the fetus through an abdominal incision; the uterine incision may be classical (vertical, cutting through both the contractile and non-contractile segments) or confined to the non-contractile lower uterine segment (either vertical or transverse incision).

Caput Succedaneum: Localized edema occurring just under the presenting part of the fetal scalp during labor; disappears within 36 to 48 hours of life.

Cardinal Movements: The predictable sequence of movements through the birth canal that the fetus will go through during labor and birth; descent, flexion, internal rotation, extension, external rotation and expulsion.

Cephalhematoma: A collection of blood between the newborn's skull bone and periosteum resulting from pressure or trauma during labor or delivery; does not cross suture lines.

Cephalic Presentation: When the head of the fetus is the presenting part; may be vertex, face, sinciput or brow presentation.

Cervical Dilatation: The opening or enlargement of the external cervical os from a few mm to 10 centimeters when completely dilated.

Cervical Effacement: The thinning or shortening of the cervix during labor from 0 to 100 percent when completely effaced.

Chadwick's Sign: The bluish or purple coloration of the vagina and cervix when pregnancy is presumed.

Chest Compressions: Artificial pumping of the blood through the heart by a bellows effect created from intermittent compression of the sternum, over the heart, during resuscitation.

Chloasma: Irregular, brownish discolorations of the forehead, nose, cheeks and neck during pregnancy (the mask of pregnancy).

Choanal Atresia: Congenital obstruction of the posterior nares (between the nose and throat). Since babies breath mainly through their noses, a baby with choanal atresia will have severe respiratory distress at birth. The immediate treatment is insertion of an oral airway.

Chromosome: The microscopic, rod-shaped bodies (46 in man), which develop from cell nucleus material and contain the genes.

Chorionic Villus Sampling: A procedure to obtain a sample of the chorionic villi from the placenta via aspiration; tests for chromosomal and biochemical disorders during early pregnancy.

Coach: A person who assumes the role of advocate and support person for the laboring woman; assists with conditioned techniques for relaxation and breathing.

Colostrum: The "first milk" secreted from the lactiferous glands.

Conceptional Age: Age of the fetus calculated from the day of fertilization.

Congenital: Refers to conditions that are present at birth, regardless of cause. Congenital defects may result from a variety of causes, including genetic factors, chromosomal factors, diseases affecting the mother, or drugs taken by the mother. The cause of most congenital defects is unknown.

Conjugation of Bilirubin: Process that occurs in the liver and combines bilirubin with another chemical so it may be removed from the blood and pass out of the body in the feces. Failure of bilirubin conjugation is one of the causes of jaundice.

Continuous Positive Airway Pressure (CPAP): A steady pressure delivered to the baby's lungs by means of a special apparatus or mechanical ventilator. CPAP may be used for babies with respiratory distress syndrome to prevent alveoli from collapsing during expiration.

Contraction Stress Test (CST): A procedure to help measure fetal well-being by stimulating the uterus to contract with oxytocin administration or nipple stimulation and measuring the response of the fetus to the contractions, can be interpreted as positive, negative or equivocal (suspicious) (see also Oxytocin challenge test).

Coombs Test: Test to determine the presence of antibodies in blood or on red cells. It is used, e.g. to detect antibodies against the red cells of Rh-positive babies born to Rh-negative sensitized mothers.

Couplet Care: A system in which one-nurse cares for the postpartum mother and her newborn as a single unit; also known as mother-baby dyad.

Denominator: The name of the part of the presentation, which is used when referring to fetal position.

Diaphragmatic Hernia: A condition when the diaphragm does not close completely and the abdominal contents slip into the thoracic cavity; causes respiratory distress in the newborn.

Dilatation of Cervix: The enlargement of the external os from an orifice a few millimeters in size to an opening large enough to allow the passage of the infant, a cervical opening approximately 10 cm in diameter is usually considered complete dilatation.

Doppler Monitor: Uses ultrasound to detect audible fetal heart sounds; an intermittent and simple monitoring technique.

Down Syndrome: A chromosomal abnormality resulting in a typical facial appearance, mental retardation and sometimes other congenital defects—it is also called mongolism or trisomy 21. Down syndrome individuals have 47 instead of the normal 46 chromosomes.

Ductus Arteriosus: A connection between the main pulmonary artery and the aorta of the fetus; closes after birth and becomes a ligament.

Ductus Venosus: A fetal blood vessel that connects the umbilical vein and the inferior vena cava.

Dysfunctional Labor: Occurs when there is a problem with the frequency, duration and intensity of uterine contractions, and/or the resting tone of the uterus between contractions.

Dyspareunia: Painful sexual intercourse experienced by females.

Dystocia: Abnormal or difficult labor or delivery. Used to refer to weak or ineffective uterine contractions; may also be used to describe the situation in which the shoulders of a baby in vertex presentation become trapped after delivery of the head (shoulder dystocia).

Early Deceleration: A transitory decrease in the fetal heart rate caused by head compression, which stimulates the vagus nerve to slow down the heart rate.

Eclampsia: A pregnancy-induced hypertensive disease associated with hypertension, proteinuria, edema, tonic and clonic seizures and coma.

Effacement: A thinning and shortening of the cervix, which occurs during pregnancy and/or labor.

Effleurage: A stroke used in massage.

Electronic Fetal Monitoring: A type of monitoring in which information about the fetal heart rate and the laboring woman's uterine contraction pattern is continually assessed; can be either direct (invasive or internal) or indirect (noninvasive or external).

Embryo: The term used for the conceptus from four to eight weeks following conception.

Encephalocele: Protrusion of the brain through a cranial fissure generally in the occipital area.

Engagement: Also referred to as lightening, when the widest fetal presenting diameter has passed through the brim of the pelvis, engagement is said to have occurred.

Engorgement: The swelling and distention of the breasts, usually during the early days of initiation of lactation due to vascular dilatation as well as the arrival of the early milk.

Epicanthus: A fold of skin extending from the root of the nose to the median end of the eyebrow and covering the inner canthus and caruncle.

Epidural Block: A type of regional anesthesia used to produce relief from pain during labor and delivery.

Epinephrine: A natural body hormone that is released into the blood during stressful activity; it may also be used as a drug during resuscitation to constrict the blood vessels, increase the blood pressure and to increase the heart rate and volume of blood pumped.

Episiotomy: An incision in the perineum to facilitate delivery.

Erythema Toxicum Neonatorum: An urticarial condition affecting newborns in the first few days of life, the lesions consist of dead white papules, grainy to the touch, with or without surrounding areas of redness.

Erythroblastosis Fetalis: A blood dyscrasia of the newborn characterized by agglutination and hemolysis of erythrocytes; usually caused by incompatibility between the infant's blood and the mother's.

Esophageal Atresia: A condition in which the esophagus ends in a blind pouch or narrows into a thin cord; usually occurs between the upper, and mid-third of the esophagus.

Expected Data of Delivery (EDD): The estimated date of delivery based on Naegle's rule or ultrasound.

Epstein's Pearls: Small, white epithelial cysts along both sides of the median raphe of the hard palate; commonly found in newborn infants.

False Labor: Characterized by irregular Braxton-Hicks contractions which do not change the cervix and do not increase in intensity, duration or frequency (see also True Labor).

Facies: The expression or appearance of the face; certain congenital syndromes present with a specific facial appearance.

Family Centered Care: The maternity delivery system that emphasizes professional quality health care of the total family unit; utilizes a combined nursery and postpartum nursing staff to form one mother-baby dyad (see Couple Care).

Fetal Bradycardia: The fetal heart rate is less than 120 beats/minutes during at least a 10-minute period of continuous monitoring.

Fetal Distress: A compromise in fetal well-being; can be either acute or chronic.

Fetal Heart Rate Acceleration: An increase in the fetal heart rate that occurs during a uterine contraction, with the fetal heart rate decreasing to its previous rate as the contraction subsides.

Fetal Heart Rate Baseline: Average fetal heart rate between periodic rate changes (accelerations or decelerations). The baseline fetal heart rate is the average fetal heart rate during any 10-minute period. The normal baseline range is between 120 and 160 beats per minute.

Fetal Heart Rate Deceleration: A decrease in the fetal heart rate that occurs in response to a uterine contraction. There are three types of decelerations (early, late and variable).

Fetal Heart Rate Variability: The beat-to-beat changes that occur in the baseline fetal heart rate.

Fetal Monitoring, External: Refers to continuous electronic monitoring using leads strapped to the mother's abdomen to detect the fetal heart rate, periodic rate changes and the timing of the uterine contraction.

Fetal Monitoring, Internal: Refers to continuous electronic monitoring using a wire placed on the fetal presenting part to detect the fetal heart rate, variability and periodic rate changes and a tube placed inside the uterus to detect the onset and intensity of the uterine contractions.

Fetal Lie: The relationship of the body of the fetus to the body of the mother, which is either longitudinal or transverse.

Fetal Position: The relationship of the landmark on the presenting fetal part to the front, sides, or back of the maternal pelvis.

Fetal Presentation: The lowest part of the fetus that comes first through the maternal pelvis and birth canal; either vertex (cephalic), shoulders or breech.

Fetal Station: Refers to the relationship of the fetus's presenting part to an imaginary line drawn between the maternal ischial spines and the pelvic outlet.

Fetal Surveillance: Methods to assess and monitor the well-being of the fetus during pregnancy, labor and birth includes fetal biophysical profile, biochemical assessments, amniocentesis, genetic studies, antenatal testing, fetal movement counting, non-stress testing, contraction stress testing and clinical assessments.

Fetal Tachycardia: When the fetal heart rate is greater than 160 beats/minute during at least for a 10-minute period of continuous monitoring.

Fetus: The term applied to the conceptus from ninth week until birth.

"Floating": When the presenting part is entirely out of the maternal pelvis and can be moved by the examiner, not engaged.

Fontanelle: An unossified space or "soft spot" lying between the cranial bones of the skull of a fetus.

Foramen Ovale: The septal opening between the atria of the fetal heart that closes soon after birth.

Four P's: The four forces of labor including passage, passenger power and psyche.

Freidman Curve: A method of evaluating the relationship of three factors to help determine normal or abnormal labor patterns over time; these three factors are uterine activity, cervical dilatation and fetal descent; can be plotted on a graph.

Gastroschisis: Congenital opening of the abdominal wall allowing the abdominal organs to protrude.

Gene: A factor responsible for the transmission of hereditary characteristics of offspring.

Generative: Capable of reproducing.

Genotype: The hereditary combination of genes, which makes up a person.

Gestational Age: The number of completed weeks of fetal development calculated from the first day of the last menstrual cycle.

Gestational Diabetes Mellitus (GDM): Glucose or carbohydrate intolerance of variable severity which develops or is discovered during the present pregnancy; the condition subsides at the completion of the pregnancy.

Gestational Period: The number of completed weeks of pregnancy calculated from the first day of the last menstrual period.

Grand Multipara: A woman who has given birth five times or more.

Gravida: The number of times a woman has been pregnant or a pregnant woman.

Gravidity: Refers to the total number of a woman's pregnancies regardless of their duration.

Grunting: Audible sound made by the newborn on expiration often indicating respiratory distress.

Hematoma: Occurs when blood escapes into the connective tissue of a traumatized area; can be life-threatening; may or may not cause severe pain.

Hemoconcentration: An increase in the number of red blood cells resulting from a decrease in the volume of plasma.

Hemorrhage: Blood volume loss of more than 500 cc or blood loss of more than 15 percent of the total estimated blood volume.

Hegar's Sign: Softness and compressibility of the uterine isthmus during the 2nd and 3rd month of pregnancy.

HELLP Syndrome: This syndrome refers to a severe and potentially fatal complication of pregnancy-induced hypertension involving hemolysis of red blood cells, elevated liver enzyme levels, and a low platelet count.

Homan's Sign: A method for detecting thrombophlebitis in which the leg is held straight and the foot flexed back; if the manoeuvre produces pain upon dorsiflexion of the foot, the test is positive and thrombophlebitis should be suspected.

Hydatidiform Mole: Cystic proliferation of chorionic villi resembling a cluster of grapes.

Hydrocephalus: The increased accumulation of cerebrospinal fluid within the ventricles of the brain; may result from congenital anomalies, infection, injury or brain tumor.

Hyperbilirubinemia: A condition when there is an excessive amount of bilirubin in the blood; excessive levels can lead to brain damage.

Hyperemesis Gravidarum: Excessive vomiting during pregnancy.

Hypospadias: A condition in which the urethral orifice is at some point between the scrotal raphe and the base of the glans penis.

Hypertonic Uterus: Labor contractions lasting longer than 90 seconds, caused by too much stimulation of the uterus.

Hypotonic Labor: Occurs during the active phase of labor causing ineffectual contractions and a lack of progression of labor.

Hypoxia: A broad term meaning diminished availability of oxygen to the body tissues.

Idiopathic Respiratory Distress Syndrome (Hyaline Membrane Disease): A severe respiratory condition found almost exclusively in preterm infants.

Inborn Error of Metabolism: A hereditary disease caused by a deficiency of a specific enzyme.

Incompetent Cervix: A condition in which the cervix dilates prematurely, causing a spontaneous abortion or preterm delivery.

Intrapartum Period: The time from the onset of labor to the delivery of the newborn and the placenta.

In Utero *(Latin):* Inside the uterus.

Jacquemiers Sign: The violet-blue discoloration of the vulva and vaginal mucosa including the vaginal portion of the cervix.

Jaundice: A condition characterized by a yellow color of the skin, the whites of the eyes, the mucous membranes, and body fluids that is due to deposition of bile pigment resulting from excess bilirubin in the blood.

Kernicterus: A clinical syndrome in newborn infants manifested by pathological changes in the central nervous system resulting from deposition of unconjugated bilirubin in certain nuclei of the brain.

Labor: A process that involves a series of integrated uterine contractions that occur over time, and work to propel the fetus from the birth canal; relies on the uterine muscles and cervical compliance.

Labor Delivery Recovery and Postpartum Care (LDRP): A system of health care delivery in which a woman labors, delivers, recovers, and is discharged for home from the same room and cared for by a primary care nurse; in home-like environment within a hospital setting.

Lactation: The process of preparing for and maintaining the production and secretion of milk including mammogenesis, lactogenesis, and galactopoiesis.

Lamaze Method: An approach to childbirth emphasizing relaxation and breathing techniques to allow for a "painless childbirth"; also known as psychoprophylaxis method.

Lanugo: A fine, downy hair covering the fetus between the 17th week of gestation and soon after birth.

Late Deceleration: A periodic decrease in the fetal heart rate below baseline occurring after the peak of the contraction; due to uteroplacental insufficiency and a sign of fetal distress.

Lecithin: One of the surfactant substances produced in the lungs; the amount of lecithin produced increases with increasing gestational age of the fetus. Therefore, the ratio of lecithin to sphingomyelin (LS ratio) in the amniotic fluid is used to estimate the lung maturity of the fetus.

Leopold's Manoeuvres: A system of evaluating the position and presentation of the fetus by palpating the maternal abdomen in four distinct locations.

Lie: The relationship of the long axis of the fetus to the long axis of the mother.

Lightening: The movement of the fetus and uterus downward into the pelvic cavity, an early sign of impending labor (see also Engagement) / A reduction in fundal height due to the fetus sinking into the lower uterine segment, which may occur at the end of pregnancy.

Lochia: The discharge from the uterus of blood, mucus, and tissue during the postpartum period; changes from rubra to serosa, to alba.

Lochia Alba: The thin, colorless discharge, which follows lochia serosa.

Lochia Rubra: The color description of the red, sanguinous vaginal flow, which follows delivery and which lasts two to four days postpartum.

Lochia Serosa: The serous, pinkish-brown watery discharge which follows lochia rubra.

Low Birth Weight (LBW): Infant weighing less than 2,500 grams.

Low Forceps: Application of forceps when the leading point of the fetal skull is at + 2 station or lower with further specification as to whether the rotation of the fetal head is less than 45°or more than 45°.

Lysozyme: An enzyme with antiseptic qualities, which destroys foreign protein.

Macrosomia: Large body size; newborn at term weighing more than 4,000 grams or is large for his or her gestational age.

Mastitis: Breast infection because of milk in the ducts.

Maternity Care: Complete care of the pregnant, laboring and newly delivered woman and her newborn; also includes pre-pregnancy counseling, infertility counseling, and parenting education.

Meconium: The first stool passed by the newborn; dark green or black material passed from the large intestine from the term or near-term fetus.

Midforceps: Application of forceps when the head is engaged but the leading part of the fetal head is above +2 station.

Milia: Distended sebaceous glands, which produce tiny pinpoint papules on the skin of newborn infants, commonly found over the bridge of the nose, chin, and cheeks.

Moulding: Normal overlapping of the skull bones of the baby to allow the fetal head to fit through the pelvis during labor.

Mongolian Spots: Benign bluish pigmentation over the lower back, buttocks or occasionally over the extensor surfaces may be present at birth, particularly in dark-skinned races.

Morbidity: Any form of permanent damage that results from an illness or accident.

Mucus-trap Suction Apparatus: A type of suction apparatus used in aspirating the naso-pharynx and trachea of a newborn infant. It consists of a catheter with a mucus trap, which prevents mucus from the baby from being drawn into the operator's mouth.

Multigravida: A woman who has been pregnant two or more times.

Multipara: A woman who has given birth to two or more babies live or still excluding abortions.

Multiple Gestation: Pregnancy with more than one fetus, e.g. twins.

Naegle's Rule: Used to determine the estimated date of delivery (EDD) or delivery date by subtracting three months from the first day of the last menstrual period, then adding 7 days.

Nasal Flaring: A sign of respiratory distress; the edges of the nostrils fan outward as the baby inhales.

Necrotizing Enterocolitis: A serious disease in which sections of the intestines die and must be surgically removed; it occurs more often in preterm infants, but the cause is unclear.

Newborn Period: From birth through the first 28 days of life.

Neonatal Period: From birth to 28 days.

Neonatologist: A pediatrician who specializes in caring for newborn infants, particularly at risk and sick babies.

Neural Tube Defect: Any congenital defect in the brain or spinal cord (neural tube of the embryo), including anencephaly, encephalocele and meningomyelocele.

Neutral Thermal Environment (Thermo-Neutral Environment): The very narrow environmental temperature range that keeps a baby's body temperature normal with the baby having to use the least amount of calories and oxygen to produce heat.

Nonstress Test (NST): A noninvasive test used to determine fetal well-being, involves external fetal monitoring of the fetal heart rate and observing the response of the heart rate to fetal movement; interpreted as reactive or non-reactive.

Nuchal Cord: The presence of one or more loops of the umbilical cord around the neck of the newborn.

Nullipara: A woman who has not carried a pregnancy to the point of viability.

Nursing Process: Perceiving, assessing, planning, implementing, and evaluation.

Omphalocele: A defect resulting from failure of closure of the abdominal wall or muscles whereby abdominal viscera covered by a thin membrane protrudes and forms a sac outside the abdominal cavity.

Operculum: The thickened mucus that forms a cervical plug during pregnancy.

Ophthalmia Neonatorum Purulent: Infection of the eyes of the newborn, usually caused by gonococcus.

Ortolani's Sign: A technique for determining the presence of a congenital dislocation of the hip, performed as part of the newborn examination.

Osiander's Sign: Increased pulsation felt in the lateral vaginal fornices.

Outlet Forceps: Application of forceps when the fetal head is visible at the introitus without separating the vulva, the fetal skull has reached the pelvic floor, the sagittal suture is in the anteroposterior diameter, the fetal head is at or on the perineum and rotation of the head does not exceed 45°.

Ovulation: The release of an egg, ready for fertilization, from an ovary.

Oxytocin: A hormone occurring naturally in the body and also used to induce labor, to enhance weak labor contractions and to cause contraction of the uterus after delivery of the placenta.

Oxytocin Challenge Test (OCT): A test to assess fetal well-being by administering oxytocin via intravenous infusion to induce uterine contractions and assessing the fetus's response; can be interpreted as positive (abnormal), negative (normal), or suspicious (inconclusive) (see also Contraction Stress Test).

Palmar Erythema: Reddening of the palms seen in pregnant women.

Parity: Refers to the number of viable infants live or dead that a woman has delivered regardless of the number of children involved (e.g., the birth of triplets increases the parity by only one).

Parturient: A woman in labor.

Perinatal: The time surrounding the baby's birth; denotes a period between 20 weeks of gestational age to 28 days after birth.

Phenylketonuria: A congenital disease caused by a defect in the metabolism of the amino acid phenylalanine. The condition is hereditary and results from lack of an enzyme, phenylalanine hydroxylase, necessary for the conversion of the amino acid phenylalanine into tyrosine.

Phosphatidyl Glycerol (PG): A chemical substance produced by the mature fetal lung, which passes into the amniotic fluid with fetal breathing. Its presence in the amniotic fluid is associated with a better than 99 percent chance that the baby will not develop Respiratory Distress Syndrome (RDS).

Phototherapy: Use of fluorescent lights to treat hyperbilirubinemia in neonates by breaking down bilirubin accumulated in the skin; the color of phototherapy lights ranges from nearly white to deep blue, depending upon the brand of lights.

Pica: Craving to eat bizarre substances like coal, wall plaster, mothballs etc. in pregnancy.

Placenta: The oval or discoid spongy structure attached to the uterus through which the fetus derives its nourishment and through which waste products from the fetus pass into the mother's blood.

Placenta Abruptio: A premature separation of a normally implanted placenta.

Placental Dysfunction: A placenta that is failing to meet fetal requirements.

Placenta Previa: A placenta, which is abnormally implanted in the lower uterine segment so that it partially or fully covers the internal os of the cervix.

Polyhydramnios: Excessive volume of amniotic fluid usually greater than 1.2 liters.

Position: The relationship between the denominator and the six points on the pelvic brim.

Positive Pressure Ventilation (PPV): Artificial breathing for a person by forcing air and/or oxygen into the lungs under pressure, either by bag and mask, bag and endotracheal tube or with a mechanical respirator.

Postpartum Depression: Delayed emotional disturbance affecting the new mother sometimes one to three weeks postpartum; less commonly experienced; more intense and serious than the postpartum "baby blues".

Postpartum Period: Period after a woman gives birth until her recovery six weeks later, when all of the reproductive changes, which occur over a nine-month pregnancy, return to the pre-pregnant state.

Postterm Pregnancy: When the pregnancy continues past 42 weeks gestation.

Precipitate Delivery: When labor lasts for less than 2 hours before spontaneous delivery; unexpected, sudden, and often unattended.

Preeclampsia: Also referred to as toxemia or PIH; a hypertensive disorder of pregnancy usually occurring after the 20th week gestation; characterized by high blood pressure, proteinuria, and edema (see also Eclampsia).

Pregnancy Induced Hypertension (PIH): A hypertensive disorder during pregnancy including conditions preeclampsia and eclamp-

sia; characterized by hypertension, proteinuria, and edema (see also Eclampsia and Preeclampsia).

Premature Infant: A live born infant of less than 38 weeks' gestation (37th completed week).

Prenatal Period: The time of pregnancy from the first day of last menstrual period (LMP) to the start of true labor.

Presentation: Refers to the part of the fetus, which lies at the pelvic brim or in the lower pole of the uterus.

Preterm Labor: When labor begins before the 37th completed week of gestation from the first day of the last menstrual period.

Primigravida: A woman pregnant for the first time.

Primipara: A woman who has given birth to a fetus or fetuses that has reached the point of viability.

Prolapsed Cord: An emergent event, when the umbilical cord slips in front of the presenting part and protrudes from the cervix into the vagina, the presenting part may press against the mother's pelvis cutting off the blood and oxygen to the fetus.

Prolonged Labor: The latent phase of labor lasts longer than 24 hours without spontaneous delivery.

Pseudocyesis: False pregnancy.

Psychoprophylaxis: Term first applied to the Lamaze childbirth method, which emphasizes relaxation, breathing and positioning, to help obtain a "painless childbirth" (see also Lamaze method).

Ptyalism: Increased salvation in pregnancy.

Quickening: Sensation of the first fetal movement usually felt by the mother around the 16th week of pregnancy; a presumptive sign of pregnancy.

Regional Anesthesia: A nerve block with an anesthetic agent which ranges from local infiltration to spinal block anesthesia, the most

GLOSSARY

Resuscitation: Restoration of life or consciousness of one, apparently dead or whose respiration has ceased.

Retractions: A sign of respiratory distress; occur each time the baby breathes as the skin is pulled inward between the ribs as the baby tries to expand stiff lungs.

Retinopathy of Prematurity (Previously called retrolental fibroplacia): Partial or complete blindness that results from abnormal blood vessel growth in the eye and may lead to detachment of the retina. The blood vessel changes may result from many factors including excessively high arterial blood oxygen levels for a period of time that can be as short as a few hours. The more preterm the baby, the more likely, the baby is to develop ROP.

Rooming-in Concept: Healthy newborns are allowed to stay in their mothers' rooms where they are cared for instead of remaining in the nursery.

Rupture of the Membranes (ROM): Refers to the breaking of the amniotic membranes and the leaking of the amniotic fluid; may happen spontaneously as an early sign of the onset of labor, or artificially ruptured with a device (see Amniotomy).

Scaphoid Abdomen: Sunken or hollow-looking abdomen, occurring when there is a diaphragmatic hernia, which allows the intestines to slip out of the abdomen through a hole in the diaphragm and into the chest cavity.

Shake Test (also called bubble test): A bedside test of amniotic fluid, formerly used for rapid estimation of fetal lung maturity and now largely replaced by more refined tests.

Shirodkar's Procedure: A suturing operative procedure carried out during pregnancy for correcting an incompetent cervix.

Single Room Maternity Care: A system of caring for a woman and family during labor, delivery and recovery in one room from her admission to the hospital until her discharge for home (see also LDRP).

Small for Gestational Age (SGA): A classification for infants based on weight and gestational age at birth; refers to an infant whose birth weight is below the 10th percentile expected for that length of gestation.

Sniffing Position: Proper position of the baby's head during bag and mask ventilation or endotracheal intubation. The baby's head and back are in straight alignment and the baby's chin is pulled as if sniffing. The neck is not hyperextended.

Spermatogenesis: The process by which mature spermatozoa are formed and during which the diploid chromosome number is reduced to the haploid.

Sphingomyelin: One of the chemical substances in the lungs; the amount of sphingomyelin remains fairly constant throughout gestation. Using amniocentesis, a sample of amniotic fluid is obtained and the ratio of lecithin to sphingomyelin is compared (L/S ratio) in order to estimate the pulmonary maturity of the fetus.

Spina Bifida Occulta: A congenital defect of the walls of the spinal canal caused by the lack of union between the laminae of the vertebrae.

Stillborn: Born without life.

Striae Gravidarum: The bluish or pink streaks occurring on the abdomen, thighs and breasts during pregnancy due to the stretching of the abdomen as the uterus grows; the streaks turn silvertone in time.

Surfactant: A group of substances, including lecithin, that contributes to the compliance (elasticity) of the lungs by coating the alveoli and allowing them to stay open during exhalation; without surfactant the alveoli collapse during expiration and are difficult to open with the next breath.

Telangiectasis: The presence of small, red focal lesions, usually in the skin or mucous membrane, caused by dilation of capillaries, arterioles or venules.

Teratogenic Agent: Virus, irradiation, or drugs, the exposure to which can damage the fetus in a pregnant woman.

Term Infant: A live born infant of between 38 and 42 weeks' completed gestation.

Thermoregulation: The regulation of body temperature; prevention of heat loss by regulating the newborn's environment.

Tetralogy of Fallot: A common congenital cardiac malformation consisting of pulmonary stenosis, ventricular septal defect, dextroposed aorta and hypertrophy of the right ventricle.

Thrombocytopenic Purpura: A hematological disorder in the newborn in which the bleeding time is prolonged, platelets are greatly decreased and there is cell fragility.

Thromboembolus: A blood clot in a vein.

Thrombophlebitis: Inflammation of a vein developing before the formation of a thrombus.

Thrush: Infection of the oral membrane by a fungus, usually *Candida albicans;* it is characterized by white patches on a red, moist, inflamed surface and may occur anywhere in the mouth; commonly seen on the tongue.

Tocolytic Therapy: Medication to quiet or inhibit the smooth muscle activity of the contracting uterus.

Tonus: The amount of continuous contraction of muscle. Uterine tonus refers to how tightly the muscle of the uterus is contracted between labor contractions. Hypertonus refers to a uterus that remains excessively tense and does not relax normally between labor contractions.

TORCH Syndrome: An acronym for a group of infections, which are particularly damaging to the fetus or newborn; includes toxoplasmosis, rubella, cytomegalovirus and herpes virus type 2.

Torticollis: Wryneck; stiff neck caused by spasmodic contraction of neck muscles drawing the head to one side with the chin pointing to the other side; congenital or acquired.

Toxemia: Disorders occurring during pregnancy or early puerperium which are characterized by one or all of the following: Hypertension, edema, albuminuria and in severe cases, convulsions and coma.

Tracheoesophageal Fistula: A congenital anomaly in which there is an abnormal tube like passage between the trachea and the esophagus.

True Labor: When uterine contractions are regular with increasing intensity and occur with greater frequency; contractions that effect a change in the dilatation and effacement of the cervix (see also False Labor).

Turner Syndrome: A chromosomal defect in which there are 45 chromosomes instead of the usual 46, with the sex chromosomes identified as XO instead of XX (female) or XY (male), and may be accompanied by physical abnormalities including webbed neck, low hairline, and certain skeletal, urinary tract and cardiac abnormalities. The baby will have female external genitalia but the ovaries may be completely absent and sexual development will be severely retarded.

Ultrasound: Also called sonogram; used to visualize the uterine environment by using sound waves that pass through soft tissue until an interface between the structures of different tissue densities is reached. When this occurs, some of the energy is reflected back to the transducer, which creates an image on the screen.

Vacuum Extraction: Used to assist in the delivery of the infant instead of applying forceps; after a vacuum cup is applied to the fetal scalp, a negative pressure is exerted to help draw the fetus's head through the birth canal.

Vaginal Birth After Cesarean (VBAC): Permits patients the opportunity of a trial of labor and possibly a vaginal delivery after previously delivering by cesarean section.

Variability: The change in the baseline fetal heart rate caused by the interplay of the sympathetic and parasympathetic nervous systems; may vary from 5 to 10 beats/minute with contractions and fetal or maternal movement.

Variable Deceleration: A periodic slowing of the fetal heart rate either with a contraction or between contractions, due to umbilical cord compression; variable in duration, intensity and timing of the deceleration.

Vernix Caseosa: A protective cheese-like substance found on the newborn to protect the skin from the drying effect of the amniotic fluid.

Vertex Presentation: The fetal head or cranium is the presenting part with the head flexed on the chest and the chin in contact with the thorax; also called cephalic presentation.

Very Low Birth Weight Infant (VLBW): When an infant weighs between 500 to 1499 grams.

Zygote: The term used for a fertilized ovum for the first three weeks following conception.

Index

Page numbers followed by *f* refer to figure

F — Favorable head position and cervix

O — Open os

R — Ruptured Membranes.

C — Contractions present.

E — Engage head & empty bladder.

P — pelvimetry (no obvious CPD)

S — Stirrups (Lithotomy position)